AF358487

Coronaviruses: Past, Present, and Future

Coronaviruses: Past, Present, and Future

Guest Editor

Qibin Geng

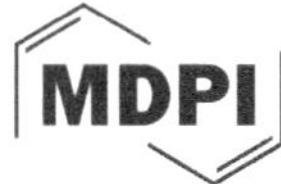Basel • Beijing • Wuhan • Barcelona • Belgrade • Novi Sad • Cluj • Manchester

Guest Editor
Qibin Geng
Department of Diagnostic
and Biological Sciences
University of Minnesota
Minneapolis
United States

Editorial Office
MDPI AG
Grosspeteranlage 5
4052 Basel, Switzerland

This is a reprint of the Special Issue, published open access by the journal *Microorganisms* (ISSN 2076-2607), freely accessible at: www.mdpi.com/journal/microorganisms/special_issues/ B7870213BA.

For citation purposes, cite each article independently as indicated on the article page online and using the guide below:

Lastname, A.A.; Lastname, B.B. Article Title. *Journal Name* **Year**, *Volume Number*, Page Range.

ISBN 978-3-7258-3060-2 (Hbk)
ISBN 978-3-7258-3059-6 (PDF)
https://doi.org/10.3390/books978-3-7258-3059-6

Contents

About the Editor

Qibin Geng

As a current Postdoctoral Associate in the Department of Diagnostic and Biological Sciences at the School of Dentistry, University of Minnesota, Twin Cities, Dr. Qibin Geng focuses on advancing the understanding of viral infections and developing innovative therapeutics. He holds a PhD in Molecular Biology from the University of Minnesota. Drawing on more than eleven years of research experience in protein chemistry, biochemistry, and virology, he has contributed to numerous high-impact publications and patents.

By integrating insights from protein engineering, biochemistry, and molecular biology, Dr. Geng strives to inform the advancements of diagnostic strategies and the development of next-generation vaccines and therapeutics for emerging infectious diseases.

Preface

Three years after the onset of the COVID-19 pandemic, the global scientific community continues to refine our collective understanding of SARS-CoV-2, its variants, and the disease(s) it causes. The scope of COVID-19 research has broadened, embracing various themes such as epidemiological surveillance, molecular pathophysiology, diagnostic and therapeutic breakthroughs, and the long-term clinical sequelae increasingly recognized as Long COVID.

In this compendium, thirty-two peer-reviewed articles examine the pandemic from various perspectives. The collection begins with population-level observations, including how new variants emerge and spread, and how public health interventions shape clinical outcomes. From there, readers are guided through the intricacies of viral pathophysiology. Several articles delve into immune responses, genetic predispositions, and how SARS-CoV-2 affects the human body on a cellular and molecular level.

Diagnostics are a focal point of this volume, highlighting both established and innovative detection approaches. The authors examine polymerase chain reaction (PCR) assays, rapid antigen tests, and cutting-edge microarray-based methods. The subsequent section on therapeutics showcases repurposed drugs, novel antimicrobial strategies, and natural products with the potential to mitigate infection or enhance patient recovery.

The discussion of vaccines encompasses studies evaluating vaccine efficacy, immune responses in special populations, and the interplay between chronic conditions such as tuberculosis and immunization outcomes. Finally, the compendium culminates in a dedicated exploration of Long COVID, underscoring the persistent impact of this disease, as well as emerging investigative directions for the future.

Although broad in scope, these articles share a unified commitment to translate rigorous research into meaningful insights that inform evidence-based clinical practice and public health policy. As a reference work, this reprint aims to serve both those on the front lines of patient care and researchers poised to expand the boundaries of COVID-19 science. By capturing the evolution of our knowledge to date, this volume offers a foundation from which the next wave of discovery can rise.

Qibin Geng
Guest Editor

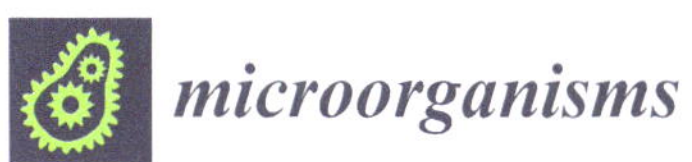

microorganisms

Perspective

COVID Variants, Villain and Victory: A Bioinformatics Perspective

Nityendra Shukla [1,†], Neha Srivastava [2,†], Rohit Gupta [1], Prachi Srivastava [2] and Jitendra Narayan [1,*]

[1] CSIR Institute of Genomics and Integrative Biology, Mall Road, Delhi 110007, India; nitinshukla218@gmail.com (N.S.); rohit.gupta.delhi1995@gmail.com (R.G.)
[2] Amity Institute of Biotechnology, Amity University, Uttar Pradesh, Lucknow Campus, Lucknow 226010, India; ns011982@gmail.com (N.S.); psrivastava@amity.edu (P.S.)
* Correspondence: jnarayan@igib.res.in
† These authors contributed equally to this work.

Abstract: The SARS-CoV-2 virus, a novel member of the Coronaviridae family, is responsible for the viral infection known as Coronavirus Disease 2019 (COVID-19). In response to the urgent and critical need for rapid detection, diagnosis, analysis, interpretation, and treatment of COVID-19, a wide variety of bioinformatics tools have been developed. Given the virulence of SARS-CoV-2, it is crucial to explore the pathophysiology of the virus. We intend to examine how bioinformatics, in conjunction with next-generation sequencing techniques, can be leveraged to improve current diagnostic tools and streamline vaccine development for emerging SARS-CoV-2 variants. We also emphasize how bioinformatics, in general, can contribute to critical areas of biomedicine, including clinical diagnostics, SARS-CoV-2 genomic surveillance and its evolution, identification of potential drug targets, and development of therapeutic strategies. Currently, state-of-the-art bioinformatics tools have helped overcome technical obstacles with respect to genomic surveillance and have assisted in rapid detection, diagnosis, and delivering precise treatment to individuals on time.

Keywords: SARS-CoV-2; genomics; immunoinformatics; drug design; bioinformatics; COVID-19

Citation: Shukla, N.; Srivastava, N.; Gupta, R.; Srivastava, P.; Narayan, J. COVID Variants, Villain and Victory: A Bioinformatics Perspective. *Microorganisms* **2023**, *11*, 2039. https://doi.org/10.3390/microorganisms11082039

Academic Editor: Qibin Geng

Received: 21 June 2023
Revised: 11 July 2023
Accepted: 11 July 2023
Published: 9 August 2023

1. Introduction

The COVID-19 pandemic, an unprecedented catastrophe, affected nearly every country on multiple levels. Since its emergence in December 2019, the pandemic has caused severe loss of human life, damage to healthcare and educational systems, and displaced economies worldwide. The scientific research community currently faces an arduous challenge since the virus undergoes frequent mutations, leading to the emergence of new variants. The high infectivity and lethality rates of the SARS-CoV-2 virus during its initial days and now, with the given propensity of the virus to mutate, further cause it to remain a major concern. To monitor and track changes in the SARS-CoV-2 genome caused by mutations and identify novel variants, various sequence-based surveillance, laboratory, and epidemiological investigations are now regularly being conducted. Continuous and vigilant genomic surveillance and analysis of viral variants in real time are crucial in the development of effective diagnostics, therapeutics, and vaccines to combat the onslaught of the pandemic.

A variant is defined as having two or more mutations that distinguish it from other variants in terms of spreading. In collaboration with the Centers for Disease Control and Prevention (CDC) and the US Department of Health and Human Services (HHS), the two institutions established an Interagency Group (SIG) to develop a classification system for SARS-CoV-2 variants. They classified them into four categories and marked them as follows: (1) variants of interest (VOI), (2) variants of concern (VOC), (3) variants of high consequences (VOHC), and 4) variants being monitored (VBM) [1,2]. Variants of interest (VOI) are variants with specific heredity marker changes characterized by alterations in the receptor-binding domain (RBD). In addition to reduced antibody neutralization generated post-infection and inoculation, variants can result in decreased efficacy of therapeutics, possible analytic effect, or anticipated expansion in contagiousness or chronic illness. During different peaks of the pandemic, certain variants emerged as notable players. In the spring of 2021, the Iota variant (B.1.526) took the spotlight in the United States, while in the summer of the same year, the Epsilon variant (B.1.427 & B.1.429) gained prominence in the region, exhibiting an approximate 20% increase in transmission rate. In the United Kingdom (UK), the Eta variant (B.1.525) emerged during the spring of 2021. In India, the Kappa variant (B.1.617.1 & B.1.617.3) made its presence known, eventually giving rise to the highly infectious Delta variant. As of June 2023, the VOIs circulating in the population are XBB.1.5 and XBB.1.16, both of which are suspected to possess increased immune escape potential and continue to cause surges in infection rates (Figure 1) [3].

SARS-CoV-2 cases per million

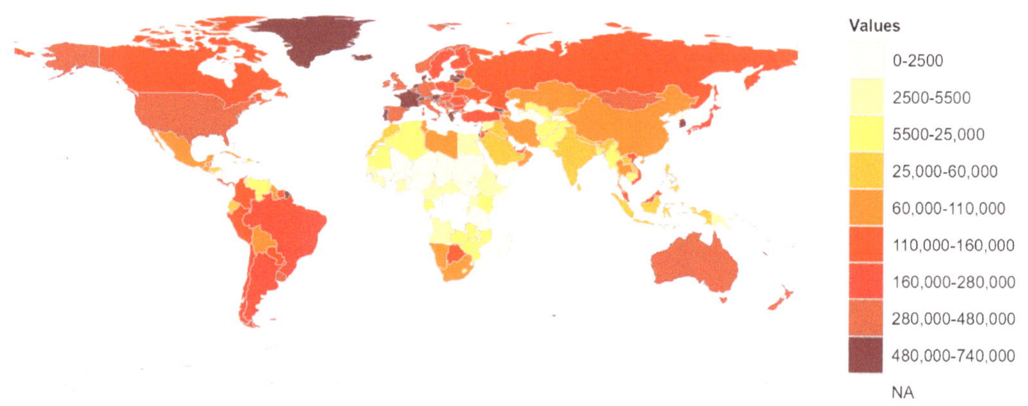

Figure 1. Frequency of confirmed COVID-19 cases per million across the world as of June 2023 [4].

Lineages classified as VOC have been the most devastating during the course of the pandemic, leading to high hospitalization and mortality rates, in addition to the development of chronic health issues such as post-acute sequelae of COVID-19 (PASC), more commonly known as long COVID, type 2 diabetes, fatigue, and dyslipidemia, among others, resulting in lifelong disability and medical care [5]. The hallmarks of VOCs are their increased rates of transmission and immune escape potential, leading to a significant reduction in neutralization antibodies in addition to decreased effectiveness of therapeutics and vaccines, resulting in high rates of hospitalization and death. The major VOCs throughout the course of the pandemic included the Alpha (B.1.1.7) variant, identified in the UK in December 2020 [6], possessing 23 mutations as compared to the wild-type variant, with an extremely high transmissibility rate of ~70% [7]; it had become dominant in 21 countries by March 2021. The Beta (B.1.351) variant was first identified in South Africa in October 2020, defined by 12 mutations in its genome compared to the wild-type, and was the first VOC to display decreased vaccine efficacy and monoclonal antibody resistance [8]; it was responsible for pandemic waves across the African continent. The Delta (B.1.617.2), first identified in India in October 2020, was the most devastating out of all VOCs so far. It was considered to be 50% more transmissible than the Alpha variant and was the dominant lineage during India's second wave, and it contributed to third waves in the UK and South Africa and eventually became the dominant variant worldwide. The Delta variant possessed 13 mutations, 8 of which were in the spike (S) protein [9], thus increasing its transmissibility and ability to infect the lower respiratory tract, causing severe disease conditions such as acute respiratory distress syndrome (ARDS) [10]. The current

VOC, Omicron (B.1.1.529), identified in November 2021 in South Africa, is the most diverse variant of all the VOCs before it, carrying approximately 50 mutations, and has since continuously evolved into subvariants, leading to WHO changing their classification system; thus, Omicron subvariants are tracked independently [11]. Omicron and its subvariants possess significant immune escape potential, with Omicron subvariants such as BA.1, BA.2, BA.4, and BA.5 being poorly neutralized by first-generation vaccines, in addition to being resistant against most monoclonal antibodies except bebtelovimab [3]. However, Omicron seems to display a bias for infecting the upper respiratory tract over the lower respiratory tract [12], possibly due to lower fusogenicity and possibly altered tissue tropism due to its ability to be primed by endosomal proteases, such as cathepsins, a phenomenon seen in SARS-CoV [13–15]. This mechanism is hypothesized to somewhat play a role in the decreased severity of disease, though all current evidence that supports this is limited to rodent models [15,16].

Thus, these variants play the role of a villain, causing serious health complications in people who are infected and post-infection as well. Delta variants have been found to be significantly more virulent as well as contagious as compared to other variants and were mainly responsible for the global surges in 2021, particularly in India, South Africa, and the United Kingdom. The high transmission rates expose the population to repeat infections, potentially leading to a higher risk of developing long COVID [17], whose symptoms can last for years and in some cases, lifelong. Additionally, repeat COVID-19 infections heighten the risk of developing adverse comorbidities such as cardiovascular disease, type 2 diabetes [18], or myalgic encephalomyelitis/chronic fatigue syndrome (ME/CFS) [19]. Furthermore, the Delta variant displayed increased lethality as compared to the Omicron variant, with a median case-fatality rate (CFR) of 8.56 as compared to 3.04, respectively [20], probably due to increased vaccine coverage and decreasing pathogenicity as the virus continues to evolve. As the virus evolves, the effect of medical therapeutics and available interventions continues to decrease, leading to an increased risk of hospitalization, particularly in high-risk groups. New mutations drive a strong increase in transmission rates, and a constantly evolving machinery of SARS-CoV-2 means decreased drug response to new symptoms that the virus may give rise to. Therefore, mutations and variants impeded research; as a result, universal inoculation was the effective long-term solution to thwart the growing risk of an evolving SARS-CoV-2 virus and assist in decreasing mortality and hospitalization rates [21].

Bioinformatics has created a milestone and has played an essential role in COVID-19 research since the emergence of the pandemic [22], especially in detecting and tracking new variants, as well as in allowing for open data-sharing across the world. Wide varieties of bioinformatics tools and techniques have been used successfully in the interpretation of the genomic architecture of SARS-CoV-2 and its variants, as well as in the creation of mathematical models used to predict infection spread, design containment methods, and drive public health policy decisions [23,24]. They have been utilized in analyzing the data generated from genomics, transcriptomics, proteomics, and structural omics, as well as single-cell data. They have contributed to a better understanding of the underlying molecular mechanisms of viral pathogenesis, allowing for the rapid identification of vaccine and drug candidates [25], particularly for the rapid deployment of repurposed drugs during the pandemic [24,26] for clinical research and eventually, for clinical trials. From this perspective, we highlight the strong contributions and achievements of bioinformatics tools and techniques in combating the COVID-19 pandemic.

2. Tracking of SARS-CoV-2

Next-generation sequencing (NGS), also defined as high-throughput sequencing technology, has become a widely adopted approach in genomics research to identify virus origins, delineate mechanistically phenotypic causative pathophysiology, and elucidate genotypic ramifications in infected individuals. These technologies have further led to the development of novel bioinformatics tools, pipelines, algorithms, and machine-learning approaches that have now become robust practices in understanding the virus genome [27].

Advancements made in metagenomics have aided in the identification of plausible co-occurring pathogens that may play a role in the clinical outcome of SARS-CoV-2 infections. Thus, studying host–pathogen interactions also become important in this context. Augmenting this with different analytical strategies that bioinformatics tools offer allows us to unravel the same genomic data via different lenses to uncover the underlying layers of host–pathogen interactions, which may modulate disease severity as well as clinical outcome [28]. Various metagenomics tools such as Kraken2 [29], MOTHUR [30], and QIIME2 [31] provide deep insights into genomic data as well as provide ways to visualize data; thus, meaningful insights can be extracted. Further, this is combined with Seurat [32], a single-cell analysis R library, which allows for spatial visualization of multiple clusters of cells that may themselves be strongly implicated in disease pathophysiology. The analysis is then extended further with downstream machine-learning tools, such as singleR [33] and clustifyr [34]. These can be leveraged to annotate cell clusters with public data libraries with high confidence and further identify causal gene–pathway relationships with respect to the cell types that may be contributing factors in disease pathophysiology.

In this context, an opportunity exists to develop a cohesive and well-developed workflow that takes into account distinct steps that occur in the data analysis, thus streamlining the process of variant discovery. Typically, an NGS data analysis pipeline consists of various integral steps, such as quality control of the data, deletion of extraneous host data, and read assembly, followed by taxonomic classification (of pathogens) and, lastly, supplemented by virus genome verification. Due to the wide adoption, use, and build of various open-source methods, various tools exist that help in further carrying out each step elucidated above.

Bioinformatics tools have accelerated efforts in unwinding the mutations and genetic variation of the SARS-CoV-2 virus. Undoubtedly, SARS-CoV-2 has the potential to adapt during the current pandemic because of its high and rapid mutation rate. How this evolution has an impact on the transmission, duration, and gravity of disease is still under study. The increasing amount of evidence of human–wildlife interactions has facilitated the zoonotic transmission from animals to humans.

In SARS-CoV-2, the spike protein of the virus has sufficient binding affinity with the receptor of angiotensin-converting enzyme 2 (ACE2), which is crucial for host cell entry and human infection. Several computational models and data have also indicated that additional mutations at the binding site strengthen the binding affinity [35,36]. According to Nextstrain [37], SARS-CoV-2 underwent roughly one genetic change per week based on the substitution rate. The mutation rate of the SARS-CoV-2 virus is estimated at 1×10^{-6}–2×10^{-6} mutations per nucleotide per replication cycle [38]. The availability of abundant data and resources on the viral genome exhibited the intense response to the pandemic by tracking and tracing of infection to drug and vaccine development. Nextstrain collects, analyzes, visualizes, and maintains metadata of SARS-CoV-2 from various public data repositories, including NCBI (www.ncbi.nlm.nih.gov, accessed 9 July 2023), GISAID (www.gisaid.org, accessed 9 July 2023), and GitHub repositories.

The genomic data allows us to understand the dynamics of the genome evolution of viruses, including mutations and natural selection, which are very important aspects for detecting clinical variants and their epidemiological significance, understanding viral evolution and responses of the immune system to mutations, and vaccine and drug development. The graphical display of sequence data is also available for a better understanding of the genomic epidemiology of SARS-CoV-2 (Figure 2). Bioinformatics strategies play a key role in the rapid detection, tracing, understanding, analysis, evaluation, and treatment of COVID-19. With the sheer amount of available data, scientists are globally investigating evolution at the genome and protein level to tackle the pandemic [39]. For early detection, tracking, tracing, sequencing, and the creation of therapeutic methods, a variety of bioinformatics workflows and tools have been developed. Interestingly, we have seen a more than four-fold increase in drug designing tools and software in the last few years, while ML tools have increased by two-fold (Figure 3). To avoid the false-positive and false-negative detection of qRT-PCR [40], a computation-based primer PriSeT has been developed for detecting the specificity and sensitivity of the qRT-PCR test [41].

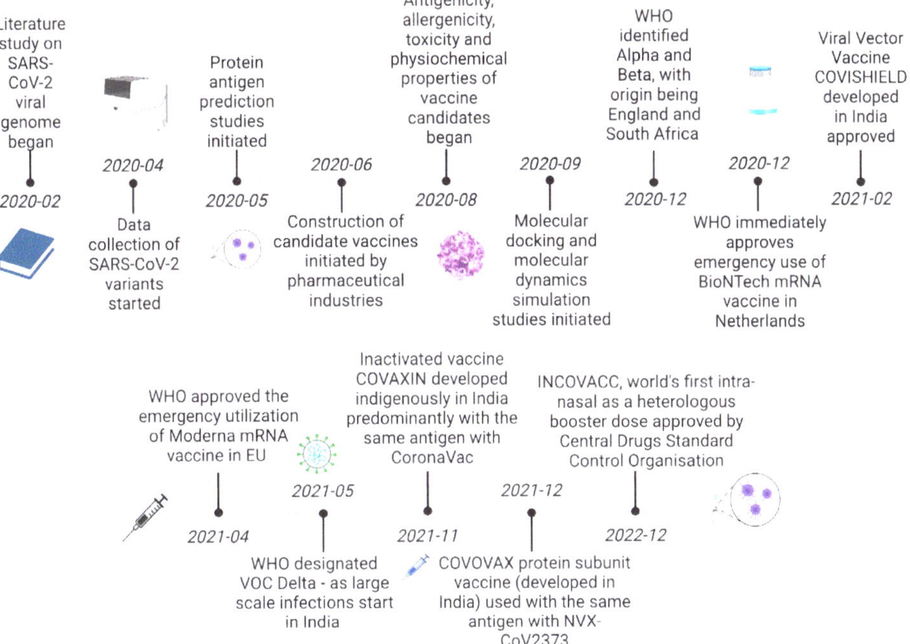

Figure 2. In silico vaccine development timeline [42,43].

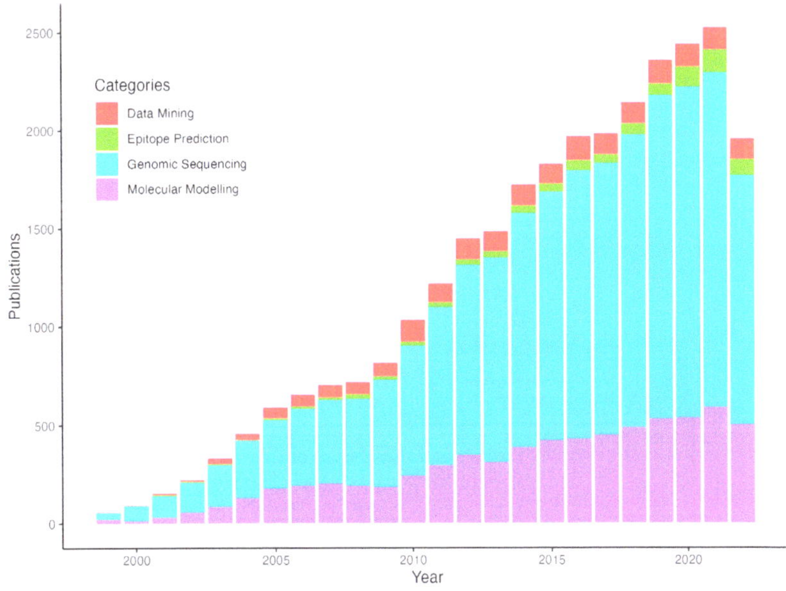

Figure 3. Stacked bar chart displaying the rising rate of published computational methods across various domains over the years.

Next-generation sequencing workflow V-Pipe [44] and Haploflow [45] are developed to evaluate and monitor genetic diversity and mutation. Amplicon-based metagenomics sequencing has been prevalent throughout the pandemic and has been extensively used to study sequence divergence [46,47]. Several open-source databases, such as GISAID, NCBI, and EMBL-EBI, provide easy access and submission for high-quality SARS-CoV-2 genome sequence metadata globally. For the detection and annotation of viral genomes, numerous bioinformatics tools, software, and pipelines have been developed, including VADR [48], VBRC tools (https://4virology.net/virology-ca-tools/, accessed 4 July 2023), and VIRULIGN [49]. Various databases, such as UniProt, Pfam, and Rfam [50], are available to allow users to investigate coding and non-coding sequence evolution and diversity to understand viral epidemiology and evolution.

Besides this, numerous platforms and models were developed to study the fundamentals of evolutionary, epidemiology, and phylogenetic divergence of viruses. The phylodynamic models include BEAST 2 [51] for phylogeographic reconstruction; epidemic-mathematical models such as COPASI [52] and COVIDSIM [53]; and evolutionary tracking models like CoV-GLUE [54] and CoVe-Tracker are available [55]. The machine-learning model Covidex [56] is an open-source alignment tool based on Nextstrain and GISAID data used for the rapid classification of viral genomes in pre-defined clusters isolated from the population. Pangolin [57] rapidly assigns the most likely classification for a large number of genome sequences, which is particularly useful for local and global surveillance. All of these tools are freely available around the world for users. Thus, bioinformaticians are quickly responding to the pandemic and have provided easy and rapid access to COVID-19-specific tools and techniques for tracking and tracing the virus.

Certain limitations do currently exist in the space of NGS; bottlenecks continue to plague the efficacy of bioinformatics tools that could otherwise be leveraged to their full potential. More often than not, the virus reads (e.g., SARS-CoV-2 reads) are usually low in genomic data; this extends to single-cell data as well. In this case, to perform detailed analysis, different approaches need to be utilized; for instance, a homology-based approach or a protein structure-based method. Furthermore, robust and time-sensitive analysis becomes a challenge with the ever-increasing magnitude of availability of full-length genome sequences of SARS-CoV-2, spanning hundreds of gigabytes. One approach is to randomly subsample data and analyses rather than performing a full phylogenetic analysis on the entire genome data, which would be time-consuming and produce extremely complex results that may not lead to mechanistic insights critical to understanding virus transmission mechanisms. Thus, it is critical to continue developing bioinformatics tools with long-term strategic applications in mind so that researchers can perform efficient and rapid data analysis and clinical trial deployment.

3. Vaccine Status and Development

At least eighty infectious agents that manifest on a regular basis are known to be pathogenic in humans. Out of these eighty, more than thirty have licensed individual vaccines that target 26 of these infectious diseases—most of which are either viral or bacterial in nature. Given that vaccines have been instrumental in reducing mortality rates across the world at tremendous rates, it is also important to note that some of these vaccines are being used regularly and have been deployed to primarily circumvent childhood infections. Vaccination programs have been instrumental in reducing morbidity and mortality and inferring immunity to immunocompromised individuals and to children [58].

SARS-CoV-2 rapid evolution and transmission that continued unabated due to lack of herd immunity and lack of clinical drugs that could provide effective treatment meant that a mass vaccination program needed to be dispositioned immediately. Bioinformatics databases—which contain data with respect to nucleic acid sequences, protein sequences, ontologies, host databases, pathogen databases, and functional immunological databases (to name a few)—played a pivotal role in accelerating the development of novel mRNA vaccines that could shift the momentum that SARS-CoV-2 infection was gaining at a rapid pace. Further, the combined use of bioinformatics tools and machine-learning tools to make use of these databases was further monumental in guiding the precise development of the vaccines [38]. Further, accelerated research in these areas proved instrumental in the development of candidate vaccines (Figure 3). A variety of AI modalities were utilized for effective vaccine development and for evaluating the safety of such vaccines. A few of the vaccines that gained emergency use approval during the pandemic included: BNT162b2 from Pfizer-BioNTech, mRNA-1273 from Moderna, ChAdOx1 nCoV-19 from Oxford-AstraZeneca, and JNJ-78436735 from Johnson and Johnson [59].

Multipronged in silico approaches, including bioinformatics, vaccino-genomics, immunoinformatics, structural biology, and molecular dynamic simulations, are freely available to support precise vaccine design (Table 1). The sequenced SARS-CoV-2 genome is widely used in computational tools and databases for predicting novel B-cell and T-cell epitopes in vaccine development, immunity protein analysis, and immunization modeling. It deserves to be mentioned that immunoinformatics continues to be challenged by the accurate prediction of B-cell epitopes (BCE) and T-cell epitopes (TCE), which form the basis of the development of epitope-based vaccines [60].

Table 1. Categories with numerous bioinformatics tools have elucidated and assisted in the design, development, and deployment of potential vaccines in the fight against SARS-CoV-2 and its variants [27,39].

Areas Supporting Candidate Vaccine Development	Description	Examples
Genome Sequencing	Rapid processing and analysis of sequenced SARS-CoV-2 genomes aid in the rapid identification of mutations and thus aid in developing potential therapeutic targets and surveillance.	Trimmomatic, BWA, SAMTools, Seurat, GATK, SPAdes, Pangolin, IGV, Deseq2/EdgeR
Molecular Modeling	Various computational tools for molecular docking and molecular dynamics simulations facilitate the design and optimize therapeutic candidates.	PyMOL, Chimera, GROMACS, CHARMM, AMBER
Epitope Prediction	Numerous bioinformatics tools are being used to predict potential epitopes (antigenic determinants) that could be used to induce an immune response in the host and accelerate research/development.	NetMHC, IEDB, BepiPred, DiscoTope, Ellipro, ABCpred
Data Mining	Large-scale data mining and synthesizing of large-scale databases and information have speeded up the process of understanding virulence factors of new mutations, predicting their behavior, and creating appropriate drugs/vaccines to mitigate severe illness and curb spread, and inform public health policy.	Weka, Orange, KNIME, Cytoscape, TANGARA

During early March 2020, when the pandemic was gaining a foothold, a structure-based immunoinformatics methodology was employed to determine epitopes in SARS-CoV-2 for potential peptide-based vaccine design initiation. Wang and colleagues predicted 9 highly antigenic B-cell epitopes on the Spike (S) protein as well as 62 T-cell epitopes [61]. Reverse vaccinology (RV) is also a broadly used technique that employs computational methods to identify open reading frames (ORFs) from viral genomes, resulting in the discovery of new antigens [62]. The VaxiJen [63] server is used to study the physicochemical properties of antigen epitopes. Various machine-learning, as well as deep-learning models, have been employed to predict novel immunogenic subunits. These models have been crucial in identifying the epitopes for cytotoxic and helper T lymphocytes as well as in exploring the genetic polymorphism in the target human population [64,65]. Structural vaccinology techniques play a prominent role in identifying structurally stable, safe, and potent peptides as novel vaccine candidates [66]. Current bioinformatics tools such as Sprint [67], ModlAMP [68], pepATTRACT [69], PEPFOLD3 [70], IEDB [71], MHCPRED [72], SVMtrip [73], and AllerTop [42] have now been integrated into the programs for vaccine development.

It has to be noted, though, the drop in values across all categories in 2022 is due to a multitude of factors, such as a significant decrease in publications due to delays in peer-review processes and timelines due to a lack of manpower/staff, since an overwhelming number of COVID-19-related studies were submitted. Furthermore, financial resources were diverted from genomic sequencing to more clinical measures of control for the pandemic—such as support for healthcare infrastructure, vaccine development, and medical supplies/equipment costs to mitigate impact [74,75]. The future of immunoinformatics is important, as it will determine the pace with which we will overcome the next pandemic, in case it manifests. The rapid design, development, and deployment pipelines for vaccines will need to be refined with iterative use, reuse, and refinement of existing open-source bioinformatics databases and tools, as well as the development of new tools/pipelines that will be created in the future. Thus, bioinformatics shows a promising role in the rapid development of potent vaccine candidates against SARS-CoV-2, fighting the global mortality of COVID-19.

4. Discussion and Conclusions

Finally, a major milestone in the fight against the pandemic was reached on 5 May 2023, when the Director-General of the World Health Organization (WHO) declared that COVID-19 was no longer classified as a 'global health emergency' but rather an ongoing health concern [76]. While this announcement marked a significant achievement, it is important to acknowledge that SARS-CoV-2, the virus responsible for COVID-19, continues to undergo rapid evolution, adapting to its environment and potentially enhancing its ability to evade immune responses and spread. However, there are indications that these changes in the virus may come at the expense of its severity. The development of effective vaccines in record time has played a major role in modifying the evolutionary landscape and weakening the severe effects of the virus. While predicting the evolutionary path of the virus is still hard, consistent genomic surveillance will allow for early prediction of its transition. Vaccines and therapeutics still need to be updated to maintain immunity in the population and prevent hospitalization and death, especially in high-risk groups and children, while also preparing to put systems in place so that states are better prepared for future pandemics and global health emergencies.

Bioinformatics has played a transformational role in SARS-CoV-2 diagnosis and treatment through high-quality, well-curated pipelines, software, and datasets, allowing for rapid design, development, and deployment. These are important not only in drug discovery but also in drug development and allied processes. It entails using informatics to gain new insights into health and disease, managing data during clinical trials, and reusing clinical data. We discovered that bioinformatics tools were critical in bolstering efforts to combat the COVID-19 pandemic, identifying and informing the public about emerging variants and their potential phenotypic manifestations and analyzing the virus at both the sequence and structural levels, and resulting in the rapid development of vaccines and other effective therapeutics to combat severe complications and, more importantly, develop vaccines. Thus, bioinformatics will continue to play a pivotal role in shaping the next paradigm of health, advancing personalized medicine and pushing the boundaries of elucidating the genomic architecture of infectious diseases, and ensuring we emerge victorious in safeguarding public health against unprecedented infectious diseases.

Author Contributions: Conceptualization, N.S. (Nityendra Shukla), J.N. and P.S.; resources, J.N., N.S. (Nityendra Shukla) and P.S.; data curation, J.N., N.S. (Nityendra Shukla), N.S. (Neha Srivastava) and R.G.; writing—original draft preparation, N.S. (Nityendra Shukla), N.S. (Neha Srivastava), P.S. and J.N.; writing—review and editing, N.S. (Nityendra Shukla), N.S. (Neha Srivastava), P.S. and J.N.; visualization, N.S. (Nityendra Shukla) and R.G.; supervision, P.S. and J.N.; project administration, J.N. All authors have read and agreed to the published version of the manuscript.

Funding: The Rockefeller Foundation provided funding for this work. The CSIR Institute of Genomics and Integrative Biology received this grant, which enabled them to carry out the research and complete the study.

Data Availability Statement: Please visit the following GitHub page https://github.com/ns012/dr-ns (accessed 2 July 2023) to find scripts utilized for construction of the plots as well as data used in the process.

Conflicts of Interest: The authors declare no conflict of interest.

References

1. Centers for Disease Control Control and Prevention. SARS-CoV-2 Variant Classifications and Definitions. 2023. Available online: https://www.cdc.gov/coronavirus/2019-ncov/variants/variant-classifications.html (accessed on 25 March 2023).
2. WHO. Updated Working Definitions and Primary Actions for SARS-CoV-2 Variants. 2023. Available online: https://www.who.int/publications/m/item/updated-working-definitions-and-primary-actions-for{-}{-}sars-cov-2-variants (accessed on 14 June 2023).
3. World Health Organization. Statement on the Update of WHO's Working Definitions and Tracking System for SARS-CoV-2 Variants of Concern and Variants of Interest. 2023. Available online: https://www.who.int/news/item/16-03-2023-statement-on-the-update-of-who-s-working-definitions-and-tracking-system-for-sars-cov-2-variants-of-concern-and-variants-of-interest (accessed on 14 June 2023).
4. Mathieu, E.; Ritchie, H.; Rodés-Guirao, L.; Appel, C.; Gavrilov, D.; Giattino, C.; Hasell, J.; Macdonald, B.; Dattani, S.; Beltekian, D.; et al. Coronavirus Pandemic (COVID-19). 2020. Available online: https://ourworldindata.org/covid-cases/ (accessed on 16 June 2023).
5. Davis, H.E.; Assaf, G.S.; McCorkell, L.; Wei, H.; Low, R.J.; Re'Em, Y.; Redfield, S.; Austin, J.P.; Akrami, A. Characterizing long COVID in an international cohort: 7 months of symptoms and their impact. *Eclinicalmedicine* **2021**, *38*, 101019. [CrossRef]
6. Rambaut, A.; Loman, N.; Pybus, O.; Barclay, W.; Barrett, J.; Carabelli, A.; Connor, T.; Peacock, T.; Robertson, D.L.; Volz, E. Preliminary Genomic Characterisation of an Emergent SARS-CoV-2 Lineage in the UK Defined by a Novel Set of Spike Mutations. 2020. Available online: https://virological.org/t/preliminary-genomic-characterisation-of-an-emergent-sars-cov-2-lineage-in-the-uk-defined-by-a-novel-set-of-spike-mutations/563 (accessed on 3 July 2023).
7. Volz, E.; Mishra, S.; Chand, M.; Barrett, J.C.; Johnson, R.; Geidelberg, L.; Ferguson, N.M. Assessing transmissibility of SARS-CoV-2 lineage B.1.1.7 in England. *Nature* **2021**, *593*, 266–269. [CrossRef] [PubMed]
8. Weisblum, Y.; Schmidt, F.; Zhang, F.; DaSilva, J.; Poston, D.; Lorenzi, J.C.; Bieniasz, P.D. Escape from neutralizing antibodies by SARS-CoV-2 spike protein variants. *eLife* **2020**, *9*, e61312. [CrossRef] [PubMed]
9. Mlcochova, P.; Kemp, S.A.; Dhar, M.S.; Papa, G.; Meng, B.; Ferreira, I.A.T.M.; Datir, R.; Collier, D.A.; Albecka, A.; Singh, S.; et al. SARS-CoV-2 B.1.617.2 Delta variant replication and immune evasion. *Nature* **2021**, *599*, 114–119. [CrossRef] [PubMed]
10. Li, X.; Ma, X. Acute respiratory failure in COVID-19: Is it "typical" ARDS? *Crit. Care* **2020**, *24*, 198. [CrossRef] [PubMed]
11. Khandia, R.; Singhal, S.; Alqahtani, T.; Kamal, M.A.; El-Shall, N.A.; Nainu, F.; Desingu, P.A.; Dhama, K. Emergence of SARS-CoV-2 Omicron (B.1.1.529) variant, salient features, high global health concerns and strategies to counter it amid ongoing COVID-19 pandemic. *Environ. Res.* **2022**, *209*, 112816. [CrossRef]
12. Hyams, C.; Challen, R.; Marlow, R.; Nguyen, J.; Begier, E.; Southern, J.; Szasz-Benczur, Z. Severity of Omicron (B.1.1.529) and Delta (B.1.617.2) SARS-CoV-2 infection among hospitalised adults: A prospective cohort study in Bristol, United Kingdom. *Lancet Reg. Health Eur.* **2023**, *25*, 100556. [CrossRef]
13. Carabelli, A.M.; Peacock, T.P.; Thorne, L.G.; Harvey, W.T.; Hughes, J. SARS-CoV-2 variant biology: Immune escape, transmission and fitness. *Nat. Rev. Microbiol.* **2023**, *21*, 162–177. [CrossRef]
14. Willett, B.J.; Grove, J.; MacLean, O.A.; Wilkie, C.; De Lorenzo, G.; Furnon, W.; Thomson, E.C. SARS-CoV-2 Omicron is an immune escape variant with an altered cell entry pathway. *Nat. Microbiol.* **2022**, *7*, 1161–1179. [CrossRef]
15. Meng, B.; Abdullahi, A.; Ferreira, I.A.; Goonawardane, N.; Saito, A.; Kimura, I.; Gupta, R.K. Altered TMPRSS2 usage by SARS-CoV-2 Omicron impacts infectivity and fusogenicity. *Nature* **2022**, *603*, 706–714. [CrossRef] [PubMed]
16. Suzuki, R.; Yamasoba, D.; Kimura, I.; Wang, L.; Kishimoto, M.; Ito, J.; Sato, K. Attenuated fusogenicity and pathogenicity of SARS-CoV-2 Omicron variant. *Nature* **2022**, *603*, 700–705. [CrossRef]
17. Bentley, E.G.; Kirby, A.; Sharma, P.; Kipar, A.; Mega, D.F.; Bramwell, C.; Stewart, J.P. SARS-CoV-2 Omicron-B.1.1.529 Variant leads to less severe disease than Pango B and Delta variants strains in a mouse model of severe COVID-19. *BioRxiv* **2021**, *Preprint*. [CrossRef]
18. Bowe, B.; Xie, Y.; Al-Aly, Z. Acute and postacute sequelae associated with SARS-CoV-2 reinfection. *Nat. Med.* **2022**, *28*, 2398–2405. [CrossRef] [PubMed]
19. Kedor, C.; Freitag, H.; Meyer-Arndt, L.; Wittke, K.; Hanitsch, L.G.; Zoller, T.; Scheibenbogen, C. A prospective observational study of post-COVID-19 chronic fatigue syndrome following the first pandemic wave in Germany and biomarkers associated with symptom severity. *Nat. Commun.* **2022**, *13*, 5104. [CrossRef] [PubMed]

20. Wang, C.; Liu, B.; Zhang, S.; Huang, N.; Zhao, T.; Lu, Q.B.; Cui, F. Differences in incidence and fatality of COVID-19 by SARS-CoV-2 Omicron variant versus Delta variant in relation to vaccine coverage: A world-wide review. *J. Med. Virol.* **2023**, *95*, e28118. [CrossRef] [PubMed]

21. Yang, W.; Shaman, J.L. Author response: COVID-19 pandemic dynamics in South Africa and epidemiological characteristics of three variants of concern (Beta, Delta, and Omicron). *eLife* **2022**, *11*, e78933. [CrossRef]

22. Ray, M.; Sable, M.N.; Sarkar, S.; Hallur, V. Essential interpretations of bioinformatics in COVID-19 pandemic. *Meta Gene* **2020**, *27*, 100844. [CrossRef]

23. Guzzi, P.H.; Petrizzelli, F.; Mazza, T. Disease spreading modeling and analysis: A survey. *Brief. Bioinform.* **2022**, *23*, bbac230. [CrossRef]

24. Kumar Das, J.; Tradigo, G.; Veltri, P.; Guzzi, P.H.; Roy, S. Data science in unveiling COVID-19 pathogenesis and diagnosis: Evolutionary origin to drug repurposing. *Brief. Bioinform.* **2021**, *22*, 855–872. [CrossRef]

25. Ma, J.; Deng, Y.; Zhang, M.; Yu, J. The role of multi-omics in the diagnosis of COVID-19 and the prediction of new therapeutic targets. *Virulence* **2022**, *13*, 1101–1110. [CrossRef]

26. Siminea, N.; Popescu, V.; Martin, J.A.S.; Florea, D.; Gavril, G.; Gheorghe, A.-M.; Iţcuş, C.; Kanhaiya, K.; Pacioglu, O.; Popa, L.I.; et al. Network analytics for drug repurposing in COVID-19. *Brief. Bioinform.* **2021**, *23*, bbab490. [CrossRef]

27. Hu, T.; Li, J.; Zhou, H.; Li, C.; Holmes, E.C.; Shi, W. Bioinformatics resources for SARS-CoV-2 discovery and surveillance. *Brief. Bioinform.* **2021**, *22*, 631–641. [CrossRef]

28. Mehta, P.; Swaminathan, A.; Yadav, A.; Chattopadhyay, P.; Shamim, U.; Pandey, R. Integrative genomics important to understand host–pathogen interactions. *Brief. Funct. Genom.* **2022**, elac021. [CrossRef]

29. Wood, D.E.; Lu, J.; Langmead, B. Improved metagenomic analysis with Kraken 2. *Genome Biol.* **2019**, *20*, 257. [CrossRef]

30. Schloss, P.D.; Westcott, S.L.; Ryabin, T.; Hall, J.R.; Hartmann, M.; Hollister, E.B.; Lesniewski, R.A.; Oakley, B.B.; Parks, D.H.; Robinson, C.J.; et al. Introducing mothur: Open-Source, Platform-Independent, Community-Supported Software for Describing and Comparing Microbial Communities. *Appl. Environ. Microbiol.* **2009**, *75*, 7537–7541. [CrossRef] [PubMed]

31. Bolyen, E.; Rideout, J.R.; Dillon, M.R.; Bokulich, N.A.; Abnet, C.C.; Al-Ghalith, G.A.; Alexander, H.; Alm, E.J.; Arumugam, M.; Asnicar, F.; et al. Reproducible, Interactive, Scalable and Extensible Microbiome Data Science using QIIME 2. *Nat. Biotechnol.* **2019**, *37*, 852–857. [CrossRef] [PubMed]

32. Hao, Y.; Hao, S.; Andersen-Nissen, E.; Mauck, W.M., 3rd; Zheng, S.; Butler, A.; Lee, M.J.; Wilk, A.J.; Darby, C.; Zager, M.; et al. Integrated analysis of multimodal single-cell data. *Cell* **2021**, *184*, 3573–3587.e29. [CrossRef] [PubMed]

33. Aran, D.; Looney, A.P.; Liu, L.; Wu, E.; Fong, V.; Hsu, A.; Chak, S.; Naikawadi, R.P.; Wolters, P.J.; Abate, A.R.; et al. Reference-based analysis of lung single-cell sequencing reveals a transitional profibrotic macrophage. *Nat. Immunol.* **2019**, *20*, 163–172. [CrossRef]

34. Fu, R.; Gillen, A.E.; Sheridan, R.M.; Tian, C.; Daya, M.; Hao, Y.; Riemondy, K.A. clustifyr: An R package for automated single-cell RNA sequencing cluster classification. *F1000Research* **2020**, *9*, 223. [CrossRef]

35. Chen, J.; Wang, R.; Wang, M.; Wei, G.W. Mutations Strengthened SARS-CoV-2 Infectivity. *J. Mol. Biol.* **2020**, *432*, 5212–5226. [CrossRef]

36. Bate, N.; Savva, C.G.; Moody, P.C.; Brown, E.A.; Evans, S.E.; Ball, J.K.; Brindle, N.P. In vitro evolution predicts emerging SARS-CoV-2 mutations with high affinity for ACE2 and cross-species binding. *PLoS Pathog.* **2022**, *18*, e1010733. [CrossRef]

37. Hadfield, J.; Megill, C.; Bell, S.M.; Huddleston, J.; Potter, B.; Callender, C.; Sagulenko, P.; Bedford, T.; Neher, R.A. Nextstrain: Real-time tracking of pathogen evolution. *Bioinformatics* **2018**, *34*, 4121–4123. [CrossRef] [PubMed]

38. Markov, P.V.; Ghafari, M.; Beer, M.; Lythgoe, K.; Simmonds, P.; Stilianakis, N.I.; Katzourakis, A. The evolution of SARS-CoV-2. *Nat. Rev. Microbiol.* **2023**, *21*, 361–379. [CrossRef]

39. Hufsky, F.; Lamkiewicz, K.; Almeida, A.; Aouacheria, A.; Arighi, C.; Bateman, A.; Marz, M. Computational strategies to combat COVID-19: Useful tools to accelerate SARS-CoV-2 and coronavirus research. *Brief. Bioinform.* **2021**, *22*, 642–663. [CrossRef] [PubMed]

40. Corman, V.M.; Landt, O.; Kaiser, M.; Molenkamp, R.; Meijer, A.; Chu, D.K.W.; Bleicker, T.; Brünink, S.; Schneider, J.; Schmidt, M.L.; et al. Detection of 2019 novel coronavirus (2019-nCoV) by real-time RT-PCR. *Eurosurveillance* **2020**, *25*, 2000045. [CrossRef] [PubMed]

41. Hoffmann, M.; Monaghan, M.T.; Reinert, K. PriSeT: Efficient de novo primer discovery. In Proceedings of the 12th ACM Conference on Bioinformatics, Computational Biology, and Health Informatics, Gaineswille, FL, USA, 1–4 August 2021; pp. 1–12.

42. Sumon, T.A.; Hussain, A.; Hasan, T.; Hasan, M.; Jang, W.J.; Bhuiya, E.H.; Chowdhury, A.A.M.; Sharifuzzaman, S.M.; Brown, C.L.; Kwon, H.-J.; et al. A Revisit to the Research Updates of Drugs, Vaccines, and Bioinformatics Approaches in Combating COVID-19 Pandemic. *Front. Mol. Biosci.* **2021**, *7*, 585899. [CrossRef]

43. Kumar, V.M.; Pandi-Perumal, S.R.; Trakht, I.; Thyagarajan, S.P. Strategy for COVID-19 vaccination in India: The country with the second highest population and number of cases. *NPJ Vaccines* **2021**, *6*, 60. [CrossRef] [PubMed]

44. Posada-Céspedes, S.; Seifert, D.; Topolsky, I.; Jablonski, K.P.; Metzner, K.J.; Beerenwinkel, N. V-pipe: A computational pipeline for assessing viral genetic diversity from high-throughput data. *Bioinformatics* **2021**, *37*, 1673–1680. [CrossRef]

45. Fritz, A.; Bremges, A.; Deng, Z.L.; Lesker, T.R.; Götting, J.; Ganzenmueller, T.; McHardy, A.C. Haploflow: Strain-resolved de novo assembly of viral genomes. *Genome Biol.* **2021**, *22*, 212. [CrossRef]

46. Gohl, D.M.; Garbe, J.; Grady, P.; Daniel, J.; Watson, R.H.; Auch, B.; Beckman, K.B. A rapid, cost-effective tailed amplicon method for sequencing SARS-CoV-2. *BMC Genom.* **2020**, *21*, 863. [CrossRef]

47. Rosenthal, S.H.; Gerasimova, A.; Ruiz-Vega, R.; Livingston, K.; Kagan, R.M.; Liu, Y.; Lacbawan, F. Development and validation of a high throughput SARS-CoV-2 whole genome sequencing workflow in a clinical laboratory. *Sci. Rep.* **2022**, *12*, 2054. [CrossRef]

48. Schäffer, A.A.; Hatcher, E.L.; Yankie, L.; Shonkwiler, L.; Brister, J.R.; Mizrachi, I.K.; Nawrocki, E.P. VADR: Validation and annotation of virus sequence submissions to GenBank. *BMC Bioinform.* **2020**, *21*, 211. [CrossRef]

49. Libin, P.J.K.; Deforche, K.; Abecasis, A.B.; Theys, K. VIRULIGN: Fast codon-correct alignment and annotation of viral genomes. *Bioinformatics* **2018**, *35*, 1763–1765. [CrossRef]

50. Kalvari, I.; Argasinska, J.; Quinones-Olvera, N.; Nawrocki, E.P.; Rivas, E.; Eddy, S.R.; Bateman, A.; Finn, R.D.; I Petrov, A. Rfam 13.0: Shifting to a genome-centric resource for non-coding RNA families. *Nucleic Acids Res.* **2018**, *46*, D335–D342. [CrossRef] [PubMed]

51. Bouckaert, R.; Heled, J.; Kühnert, D.; Vaughan, T.; Wu, C.-H.; Xie, D.; Suchard, M.A.; Rambaut, A.; Drummond, A.J. BEAST 2: A Software Platform for Bayesian Evolutionary Analysis. *PLoS Comput. Biol.* **2014**, *10*, e1003537. [CrossRef]

52. Hoops, S.; Sahle, S.; Gauges, R.; Lee, C.; Pahle, J.; Simus, N.; Kummer, U. COPASI—A COmplex PAthway SImulator. *Bioinformatics* **2006**, *22*, 3067–3074. [CrossRef] [PubMed]

53. Adam, D. Special report: The simulations driving the world's response to COVID-19. *Nature* **2020**, *580*, 316–318. [CrossRef] [PubMed]

54. Singer, J.; Gifford, R.; Cotten, M.; Robertson, D. CoV-GLUE: A Web Application for Tracking SARS-CoV-2 Genomic Variation. *Preprints.org* **2020**, 2020060225. [CrossRef]

55. Sathyaseelan, C.; Magateshvaren Saras, M.A.; Prasad Patro, L.P.; Uttamrao, P.P.; Rathinavelan, T. CoVe-Tracker: An Interactive SARS-CoV-2 Pan Proteome Evolution Tracker. *J. Proteome Res.* **2023**, *22*, 1984–1996. [CrossRef]

56. Cacciabue, M.; Aguilera, P.; Gismondi, M.I.; Taboga, O. Covidex: An ultrafast and accurate tool for SARS-CoV-2 subtyping. *Infect Genet. Evol.* **2022**, *99*, 105261. [CrossRef]

57. O'Toole, Á.; Scher, E.; Underwood, A.; Jackson, B.; Hill, V.; McCrone, J.T.; Colquhoun, R.; Ruis, C.; Abu-Dahab, K.; Taylor, B.; et al. Assignment of Epidemiological Lineages in an Emerging Pandemic Using the Pangolin Tool. *Virus Evol.* **2021**, *7*, veab064. [CrossRef]

58. Flower, D.R. *Bioinformatics for Vaccinology*; John Wiley & Sons: Hoboken, NJ, USA, 2008; ISBN 9780470027110.

59. WHO. COVID-19 Vaccines with WHO Emergency Use Listing. Available online: https://extranet.who.int/pqweb/vaccines/vaccinescovid-19-vaccine-eul-issued (accessed on 15 June 2023).

60. Wang, D.; Mai, J.; Zhou, W.; Yu, W.; Zhan, Y.; Wang, N.; Yang, Y. Immunoinformatic Analysis of T- and B-Cell Epitopes for SARS-CoV-2 Vaccine Design. *Vaccines* **2020**, *8*, 355. [CrossRef] [PubMed]

61. Ullah, A.; Sarkar, B.; Islam, S.S. Exploiting the reverse vaccinology approach to design novel subunit vaccines against Ebola virus. *Immunobiology* **2020**, *225*, 151949. [CrossRef] [PubMed]

62. Doytchinova, I.A.; Flower, D.R. VaxiJen: A server for prediction of protective antigens, tumour antigens and subunit vaccines. *BMC Bioinform.* **2007**, *8*, 4. [CrossRef]

63. Bukhari SN, H.; Jain, A.; Haq, E.; Mehbodniya, A.; Webber, J. Machine Learning Techniques for the Prediction of B-Cell and T-Cell Epitopes as Potential Vaccine Targets with a Specific Focus on SARS-CoV-2 Pathogen: A Review. *Pathogens* **2022**, *11*, 146. [CrossRef] [PubMed]

64. Yang, X.; Zhao, L.; Wei, F.; Li, J. DeepNetBim: Deep learning model for predicting HLA-epitope interactions based on network analysis by harnessing binding and immunogenicity information. *BMC Bioinform.* **2021**, *22*, 231. [CrossRef]

65. Kames, J.; Holcomb, D.D.; Kimchi, O.; DiCuccio, M.; Hamasaki-Katagiri, N.; Wang, T.; Kimchi-Sarfaty, C. Sequence analysis of SARS-CoV-2 genome reveals features important for vaccine design. *Sci. Rep.* **2020**, *10*, 15643. [CrossRef]

66. Taherzadeh, G.; Yang, Y.; Zhang, T.; Liew, A.W.; Zhou, Y. Sequence-based prediction of protein–peptide binding sites using support vector machine. *J. Comput. Chem.* **2016**, *37*, 1223–1229. [CrossRef]

67. Müller, A.T.; Gabernet, G.; Hiss, J.A.; Schneider, G. modlAMP: Python for antimicrobial peptides. *Bioinformatics* **2017**, *33*, 2753–2755. [CrossRef]

68. De Vries, S.J.; Rey, J.; Schindler, C.E.M.; Zacharias, M.; Tuffery, P. The pepATTRACT web server for blind, large-scale peptide–protein docking. *Nucleic Acids Res.* **2017**, *45*, W361–W364. [CrossRef]

69. Lamiable, A.; Thévenet, P.; Rey, J.; Vavrusa, M.; Derreumaux, P.; Tufféry, P. PEP-FOLD3: Faster de novo structure prediction for linear peptides in solution and in complex. *Nucleic Acids Res.* **2016**, *44*, W449–W454. [CrossRef]

70. Vita, R.; Mahajan, S.; Overton, J.A.; Dhanda, S.K.; Martini, S.; Cantrell, J.R.; Wheeler, D.K.; Sette, A.; Peters, B. The Immune Epitope Database (IEDB): 2018 update. *Nucleic Acids Res.* **2019**, *47*, D339–D343. [CrossRef] [PubMed]

71. Guan, P.; Hattotuwagama, C.K.; Doytchinova, I.A.; Flower, D.R. MHCPred 2.0: An updated quantitative T-cell epitope prediction server. *Appl. Bioinform.* **2006**, *5*, 55–61. [CrossRef] [PubMed]

72. Yao, B.; Zhang, L.; Liang, S.; Zhang, C. SVMTriP: A Method to Predict Antigenic Epitopes Using Support Vector Machine to Integrate Tri-Peptide Similarity and Propensity. *PLoS ONE* **2012**, *7*, e45152. [CrossRef]

73. Dimitrov, I.; Bangov, I.; Flower, D.R.; Doytchinova, I. AllerTOP v.2—A server for in silico prediction of allergens. *J. Mol. Model.* **2014**, *20*, 2278. [CrossRef]

74. Harper, L.; Kalfa, N.; Beckers, G.; Kaefer, M.; Nieuwhof-Leppink, A.; Fossum, M.; Herbst, K.; Bagli, D. The impact of COVID-19 on research. *J. Pediatr. Urol.* **2020**, *16*, 715–716. [CrossRef]

75. Venkatesh, V. Impacts of COVID-19: A research agenda to support people in their fight. *Int. J. Inf. Manag.* **2020**, *55*, 102197. [CrossRef] [PubMed]
76. WHO. Statement on the Fifteenth Meeting of the IHR (2005) Emergency Committee on the COVID-19 Pandemic. Available online: https://www.who.int/news/item/05-05-2023-statement-on-the-fifteenth-meeting-of-the-international-health-regulations-(2005)-emergency-committee-regarding-the-coronavirus-disease-(covid-19)-pandemic (accessed on 6 July 2023).

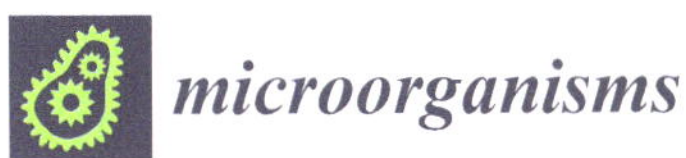

Article

Introduction, Dispersal, and Predominance of SARS-CoV-2 Delta Variant in Rio Grande do Sul, Brazil: A Retrospective Analysis

Thaís Regina y Castro [1,†], Bruna C. Piccoli [1,†], Andressa A. Vieira [1], Bruna C. Casarin [1], Luíza F. Tessele [1], Richard S. Salvato [2], Tatiana S. Gregianini [2], Leticia G. Martins [2], Paola Cristina Resende [3], Elisa C. Pereira [3], Filipe R. R. Moreira [4], Jaqueline G. de Jesus [5], Ana Paula Seerig [6], Marcos Antonio O. Lobato [7], Marli M. A. de Campos [8], Juliana S. Goularte [9], Mariana S. da Silva [9], Meriane Demoliner [9], Micheli Filippi [9], Vyctoria M. A. Góes Pereira [9], Alexandre V. Schwarzbold [10], Fernando R. Spilki [9] and Priscila A. Trindade [1,*]

1   Laboratório de Biologia Molecular e Bioinformática Aplicadas a Microbiologia Clínica, Departamento de Análises Clínicas e Toxicológicas, Universidade Federal de Santa Maria, Santa Maria 97105-900, Brazil
2   Centro Estadual de Vigilância em Saúde, Secretaria Estadual da Saúde do Rio Grande do Sul (CEVS/SES-RS), Porto Alegre 90610-000, Brazil
3   Laboratório de Vírus Respiratórios e Sarampo, Instituto Oswaldo Cruz Institute, Fundação Oswaldo Cruz (FIOCRUZ), Rio de Janeiro 21040-360, Brazil
4   Departamento de Genética, Instituto de Biologia, Universidade Federal do Rio de Janeiro, Rio de Janeiro 21941-853, Brazil
5   Instituto de Medicina Tropical, Faculdade de Medicina da Universidade de São Paulo, São Paulo 05508-220, Brazil
6   Vigilância em Saúde, Secretaria Municipal da Saúde de Santa Maria, Santa Maria 97060-001, Brazil
7   Departamento de Saúde Coletiva, Universidade Federal de Santa Maria, Santa Maria 97105-900, Brazil
8   Departamento de Análises Clínicas e Toxicológicas, Universidade Federal de Santa Maria, Santa Maria 97105-900, Brazil
9   Laboratório de Microbiologia Molecular, Universidade FEEVALE, Novo Hamburgo 93510-235, Brazil
10 Departamento de Clínica Médica, Universidade Federal de Santa Maria, Santa Maria 97105-900, Brazil
*   Correspondence: priscila.trindade@ufsm.br; Tel.: +55-55991360082
†   These authors contributed equally to this work.

Citation: y Castro, T.R.; Piccoli, B.C.; Vieira, A.A.; Casarin, B.C.; Tessele, L.F.; Salvato, R.S.; Gregianini, T.S.; Martins, L.G.; Resende, P.C.; Pereira, E.C.; et al. Introduction, Dispersal, and Predominance of SARS-CoV-2 Delta Variant in Rio Grande do Sul, Brazil: A Retrospective Analysis. *Microorganisms* **2023**, *11*, 2938. https://doi.org/10.3390/microorganisms11122938

Academic Editors: Ahmed Atef Mesalam and Qibin Geng

Received: 28 September 2023
Revised: 14 November 2023
Accepted: 24 November 2023
Published: 7 December 2023

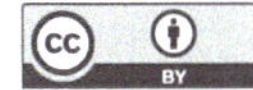

Abstract: Mutations in the SARS-CoV-2 genome can alter the virus' fitness, leading to the emergence of variants of concern (VOC). In Brazil, the Gamma variant dominated the pandemic in the first half of 2021, and from June onwards, the first cases of Delta infection were documented. Here, we investigate the introduction and dispersal of the Delta variant in the RS state by sequencing 1077 SARS-CoV-2-positive samples from June to October 2021. Of these samples, 34.7% were identified as Gamma and 65.3% as Delta. Notably, 99.2% of Delta sequences were clustered within the 21J lineage, forming a significant Brazilian clade. The estimated clock rate was 5.97×10^{-4} substitutions per site per year. The Delta variant was first reported on 17 June in the Vinhedos Basalto microregion and rapidly spread, accounting for over 70% of cases within nine weeks. Despite this, the number of cases and deaths remained stable, possibly due to vaccination, prior infections, and the continued mandatory mask use. In conclusion, our study provides insights into the Delta variant circulating in the RS state, highlighting the importance of genomic surveillance for monitoring viral evolution, even when the impact of new variants may be less severe in a given region.

Keywords: genomic surveillance; viral lineages; variants of concern; genome analysis; phylogeny

1. Introduction

At the end of January 2021, new cases of COVID-19 emerged in various districts of Maharashtra, India, after a four-month hiatus. Subsequently, India experienced a second wave of the COVID-19 pandemic, resulting in more than 400,000 deaths. This surge was attributed to the emergence of lineage B.1.617 [1], primarily sublineages B.1.617.1 (Kappa variant) and B.1.617.2 (Delta variant). The Delta variant swiftly spread worldwide [2].

In May 2021, the World Health Organization (WHO) designated the Delta variant as a VOC [3]. Additionally, four other SARS-CoV-2 VOCs have been identified: Alpha [4], Beta [5], Gamma [6], and Omicron [7]. Due to global travel and transit, VOCs have been both imported into and exported from their countries of origin, circulating worldwide. Delta was detected in Brazil in May 2021 by a ship crew of Asian origin that had docked in the state of Maranhão [8]. By July 2021, autochthonous transmission of this variant was evidenced in Rio de Janeiro [9]. This marked the first of several independent importation events involving Delta. By September 2021, Delta had become the dominant lineage in the pandemic landscape across the southeast, northeast, and south regions of Brazil [10].

The first case of SARS-CoV-2 infection in Rio Grande do Sul (RS) was reported on 10 March 2020. RS, located in the southernmost region of Brazil, occupies 3% of the nation's total land area. It ranks as the ninth-largest state in Brazil and shares its borders with two neighboring countries, Uruguay and Argentina [11]. Among its 497 cities, 196 are situated along the border strip, including 11 twin cities [12]. RS is the fifth most populous state in the country, trailing behind São Paulo, Minas Gerais, Rio de Janeiro, and Bahia [13]. The state's economy is based primarily on agriculture, livestock, and industry, positioning RS as the fourth-largest economic contributor in Brazil [14]. Moreover, RS has notable social indicators, including low infant mortality rates and high life expectancy and literacy rates, all of which contribute to its status as one of the states with the highest quality of life in Brazil [15]. Up until the study period, the state had confirmed over 1,436,734 cases of SARS-CoV-2 infection, with an incidence rate of 12,725.72 per 100,000 inhabitants and more than 35,203 deaths attributed to complications of the COVID-19 [16].

Mutations and genetic recombination events within the SARS-CoV-2 genome, particularly in the spike protein (S), have the potential to impact the virus' fitness. These events may result in increased transmissibility, evasion of the host's immune response, and reduced effectiveness of certain vaccines and treatments [17]. The Delta variant, in particular, harbors a set of mutations in the S protein, including L452R, T478K, and P681R, all of which have contributed to the increased transmissibility of this variant [18]. Notably, the L452R mutation within the S receptor-binding motif (RBM) [19] has been shown to enhance infectivity while reducing sensitivity to neutralizing responses [1]. These cumulative mutations have raised the S protein's affinity for angiotensin-converting enzyme 2 (ACE2), resulting in decreased vaccine efficacy compared to the Alpha and Beta variants that were prevalent before the emergence of Delta [18]. As the Delta variant continued to evolve, it gave rise to subvariants, such as AY.1, characterized by an additional mutation in the S protein, K417N. This mutation confers heightened antibody escape properties, increased transmissibility, and a strong affinity for lung epithelial cells [20]. Subsequently, numerous Delta subvariants have emerged, potentially carrying altered biological characteristics and clinical manifestations [21].

Detection and genomic surveillance of infectious diseases, such as COVID-19, are crucial for responding to the pandemic. Next-generation sequencing (NGS) technologies, which enable timely whole-genome sequencing (WGS), have become one of the most commonly used tools in virus research. They serve as a common approach for pathogen identification and tracking, establishing transmission routes, monitoring virus evolution, and controlling outbreaks [22,23]. In Brazil, less than 1% of SARS-CoV-2-positive cases are sequenced [24]. Furthermore, the vast territorial expanse of the country and the decentralized health surveillance system pose challenges in monitoring, expanding, and connecting regional genomic data. In this study, we conducted an extensive and robust analysis of the introduction and dispersal of the Delta variant in the RS state. To achieve this, we sequenced 1077 SARS-CoV-2-positive samples collected from June to October 2021 and analyzed the whole-genome sequences with regard to phylogenetic profiles and polymorphisms, as well as the dispersion of the variant across the state.

2. Materials and Methods

2.1. Study Population

The study population consisted of SARS-CoV-2-positive patients in the state of RS, Brazil, from 13 June to 9 October 2021, spanning epidemiological weeks (EW) 24 to 40. The study received approval from the Research Ethics Committee of the Universidade Federal de Santa Maria (Certificado de Apresentação de Apreciação Ética—CAAE: 51019821.0.0000.5346) and Universidade FEEVALE (Certificado de Apresentação de Apreciação Ética—CAAE: 33202820.7.1001.5348).

2.2. Epidemiological and Clinical Data

Epidemiological data for SARS-CoV-2-positive patients were obtained from DATASUS, in accordance with patient data protection laws. We assessed data related to age, gender, city, and the date of the SARS-CoV-2 positive test. Additionally, the number of confirmed cases and deaths and vaccination data were retrieved from public government databases [16,25].

2.3. Sample Screening and Genome Sequencing

SARS-CoV-2-positive samples from public and private laboratories in the RS state were sent to the Laboratório de Biologia Molecular e Bioinformática Aplicada a Microbiologia Clínica (LABIOMIC), Universidade Federal de Santa Maria, Santa Maria ($n = 260$); the Laboratório de Microbiologia Molecular (LMM), Universidade FEEVALE, Novo Hamburgo ($n = 263$); or Fundação Oswaldo Cruz (FIOCRUZ), Rio de Janeiro ($n = 554$), Brazil. Samples with a cycle threshold (Ct) ≤ 30 were pre-selected for sequencing. Due to the high number of SARS-CoV-2-positive patients, the pre-selected samples were randomly chosen, taking into account the sequencing capacity of the laboratories. Library construction was performed as described in the ARTIC protocol version 3 [26], the QIAseq SARS-CoV-2 Primer Panel (QIAGEN, Hilden, Germany) for paired library enrichment and QIAseq FX DNA Library UDI Kit (QIAGEN, Hilden, Germany), or the Illumina COVIDSeq Test (Illumina, San Diego, CA, USA). Genomes were sequenced using the MinION device (Oxford Nanopore Technologies, Oxford, UK) or Illumina MiSeq (Illumina, San Diego, CA, USA). MinKNOW v.21.05.12 was used to collect raw data from the MinION, which underwent high-accuracy base-calling and quality control analyses using Guppy v5.0.12. Illumina raw data were processed in Basespace (https://basespace.illumina.com, accessed on 17 October 2022).

2.3.1. Viral Genome Assembly

The assembly of the consensus sequence was conducted using the nCoV-2019 novel coronavirus bioinformatics protocol [27] along with Minimap2 version 2.8.3 [28] and BCFtools version 1.7-2 [29], Geneious Prime™ version 2022.2 [30], or ViralFlow 0.0.6 [31]. To compare the sequences in subsequent analyses, those with over 75% genomic coverage, fewer than 3000 undetermined nucleotides (N), and those rated as either good or mediocre by Nextclade were selected. Sequences failing to meet these standards were excluded from our analysis.

2.3.2. Lineage Identification

The clade and the number of gap regions in the viral consensus sequences were analyzed using Nextclade version 2.4.1 [32]. The lineages of the viral consensus sequences were also determined using Pangolin version 4.1.1 and pangolin-data version 1.13 [33].

2.3.3. Single Nucleotide Polymorphism Identification

To identify SNPs, insertions, and deletions, Geneious Prime™ [30] was employed. In brief, the FASTA-assembled consensus sequences were imported and aligned with the reference genome (NC_045512.2). The 'Find Variations/SNPs' tool was configured with a minimum variant frequency of 0.25.

2.4. Spatio-Temporal Analysis

For the spatio-temporal analysis, we searched for sequences that had location indications in metadata deposited in GISAID [34,35] between 13 June and 9 October 2021. However, only the samples sequenced in this study met this criterion. The coordinates of the 30 health microregions (Verdes Campos, Entre Rios, Fronteira Oeste, Belas Praias, Bons Ventos, Paranhana, Vale dos Sinos, Vale do Caí, Carbonífera, Capital/Vale do Gravataí, Sete Povos das Missões, Portal das Missões, Região da Diversidade, Fronteira Noroeste, Caminho das Águas, Alto Uruguai Gaúcho, Região do Planalto, Região das Araucárias, Região do Botucaraí, Rota da Produção, Região Sul, Pampa, Caxias, Campos de Cima da Serra, Vinhedos, Uvas e Vales, Jacuí/Centro, Santa Cruz do Sul, Vale das Montanhas, and Vale da Luz) [36] (Figure S1) were combined with the results of the genotyped samples, and a model of the Gamma variant replacement and Delta variant dispersal in the RS state was built. Kernel density analysis was performed using QGIS v3.26 software [37]. The cartographic base was provided by the Instituto Brasileiro de Geografia e Estatística (IBGE) [38].

2.5. Phylogenetic Analysis

2.5.1. Data Sets

Two data sets were compiled in accordance with Fonseca et al. [39]. Both data sets encompassed all Delta variant sequences (Pango lineage AY.*, NextStrain clade 21J) captured on 20 October 2022 (n = 5006) from GISAID. For the proportional target data set, samples from all Brazilian states were randomly selected in proportion to the estimated number of Delta variant cases per week in each state during EW 24 to 40. To achieve this, all high-quality complete genome sequences from Brazil between 13 June and 9 October 2021 were downloaded and categorized by variant and state. Using this categorization, we calculated the frequency of Delta infection cases by dividing the total number of SARS-CoV-2 sequences by the number of Delta variant sequences per week in each state. Estimates of Delta variant infection cases were determined by multiplying the frequency by the corresponding total number of confirmed cases per week in each state, as provided by the government [40]. The estimated numbers of Delta variant cases per week in each state were then divided by the total estimated cases of this variant and multiplied by 5000 (approximately the number of NextStrain clade 21J sequences) to obtain the number of target samples. In cases where a state had more Delta variant sequences than the target number, we generated a selection of random numbers using the random() function in Python. Sequences were manually inspected using AliView v.1.28 [41], and duplicate sequences were removed. Conversely, when the target number exceeded the number of Delta variant sequences available, we included all of them (detailed calculations are available in Table S1). This selection resulted in 5008 samples, including 1077 from RS, totaling 10,014 sequences. For the uniform targets data set, we used the median of weekly Delta variant sequences for RS over the study period. This corresponded to selecting 40 targets per week in each state, either randomly or by including all available sequences, as in the previous data set. This selection resulted in 7025 samples, including 1077 from RS, totaling 12,031 sequences.

2.5.2. Analysis of Temporal Signal and Identification of Brazilian Clades

Each data set, along with the Wuhan-Hu reference genome (EPI_ISL_402124), was aligned using Pangolin with default settings. A maximum-likelihood phylogenetic construction was conducted using IQ-Tree v2.1.2 [42] under the GTR+F+I+G4 nucleotide substitution model [43,44] and a Shimodaira–Hasegawa-like approximate likelihood ratio (SH-aLRT) branch test [45]. The constructed tree was manually rooted with the oldest sequence in FigTree [46]. The maximum-likelihood tree was examined in TempEst v1.5.3 [47] to identify samples with inconsistent temporal signals, i.e., in the root-to-tip regression, sequences that deviated more than 1.5 times the interquartile range of the residual distribution were considered outliers. The outliers were removed, and the rooted tree was evaluated with the TreeTime [48] mugration method using a discrete asymmetric two-state model (Brazil/International). Figure 1 provides a comprehensive diagram of the study methodology.

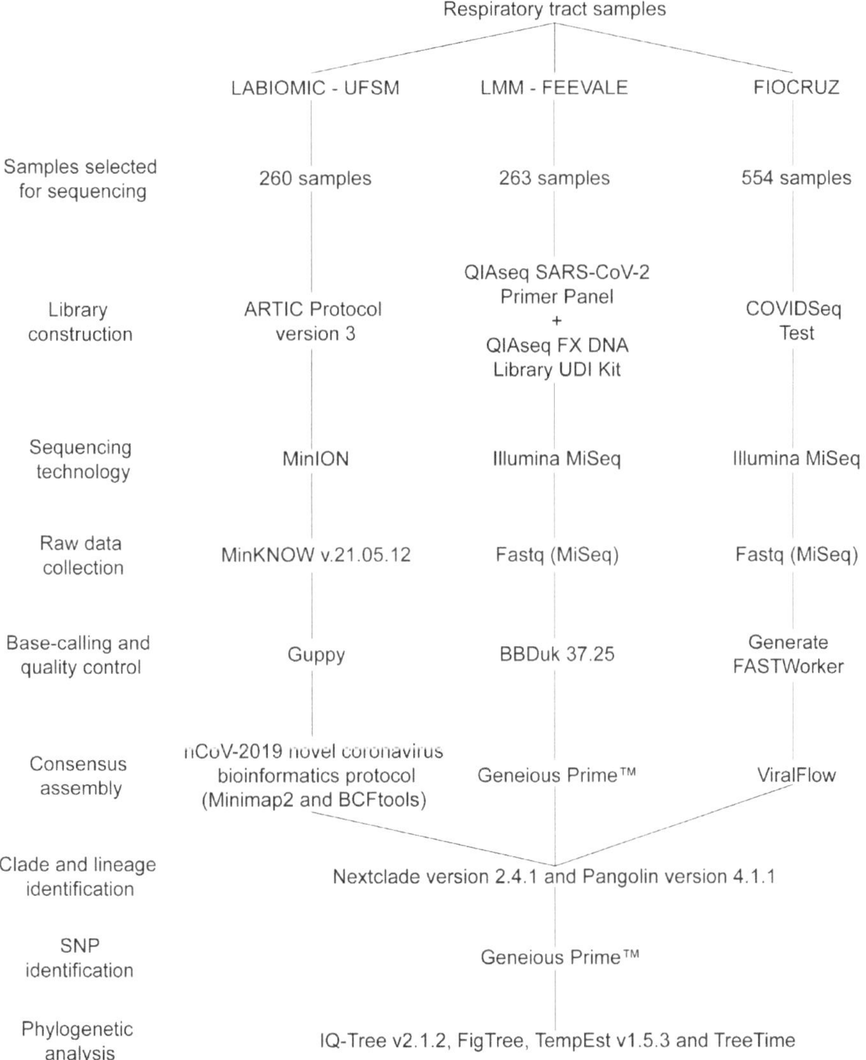

Figure 1. Diagram of the study methodology.

3. Results

3.1. COVID-19 Overview

We analyzed the dispersal of the Delta variant in the RS state between EW 24 and 40 (June to October 2021). During this period, the RS state government registered 164,194 new confirmed cases of SARS-CoV-2 infection. There was a mean of 7440 ± 5143 confirmed cases and 181 ± 188 deaths (Figure 2A). Despite the introduction of the Delta variant in the state, the data do not indicate an increase in confirmed cases or deaths from COVID-19.

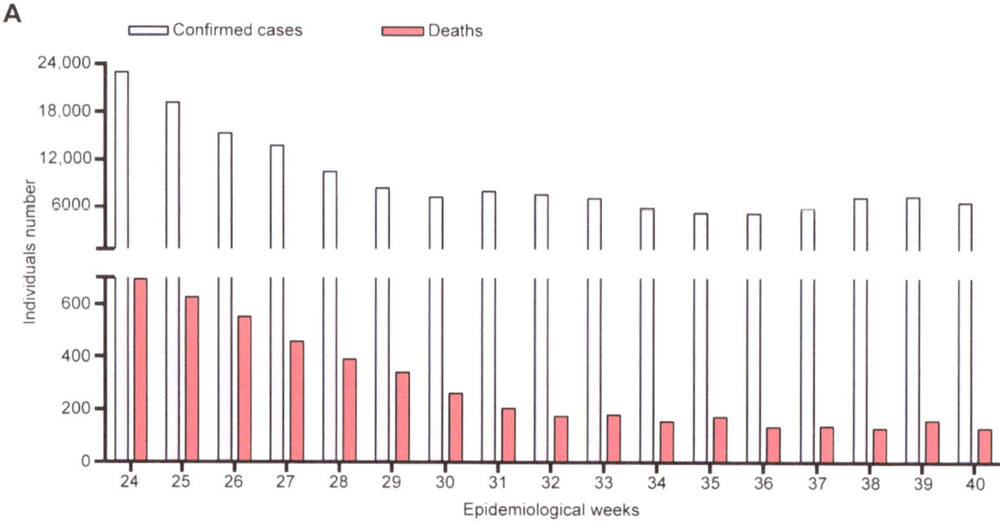

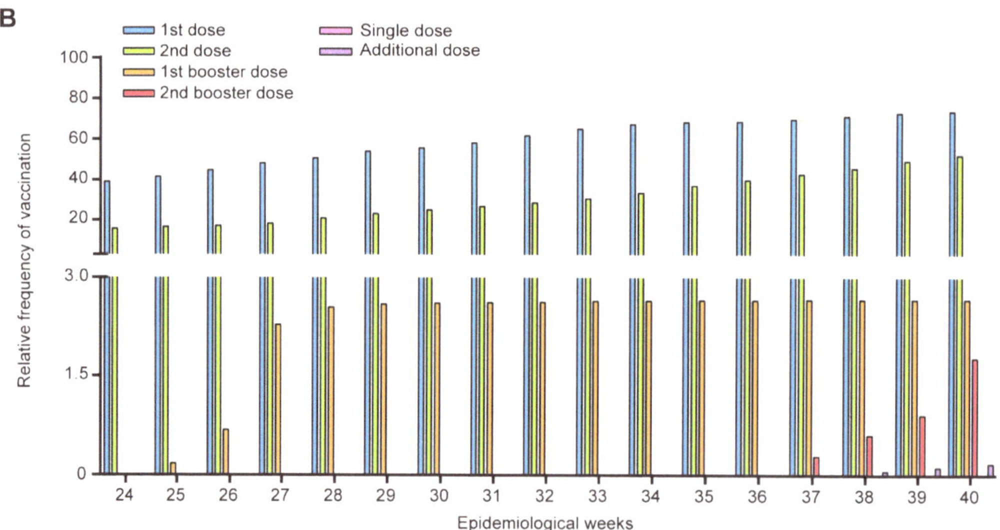

Figure 2. COVID-19 overview in the Rio Grande do Sul state, Brazil, during epidemiological weeks 26 to 40 of 2021. (**A**) number of confirmed cases, deaths, and (**B**) vaccinated individuals.

The introduction of the previous VOC was accompanied by mandatory mask use and large-scale population SARS-CoV-2 vaccination (Figure 2B). It is estimated that on 13 June 2021, 6,305,296 vaccines were administered, and by 9 October, this number reached 15,033,655. These numbers represent 39.17% and 15.82% of the total RS population vaccinated with the first and second doses, respectively (EW 24). In addition, 0.0009% received a single dose. Starting from EW 27, the percentage of individuals vaccinated with the third dose increased significantly, and from EW 37 onwards, the number of those who received the additional dose (previously vaccinated with the single dose) also increased. Moreover, during the evaluated period, 19 individuals received a fourth dose.

3.2. Epidemiological Aspects of Delta Introduction Period

Among the SARS-CoV-2-positive samples, a total of 1077 were sequenced to delineate the introduction, dispersal, and prevalence of the Delta variant. The mean genome coverage achieved in our analysis was 98.1%, encompassing a range from 75.1 to 100%, relative to the 29,903 bp of the NC_045512 reference genome. The average depth of our sequencing was 1159×, with a variability spectrum extending from 20 to 8019 (Table S2). Within this sample set, 422 genomes were classified as Gamma and 648 genomes were designated as Delta (Table S3 for further details). Additionally, our analysis identified one case of Alpha, two cases of Lambda, as well as one case each of B and B.1 variants. Patients infected with the Gamma variant exhibited a median age of 43, whereas those infected with the Delta variant had a slightly lower median age of 41, as detailed in Table 1. The majority of these patients were adults, comprising 76.8% for the Gamma variant and 66.7% for the Delta variant, with a female predominance.

Table 1. Epidemiological data of SARS-CoV-2-positive patients infected with SARS-CoV-2.

	Gamma Positive ($n = 422$)	Delta Positive ($n = 648$)	Others ($n = 7$)
Age (median)	43	41	37
<18 (number)	17	48	0
18–60	324	432	5
>60	81	167	2
Female (%)	237 (56%)	340 (52%)	5 (71%)

3.3. SARS-CoV-2 Delta Introduction and Dispersal

The first case of infection with the Delta variant was pinpointed on 17 June, during EW 24 (Figure 3). The Gamma variant exhibited a prominent presence, constituting more than 70% of the reported cases in the RS state during the period spanning EW 24 to 28. Nevertheless, there was a gradual increase in cases attributed to the Delta variant. By the time EW 32 arrived, a total of 26 cases of the Gamma variant were documented, accounting for 41.9% of the overall caseload. Into EW 33, a shift in the viral landscape became evident, marked by a transition in the predominant variants. The Delta variant established itself as the predominant variant, representing more than 70% of all SARS-CoV-2-positive cases.

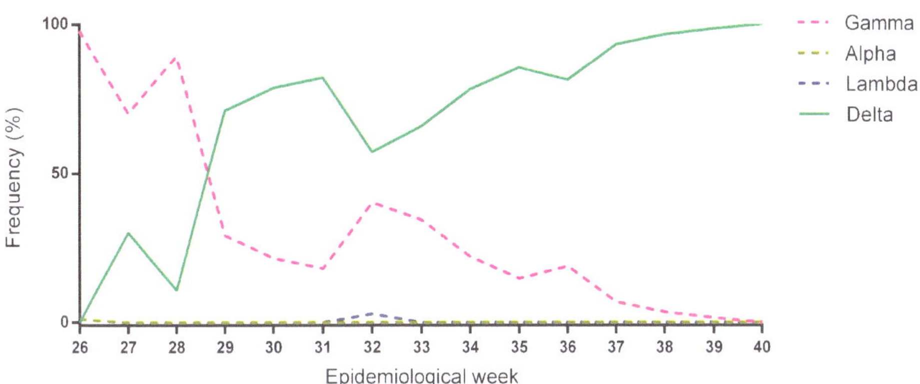

Figure 3. Replacement of Gamma variant by Delta variant considering the sequenced samples in this study.

When we detailed the genetic composition of the 1077 sequenced samples, twenty-four Pangolin lineages were identified (Figure 4). The most frequently detected lineage was AY.99.2 (440 sequences, 40.85%), followed by P.1 (356 sequences, 33.05%), AY.101 (162 sequences, 15.04%), P.1.2 (35 sequences, 3.25%), AY.43.2 (22 sequences, 2.04%), P.1.7 (13 sequences, 1.21%), and AY.100 (12 sequences, 1.11%) (Figure 4B). The remaining ten lineages had a frequency lower than 1%, collectively representing less than 3.5% of the sequences.

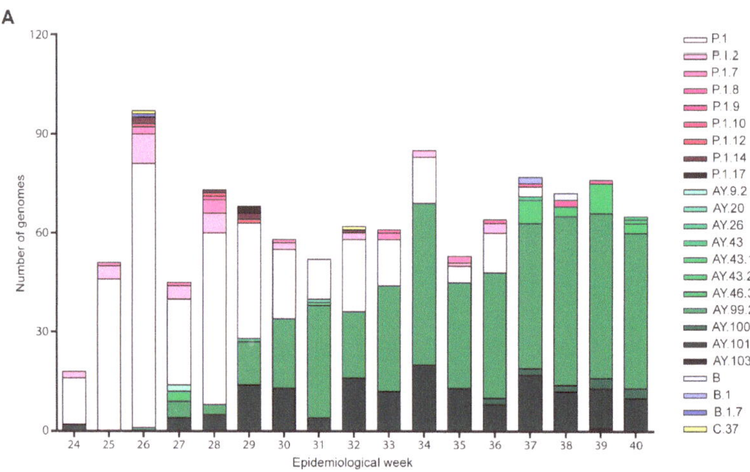

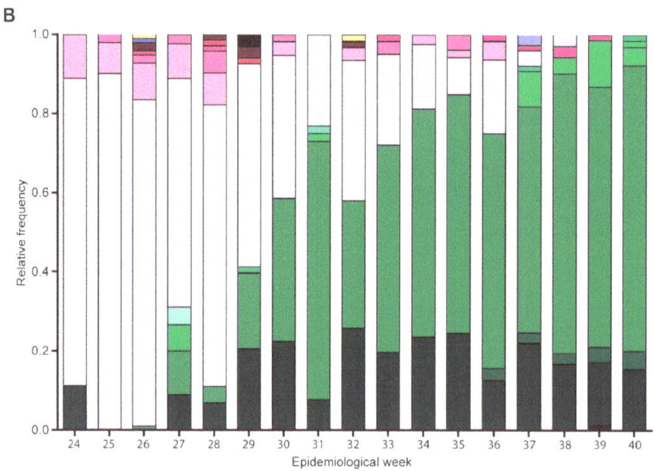

Figure 4. Genetic composition of SARS-CoV-2 lineages in Rio Grande do Sul from June to October 2021. (**A**) absolute variation number in lineages' frequencies across epidemiological weeks, as classified by Pangolin version 4.1.1; (**B**) lineages' variation frequencies in relative terms.

3.4. Single Nucleotide Polymorphism

The genome-wide mutation profile of the Gamma and Delta variants sequenced in the RS state is depicted in Figure 5. The Gamma variant exhibited 38 mutations, comprising 30 single nucleotide polymorphisms (SNPs—18 transitions and 12 transversions), 2 substitutions, 1 insertion, and 5 deletions (Table S4). Of these, 5.3% (2) were located in the 5'-UTR, 36.8% (14) in the ORF1ab, 31.6% (12) in the S gene, 2.6% (1) in ORF3a, 2.6% (1) in ORF8, 7.9% (3) in the N gene, 2.6% (1) in the intergenic UTR, and 10.5% (4) in the 3'-UTR (Figure 5A and Table S4). The Delta variant presented a higher number of mutations, amounting to 45, including 42 SNPs (32 transitions and 10 transversions) and 3 deletions (Table S5). Among these, 4.4% (2) were found in the 5'-UTR, 48.9% (22) in the ORF1ab, 17.8% (8) in the S gene, 4.42% (2) in ORF3a, 2.2% (1) in the M gene, 6.7% (3) in ORF7a, 2.2% (1) in ORF7b, 2.2% (1) in ORF8, 8.9% (4) in the N gene, and 2.2% (1) in the intergenic UTR (Figure 5B and Table S5). Notably, 74.2% (23) and 73.8% (31) of the SNPs occurring in the Gamma and Delta variant coding regions, respectively, were non-synonymous, particularly those occurring in the S gene (Tables S3 and S4). The Gamma variant circulating in RS did not possess the S84L mutation (ORF8) characteristic of this variant (Table S6). The Delta variant circulating in RS did not exhibit the E156G (S gene), S84L (ORF8), and T60A (ORF9b) mutations. However, it did have the additional mutations I1091V (ORF1a), T4087I (ORF1a), and A23V (ORF3a).

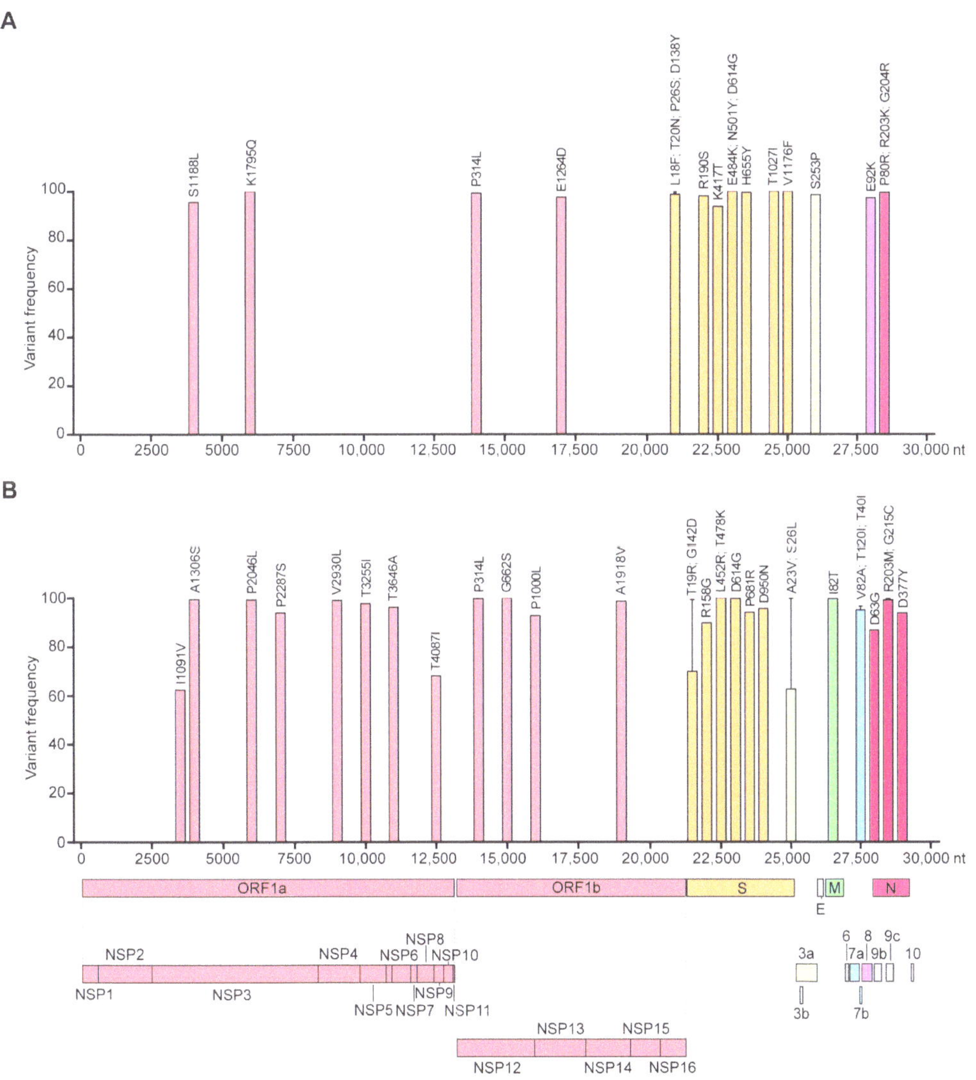

Figure 5. Mutational profile and variant frequency in the coding region of SARS-CoV-2 Gamma (**A**) and Delta (**B**) variants.

3.5. Phylogenetic Analysis

To compare the SARS-CoV-2 strains circulating in RS with those in the rest of Brazil and the world, we conducted phylogenetic analyses. Firstly, we conducted a maximum likelihood phylogenetic analysis using the proportional data set (Figure 6A). Within this analysis, 63.9% of the Delta sequences clustered in a large Brazilian clade, encompassing a total of 3025 sequences. The remaining sequences were distributed throughout the tree. Subsequently, we isolated the large Brazilian clade and generated a new maximum likelihood tree. This tree exhibited a significant temporal signal ($R^2 = 0.21$; $\beta = 9.09 \times 10^{-4}$) (Figure 6B). A Bayesian analysis, utilizing 10% of these sequences, estimated a rate of 5.43×10^{-4} substitutions/site/year (95 per cent HPD median: 4.41×10^{-4}–6.42×10^{-4}) (Figure 6C). These analyses were replicated with a uniform data set, yielding similar results (Figure S2).

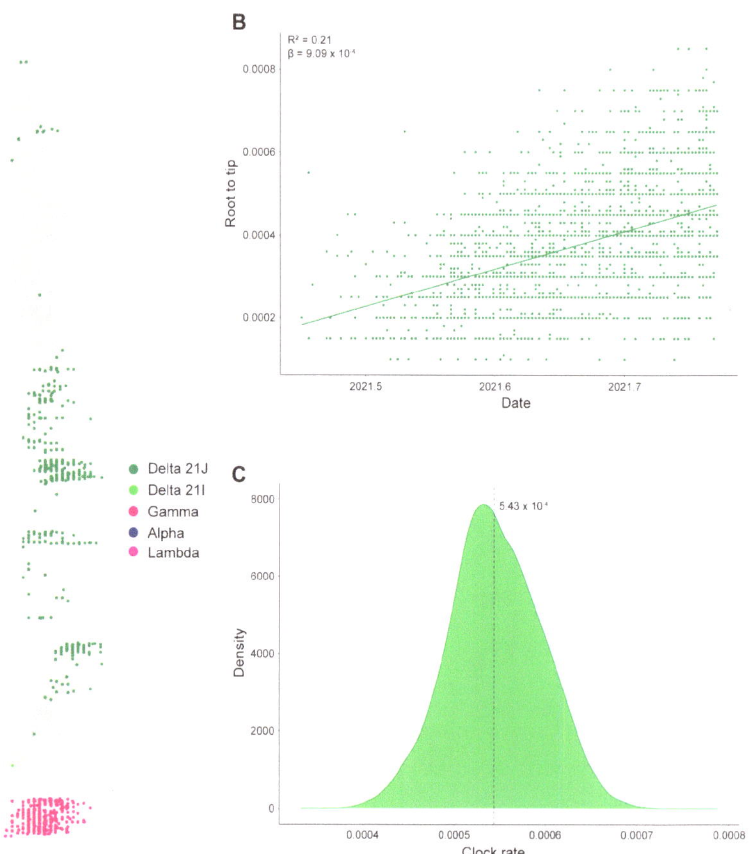

Figure 6. Maximum likelihood phylogeny constructed with proportional data set ($n = 10,013$). In this study, 63.9% of the Delta cases sequenced clustered into a large Brazilian clade (highlighted in gray), covering 3025 sequences (**A**). Temporal signal analysis of the large Brazilian clade through root-to-tip regression (**B**). Clock rate distribution using 10% of the large Brazilian clade sequences (**C**).

We assessed the retraction of the Gamma variant and the dispersal of the Delta variant within the state of RS by analyzing the locations of infected patients' residences (Figure 7). The pandemic landscape was predominantly characterized by the Gamma variant. Within the EWs under scrutiny in this study, EW 26 recorded the highest percentage of territories with the presence of the Gamma variant, accounting for 63.3%. On average, Gamma variant samples were identified across 25.88% of the state. A turning point occurred on 17 June during EW 24 when the first case of Delta variant infection was documented in a patient originating from the city of Garibaldi, within the Vinhedos e Basalto Microregion (Figure 7B). Interestingly, the subsequent week (EW 25) showed no instances of Delta variant infection reported. Starting from the onset of EW 26, the incidence of Delta variant infections experienced a steady ascent, permeating throughout the entirety of RS. In EW 27, an additional 13 cases of Delta variant infections were identified, spanning multiple health microregions, including Capital/Vale do Gravataí, Caxias, Fronteira Oeste, Região da Diversidade, Região do Planalto, and Vale do Caí (Figure 7B). The majority of Delta cases was observed in the Capital/Vale do Gravataí region (23.64%), closely followed by Alto Uruguai Gaúcho (17.57%), with Vale dos Sinos (11.51%) and Vale do Caí (11.2%) also reporting significant numbers (Figure 7B). By EW 39, the Delta variant had reached a maximum presence of 63.3% across the state's territory, with an average of 26.3% coverage. These data highlight the presence of gaps in the state's surveillance system as all municipalities in the region reported individuals infected with SARS-CoV-2, yet the specific variant and/or subvariant remained unidentified. Predominantly, the south and west regions accounted for the most uncovered in this regard.

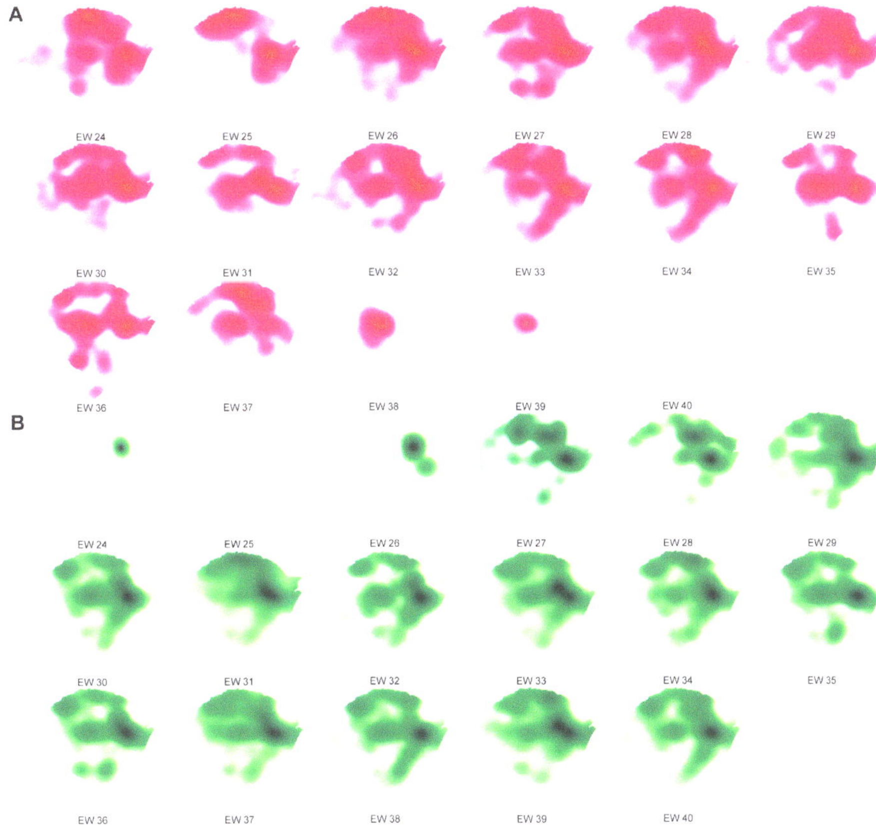

Figure 7. SARS-CoV-2 genomic surveillance in Rio Grande do Sul, Brazil, from June to October 2021. Gamma retraction (**A**) and Delta variant dispersal (**B**) across the state of Rio Grande do Sul considering the H = health microregions in each epidemiological week sampled in our study.

4. Discussion

In this study, we conducted a retrospective analysis using a large data set to identify the introduction and dispersal of the Delta variant in the RS state. The previously circulating Gamma variant led to approximately a 4-fold increase in the number of SARS-CoV-2-positive cases and approximately a 6.7-fold increase in deaths [16]. However, the replacement of Gamma with Delta did not result in an alteration in the incidence of cases and deaths. This stability likely resulted from natural and/or vaccinated immunity, particularly in the RS population [25,49]. When the Delta variant was introduced in the RS state on 17 June, 39.16% of the total population had received the first dose of the vaccine. The RS state had already experienced COVID-19 waves, leading a significant portion of the population to acquire natural immunity against SARS-CoV-2. Of particular note, the use of masks became mandatory on 20 March 2020 [50] and remained in effect during the period of the introduction and spread of the Delta variant. This situation differed from that of many European and Asian countries facing the third wave of SARS-CoV-2 (previous VOC Delta) [51–53]. The Brazilian government faces challenges in the domain of Public Health Surveillance. During our study period, we documented eight individuals who had received a fourth vaccine dose, even though the official campaign only began in December 2021.

The Delta variant rapidly dispersed, comprising 71% of the SARS-CoV-2-positive cases by EW 33 (15–21 August 2021), nine weeks after the first case. This finding aligns with a study involving 183 SARS-CoV-2-positive samples, which reported that the RS state reached this milestone in August [49]. Based on sequences accessible through GISAID, Mayer et al. have further substantiated these findings [54]. Utilizing phylogeographic analysis, it has been determined that the RS state imported the AY.99.1 and AY.99.2 sublineages from Brazil's southeast region, as well as the AY.101 sublineage from Paraná, which is also part of the southern region of the country [55]. The state of Rio de Janeiro, located in Brazil's southeast region, reported the first autochthonous transmission of the Delta variant in July. By August, it had become the dominant variant in the state [56]. Minas Gerais, a state bordering Rio de Janeiro, reported 73% of Delta variant infections in September, specifically during EW 37 [39]. In October, the Tocantins [57] and Rondônia [58] states in the northern region of Brazil also reached the same percentage mark. Interestingly, the state of Pará, situated along the border with Tocantins, registered infection with the Gamma variant up until July 2022 [59]. To our knowledge, it was only these five Brazilian states that investigated the replacement of Gamma by the Delta variant. Comprehensive studies analyzing data from across Brazil have established that by September 70% of SARS-CoV-2 positive cases were of the Delta variant [60,61].

The Delta variant exhibits greater transmissibility and lower sensitivity to neutralizing antibodies derived from vaccination or prior infection [17]. Our sequences revealed the presence of 90.6% of the distinctive mutations associated with the Delta variant, along with two additional mutations, specifically I1091V and T4087I [49]. These mutations were identified within the ORF1ab region of the Delta variant, which was introduced into Brazil via the state of Rio de Janeiro [9]. The T4087I mutation involves the substitution of a hydrophilic amino acid, threonine, with a hydrophobic amino acid, isoleucine. This change could exert an influence on viral replication and infection rates [62]. Mutations in the spike protein have a significant influence on immune evasion and infectivity. The T19R mutation is associated with a reduction in the efficacy of monoclonal antibodies [63]. The G142D mutation is linked to a higher viral load [64]. The L452R mutation, in combination with T478K, stabilizes the RBD-ACE2 complex, enhancing infectivity, improving the ability to evade the host's immune response, and increasing transmissibility. The D614G mutation, present in various SARS-CoV-2 variants, is associated with increased virulence and enhances the cleavage rate at the S1/S2 site [65–73]. Finally, the P681R mutation, located at the furin cleavage site S1/S2, augments the cleavage rate and cell invasion, thereby increasing infectivity and transmissibility [65,74–76]. It is worth noting that there is a lack of consensus among the Covariants, Outbreak.info, and WHO databases regarding defining mutations of this variant. Consequently, it was classified as a non-characteristic mutation, meaning it was not present in any of the databases.

The majority of the sequenced Delta variants in our study were clustered within the 21J lineage, while three variants were clustered in 21I. Employing a Bayesian analysis, we determined a substitution rate of 5.43×10^{-4} substitutions per site per year, which translates to approximately 16.24 substitutions per year. Notably, by utilizing a comprehensive data set, we mitigated sampling bias in comparison to the study conducted by Gularte et al., which reported a higher substitution rate of 34.5 substitutions per year due to their smaller sample size of 183 sequences [49]. Ferrareze et al. estimated a substitution rate per site for the AY.99/AY.99.1, AY.99.2, and AY.101 sublineages circulating in RS, revealing rates ranging from 4.0612 to 6.6080×10^{-4}, which align closely with the values obtained in the current study [55].

The first case of Delta variant infection was documented on 17 June (EW 24) in a patient from Garibaldi city, within the Vinhedos e Basalto health microregion. This finding diverges from the typical pattern of introducing new variants, which often happens in capital cities, metropolitan areas, or cities with major airports [77]. In RS, the introduction of the Delta variant occurred within the Vinhedos e Basalto region, a tourist destination, primarily during the winter season. We postulate that the progress in vaccination and the partial relaxation of COVID-19 prevention and control measures in Brazil facilitated tourism, ultimately leading to the introduction and dispersal of the Delta variant in this region, spanning from EW 24 to 33 of 2021. It is important to highlight the shortcomings in genomic surveillance and the reporting of SARS-CoV-2 infection cases. The COVID-19 pandemic presented an unprecedented challenge for the Brazilian healthcare system and likely for healthcare systems worldwide. Whole-genome sequencing was not readily available to the majority of institutions, and while there has been an increase in the number of institutions adopting this technique, it still falls short of enabling effective genomic surveillance. The absence of coordination and standardized criteria for sample sequencing, resulting in some health microregions being underrepresented or not represented at all. This limitation is evident in our study, where we encountered a scarcity of samples from the west and south regions of the state, hampering our ability to accurately identify the circulating variants in those areas. Despite the absence of data from various regions, our study compiled samples from 140 municipalities within the state, surpassing the previously recorded figures of 44 [55] and 20 municipalities [49].

Although the Delta variant is no longer in active circulation, it remains essential to retrospectively analyze the progression of the COVID-19 pandemic. Such analysis is crucial for the scientific community and governmental authorities to understand the behavior of an emerging virus, identify the most effective control and prevention strategies to mitigate transmission, discern the factors that contributed to the reduction in hospitalizations and deaths, and recognize which approaches were ineffective. This information is vital for understanding how emerging pathogens may behave within the state and for guiding the government in the development of more targeted control and prevention measures for the future.

5. Conclusions

Our study provides insights into the introduction and dispersal of the Delta variant in the RS state of Brazil. We observed the replacement of the previously dominant Gamma variant by Delta, which exhibited greater transmissibility and reduced sensitivity to neutralizing antibodies. Despite this shift, the incidence of COVID-19 cases and deaths remained stable, likely due to a combination of natural and vaccinated immunity, as well as the continued mandatory mask use. Sequencing data revealed the presence of characteristic Delta variant mutations, along with additional ones. However, the lack of consensus among different databases regarding defining characteristic mutations underscores the complexity of variant characterization. Phylogenetic analysis and substitution rate estimation provide valuable insights into the viral evolution of the Delta variant in the RS state, addressing previous sampling biases. In summary, our study underscores the need for ongoing genomic surveillance and the importance of maintaining public health measures in the face of emerging SARS-CoV-2 variants. Monitoring and understanding the dynamics of these variants are crucial for effective pandemic response and control.

Supplementary Materials: The following supporting information can be downloaded at: https://www.mdpi.com/article/10.3390/microorganisms11122938/s1, Figure S1: Rio Grande do Sul Health Microregions; Figure S2: Maximum likelihood phylogeny constructed with proportional data set (*n* = 12,031). Delta sequenced in this study clustered into a large Brazilian clade (highlighted in gray) covering 3025 sequences (A). Temporal signal analysis of the large Brazilian clade through root-to-tip regression (B). Clock rate distribution using 10% of the large Brazilian clade sequences (C). Table S1: Calculation of the frequency of SARS-CoV-2 infection per epidemiological week and per Brazilian state to construct proportional and uniform data sets; Table S2: Assessment of quality parameters in SARS-CoV-2-positive samples sequenced. Table S3: Epidemiological information regarding individuals infected with SARS-CoV-2; Table S4: Mutational profile of Gamma variant; Table S5: Mutational profile of Delta variant; Table S6: Characteristic mutations of Gamma and Delta variants. References [78–97] are cited in the Supplementary Materials.

Author Contributions: Conceptualization, T.R.y.C., A.A.V., B.C.P. and P.A.T.; methodology, T.R.y.C., B.C.P., A.A.V., L.F.T., B.C.C. and P.A.T.; formal analysis, T.R.y.C., B.C.P., A.A.V., B.C.C. and L.F.T.; investigation, T.R.y.C., B.C.P., A.A.V., L.F.T., R.S.S., T.S.G., L.G.M., P.C.R., E.C.P., F.R.R.M., A.P.S., M.A.O.L., J.S.G., M.S.d.S., M.D., M.F., V.M.A.G.P., J.G.d.J. F.R.S. and P.A.T.; resources, A.V.S. and P.A.T.; data curation, T.R.y.C., B.C.P., A.A.V., B.C.C. and L.F.T.; writing—original draft preparation, T.R.y.C. and B.C.P.; writing—review and editing, F.R.S. and P.A.T.; visualization, T.R.y.C. and B.C.P.; supervision, M.M.A.d.C. and P.A.T.; project administration, A.V.S. and P.A.T.; funding acquisition, A.V.S., F.R.S. and P.A.T. All authors have read and agreed to the published version of the manuscript.

Funding: This research was funded by Coordenação de Aperfeiçoamento de Pessoal de Nível Superior (CAPES), grant numbers 88887.502716/2020-00 and 88882.461702/2019-01, Rede Corona-omica BR MCTI/FINEP affiliated to RedeVírus/MCTI (FINEP grant 01.20.0029.000462/20, CNPq 404096/2020-4), and FAPERGS (grant 21/2551-0000081-3); AstraZeneca (grant numbers 28186 and 28186*1), and Bill e Melinda Gates Foundation (grant number 28098).

Data Availability Statement: All SARS-CoV-2 genomic sequences used in this study are available on GISAID (https://gisaid.org/). The list of epicodes is available in Table S2.

Acknowledgments: Authors would like to thank all the participants in this study, the Universidade Federal de Santa Maria, the Hospital Universitário de Santa Maria, the Secretaria de Município da Saúde de Santa Maria/Rio Grande do Sul, Brazil, and the financial support.

Conflicts of Interest: The authors declare no conflict of interest. The funders had no role in the design of the study; in the collection, analyses, or interpretation of data; in the writing of the manuscript; or in the decision to publish the results.

References

1. Cherian, S.; Potdar, V.; Jadhav, S.; Yadav, P.; Gupta, N.; Das, M.; Rakshit, P.; Singh, S.; Abraham, P.; Panda, S. SARS-CoV-2 Spike Mutations, L452R, T478K, E484Q and P681R, in the Second Wave of COVID-19 in Maharashtra, India. *Microorganisms* **2021**, *9*, 1542. [CrossRef] [PubMed]
2. CoVariants. Overview of Variants in Countries. Available online: https://covariants.org/per-country?variant=21A+%252 8Delta%2529&variant=21I+%2528Delta%2529&variant=21J+%2528Delta%2529 (accessed on 1 November 2023).
3. World Health Organization. Tracking SARS-CoV-2 Variants. Available online: https://www.who.int/publications/m/item/historical-working-definitions-and-primary-actions-for-sars-cov-2-variants (accessed on 1 November 2023).
4. Volz, E.M.; Mishra, S.; Chand, M.; Barrett, J.C.; Johnson, R.; Geidelberg, L.; Hinsley, W.R.; Laydon, D.J.; Dabrera, G.; O'Toole, Á.; et al. Assessing Transmissibility of SARS-CoV-2 Lineage B.1.1.7 in England. *Nature* **2021**, *593*, 266–269. [CrossRef] [PubMed]
5. Tegally, H.; Wilkinson, E.; Giovanetti, M.; Iranzadeh, A.; Fonseca, V.; Giandhari, J.; Doolabh, D.; Pillay, S.; San, E.J.; Msomi, N.; et al. Detection of a SARS-CoV-2 Variant of Concern in South Africa. *Nature* **2021**, *592*, 438–443. [CrossRef] [PubMed]
6. Naveca, F.G.; Nascimento, V.; de Souza, V.C.; de Lima Corado, A.; Nascimento, F.; Silva, G.; Costa, Á.; Duarte, D.; Pessoa, K.; Mejía, M.; et al. COVID-19 in Amazonas, Brazil, Was Driven by the Persistence of Endemic Lineages and P.1 Emergence. *Nat. Med.* **2021**, *27*, 1230–1238. [CrossRef] [PubMed]

7.   Viana, R.; Moyo, S.; Amoako, D.G.; Tegally, H.; Scheepers, C.; Althaus, C.L.; Anyaneji, U.J.; Bester, P.A.; Boni, M.F.; Chand, M.; et al. Rapid Epidemic Expansion of the SARS-CoV-2 Omicron Variant in Southern Africa. *Nature* **2022**, *603*, 679–686. [CrossRef]
8.   Dos Santos, M.C.; Júnior, E.C.; Ferreira, J.A.; Barbagelata, L.S.; Da Silva, S.P.; Silva, A.M.; Cardoso, J.; Bedran, R.L.S.; Júnior, W.D.C.; Bezerra, D.A.M.; et al. First Reported Cases of SARS-CoV-2 Sub-Lineage B.1.617.2 in Brazil: An Outbreak in a Ship and Alert for Spread. Available online: https://virological.org/t/first-reported-cases-of-sars-cov-2-sub-lineage-b-1-617-2-in-brazil-an-outbreak-in-a-ship-and-alert-for-spread/706 (accessed on 3 October 2022).
9.   Lamarca, A.P.; de Almeida, L.G.P.; da Silva Francisco, R.; Cavalcante, L.; Machado, D.T.; Brustolini, O.; Gerber, A.L.; de C Guimarães, A.P.; Policarpo, C.; da Silva de Oliveira, G.; et al. Genomic Surveillance Tracks the First Community Outbreak of the SARS-CoV-2 Delta (B.1.617.2) Variant in Brazil. *J. Virol.* **2022**, *96*, e01228-21. [CrossRef]
10. Arantes, I.; Naveca, F.G.; Gräf, T.; Miyajima, F.; Faoro, H.; Wallau, G.L.; Delatorre, E.; Appolinario, L.R.; Pereira, E.C.; Venas, T.M.M.; et al. Emergence and Spread of the SARS-CoV-2 Variant of Concern Delta across Different Brazilian Regions. *Microbiol. Spectr.* **2022**, *10*, e02641-21. [CrossRef]
11. Rio Grande do Sul State Government. Geography of Rio Grande Do Sul State. Available online: https://www.estado.rs.gov.br/geografia (accessed on 10 August 2022).
12. Instituto Brasileiro de Geografia e Estatística (IBGE). Border Strip Municipalities and Twin Cities. Available online: https://www.ibge.gov.br/geociencias/organizacao-do-territorio/estrutura-territorial/24073-municipios-da-faixa-de-fronteira.html?=&t=acesso-ao-produto (accessed on 10 August 2022).
13. Instituto Brasileiro de Geografia e Estatística (IBGE). Demographic Census 2010. Available online: https://cidades.ibge.gov.br/brasil/rs/pesquisa/23/25207?tipo=ranking (accessed on 10 August 2022).
14. Parana State Govenment. Com 6412%, Paraná Alcança Maior Participação Da História No PIB Nacional. Available online: https://www.aen.pr.gov.br/Noticia/Com-6412-Parana-alcanca-maior-participacao-da-historia-no-PIB-nacional (accessed on 26 September 2023).
15. Rio Grande do Sul State Government. Características Gerais—Atlas Socioeconômico Do Rio Grande Do Sul. Available online: https://atlassocioeconomico.rs.gov.br/caracteristicas-gerais (accessed on 26 September 2023).
16. State Health Department of Rio Grande do Sul. Coronavirus Dashboard. Available online: https://ti.saude.rs.gov.br/covid19/ (accessed on 26 September 2023).
17. Long, S.W.; Olsen, R.J.; Christensen, P.A.; Subedi, S.; Olson, R.; Davis, J.J.; Saavedra, M.O.; Yerramilli, P.; Pruitt, L.; Reppond, K.; et al. Sequence Analysis of 20,453 Severe Acute Respiratory Syndrome Coronavirus 2 Genomes from the Houston Metropolitan Area Identifies the Emergence and Widespread Distribution of Multiple Isolates of All Major Variants of Concern. *Am. J. Pathol.* **2021**, *191*, 983–992. [CrossRef]
18. Dhawan, M.; Sharma, A.; Priyanka; Thakur, N.; Rajkhowa, T.K.; Choudhary, O.P. Delta Variant (B.1.617.2) of SARS-CoV-2: Mutations, Impact, Challenges and Possible Solutions. *Hum. Vaccin. Immunother.* **2022**, *18*, 2068883. [CrossRef]
19. Ferreira, I.A.T.M.; Kemp, S.A.; Datir, R.; Saito, A.; Meng, B.; Rakshit, P.; Takaori-Kondo, A.; Kosugi, Y.; Uriu, K.; Kimura, I.; et al. SARS CoV 2 B.1.617 Mutations L452R and E484Q Are Not Synergistic for Antibody Evasion. *J. Infect. Dis.* **2021**, *224*, 989–994. [CrossRef]
20. Arora, P.; Kempf, A.; Nehlmeier, I.; Graichen, L.; Sidarovich, A.; Winkler, M.S.; Schulz, S.; Jäck, H.M.; Stankov, M.V.; Behrens, G.M.N.; et al. Delta Variant (B.1.617.2) Sublineages Do Not Show Increased Neutralization Resistance. *Cell. Mol. Immunol.* **2021**, *18*, 2557–2559. [CrossRef] [PubMed]
21. Planas, D.; Veyer, D.; Baidaliuk, A.; Staropoli, I.; Guivel-Benhassine, F.; Rajah, M.M.; Planchais, C.; Porrot, F.; Robillard, N.; Puech, J.; et al. Reduced Sensitivity of SARS-CoV-2 Variant Delta to Antibody Neutralization. *Nature* **2021**, *596*, 276–280. [CrossRef] [PubMed]
22. Lo, S.W.; Jamrozy, D. Genomics and Epidemiological Surveillance. *Nat. Rev. Microbiol.* **2020**, *18*, 478. [CrossRef]
23. Hu, T.; Li, J.; Zhou, H.; Li, C.; Holmes, E.C.; Shi, W. Bioinformatics Resources for SARS-CoV-2 Discovery and Surveillance. *Brief. Bioinform.* **2021**, *22*, 631–641. [CrossRef] [PubMed]
24. Chen, Z.; Azman, A.S.; Chen, X.; Zou, J.; Tian, Y.; Sun, R.; Xu, X.; Wu, Y.; Lu, W.; Ge, S.; et al. Global Landscape of SARS-CoV-2 Genomic Surveillance and Data Sharing. *Nat. Genet.* **2022**, *54*, 499–507. [CrossRef]
25. State Health Department of Rio Grande do Sul. COVID-19 Immunization Monitoring. Available online: https://vacina.saude.rs.gov.br/ (accessed on 5 October 2022).
26. Artic Network. nCov-2019 Sequencing Protocol v3 (LoCost). Available online: https://www.protocols.io/view/ncov-2019-sequencing-protocol-v3-locost-bp2l6n26rgqe/v3?version_warning=no (accessed on 18 August 2022).
27. Artic Network. nCoV-2019 Novel Coronavirus Bioinformatics Protocol. Available online: https://artic.network/ncov-2019/ncov2019-bioinformatics-sop.html (accessed on 18 August 2022).
28. Li, H. Minimap2: Pairwise Alignment for Nucleotide Sequences. *Bioinformatics* **2018**, *34*, 3094–3100. [CrossRef] [PubMed]
29. Danecek, P.; Bonfield, J.K.; Liddle, J.; Marshall, J.; Ohan, V.; Pollard, M.O.; Whitwham, A.; Keane, T.; McCarthy, S.A.; Davies, R.M.; et al. Twelve Years of SAMtools and BCFtools. *Gigascience* **2021**, *10*, giab00. [CrossRef]
30. Kearse, M.; Moir, R.; Wilson, A.; Stones-Havas, S.; Cheung, M.; Sturrock, S.; Buxton, S.; Cooper, A.; Markowitz, S.; Duran, C.; et al. Geneious Basic: An Integrated and Extendable Desktop Software Platform for the Organization and Analysis of Sequence Data. *Bioinformatics* **2012**, *28*, 1647–1649. [CrossRef]

31. Dezordi, F.Z.; da Silva Neto, A.M.; de Lima Campos, T.; Jeronimo, P.M.C.; Aksenen, C.F.; Almeida, S.P.; Wallau, G.L. ViralFlow: A Versatile Automated Workflow for SARS-CoV-2 Genome Assembly, Lineage Assignment, Mutations and Intrahost Variant Detection. *Viruses* **2022**, *14*, 217. [CrossRef]

32. Aksamentov, I.; Roemer, C.; Hodcroft, E.B.; Neher, R.A. Nextclade: Clade Assignment, Mutation Calling and Quality Control for Viral Genomes. *J. Open Source Softw.* **2021**, *6*, 3773. [CrossRef]

33. O'Toole, Á.; Scher, E.; Underwood, A.; Jackson, B.; Hill, V.; McCrone, J.T.; Colquhoun, R.; Ruis, C.; Abu-Dahab, K.; Taylor, B.; et al. Assignment of Epidemiological Lineages in an Emerging Pandemic Using the Pangolin Tool. *Virus Evol.* **2021**, *7*, veab064. [CrossRef] [PubMed]

34. Shu, Y.; McCauley, J. GISAID: Global Initiative on Sharing All Influenza Data—From Vision to Reality. *Euro Surveill.* **2017**, *22*, 30494. [CrossRef] [PubMed]

35. GISAID EpiCoV Database. Available online: https://gisaid.org/ (accessed on 20 October 2022).

36. Council of Municipal Health Departments of Rio Grande do Sul. Health Regions. Available online: https://www.cosemsrs.org.br/regioes-de-saude (accessed on 3 October 2022).

37. QGIS Development Team. QGIS: A Free and Open Source Geographic Information System. Available online: https://qgis.org/en/site/ (accessed on 3 October 2022).

38. Instituto Brasileiro de Geografia e Estatística (IBGE). Rio Grande Do Sul Cartographic Base. Available online: https://geoftp.ibge.gov.br/cartas_e_mapas/bases_cartograficas_continuas/bc100/rio_grande_do_sul/ (accessed on 3 October 2022).

39. Fonseca, P.L.C.; Moreira, F.R.R.; De Souza, R.M.; Guimarães, N.R.; Carvalho, N.O.; Adelino, T.E.R.; Alves, H.J.; Alvim, L.B.; Candido, D.S.; Coelho, H.P.; et al. Tracking the Turnover of SARS-CoV-2 VOCs Gamma to Delta in a Brazilian State (Minas Gerais) with a High-Vaccination Status. *Virus Evol.* **2022**, *8*, veac064. [CrossRef] [PubMed]

40. Brazilian Government. Coronavirus Dashboard. Available online: https://covid.saude.gov.br/ (accessed on 20 October 2022).

41. Larsson, A. AliView: A Fast and Lightweight Alignment Viewer and Editor for Large Datasets. *Bioinformatics* **2014**, *30*, 3276–3278. [CrossRef] [PubMed]

42. Minh, B.Q.; Schmidt, H.A.; Chernomor, O.; Schrempf, D.; Woodhams, M.D.; Von Haeseler, A.; Lanfear, R.; Teeling, E. IQ-TREE 2: New Models and Efficient Methods for Phylogenetic Inference in the Genomic Era. *Mol. Biol. Evol.* **2020**, *37*, 1530–1534. [CrossRef]

43. Kirkwood, T.B.L. Some Mathematical Questions in Biology: DNA Sequence Analysis. *Stat. Med.* **1989**, *8*, 523–524. [CrossRef]

44. Yang, Z. Maximum Likelihood Phylogenetic Estimation from DNA Sequences with Variable Rates over Sites: Approximate Methods. *J. Mol. Evol.* **1994**, *39*, 306–314. [CrossRef]

45. Guindon, S.; Dufayard, J.F.; Lefort, V.; Anisimova, M.; Hordijk, W.; Gascuel, O. New Algorithms and Methods to Estimate Maximum-Likelihood Phylogenies: Assessing the Performance of PhyML 3.0. *Syst. Biol.* **2010**, *59*, 307–321. [CrossRef]

46. Rambaut, A. FigTree. Available online: http://tree.bio.ed.ac.uk/software/figtree/ (accessed on 20 October 2022).

47. Rambaut, A.; Lam, T.T.; Carvalho, L.M.; Pybus, O.G. Exploring the Temporal Structure of Heterochronous Sequences Using TempEst (Formerly Path-O-Gen). *Virus Evol.* **2016**, *2*, vew007. [CrossRef]

48. Sagulenko, P.; Puller, V.; Neher, R.A. TreeTime: Maximum-Likelihood Phylodynamic Analysis. *Virus Evol.* **2018**, *4*, vex042. [CrossRef]

49. Gularte, J.S.; da Silva, M.S.; Mosena, A.C.S.; Demoliner, M.; Hansen, A.W.; Filippi, M.; de Abreu Góes Pereira , V.M.; Heldt, F.H.; Weber, M.N.; de Almeida, P.R.; et al. Early Introduction, Dispersal and Evolution of Delta SARS-CoV-2 in Southern Brazil, Late Predominance of AY.99.2 and AY.101 Related Lineages. *Virus Res.* **2022**, *311*, 198702. [CrossRef]

50. Presidency of the Federative Republic of Brazil. Law Number 13,979, of 6 February 2020. Available online: http://www.planalto.gov.br/ccivil_03/_ato2019-2022/2020/lei/L13979.htm (accessed on 3 October 2022).

51. Elliott, P.; Haw, D.; Wang, H.; Eales, O.; Walters, C.E.; Ainslie, K.E.C.; Atchison, C.; Fronterre, C.; Diggle, P.J.; Page, A.J.; et al. Exponential Growth, High Prevalence of SARS-CoV-2, and Vaccine Effectiveness Associated with the Delta Variant. *Science* **2021**, *374*, eabl9551. [CrossRef]

52. Umair, M.; Ikram, A.; Salman, M.; Haider, S.A.; Badar, N.; Rehman, Z.; Ammar, M.; Rana, M.S.; Ali, Q. Genomic Surveillance Reveals the Detection of SARS-CoV-2 Delta, Beta, and Gamma VOCs during the Third Wave in Pakistan. *J. Med. Virol.* **2022**, *94*, 1115–1129. [CrossRef]

53. Yakovleva, A.; Kovalenko, G.; Redlinger, M.; Liulchuk, M.G.; Bortz, E.; Zadorozhna, V.I.; Scherbinska, A.M.; Wertheim, J.O.; Goodfellow, I.; Meredith, L.; et al. Tracking SARS-COV-2 Variants Using Nanopore Sequencing in Ukraine in 2021. *Sci. Rep.* **2022**, *12*, 15749. [CrossRef]

54. de Menezes Mayer, A.; Gröhs Ferrareze, P.A.; de Oliveira, L.F.V.; Gregianini, T.S.; Neves, C.L.A.M.; Caldana, G.D.; Kmetzsch, L.; Thompson, C.E. Genomic Characterization and Molecular Evolution of SARS-CoV-2 in Rio Grande Do Sul State, Brazil. *Virology* **2023**, *582*, 1–11. [CrossRef] [PubMed]

55. Ferrareze, P.A.G.; Cybis, G.B.; de Oliveira, L.F.V.; Zimerman, R.A.; Schiavon, D.E.B.; Peter, C.; Thompson, C.E. Intense P.1 (Gamma) Diversification Followed by Rapid Delta Substitution in Southern Brazil: A SARS-CoV-2 Genomic Epidemiology Study. *Microbes Infect.* **2023**, *10*, 105216. [CrossRef] [PubMed]

56. Moreira, F.R.R.; D'Arc, M.; Mariani, D.; Herlinger, A.L.; Schiffler, F.B.; Rossi, Á.D.; Leitão, I.D.C.; Miranda, T.D.S.; Cosentino, M.A.C.; Tôrres, M.C.D.P.; et al. Epidemiological Dynamics of SARS-CoV-2 VOC Gamma in Rio de Janeiro, Brazil. *Virus Evol.* **2021**, *7*, 1–11. [CrossRef] [PubMed]

57. de Souza, U.J.B.; Dos Santos, R.N.; de Melo, F.L.; Belmok, A.; Galvão, J.D.; de Rezende, T.C.V.; Cardoso, F.D.P.; Carvalho, R.F.; da Silva Oliveira, M.; Junior, J.C.R.; et al. Genomic Epidemiology of SARS-CoV-2 in Tocantins State and the Diffusion of P.1.7 and AY.99.2 Lineages in Brazil. *Viruses* **2022**, *14*, 659. [CrossRef] [PubMed]

58. Sgorlon, G.; da Silva Queiroz, J.A.; Roca, T.P.; da Silva, A.M.P.; Gasparelo, N.W.F.; Teixeira, K.S.; da Nóbrega Oliveira, A.S.; de Melo Mendonça, A.L.F.; Maia, A.C.S.; Pereira, S.D.S.; et al. Clinical and Epidemiological Aspects of Delta and Gamma SARS-CoV-2 Variant of Concern from the Western Brazilian Amazon. *Mem. Inst. Oswaldo Cruz* **2022**, *117*, 117. [CrossRef] [PubMed]

59. Pinho, C.T.; Vidal, A.F.; Costa Negri Rocha, T.; Oliveira, R.R.M.; Clara da Costa Barros, M.; Closset, L.; Azevedo-Pinheiro, J.; Braga-da-Silva, C.; Santos Silva, C.; Magalhães, L.L.; et al. Transmission Dynamics of SARS-CoV-2 Variants in the Brazilian State of Pará. *Front. Public Health* **2023**, *11*, 11. [CrossRef]

60. Silva, J.P.; de Lima, A.B.; Alvim, L.B.; Malta, F.S.V.; Mendonça, C.P.T.B.; Fonseca, P.L.C.; Moreira, F.R.R.; Queiroz, D.C.; Ferreira, J.G.G.; Ferreira, A.C.S.; et al. Delta Variant of SARS-CoV-2 Replacement in Brazil: A National Epidemiologic Surveillance Program. *Viruses* **2022**, *14*, 847. [CrossRef]

61. Giovanetti, M.; Fonseca, V.; Wilkinson, E.; Tegally, H.; San, E.J.; Althaus, C.L.; Xavier, J.; Slavov, S.N.; Viala, V.L.; Lima, A.R.J.; et al. Replacement of the Gamma by the Delta Variant in Brazil: Impact of Lineage Displacement on the Ongoing Pandemic. *Virus Evol.* **2022**, *8*, veac024. [CrossRef]

62. Patané, J.; Viala, V.; Lima, L.; Martins, A.; Barros, C.; Bernardino, J.; Moretti, D.; Slavov, S.; Santos, R.; Rodrigues, E.; et al. SARS-CoV-2 Delta Variant of Concern in Brazil—Multiple Introductions, Communitary Transmission, and Early Signs of Local Evolution. *medRxiv* **2021**. [CrossRef]

63. Saifi, S.; Ravi, V.; Sharma, S.; Swaminathan, A.; Chauhan, N.S.; Pandey, R. SARS-CoV-2 VOCs, Mutational Diversity and Clinical Outcome: Are They Modulating Drug Efficacy by Altered Binding Strength? *Genomics* **2022**, *114*, 110466. [CrossRef]

64. Shen, L.; Triche, T.J.; Dien Bard, J.; Biegel, J.A.; Judkins, A.R.; Gai, X. Spike Protein NTD Mutation G142D in SARS-CoV-2 Delta VOC Lineages Is Associated with Frequent Back Mutations, Increased Viral Loads, and Immune Evasion. *medRxiv* **2021**. [CrossRef]

65. Rahimi, A.; Mirzazadeh, A.; Tavakolpour, S. Genetics and Genomics of SARS-CoV-2: A Review of the Literature with the Special Focus on Genetic Diversity and SARS-CoV-2 Genome Detection. *Genomics* **2021**, *113*, 1221–1232. [CrossRef]

66. Daniloski, Z.; Jordan, T.X.; Ilmain, J.K.; Guo, X.; Bhabha, G.; Tenoever, B.R.; Sanjana, N.E. The Spike D614G Mutation Increases SARS-CoV-2 Infection of Multiple Human Cell Types. *Elife* **2021**, *10*, e65365. [CrossRef]

67. Groves, D.C.; Rowland-Jones, S.L.; Angyal, A. The D614G Mutations in the SARS-CoV-2 Spike Protein: Implications for Viral Infectivity, Disease Severity and Vaccine Design. *Biochem. Biophys. Res. Commun.* **2021**, *538*, 104–107. [CrossRef] [PubMed]

68. Ozono, S.; Zhang, Y.; Ode, H.; Sano, K.; Tan, T.S.; Imai, K.; Miyoshi, K.; Kishigami, S.; Ueno, T.; Iwatani, Y.; et al. SARS-CoV-2 D614G Spike Mutation Increases Entry Efficiency with Enhanced ACE2-Binding Affinity. *Nat. Commun.* **2021**, *12*, 848. [CrossRef]

69. Volz, E.; Hill, V.; McCrone, J.T.; Price, A.; Jorgensen, D.; O'Toole, Á.; Southgate, J.; Johnson, R.; Jackson, B.; Nascimento, F.F.; et al. Evaluating the Effects of SARS-CoV-2 Spike Mutation D614G on Transmissibility and Pathogenicity. *Cell* **2021**, *184*, 64–75. [CrossRef]

70. Hou, Y.J.; Chiba, S.; Halfmann, P.; Ehre, C.; Kuroda, M.; Dinnon, K.H.; Leist, S.R.; Schäfer, A.; Nakajima, N.; Takahashi, K.; et al. SARS-CoV-2 D614G Variant Exhibits Efficient Replication Ex Vivo and Transmission in vivo. *Science* **2020**, *370*, 1464–1468. [CrossRef]

71. Plante, J.A.; Liu, Y.; Liu, J.; Xia, H.; Johnson, B.A.; Lokugamage, K.G.; Zhang, X.; Muruato, A.E.; Zou, J.; Fontes-Garfias, C.R.; et al. Spike Mutation D614G Alters SARS-CoV-2 Fitness. *Nature* **2020**, *592*, 116–121. [CrossRef]

72. Ogawa, J.; Zhu, W.; Tonnu, N.; Singer, O.; Hunter, T.; Ryan, A.L.; Pao, G.M. The D614G Mutation in the SARS-CoV2 Spike Protein Increases Infectivity in an ACE2 Receptor Dependent Manner. *bioRxiv* **2020**, 1–10. [CrossRef]

73. Zhang, L.; Jackson, C.B.; Mou, H.; Ojha, A.; Peng, H.; Quinlan, B.D.; Rangarajan, E.S.; Pan, A.; Vanderheiden, A.; Suthar, M.S.; et al. SARS-CoV-2 Spike-Protein D614G Mutation Increases Virion Spike Density and Infectivity. *Nat. Commun.* **2020**, *11*, 6013. [CrossRef] [PubMed]

74. Winger, A.; Caspari, T. The Spike of Concern-The Novel Variants of SARS-CoV-2. *Viruses* **2021**, *13*, 1002. [CrossRef]

75. Peacock, T.P.; Goldhill, D.H.; Zhou, J.; Baillon, L.; Frise, R.; Swann, O.C.; Kugathasan, R.; Penn, R.; Brown, J.C.; Sanchez-David, R.Y.; et al. The Furin Cleavage Site in the SARS-CoV-2 Spike Protein Is Required for Transmission in Ferrets. *Nat. Microbiol.* **2021**, *6*, 899–909. [CrossRef]

76. Hoffmann, M.; Kleine-Weber, H.; Pöhlmann, S. A Multibasic Cleavage Site in the Spike Protein of SARS-CoV-2 Is Essential for Infection of Human Lung Cells. *Mol. Cell* **2020**, *78*, 779–784. [CrossRef]

77. Lamarca, A.P.; de Almeida, L.G.P.P.; da Silva Francisco, R.; Cavalcante, L.; Brustolini, O.; Gerber, A.L.; de C Guimarães, A.P.; de Oliveira, T.H.; Nascimento, É.R.D.S.; Policarpo, C.; et al. Phylodynamic Analysis of SARS-CoV-2 Spread in Rio de Janeiro, Brazil, Highlights How Metropolitan Areas Act as Dispersal Hubs for New Variants. *Microb. Genom.* **2022**, *8*, 000859. [CrossRef]

78. te Velthuis, A.J.W.; Arnold, J.J.; Cameron, C.E.; van den Worm, S.H.E.; Snijder, E.J. The RNA Polymerase Activity of SARS-Coronavirus Nsp12 Is Primer Dependent. *Nucleic Acids Res.* **2010**, *38*, 203–214. [CrossRef]

79. Zhang, B.Z.; Hu, Y.; Chen, L.; Yau, T.; Tong, Y.; Hu, J.; Cai, J.; Chan, K.H.; Dou, Y.; Deng, J.; et al. Mining of Epitopes on Spike Protein of SARS-CoV-2 from COVID-19 Patients. *Cell Res.* **2020**, *30*, 702–704. [CrossRef] [PubMed]

80. Mishra, T.; Dalavi, R.; Joshi, G.; Kumar, A.; Pandey, P.; Shukla, S.; Mishra, R.K.; Chande, A. SARS-CoV-2 Spike E156G/Δ157-158 Mutations Contribute to Increased Infectivity and Immune Escape. *Life Sci. Alliance* **2022**, *5*, 1–14. [CrossRef] [PubMed]
81. Dejnirattisai, W.; Zhou, D.; Supasa, P.; Liu, C.; Mentzer, A.J.; Ginn, H.M.; Zhao, Y.; Duyvesteyn, H.M.E.; Tuekprakhon, A.; Nutalai, R.; et al. Antibody Evasion by the P.1 Strain of SARS-CoV-2. *Cell* **2021**, *184*, 2939–2954. [CrossRef]
82. Padilha, D.A.; Filho, V.B.; Moreira, R.S.; Soratto, T.A.T.; Maia, G.A.; Christoff, A.P.; Barazzetti, F.H.; Schörner, M.A.; Ferrari, F.L.; Martins, C.L.; et al. Emergence of Two Distinct SARS-CoV-2 Gamma Variants and the Rapid Spread of P.1-like-II SARS-CoV-2 during the Second Wave of COVID-19 in Santa Catarina, Southern Brazil. *Viruses* **2022**, *14*, 695. [CrossRef]
83. Fratev, F. N501Y and K417N Mutations in the Spike Protein of SARS-CoV-2 Alter the Interactions with Both HACE2 and Human-Derived Antibody: A Free Energy of Perturbation Retrospective Study. *J. Chem. Inf. Model.* **2021**, *61*, 6079–6084. [CrossRef]
84. Mohammadi, M.; Shayestehpour, M.; Mirzaei, H. The Impact of Spike Mutated Variants of SARS-CoV2 [Alpha, Beta, Gamma, Delta, and Lambda] on the Efficacy of Subunit Recombinant Vaccines. *Braz. J. Infect. Dis.* **2021**, *25*, 1–9. [CrossRef]
85. Deng, X.; Garcia-Knight, M.A.; Khalid, M.M.; Servellita, V.; Wang, C.; Morris, M.K.; Sotomayor-González, A.; Glasner, D.R.; Reyes, K.R.; Gliwa, A.S.; et al. Transmission, Infectivity, and Neutralization of a Spike L452R SARS-CoV-2 Variant. *Cell* **2021**, *184*, 3426–3437. [CrossRef] [PubMed]
86. Adam, D. What Scientists Know about New, Fast-Spreading Coronavirus Variants. *Nature* **2021**, *594*, 19–20. [CrossRef] [PubMed]
87. Motozono, C.; Toyoda, M.; Zahradnik, J.; Saito, A.; Nasser, H.; Tan, T.S.; Ngare, I.; Kimura, I.; Uriu, K.; Kosugi, Y.; et al. SARS-CoV-2 Spike L452R Variant Evades Cellular Immunity and Increases Infectivity. *Cell Host Microbe* **2021**, *29*, 1124–1136. [CrossRef] [PubMed]
88. Hirabara, S.M.; Serdan, T.D.A.; Gorjao, R.; Masi, L.N.; Pithon-Curi, T.C.; Covas, D.T.; Curi, R.; Durigon, E.L. SARS-COV-2 Variants: Differences and Potential of Immune Evasion. *Front. Cell. Infect. Microbiol.* **2021**, *11*, 1401. [CrossRef] [PubMed]
89. Khan, A.; Zia, T.; Suleman, M.; Khan, T.; Ali, S.S.; Abbasi, A.A.; Mohammad, A.; Wei, D.Q. Higher Infectivity of the SARS-CoV-2 New Variants Is Associated with K417N/T, E484K, and N501Y Mutants: An Insight from Structural Data. *J. Cell. Physiol.* **2021**, *236*, 7045–7057. [CrossRef]
90. Zhou, D.; Dejnirattisai, W.; Supasa, P.; Liu, C.; Mentzer, A.J.; Ginn, H.M.; Zhao, Y.; Duyvesteyn, H.M.E.; Tuekprakhon, A.; Nutalai, R.; et al. Evidence of Escape of SARS-CoV-2 Variant B.1.351 from Natural and Vaccine-Induced Sera. *Cell* **2021**, *184*, 2348–2361. [CrossRef]
91. Golubchik, T.; Lythgoe, K.A.; Hall, M.; Ferretti, L.; Fryer, H.R.; MacIntyre-Cockett, G.; de Cesare, M.; Trebes, A.; Piazza, P.; Buck, D.; et al. Early Analysis of a Potential Link between Viral Load and the N501Y Mutation in the SARS-COV-2 Spike Protein. *medRxiv* **2021**. [CrossRef]
92. Islam, S.R.; Prusty, D.; Manna, S.K. Structural Basis of Fitness of Emerging SARS-COV-2 Variants and Considerations for Screening, Testing and Surveillance Strategy to Contain Their Threat. *medRxiv* **2021**. [CrossRef]
93. Grubaugh, N.D.; Hanage, W.P.; Rasmussen, A.L. Making Sense of Mutation: What D614G Means for the COVID-19 Pandemic Remains Unclear. *Cell* **2020**, *182*, 794–795. [CrossRef] [PubMed]
94. Escalera, A.; Gonzalez-Reiche, A.S.; Aslam, S.; Mena, I.; Laporte, M.; Pearl, R.L.; Fossati, A.; Rathnasinghe, R.; Alshammary, H.; van de Guchte, A.; et al. Mutations in SARS-CoV-2 Variants of Concern Link to Increased Spike Cleavage and Virus Transmission. *Cell Host Microbe* **2022**, *30*, 373–387. [CrossRef] [PubMed]
95. Cruz, C.A.; Medina, P.M. Temporal Changes in the Accessory Protein Mutations of SARS-CoV-2 Variants and Their Predicted Structural and Functional Effects. *J. Med. Virol.* **2022**, *94*, 5189–5200. [CrossRef] [PubMed]
96. Johnson, B.A.; Zhou, Y.; Lokugamage, K.G.; Vu, M.N.; Bopp, N.; Crocquet-Valdes, P.A.; Kalveram, B.; Schindewolf, C.; Liu, Y.; Scharton, D.; et al. Nucleocapsid Mutations in SARS-CoV-2 Augment Replication and Pathogenesis. *PLoS Pathog.* **2022**, *18*, e1010627. [CrossRef]
97. Wu, H.; Xing, N.; Meng, K.; Fu, B.; Xue, W.; Dong, P.; Tang, W.; Xiao, Y.; Liu, G.; Luo, H.; et al. Nucleocapsid Mutations R203K/G204R Increase the Infectivity, Fitness, and Virulence of SARS-CoV-2. *Cell Host Microbe* **2021**, *29*, 1788–1801. [CrossRef]

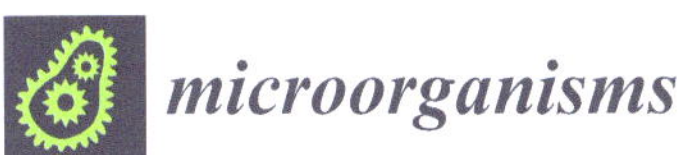

Article

Characterization of SARS-CoV-2 Variants in Military and Civilian Personnel of an Air Force Airport during Three Pandemic Waves in Italy

Michele Equestre [1], Cinzia Marcantonio [2], Nadia Marascio [3,*], Federica Centofanti [2], Antonio Martina [4], Matteo Simeoni [4], Elisabetta Suffredini [5], Giuseppina La Rosa [6], Giusy Bonanno Ferraro [6], Pamela Mancini [6], Carolina Veneri [6], Giovanni Matera [3], Angela Quirino [3], Angela Costantino [2], Stefania Taffon [2], Elena Tritarelli [2], Carmelo Campanella [7], Giulio Pisani [4], Roberto Nisini [2], Enea Spada [2], Paola Verde [8], Anna Rita Ciccaglione [2] and Roberto Bruni [2]

[1] Department of Neurosciences, Istituto Superiore di Sanità, 00161 Rome, Italy; michele.equestre@iss.it
[2] Department of Infectious Diseases, Istituto Superiore di Sanità, 00161 Rome, Italy; cinzia.marcantonio@iss.it (C.M.); centofantifederica@outlook.it (F.C.); angela.costantino@iss.it (A.C.); stefania.taffon@iss.it (S.T.); elena.tritarelli@iss.it (E.T.); roberto.nisini@iss.it (R.N.); enea.spada@iss.it (E.S.); annarita.ciccaglione@iss.it (A.R.C.); roberto.bruni@iss.it (R.B.)
[3] Clinical Microbiology Unit, Department of Health Sciences, "Magna Grecia" University, 88100 Catanzaro, Italy; mmatera@unicz.it (G.M.); quirino@unicz.it (A.Q.)
[4] Center for Immunobiologicals Research and Evaluation, Istituto Superiore di Sanità, 00161 Rome, Italy; antonio.martina@iss.it (A.M.); matteo.simeoni@iss.it (M.S.); giulio.pisani@iss.it (G.P.)
[5] Department of Food Safety, Nutrition and Veterinary Public Health, Istituto Superiore di Sanità, 00161 Rome, Italy; elisabetta.suffredini@iss.it
[6] Department of Environment and Health, Istituto Superiore di Sanità, 00161 Rome, Italy; giuseppina.larosa@iss.it (G.L.R.); giusy.bonannoferraro@iss.it (G.B.F.); pamela.mancini@iss.it (P.M.); carolina.veneri@iss.it (C.V.)
[7] Clinical Analysis and Molecular Biology Laboratory Rome, Institute of Aerospace Medicine, 00185 Rome, Italy; carmelocampanella21@gmail.com
[8] Aerospace Medicine Department, Aerospace Test Division, Militay Airport Mario De Bernardi, Pratica di Mare, 00040 Rome, Italy; paolaverde26@gmail.com
* Correspondence: nmarascio@unicz.it; Tel.: +39-096-1369-7742; Fax: +39-096-1369-7760

Citation: Equestre, M.; Marcantonio, C.; Marascio, N.; Centofanti, F.; Martina, A.; Simeoni, M.; Suffredini, E.; La Rosa, G.; Bonanno Ferraro, G.; Mancini, P.; et al. Characterization of SARS-CoV-2 Variants in Military and Civilian Personnel of an Air Force Airport during Three Pandemic Waves in Italy. *Microorganisms* **2023**, *11*, 2711. https://doi.org/10.3390/microorganisms11112711

Academic Editor: Qibin Geng

Received: 7 October 2023
Revised: 1 November 2023
Accepted: 3 November 2023
Published: 5 November 2023

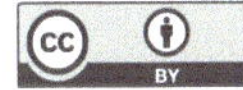

Abstract: We investigated SARS-CoV-2 variants circulating, from November 2020 to March 2022, among military and civilian personnel at an Air Force airport in Italy in order to classify viral isolates in a potential hotspot for virus spread. Positive samples were subjected to Next-Generation Sequencing (NGS) of the whole viral genome and Sanger sequencing of the spike coding region. Phylogenetic analysis classified viral isolates and traced their evolutionary relationships. Clusters were identified using 70% cut-off. Sequencing methods yielded comparable results in terms of variant classification. In 2020 and 2021, we identified several variants, including B.1.258 (4/67), B.1.177 (9/67), Alpha (B.1.1.7, 9/67), Gamma (P.1.1, 4/67), and Delta (4/67). In 2022, only Omicron and its sub-lineage variants were observed (37/67). SARS-CoV-2 isolates were screened to detect naturally occurring resistance in genomic regions, the target of new therapies, comparing them to the Wuhan Hu-1 reference strain. Interestingly, 2/30 non-Omicron isolates carried the G15S 3CLpro substitution responsible for reduced susceptibility to protease inhibitors. On the other hand, Omicron isolates carried unusual substitutions A1803V, D1809N, and A949T on PLpro, and the D216N on 3CLpro. Finally, the P323L substitution on RdRp coding regions was not associated with the mutational pattern related to polymerase inhibitor resistance. This study highlights the importance of continuous genomic surveillance to monitor SARS-CoV-2 evolution in the general population, as well as in restricted communities.

Keywords: SARS-CoV-2 variant; 3CLpro; RdRp; Plpro; spike; nucleocapsid; mutations; Sanger; Next-Generation Sequencing

1. Introduction

Italy was one of the worst afflicted countries during the Severe Acute Respiratory Syndrome Coronavirus 2 (SARS-CoV-2) pandemic, with 101,739 infected cases and more than 10,000 people deceased by March 2020. Due to rapid decision making, on 27 December 2020, the Italian Medicines Agency approved the BioNTech/Pfizer mRNA BNT162b2 Comirnaty vaccine and started the first stage of the vaccination campaign, initially targeting healthcare workers [1]. By 1 May 2021, over 20,000,000 single doses of vaccine had been administered. By March 2023, 40,478,062 people had been administered with a booster dose of vaccine [2]. To control and monitor the SARS-CoV-2 pandemic, the World Health Organization (WHO) and the European Centre for Disease Prevention and Control (ECDC) recommend Whole Genome Sequencing (WGS), or complete/partial spike (S) gene sequencing to detect new variants with variable severity and infectivity, as well as immune escape potential [3–5]. During the pandemic, several variants were identified and subsequently designated by WHO as Variants Being Monitored (VBMs), Variants of Interest (VOIs) or of Concern (VOCs), characterized by greater transmissibility, virulence, and resistance, and finally, Variants of High Consequence (VOHCs), which are highly dangerous and epidemic [5,6].

The first VOCs to emerge in Italy were the Alpha (B.1.1.7) VOC, first identified in the UK (September 2020) and around 30–40% more transmissible than the original wild-type, the Beta (B.1.351) VOC, first documented in South Africa (May 2020), and the Gamma (P1) VOC, first identified in Manaus, Brazil (November 2020), 1.7–2.4 times more transmissible than wild-type [7]. From June 2020, two novel SARS-CoV-2 variants were detected in the Italian territory, the B.1.177 (20A.EU1) and the B.1.258 (20A) variants [7]. The latter represented an example of a nationally prevailing variant not commonly detected in other countries at that time, but later spread globally, likely due to the acquisition of beneficial mutations including ΔH69/V70 deletions, N439K, and D614G, all concentrated in the S1 subunit, specifically at the start of the N-terminal domain (NTD) and in the receptor-binding domain (RBD) [8]. The detection of S gene mutations is of particular importance in monitoring emerging variants able to enhance virus transmission, reinfection, and vaccine escape [9]. Additionally, recent data highlight the high mutational rate of the nucleocapsid (N) gene and its implication on pathogenesis and on diagnosis failure by commercial assays [10,11].

Based on genomic surveillance, surveys conducted across the whole Italian territory during the first month of 2021 highlighted the Alpha variant as dominant, followed by a substantial proportion of cases of the Gamma variant, almost exclusively in central Italy [12]. These two variants decreased during the summer of 2021, when the number of reported cases caused by the Delta variant (B.1.617.2) exceeded those caused by the Alpha. More than 80% of cases in all age groups were caused by the Delta variant, with the highest percentage in subjects aged between 10 and 29 years [13]. The Delta variant was characterized by higher transmissibility, viral RNA loads, and infectivity than the Alpha in both vaccinated and unvaccinated individuals [14]. On 27 November 2021, the Omicron variant was identified for the first time in Italy. Nine cases were reported in four regions, and all patients were either asymptomatic or with mild or cured symptoms [13]. The Omicron variant (BA) rapidly spread across the country, and its prevalence increased from 1.0% to 65.9% in only three weeks, reaching 80% in the first week of January, when it became predominant [15]. Recently, the XBB.1.5 (also known as Kraken), plus F456L substitution VOI and the EG.5 (also known as Eris), and BA.2.86 (also known as Pirola), VBMs were detected globally [16]. These new SARS-CoV-2 variants are potentially able to cause breakthrough infections in people with previous immunity (infected or vaccinated) [16]. Even if hospitalization rates and severe illness have not yet increased, the COVID-19 vaccine targeting the XBB.1.5 VOC is ongoing [17]. It is expected to be effective against the new variants identified during the current international epidemiological surveillance [17]. The large number of published papers and available sequences were, and still are, very useful for monitoring SARS-CoV-2 spread direction, noting each new mutation and its potential role on transmissibility and disease severity [9,18–20].

Since 2021, some antivirals are available for treating viral infection in combination or not with monoclonal antibodies (mAbs), most of which are ineffective due to immune escape [9,21]. New antivirals target viral enzymes involved in replication, such as 3-Chymotrypsin-like protease (3CLpro), RNA-dependent RNA polymerase (RdRp), and the papain-like protease (PLpro) [22]. Naturally occurring resistance mutations, already fixed in the viral population, or selected resistance under drug pressure could be responsible for treatment failure [23]. In this regard, SARS-CoV-2 molecular characterization, used to monitor antiviral resistance of different variants, can help prioritize healthcare resources and optimize patient management strategies. The most at-risk patients treated by a combination therapy were not hospitalized and had no adverse events [22,24]. Furthermore, this treatment could reduce selection of SARS-CoV-2 resistant isolates [24].

Since the beginning of the pandemic, the Italian Government, in order to cope with the transmission of COVID-19, enacted a series of control measures that limited interaction between people, such as social distancing, closure of many commercial activities, and implementation of home working. Simultaneously, public health services were improved to control any outbreak occurring in restricted areas by contact tracing [25]. In the globalized era, air transport and passenger mobility are essential for economic development, but they also increase risks associated with the transmission of COVID-19 disease in airport areas due to the provenance of travelers from different countries and latitudes, making early identification and isolation of asymptomatic carriers necessary to avoid possible outbreaks [25]. Similarly, Air Force personnel deployed to military bases abroad may be a hotspot for virus transmission, due to interaction with both military and civilian personnel from different nations. The screening program and molecular epidemiology studies can help to monitor and limit the spread of the virus within these communities by identifying potential outbreaks and implementing appropriate control measures [3–5,26].

In this scenario, from November 2020 to March 2022, a COVID-19 screening program and surveillance testing was conducted among the military and civilian personnel of the "Mario De Bernardi" military airport, within the framework of the Scientific Collaboration Protocol signed by the Experimental Flight Center—Italian Air Force Logistic Command—and the Istituto Superiore di Sanità, with the aim of reducing viral transmission among personnel attending the military airport base [27].

Herein, we analyzed SARS-CoV-2 positive nasopharyngeal swabs using Next-Generation Sequencing and Sanger methods to characterize variants spread in the restricted community of the military airport during three pandemic waves in Italy. We focused attention on known and unusual mutations in genomic regions, the target for new therapies (3CLpro, RdRp, PLpro), and N and S coding regions, both important genomic hotspots, also involved in routine diagnosis. In addition, as a secondary objective, we evaluated the performance of partial sequencing of the spike coding region in identifying different variants accurately by comparison with results from whole genome sequencing.

2. Materials and Methods

2.1. Ethical Statement

The study protocol was approved and signed by the Scientific Collaboration Partners (i.e., Experimental Flight Center, Italian Air Force Logistic Command and Istituto Superiore di Sanità) on 30 November 2020. Personal data were collected and processed in compliance with EU and Italian legislation [28–30]. Written informed consent was obtained from all participants or their legal representative. All activities were carried out as public health activities to improve the tracing of infected individuals and contacts with the aim of reducing virus transmission among personnel attending the military airport base.

2.2. Study Design

From November 2020 to March 2022, the military and civilian personnel of the "Mario De Bernardi" military airport, located in the metropolitan area of Rome, underwent a screening program to control workplace transmission of SARS-CoV-2 infection. According to the national legislation [31–33], testing was performed locally by a first-line rapid antigen test, then positive and negative nasopharyngeal swabs (NPSs) were sent to the Istituto Superiore di Sanità (ISS) for confirmation of results by Nucleic Acid Amplification (NAAT) (overall, 1294 samples were included) [27]. From May 2021 to March 2022, only rapid antigen test positive samples were sent to ISS for confirmation by NAAT (43 samples in total). The subjects with confirmed SARS-CoV-2 positive test by gold standard real-time reverse transcription-polymerase chain reaction (RT-PCR) were included in the study. Positive samples were subjected to Next-Generation Sequencing (NGS) of the whole viral genome and Sanger sequencing of the spike coding region. Newly generated sequences were analyzed by molecular analyses. The study design is reported in Figure 1.

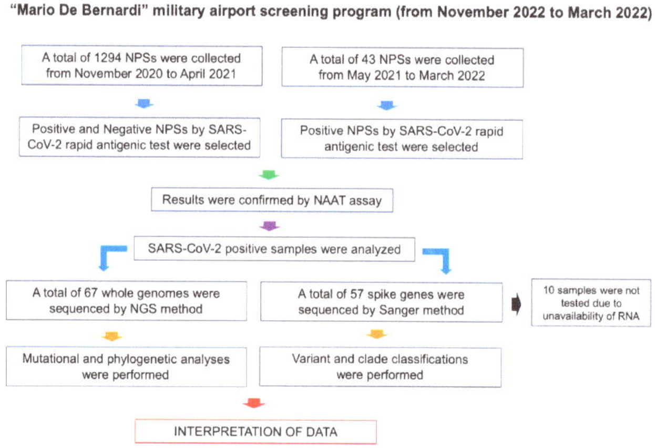

Figure 1. Study design. NPSs, nasopharyngeal swabs; NAAT, Nucleic Acid Amplification; NGS, Next-Generation Sequencing.

The study was part of the public health response to control any outbreak occurring in the military airport as soon as possible (as reported in the Scientific Collaboration Protocol, see above). All participants were asked to complete a questionnaire including demographic data, symptoms (if any), and potential exposure to infection (previous COVID-19, contact with proven COVID-19 cases, or contact with persons who tested positive for SARS-CoV-2 by molecular or antigenic tests). Subsequently, the data collected for the screening purpose were linked to the SARS-CoV-2 variants resulting from sequencing to better characterize the positive cohort.

2.3. Diagnostic Reverse Transcription (RT) Real-Time PCR

The confirmation of rapid antigen test results was based on a RT-qPCR assay (RealStar® SARS-CoV-2 RT-PCR Kit 1.0, Altona Diagnostics, Hamburg, Germany) for the detection of envelope (E) and spike (S) genes. According to manufacturer's procedures, 10 μL of RNA was used for a one step reaction to synthetize cDNA and amplify viral genome. The cDNA was used as a template with the following PCR conditions: 95 °C for 2 min, 45 cycles of 95 °C for 15 s, 55 °C for 45 s, and 72 °C for 15 s. RNA was extracted using the QIAamp® MinElute® Virus Spin Kit (QIAGEN, Hilden, Germany). Nucleic acid purification was performed using the QIAcube instrument (QIAGEN Biotechnology & Life Science). The purified RNA was amplified by RT-qPCR technology on the Rotor-Gene® instrument (QIAGEN, Hilden, Germany) [27].

2.4. SARS-CoV-2 NGS Sequencing

Sixty-seven SARS-CoV-2 sequences were collected from positive individuals by real-time RT-PCR assay. Viral nucleic acids were extracted from swab samples using QIAamp MinElute Virus Spin Kit (Qiagen, GmbH, Hilden, Germany). To generate complete genome sequences, a targeted amplicon-based approach was utilized, employing the Illumina COVIDSeq Assay (96 samples). This assay incorporates a pool of primers whose design was based on the well-established and publicly accessible ARTIC consortium multiplex PCR protocol, specifically developed for the detection and characterization of SARS-CoV-2 RNA [34]. The Illumina COVIDSeq Assay involved the multiplex amplification of overlapping PCR products, preceded by a reverse transcription step to convert SARS-CoV-2 RNA into cDNA. The resulting amplified fragments were used to construct a library for Illumina deep sequencing, utilizing the Nextera XT DNA Library Preparation and Index kits (Illumina, San Diego, CA, USA). Sequencing was performed with a pair end approach on the Illumina MiSeq platform using the MiSeq Reagent Kit v3 [35].

The obtained sequence data were subjected to analysis using the Illumina® DRAGEN COVID Lineage App [35]. Briefly, following base calling and quality scoring, the resulting sequence reads underwent adapter removal and trimming of ends with low-quality scores. The remaining high-quality reads were then mapped and aligned to the Wuhan-hu-1 reference sequence (Accession Number MN908947.3). Sequence variants were identified using the DRAGEN Somatic caller and the high confident ones incorporated into the reference genome to generate a consensus genome for the sequences based on the selected reference [35]. The first lineage/clade analysis on the consensus genomes was run using Pangolin [36] and/or NextClade [37].

2.5. SARS-CoV-2 Sanger Sequencing

Overall, of the 67 samples that underwent whole genome sequencing, 57 were also subjected to long PCR and Sanger sequencing for the purpose of comparison [38]. The remaining 10 samples could not be tested using PCR due to the unavailability of RNA.

The long-nested RT-PCR assay amplifies approximately 1600 bps spanning the region coding for amino acids 58 to 573 of the spike protein, allowing for the detection of multiple nucleotide changes resulting in key spike protein mutations distinctive of circulating SARS-CoV-2 variants. This assay has been successfully used for the screening of both clinical and environmental samples [39,40]. After amplification, the products were run on a QIAxcel Connect System, a capillary electrophoresis instrument for easy and cost-effective fragment analysis (Qiagen). The PCR products of the expected size were purified using a Montage PCRm96 Microwell Filter Plate (Millipore, Billerica, MA, USA) and sequenced by Sanger sequencing through an external service (Bio-Fab Research, Rome, Italy) [39,40]. Consensus sequences were generated using Molecular Evolutionary Genetics Analysis (MEGA X) software version 10 [41,42]. CoVsurver, enabled on the GISAID website, was used to analyze SARS-CoV-2 mutations by comparison with the reference strain hCov-19/Wuhan/WIV04/2019 [43].

2.6. Classification and Mutational Analysis

SARS-CoV-2 viral isolates were classified by Pangolin COVID-19 Lineage Assigner v.4.0.6 [36]. The following genomic regions were analyzed: ORF1ab (21,289 nucleotides, nt), S (3821 nt), ORF3a (827 nt), E (Envelope, 227 nt), M (Membrane, 668 nt), ORF6a (185 nt), ORF7a (365 nt), ORF7b (131 nt), ORF8 (365 nt), N (1259 nt), and ORF10 (116 nt). Amino acid changes of the whole genome were submitted to CoVsurver, Stanford Coronavirus Resistance Database (CoV-RDB), and Nextclade web servers [18,37,41]. The amino acid (aa) changes were further confirmed by comparing newly identified isolates with the SARS-CoV-2 Wuhan-Hu-1 reference sequence (accession NC_045512) downloaded from the GenBank® database [44]. Mutations were noted on the following predicted proteins: non-structural protein 1 (nsp1, 180 aa), nsp2 (638 aa), nsp3 (PLpro, 1944 aa), nsp4 (499 aa), nsp5 (3CLpro, 605 aa), nsp6 (289 aa), nsp7 (82 aa), nsp8 (197 aa), nsp9 (112 aa), nsp10 (138 aa), nsp12 (RdRp, 931 aa), nsp13 (600 aa), nsp14 (526 aa), nsp15 (345 aa), nsp16 (297 aa), S (1273 aa) NS3a (275 aa), E (75 aa), M (222 aa), NS6 (61 aa), NS7a (121 aa), NS7b (43 aa), NS8 (121 aa), N (419 aa), NS10 (38 aa).

2.7. Phylogenetic Analysis

The 67 final assembled whole genome sequences were aligned by ClustalW in BioEdit alongside 17 reference sequences (including the Wuhan-hu-1 reference and representatives of the major SARS-CoV-2 strains/VOCs) [45,46]. Then, the aligned sequences were checked and, wherever needed, manually edited to optimize alignment accuracy. The best substitution model for the dataset under analysis was evaluated by the Models tool available in MEGA software version 10 [41,42]. A phylogenetic tree was constructed using the Maximum Likelihood approach implemented in MEGA, with the estimated best substitution model (GTR + G + I). Statistical reliability of the phylogenetic tree was assessed by bootstrap analysis (1000 replicates); a bootstrap value > 70 was considered significant [47].

3. Results

3.1. Demographic Characteristics of the Cohort

Overall, 67 SARS-CoV-2 sequences were collected from individuals who were positive by real-time RT-PCR assay. Thirty sequences were classified as non-Omicron variants and thirty-seven as Omicron or its sub-lineages. Table 1 reports information about these two groups of the studied cohort, including referred symptoms.

Table 1. Demographic data, clinical manifestation, and contact tracing of sixty-seven positive people.

SARS-CoV-2 Variant	Non-Omicron			Omicron and Sub-Lineages		
Total Cases (n)	30			37		
Gender	Male	Female	Male (%)	Male	Female	Male (%)
	22	7	75.9	23	14	62.2
Age (years old)						
10–19	2	2	50.0	0	3	0.0
20–29	3	0	100.0	4	2	66.7
30–39	2	2	50.0	2	1	66.7
40–49	8	3	72.7	5	4	55.6
50–59	6	0	100.0	11	3	78.6
60–69	0	0	-	0	1	0.0
$\geq$70	0	0	-	1	0	100.0
not available	1					
Clinical manifestations						
Non-specific symptoms of infection	7	3	70.0	17	12	58.6
COVID-19 symptoms	12	5	70.6	18	13	58.1
Previous COVID-19 diagnosis	6	0	100.0	4	7	36.4
Previous SARS-CoV-2 positive swab	5	1	83.3	4	7	36.4
Chronic diseases	3	0	100.0	7	8	46.7
Contact tracing						
Contact with COVID-19 sick people in the previous 14 days	9	4	69.2	13	12	52.0
Contact with positive people to the SARS-CoV-2 swab in the previous 14 days	11	4	73.3	14	13	51.9
not available	1					

The median age of the 30 non-Omicron subjects was 38.1 years old (range 13–55) and there was a greater proportion of males (75.9%) than females (24.1%). The reported COVID-19 symptoms at the time of diagnosis were typical in 17 subjects, while atypical in 10 individuals (70% males). Interestingly, chronic co-morbidities were reported in three male individuals. Previous SARS-CoV-2 positive swab or COVID-19 diagnosis was reported by 12 subjects.

Among the 37 individuals infected by Omicron and its sub-lineages, the median age was 43.4 years (range 15–74) and the percentage of females was 37.8%. All individuals presented specific COVID-19 symptoms except six subjects; chronic diseases were reported in 15 cases. Most of the subjects had been in contact with SARS-CoV-2 swab-positive individuals or had contact with COVID-19 sick people.

3.2. Classification and Timing of Detected Variants

In Italy, three pandemic waves were observed between December 2020 and March 2022. In the same time span, we sequenced 67 SARS-CoV-2 genomes during the screening program in the "Mario De Bernardi" military airport. Since the end of December 2020, several variants became dominant, leading up to the beginning of the Omicron era; this latter variant became continuously dominant in the first months of 2022 (Figure 2). In our cohort, we identified the B.1.258 and sub-lineages (4/67), B.1.177 variant (9/67), Alpha (B.1.1.7) VOC (8/67), Gamma (P.1.1) VOC (4/67), Delta VOC and AY.125, AY.4, AY.4.2.3, AY.5 sub-lineages (4/67), finally Omicron VOC and BA.1.1, BA.1.1.1, BA.1.15, BA.1.17, BA.1.18, BA.1.8, BA.2 sub-lineages (37/67).

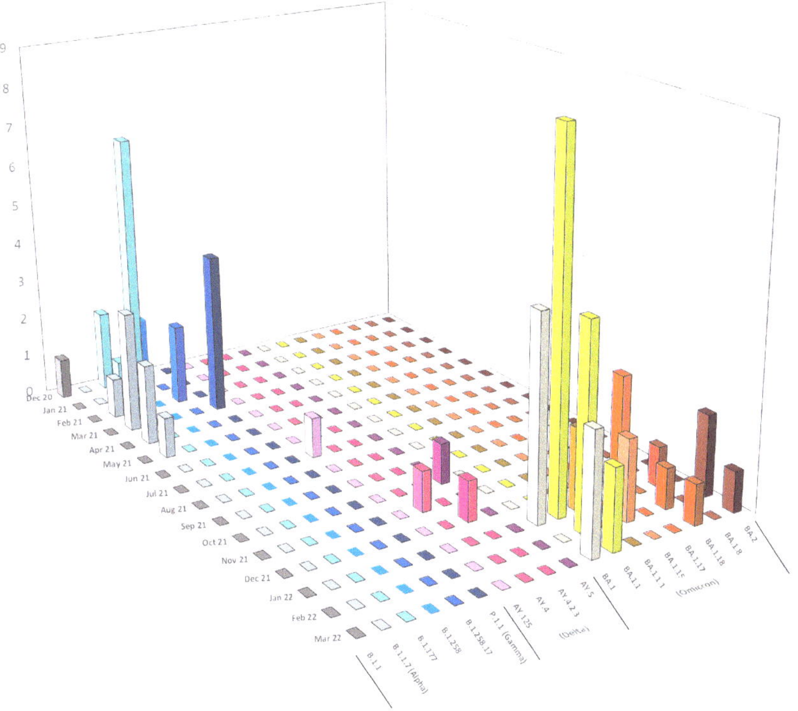

Figure 2. SARS-CoV-2 variants dynamic distribution between December 2020 and March 2022 in the military airport. The colors identify the different SARS-CoV-2 variants during the time span.

3.3. Whole Genome Analysis

Genomic analysis of 67 isolates showed a high number of amino acid (aa) changes in whole genomes (Supplementary Tables S1 and S2). The substitutions with low prevalence (unusual) among newly generated sequences, detected on the whole genome of non-Omicron (Figure 3) and Omicron (Figure 4) variants were noted.

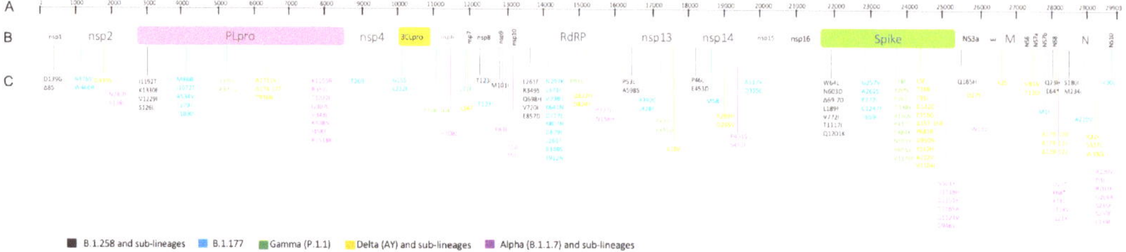

Figure 3. (A) SARS-CoV-2 whole genome length. (B) Polyprotein subdivided in structural and non-structural proteins. (C) Amino acid substitutions of non-Omicron variants and their sub-lineages were reported for each variant with a different color according to the viral isolates (little square). The * symbol identified the stop codon.

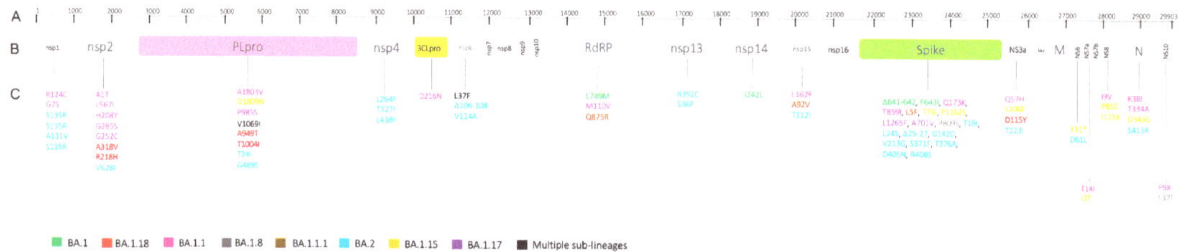

Figure 4. (A) SARS-CoV-2 whole genome length. (B) Polyprotein subdivided in structural and non-structural proteins. (C) Amino acid substitutions of Omicron VOC and its sub-lineages were reported for each variant with a different color according to the viral isolates (little square). The * symbol identified the stop codon.

3.3.1. PLpro Protein

The PLpro showed the highest number of mutations considering the whole ORF1 region. We found a total of 22 unusual aa substitutions among the 30 non-Omicron isolates, most of which related to the Alpha. A total of two B.1.258 isolates displayed the K1330E, two B.1.177 isolates showed the same three mutations (A534V, T1797I and T1830I), three Gamma VOC carried the substitution S370L, plusK977Q on two isolates, two Delta VOC displayed the A1711V substitution, and three Alpha VOC carried the G307C, V348L, and K408N mutations. Unique mutations detected on PLpro protein of non-Omicron isolates were: I1192T, V1229F, S126L, M988I, I1672T, Δ174-177, T936N, K1155R, R352C, T1022I, I458T, and R1518K (Supplementary Table S1). Among Omicron isolates, we found eight unusual aa substitutions. In particular, the A1803V, D1809N, and A949T substitutions were present in one out of 37 isolates, respectively. All three isolates belonging to BA.1.17 sub-lineage and one BA.1.18 isolate showed the V1069I aa change, while all BA.2 isolates carried the double mutation T24I and G489S (Supplementary Table S2).

3.3.2. 3CLpro Protein

Two major mutations characterize this protease in non-Omicron VOC isolates: G15S and L232F, both belonging to B.1.177 (Supplementary Table S1). An Omicron VOC isolate related to the BA.1.1 sub-lineage carried the amino acidic substitution D216N, which is very uncommon worldwide (Supplementary Table S2).

3.3.3. RdRp Protein

Eighteen unusual mutations were observed in the RdRp protein of non-Omicron VOC isolates. Seven (N297K, L371F, V398IL, K641N, D717E, K807N, and D879E) were carried by the same B.1.177 isolate. The L261F and R349S substitutions were both shown by B.1.177 and B.1.258 isolates, the latter also carrying Q698H and E857D mutations. Other unusual mutations were found in the genomic region of different isolates: V720I (1/30), T912N (1/30), P94S (3/30), Q822H (1/30), D824Y (1/30), P227L (1/30), and N158H (2/30) (Supplementary Table S1). Similarly, genomic analysis of Omicron VOC isolates showed three uncommon aa changes in BA.1, BA.1.1, and BA.1.1.1 sub-lineages: L749M (1/37), M110V (1/37), and Q875R (2/37), respectively (Supplementary Table S2).

3.3.4. Spike Protein

In the S glycoprotein of non-Omicron isolates, we found 12 unusual mutations, which were related to both B.1.258 and B.1.177 variants. The N603D, G257V, and T859I were detected only in single isolates. Six unusual mutations were observed in Alpha isolates, including D1153Y (1/30), G1124V (1/30), G946V (1/30), and the unique D1165A substitution. Furthermore, a total of 21 unusual mutations were observed in Gamma and Delta isolates, among which L5F, Y145H, and V1104L (each one present in 1/30) and G142D (carried by 2/20 isolates) (Supplementary Table S1).

A higher number of aa substitutions was observed in Omicron isolates, including 19 unusual mutations such as Q173K (1/37), T859I (1/37), L1265F (2/37), A701V (1/37), P809S (1/37), and L5F (1/37) already present in the Delta VOC. One isolate (BA.1) carried the Δ641–642 deletion and F643I substitution. One isolate (BA.1.15) showed the T73I plus P1162S change, while the three isolates belonging to BA.2 sub-lineage carried the T19I, L24S, Δ25–27, G142D, V213G, S371F, T376A, D405N, and R408S mutations (Supplementary Table S2).

3.3.5. Nucleocapsid Protein

The analysis of the N protein of non-Omicron isolates showed the presence of 12 unusual mutations among the non-Omicron VOC isolates, of which the S250F substitution deserves special attention. Eleven Alpha isolates carried the double amino acid change R203K and G204R plus S235F in 6/9 isolates. One Delta isolate showed both the S327L and W330L substitutions. Other observed mutations were S180I and M234I, detected in two and one B.1.258 isolates, respectively. The A220V was carried by seven B.1.177 variant isolates and by one Alpha. The R32H was detected in one Delta. The L139F (2/30) and D3L (8/30) were detected in Alpha isolates (Supplementary Table S1).

Among non-Omicron VOCs, two subjects who were SARS-CoV-2 positive by real-time RT-PCR (median Ct: 24) had tested negative by the first-line rapid antigen test used for the screening, targeting the N protein: one of them (AM-0607 isolate, belonging to B.1.258) displayed the S180I substitution, while the other (AM-0143 isolate, belonging to Alpha VOC) carried the A220V substitution.

Among Omicron isolates, the BA.1.1 sub-lineage showed uncommon mutations, such as K38I and T334A. Both BA.1.15 isolates carried the amino acid substitution D343G, while all BA.2 isolates showed the mutation S413R (Supplementary Table S2). In five cases, the SARS-CoV-2 isolates AM-0074, AM-0080, AM-0258, AM-0953, and AM-1185 were detected by real-time RT-PCR but not by rapid antigen testing. The median Ct values were 32, 31, 29, 15, and 23, respectively.

3.4. Phylogenetic and Clustering Analyses

The phylogenetic relationship of SARS-CoV-2 circulating strains within the military airport was performed by molecular analysis of the sequences aligned to Wuhan Hu-1 and to several VOC reference sequences, to designate clades and lineages (Figure 5).

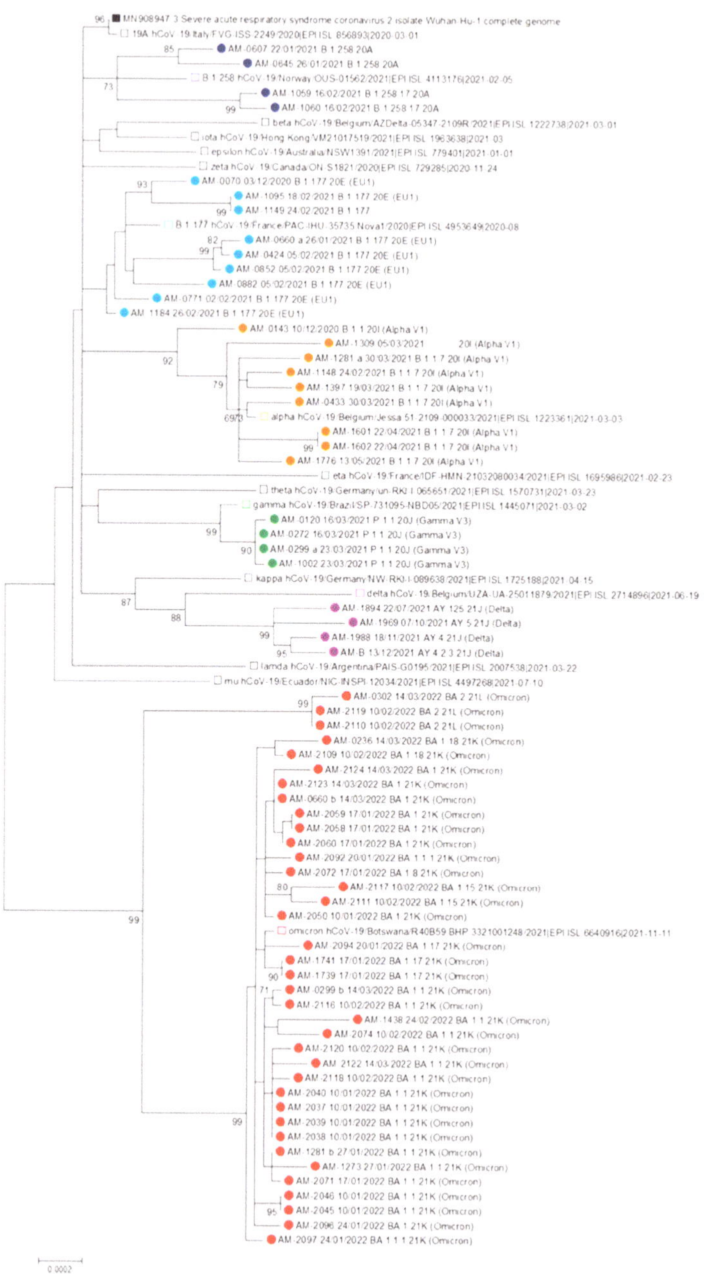

Figure 5. ML phylogenetic tree was estimated using 17 reference sequences and 67 SARS-CoV-2 newly generated sequences. The reliability of the phylogenetic clustering was evaluated using bootstrap analysis with 1000 replicates. The bootstrap support values > 70% are shown. The scale bar at the bottom of the figure represents genetic distance. The colors identify the several clusters of SARS-CoV-2 variants. The circles show the newly generated sequences, while the squares the reference sequences.

In our samples, we identified seven clades according to specific time span: clade 20E (12.1%) between December 2020–February 2021; clade 20I (13.6%) December 2020–March 2021; clade 20A (6.1%) between January–February 2021; clade 20J (6.1%) in March 2021; clade 21J (6.1%) between July–December 2021; clade 21K (51.5%) between January–March 2022; finally, clade 21L (4.5%) between January–February 2022. One viral strain, classified as B.1.177 by Pango lineage, was unclassified by Nextstrain nomenclature. The clades 21K and 21L, related to Omicron VOC, represented most of the sequences (56.0%) included in the phylogenetic tree, according to their high prevalence in 2022. Additionally, the ML phylogenetic tree showed the presence of six clusters: B.1.258 and sub-lineages, B.1.177, Alpha (B.1.1.7) and sub-lineages, Gamma (P.1.1), Delta (AY) and sub-lineages, Omicron (BA.1) and sub-lineages (Figure 5).

Interestingly, the viral strains from the married couple AM-1149 and AM-1184 (light blue dots) did not cluster with a significant bootstrap support. The B.1.177 isolates displayed different aa substitution on nsp2, PLpro, nsp7, nsp8, nsp13, and nsp15 regions (Supplementary Table S1). On the contrary, the viral strains isolated from the married couple AM-0607 and AM-0645 (dark blue dots) clustered with a good bootstrap value (bootstrap = 85). Both these B.1.258 isolates carried the same substitutions on whole genome, except for mutations I1192T on PLpro protein and N603D on S protein (Supplementary Table S1).

During the pandemic wave from January to March 2022, three subjects previously infected by B.1.177 (light blue dot: AM-0660a), Alpha (orange dot: AM-1281a), and Gamma (dark green dot: AM-0299a) acquired reinfection by Omicron or its sub-lineages (red dots: AM-0660b, AM-1281b and AM-0299b, respectively) (Figure 5).

3.5. Sanger Sequencing of Partial Spike Coding Region

The results obtained by sequencing the long amplicon of the spike protein are presented in Table 2. Fifty-seven partial sequences of the spike coding region yielded comparable results to whole genome sequencing. Specifically, in 2020, clade 20E (EU1) was detected in one sample, while in 2021, clades 20A, 20E, 20I (Alpha), and 20J (Gamma) were found in 19 samples. In 2022, all 37 samples belonged to the Omicron variant (clade 21K: BA.1, BA.1.1, BA.2).

Table 2. Variant and clade classification using Sanger sequencing of the spike region.

Sampling Period		ID Sample	Variant/Clade
2020	3 December	AM-70	20E (EU1)
	22 January	AM-607	20A
	26 January	AM-660	20E (EU1)
	02 February	AM-771	20E (EU1)
	05 February	AM-424	20E (EU1)
	09 February	AM-882	20E (EU1)
	16 February	AM-1059	20A
	16 February	AM-1060	20A
	18 February	AM-1095	20E (EU1)
	24 February	AM-1148	20I (Alpha, V1)
2021	26 February	AM-1184	20E (EU1)
	05 March	AM-1309	20I (Alpha, V1)
	16 March	AM-272	20J (Gamma, V3)
	19 March	AM-1397	20I (Alpha, V1)
	23 March	AM-299	20J (Gamma, V3)
	30 March	AM-433	20I (Alpha, V1)
	30 March	AM-1281	20I (Alpha, V1)
	22 April	AM-1601	20I (Alpha, V1)
	22 April	AM-1602	20I (Alpha, V1)
	13 December	AM-B	21J (Delta)

Table 2. *Cont.*

Sampling Period		ID Sample	Variant/Clade
	10 January	AM-2037	Omicron BA.1.1
	10 January	AM-2038	Omicron BA.1.1
	10 January	AM-2039	Omicron BA.1.1
	10 January	AM-2040	Omicron BA.1.1
	10 January	AM-2045	Omicron BA.1.1
	10 January	AM-2046	Omicron BA.1.1
	10 January	AM-2050	Omicron BA.1
	17 January	AM-1739	Omicron BA.1
	17 January	AM-1741	Omicron BA.1
	17 January	AM-2058	Omicron BA.1
	17 January	AM-2059	Omicron BA.1
	17 January	AM-2060	Omicron BA.1
	17 January	AM-2071	Omicron BA.1.1
	17 January	AM-2072	Omicron BA.1
	20 January	AM-2092	Omicron
	20 January	AM-2094	Omicron
	24 January	AM-2096	Omicron
	24 January	AM-2097	Omicron
2022	27 January	AM-1273	Omicron
	27 January	AM-1281	Omicron
	10 February	AM-2074	Omicron
	10 February	AM-2109	Omicron
	10 February	AM-2110	Omicron
	10 February	AM-2111	Omicron
	10 February	AM-2116	Omicron
	10 February	AM-2117	Omicron
	10 February	AM-2118	Omicron
	10 February	AM-2119	Omicron
	10 February	AM-2120	Omicron
	24 February	AM-1438	Omicron
	14 March	AM-0236	Omicron
	14 March	AM-0299/B	Omicron
	14 March	AM-0302	Omicron
	14 March	AM-0660	Omicron
	14 March	AM-2122	Omicron
	14 March	AM-2123	Omicron
	14 March	AM-2124	Omicron

4. Discussion

Rapid identification and characterization of emerging variants can inform public health strategies, such as implementing targeted interventions and adapting vaccination efforts to address the changing viral epidemiology [5,6]. The present study aimed to comprehensively investigate the characteristics of SARS-CoV-2 variants circulating among military and civilian personnel at an Air Force airport in Italy during three pandemic waves, spanning from November 2020 to March 2022. Military bases may be a hotspot for virus transmission and monitoring outbreaks is important to prevent spread to the general population. By analyzing a set of viral samples collected from the study population, we employed NGS and Sanger sequencing techniques to identify and to analyze various SARS-CoV-2 variants.

The results of the sequencing analysis revealed the presence of multiple SARS-CoV-2 variants circulating within the study population. Among several variants, the B.1.1.7 (Alpha, 9/67), the P.1 (Gamma, 4/67), and the B.1.617.2 (Delta, 4/67) VOCs were identified in 2020 and 2021. All these VOCs were previously characterized by the reduced susceptibility (potential immune escape) to antibodies generated during natural infection or after vaccination, as well as to mAbs therapies [9]. Additionally, each new VOC increased its transmissibility compared to the previous one, enhancing the number of new cases in the epidemiological landscape [9]. In December 2020, we detected B.1.177 (20E) and the B.1.1. B.1.258, B1.1.177, and Alpha were observed from January to February 2021. Between February and May 2021, Alpha was the major prevalent VOC in this community. In March 2021, we revealed the co-circulation of Alpha and Gamma VOCs. Delta VOC was detected from July 2021 to the end of the year. In 2022, only the Omicron (37/67) VOC, with its subvariants BA.1 (8/37), BA.1.1 (16/37), BA.1.1.1 (2/37), BA.1.15 (2/37), BA.1.17 (3/37), BA.1.18 (2/37), BA.1.8 (1/37), and BA.2 (3/37), were detected. Notably, BA.1 and BA.1.1 sub-lineages co-circulated during the first three months of 2022. Overall, this data agrees with the global epidemiology of SARS-CoV-2, since Omicron and its sub-lineages are extremely transmissible with a high infectivity rate, spreading much quicker than any other VOCs [9]. In the same time span, the Ministry of Health reduced public health restrictions in Italy, according to WHO guidelines [48]. Comparing our results with the overall Italian epidemiology, the appearance of VOCs and VOIs showed a similar trend at the military airport, suggesting that this community reflects the general population [12,49,50].

The genomic analysis of the 67 isolates highlighted a high number of aa changes in different regions of whole genomes. Starting from non-Omicron isolates, two major mutations characterize 3CLpro protein: G15S (2/30) and L232F (1/30). G15S was one of the most frequently identified missense mutations associated with 3cLpro inhibitor resistance, conferring reduced susceptibility to nirmatrelvir and ensitrelvir activity [21]. This mutation was fixed in some lineages, present in almost all strains in the lineages B.1.1.1, B.1.1.369, B.1.1.372, B.1.1.375, and lineage C, including the Lambda VOI [21]. Eighteen mutations were observed in the RdRp protein of non-Omicron VOC isolates. Some of the substitutions in nsp12 (polymerase) predict positive or negative functional effects. For example, Q822H predicts increased stability of the loop in the thumb domain [51]. The mutation at P227L influenced the tertiary Structure of nsp12, decreasing molecular flexibility on the protein structure. This substitution modifies the side chain, resulting in the alteration of intramolecular bonds in the pocket, which could lead to instability in co-factor binding (nsp7 and nsp8), ultimately modifying the proofreading complex and losing the structural integrity provided by proline [52]. Interestingly, the P323L substitution, emerging together with D614G, was found in all non-Omicron and Omicron new isolates. Very recently, structural analysis of P323L, G671S, and F694Y mutational patterns showed susceptibility to remdesivir, supporting the continued clinical use of this drug [53]. In the S glycoprotein of non-Omicron isolates, we found 12 unusual mutations, which were related to both B.1.258 and B.1.177 variants. Among these, the ΔH69–V70 deletion, observed in ten isolates, has been associated with increased infectivity and decreased susceptibility to neutralizing antibodies [54,55]. Furthermore, it has been identified in variants associated with immune escape in immunocompromised individuals treated with convalescent plasma [56]. Different changes were found in the function of the S protein. The T1117I substitution (AM-1059, AM-1060) determined a more stable interaction with a ligand (nelfinavir drug), but no differences with other genomes on transmissibility, severity, immune response, nor vaccine effectiveness were predicted [57,58]. Two isolates (AM-0424, AM-0882) carried the A262S mutation, which has demonstrated a slight increase of infectivity and decreased reactivities to mAb [59]. The P272L mutation carried by AM-0771, AM-0424, AM-0852, and AM-0882 allows evasion of T-cell responses in convalescent patients, and escape recognition by killer T-cells in vaccinated individuals [60,61]. Six unusual mutations were observed in Alpha isolates, including G1124V mutation, that appears to reduce epitope binding affinity of Human Leukocyte Antigen (HLA) alleles to a level that some are no longer able to bind, leading to virus escape from immune recognition [62]. Additionally, a total of 21 unusual mutations were observed in Gamma and Delta isolates, among which were L5F (AM-1988), L18F (AM-1059, AM-1060), and H655Y (AM-0272, AM-0299_a, AM-1002, AM-0120). The L5F mutation is in sites recognized by HLA, and it is seen to increase the epitope binding affinity for different HLA alleles [63]. Thus, the L5F is disadvantageous for the SARS-CoV-2 virus because the mutated epitope could enhance CD8 T cell recognition and killing through this improved interaction [63]. Additionally, it was the only unusual substitution to appear in BA.2 and BA.5 sub-lineages among 272 positive samples isolated in Southern Italy [64]. The L18F substitution is of significance because it has been found to compromise binding of neutralizing antibodies, allowing a much faster propagation in the presence of plasma antibodies collected from donors infected in the previous wave of the epidemic [65]. H655Y is responsible for alteration of entry properties and fusogenicity, using the preferential entry pathway without affecting the S cleavage status, and leading to modulations of tissue and cell tropism, and reduced pathogenicity [66]. V1176F (AM-0299a, AM-1002, AM-0120) is a recurrent S substitution that is frequently acquired by SARS-CoV-2 variants to increase viral fitness, improving interaction with heptad repeat 1 and enhance virus entry [67]. Three significant mutations in RBD (K417T/N, E484K and N501Y) are responsible for the escape from neutralizing mAbs and they could escape from both vaccine-induced sera and natural sera [68]. In particular, the glutamate to lysine substitution at position 484 (E484K) in the RBD of the spike protein is a single point mutation that affects binding by neutralizing antibodies, reducing the neutralizing activity of human polyclonal sera and thereby potentially rendering vaccine-induced immunity less protective [69]. The N501Y substitution also improved the affinity of the viral spike protein for cellular receptors, determining enhanced infection of the upper airway and viral transmission [70]. Other mutations that have been shown to potentially confer resistance to neutralization by mAbs are T20N, only detected in the Gamma P.1 VOC [71], and D138Y, which has higher binding affinity for human ACE2; as such, it could contribute to reduced neutralization by some mAbs, convalescent plasma, and sera from vaccines [72]. The G142D mutation (AM-1988, AM-B) at amino acid position 142 in the NTD of the spike protein was observed at multiple time points and across Delta VOC sub-lineages. This mutation is associated with higher viral load, further enhanced in the presence of another NTD mutation (T95I). The G142D mutation alters the surface topography of the NTD, more specifically, it disturbs the 'super site' epitope that binds NTD-directed neutralizing antibodies (nAbs) [73]. The T95I mutation occurs in the Delta variant and helps increase SARS-CoV-2 virulence [74]. T95I is a replacement of neutral and polar threonine by an acidic polar aspartic acid, enhancing viral load and adaptation by inducing the transition of a β-strand to an α-helix [74]. The same three isolates that showed the T95I mutation (AM-1894, AM-1988, AM-B) also carried three other amino acid changes: T19R, E156G/Δ157–158. T19R mutation was detected in the N terminal domain of the S protein and this mutation is plausible for increased infectivity, elevated transmissibility, and reduced sensitivity to anti-NTD neutralizing antibodies [75]. The NTD-specific E156G/Δ157–158 are, respectively, a change of glutamic acid to glycine at position 156 and a loss of two amino acids at positions 157 and 158. These mutations conferred an infectivity advantage, allowed immune escape, and reduced sensitivity to vaccine-induced antibodies [76]. Three isolates (AM-1988, AM-B, AM-1969) possessed two unique amino acid substitutions in their spike protein: S-P681R and S-D950N. P681R plays a key role in the Alpha-to-Delta variant replacement. This mutation is located at a furin cleavage site that separates the spike 1 (S1) and S2 subunits and it enhances the cleavage of the full-length spike to S1 and S2, which could improve cell-surface-mediated virus entry, increasing Delta-variant replication [77]. The D950N is a missense mutation that slightly promoted membrane fusion. It is located in the heptad repeat 1 (HR1) of the S2 subunit and is essential for the conformational change for virus fusogenicity [78]. A sub-lineage of the Delta variant, AY.4.2, exhibits distinguishing spike mutations Y145H (AM-B isolate) and A222V (found in nine isolates) that lie within the NTD of the spike. Through modelling, the Y145H substitution seems to decrease spike stability, but this has not been experimentally demonstrated [79].

On the other hand, a higher number of aa substitutions was observed in Omicron isolates, including 19 mutations such as Q173K (AM-0299_b) and A701V (AM-2094) already present in the Delta VOC. The Q173K resides within the N-terminal S1A that exhibits low conservation, which helps SARS-CoV-2 adapt to host cells and host immunity. This domain is bound very tightly by antibodies isolated from COVID-19 convalescent patients and conversion from a neutral to charged amino acid have the potential to alter interaction for antibody recognition [80]. A701V is near the furin cleavage site and seems to affect viral transmission, raising the affinity of protein interactions by enhancing the spike protein's binding affinity and impacting antibody neutralization [74]. Three isolates belonging to BA.2 sub-lineage (AM-2110, AM-2119, AM-0302) carried the T19I, G142D, S371F, T376A, D405N, and R408S mutations. T19I in NTD spike was found to be significantly associated with Omicron mortality [81]. It caused significant evasion from NTD-targeted neutralizing mAbs [82], as well as R408S mutation that may reduce the efficacy of many antibodies [83]. G142D was located on the N-terminal domain of the spike protein and is involved in host cell attachment through diverse polysaccharide moieties. This mutation is known to be involved in increasing viral pathogenicity, vaccine breakthrough, and showed resistance to the mAbs [84]. S371F, in the ACE2-receptor-binding domain as well as the adjacent BA.2 specific T376A change, is reported to bear a significant fitness cost and impaired S infectivity, whilst also reducing processing efficiency and/or incorporation into viral pseudo particles [85]. The D405N mutation showed a dramatic loss of function by inhibiting spike/integrins interactions and consequently the virus ability to infect human lung microvascular endothelial cells, thus providing protection against virus-induced endothelial cell dysfunction [86].

Analysis of the N protein of non-Omicron isolates showed the presence of 12 unusual mutations among the non-Omicron VOC isolates, of which the A220V mutation, carried by seven B.1.177 variant isolates and one Alpha variant, stabilized the mutated N protein's linker region, affecting RNA binding affinity [87], and L139F (AM-1601, AM-1602) localized in NTD of N protein that is most likely to affect the structure and stability of the N protein [88]. Eleven Alpha isolates also carried the double amino acid change (R203K and G204R plus S235F) in 6/9 isolates. The R203K/G204R are co-occurring mutations in the N protein responsible for the high transmissibility of lineages B.1.1.7 (Alpha) and P.1 (Gamma) due to their conferment of a replication advantage over preceding variants and increase virus fitness and virulence [89]. The S235F was seen to alter virus epitopes, causing changes in the specificity of certain antibodies, and altering vaccine-induced protection [90]. One B.1.258 isolate (AM-1059) showed the M234I mutation located in the link region between the RNA-binding domain and the dimerization domain of the N protein [91]. In particular, the S180I and A220V substitutions detected in two SARS-CoV-2 isolates, did not affect the negative results by the first-line rapid antigen test used for screening, targeting the N protein. Indeed, these substitutions were also carried by several isolates. The performance of this specific antigenic test is related to different features as already reported [27]. Among Omicron isolates, BA.1.1 sub-lineage showed uncommon mutations, such as K38I and T334A, while all BA.2 isolates showed the mutation S413R (serine→arginine) residing in the C-terminal end with no apparent effect on dimerization [92].

As discussed above, several known, unusual, and new mutations were studied by in vitro and/or in silico experiments to better define their function on pathogenicity, transmissibility, and disease severity of SAR-CoV-2 [53,57,66,73]. However, among the new isolates, we identified aa changes with a very low prevalence worldwide, carried on key regions, such as nsp3 (PLpro), nsp5 (3CLpro), nsp12 (RdRp), and ORF8 by non-Omicron and Omicron variants. In particular, we detected A1803V, D1809N, and A949T on PLpro and D216N on 3CLpro and P323L on RdRp Omicron coding regions, which are targets for new antiviral drugs. Very recently, a retrospective study regarding Delta VOC in Italy identified the aa changes with a positive selected pressure along the whole genome in order to evaluate the recurrent mutations for potential implications in the SARS-CoV-2 evolution. Comparing the newly generated sequences, we found several aa substitutions fixed in the viral population, offering a selective advantage: A318V and G339S (nsp2); P1228L (PLpro); L37F (nsp6); P323L (RdRp); P77L (nsp13); R289H (nsp14); L5F, T95I, G142D, N501Y, D614G, P681R, and D950N (S) [93]. In this paper, the G142D, L452R, D614G, P681R, and D950N substitutions (S region) and the P323L (RdRp region) were detected with higher frequency, identifying these substitutions as favoring viral adaptation [93]. In the Omicron era, it is important to monitor each new and known mutation already carried by previous VOCs, potentially involved in treatment, and in viral fitness.

To better characterize the positive cohort, we explored the demographic and referred clinical characteristics of individuals infected with different SARS-CoV-2 variants. The most infected people were male, 75.9% by non-Omicron variants and 62.2% by Omicron and sub-lineages, both group older than 50 years (100.0% versus 78.6%). Male and female subjects were not hospitalized even though 19/67 referred chronic diseases, therefore vaccines were certainly successful in preventing critical illness [94] Several studies have reported a higher risk of mortality or hospitalization in male than female COVID-19 patients [9]. Non-specific symptoms of infection were reported more by people infected with Omicron and its sub-lineages (29/39) than individuals infected (10/39) in previous waves. COVID-19 symptoms and disease severity are directly related to interaction between SARS-CoV-2 variants and the human genome [95]. A total of 34/67 subjects had a previous diagnosis of COVID-19 or SARS-CoV-2 positivity, suggesting a second infection in the non-Omicron (12/67) time span, as well as in the Omicron era (22/67). The ML phylogenetic analysis clearly identified reinfections in people with available sequences during both infections. Three subjects previously infected by B.1.177 (AM-0660a), Alpha (AM-1281a) and Gamma (AM-0299a) acquired reinfection by Omicron or its sub-lineages (AM-0660b, AM-1281b and AM-0299b). Reinfection also occurred in people with two or three doses of vaccine. Alpha and Gamma VOCs manifested relatively mild escape from vaccination, while Omicron VOC showed a decrease in vaccine protection [20].

Phylogenetic analysis identified six clusters, with a bootstrap support >70, according to SARS-CoV-2 variants, such as B.1.258 and sub-lineages, B.1.177, Alpha and sub-lineages, Gamma, Delta and sub-lineages, Omicron and sub-lineages. Among these clusters, viral isolates from the couple AM-1149 and AM-1184 clustered with a low bootstrap support, suggesting two independent routes of transmission. On the other hand, the viral strains isolated from the couple AM-0607 and AM-0645 clustered with a bootstrap value of 85. Even if viral isolates were closely related, one of the two carried the additional I1192T and N603D substitutions on PLpro and S proteins, respectively, highlighting a continuous variability of the virus.

This study has some limitations. Symptoms and previous exposure to infection were noted from a questionnaire. The description and stratification of the cases based on the severity of symptoms was not applied due to the self-reporting of symptoms. Vaccination status was not available for all participants. From May 2021 to March 2022 only positive antigenic tests were confirmed by real-time RT-PCR. Finally, 57/67 samples were characterized using both NGS and Sanger methods due to unavailability of 10 viral RNA.

5. Conclusions

We provided valuable insights into the characteristics of SARS-CoV-2 variants circulating among military and civilian personnel at an Air Force airport as an important hotspot for viral spread. Our results indicated that partial sequencing of the spike coding region could yield comparable outcomes to whole genome sequencing, presenting itself as a rapid and cost-effective approach for identifying variants. In conditions of limited resources or when a result is urgently needed, a sequencing approach targeting a portion of the spike coding region can be used as an alternative to whole genome sequencing. However, while long PCR targeting the S gene may offer a quicker and targeted approach, it may miss important known, new, or unusual mutations in other genomic regions. These mutations could impact the virus spread, such as V1176F and T19R, the potential immune escape (i.e., well known E484K), the antiviral resistance, such as G15S, or the greater viral adaptation (P323L). It is noteworthy that the A1803V, D1809N, A949T, and the D216N substitutions (not yet characterized) were detected in target regions for new antiviral drugs. Finally, screening of the N region revealed the presence of S180I and A220V, which does not result in diagnostic failure by antigenic tests. The study's findings highlight the importance of continuous genomic surveillance to monitor the evolution and spread of SARS-CoV-2 variants in the general population, as well as in restricted communities.

Supplementary Materials: The following supporting information can be downloaded at: https://www.mdpi.com/article/10.3390/microorganisms11112711/s1, Table S1: Major amino acidic changes along the proteins of non-Omicron VOCs isolates; Table S2: Major amino acidic changes along the proteins of Omicron VOC and its sub-lineage isolates.

Author Contributions: Conceptualization, M.E., R.B. and A.R.C.; methodology, M.E., R.B., A.R.C. and G.L.R.; formal analysis, M.E., R.B., C.M., N.M., F.C., G.L.R. and A.R.C.; investigation, M.E., C.M., A.M., M.S., G.B.F., P.M., C.V., E.S. (Elisabetta Suffredini), A.C., S.T., E.T. and C.C.; resources, A.R.C. and G.L.R.; data curation, M.E., C.M., R.B. and G.L.R.; writing—original draft preparation, N.M. and F.C.; writing—review and editing, R.B., A.R.C., M.E., E.S. (Enea Spada), P.V., R.N., G.P., G.M. and A.Q.; visualization, N.M., F.C. and R.B.; supervision, M.E., R.B., A.R.C., N.M. and G.L.R.; project administration, A.R.C.; funding acquisition, A.R.C. All authors have read and agreed to the published version of the manuscript.

Funding: The study was supported in part by institutional funds of the Istituto Superiore di Sanità and in part by Project N°7S06 by the Italian Ministry of Health.

Data Availability Statement: All sequences can be retrieved from GenBank under accession numbers: OR761892–OR761958.

Acknowledgments: The authors would like to thank Neill J. Adams for his valuable scientific and language editing of the manuscript.

Conflicts of Interest: The authors declare no conflict of interest.

References

1. Fabiani, M.; Ramigni, M.; Gobbetto, V.; Mateo-Urdiales, A.; Pezzotti, P.; Piovesan, C. Effectiveness of the Comirnaty (BNT162b2, BioNTech/Pfizer) vaccine in preventing SARS-CoV-2 infection among healthcare workers, Treviso province, Veneto region, Italy, 27 December 2020 to 24 March 2021. *Euro Surveill.* **2021**, *26*, 2100420. [CrossRef]
2. Oliani, F.; Savoia, A.; Gallo, G.; Tiwana, N.; Letzgus, M.; Gentiloni, F.; Piatti, A.; Chiappa, L.; Bisceti, A.; Laquintana, D.; et al. Italy's rollout of COVID-19 vaccinations: The crucial contribution of the first experimental mass vaccination site in Lombardy. *Vaccine* **2022**, *40*, 1397–1403. [CrossRef] [PubMed]
3. Dhanasooraj, D.; Viswanathan, P.; Saphia, S.; Jose, B.P.; Parambath, F.C.; Sivadas, S.; Akash, N.P.; Vlmisha, T.V.; Nair, P.R.; Mohan, A.; et al. Genomic surveillance of SARS-CoV-2 by sequencing the RBD region using Sanger sequencing from North Kerala. *Front. Public Health* **2022**, *10*, 974667. [CrossRef]
4. Guthrie, J.L.; Teatero, S.; Zittermann, S.; Chen, Y.; Sullivan, A.; Rilkoff, H.; Joshi, E.; Sivaraman, K.; de Borja, R.; Sundaravadanam, Y.; et al. Detection of the novel SARS-CoV-2 European lineage B.1.177 in Ontario, Canada. *J. Clin. Virol. Plus* **2021**, *1*, 100010. [CrossRef] [PubMed]
5. European Centre for Disease Prevention and Control ECDC. Available online: https://www.ecdc.europa.eu/en (accessed on 11 September 2023).
6. World Health Organization Tracking SARS-CoV-2 Variants. Available online: https://www.who.int/activities/tracking-SARS-CoV-2-variants (accessed on 11 September 2023).
7. De Marco, C.; Veneziano, C.; Massacci, A.; Pallocca, M.; Marascio, N.; Quirino, A.; Barreca, G.S.; Giancotti, A.; Gallo, L.; Lamberti, A.G.; et al. Dynamics of Viral Infection and Evolution of SARS-CoV-2 Variants in the Calabria Area of Southern Italy. *Front. Microbiol.* **2022**, *13*, 934993. [CrossRef] [PubMed]
8. Chrysostomou, A.C.; Vrancken, B.; Haralambous, C.; Alexandrou, M.; Aristokleous, A.; Christodoulou, C.; Gregoriou, I.; Ioannides, M.; Kalakouta, O.; Karagiannis, C.; et al. Genomic Epidemiology of the SARS-CoV-2 Epidemic in Cyprus from November 2020 to October 2021: The Passage of Waves of Alpha and Delta Variants of Concern. *Viruses* **2023**, *15*, 108. [CrossRef]
9. Hoteit, R.; Yassine, H.M. Biological Properties of SARS-CoV-2 Variants: Epidemiological Impact and Clinical Consequences. *Vaccines* **2022**, *10*, 919. [CrossRef] [PubMed]
10. Zhao, H.; Nguyen, A.; Wu, D.; Li, Y.; Hassan, S.A.; Chen, J.; Shroff, H.; Piszczek, G.; Schuck, P. Plasticity in structure and assembly of SARS-CoV-2 nucleocapsid protein. *PNAS Nexus* **2022**, *1*, pgac049. [CrossRef]
11. Alkhatib, M.; Bellocchi, M.C.; Marchegiani, G.; Grelli, S.; Micheli, V.; Stella, D.; Zerillo, B.; Carioti, L.; Svicher, V.; Rogliani, P.; et al. First Case of a COVID-19 Patient Infected by Delta AY.4 with a Rare Deletion Leading to a N Gene Target Failure by a Specific Real Time PCR Assay: Novel Omicron VOC Might Be Doing Similar Scenario? *Microorganisms* **2022**, *10*, 268. [CrossRef]
12. Stefanelli, P.; Trentini, F.; Guzzetta, G.; Marziano, V.; Mammone, A.; Sane Schepisi, M.; Poletti, P.; Molina Grané, C.; Manica, M.; Del Manso, M.; et al. Co-circulation of SARS-CoV-2 Alpha and Gamma variants in Italy, February and March 2021. *Euro Surveill.* **2022**, *27*, 2100429. [CrossRef]

13. Monitoraggio delle Varianti del Virus SARS-CoV-2 di Interesse in Sanità Pubblica in Italia. Available online: https://www.epicentro.iss.it/coronavirus/sars-cov-2-monitoraggio-varianti-rapporti-periodici (accessed on 11 September 2023).

14. Luo, C.H.; Morris, C.P.; Sachithanandham, J.; Amadi, A.; Gaston, D.C.; Li, M.; Swanson, N.J.; Schwartz, M.; Klein, E.Y.; Pekosz, A.; et al. Infection with the Severe Acute Respiratory Syndrome Coronavirus 2 (SARS-CoV-2) Delta Variant Is Associated with Higher Recovery of Infectious Virus Compared to the Alpha Variant in Both Unvaccinated and Vaccinated Individuals. *Clin. Infect. Dis.* **2022**, *75*, e715–e725. [CrossRef] [PubMed]

15. La Rosa, G.; Iaconelli, M.; Veneri, C.; Mancini, P.; Bonanno Ferraro, G.; Brandtner, D.; Lucentini, L.; Bonadonna, L.; Rossi, M.; Grigioni, M.; et al. The rapid spread of SARS-COV-2 Omicron variant in Italy reflected early through wastewater surveillance. *Sci. Total Environ.* **2022**, *837*, 155767. [CrossRef] [PubMed]

16. Harris, E. CDC Assesses Risk From BA.2.86, Highly Mutated COVID-19 Variant. *JAMA*, 2023; *epub ahead of print*. [CrossRef]

17. Mohapatra, R.K.; Mishra, S.; Kandi, V.; Branda, F.; Ansari, A.; Rabaan, A.A.; Kudrat-E-Zahan, M. Analyzing the emerging patterns of SARS-CoV-2 Omicron subvariants for the development of next-gen vaccine: An observational study. *Health Sci. Rep.* **2023**, *6*, e1596. [CrossRef] [PubMed]

18. Stanford Coronavirus Resistance Database CoV-RDB. Available online: https://covdb.stanford.edu (accessed on 20 June 2023).

19. Bloom, J.D.; Neher, R.A. Fitness effects of mutations to SARS-CoV-2 proteins. *Virus Evol.* **2023**, *9*, vead055. [CrossRef]

20. Sun, C.; Xie, C.; Bu, G.L.; Zhong, L.Y.; Zeng, M.S. Molecular characteristics, immune evasion, and impact of SARS-CoV-2 variants. *Signal Transduct. Target. Ther.* **2022**, *7*, 202. [CrossRef]

21. Ip, J.D.; Wing-Ho Chu, A.; Chan, W.M.; Cheuk-Ying Leung, R.; Umer Abdullah, S.M.; Sun, Y.; Kai-Wang To, K. Global prevalence of SARS-CoV-2 3CL protease mutations associated with nirmatrelvir or ensitrelvir resistance. *EBioMedicine* **2023**, *91*, 104559. [CrossRef]

22. Andrews, H.S.; Herman, J.D.; Gandhi, R.T. Treatments for COVID-19. *Annu. Rev. Med.* **2023**, *75*, 25. [CrossRef]

23. de Oliveira, V.M.; Ibrahim, M.F.; Sun, X.; Hilgenfeld, R.; Shen, J. H172Y mutation perturbs the S1 pocket and nirmatrelvir binding of SARS- CoV-2 main protease through a non native hydrogen bond. *bioRxiv* **2022**. [CrossRef]

24. Scaglione, V.; Rotundo, S.; Marascio, N.; De Marco, C.; Lionello, R.; Veneziano, C.; Berardelli, L.; Quirino, A.; Olivadese, V.; Serapide, F.; et al. Lessons learned and implications of early therapies for coronavirus disease in a territorial service centre in the Calabria region: A retrospective study. *BMC Infect. Dis.* **2022**, *22*, 793. [CrossRef]

25. Malagón Rojas, J.N.; Mercado, M.; Gómez Rendón, C.P. SARS-CoV-2 and work-related transmission: Results of a prospective cohort of airport workers, 2020. *Rev. Bras. Med. Trab.* **2020**, *18*, 371–380. [CrossRef] [PubMed]

26. De Marco, C.; Marascio, N.; Veneziano, C.; Biamonte, F.; Trecarichi, E.M.; Santamaria, G.; Leviyang, S.; Liberto, M.C.; Mazzitelli, M.; Quirino, A.; et al. Whole-genome analysis of SARS-CoV-2 in a 2020 infection cluster in a nursing home of Southern Italy. *Infect. Genet. Evol.* **2022**, *99*, 105253. [CrossRef] [PubMed]

27. Verde, P.; Marcantonio, C.; Costantino, A.; Martina, A.; Simeoni, M.; Taffon, S.; Tritarelli, E.; Campanella, C.; Cresta, R.; Bruni, R.; et al. Diagnostic accuracy of a SARS-CoV-2 rapid antigen test among military and civilian personnel of an Air Force airport in central Italy. *PLoS ONE* **2022**, *17*, e0277904. [CrossRef]

28. European Regulation (UE) 2016/679. Available online: https://eur-lex.europa.eu/eli/reg/2016/679/oj (accessed on 2 May 2022).

29. Italian Decree n. 196 of 2003. Available online: https://web.camera.it/parlam/leggi/deleghe/Testi/03196dl.htm (accessed on 2 May 2022).

30. Italian Decree n. 101 of 2018. Available online: https://www.gazzettaufficiale.it/eli/id/2018/09/04/18G00129/sg (accessed on 2 May 2022).

31. Ministry of Health Note n. 31400 of 29 September 2020. Available online: https://www.trovanorme.salute.gov.it/norme/renderNormsanPdf?anno=2020&codLeg=76433&parte=1%20&serie=null (accessed on 2 May 2022).

32. Ministry of Health Note n. 35324 of 30 October 2020. Available online: https://www.trovanorme.salute.gov.it/norme/renderNormsanPdf?anno=2020&codLeg=76939&parte=1%20&serie=null (accessed on 2 May 2022).

33. Ministry of Health Note n. 705 of 8 January 2021. Available online: https://www.trovanorme.salute.gov.it/norme/renderNormsanPdf?anno=2021&codLeg=78155&parte=1%20&serie=null (accessed on 2 May 2022).

34. ARTIC Network. Real-Time Molecular Epidemiology for Outbreak Response. Available online: https://artic.network/ncov-2019 (accessed on 2 April 2022).

35. Carpenter, R.E.; Tamrakar, V.K.; Almas, S.; Sharma, A.; Sharma, R. SARS-CoV-2 Next Generation Sequencing (NGS) data from clinical isolates from the East Texas Region of the United States. *Data Brief* **2023**, *49*, 109312. [CrossRef]

36. Pangolin COVID-19 Lineage Assigner. Available online: https://pangolin.cog-uk.io (accessed on 5 June 2023).

37. Nextclade v2.12.0. Available online: https://clades.nextstrain.org/ (accessed on 6 June 2023).

38. La Rosa, G.; Mancini, P.; Bonanno Ferraro, G.; Veneri, C.; Iaconelli, M.; Lucentini, L.; Bonadonna, L.; Brusaferro, S.; Brandtner, D.; Fasanella, A.; et al. Rapid screening for SARS-CoV-2 variants of concern in clinical and environmental samples using nested RT-PCR assays targeting key mutations of the spike protein. *Water Res.* **2021**, *197*, 11714. [CrossRef]

39. La Rosa, G.; Brandtner, D.; Mancini, P.; Veneri, C.; Bonanno Ferraro, G.; Bonadonna, L.; Lucentini, L.; Suffredini, E. Key SARS-CoV-2 Mutations of Alpha, Gamma, and Eta Variants Detected in Urban Wastewaters in Italy by Long-Read Amplicon Sequencing Based on Nanopore Technology. *Water* **2021**, *13*, 2503. [CrossRef]

40. La Rosa, G.; Brandtner, D.; Bonanno Ferraro, G.; Veneri, C.; Mancini, P.; Iaconelli, M.; Lucentini, L.; Del Giudice, C.; Orlandi, L.; SARI Network; et al. Wastewater surveillance of SARS-CoV-2 variants in October-November 2022 in Italy: Detection of XBB.1, BA.2.75 and rapid spread of the BQ.1 lineage. *Sci. Total Environ.* **2023**, *873*, 162339. [CrossRef] [PubMed]

41. MEGA Software. Available online: https://www.megasoftware.net/ (accessed on 14 June 2023).

42. Tamura, K.; Stecher, G.; Kumar, S. MEGA 11: Molecular Evolutionary Genetics Analysis Version 11. *Mol. Biol. Evol.* **2021**, *38*, 3022–3027. [CrossRef]

43. GISAID-CoVsurver Mutations App. Available online: https://www.gisaid.org/epiflu-applications/covsurver-mutations-app/ (accessed on 15 June 2023).

44. Benson, D.A.; Clark, K.; Karsch-Mizrachi, I.; Lipman, D.J.; Ostell, J.; Sayers, E.W. GenBank. *Nucleic Acids Res.* **2014**, *42*, 32–37. [CrossRef] [PubMed]

45. Thompson, J.D.; Higgins, D.G.; Gibson, T.J. CLUSTAL W: Improving the sensitivity of progressive multiple sequence alignment through sequence weighting, position-specific gap penalties and weight matrix choice. *Nucleic Acids Res.* **1994**, *22*, 4673–4680. [CrossRef] [PubMed]

46. Hall, T.A. BioEdit: A User-Friendly Biological Sequence Alignment Editor and Analysis Program for Windows 95/98/NT. *Nucleic Acids Symp. Ser.* **1999**, *41*, 95–98.

47. Marascio, N.; Cilburunoglu, M.; Torun, E.G.; Centofanti, F.; Mataj, E.; Equestre, M.; Bruni, R.; Quirino, A.; Matera, G.; Ciccaglione, A.R.; et al. Molecular Characterization and Cluster Analysis of SARS-CoV-2 Viral Isolates in Kahramanmaraş City, Turkey: The Delta VOC Wave within One Month. *Viruses* **2023**, *15*, 802. [CrossRef] [PubMed]

48. World Health Organization (WHO). Available online: https://www.who.int/ (accessed on 6 September 2023).

49. Bellocchi, M.C.; Scutari, R.; Carioti, L.; Iannetta, M.; Marchegiani, G.; Piermatteo, L.; Coppola, L.; Tedde, S.; Duca, L.; Malagnino, V.; et al. Frequency of Atypical Mutations in the Spike Glycoprotein in SARS-CoV-2 Circulating from July 2020 to July 2022 in Central Italy: A Refined Analysis by Next Generation Sequencing. *Viruses* **2023**, *15*, 1711. [CrossRef]

50. Dolci, M.; Signorini, L.; Cason, C.; Campisciano, G.; Kunderfranco, P.; Pariani, E.; Galli, C.; Petix, V.; Ferrante, P.; Delbue, S.; et al. Circulation of SARS-CoV-2 Variants among Children from November 2020 to January 2022 in Trieste (Italy). *Microorganisms* **2022**, *10*, 612. [CrossRef] [PubMed]

51. Martínez González, B.; Soria, M.E.; Vázquez Sirvent, L.; Ferrer Orta, C.; Lobo Vega, R.; Mínguez, P.; de la Fuente, L.; Llorens, C.; Soriano, B.; Ramos, R.; et al. SARS-CoV-2 Point Mutation and Deletion Spectra and Their Association with Different Disease Outcomes. *Microbiol. Spectr.* **2022**, *10*, e0022122. [CrossRef] [PubMed]

52. Mazhari, S.; Alavifard, H.; Rahimian, K.; Karimi, Z.; Mahmanzar, M.; Sisakht, M.M.; Bitaraf, M.; Arefian, E. SARS-CoV-2 NSP-12 mutations survey during the pandemic in the world. *Res. Sq.* **2021**, *preprint*. [CrossRef]

53. Pitts, J.; Li, J.; Perry, J.K.; Du Pont, V.; Riola, N.; Rodriguez, L.; Lu, X.; Kurhade, C.; Xie, X.; Camus, G.; et al. Remdesivir and GS-441524 Retain Antiviral Activity against Delta, Omicron, and Other Emergent SARS-CoV-2 Variants. *Antimicrob. Agents Chemother.* **2022**, *66*, e0022222. [CrossRef]

54. Harvey, W.T.; Carabelli, A.M.; Jackson, B.; Gupta, R.K.; Thomson, E.C.; Harrison, E.M.; Ludden, C.; Reeve, R.; Rambaut, A.; COVID-19 Genomics UK (COG-UK) Consortium; et al. SARS-CoV-2 variants, spike mutations and immune escape. *Nat. Rev. Microbiol.* **2021**, *19*, 409–424. [CrossRef] [PubMed]

55. Kemp, S.A.; Harvey, W.T.; Datir, R.P.; Collier, D.A.; Ferreira, I.A.; Carabelli, A.M.; Gupta, R.K.; Meng, B. Recurrent emergence and transmission of a SARS-CoV-2 spike deletion ΔH69/V70. *bioRxiv* **2020**, preprint. [CrossRef]

56. Mlcochova, P.; Kemp, S.A.; Dhar, M.S.; Papa, G.; Meng, B.; Ferreira, I.A.T.M.; Datir, R.; Collier, D.A.; Albecka, A.; Singh, S.; et al. SARS-CoV-2 B.1.617.2 Delta variant replication and immune evasion. *Nature* **2021**, *599*, 114–119. [CrossRef]

57. Molina Mora, J.A.; Cordero Laurent, E.; Godinez, A.; Calderon Osorno, M.; Brenes, H.; Soto Garita, C.; Perez Corrales, C.; COINGESA-CR Consorcio Interinstitucional de Estudios Genomicos del SARS-CoV-2 Costa Rica; Drexler, J.F.; Moreira Soto, A.; et al. SARS-CoV-2 Genomic Surveillance in Costa Rica: Evidence of a Divergent Population and an Increased Detection of a Spike T1117I Mutation. *Infect. Genet. Evol.* **2021**, *92*, 104872. [CrossRef]

58. Molina Mora, J.A. Insights into the mutation T1117I in the spike and the lineage B.1.1.389 of SARS-CoV-2 circulating in Costa Rica. *Gene Rep.* **2022**, *27*, 101554. [CrossRef]

59. Zhang, L.; Li, Q.; Nie, J.; Ding, R.; Wang, H.; Wu, J.; Li, X.; Yang, X.; Huang, W.; Wang, Y. Cellular tropism and antigenicity of mink-derived SARS-CoV-2 variants. *Signal Transduct. Target. Ther.* **2021**, *6*, 196. [CrossRef] [PubMed]

60. Wang, Y.; Wang, B.; Zhao, Z.; Xu, J.; Zhang, Z.; Zhang, J.; Chen, Y.; Song, X.; Zheng, W.; Hou, L.; et al. Effects of SARS-CoV-2 Omicron BA.1 Spike Mutations on T-Cell Epitopes in Mice. *Viruses* **2023**, *15*, 763. [CrossRef]

61. Dolton, G.; Rius, C.; Hasan, M.S.; Wall, A.; Szomolay, B.; Behiry, E.; Whalley, T.; Southgate, J.; Fuller, A.; COVID-19 Genomics UK (COG-UK) consortium; et al. Emergence of immune escape at dominant SARS-CoV-2 killer T cell epitope. *Cell* **2022**, *185*, 2936–2951.e19. [CrossRef]

62. Guo, E.; Guo, H. CD8 T cell epitope generation toward the continually mutating SARS-CoV-2 spike protein in genetically diverse human population: Implications for disease control and prevention. *PLoS ONE* **2020**, *15*, e0239566. [CrossRef] [PubMed]

63. Martins, Y.; Silva, R. The impact of non-lineage defining mutations in the structural stability for variants of concern of SARS-CoV-2. *bioRxiv*, 2023; *preprint*. [CrossRef]

64. Veneziano, C.; Marascio, N.; De Marco, C.; Quaresima, B.; Biamonte, F.; Trecarichi, E.M.; Santamaria, G.; Quirino, A.; Torella, D.; Quattrone, A.; et al. The Spread of SARS-CoV-2 Omicron Variant in CALABRIA: A Spatio-Temporal Report of Viral Genome Evolution. *Viruses* **2023**, *15*, 408. [CrossRef]

65. Grabowski, F.; Preibisch, G.; Giziński, S.; Kochańczyk, M.; Lipniacki, T. SARS-CoV-2 Variant of Concern 202012/01 Has about Twofold Replicative Advantage and Acquires Concerning Mutations. *Viruses* **2021**, *13*, 392. [CrossRef]

66. Yamamoto, M.; Tomita, K.; Hirayama, Y.; Inoue, J.; Kawaguchi, Y.; Gohda, J. SARS-CoV-2 Omicron spike H655Y mutation is responsible for enhancement of the endosomal entry pathway and reduction of cell surface entry pathways. *biorxiv* 2022, *preprint*. [CrossRef]

67. Yang, X.J. δ1 variant of SARS-COV-2 acquires spike V1176F and yields a highly mutated subvariant in Europe. *biorxiv* 2021, *preprint*. [CrossRef]

68. Chakraborty, C.; Bhattacharya, M.; Sharma, A.R. Present variants of concern and variants of interest of severe acute respiratory syndrome coronavirus 2: Their significant mutations in S-glycoprotein, infectivity, re-infectivity, immune escape and vaccines activity. *Rev. Med. Virol.* **2022**, *32*, e2270. [CrossRef]

69. Jangra, S.; Ye, C.; Rathnasinghe, R.; Stadlbauer, D.; Krammer, F.; Simon, V.; Martinez-Sobrido, L.; Garcia-Sastre, A.; Schotsaert, M. The E484K mutation in the SARS-CoV-2 spike protein reduces but does not abolish neutralizing activity of human convalescent and post-vaccination sera. *medRxiv* 2021, *preprint*. [CrossRef]

70. Liu, Y.; Liu, J.; Plante, K.S.; Plante, J.A.; Xie, X.; Zhang, X.; Ku, Z.; An, Z.; Scharton, D.; Schindewolf, C.; et al. The N501Y spike substitution enhances SARS-CoV-2 transmission. *bioRxiv* 2021, *preprint*. [CrossRef]

71. Alkhatib, M.; Svicher, V.; Salpini, R.; Ambrosio, F.A.; Bellocchi, M.C.; Carioti, L.; Piermatteo, L.; Scutari, R.; Costa, G.; Artese, A.; et al. SARS-CoV-2 Variants and Their Relevant Mutational Profiles: Update Summer 2021. *Microbiol. Spectr.* **2021**, *9*, e0109621. [CrossRef] [PubMed]

72. Eslami, S.; Glassy, M.C.; Ghafouri Fard, S. A comprehensive overview of identified mutations in SARS CoV-2 spike glycoprotein among Iranian patients. *Gene* **2022**, *813*, 146113. [CrossRef] [PubMed]

73. Shen, L.; Triche, T.J.; Bard, J.D.; Biegel, J.A.; Judkins, A.R.; Gai, X. Spike protein NTD mutation G142D in SARS-CoV-2 Delta VOC lineages is associated with frequent back mutations, increased viral loads, and immune evasion. *medRxiv* 2021, *preprint*. [CrossRef]

74. Asif, A.; Ilyas, I.; Abdullah, M.; Sarfraz, S.; Mustafa, M.; Mahmood, A. The Comparison of Mutational Progression in SARS-CoV-2: A Short Updated Overview. *J. Mol. Pathol.* **2022**, *3*, 201–218. [CrossRef]

75. Mahmood, T.B.; Hossan, M.I.; Mahmud, S.; Shimu, M.S.S.; Alam, M.J.; Bhuyan, M.M.R.; Emran, T.B. Missense mutations in spike protein of SARS-CoV-2 delta variant contribute to the alteration in viral structure and interaction with hACE2 receptor. *Immunity Inflamm. Dis.* **2022**, *10*, e683. [CrossRef]

76. Mishra, T.; Dalavi, R.; Joshi, G.; Kumar, A.; Pandey, P.; Shukla, S.; Mishra, R.K.; Chande, A. SARS-CoV-2 spike E156G/Δ157-158 mutations contribute to increased infectivity and immune escape. *Life Sci. Alliance* **2022**, *5*, e202201415. [CrossRef] [PubMed]

77. Liu, Y.; Liu, J.; Johnson, B.A.; Xia, H.; Ku, Z.; Schindewolf, C.; Widen, S.G.; An, Z.; Weaver, S.C.; Menachery, V.D.; et al. Delta spike P681R mutation enhances SARS-CoV-2 fitness over Alpha variant. *Cell Rep.* **2022**, *39*, 110829. [CrossRef] [PubMed]

78. Furusawa, Y.; Kiso, M.; Iida, S.; Uraki, R.; Hirata, Y.; Imai, M.; Suzuki, T.; Yamayoshi, S.; Kawaoka, Y. In SARS-CoV-2 delta variants, Spike-P681R and D950N promote membrane fusion, Spike-P681R enhances spike cleavage, but neither substitution affects pathogenicity in hamsters. *EBioMedicine* **2023**, *91*, 104561. [CrossRef] [PubMed]

79. Saunders, N.; Planas, D.; Bolland, W.H.; Rodriguez, C.; Fourati, S.; Buchrieser, J.; Planchais, C.; Prot, M.; Staropoli, I.; Guivel-Benhassine, F.; et al. Fusogenicity and neutralization sensitivity of the SARS-CoV-2 Delta sublineage AY.4.2. *EBioMedicine* **2022**, *77*, 103934. [CrossRef] [PubMed]

80. Pater, A.A.; Bosmeny, M.S.; Barkau, C.L.; Ovington, K.N.; Chilamkurthy, R.; Parasrampuria, M.; Eddington, S.B.; Yinusa, A.O.; White, A.A.; Metz, P.E.; et al. Emergence and Evolution of a Prevalent New SARS-CoV-2 Variant in the United States. *bioRxiv* 2021, *preprint*. [CrossRef]

81. Saifi, S.; Ravi, V.; Sharma, S.; Swaminathan, A.; Chauhan, N.S.; Pandey, R. SARS-CoV-2 VOCs, Mutational diversity and clinical outcome: Are they modulating drug efficacy by altered binding strength? *Genomics* **2022**, *114*, 110466. [CrossRef]

82. Xia, S.; Wang, L.; Zhu, Y.; Lu, L.; Jiang, S. Origin, virological features, immune evasion and intervention of SARS-CoV-2 Omicron sublineages. *Signal Transduct. Target. Ther.* **2022**, *7*, 241. [CrossRef] [PubMed]

83. Chen, J.; Wei, G.W. Omicron BA.2 (B.1.1.529.2): High potential to becoming the next dominating variant. *arXiv* 2022, *preprint*.

84. Muttineni, R.; Binitha, R.N.; Putty, K.; Marapakala, K.; Sandra, K.P.; Panyam, J.; Vemula, A.; Singh, S.M.; Balachandran, S.; Viroji Rao, S.T.; et al. SARS-CoV-2 variants and spike mutations involved in second wave of COVID-19 pandemic in India. *Transbound. Emerg. Dis.* **2022**, *69*, e1721–e1733. [CrossRef]

85. Pastorio, C.; Zech, F.; Noettger, S.; Jung, C.; Jacob, T.; Sanderson, T.; Sparrer, K.M.J.; Kirchhoff, F. Determinants of Spike infectivity, processing, and neutralization in SARS-CoV-2 Omicron subvariants BA.1 and BA.2. *Cell Host Microbe* **2022**, *30*, 1255–1268.e5. [CrossRef]

86. Bugatti, A.; Filippini, F.; Messali, S.; Giovanetti, M.; Ravelli, C.; Zani, A.; Ciccozzi, M.; Caruso, A.; Caccuri, F. The D405N Mutation in the Spike Protein of SARS-CoV-2 Omicron BA.5 Inhibits Spike/Integrins Interaction and Viral Infection of Human Lung Microvascular Endothelial Cells. *Viruses* **2023**, *15*, 332. [CrossRef]

87. Alam, A.S.M.R.U.; Islam, O.K.; Hasan, M.S.; Islam, M.R.; Mahmud, S.; Al-Emran, H.M.; Jahid, I.K.; Crandall, K.A.; Hossain, M.A. Dominant clade-featured SARS-CoV-2 co-occurring mutations reveal plausible epistasis: An in silico based hypothetical model. *J. Med. Virol.* **2022**, *94*, 1035–1049. [CrossRef] [PubMed]

88. Azad, G.K. The molecular assessment of SARS-CoV-2 Nucleocapsid Phosphoprotein variants among Indian isolates. *Heliyon* **2021**, *7*, e06167. [CrossRef] [PubMed]

89. Wu, H.; Xing, N.; Meng, K.; Fu, B.; Xue, W.; Dong, P.; Tang, W.; Xiao, Y.; Liu, G.; Luo, H.; et al. Nucleocapsid mutations R203K/G204R increase the infectivity, fitness, and virulence of SARS-CoV-2. *Cell Host Microbe* **2021**, *29*, 1788–1801.e6. [CrossRef]

90. Mohammad, T.; Choudhury, A.; Habib, I.; Asrani, P.; Mathur, Y.; Umair, M.; Anjum, F.; Shafie, A.; Yadav, D.K.; Hassan, M.I. Genomic Variations in the Structural Proteins of SARS-CoV-2 and Their Deleterious Impact on Pathogenesis: A Comparative Genomics Approach. *Front. Cell. Infect. Microbiol.* **2021**, *11*, 765039. [CrossRef] [PubMed]

91. Díaz, Y.; Ortiz, A.; Weeden, A.; Castillo, D.; González, C.; Moreno, B.; Martínez-Montero, M.; Castillo, M.; Vasquez, G.; Sáenz, L.; et al. SARS-CoV-2 reinfection with a virus harboring mutation in the Spike and the Nucleocapsid proteins in Panama. *Int. J. Infect. Dis.* **2021**, *108*, 588–591. [CrossRef] [PubMed]

92. Hossain, A.; Akter, S.; Rashid, A.A.; Khair, S.; Alam, A.S.M.R.U. Unique mutations in SARS-CoV-2 Omicron subvariants' non-spike proteins: Potential impacts on viral pathogenesis and host immune evasion. *Microb. Pathog.* **2022**, *170*, 105699. [CrossRef] [PubMed]

93. Lo Presti, A.; Di Martino, A.; Ambrosio, L.; De Sabato, L.; Knijn, A.; Vaccari, G.; Di Bartolo, I.; Morabito, S.; Terregino, C.; Fusaro, A.; et al. Tracking the Selective Pressure Profile and Gene Flow of SARS-CoV-2 Delta Variant in Italy from April to October 2021 and Frequencies of Key Mutations from Three Representative Italian Regions. *Microorganisms* **2023**, *11*, 2644. [CrossRef]

94. Forchette, L.; Sebastian, W.; Liu, T. A comprehensive review of COVID-19 virology, vaccines, variants, and therapeutics. *Curr. Med. Sci.* **2021**, *41*, 1037–1051. [CrossRef] [PubMed]

95. Asgari, S.; Pousaz, L.A. Human genetic variants identified that affect COVID susceptibility and severity. *Nature* **2021**, *600*, 390–391. [CrossRef]

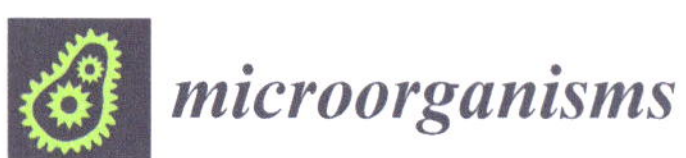 *microorganisms*

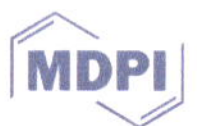

Article

Anomaly Detection Models for SARS-CoV-2 Surveillance Based on Genome *k*-mers

Haotian Ren [1], Yixue Li [1,2,3,4,5,*] and Tao Huang [1,*]

1   Bio-Med Big Data Center, CAS Key Laboratory of Computational Biology, Shanghai Institute of Nutrition and Health, University of Chinese Academy of Sciences, Chinese Academy of Sciences, Shanghai 200031, China; renhaotian2021@sibs.ac.cn
2   Key Laboratory of Systems Health Science of Zhejiang Province, School of Life Science, Hangzhou Institute for Advanced Study, University of Chinese Academy of Sciences, Hangzhou 310024, China
3   Guangzhou Laboratory, Guangzhou 510005, China
4   School of Life Sciences and Biotechnology, Shanghai Jiao Tong University, Shanghai 200240, China
5   Collaborative Innovation Center for Genetics and Development, Fudan University, Shanghai 200433, China
*   Correspondence: yxli@sibs.ac.cn (Y.L.); huangtao@sibs.ac.cn (T.H.)

Abstract: Since COVID-19 has brought great challenges to global public health governance, developing methods that track the evolution of the virus over the course of an epidemic or pandemic is useful for public health. This paper uses anomaly detection models to analyze SARS-CoV-2 virus genome *k*-mers to predict possible new critical variants in the collected samples. We used the sample data from Argentina, China and Portugal obtained from the Global Initiative on Sharing All Influenza Data (GISAID) to conduct multiple rounds of evaluation on several anomaly detection models, to verify the feasibility of this virus early warning and surveillance idea and find appropriate anomaly detection models for actual epidemic surveillance. Through multiple rounds of model testing, we found that the LUNAR (learnable unified neighborhood-based anomaly ranking) and LUNAR+LUNAR stacking model performed well in new critical variants detection. The results of simulated dynamic detection validate the feasibility of this approach, which can help efficiently monitor samples in local areas.

Keywords: anomaly detection; virus surveillance; SARS-CoV-2; *k*-mer; machine learning

Citation: Ren, H.; Li, Y.; Huang, T. Anomaly Detection Models for SARS-CoV-2 Surveillance Based on Genome *k*-mers. *Microorganisms* **2023**, *11*, 2773. https://doi.org/10.3390/microorganisms11112773

Academic Editor: Qibin Geng

Received: 26 September 2023
Revised: 6 November 2023
Accepted: 10 November 2023
Published: 15 November 2023

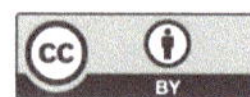

1. Introduction

Ever since the COVID-19 outbreak, the SARS-CoV-2 virus has undergone numerous mutations, leading to the emergence of different variants [1]. Towards the end of 2020, the World Health Organization (WHO) classified certain variants as variants of interest (VOI) and variants of concern (VOC) due to their significant impact on the transmission, severity and effectiveness of vaccines and prevention strategies [2]. One notable variant is the Omicron variant, whose parent lineage was listed as a VOC by the WHO on 6 November 2021, which did not end until 14 March 2023. In addition, the subvariants of Omicron, XBB.1.5 and XBB.1.16, were defined as VOI on 11 January 2023 and 17 April 2023, respectively, and both remain VOI as of 6 November 2023 [2–4].

It is crucial to swiftly identify samples of new virus variants that pose challenges to epidemic prevention and control. By detecting them in a timely manner, we can promptly implement appropriate measures, such as isolation and treatment, to effectively address new virus outbreaks in the region.

In China, nasal and throat swabs are predominantly used for collecting human virus samples. Additional techniques like saliva sampling are also employed [5]. These samples are then subjected to genome sequencing technologies to obtain the genetic code of the virus variants [6,7]. This is just the beginning of understanding this virus variant. The virus genome sequence is usually utilized for phylogenetic analysis, which helps researchers gain more insights into the virus lineage, expression proteins and mutation sites. This valuable information aids in further studying the various features of the virus [8,9]. Sequence alignment [10] plays a significant role in the phylogenetic workflow. However, due to the vast number of COVID-19 sequence samples and the large size of the SARS-CoV-2 virus genome (approximately 30 kb) [11], performing multiple sequence alignment [10,12] becomes computationally complex and time-consuming [13]. This impedes the swift detection of variants. Despite the existence of excellent multiple sequence alignment tools like UShER [14] for SARS-CoV-2, they still do not meet the speed requirements for frontline workers.

Therefore, our approach involves utilizing an alignment-free method [13] that relies on the numerical properties of sequences to compare them. This allows us to bypass issues associated with sequence alignment. One widely used method in this category is k-mer analysis [15–17]. A common step is to break a reference sequence into k-mers and use them to create a hash table. Then, target sequences are broken into k-mers and queried against the hash table to check for shared k-mers [18]. Several tools, such as VirFinder [19], CAFE [20], kmer2vec [21] and KINN [22], are built upon the concept of k-mer analysis. Various k-mer models have been developed to optimize sequence analysis and comparison. For example, Jia Wen et al. [23] proposed a k-mer sparse matrix model for sequence comparison. Furthermore, rather than utilizing phylogenetic methods focused on virus evolution and structural characteristics, we have opted for an anomaly detection algorithm widely employed in diverse industries [24]. By employing machine learning techniques, our intention is to swiftly identify noteworthy new variants from a substantial collection of virus sequence samples.

Anomaly detection is an important research direction in the field of machine learning, whose purpose is to identify "outliers" in data, as the name suggests. Anomaly detection can be further classified into outlier detection [25] and novelty detection [26], which have certain conceptual differences. The former refers to determining whether a certain data point is abnormal in the case of known data distribution, while the latter refers to finding novel data points different from the existing data in unknown datasets [27,28]. In our case, we aim to detect the emergence of VOC in a specific region during a certain period, aligning with the principles of novelty detection. To accomplish this, we have selected six different types of anomaly detection models from the PyOD [29] toolkit to conduct a variety of test evaluations on this detection task, which are as follows: empirical cumulative distribution based outlier detection (ECOD) [30], one-class support vector machines (OCSVM) [31], k nearest neighbors (KNN) [32], isolation forest (IForest) [33], AutoEncoder [34] and learnable unified neighborhood-based anomaly ranking (LUNAR) [35]. Additionally, we propose a method for stacking models to make predictions for new critical variants. Stacking is an ensemble learning technique where multiple base learners are combined with a meta learner, using the base learners' outputs as input to the meta learner [36]. In these prediction tasks, the models will train the known "normal samples" to determine whether there are "abnormal samples" in the new dataset, which is actually semi-supervised learning [37].

Giovanna Nicora et al. [38] also had a similar idea, but they used one class SVM to analyze the spike protein sequence of SARS-CoV-2. However, this method still requires the support of phylogenetic techniques, making the data processing more complex in practical applications. Additionally, this approach may not be suitable for situations where a specific virus variant remains dominant in a particular region over time. Because, even if the virus variant is VOC/VOI, it is just a "normal" circulating strain, since it has been popular in the region during this period. Hence, identifying the strain as "abnormal" in such cases lacks practical significance.

Based on the above considerations, this study aims to detect new critical variants that may appear in the samples collected over a period. We evaluate the efficacy of different anomaly detection algorithms on the k-mers of the SARS-CoV-2 genome to determine a suitable model for real-world epidemic surveillance. In this work, we consider variants that were once defined as VOC as critical variants, and the variants that were never defined as VOC are not critical variants. The reason why a VOC is only used as a critical variant is that the public health impact of a VOI is significantly smaller than that of a VOC, and many VOIs turned out to be benign. We selected six independent anomaly detection models. At the same time, we proposed that these independent models could be stacked to complete the prediction task of new variant detection and critical variant detection, so as to improve the interpretability of the prediction process of new critical variant detection (Figure 1). We tested and evaluated these models in various ways using public datasets and simulated their use in real world scenarios.

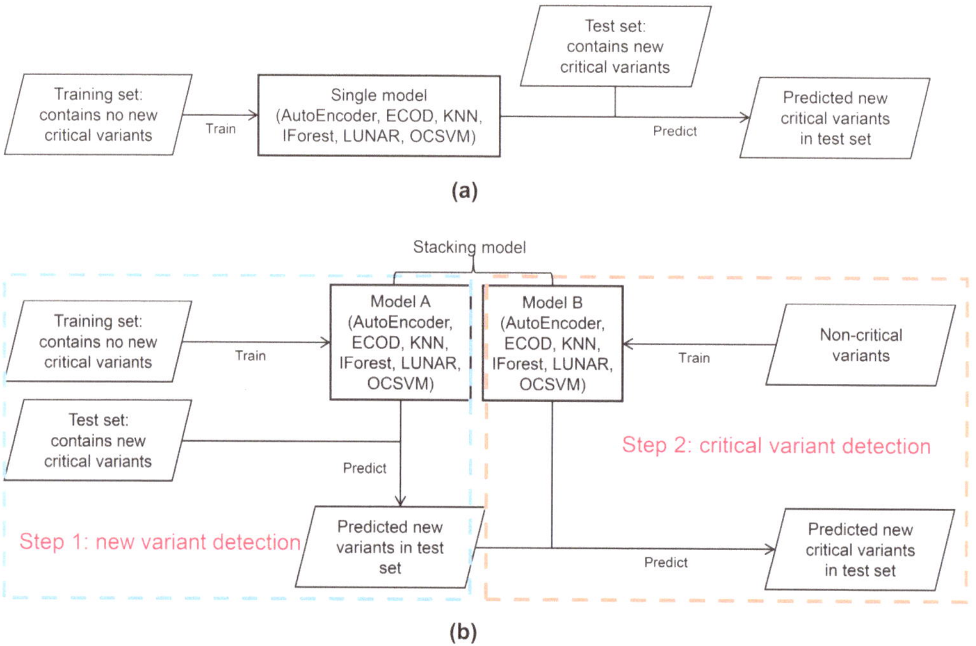

Figure 1. An overview of the models used to detect new critical variants in this work. (**a**) Detect new critical variants using a single outlier detection model; (**b**) detect new critical variants using the stacking model.

2. Materials and Methods

2.1. Data Source

From the EpiCoV database, which is a repository of information on SARS-CoV-2 in the Global Initiative on Sharing All Influenza Data (GISAID) [39], we obtained the sample sequences of complete SARS-CoV-2 genome sequences from human hosts and their metadata in Argentina, China and Portugal between 2020 and 2022. These countries, situated on different continents, have each implemented national epidemic control measures, although the timing and intensity of these policies varied. China gradually liberalized epidemic control until the end of 2022 [40]. Portugal was cited as a COVID-19 success story due to the low number of deaths in the early stages of the pandemic [41]. Argentina also implemented strict nationwide lockdown measures in phases during the year 2020 [42]. Moreover, all three countries achieved high rates of vaccinations [43]. We selected samples of these three countries as model test data to simulate the implementation of new critical variant anomaly detection under reasonable and effective epidemic prevention and control policies, so as to evaluate the feasibility of this surveillance approach.

2.2. Data Processing

We input the sequence file into the pipeline of Nextclade [44] to obtain the table file including the Nextstrain lineage information for each sample. Next, we calculated the *k*-mers for all sequences. A set of subsequences of length k in a biological sequence is called *k*-mer, and a sequence of length N has N–k+1 *k*-mers. RNA sequence contains 4 ribonucleotides, so there are up to 4 k types of *k*-mers. To control the number of *k*-mers and ensure that valid sequence characteristic information can be retained, we set k to 5, so there were 1024 *k*-mers. The table of each sequence *k*-mers was combined with its sample name, serial number, collection time, lineage and other information. And the samples with incomplete information were filtered out. In the end, we obtained a total of 74,885 sample data, including 9485 sequence samples that were consistently excluded from VOC. The sample statistics of each country are shown in Figure 2.

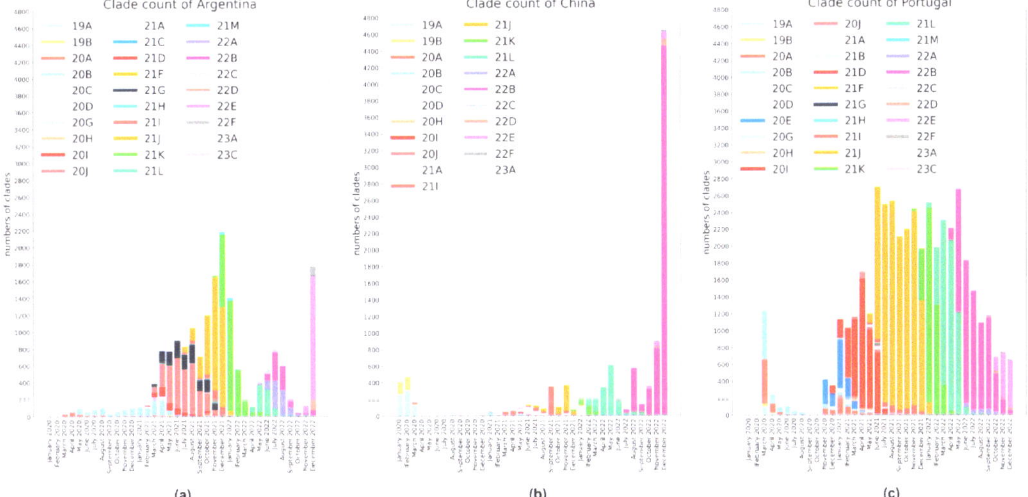

Figure 2. An overview of complete SARS-CoV-2 genome sequences in human hosts from three countries in the years from 2020 to 2022. (**a**) Statistics of SARS-CoV-2 variants in Argentina; (**b**) statistics of SARS-CoV-2 variants in China; (**c**) statistics of SARS-CoV-2 variants in Portugal.

2.3. Anomaly Detection Models

There are many types of existing anomaly detection models. According to the classification of individual anomaly detection models by PyOD [29], we selected six different types of anomaly detection models for research, which are as follows: ECOD [30] based on probability, OCSVM [31] based on linear model, KNN [32] based on proximity, IForest [33] based on outlier ensembles, AutoEncoder [34] based on neural networks and LUNAR [35] based on graphs. We used these six anomaly detection models to simulate the monitoring of samples from three countries to explore the potential of these models in the detection of new critical variants. At the same time, to improve the interpretability of the anomaly detection process, we have divided the task of new critical variant detection into two steps, namely, new variant detection and critical variant detection. We combined these six anomaly detection models to match two different steps, resulting in a total of 36 stacking models. We describe the stacking model in the form of "model A + model B", where model A is the model used in the new variant detection and model B is the model used in the critical variant detection. We conducted a comprehensive evaluation of the performance of these single models and stacking models on the task of detecting new critical variants. To be specific, it includes the following tasks: model evaluation of new variant detection; model evaluation of critical variant detection; model evaluation of new critical variant detection; comparison of the ability of these models to detect all critical variants on the day they first appear in the three countries; and analog dynamic monitoring. The source code of our work is available at https://github.com/sweety919/Anomaly-detection-models-for-SARS-CoV-2-surveillance-based-on-genome-k-mers (accessed on 12 November 2023).

2.4. Dataset Preparation

2.4.1. Datasets for Model Evaluation of New Variant Detection

To evaluate the performance of various anomaly detection models for identifying new variants, we conducted experiments using three distinct datasets (Figure 3a). The first dataset consists of a training set of 4914 samples in three countries from January 2020 to November 2020 and a test set of 506 samples in three countries from December 2020. The second dataset consists of a training set of 30,655 samples in three countries from January 2021 to November 2021 and a test set of 4216 samples in three countries from December 2021. The third dataset consists of a training set of 27,475 samples in three countries from January 2022 to November 2022 and a test set of 7119 samples in three countries from December 2022. During these tests, the training set exclusively comprised "normal samples", representing variants that have previously occurred. Conversely, any variants present in the test set that were not observed in the training set were classified as "abnormal samples".

2.4.2. Datasets for Model Evaluation of Critical Variant Detection

To test the ability of different anomaly detection models in the step of critical variant detection (Figure 3b), we conducted a random sampling process from a dataset containing 74,885 samples. From this sampling, we obtained 3000 sequence samples ("normal samples") that always did not belong to VOC as the training set. In other words, the samples in the training set are not critical variants. At the same time, 150 different sequence samples which are not critical variants ("normal samples") and 150 VOC sequence samples which are critical variants ("abnormal samples") were selected to form a test set. This process was repeated five times to create five different datasets.

2.4.3. Datasets for Model Evaluation of New Critical Variant Detection

This test step (Figure 3c) used the datasets which were used in the model evaluation of new variant detection, that is, a total of three datasets. When evaluating a single model, the new critical variant in the test set was considered an abnormal sample. However, when evaluating stacking models, we needed to define abnormal and normal samples in multiple steps. In the first step, samples in the test set that were not included in the training set were considered abnormal samples. Then, the samples that were classified as abnormal in this step were used as the test set in the second step, which aimed to detect critical variants. The training set in this step consisted of all non-VOC sequence samples originally input into the entire stacking model. The samples that were identified as abnormal in the final output represented the model's decision on new critical variants.

2.4.4. Datasets for Comparing the Detection of All Critical Variants on the Days They First Appeared in Three Countries

In our research, we focused on analyzing VOC in Argentina, China and Portugal from 2020 to 2022. We took all samples collected in the country on the day these critical variants appeared as the test sets (Figure 3d). These critical variants were the real abnormal samples in the test sets. All samples collected in the country during the 30 days before this day were training sets, and all non-VOC occurring in the country before this day were training sets for the critical variant detection step in the stacking models.

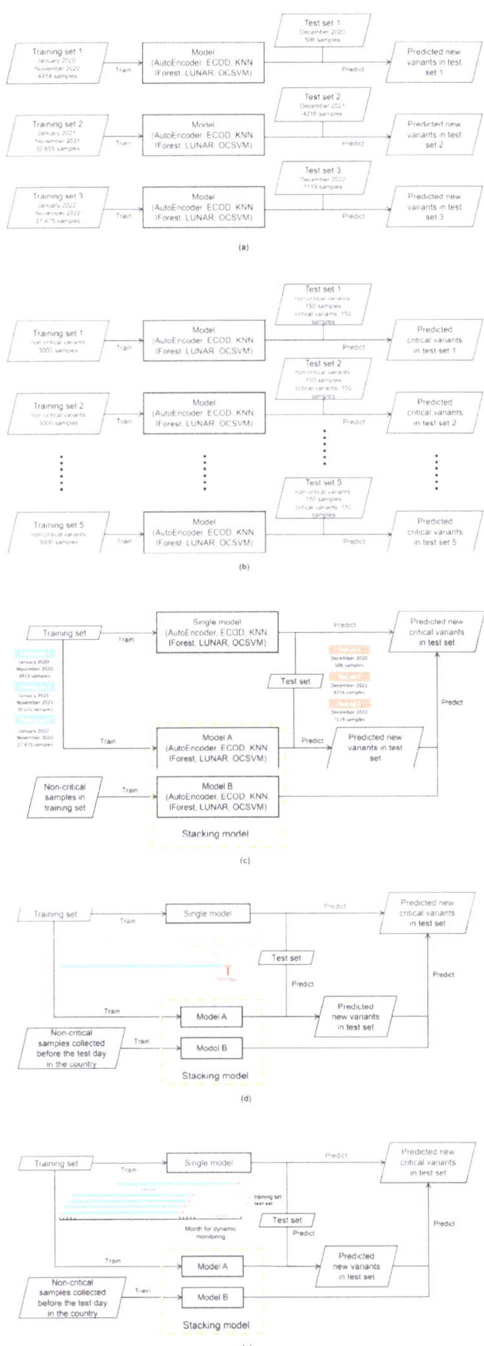

Figure 3. Five rounds of evaluation of anomaly detection models for SARS-CoV-2 surveillance based on genome *k*-mers. (**a**) Evaluation of new variant detection; (**b**) evaluation of critical variant detection; (**c**) evaluation of new critical variant detection; (**d**) compare the detection of all critical variants on the days they first appeared in three countries; (**e**) analog dynamic monitoring.

2.4.5. Datasets for Analog Dynamic Monitoring

To simulate dynamic monitoring, we selected one month from different time periods for each of the three countries (Figure 3e). For each selected day, the samples collected in that country formed the test set. The corresponding training set for that day consisted of all the samples collected in that country during the previous 30 days. Similarly, any non-VOC samples present in the country prior to that day were included as training sets for the critical variant detection step in the stacking models.

3. Results

3.1. Evaluation of New Variant Detection

In this section, we conducted performance testing on six anomaly detection models using three different datasets. All models utilized the default parameters provided by PyOD [29]. We evaluated the models using various metrics, such as the Matthews correlation coefficient (MCC) [45], f1-score, accuracy, recall, accuracy, specificity and area under the curve (AUC). The average values of these metrics were calculated (Tables 1 and S1). The recall metric indicates the model's ability to identify correct "abnormal samples", while the AUC reflects the model's classification performance. The MCC is a comprehensive indicator that assesses the model's classification ability in the presence of imbalanced sample categories. Thus, our focus was on these three metrics. From our analysis, we observed that both KNN and LUNAR models outperformed other models in terms of their capability to detect "abnormal samples" accurately. However, it is worth noting that most models struggled with the MCC, particularly those with MCC values below 0, indicating poorer performance in classifying imbalanced datasets.

Table 1. Evaluation of new variant detection.

Model	MCC	F1-Score	Precision	Recall	Accuracy	Specificity	AUC
AutoEncoder [34]	−0.016	0.004	0.002	0.078	0.838	0.842	0.460
ECOD [30]	−0.005	0.008	0.004	0.078	0.887	0.891	0.485
IForest [33]	−0.012	0.005	0.003	0.078	0.857	0.860	0.469
KNN [32]	0.092	0.035	0.018	0.741	0.793	0.792	0.767
LUNAR [35]	0.080	0.036	0.019	0.556	0.837	0.838	0.697
OCSVM [31]	0.006	0.010	0.005	0.207	0.874	0.878	0.543

3.2. Evaluation of Critical Variant Detection

We also tested the ability of the six models to detect critical variants. We calculated the evaluation metrics of the models' predictions over five prepared datasets and then took their average (Tables 2 and S2). Compared with the poor performance of many models in the step of new variant detection, the prediction effect of most models in critical variant detection appears to be quite good, because these models have learned the non-VOC sequence features well in the training set. This indicates that anomaly detection methods hold significant potential for detecting critical variants. Notably, the AutoEncoder and LUNAR models, both of which are anomaly detection methods based on deep learning, exhibited superior performance. This highlights the advantages of deep learning methods in handling complex relationships and features within sequences. We know that k-mers carry sequence information. Each k-mer does not exist alone, and there may be complex correlations among them which are also very likely to contain sequence characteristics. While conventional machine learning methods struggle to handle such high-dimensional information, deep learning methods can extract crucial features that contribute to excellent classification abilities.

Table 2. Evaluation of critical variant detection.

Model	MCC	F1-Score	Precision	Recall	Accuracy	Specificity	AUC
AutoEncoder [34]	0.539	0.722	0.855	0.625	0.759	0.893	0.759
ECOD [30]	0.122	0.303	0.643	0.200	0.544	0.889	0.544
IForest [33]	0.192	0.372	0.697	0.257	0.576	0.895	0.576
KNN [32]	0.171	0.345	0.691	0.231	0.564	0.897	0.564
LUNAR [35]	0.663	0.811	0.891	0.745	0.827	0.908	0.827
OCSVM [31]	−0.009	0.174	0.487	0.107	0.497	0.888	0.497

3.3. Evaluation of New Critical Variant Detection

In this round of evaluation, we tested the ability of 6 single models and 36 stacking models to detect new critical variants, calculated the metrics and averaged them (Tables 3 and S3). We found that the effects of KNN, LUNAR and three stacking models, which are KNN+KNN, KNN+LUNAR and LUNAR+LUNAR, were relatively outstanding among all models, with recall rates exceeding 0.5 and AUC scores surpassing 0.6. However, our findings also indicate that, similar to the evaluation outcomes for new variant detection, the low MCC values highlight room for improvement in the models' classification abilities, particularly when dealing with imbalanced datasets.

3.4. Comparing the Detection of All Critical Variants on the Days They First Appeared in Three Countries

For all VOCs that occurred in Argentina, China and Portugal between 2020 and 2022, we investigated the days they first appeared in each country. And we calculated the number of samples collected on the days the critical variants first appeared, as well as the samples collected in the 30 days before the critical variants appeared (Table S4). After a preliminary model evaluation of the new critical variant detection, we found that KNN, LUNAR, KNN+KNN, KNN+LUNAR and LUNAR+LUNAR performed better than other models, so we used these models for further testing. They were used to predict samples collected on the day all critical variants first appeared in the three countries. Although the training set entered by the stacking model in the new variant detection is the samples collected in the 30 days before the critical variant appeared, the training set used in the critical variant detection is all the non-VOC samples recorded in this country before the day when the critical variant appeared. We calculated the MCC, f1-score, accuracy, recall, accuracy, specificity and AUC for each round of testing, then compared and counted them (Figure 4). Since on the day that each new critical variant appeared, and usually only the variant sample was an anomaly, this accounts for a small proportion of the test set. So, this is a very unbalanced data set, and this is the reason why the models performed poorly on the MCC evaluation index. We believe that, if the MCC is greater than 0, the classification ability of the model is stronger than that of random classification. As shown in Figure 4, the median of the MCC is around 0, while the average is greater than 0. Combined with the distribution of the AUC, these models have a certain ability to detect new critical variants. In addition to the MCC and AUC, we also paid special attention to the recall. According to Table S4, we can see that the number of new critical variants in the test sets is mostly 1, which caused the model to display a recall of 0 when the critical variants were not correctly identified, and a recall of 1 when they were identified. This explains why the distribution of recall in Figure 4 is from 0 to 1. In this case, though, we can look at the median and average of the recall to compare the performance of the different models. As you can see from Figure 4, LUNAR and LUNAR+LUNAR performed better than the other models. What is more, we further compared the performance of the three stacking models in the new variant detection step. In this step, only KNN and LUNAR play a role. We found that LUNAR was superior to KNN in this step (Figure 5). At the same time, comparing the results of the new variant detection step (Figure 5) with the results of the stacking models after two steps (Figure 4), in terms of the stacking model, the new variant detection step has a great impact on the overall new critical variant detection. And the effect of LUNAR in the first step is better than that of KNN.

Table 3. Evaluation of new critical variant detection.

Model	MCC	F1-Score	Precision	Recall	Accuracy	Specificity	AUC
AutoEncoder [34]	−0.014	0.004	0.002	0.078	0.839	0.842	0.460
ECOD [30]	−0.003	0.008	0.004	0.078	0.888	0.891	0.485
IForest [33]	−0.008	0.006	0.003	0.098	0.850	0.853	0.476
KNN [32]	0.105	0.035	0.018	0.852	0.794	0.793	0.822
LUNAR [35]	0.104	0.046	0.024	0.722	0.811	0.811	0.767
OCSVM [31]	0.008	0.010	0.005	0.207	0.875	0.878	0.543
AutoEncoder+AutoEncoder	−0.011	0.004	0.002	0.078	0.860	0.862	0.470
AutoEncoder+ECOD	−0.016	0.001	0.001	0.010	0.920	0.924	0.467
AutoEncoder+IForest	−0.005	0.006	0.003	0.078	0.890	0.893	0.486
AutoEncoder+KNN	−0.010	0.004	0.002	0.078	0.864	0.867	0.473
AutoEncoder+LUNAR	−0.011	0.004	0.002	0.078	0.861	0.864	0.471
AutoEncoder+OCSVM	−0.006	0.007	0.004	0.069	0.887	0.891	0.480
ECOD+AutoEncoder	0.000	0.008	0.004	0.078	0.907	0.910	0.494
ECOD+ECOD	−0.013	0.003	0.002	0.020	0.919	0.923	0.471
ECOD+IForest	0.000	0.008	0.004	0.078	0.906	0.909	0.494
ECOD+KNN	0.000	0.008	0.004	0.078	0.908	0.911	0.495
ECOD+LUNAR	0.000	0.008	0.004	0.078	0.907	0.910	0.494
ECOD+OCSVM	−0.005	0.007	0.004	0.069	0.894	0.897	0.483
IForest+AutoEncoder	−0.002	0.007	0.004	0.078	0.902	0.905	0.492
IForest+ECOD	−0.015	0.001	0.001	0.010	0.921	0.925	0.467
IForest+IForest	−0.003	0.007	0.004	0.069	0.905	0.909	0.489
IForest+KNN	−0.004	0.007	0.003	0.098	0.878	0.881	0.489
IForest+LUNAR	0.000	0.008	0.004	0.088	0.900	0.903	0.496
IForest+OCSVM	−0.006	0.007	0.004	0.069	0.888	0.891	0.480
KNN+AutoEncoder	−0.002	0.007	0.004	0.108	0.876	0.879	0.493
KNN+ECOD	−0.016	0.001	0.001	0.010	0.920	0.924	0.467
KNN+IForest	−0.006	0.006	0.003	0.078	0.888	0.891	0.485
KNN+KNN	0.081	0.031	0.016	0.578	0.864	0.864	0.721
KNN+LUNAR	0.064	0.025	0.013	0.500	0.845	0.845	0.672
KNN+OCSVM	0.011	0.010	0.005	0.254	0.861	0.864	0.559
LUNAR+AutoEncoder	0.008	0.012	0.006	0.108	0.907	0.910	0.509
LUNAR+ECOD	−0.010	0.005	0.002	0.029	0.918	0.921	0.475
LUNAR+IForest	−0.004	0.006	0.003	0.069	0.901	0.904	0.486
LUNAR+KNN	0.075	0.037	0.020	0.412	0.909	0.910	0.661
LUNAR+LUNAR	0.110	0.047	0.025	0.637	0.891	0.891	0.764
LUNAR+OCSVM	0.012	0.011	0.006	0.291	0.834	0.837	0.564
OCSVM+AutoEncoder	−0.005	0.006	0.003	0.059	0.909	0.913	0.486
OCSVM+ECOD	−0.013	0.003	0.002	0.020	0.921	0.925	0.472
OCSVM+IForest	−0.005	0.006	0.003	0.059	0.910	0.913	0.486
OCSVM+KNN	−0.005	0.006	0.003	0.059	0.911	0.914	0.486
OCSVM+LUNAR	−0.005	0.006	0.003	0.059	0.910	0.913	0.486
OCSVM+OCSVM	0.008	0.010	0.005	0.207	0.875	0.878	0.543

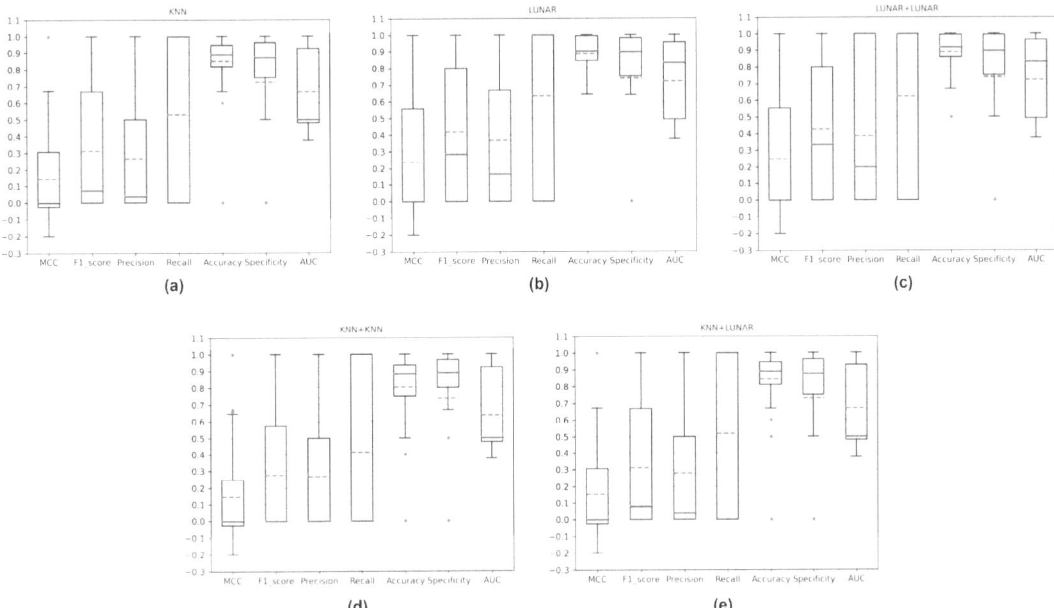

Figure 4. Compare the detection of all critical variants on the days they first appeared in three countries. (**a**) The evaluation metrics of KNN; (**b**) the evaluation metrics of LUNAR; (**c**) the evaluation metrics of LUNAR+LUNAR; (**d**) the evaluation metrics of KNN+KNN; (**e**) the evaluation metrics of KNN+LUNAR. The red lines in the boxplots indicate the medians, the blue lines indicate the mean values and the pink dots indicate the outliers.

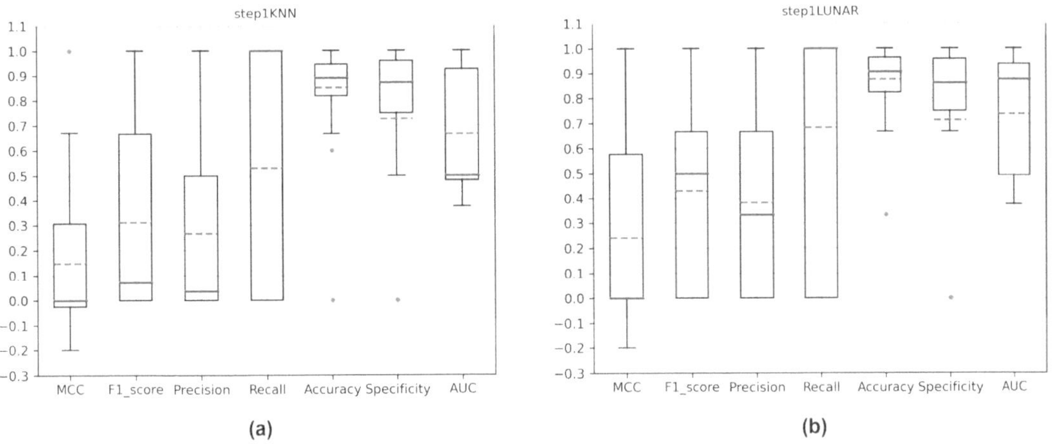

Figure 5. Compare the new variant detection of all critical variants on the days they first appeared in three countries. (**a**) The evaluation metrics of KNN; (**b**) the evaluation metrics of LUNAR. The red lines in the boxplots indicate the medians, the blue lines indicate the mean values and the pink dots indicate the outliers.

3.5. Analog Dynamic Monitoring

In addition to comparing the detection capabilities of models on the day the critical variants first appeared in the three countries, we also used these five relatively reliable models to simulate real dynamic detection scenarios. We selected a month in different time periods for the three countries and analyzed the samples with the models every day. We compared the number of new critical variants predicted by the models with the actual number of new critical variants (Figure 6). In fact, the days that a new critical variant appeared were a few, and so were the new critical variants. And our models, despite their ability to spot critical new variants on the day they appear, still produced false positives most of the time (Table S5). We used the specificity in Table S5 to calculate the false positive rate (FPR) (FPR = 1 − specificity) According to the bootstrap interval estimation [46], we calculated the 95% confidence interval of the false positive rate of each model: KNN was (0.072, 0.142), LUNAR was (0.100, 0.187), KNN+LUNAR was (0.075, 0.146), KNN+KNN was (0.076, 0.145) and LUNAR+LUNAR was (0.068, 0.136). Summing over all three countries, there were six days on which a new VOC occurred. On three of those six days, all five models predicted at least one new critical variant, but on only two days did all five models correctly predict the real new critical variant. And all five models failed to predict any new variant on two of these six days. On one of these six days, LUNAR correctly predicted one new variant, while the other models did not. Of the 81 days in which no new critical variant appeared, only on 19 of these days did all five models predict no new critical variants. Therefore, at least in the context evaluated, this approach would need to be considerably improved before deployment in a real-world situation. This is because the existing models still have many shortcomings in the case of conditional anomaly detection.

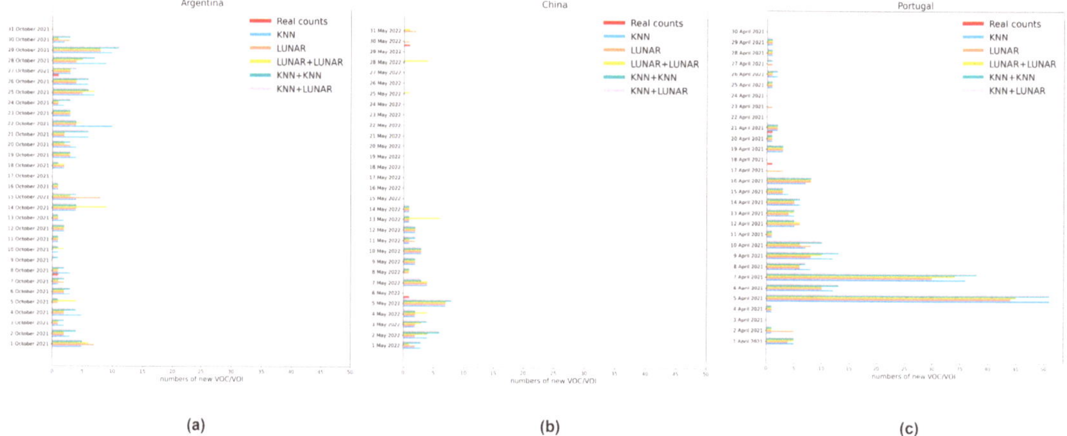

Figure 6. Analog dynamic monitoring of the new critical variants in three countries during a certain period. (**a**) Comparison of the predicted quantity with the actual quantity in Argentina; (**b**) comparison of the predicted quantity with the actual quantity in China; (c) comparison of the predicted quantity with the actual quantity in Portugal.

When we tested the method of Giovanna Nicora et al. [38] on the data sets used here, we found that their model had much better precision, although there were cases where some VOCs were not identified (Figure 7). This is because the method of Giovanna Nicora et al. [38] was used for VOC detection. For recurring VOCs over a period, the model also considered them abnormal samples. This anomaly detection method is based on the difference of sequence features between VOC and non-VOC. According to the evaluation results of the ability of each anomaly detection model in the critical variant detection, this is reasonable, since many anomaly detection models are fully capable of doing so.

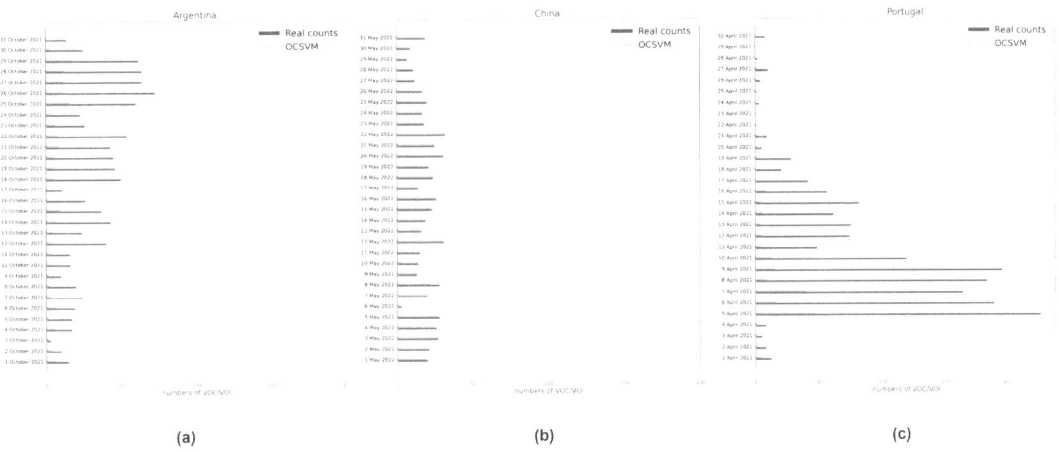

(a)   (b)   (c)

Figure 7. Analog dynamic monitoring of the critical variants in three countries during a certain period using OCSVM. (**a**) Comparison of the predicted quantity with the actual quantity in Argentina; (**b**) comparison of the predicted quantity with the actual quantity in China; (**c**) comparison of the predicted quantity with the actual quantity in Portugal.

4. Discussion

For infectious viruses such as SARS-CoV-2, which are highly transmissible and mutate frequently [47], it is important to detect new and noteworthy variants in a region in good time. These variants may have increased transmissibility and pathogenicity, posing a significant threat to global or regional public health security. Therefore, detecting these variants promptly can assist relevant agencies in rapidly developing prevention and control strategies. We proposed the use of the anomaly detection models to analyze SARS-CoV-2 virus genome k-mers and predict the new critical variants that may exist in the collected samples. Multiple rounds of testing and evaluation were conducted on several anomaly detection models, aiming to assess the feasibility of this early warning concept and identify suitable models for real-life epidemic surveillance.

For the performance evaluation of anomaly detection models in detecting new critical variants, we carried out five tests using sample sequences obtained from Argentina, China and Portugal between 2020 and 2022, sourced from GISAID. Throughout the testing rounds, which included new variant detection, critical variant detection and new critical variant detection, we observed that the comprehensive performance of the five models (KNN, LUNAR, KNN+LUNAR, LUNAR+LUNAR and KNN+KNN) surpassed that of the other 4 single models and 33 stacking models examined in this study. Additionally, indicators such as the MCC and AUC demonstrated the models' capacity to classify samples, even when the categories were highly imbalanced. Subsequently, we employed these five models to assess their ability to detect variants on the day when all critical variants first appeared in the aforementioned three countries. Based on the test results, we have determined that the new variant detection step is crucial in the overall identification of new critical variants for the stacking model. Additionally, LUNAR, as a deep learning method, outperformed KNN in both the independent detection of new critical variants and prediction as part of the stacking models. This demonstrates the significant advantages of LUNAR, which falls under the graph neural network method, in handling complex relationships between features. To assess the feasibility of our approach in real-time epidemic surveillance, we utilized these five models to predict daily samples from three different countries during various periods. Apart from evaluating VOC as a crucial variant, we also conducted tests on both VOC and VOI as crucial variants (Tables S6–S9, Figures S1–S4). Although the models all have certain false positive rates, we pay more attention to the recall of the models because, in virus surveillance, we are more worried about missing abnormal samples. The test results

63

further confirm that LUNAR exhibits the highest level of comprehensive performance among all the models tested across multiple rounds. We compared the performance of our proposed method to the method proposed by Giovanna Nicora et al. [38] on the same data. The results revealed that our method, unlike the method of Giovanna Nicora et al. [38], which solely predicts VOC in samples, incorporates the ability to detect new variants, enabling the identification of new critical variants. This helps reduce the workload of personnel involved in inspecting "key" samples and enhances the efficiency of epidemic prevention and control. However, the detection capability of the five models currently used still has some room for improvement. Therefore, phylogenetic approaches continue to play a crucial role in virus surveillance and early warning. Laboratories equipped with high-performance computing and programming resources may benefit from utilizing analysis pipelines that incorporate phylogenetic considerations.

We propose using anomaly detection models to analyze SARS-CoV-2 virus genome k-mers and predict new critical variants that may exist in collected samples, and evaluate some models in various aspects. This approach could be extended to other infectious viruses, such as seasonal influenza viruses [48]. The study in this paper is an attempt to apply machine learning to epidemic surveillance. Despite the limitations of the models tested in this paper, it demonstrates the feasibility of using anomaly detection in epidemic surveillance, even when dealing with large volumes of unanalyzed genomic data. In the future, we have the option to optimize the feature extraction of a viral genome. We observe that a current package, named MathFeature [49], integrates the methods for deriving numerical data from biological sequences. The performance of downstream model predictions may be enhanced by the introduction of these efficient feature extraction methods. Furthermore, we can introduce incremental learning to enable the model to quickly detect real-time data [50], thereby improving its practicality in real-world scenarios.

5. Conclusions

This work proposed using anomaly detection models to analyze SARS-CoV-2 virus genome k-mers and predict new critical variants that may exist in collected samples. Several anomaly detection models were evaluated through multiple rounds of tests. To verify the feasibility of this virus early warning idea and find a suitable anomaly detection model for actual epidemic surveillance, the dynamic monitoring of SARS-CoV-2 in a real-world scenario was simulated in this work.

Supplementary Materials: The following supporting information can be downloaded at: https://www.mdpi.com/article/10.3390/microorganisms11112773/s1. Table S1: Evaluation metrics of new variant detection; Table S2: Evaluation metrics of critical variant detection: Table S3: Evaluation metrics of new critical variant detection; Table S4: Evaluation metrics of the detection of all critical variants on the days they first appeared in three countries; Table S5: Results of analog dynamic monitoring of new critical variant detection; Table S6: Evaluation of new variant detection (consider VOC/VOI as critical variants); Table S7: Evaluation of critical variant detection (consider VOC/VOI as critical variants); Table S8: Evaluation of new critical variant detection (consider VOC/VOI as critical variants); Table S9: Results of analog dynamic monitoring of new critical variant detection (consider VOC/VOI as critical variants); Figure S1: Compare the detection of all critical variants on the days they first appeared in three countries (consider VOC/VOI as critical variants); Figure S2: Compare the new variant detection of all critical variants on the days they first appeared in three countries (consider VOC/VOI as critical variants); Figure S3: Analog dynamic monitoring of the new critical variants in three countries during a certain period (consider VOC/VOI as critical variants); Figure S4: Analog dynamic monitoring of the critical variants in three countries during a certain period using OCSVM (consider VOC/VOI as critical variants).

Author Contributions: Conceptualization, T.H. and Y.L.; methodology, H.R. and T.H.; formal analysis, H.R.; data curation, H.R.; writing—original draft preparation, H.R.; writing—review and editing, T.H. and Y.L. funding acquisition, T.H. and Y.L. All authors have read and agreed to the published version of the manuscript.

Funding: This work was supported by the National Key R&D Program of China (2022YFF1203202, 2018YFC2000205), the Strategic Priority Research Program of Chinese Academy of Sciences (XDB38050200, XDA26040304) and the Self-supporting Program of Guangzhou Laboratory (SRPG22-007).

Institutional Review Board Statement: Not applicable.

Informed Consent Statement: Informed consent was obtained from all subjects involved in the study.

Data Availability Statement: All scripts are available at https://github.com/sweety919/Anomaly-detection-models-for-SARS-CoV-2-surveillance-based-on-genome-k-mers (accessed on 12 November 2023). The data are available in the EpiCoV and GISAID databases.

Conflicts of Interest: The authors declare no conflict of interest.

References

1. Li, T.; Huang, T.; Guo, C.; Wang, A.; Shi, X.; Mo, X.; Lu, Q.; Sun, J.; Hui, T.; Tian, G.; et al. Genomic Variation, Origin Tracing, and Vaccine Development of SARS-CoV-2: A Systematic Review. *Innovation* **2021**, *2*, 100116. [CrossRef] [PubMed]
2. WHO. Tracking SARS-CoV-2 Variants. Available online: https://www.who.int/en/activities/tracking-SARS-CoV-2-variants/ (accessed on 8 May 2023).
3. Ren, S.Y.; Wang, W.B.; Gao, R.D.; Zhou, A.M. Omicron Variant (B.1.1.529) of SARS-CoV-2: Mutation, Infectivity, Transmission, and Vaccine Resistance. *World J. Clin. Cases* **2022**, *10*, 1–11. [CrossRef] [PubMed]
4. Khan, N.A.; Al-Thani, H.; El-Menyar, A. The Emergence of New SARS-CoV-2 Variant (Omicron) and Increasing Calls for COVID-19 vaccine boosters-The debate continues. *Travel Med. Infect. Dis.* **2022**, *45*, 102246. [CrossRef] [PubMed]
5. Yan, Y.; Chang, L.; Wang, L.N. Laboratory testing of SARS-CoV, MERS-CoV, and SARS-CoV-2 (2019-nCoV): Current Status, Challenges, and Countermeasures. *Rev. Med. Virol.* **2020**, *30*, e2106. [CrossRef] [PubMed]
6. Goswami, C.; Sheldon, M.; Bixby, C.; Keddache, M.; Bogdanowicz, A.; Wang, Y.H.; Schultz, J.; McDevitt, J.; LaPorta, J.; Kwon, E.; et al. Identification of SARS-CoV-2 Variants Using Viral Sequencing for the Centers for Disease Control and Prevention Genomic Surveillance Program. *BMC Infect. Dis.* **2022**, *22*, 1–12. [CrossRef]
7. Berno, G.; Fabeni, L.; Matusali, G.; Gruber, C.E.M.; Rueca, M.; Giombini, E.; Garbuglia, A.R. SARS-CoV-2 Variants Identification: Overview of Molecular Existing Methods. *Pathogens* **2022**, *11*, 1058. [CrossRef]
8. Caputo, E.; Mandrich, L. Structural and Phylogenetic Analysis of SARS-CoV-2 Spike Glycoprotein from the Most Widespread Variants. *Life* **2022**, *12*, 1245. [CrossRef]
9. Ren, H.; Ling, Y.; Cao, R.; Wang, Z.; Li, Y.; Huang, T. Early Warning of Emerging Infectious Diseases Based on Multimodal Data. *Biosaf. Health* **2023**. *online ahead of print*. [CrossRef]
10. Chao, J.N.; Tang, F.R.; Xu, L. Developments in Algorithms for Sequence Alignment: A Review. *Biomolecules* **2022**, *12*, 546. [CrossRef]
11. Zhou, P.; Yang, X.L.; Wang, X.G.; Hu, B.; Zhang, L.; Zhang, W.; Si, H.R.; Zhu, Y.; Li, B.; Huang, C.L.; et al. A Pneumonia Outbreak Associated with a New Coronavirus of Probable Bat Origin. *Nature* **2020**, *579*, 270–273. [CrossRef]
12. Chatzou, M.; Magis, C.; Chang, J.M.; Kemena, C.; Bussotti, G.; Erb, I.; Notredame, C. Multiple Sequence Alignment Modeling: Methods and Applications. *Brief. Bioinform.* **2016**, *17*, 1009–1023. [CrossRef] [PubMed]
13. Zielezinski, A.; Vinga, S.; Almeida, J.; Karlowski, W.M. Alignment-Free Sequence Comparison: Benefits, Applications, and Tools. *Genome Biol.* **2017**, *18*, 186. [CrossRef] [PubMed]
14. Turakhia, Y.; Thornlow, B.; Hinrichs, A.S.; De Maio, N.; Gozashti, L.; Lanfear, R.; Haussler, D.; Corbett-Detig, R. Ultrafast Sample placement on Existing tRees (UShER) Enables Real-Time Phylogenetics for the SARS-CoV-2 Pandemic. *Nat. Genet.* **2021**, *53*, 809–816. [CrossRef] [PubMed]
15. Forsdyke, D.R. Success of Alignment-Free Oligonucleotide (k-mer) Analysis Confirms Relative Importance of Genomes not Genes in Speciation and Phylogeny. *Biol. J. Linn. Soc.* **2019**, *128*, 239–250. [CrossRef]
16. Li, W.T.; Freudenberg, J.; Freudenberg, J. Alignment-Free Approaches for Predicting Novel Nuclear Mitochondrial Segments (NUMTs) in the Human Genome. *Gene* **2019**, *691*, 141–152. [CrossRef] [PubMed]
17. Ma, Y.L.; Yu, Z.G.; Tang, R.B.; Xie, X.H.; Han, G.H.; Anh, V.V. Phylogenetic Analysis of HIV-1 Genomes Based on the Position-Weighted K-mers Method. *Entropy* **2020**, *22*, 255. [CrossRef]
18. Petrucci, E.; Noé, L.; Pizzi, C.; Comin, M. Iterative Spaced Seed Hashing: Closing the Gap Between Spaced Seed Hashing and k-mer Hashing. *Bioinform. Res. Appl. Isbra* **2019**, *11490*, 208–219. [CrossRef]
19. Ren, J.; Ahlgren, N.A.; Lu, Y.Y.; Fuhrman, J.A.; Sun, F.Z. VirFinder: A Novel k-mer Based Tool for Identifying Viral Sequences from Assembled Metagenomic Data. *Microbiome* **2017**, *5*, 1–20. [CrossRef]
20. Lu, Y.Y.; Tang, K.J.; Ren, J.; Fuhrman, J.A.; Waterman, M.S.; Sun, F.Z. CAFE: Accelerated Alignment-FrEe Sequence Analysis. *Nucleic Acids Res.* **2017**, *45*, W554–W559. [CrossRef]
21. Ren, R.H.; Yin, C.C.; Yau, S.S.T. kmer2vec: A Novel Method for Comparing DNA Sequences by word2vec Embedding. *J. Comput. Biol.* **2022**, *29*, 1001–1021. [CrossRef]

22. Tang, R.B.; Yu, Z.G.; Li, J.Y. KINN: An Alignment-Free Accurate Phylogeny Reconstruction Method Based on Inner Distance Distributions of k-mer Pairs in Biological Sequences. *Mol. Phylogenet Evol.* **2023**, *179*, 107662. [CrossRef] [PubMed]
23. Wen, J.; Zhang, Y.; Yau, S.S. k-mer Sparse Matrix Model for Genetic Sequence and Its Applications in Sequence Comparison. *J. Theor. Biol.* **2014**, *363*, 145–150. [CrossRef] [PubMed]
24. Nassif, A.B.; Talib, M.A.; Nasir, Q.; Dakalbab, F.M. Machine Learning for Anomaly Detection: A Systematic Review. *IEEE Access* **2021**, *9*, 78658–78700. [CrossRef]
25. Zimek, A.; Filzmoser, P. There and Back Again: Outlier Detection between Statistical Reasoning and Data Mining Algorithms. *Wires Data Min. Knowl.* **2018**, *8*, e1280. [CrossRef]
26. Pimentel, M.A.F.; Clifton, D.A.; Clifton, L.; Tarassenko, L. A Review of Novelty Detection. *Signal Process.* **2014**, *99*, 215–249. [CrossRef]
27. Chandola, V.; Banerjee, A.; Kumar, V. Anomaly Detection: A survey. *ACM Comput. Surv.* **2009**, *41*, 1–58. [CrossRef]
28. Pang, G.S.; Shen, C.H.; Cao, L.B.; Van den Hengel, A. Deep Learning for Anomaly Detection: A Review. *ACM Comput. Surv.* **2021**, *54*, 1–38. [CrossRef]
29. Zhao, Y.; Nasrullah, Z.; Li, Z. PyOD: A Python Toolbox for Scalable Outlier Detection. *Comput. Sci.* **2019**, *20*, 1–7.
30. Li, Z.; Zhao, Y.; Hu, X.; Botta, N.; Ionescu, C.; Chen, G. ECOD: Unsupervised Outlier Detection Using Empirical Cumulative Distribution Functions. *IEEE Trans. Knowl. Data Eng.* **2022**, *35*, 12181–12193. [CrossRef]
31. Schölkopf, B.; Williamson, R.; Smola, A.; Shawe-Taylor, J.; Platt, J. Support Vector Method for Novelty Detection. In Proceedings of the 12th International Conference on Neural Information Processing Systems, Denver, CO, USA, 29 November–4 December 1999; pp. 582–588.
32. Angiulli, F.; Pizzuti, C. Fast Outlier Detection in High Dimensional Spaces. In *Principles of Data Mining and Knowledge Discovery*; Springer: Berlin/Heidelberg, Germany, 2002; pp. 15–27.
33. Liu, F.T.; Ting, K.M.; Zhou, Z.-H. Isolation-Based Anomaly Detection. *ACM Trans. Knowl. Discov. Data* **2012**, *6*, 1–39. [CrossRef]
34. Michelucci, U. Autoencoders. In *Applied Deep Learning with TensorFlow 2: Learn to Implement Advanced Deep Learning Techniques with Python*; Apress: Berkeley, CA, USA, 2022; pp. 257–283. [CrossRef]
35. Goodge, A.; Hooi, B.; Ng, S.K.; Ng, W.S. LUNAR: Unifying Local Outlier Detection Methods via Graph Neural Networks. *AAAI Conf. Artif. Intell.* **2022**, *36*, 6737–6745. [CrossRef]
36. Zhang, Y.Z.; Liu, J.J.; Shen, W.J. A Review of Ensemble Learning Algorithms Used in Remote Sensing Applications. *Appl. Sci.* **2022**, *12*, 8654. [CrossRef]
37. van Engelen, J.E.; Hoos, H.H. A Survey on Semi-Supervised Learning. *Mach. Learn.* **2020**, *109*, 373–440. [CrossRef]
38. Nicora, G.; Salemi, M.; Marini, S.; Bellazzi, R. Predicting Emerging SARS-CoV-2 Variants of Concern through a One Class Dynamic Anomaly Detection Algorithm. *BMJ Health Care Inform.* **2022**, *29*, e100643. [CrossRef]
39. Elbe, S.; Buckland-Merrett, G. Data, Disease and Diplomacy: GISAID's Innovative Contribution to Global Health. *Glob. Chall.* **2017**, *1*, 33–46. [CrossRef]
40. Taskforce for Joint Prevention and Control Mechanism for COVID-19 under the State Council and the National Health Commission of P.R. China. Scientific and Targeted Prevention and Control Measures to Optimize COVID-19 Response. *Health Care Sci.* **2023**, *2*, 1–6. [CrossRef]
41. Milhinhos, A.; Costa, P.M. On the Progression of COVID-19 in Portugal: A Comparative Analysis of Active Cases Using Non-linear Regression. *Front. Public Health* **2020**, *8*, 495. [CrossRef]
42. Larrosa, J.M.C. SARS-CoV-2 in Argentina: Lockdown, Mobility, and Contagion. *J. Med. Virol.* **2021**, *93*, 2252–2261. [CrossRef]
43. Data, Our World in "Coronavirus (COVID-19)" Vaccinations. Available online: https://ourworldindata.org/covid-vaccinations (accessed on 21 October 2023).
44. Hadfield, J.; Megill, C.; Bell, S.M.; Huddleston, J.; Potter, B.; Callender, C.; Sagulenko, P.; Bedford, T.; Neher, R.A. Nextstrain: Real-Time Tracking of Pathogen Evolution. *Bioinformatics* **2018**, *34*, 4121–4123. [CrossRef]
45. Chicco, D.; Jurman, G. The Advantages of the Matthews Correlation Coefficient (MCC) over F1 Score and Accuracy in Binary Classification Evaluation. *BMC Genom.* **2020**, *21*, 6. [CrossRef]
46. Markus, M.T.; Groenen, P.J.F. An Introduction to the Bootstrap. *Psychometrika* **1998**, *63*, 97–101.
47. Harrison, A.G.; Lin, T.; Wang, P.H. Mechanisms of SARS-CoV-2 Transmission and Pathogenesis. *Trends Immunol.* **2020**, *41*, 1100–1115. [CrossRef] [PubMed]
48. Brammer, L.; Budd, A.; Cox, N. Seasonal and Pandemic Influenza Surveillance Considerations for Constructing Multicomponent Systems. *Influenza Other Respir. Viruses* **2009**, *3*, 51–58. [CrossRef] [PubMed]
49. Bonidia, R.P.; Domingues, D.S.; Sanches, D.S.; de Carvalho, A. MathFeature: Feature Extraction Package for DNA, RNA and Protein Sequences Based on Mathematical Descriptors. *Brief. Bioinform.* **2022**, *23*, bbab434. [CrossRef] [PubMed]
50. Tan, C.H.; Lee, V.C.; Salehi, M. MIR_MAD: An Efficient and On-line Approach for Anomaly Detection in Dynamic Data Stream. In Proceedings of the 20th IEEE International Conference on Data Mining (ICDM), Electr Network, Sorrento, Italy, 17–20 November 2020; pp. 424–431.

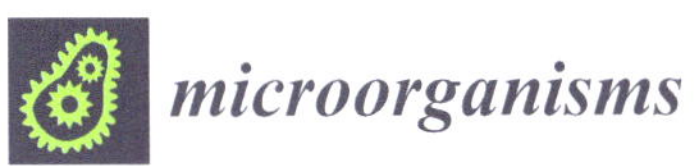 *microorganisms*

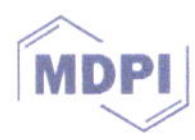

Article

Assessing Continuity of Adherence to Precautionary Measures for COVID-19 among Vaccinated People in Jazan, Saudi Arabia

Anwar Alameer [1], Yahya Maslamani [1], Ibrahim M. Gosadi [2,*], Mohammed Y. Elamin [1], Mohammed A. Muaddi [2], Ahmad Y. Alqassim [2], Abrar Doweri [1], Ibrahim Namis [3], Fatimah Busayli [4], Hussam Ahmadini [1], Yehya Hejri [1] and Abdu Dahlan [1]

[1] Public Health Administration, Jazan Health Directorate, Jazan 82611, Saudi Arabia
[2] Department of Family and Community Medicine, Faculty of Medicine, Jazan University, Jazan 45142, Saudi Arabia
[3] Endocrinology and Diabetic Center, Jazan Health Directorate, Jazan 82611, Saudi Arabia
[4] Sabya General Hospital, Jazan Health Directorate, Jazan 82611, Saudi Arabia
* Correspondence: gossady@hotmail.com

Abstract: Background: Adherence to behavioral respiratory hygiene practices is essential in preventing the transmission of COVID-19, especially given the appearance of new variants of the COVID-19 virus. This study estimated the pre- and post-vaccination levels of adherence to COVID-19 preventive behavioral measures among vaccinated people. Methods: This cross-sectional study assessed the sociodemographics and preventive behavioral measures, and pre- and post-vaccination data, via a questionnaire. Paired t-tests and Chi-squared tests were used to assess the variation in adherence levels. Results: Of the 480 participants, 57.9% were male, and 30.4% were aged between 30 and 39 years of age. After vaccination, there was a statistically significant decline in adherence to all the assessed behavioral protective measures ($p < 0.05$). Being 50 years old or older, female, a healthcare worker, and a smoker were associated with higher adherence levels compared with other groups in the same categories. Conclusions: A change in the behavior of the community members regarding COVID-19 after receiving the vaccination and a reduction in adherence to respiratory hygiene practices was observed. This indicates the importance of raising awareness about the possibility of reinfection with COVID-19 despite the vaccination, and the importance of behavioral respiratory hygiene for the prevention and control of COVID-19.

Keywords: COVID-19; respiratory hygiene; variants; post-vaccination; adherence; prevention

Citation: Alameer, A.; Maslamani, Y.; Gosadi, I.M.; Elamin, M.Y.; Muaddi, M.A.; Alqassim, A.Y.; Doweri, A.; Namis, I.; Busayli, F.; Ahmadini, H.; et al. Assessing Continuity of Adherence to Precautionary Measures for COVID-19 among Vaccinated People in Jazan, Saudi Arabia. *Microorganisms* **2023**, *11*, 800. https://doi.org/10.3390/microorganisms11030800

Academic Editor: Qibin Geng

Received: 13 February 2023
Revised: 18 March 2023
Accepted: 20 March 2023
Published: 21 March 2023

1. Introduction

Coronavirus disease 2019 (COVID-19) was first discovered in Wuhan, China, in December 2019. The World Health Organization (WHO) declared a pandemic in March 2020 after it had spread to more than 200 territories. As of 5 February 2023, 754 million confirmed cases and 6.8 million deaths have been reported globally [1]. About 829,388 confirmed coronavirus cases and 9614 deaths were recorded in Saudi Arabia by February 2023. The curve of the coronavirus epidemic, which fluctuates across years and seasons, is closely monitored by the Saudi Ministry of Health in terms of recorded cases and deaths for the sake of urgent intervention and control. To date, more than 68 million coronavirus vaccine doses have been administered in Saudi Arabia [2].

As of the start of 2023, despite the preventive and control measures applied against COVID-19, infections with the virus are ongoing. In the period between 12 and 19 January 2023, 1.3 million new cases of COVID-19 were reported in the Western Pacific region. Similarly, 649,000 and 234,000 new cases of COVID-19 were reported in the same week in the Americas and Europe, respectively [3]. These infection rates are augmented by the likely appearance of new variants of the virus due to the constant changes in its properties. The WHO recommended the use of letters of the Greek alphabet to indicate new variants of concern of SARS-CoV-2, which causes COVID-19. Currently, there are five main variants of concern, namely, alpha, beta, gamma, delta, and omicron. Each variant's first appearance was linked to a specific country, while the first detected cases of the omicron variant were documented in several countries [4].

Although vaccines are among the interventions that have saved millions of lives since their development, behavioral precautions are still considered a cornerstone in suppressing the exponential growth in COVID-19 cases [5]. Additionally, strict policies (e.g., behavioral precautions, travel restrictions, lockdowns, and curfews) for the prevention and control of COVID-19 have been applied to several populations. Many regulations have diminished as a response to an improvement in the epidemic curve of COVID-19 cases, with careful continuation of regular assessments of the epidemiological situation. For example, on 23 March 2020, the United Kingdom's government announced the first lockdown in the UK, which was followed by conditional lifting of the lockdown in the subsequent months, until the final removal of most legal limits on social contact by July 2021 [6]. Nonetheless, the ongoing incidence of COVID-19 infections despite vaccinations indicates the importance of adhering to respiratory hygiene practices for the prevention and control of respiratory illnesses, including COVID-19.

Respiratory hygiene is a preventive behavioral precaution that limits the transmission of respiratory pathogens, including COVID-19, via airborne or droplet routes. Respiratory hygiene includes several elements, such as covering the nose and mouth when coughing or sneezing, using and appropriately disposing of tissues, practicing appropriate hand washing and sanitization, avoiding touching the nose and mouth, and wearing face masks in individuals exhibiting respiratory symptoms [7].

Despite the reported effectiveness of COVID-19 vaccinations in preventing infection, the risk of breakthrough infections is considerable, elevating the importance of adhering to behavioral precautions against COVID-19. Adherence to behavioral precautions is essential for preventing the transmission of COVID-19 because it helps the population return to normal activities [8,9]. Vaccinations and adherence to behavioral precautions synergize to achieve a professional control strategy.

There are multiple conceptual frameworks that can be correlated with the changes in personal protective behavior concerning COVID-19. Nonetheless, due to the nature of the disease and the associated factors influencing adherence to personal protective behavior, the conceptual framework of the current investigation was associated with the health belief model. The model assumes that optimal behavior toward a particular disease is affected by perceived susceptibility, severity, barriers, and benefits.

Studies assessing the adherence of individuals vaccinated against COVID-19 to respiratory behavioral precautions are limited in Saudi Arabia. The main objective of this study was to estimate the pre- and post-vaccination levels of adherence to COVID-19 preventive measures among vaccinated people in the Jazan area, and to explore the associated factors. This estimation is essential for assessing and analyzing the current situation and for determining beneficial control strategies for future prevention. The assessment of the factors associated with the adherence of the participants concerning personal protective behavior is followed by the correlation of the findings with the health belief model to allow a better explanation of the factors that might predict the continuity of adherence to precautionary measures, especially regarding diseases of a respiratory nature.

2. Materials and Methods

2.1. Study Design and Settings

This cross-sectional study was conducted in the Jazan region of southwest Saudi Arabia. Jazan Health Affairs offers its services to more than almost 1.4 million people in 14 cities and numerous villages. Figure 1 illustrates the timeline of COVID-19 in the region and the performance of the assessment in the current investigation. The target population included all vaccinated people from February 2021 to July 2021. This investigation was performed after securing ethical approval from the Jazan Health Ethics Committee (approval number 2184, dated October 2021). Informed consent was secured from the study participants before enrolment, and the study was performed according to the principles of the Declaration of Helsinki.

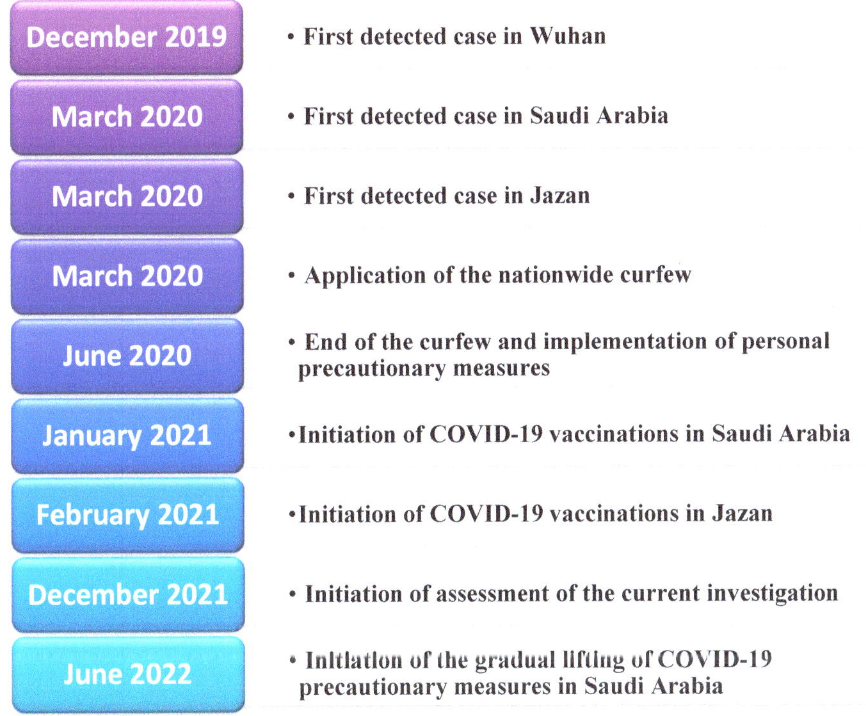

Figure 1. Timeline of COVID-19 prevention and control measures in the setting of Jazan, Saudi Arabia.

2.2. Study Population and Data Collection Procedures

In total, there were approximately 715,579 vaccinated people in the 14 administrative areas at the start of the study. The participants were chosen according to the following eligibility criteria: aged $\geq$ 18 years, living in the Jazan region, and having taken the COVID-19 vaccine. Participants were excluded if they refused to give informed consent, were younger than 18 years, did not take the vaccine, and did not reside in the Jazan region.

Participants were chosen randomly from eight vaccination data banks of the public health sector, and the desired sample size was proportional to the size of each area's vaccinated population; therefore, eligible participants were recruited by a simple randomization method proportional to the number of vaccinated people in each city. Participants were contacted by mobile phone and recruited voluntarily after receiving a complete description of the study. Then they were filtered by the study's inclusion and exclusion criteria. On average, it took 20 min to complete the questionnaire. Data collection was completed within a period of 2 months from the study's initiation. According to the following parameters, there was an estimated adherence level of 50% among the population of Jazan, a 0.05 margin of error, and a 95% confidence interval. The sample size was calculated using the method of Swanson and Cohen (N = Z2P (1 − P)/d2). The calculated sample size was 384 subjects, which was adjusted to 422 to account for a 10% non-response rate.

2.3. Measures

This study evaluated differences in pre- and post-vaccination levels of adherence to COVID-19 preventive measures among vaccinated people and explored the associated factors. The dependent variables were differences between pre- and post-vaccination levels of adherence to COVID-19 preventive measures among vaccinated people in the Jazan area. Data concerning adherence during the pre- and post-vaccination stages were collected at one time point. The independent variables were age, gender, area of residence, economic status, social status, education level, employment type (medical vs. non-medical), smoking status, and having a chronic illness.

The data collection tool of the International Citizen Project COVID-19 general questionnaire was used in this study. It comprised three parts that assessed the level of adherence to COVID-19 preventive measures and the associated factors according to the WHO guidelines and the Saudi national guidelines on COVID-19 prevention [10]. The first part of the questionnaire collected sociodemographic information about each participant. The second part assessed daily and professional life during the coronavirus epidemic, while the third part considered personal and community preventive measures. Adherence to preventive measures was evaluated using 10 "yes" or "no" questions. It included the following: the use of a face mask, physical distancing, coughing or sneezing into the crease of the elbow or covering the mouth and nose with a disposable handkerchief, hand washing/sanitizing immediately after coughing or sneezing, checking body temperature at least twice a week, regular hand washing during the day, using alcohol-based hand sanitizer during the day, avoiding touching the face (eyes, nose, mouth), sanitizing phones when returning home, and staying at home when experiencing influenza-like symptoms. The internal consistency of the items was tested via a Cronbach's alpha test, revealing a value of 0.85. Additionally, the external consistency of the items was tested via the kappa test, revealing an overall value of 0.86.

2.4. Statistical Analysis

Data were analyzed using the Statistical Package for the Social Sciences, version 23. The analysis of the data was performed via three main steps. The first step included performing descriptive statistics. The descriptive statistics were used to summarize the main findings of the study, including the frequencies, proportions, means, and standard deviations. The descriptive analysis was followed up by conducting inferential statistics to identify the factors associated with adherence levels. Finally, factors identified to be associated with adherence levels were further assessed via the health belief model.

A scoring system was utilized for the assessment of adherence. Each adherence item scored 1 if the study participant confirmed that they adhered to the measure and 0 otherwise. Adherence scores were calculated by summing the responses to the 10 questions related to adherence to the preventive measures against COVID-19. A cut-off point was used to classify the practices into two levels: inadequate (<6) and adequate ($\geq$6). This cut-off point was decided after identifying a mean adherence score value of 6, where those who scored lower values were indicated as having inadequate adherence and those who scored higher values were indicated as having adequate adherence.

Subsequently, inferential statistics were performed in two steps to test the variation in the level of adherence according to the sample characteristics. The first step included performing a paired t-test to assess the variations in the overall adherence levels as continuous variables before and after receiving the vaccines according to the measured sample's sociodemographic characteristics. Additionally, the Chi-squared test was used to assess the variations in adherence to each practice item as a binary variable before and after receiving the vaccines. A value of $p = 0.05$ was considered statistically significant for the applied statistical tests.

Factors associated with adherence levels among the studied community were correlated with the health belief model to allow for the possible understanding of the barriers, norms, and drivers of adherence to personal protective behavior; disease-based factors that may affect adherence; population-based adherence, which may influence adherence; and finally, geography-based factors that might influence adherence.

3. Results

In total, 480 participants agreed to participate in the current investigation, with a total response rate of 97.6%. Table 1 illustrates the sociodemographic characteristics of the recruited sample. It may be noted that nearly 50% of the sample were above the age of 40, more than half were males (57.9%), and the majority were married and living with their spouses (78.1%). Furthermore, the majority of the sample indicated receiving a university education (74%) and reported living in urban areas of the Jazan region (67.9%). Nearly one-third of the sample indicated that they were healthcare workers (31.5%). The majority of the sample reported living with other persons in their residences (97.1%). Finally, less than half of the sample reported having a diagnosed chronic disease (43.5%), and a minority indicated that they were current smokers at the time of recruitment (13.8%).

Table 1. Sociodemographic characteristics of a sample of 480 participants from Jazan, Saudi Arabia.

Item	Frequency (Proportion)
Age (years)	
18–29	93 (19.4%)
30–39	146 (30.4%)
40–49	118 (24.6%)
≥50	123 (25.6%)
Gender	
Male	278 (57.9%)
Female	202 (42.1%)
Marital status	
Single/divorced/widowed	105 (21.9%)
Married/living together	375 (78.1%)
Education	
≤Secondary	122 (25.4%)
≥University	358 (74.6%)
Belonging to the health sector	
No	329 (68.5%)
Yes	151 (31.5%)
Area of residency	
Urban	326 (67.9%)
Rural	154 (32.1%)
Living conditions	
Living with others	466 (97.1%)
Living alone	14 (2.9%)
Smoking	
Smoker	66 (13.8%)
Non-smoker	414 (86.3%)
Having a chronic disease	
With a chronic disease	209 (43.5%)
No chronic disease	271 (56.5%)

Table 2 displays the distribution of the estimated levels of adherence to personal protective measures before and after receiving the COVID-19 vaccination, according to the measured study characteristics. The overall mean adherence score was 6.62 (SD: 2.9) before receiving the vaccine and 3.96 (SD: 2.2) after receiving the vaccine. The reduction in the mean of overall levels of adherence reached 2.66, and this reduction was statistically significant (p value < 0.001). This reduction in the overall mean adherence score suggests lower adherence among adults living in the Jazan region to the personal protective measures against COVID-19 after receiving the vaccination.

Table 2. Comparison of pre- and post-COVID-19 vaccination levels of adherence to personal protective measures among 480 participants in the Jazan region according to their sociodemographic characteristics.

Item	N (%)	Adherence Level		Mean Reduction	p Value *
		Pre-Vaccination	Post-Vaccination		
		Mean ± SD	Mean ± SD		
Age (years)					
18–29	93 (19.4)	6.47 ± 2.89	3.75 ± 2.37	−2.72	$p < 0.001$
30–39	146 (30.4)	6.68 ± 2.93	3.78 ± 2.11	−2.9	$p < 0.001$
40–49	118 (24.6)	6.59 ± 3.17	3.88 ± 2.43	−2.71	$p < 0.001$
≥50	123 (25.6)	6.70 ± 2.65	4.44 ± 2.08	−2.26	$p < 0.001$
Gender					
Male	278 (57.9)	6.21 ± 2.95	3.73 ± 2.26	−2.48	$p < 0.001$
Female	202 (42.1)	7.20 ± 2.76	4.29 ± 2.19	−2.91	$p < 0.001$
Marital status					
Single/divorced/widowed	105 (21.9)	6.52 ± 2.80	4.10 ± 2.58	−2.42	$p < 0.001$
Married/living together	375 (78.1)	6.65 ± 2.94	3.93 ± 2.15	−2.72	$p < 0.001$
Education					
≤Secondary	122 (25.4)	6.17 ± 2.98	3.98 ± 2.04	−2.19	$p < 0.001$
≥University	358 (74.6)	6.77 ± 2.87	3.96 ± 2.31	−2.81	$p < 0.001$
Belonging to the health sector					
No	329 (68.5)	6.38 ± 2.96	3.75 ± 2.22	−2.63	$p < 0.001$
Yes	151 (31.5)	7.15 ± 2.71	4.44 ± 2.23	−2.71	$p < 0.001$
Area of residency					
Urban	326 (67.9)	7.02 ± 2.69	4.24 ± 2.23	−2.78	$p < 0.001$
Rural	154 (32.1)	5.77 ± 3.17	3.40 ± 2.17	−2.37	$p < 0.001$
Live alone or with other people					
Live alone	14 (2.9)	6.86 ± 3.41	5.78 ± 2.51	−1.08	$p = 0.119$
Smoking					
Smoker	66 (13.8)	7.80 ± 2.18	4.44 ± 2.44	−3.36	$p < 0.001$
Non-smoker	414 (86.3)	6.44 ± 2.96	3.89 ± 2.2	−2.55	$p < 0.001$
Having a chronic disease					
With a chronic disease	209 (43.5)	6.33 ± 3.14	3.60 ± 2.34	−2.73	$p < 0.001$
No chronic disease	271 (56.5)	6.84 ± 2.7	4.25 ± 2.13	−2.59	$p < 0.001$
Overall adherence score (OALS)		6.62 ± 2.9	3.96 ± 2.2	−2.66	2.66

* Paired t test.

Before people received the COVID-19 vaccination, the mean level of adherence varied between 7.8 (the highest mean adherence level, found among smokers) and 5.77 (the lowest mean adherence level, found among the participants residing in rural areas). Although the current investigation did not investigate why smokers were more likely to report higher adherence scores, it can be postulated that the awareness of the smokers that they were at higher risk of developing serious respiratory complications of COVID-19 might encourage them to adhere to personal protective measures. Similarly, the lower adherence level score identified in rural areas can be partially explained by the lower probability of adults living in rural areas of the Jazan region being exposed to the enforcement of the precautionary measures applied by official institutions in the region (including nationwide precautionary measures, as indicated in Figure 1).

After people received the COVID-19 vaccination, the mean level of adherence varied between 5.78 (the highest mean adherence score, found among people who reported living alone) and 3.4 (the lowest mean adherence level, found among participants residing in rural areas). The reason for the higher adherence scores among those who lived alone, though not measured in the current investigation, can be postulated to be the fact that adults living alone might exhibit higher adherence to measures related to social isolation when experiencing symptoms suggesting COVID-19 infection, in comparison with those who are living with other family members.

A comparison of the adherence scores before and after receiving the COVID-19 vaccination, according to the measured sample's sociodemographic characteristics, indicated a reduction in the adherence levels after receiving the vaccination in all comparison groups (p values < 0.001), except for the comparison made according to whether people lived alone or shared the residence with others, which did not exhibit a statistically significant change. When the reductions in the means of the adherence scores were compared according to the study population's characteristics, a variation in the reduction in the means was noted.

The age group of 30–39 years displayed the largest reduction in the mean adherence level compared with other age groups. Females exhibited larger reductions in the mean adherence scores in comparison with males. Those who were not married showed lower reductions in the mean adherence levels in comparison with those who were married. Adults with university-level education showed larger reductions in comparison with those with lower than university-level education.

Adults working in the health sector exhibited greater reductions in the mean adherence scores in comparison with those not working in the health sector. Similarly, those living in rural areas showed greater reductions in comparison with those residing in urban areas. Smokers exhibited greater reductions in the means in comparison with non-smokers. Finally, adults diagnosed with a chronic disease showed greater reductions in comparison with those who reported not being diagnosed with a chronic disease.

Table 3 displays a comparison of the reported adherence to specific personal preventive measures before and after receiving the COVID-19 vaccine among the study's participants. Overall, there was a statistically significant reduction (p < 0.05) in the level of adherence to behavioral personal preventive measures according to pre- and post-vaccination status in all 10 aspects. Before the vaccination, there was a higher level of adherence to most of the preventive behavioral measures in comparison with after receiving the vaccine.

The highest levels of adherence were reported to be associated with using a tissue, handkerchief, or elbow to cover coughs (83.5%); staying at home in the case of contact with a confirmed COVID-19 case (77.7%); staying at home in the case of experiencing influenza-like symptoms (75.2%); correctly using face masks (73.5%); and using face masks (72.7%). Lower adherence levels were reported to the remaining measures, including avoiding mass gatherings (66.7%), practicing social distancing (61.7%), performing regular hand washing/sanitizing (58.3%), and avoiding touching the mouth, eyes, and nose (47.1%). The lowest level of adherence was related to avoiding shaking hand (46.0%).

After receiving the vaccination, there was a statistically significant decline in the level of adherence to all preventive behavioral measures (Figure 2). However, the highest levels of adherence were reported to be associated with using a tissue, handkerchief, or elbow to cover coughs (76.9%); staying at home in the case of contact with a confirmed COVID-19 case (65.8%); using a face mask (53.5%); correctly using a face mask (51.7%); and staying at home in the case of having influenza-like symptoms (42.9%). Lower adherence levels were indicated for practicing social distancing (40.4%); avoiding mass gatherings (28.3%);

avoiding touching the mouth, eyes, and nose (25.0%); and avoiding shaking hand (8.8%). The lowest level of adherence was associated with regular hand washing/sanitizing (3.5%).

Table 3. Comparison of pre- and post-COVID-19 vaccination levels of adherence to personal protective measures among 480 participants in the Jazan region.

Item	Pre-Vaccination	Post-Vaccination	% Change	*p* Value *
	N (%)	N (%)		
Physical distancing 1.5–2 m				
Yes	296 (61.7)	194 (40.4)	−21.3	$p < 0.001$
No	184 (38.3)	286 (59.6)		
Use of face mask				
Yes	349 (72.7)	257 (53.5)	−19.2	$p < 0.001$
No	131 (27.3)	223 (46.5)		
Correct mask use				
Yes	353 (73.5)	248 (51.7)	−21.8	$p < 0.001$
No	127 (26.5)	232 (48.3)		
Regular hand washing and alcohol-based hand sanitizer use				
Yes	280 (58.3)	17 (3.5)	−54.8	$p = 0.002$
No	200 (41.7)	463 (96.5)		
Avoiding handshakes				
Yes	221 (46)	42 (8.8)	−37.2	$p < 0.001$
No	259 (54)	438 (91.3)		
Avoiding touching the mouth, eyes, and nose				
Yes	226 (47.1)	120 (25)	−22.1	$p < 0.001$
No	254 (52.9)	360 (75)		
Coughing by covering mouth/nose with a disposable handkerchief or coughing into the crease of the elbow				
Yes	401 (83.5)	369 (76.9)	−6.6	$p < 0.001$
No	79 (16.5)	111 (23.1)		
Staying at home in the case of influenza-like symptoms				
Yes	361 (75.2)	206 (42.9)	−32.3	$p < 0.001$
No	119 (24.8)	274 (57.1)		
Stay at home in the case of contact with a COVID-19 case				
Yes	373 (77.7)	316 (65.8)	−11.9	$p < 0.001$
No	107 (22.3)	164 (34.2)		
Avoiding mass gathering				
Yes	320 (66.7)	136 (28.3)	−38.4	$p < 0.001$
No	160 (33.3)	344 (71.7)		

* Chi-squared test.

Although a high level of adherence remained for using a tissue, handkerchief, or elbow to cover coughs (76.9%), the level of adherence decreased sharply, by around 20% to 55%, for the remaining personal protective behaviors. The highest percentage of decrease in the level of adherence was related to regular hand washing/sanitizing (54.8%), followed by avoiding mass gatherings (38.4%), avoiding shaking hands (37.2%), and staying at home in the case of experiencing influenza-like symptoms (32.3%). Lower reductions were identified for avoiding touching the mouth, eyes, and nose (22.1%); correctly using a face mask (21.8%); practicing social distancing (21.3%); using a face mask (19.2%); and staying at home in the case of contact with a confirmed COVID-19 case (11.9%). The lowest percentage of decrease in the level of adherence (6.6%) was reported to be associated with using a tissue, handkerchief, or elbow to cover coughs.

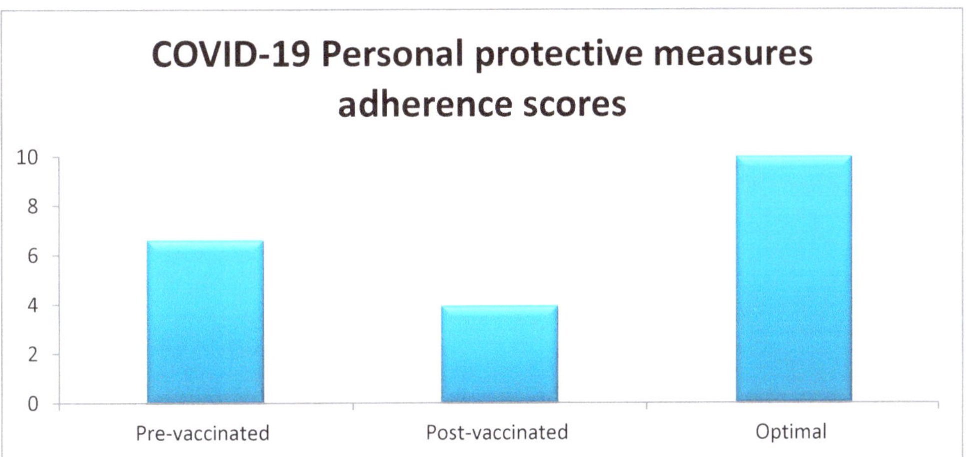

Figure 2. Optimal adherence scores regarding personal protective measures against COVID-19 and comparisons between the scores of pre-vaccinated and post-vaccinated participants in the Jazan region of Saudi Arabia.

Table 4 illustrates the correlations among the factors associated with adherence to personal protective measures against COVID-19 according to vaccination status and the health belief model. Vaccination status was associated with lower adherence to some preventive behavioral measures, including hand hygiene and avoiding close contact with sick people, possibly due to a false sense of security among vaccinated individuals. The factors identified by the current investigation as being associated with a reduction in adherence were classified into two domains. The first domain was related to predictors of behavioral change according to the health belief model, namely, perceived susceptibility, perceived severity, perceived benefits, and perceived barriers. Furthermore, the second domain was related to the nature of the determinants of adherence, classified according to the disease, the population, and the geography.

Table 4. Correlations among factors associated with adherence to personal protective measures against COVID-19 according to vaccination status and the health belief model.

Behaviour Predictors	Nature of the Determinants of Adherence			Factors Assessed According to Vaccination Status	
	Disease	Population	Geography	Pre-Vaccination	Post-Vaccination
Perceived susceptibility	√	√	√	↑ Females ↑ People in urban areas ↑ Healthcare workers	↑ Females ↑ People in urban areas ↑ Healthcare workers
Perceived severity	√	√		↑ Smokers ↑ Older age groups ↓ People with chronic diseases	↑ Smokers ↑ Older age groups ↓ People with chronic diseases
Perceived benefits	√	√		↓ People with higher education ↑ People in relationships	↔ People with higher education ↓ People in relationships

↑: suggests higher motivation. ↓: suggests lower motivation. ↔: suggests no effect on motivation.

After applying the health belief model to the constructs of the current investigation, we presumed that disease-based factors and population-based factors were associated with the perceived susceptibility, the perceived severity, and perceived health benefits. However, geography-based factors can be postulated to be associated with the perceived susceptibility only. The majority of the factors displayed in Table 4 can assumed to be motivators for adherence to personal protective measures against COVID-19, both before and after receiving the vaccine. However, being diagnosed with a chronic disease appeared to produce lower motivation for adherence, while education seemed to offer produce motivation or had no effect on the adherence level. Only the factor of being in a relationship seemed to have a motivating effect on adherence during the pre-vaccination stage but not after the vaccination, indicating the modifying effect of receiving the vaccine on the motivation for adherence.

4. Discussion

This study involved a cross-sectional investigation conducted in Jazan, Saudi Arabia, to assess adherence levels to preventive behavioral measures against COVID-19 among the community, according to their COVID-19 vaccination status. The findings indicated that the adherence to preventive measures by the participants was higher before receiving the vaccination than after. This suggests a change in the behavior of the community members toward COVID-19 due to receiving the vaccination and a reduction in adherence to respiratory hygiene practices.

The findings of our current investigation can be compared with those of similar assessments. Some previous studies have shown that vaccinated people may reduce their precautionary behavior regarding COVID-19 [11]. This would represent a real threat to controlling this epidemic and justifies investment into health education endeavors. Feeling safe and avoiding danger may induce a desire to let go of precautionary measures [12]. A comparison of this study's findings to those of similar studies assessing adherence to COVID-19 preventive measures according to vaccination status revealed similarities. In a study in India by Nizam et al., it was concluded that adherence to COVID-19 preventive measures was reduced after vaccination [13]. On the other hand, a study by Wright et al. conducted in the UK revealed contradictory findings, where an increase in the adherence level was noted even after receiving the COVID-19 vaccination [14]. Nonetheless, it can be postulated that the epidemiology of COVID-19 in the UK and the occurrence of a second wave of the disease might partially explain the extended period of adherence, even after receiving the vaccine.

All preventive behavioral practices were reduced post-vaccination, where the largest reduction was related to the practice of hand washing and the use of sanitizers, followed by the avoidance of mass gatherings and shaking hands. These results are compatible with those of previous studies in Egypt, Nigeria, and Ethiopia [15,16]. This indicates that not all COVID-19 preventive measures are given equal attention. Long-term commitment is vital to mitigate the spread of the disease and reduce its impact.

The assessment of factors associated with adherence to COVID-19 preventive behavioral measures in the current investigation after vaccination suggested that being 50 years old or older, female, a healthcare worker, and a smoker were associated with higher adherence levels compared with other groups in the same categories. Elderly people are more vulnerable to complications from COVID-19 and are thus more committed to preventive precautions, as expected [17].

A survey by Almalki recruited a sample of 597 respondents from Jazan and assessed their knowledge, attitudes, and practices concerning COVID-19 during May 2020, indicating an adequate level of knowledge, a good attitude, and acceptable practices regarding the disease [18]. However, an assessment of practices revealed that females had greater odds of reporting wearing a face mask compared with males. Considering the differences in the scope of Almalki's study and the current study, Almalki did not assess the influence of vaccination status, unlike in our research, and females exhibited higher adherence levels in the current investigation both before and after vaccination against COVID-19.

Previous studies have shown that low levels of education, occupation, and income are associated with reduced adherence to preventive measures [19,20]. The high level of knowledge among healthcare workers may be a crucial factor contributing to the high levels of adherence to preventive measures [21]. Smokers are probably more adherent to preventive measures, since their lungs are already compromised by smoking; therefore, they have a lower chance of surviving COVID-19 than healthy people [22].

According to a review by Sabaté, lack of access to healthcare, financial constraints, side effects of medication, forgetfulness, and competing priorities can act as barriers to adherence to medication. Other factors such as cultural, social, and family beliefs, attitudes, and values can influence adherence norms. In addition, the perceived benefits of treatment, social support, and healthcare–provider communication and trust are some of the drivers of adherence [23]. Disease-based factors, including the severity and chronicity of the disease, the complexity of the treatment regimen, co-morbidities, and the presence of symptoms, can all affect adherence [24]. Population-based factors, such as age, gender, race, and socioeconomic status, as well as access to healthcare and education, can also impact adherence. Health literacy and self-efficacy are other factors that may play a role in adherence [25]. Geography-based factors, including geographic location (such as rural or urban areas), and access to healthcare and transportation, as well as environmental factors such as air pollution and climate can also influence adherence [26]. Improved health outcomes and disease management, reduced healthcare costs and burden on the healthcare system, improved quality of life and productivity, increased patient satisfaction, and trust in healthcare providers are some of the positive consequences of adherence [23].

It can be noted that adherence usually refers to the uptake of a particular medication or vaccine. However, our investigation studies the effect of receiving an intervention, namely the COVID-19 vaccine, on adherence levels. As indicated in Table 4, the motivators of adherence are explained by the perceived susceptibility, perceived severity, and perceived benefit, depending on the nature of the disease, the type of the population, and the geography, whereby several explanations can be provided for the detected associations.

For example, people with relationships were noted to exhibit higher adherence levels before receiving the vaccine but not afterward. This can be associated with the reduced perceived benefit of adherence to personal protective behavior for protecting family members after receiving the vaccine. Additionally, it can be postulated that healthcare workers were more motivated to adhere to personal protective measures, both before and after receiving the vaccine, due to their perceived susceptibility and because they were at a higher risk of infection, in addition to adherence to protective measures being a requirement of their work conditions.

Perceived disease severity can partially explain the higher adherence levels among smokers and older participants, as they are at a higher risk of developing the severe consequences of the infection due to the nature of the disease and due to their personal characteristics. The higher adherence levels among those in relationships may suggest the presence of perceived benefits, as adherence to protective measures is likely to protect family members against the infection. Nonetheless, the perceived benefit of adherence was no longer present after receiving the vaccination, suggesting the presence of a behavior modification that can be partially correlated with receiving the vaccine. Nonetheless, the lower motivation among people with chronic diseases to adhere to personal preventive measures requires further assessment. Geographical determinants can be postulated to be present regarding the motivation of people in urban areas to exhibit higher adherence levels before and after receiving the vaccine due to their higher susceptibility to infection in comparison with those living in less crowded urban areas.

The current study has multiple areas of strengths and weaknesses. The main strength of the current investigation is related to the timing of the data collection and its ability to reach a sample of vaccinated individuals to enable an assessment of the adherence to preventive measures against COVID-19 before the lifting of preventive precautionary measures against COVID-19 in Saudi Arabia. Another strength area is related to the behavioral conceptualization applied in the current study and the potential ability to generalize the findings of the study to other international contexts or future pandemics of similar respiratory illnesses. The main limitation of the current investigation is related to the design, which was reliant on retrospective data collection via a cross-sectional design. Nonetheless, it is possible to argue that the practices assessed before and after receiving the vaccination were measured within a relatively short timeframe and the probability of a recall bias, though it cannot be neglected, is low.

5. Conclusions

The assessment of the levels of adherence to COVID-19 preventive measures among the community according to COVID-19 vaccination status revealed that adherence to preventive behavioral measures was higher among the participants before receiving the vaccination than afterward. All preventive behavioral practices were reduced after vaccination; the largest reduction was related to hand washing practices and the use of sanitizers, followed by the avoidance of mass gatherings and shaking hand. This indicates the importance of raising awareness about the possibility of re-infection with COVID-19 despite having been vaccinated, and increasing awareness about preventive behavioral measures, especially with the ongoing incidence of COVID-19 cases. Furthermore, this investigation indicates the need for the development of public health policies that incorporate prevention measures being maintained after exposure to a particular intervention (such as vaccination), with measures aiming to enhance overall personal hygiene (such as respiratory hygiene) in order to increase the effectiveness of the applied public health interventions in real-life situations.

Author Contributions: Conceptualization, A.A.; Validation, Y.M., M.Y.E. and M.A.M.; Investigation, A.Y.A. and Y.H.; Resources, A.D. (Abrar Doweri), I.N., F.B. and H.A.; Writing—review & editing, I.M.G.; Supervision, A.D. (Abdu Dahlan). All authors have read and agreed to the published version of the manuscript.

Funding: This research received no external funding.

Data Availability Statement: Data are available upon request due to the ethical restrictions regarding the participants' privacy. Requests for the data may be sent to the corresponding author.

Conflicts of Interest: The authors declare no conflict of interest.

References

1. World Health Organization. Weekly Epidemiological Update on COVID-19. 21 December 2022. Available online: https://www.who.int/publications/m/item/covid-19-weekly-epidemiological-update---21-december-2022 (accessed on 8 March 2023).
2. World Health Organization Saudi Arabia Situation. 2023. Available online: https://covid19.who.int/region/emro/country/sa (accessed on 8 March 2023).
3. World Health Organization. WHO Coronavirus (COVID-19) Dashboard. Available online: https://covid19.who.int/table (accessed on 8 March 2023).
4. World Health Organization. Tracking SARS-CoV-2 Variants. Available online: https://www.who.int/activities/tracking-SARS-CoV-2-variants (accessed on 8 March 2023).
5. Maier, B.F.; Brockmann, D. Effective containment explains subexponential growth in recent confirmed COVID-19 cases in China. *Science* **2020**, *368*, 742–746. [CrossRef] [PubMed]
6. Institute for Governemnt Key Lockdowns and Measure Introduced during the COVID Pandemic between March 2020 and December 2021. Available online: https://www.instituteforgovernment.org.uk/data-visualisation/timeline-coronavirus-lockdowns (accessed on 8 March 2023).
7. Centers for Disease Control and Prevention Respiratory Hygiene/Cough Etiquette. Available online: https://www.cdc.gov/oralhealth/infectioncontrol/faqs/respiratory-hygiene.html#print (accessed on 8 March 2023).
8. Betsch, C. How behavioural science data helps mitigate the COVID-19 crisis. *Nat. Hum. Behav.* **2020**, *4*, 438. [CrossRef] [PubMed]
9. Rahamim-Cohen, D.; Gazit, S.; Perez, G.; Nada, B.; Moshe, S.B.; Mizrahi-Reuveni, M.; Azuri, J.; Patalon, T. Survey of Behaviour Attitudes Towards Preventive Measures Following COVID-19 Vaccination. *medRxiv* **2021**. [CrossRef]

10. Majam, M.; Fischer, A.; Phiri, J.; Venter, F.; Lalla-Edward, S.T. International citizen project to assess early stage adherence to public health measures for COVID-19 in South Africa. *PLoS ONE* **2021**, *16*, e0248055. [CrossRef] [PubMed]
11. Desrichard, O.; Moussaoui, L.; Ofosu, N. Reduction of Precautionary Behaviour following Vaccination against COVID-19: A Test on a British Cohort. *Vaccines* **2022**, *10*, 936. [CrossRef] [PubMed]
12. World Health Organization. Mental Health and Psychosocial Considerations during the COVID-19 Outbreak. Available online: https://www.who.int/publications/i/item/WHO-2019-nCoV-MentalHealth-2020.1 (accessed on 8 March 2023).
13. Nizam, J.; Parasuramalu, B.G.; Manjunatha, S. Assessment of adherence to COVID appropriate behavior among post-vaccinated individuals in rural practice area of Raja Rajeswari medical college and hospital, Bengaluru. *Int. J. Community Med. Public Health* **2022**, *9*, 1474–1478. [CrossRef]
14. Wright, L.; Steptoe, A.; Mak, H.W.; Fancourt, D. Do people reduce compliance with COVID-19 guidelines following vaccination? A longitudinal analysis of matched UK adults. *J. Epidemiol. Community Health* **2022**, *76*, 109–115. [CrossRef] [PubMed]
15. Bante, A.; Mersha, A.; Tesfaye, A.; Tsegaye, B.; Shibiru, S.; Ayele, G.; Girma, M. Adherence with COVID-19 Preventive Measures and Associated Factors Among Residents of Dirashe District, Southern Ethiopia. *Patient Prefer. Adherence* **2021**, *15*, 237–249. [CrossRef] [PubMed]
16. Elnadi, H.; Odetokun, I.A.; Bolarinwa, O.; Ahmed, Z.; Okechukwu, O.; Al-Mustapha, A.I. Correction: Knowledge, attitude, and perceptions towards the 2019 Coronavirus Pandemic: A bi-national survey in Africa. *PLoS ONE* **2021**, *16*, e0247351. [CrossRef] [PubMed]
17. Alam, M.S.; Sultana, R.; Haque, M.A. Vulnerabilities of older adults and mitigation measures to address COVID-19 outbreak in Bangladesh: A review. *Soc. Sci. Humanit. Open* **2022**, *6*, 100336. [CrossRef] [PubMed]
18. Almalki, M.J. Knowledge, Attitudes, and Practices Toward COVID-19 Among the General Public in the Border Region of Jazan, Saudi Arabia: A Cross-Sectional Study. *Front. Public Health* **2021**, *9*, 733125. [CrossRef] [PubMed]
19. Abeya, S.G.; Barkesa, S.B.; Sadi, C.G.; Gemeda, D.D.; Muleta, F.Y.; Tolera, A.F.; Ayana, D.N.; Mohammed, S.A.; Wako, E.B.; Hurisa, M.B.; et al. Adherence to COVID-19 preventive measures and associated factors in Oromia regional state of Ethiopia. *PLoS ONE* **2021**, *16*, e0257373. [CrossRef] [PubMed]
20. Ahmed, H.M. Adherence to COVID-19 preventive measures among male medical students, Egypt. *J. Egypt. Public Health Assoc.* **2022**, *97*, 8. [CrossRef] [PubMed]
21. Alhumaid, S.; Al Mutair, A.; Al Alawi, Z.; Alsuliman, M.; Ahmed, G.Y.; Rabaan, A.A.; Al-Tawfiq, J.A.; Al-Omari, A. Knowledge of infection prevention and control among healthcare workers and factors influencing compliance: A systematic review. *Antimicrob. Resist. Infect. Control* **2021**, *10*, 86. [CrossRef]
22. He, Y.; Sun, J.; Ding, X.; Wang, Q. Mechanisms in Which Smoking Increases the Risk of COVID-19 Infection: A Narrative Review. *Iran J. Public Health* **2021**, *50*, 431–437. [CrossRef]
23. Sabaté, E.; Sabaté, E. *Adherence to Long-Term Therapies: Evidence for Action*; World Health Organization: Geneva, Switzerland, 2003.
24. Lash, T.L.; Fox, M.P.; Fink, A.K. *Applying Quantitative Bias Analysis to Epidemiologic Data*; Statistics for Biology and Health; Springer: New York, NY, USA, 2009; Volume XII, p. 192. [CrossRef]
25. Shrank, W.; Avorn, J.; Rolon, C.; Shekelle, P. Medication Safety: Effect of Content and Format of Prescription Drug Labels on Readability, Understanding, and Medication Use: A Systematic Review. *Ann. Pharmacother.* **2007**, *41*, 783–801. [CrossRef] [PubMed]
26. Galende, N.; Redondo, I.; Dosil-Santamaria, M.; Ozamiz-Etxebarria, N. Factors Influencing Compliance with COVID-19 Health Measures: A Spanish Study to Improve Adherence Campaigns. *Int. J. Environ. Res. Public Health* **2022**, *19*, 4853. [CrossRef] [PubMed]

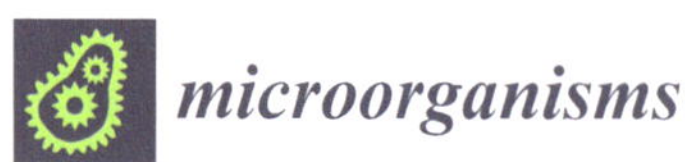 *microorganisms*

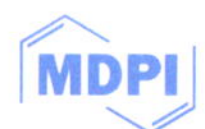

Review

Indirect Effects of the COVID-19 Pandemic on Routine Childhood Vaccination in Low-Income Countries: A Systematic Review to Set the Scope for Future Pandemics

Jessica E. Beetch [1], Amanda Janitz [1], Laura A. Beebe [1], Mary Gowin [2], Chao Xu [1], Shari Clifton [3] and Katrin Gaardbo Kuhn [1,*]

[1] Department of Biostatistics and Epidemiology, Hudson College of Public Health, University of Oklahoma Health Sciences, Oklahoma City, OK 73104, USA; jessica-beetch@ouhsc.edu (J.E.B.); amanda-janitz@ouhsc.edu (A.J.); laura-beebe@ouhsc.edu (L.A.B.); chao-xu@ouhsc.edu (C.X.)

[2] Department of Health Promotion Sciences, Hudson College of Public Health, University of Oklahoma Health Sciences, Oklahoma City, OK 73104, USA; mary-gowin@ouhsc.edu

[3] Robert M. Bird Health Sciences Library, University of Oklahoma Health Sciences, Oklahoma City, OK 73104, USA; shari-clifton@ouhsc.edu

* Correspondence: katrin-kuhn@ouhsc.edu; Tel.: +1-(405)-271-2229

Abstract: The COVID-19 pandemic halted progress in global vaccine coverage and disrupted routine childhood vaccination practices worldwide. While there is ample evidence of the vaccination decline experienced during the pandemic, it is less clear how low-income countries were affected. We executed a systematic review to synthesize the current literature on the impacts of routine childhood vaccinations in low-income countries from 1 January 2020 to 8 February 2023. We collected data using an extraction form on Covidence and assessed the quality of studies included in the review using the Risk of Bias in Non-Randomized Studies of Interventions (ROBINS-I) tool. Effect estimates for changes in vaccination during the pandemic were reported and summarized. Factors that influenced changes were grouped into descriptive themes. Thirteen studies, encompassing 18 low-income countries and evaluating 15 vaccines at varying doses, were included in the final review. We found that routine childhood vaccinations during the COVID-19 pandemic varied considerably by vaccine type, location, and phase of the pandemic. Nine different themes were identified as factors that influenced changes in vaccination. Documenting past experiences and lessons learned is crucial for informing preparedness efforts in anticipation of future public health emergencies. Failure to effectively address these things in the next public health emergency could result in a recurrence of declining routine childhood vaccinations.

Keywords: COVID-19; pandemic; vaccination; public health; children; low-income

Citation: Beetch, J.E.; Janitz, A.; Beebe, L.A.; Gowin, M.; Xu, C.; Clifton, S.; Kuhn, K.G. Indirect Effects of the COVID-19 Pandemic on Routine Childhood Vaccination in Low-Income Countries: A Systematic Review to Set the Scope for Future Pandemics. *Microorganisms* **2024**, *12*, 573. https://doi.org/10.3390/microorganisms12030573

Academic Editor: Qibin Geng

Received: 12 February 2024
Revised: 9 March 2024
Accepted: 11 March 2024
Published: 13 March 2024

1. Introduction

Global vaccination, particularly in children, has had a profound impact on public health in recent centuries. Routine childhood vaccines have prevented multiple diseases that can be fatal or cause life-long disabilities and are a catalyst for improved overall health. Vaccination programs have successfully reduced the incidence of previously virulent diseases like polio, measles, and influenza and have eradicated smallpox, one of the deadliest diseases in history [1]. Adequate vaccination coverage is essential to create herd immunity. With herd immunity, a sufficient number of individuals are vaccinated so that the disease is less likely to spread to those who cannot be vaccinated, like those who are too young or have certain health conditions. When vaccination coverage drops and herd immunity subsides, outbreaks are more likely to arise [2].

Prior to the onset of the COVID-19 pandemic, vaccination coverage had greatly improved over several decades, reducing the incidence of many vaccine-preventable diseases worldwide [3]. Although vaccines are administered for numerous diseases throughout the world, the third dose of diphtheria, tetanus, and pertussis (DTP 3) vaccine is a good indicator of access to immunization services and is therefore commonly used as a metric for global vaccination coverage [4]. DTP 3 global vaccination coverage remained at 86% from 2016 to 2019 after steadily increasing over recent decades. However, global vaccination coverage for DTP 3 decreased to 83% in 2020 (ranging from 72% in Africa to 95% in the Western Pacific) [5] and 81% in 2021 (ranging from 71% in Africa to 94% in Europe) [6]. Even a small drop in global vaccination coverage implies that millions of children did not receive the DTP 3 vaccine and other important routine vaccinations. With the emergence of COVID-19 came a shift in prioritization of services, resulting in delays in medical care and declines in vaccination coverage [7]. Although vaccine services were delayed for all ages, including adults, the largest declines in vaccination were observed in children [8]. The United Nations International Children's Emergency Fund (UNICEF) described a major backslide in childhood vaccinations caused by the pandemic [9]. In 2020, 23 million children missed routine vaccinations, almost four million more than in 2019. A majority of those children did not receive a single vaccine of any type, widening vaccine inequities. This worsened in 2021, when global vaccine coverage was the lowest it had been since 2007 [10]. Even in countries that had widespread access to the COVID-19 vaccine, other routine vaccinations slipped, leaving children at risk for preventable diseases [9]. A multitude of factors contribute to reductions in vaccination coverage, including local vaccination culture, vaccine hesitancy, and vaccine mandates, as well as access to care and adequate vaccine supply [11]. Vaccination coverage started to recover in 2022 when DTP 3 vaccine coverage increased to 84% globally (Africa = 72%, Americas = 83%, Eastern Mediterranean = 84%, Europe = 94%, South East Asia = 91%, and Western Pacific = 93%) [12]. However, millions of children were still missing out on vaccines compared to before the pandemic began. Low-income countries experienced a slower recovery, with some areas encountering ongoing declines and stagnant trends. Recovery has not been equal, even within low-income countries, due to inequitable jobs and welfare and different levels of urgency to ensure vaccine accessibility after the COVID-19 lockdowns. The speed of recovery has also been influenced by high populations of children and civil unrest within countries [13]. The pandemic has been a stark reminder that vaccine distribution has been inequitable throughout time, and the poorest children continue to be the least likely to receive vaccines [4].

While it is known that the COVID-19 pandemic impacted routine childhood vaccination, with declines in vaccine administration seen worldwide [14], these effects have not been thoroughly studied in all major population segments. Research is often heavily concentrated in high-income countries, with a lack of attention to outcomes in lower-income countries [15]. Previous reviews have identified disruptions to routine vaccination practices globally [16,17] or in both low- and middle-income countries [18,19] but have never specifically focused on the impacts to low-income countries. Although routine vaccination disruption in low-income countries has been discussed as a concern [20], the topic has not been synthesized in a systematic review. Further, no papers in the literature have studied the quantitative impacts of the pandemic on routine vaccination combined with the qualitative suspected factors influencing changes in vaccination practices in low-income countries. It is essential to study populations that are vulnerable to poverty, such as low-income countries, to gather information about their unique situations and the contributing factors to vaccine uptake. Populations vulnerable to poverty often face disproportionate outcomes in mental health, birth defects, and chronic and infectious diseases and experience systemic inequalities, like discrimination and differential resources, which increase their risk of severe health outcomes [21]. Although childhood poverty persists throughout the world, even in high-income countries, it is most prevalent in lower-income countries located throughout Sub-Saharan Africa and South Asia [22]. The pandemic has emphasized the necessity to address health inequities and conduct research on these low-income groups.

Consequences emerge when routine vaccination practices change, especially in low-income areas. When vaccination declines, there is a higher risk of contracting vaccine-preventable diseases and the potential for outbreaks increases. These adverse outcomes, along with other social and economic factors such as reduced education, employment, and safety in low-income populations, exacerbate their health risk. It is not only important to understand the extent to which the pandemic impacted routine childhood vaccinations, but also which populations bore the impacts disproportionately. To the best of our knowledge, this systematic review will be the first to address the pandemic's impact on routine childhood vaccinations in low-income countries worldwide by collecting relevant published evidence on this topic. The overall goal of this review is to increase understanding of how children in low-income countries worldwide experienced indirect impacts on their health due to the COVID-19 pandemic. It is vital to study the pandemic's impacts and identify high-risk groups to prepare for the next large outbreak or public health emergency.

The objectives of this systematic review were to identify and evaluate how the COVID-19 pandemic impacted routine childhood vaccinations in low-income countries by (i) identifying changes in vaccination rates and (ii) identifying reported factors that led to changes in vaccination rates in studies published from 1 January 2020 to 8 February 2023.

2. Materials and Methods

2.1. Protocol

We prepared the systematic review protocol using guidance from Preferred Reporting Items for Systematic Reviews and Meta-Analyses (PRISMA 2020) [23] with additional recommendations from Conducting Systematic Reviews and Meta-Analyses of Observational Studies of Etiology (COSMOS-E) [24]. We registered the protocol with the International Prospective Register of Ongoing Systematic Reviews, United Kingdom (PROSPERO CRD42023491742).

2.2. Eligibility Criteria

Studies were selected according to the following criteria:

2.2.1. Population

This review focused on the impacts of the pandemic on children in low-income countries. It only included studies focusing on persons 18 years of age and younger residing in countries with a low-income economy (USD $1085 or less as of February 2023). The 28 low-income countries worldwide include Afghanistan, Burkina Faso, Burundi, the Central African Republic, Chad, the Democratic Republic of the Congo, Eritrea, Ethiopia, Gambia, Guinea, Guinea-Bissau, Liberia, Madagascar, Malawi, Mali, Mozambique, Niger, North Korea, Rwanda, Sierra Leone, Somalia, South Sudan, Sudan, Syrian Arab Republic, Togo, Uganda, Yemen, and Zambia [25]. All genders and racial/ethnic groups were eligible for inclusion.

2.2.2. Exposure and Comparison

We included studies published from 1 January 2020, the month after the first COVID-19 case was discovered, until 8 February 2023, the day before the search took place. The exposure of interest was the three-year time period (1 January 2020 to 8 February 2023) that included COVID-19 emergence and a significant portion of the COVID-19 pandemic. The comparison time period (31 December 2019 and before) included the time prior to COVID-19 emergence. All included studies were needed to compare outcomes during the COVID-19 time period to those of the pre-COVID-19 time period.

2.2.3. Outcome

The outcomes of interest were two separate components related to routine childhood vaccination practices. These components included potential quantitative changes in vaccination rates and qualitative factors that led to the changes. The definition and calculation of changes in routine childhood vaccination vary between locations. Therefore, for this review, we considered all routine vaccinations that were reported as relevant for each study population and location.

2.2.4. Study Design

We included retrospective cohort studies, case–control studies, ecological studies, cross-sectional studies, and papers analyzing local or national surveillance data.

2.2.5. Language

We only included studies that were reported in the English language.

2.2.6. Exclusions

We excluded studies not covering routine childhood vaccinations, papers not published in English, studies that reported results from only high- or middle-income countries, and studies that did not directly relate the COVID-19 pandemic to the indirect impacts on childhood vaccinations. Further, we excluded systematic and narrative reviews, modeling studies, single case studies, laboratory studies, letters, reports, editorials, commentaries, and studies with only qualitative results, such as surveys with caregiver opinions.

2.3. Search Strategy

We searched the available literature on Ovid MEDLINE® and Epub Ahead of Print, In-Process, In-Data-Review, and Other Non-Indexed Citations. The search was executed on 9 February 2023. To focus on impacts of the COVID-19 pandemic, the search was limited to studies published from 1 January 2020 to 8 February 2023. The search used a combination of controlled vocabulary terms and keywords to incorporate the following concepts of "immunization, vaccination or vaccine, low-income, SARS-CoV-2, COVID-19, pediatric or child or infant or neonate or adolescent or teen or youth, and routine or schedule or catchup", the search functions "exploded and multi-purpose", and Boolean operators "and, or". Search strategy and keywords were discussed and finalized with the Associate Director and Head of Reference and Instructional Services at the Robert M. Bird Health Sciences Library (S.C.).

2.4. Result Screening and Selection

Screening and selection of articles were conducted using the web-based application Covidence [26]. Articles produced by the literature search were screened for inclusion using a two-step process. Firstly, articles were screened based on their title and abstract to remove duplicates and irrelevant papers. Secondly, the remaining papers required full-text review to determine eligibility. Articles were excluded if they did not meet the eligibility criteria, including those with ineligible study designs, outcomes, and/or populations. Screening and selection of articles were completed independently by two reviewers to reduce error. Discrepancies were discussed and resolved by the two-reviewer team (J.E.B. and K.G.K.).

2.5. Data Collection

Data collection was completed using a customized extraction form developed on Covidence [26]. Data collection questions were developed using data extraction guidelines from COSMOS-E. This included the collection of bibliographic information, study design, study participant characteristics, exposure(s) and outcomes, and effect measures from each included paper [24]. Data items were collected independently by one reviewer (J.E.B.) and then examined for errors by a second reviewer (K.G.K.).

2.6. Data Items

Using the customized data collection form, the data extracted from each paper are itemized in Table 1.

Table 1. Data items collected from included papers.

Type	Item
Bibliographic information	Authors
	Publication month and year
	Digital object identifier (DOI)
Study design	Assessment of the study design that was completed
Study participant characteristics	Geographic location of study
	Age groups studied
	Population description
Exposure(s) and outcomes	Time period of the study
	Vaccine(s) studied
Effect measures	Type of measure
	Effect estimate
	Measure before the COVID-19 pandemic, if available
	Measure during the COVID-19 pandemic, if available
Qualitative factors	Factors associated with changes in measurement

2.7. Risk of Bias Assessment

We appraised the methodological quality of the papers included in the review using bias domains and scoring categories from the Risk of Bias in Non-Randomized Studies of Interventions (ROBINS-I) tool by Cochrane [27]. ROBINS-I bias domains used in the assessment included bias due to confounding, bias in the selection of participants into the study, bias in the measurement of exposures and outcomes, bias due to missing data, and bias in the selection of studies or reported results. Scoring categories for risk of bias judgement for each domain were low risk, moderate risk, and high risk. The risk of bias assessment was conducted independently by two reviewers. Discrepancies were discussed and resolved by the two-reviewer team (J.E.B. and K.G.K.).

2.8. Data Synthesis

We anticipated considerable differences in study periods, vaccine types, and analyses between studies; therefore, a meta-analysis was deemed inappropriate due to substantial heterogeneity. However, effect estimates for quantitative changes in vaccination during the pandemic were reported and summarized by 'decline in vaccination' and 'increase in vaccination' groups. We also conducted a narrative synthesis of factors that influenced changes in effect estimates. We extracted these factors from results, findings, or discussion sections from each study included in the review. We entered the factors extracted from the studies verbatim into the Covidence extraction form. Finally, we manually grouped the reoccurring factors and developed descriptive themes [28].

3. Results

3.1. Study Selection

We identified 118 studies from the extended MEDLINE file from 1 January 2020 to 8 February 2023 (Supplementary Table S1). After removing one duplicate paper, we excluded 68 papers during title and abstract screening that did not meet eligibility criteria for reasons such as ineligible outcomes, population, location, and study design (Figure 1). Four of the 49 remaining papers were unable to be accessed or retrieved. We completed a full-text review on 45 papers where studies were excluded due to outcomes not pertaining to routine vaccination practices (n = 6), studies focusing on adult populations instead of children (n = 3), wrong study design (n = 22), and duplicate outcomes due to use of the same vaccine data (n = 1). The final review included 13 studies in total (Figure 1).

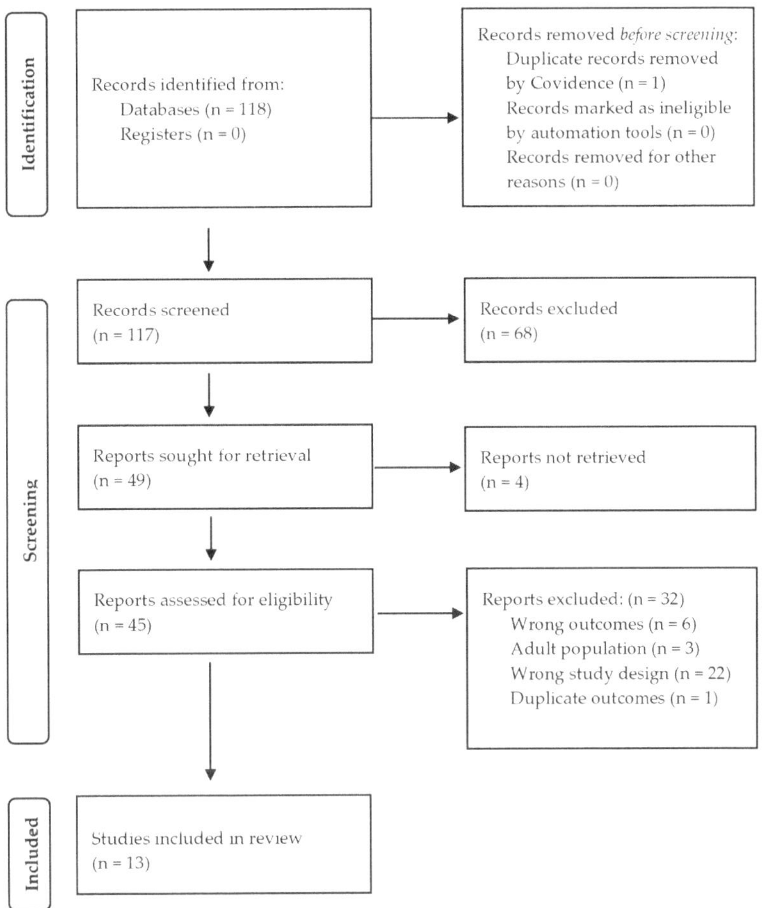

Figure 1. PRISMA 2020 flow diagram of study selection.

3.2. Study Characteristics

The 13 studies selected for inclusion assessed changes in routine vaccination in 18 low-income countries including Afghanistan, Burundi, the Central African Republic, Chad, the Democratic Republic of the Congo, Eritrea, Ethiopia, Gambia, Liberia, Malawi, Mali, Mozambique, Rwanda, Sierra Leone, Somalia, South Sudan, Uganda, and Yemen (highlighted in dark blue in Figure 2). Some studies were set in capital cities, while others examined part of a country, a single country, or a group of countries. While all 13 studies assessed routine vaccination changes in children, one paper specifically studied newborns [29], one paper studied children younger than one year of age [30], and two papers studied children younger than five years of age [31,32]. The studies assessed 15 different vaccines at varying doses including Bacillus Calmette–Guerin for tuberculosis (BCG), polio (Pol), inactivated polio vaccine (IPV), oral polio vaccine (OPV), combined diphtheria, tetanus, and pertussis, hepatitis B, Haemophilus influenzae type b (DTP Hep B Hib), diphtheria, tetanus, and pertussis (DTP), hepatitis B (Hep B), pneumococcal, pneumococcal conjugate vaccine (PCV), rotavirus (Rota), measles-containing vaccine (MCV), measles and rubella, pentavalent (Penta), malaria intermittent preventive treatment (IPTi) and yellow fever, while some studies examined overall vaccination or fully vaccinated status. The study periods ranged from January 2016 to February 2021 but were published between

September 2020 and December 2022. Methodologically, five studies used a cross-sectional study design [29,31–34], five used an interrupted time series study design [35–39], two used a cohort study design [30,40], and one used a mixed methods study design [41].

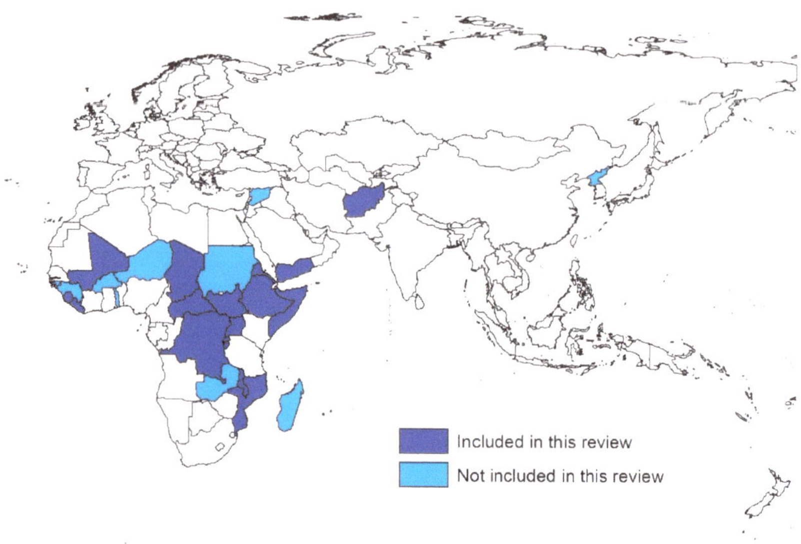

Figure 2. The 28 low-income countries worldwide, as defined by the World Bank.

3.3. Changes in Vaccination

The number of children who received routine vaccinations during the COVID-19 pandemic varied considerably by vaccine type, location, and phase of the pandemic (Table 2). Although declines in vaccination practices were seen at some point in the pandemic in every low-income country studied, some countries experienced nonsignificant changes while others observed increases in vaccination during the pandemic compared to before it began. The effect estimates captured include measures of mean values, observed values, and percent change (Table 3).

Table 2. Study characteristics of included studies, (n = 13).

Citation	Location	Time Period	Age Group	Vaccines	Key Findings *	
Abid 2022 [31]	Laghman, Afghanistan	April–July 2019 (baseline) compared to April–July 2020 (pandemic)	Children under 5	Overall vaccination, BCG, DTP, Hep B, IPV, MCV, OPV, PCV, Penta 1, Rota 1–2	Significant declines in vaccination for all vaccines studied	↓
Arsenault 2022 [39]	Ethiopia	January 2019–March 2020 (baseline) compared to April–December 2020 (pandemic)	Children	BCG, Penta, Pneumococcal, Rota, MCV	Non-significant declines in vaccination for all vaccines studied	↓

Table 2. *Cont.*

Citation	Location	Time Period	Age Group	Vaccines	Key Findings *	
Buonsenso 2020 [32]	Rural Western Area, Sierra Leone	1 March–26 April 2019 (baseline) compared to 1 March–26 April 2020 (pandemic)	Children under 5	BCG, OPV 0–2, Penta 1–3, PCV 1–3, Rota 1–2, IPTi 1–3, IPV, MCV 1–2, Yellow fever	Significant declines in vaccination for all vaccines studied	↓
Burt 2021 [38]	Kampala, Uganda	July 2019–March 2020 (baseline), April–June 2020 (pandemic)	Children	Overall vaccination	Significant decline in immunization clinic attendance	↓
Connolly 2022 [30]	Liberia and Malawi	January 2016–February 2020 (baseline) compared to March 2020–August 2020 (early pandemic) and September 2020-February 2021 (late pandemic)	Children under 1	BCG, OPV or IPV 0–3, Penta 1–3, PCV 1–3, Rota 1–2, MCV	Non-significant decline in vaccination in Malawi, and non-significant increase in vaccination in Liberia	↑↓
das Neves Martins Pires 2021 [41]	Nampula, Mozambique	March–May 2019 (baseline) compared to March–May 2020 (pandemic)	Children	Overall vaccination	Non-significant declines in vaccination	↓
Gebreegziabher 2022 [34]	Addis Ababa, Ethiopia	July–September 2019 (baseline) compared to April–June 2020 (pandemic)	Children	Penta 1, Penta 3, MCV, fully vaccinated	Non-significant decline in Penta 1 and 3 vaccination and fully vaccinated status, and non-significant increase in MCV vaccination	↑↓
Kassie 2021 [29]	South West Ethiopia	March–June 2019 (baseline) compared to March–June 2020 (pandemic)	Newborns	Penta 1, MCV 1	Significant declines in vaccination for both vaccines studied	↓
Kotiso 2022 [40]	Yemen	January–June 2019 (baseline) compared to February–June 2020 (pandemic)	Children	Penta 3	Significant decline in vaccination in February, April, May and June, and non-significant increase in March	↑↓

Table 2. *Cont.*

Citation	Location	Time Period	Age Group	Vaccines	Key Findings *	
Masresha 2020 [37]	Central African Republic, Chad, Democratic Republic of the Congo, South Sudan, Burundi, Eritrea, Rwanda	January–March 2020 (baseline) compared to April–June 2020 (pandemic)	Children	DPT 3, MCV 1	Declines and increases in vaccination for both vaccines	↑↓
Osei 2022 [36]	Rural Gambia	1 September 2019–31 March 2020 (baseline), 1 April–30 June 2020 (interruption), 1 July–30 September 2020 (initial recovery), 1 October–31 December 2020 (late recovery)	Children	Overall vaccination, BCG, Hep B, Penta 1, OPV 1, PCV 1, Rota 1	Declines in vaccination for all vaccines during interruption, and declines and increases in vaccination during initial and late recovery depending on vaccine	↑↓
Shapira 2021 [35]	Democratic Republic of the Congo, Liberia, Malawi, Mali, Sierra Leone, Somalia	January 2018–February 2020 (baseline) compared to March–July 2020 (pandemic)	Children	BCG, Penta 3	Significant declines in vaccination for Penta 3 in three countries, significant declines in vaccination for BCG in two countries, significant increase in BCG in one country, and non-significant results for vaccinations in other countries	↑↓
Wanyana 2021 [33]	Rwanda	March–April 2019 (baseline) compared to March–April 2020 (pandemic)	Children	BCG, Pol 0–3, IPV, DTP Hep B Hib 1–3, Pneumococcal 1–3, Rota 1–2, Measles + Rubella	Significant declines in 11 vaccines, non-significant declines in four vaccines, and non-significant increase in one vaccine	↑↓

Note: Significance was determined using results displayed in Table 3. * Downward pointing arrows signify declines in vaccination. Downward and upward pointing arrows signify declines and increases in vaccination.

Table 3. Vaccination change results of included studies.

Citation	Measure Type	Results
Abid 2022 [31]	Daily vaccination coverage percent change	Overall vaccination coverage: -21.4% ($p < 0.001$) * BCG: -19% ($p < 0.001$) * DTP 2: -22% ($p < 0.001$) *, 3: -23% ($p < 0.001$) * Hep B: -6% ($p < 0.001$) * IPV: -23% ($p < 0.001$) * MCV: -28% ($p < 0.001$) * OPV 0: -18% ($p < 0.001$) *, 1: -19% ($p < 0.001$) *, 2: -22% ($p < 0.001$) *, 3: -23% ($p < 0.001$) *, 4: -28% ($p < 0.001$) * PCV 1: -21% ($p < 0.001$) *, 2: -23% ($p < 0.001$) *, 3: -26% ($p < 0.001$) * Penta 1: -19% ($p < 0.001$) * Rota 1: -20% ($p < 0.001$) *, 2: -23% ($p < 0.001$) *
Arsenault 2022 [39]	Vaccination coverage percent change	Fully vaccinated by 1 year: -0.91% (95% CI: -3.91, 2.1) BCG: -5.12% (95% CI: -14.73, 4.5) MCV: -1.69% (95% CI: -6.24, 2.87) Penta: -4.02% (95% CI: -10.84, 2.83) Pneumococcal: -3.97% (95% CI: -11.19, 3.26) Rota: -2.15% (95% CI: -7.73, 3.43)
Buonsenso 2020 [32]	Vaccination coverage percent change	BCG: -52.7% ($p < 0.0005$) * OPV 0: -52.7% ($p < 0.0005$) *, 1: -70.7% ($p < 0.0005$) *, 2: -78.9% ($p < 0.0005$) *, 3: -77.6% ($p < 0.0005$) * Penta 1: -70.7% ($p < 0.0005$) *, 2: -78.9% ($p < 0.0005$) *, 3: -77.6% ($p < 0.0005$) * PCV 1: -70.7% ($p < 0.0005$) *, 2: -78.9% ($p < 0.0005$) *, 3: -77.6% ($p < 0.0005$) * Rota 1: -70.7% ($p < 0.0005$) *, 2: -78.9% ($p < 0.0005$) * IPTI 1: -69.4% ($p < 0.0005$) *, 2: -65.9% ($p < 0.0005$) *, 3: -51.1% ($p < 0.0005$) * IPV: -77.6% ($p < 0.0005$) * MCV 1: -65.6% ($p < 0.0005$) *, 2: -83.7% ($p < 0.0005$) * Yellow fever: -65.6% ($p < 0.0005$) *
Burt 2021 [38]	Vaccination clinic attendance	Baseline: 5871 (95% CI: 5643, 6094) Pandemic: 906 (95% CI: 771, 2248) ($p = 0.04$) *
Connolly 2022 [30]	Vaccination coverage percent change	*Whole period* Overall vaccination coverage: 8% (95% CI: -12.1, 15.9) for Liberia, -2% (95% CI: -14.1, 12.6) for Malawi *Early pandemic* Overall vaccination coverage: -17% (95% CI: -39.1, -8) * for Liberia, 13.7% (95% CI: 2.4, 33.6) * for Malawi *Late pandemic* Overall vaccination coverage: 27% (95% CI: -12.5, 56.5) for Liberia, -9% (95% CI: -18, -3.9) * for Malawi
das Neves Martins Pires 2021 [41]	Vaccination coverage percent change	Overall vaccination coverage: -20% ($p = 0.197$) Complete vaccination: -18% ($p = 0.544$)
Gebreegziabher 2022 [34]	Vaccination coverage percent change	Fully vaccinated: -0.6% ($p = 0.95$) Penta 1: -0.3% ($p = 0.94$), 3: -4.7% ($p = 0.27$) MCV: 1.7% ($p = 0.86$)
Kassie 2021 [29]	Vaccination coverage proportion change	Penta: -0.033 ($p = 0.011$) * MCV: -0.031 ($p = 0.008$) *
Kotiso 2022 [40]	Vaccination coverage change	*February* Penta 3: -3.46 (95% CI: -6.63, -0.29) * *March* Penta 3: 0.02 (95% CI: -4.32, 4.37) *April* Penta 3: -6.09 (95% CI: -10.36, -1.82) * *May* Penta 3: -24.47 (95% CI: -30.56, -18.38) * *June* Penta 3: -15.31 (95% CI: -20.18, -10.45) *

Table 3. *Cont.*

Citation	Measure Type	Results
Masresha 2020 [37]	Mean monthly vaccination dose percent change	Central African Republic DPT 3: −3%, MCV 1: −3% Chad DPT 3: 6%, MCV 1: 13% Democratic Republic of the Congo DPT 3: 1%, MCV 1: 2% South Sudan DPT 3: −7%, MCV 1: 9% Burundi DPT 3: −12%, MCV 1: −20% Eritrea DPT 3: −9%, MCV 1: 2% Rwanda DPT 3: −2%, MCV 1: −4%
Osei 2022 [36]	Vaccination coverage percent change	*Interruption* Vaccine administration: −38.3% BCG: −47.2% Hep B: −46.9% Penta 1: −43.1% OPV 1: −83.6% PCV 1: −42.4% Rota 1: −43.4% *Initial recovery* Vaccine administration: −15.1% BCG: −20% Hep B: −20% Penta 1: −33% OPV 1: −34% PCV 1: −33% Rota 1: −34% MCV: 79% Yellow fever: 88.9% *Late recovery* Vaccine administration: 1.9% BCG: 3% Hep B: 2.5% OPV 1: 22.7% PCV 1: −2% Rota 1: −2.6%
Shapira 2021 [35]	Vaccination coverage percent change	Democratic Republic of the Congo BCG: −1.4% (95% CI: −3.4, 0.6), Penta 3: −0.1% (95% CI: −1.2, 1) Liberia BCG: 0.3% (95% CI: −5.2, 5.8), Penta 3: −7.8% (95% CI: −13, −2.5) * Malawi BCG: 5.6% (95% CI: 0.5, 10.8) *, Penta 3: 1.2% (95% CI: −2.5, 4.9) Mali BCG: −11.8% (95% CI: −15.4, −8.2) *, Penta 3: −17.4% (95% CI: −22.6, −12.3) * Sierra Leone BCG: −7.4% (95% CI: −11.9, −2.9) *, Penta 3: −12.6% (95% CI: −19.1, −6.1) * Somalia BCG: −2.4% (95% CI: −8.9, 4.2), Penta 3: −3.6% (95% CI: −9.8, 2.6)

Table 3. *Cont.*

Citation	Measure Type	Results
Wanyana 2021 [33]	Vaccination utilization rate change	BCG: -0.104 ($p = 0.002$) * Pol 0: -0.106 ($p = 0.001$) *, 1: -0.080 ($p = 0.008$) *, 2: -0.075 ($p = 0.008$) *, 3: -0.050 ($p = 0.081$) IPV: -0.047 (0.101) DTP HepB Hib 1: -0.080 (0.007) *, 2: -0.076 (0.007) *, 3: -0.050 (0.078) Pneumococcal 1: -0.081 (0.007) *, 2: -0.076 (0.007) *, 3: -0.050 (0.079) Rota 1: -0.083 (0.006) *, 2: -0.075 (0.009) * Measles + rubella 1: 0.014 (0.642), 2: -0.011 (0.625)

Note: Estimates are listed by vaccine dose when applicable. Doses range from 0 to 4 depending on the recommended schedule for each vaccine. * Significant results, $p < 0.05$.

3.3.1. Declines in Vaccination

Laghman, Afghanistan, faced a 21.4% ($p < 0.001$) decline in overall vaccination from April to July 2020 [31]. Liberia experienced a 17.0% decline in overall vaccination coverage (95% CI: -39.1, -8.0) early in the pandemic from March to August 2020, while Malawi experienced a 9.0% decline in overall vaccination coverage (95% CI: -18.0, -3.9) later in the pandemic from September 2020 to February 2021 [30]. Other settings remained stable in children fully vaccinated by 1 year of age throughout Ethiopia (-0.9, 95% CI: -3.9, 2.1) [39], children fully vaccinated in Addis Ababa, Ethiopia (-0.6, $p = 0.95$) [34], and overall vaccination coverage (-20.0%, $p = 0.197$) and complete vaccination (-18.0%, $p = 0.544$) in Nampula, Mozambique [41]. Vaccine clinic attendance declined from pre-pandemic baseline levels in Kampala, Uganda, with almost 5000 fewer attendees during the pandemic ($p = 0.04$) [38].

Laghman, Afghanistan, reported 6.0% to 28.0% ($p < 0.001$) declines in BCG, DTP 2–3, Hep B, IPV, MCV, OPV 0–4, PCV 1–3, Penta 1, and Rota 1–2 vaccinations from April to July 2020 [31]. West Rural Area, Sierra Leone, experienced large declines in vaccinations for all vaccines studied, ranging from a 51.1% to 83.7% ($p < 0.0005$) drop in BCG, OPV 0–3, Penta 1–3, PCV 1–3, Rota 1–2, IPTI 1–3, IPV, MCV 1–2, and yellow fever vaccinations in March and April 2020 [32]. The third dose of the Penta vaccine declined in Yemen in February, April, May, and June of 2020, with the strongest declines seen in May 2020 (-24.5, 95% CI: -30.6, -18.4) and June 2020 (-15.3, 95% CI: -20.2, -10.5) [40]. Vaccinations also declined for the third dose of the Penta vaccine in Liberia (-7.8%, 95% CI: -13.0, -2.5), Mali (-17.4%, 95% CI: -22.6, -12.3), and Sierra Leone (-12.6%, 95% CI: -19.1, -6.1) and for BCG in Mali (-11.8%, 95% CI: -15.4, -8.2) and Sierra Leone (-7.4%, 95% CI: -11.9, -2.9) from March to July 2020 [35]. Utilization rates declined in Rwanda for BCG, Pol 0–2, DTP Hep B Hib 1–2, Pneumococcal 1–2, and Rota 1–2 vaccines ($p = 0.001$ to $p = 0.009$) in March and April 2020 [33]. Vaccinations remained stable for Penta 3 and BCG vaccines in the Democratic Republic of the Congo (-0.1%, 95% CI: -1.2, 1.0, and -1.4%, 95% CI: -3.4, 0.6, respectively) and Somalia (-3.6%, 95% CI: -9.8, 2.6, and -2.4%, 95% CI: -8.9, 4.2, respectively) from March to July 2020 [35]. Declines were seen in the third dose of the DPT vaccine in the Central African Republic (-3.0%), South Sudan (-7.0%), Burundi (-12.0%), Eritrea (-9.0%), and Rwanda (-2.0%) and in the first dose of MCV in the Central African Republic (-3.0%), Burundi (-20.0%), and Rwanda (-4.0%) from April to June 2020 [37]. Further, rural Gambia experienced declines in vaccination during the interruption period (April to June 2020), the initial recovery period (July to September 2020), and the late recovery period (October 2020 to December 2020) [36]. Declines were reported in vaccine administration (interruption: -38.3%, initial recovery: -15.1%) and for BCG (interruption: -47.2%, initial recovery: -20.0%), Hep B (interruption: -46.9%, initial recovery: -20.0%), Penta 1 (interruption: -43.1%, initial recovery: -33.0%), OPV 1 (interruption: -83.6%, initial recovery: -34.0%), PCV 1 (interruption: -42.4%, initial recovery: -33.0%, late recovery: -2.0%), and Rota 1 (interruption: -43.4%, initial recovery: -34.0%, late recovery: -2.6%) vaccinations [36].

3.3.2. Increases in Vaccination

While many low-income countries reported declines in routine childhood vaccination during the COVID-19 pandemic, some experienced increases in routine vaccination at differing phases throughout the pandemic. Overall vaccination coverage increased in Malawi early in the pandemic (13.7%, 95% CI: 2.4, 33.6) from March 2020 to August 2020 compared to before the pandemic began. Overall vaccination coverage was stable in Liberia late in the pandemic (27.0%, 95% CI: −12.5, 56.5) from September 2020 to February 2021 and throughout the whole pandemic study period (8.0%, 95% CI: −12.1, 15.9) [30].

In Malawi, BCG vaccination increased (5.6%, 95% CI: 0.5, 10.8), but Penta 3 vaccination was stable (1.2%, 95% CI: −2.5, 4.9) alongside BCG vaccination in Liberia (0.3%, 95% CI: −5.2, 5.8) from March to July 2020 [35]. Although declines in vaccination were experienced in other months of the pandemic in Yemen, Penta vaccinations were stable in March 2020 (0.02, 95% CI: −4.3, 4.4) [40]. In Rwanda, the vaccination utilization rate of the measles + rubella vaccine remained stable in March and April 2020 (0.014, $p = 0.642$) [33], while in Addis Ababa, Ethiopia, MCV vaccination coverage change was also stable from April to June 2020 (1.7, $p = 0.86$) [34]. Additionally, the first dose of MCV increased in Chad (13.0%), the Democratic Republic of the Congo (2.0%), and Eritrea (2.0%), and the third dose of DPT increased in Chad (6.0%) and the Democratic Republic of the Congo (1.0%) from April to June 2020 [37]. Finally, in rural Gambia, increases were observed during the initial recovery period from July to September 2020 for MCV (79.0%) and yellow fever (88.9%) vaccinations. During the late recovery period from October to December 2020, vaccine administration (1.9%), BCG (3.0%), Hep B (2.5%), and OPV 1 (22.7%) vaccination increased [36].

3.4. Factors That Influenced Changes in Vaccination Rates

We summarized the proposed factors that influenced changes in vaccination rates in low-income countries during the pandemic and grouped them into nine different themes, as shown in Table 4.

Table 4. Summary of factors that influenced changes in routine childhood vaccination during the COVID-19 pandemic.

Themes	Factors	Studies
Communication challenges (n = 3)	• Reduced communication for routine health services	Wanyana 2021 [33]
	• Risk communication increased reluctancy to leave homes and get care	Abid 2022 [31]
	• Social media misinformation	Shapira 2021 [35]
Fear of COVID-19 (n = 9)	• Fear of contracting COVID-19 or transmission of COVID-19 in health facilities	Arsenault 2022 [30], Buonsenso 2020 [32], Burt 2021 [38], Connolly 2022 [30], das Neves Martins Pires 2021 [41], Gebreegziabher 2022 [34], Kotiso 2022 [40], Osei 2022 [36], Wanyana 2021 [33]
Financial barriers (n = 2)	• Financial barriers to health services	Gebreegziabher 2022 [34]
	• Inability to pay for healthcare due to loss of employment	Arsenault 2022 [39]
Health system practices (n = 5)	• Weaker health systems were vulnerable to disruptions	Masresha 2020 [37]
	• Resilience and structure of health systems	Shapira 2021 [35] Kassie 2021 [29]
	• Inadequate immediate care practices	
	• Suspension of routine care practices for patients with COVID-19	Arsenault 2022 [39]
	• Wait times increased	das Neves Martins Pires 2021 [41]

Table 4. *Cont.*

Themes	Factors	Studies
Lockdowns and emergency measures (n = 4)	• Strict or lengthy lockdowns • State of emergency raised alarms even with no lockdowns • Closure of borders	Arsenault 2022 [39], Masresha 2020 [37] Osei 2022 [36] Abid 2022 [31]
Pre-existing factors (n = 2)	• Pre-existing poor quality of services, poor road conditions, and lack of infrastructure for production of medical supplies • Prior experiences with epidemics and restrictions	Wanyana 2021 [33] Shapira 2021 [35]
Supply shortages (n = 4)	• Vaccines out of stock • Shortages in vaccines and other supplies, and disruptions in supply chains • Inadequate supply of PPE	Connolly 2022 [30], Osei 2022 [36] Abid 2022 [31] Gebreegziabher 2022 [34]
Transportation barriers (n = 5)	• Transportation restrictions and restricted movement • Closure of public transport and increased price of transport • Motorcycle ambulances not used as often	Connolly 2022 [30], Osei 2022 [36], Wanyana 2021 [33] Burt 2021 [38] das Neves Martins Pires 2021 [41]
Workforce changes (n = 3)	• Redirected workforce to COVID-19 care • Decrease in health professionals	Gebreegziabher 2022 [34] Burt 2021 [38], das Neves Martins Pires 2021 [41]

3.4.1. Communication Challenges

In Rwanda, reduced communications on routine health services led to declines in vaccinations [33]. Conversely, increased high-risk communication during COVID-19 in Laghman, Afghanistan, made people reluctant to leave their homes and seek routine health services, leading to a decline in vaccinations [31]. The Democratic Republic of the Congo, Liberia, Malawi, Mali, Sierra Leone, and Somalia experienced false social media claims, such as voice notes on WhatsApp warning mothers not to visit immunization clinics and vaccinate their babies with Western-developed COVID-19 vaccines. Clinic attendance later began to improve with radio programs and community visits to dispel rumors [35].

3.4.2. Fear of COVID-19

Fear of COVID-19 was reported as a widespread issue during the pandemic across multiple low-income countries. Many people were hesitant to visit health facilities, hospitals, or immunization clinics due to fear of infection or transmission of the virus. Fear of contagion was suggested as a reason for vaccination declines in parts of Ethiopia [34,39], Sierra Leone [32], Uganda [38], Liberia and Malawi [30], Yemen [40], Gambia [36], and Rwanda [33].

3.4.3. Financial Barriers

Financial barriers to seeking routine health services were proposed as a factor contributing to declines in vaccination during the pandemic in Addis Ababa, Ethiopia [34]. Throughout Ethiopia, many were unable to pay for health services due to loss of employment or compensation [39].

3.4.4. Health System Practices

The differences in vaccination rates experienced between low-income countries were, in part, from differences in the resilience and structure of their health systems [35]. In the Central African Republic, Chad, the Democratic Republic of the Congo, South Sudan, Burundi, Eritrea, and Rwanda, the countries that had weaker health systems were more vulnerable to disruptions. Countries with previously high vaccination coverage did a better job maintaining those levels, but those with previously lower coverage saw larger declines [37]. In South West Ethiopia, there were inadequate newborn care practices [29], whereas, in Nampula, Mozambique, wait times for care increased during the pandemic [41]. An obstacle widely experienced was the intentional suspension of routine care to allow room for patients with COVID-19 [32]. However, in some places like the Rural Western Area, Sierra Leone, health systems maintained the same activities as before the pandemic began [32].

3.4.5. Lockdowns and Emergency Measures

Strict or lengthy lockdowns caused barriers to receiving routine health services and greatly influenced changes in vaccination during the pandemic, as reported in Ethiopia [39], the Central African Republic, Chad, the Democratic Republic of the Congo, South Sudan, Burundi, Eritrea, and Rwanda [37]. In rural Gambia, there were no lockdowns, but the state of emergency raised alarms and led to restricted movement [36]. In Laghman, Afghanistan, border closures also restricted movement to inhibit the attendance of routine health services [31]. Restrictions differed by district in Liberia and Malawi but were not strictly adhered to in rural districts [30]. Yemen did not enforce lockdowns or restrict movement [40].

3.4.6. Pre-Existing Factors

Other contributing factors that influenced vaccination were compounded by pre-existing challenges in low-income countries. Pre-existing poor-quality services, poor road conditions, and lack of infrastructure for the production of medical supplies were reported as challenges in Rwanda [33]. The Democratic Republic of the Congo, Liberia, Malawi, Mali, Sierra Leone, and Somalia differed in outcomes because of their prior experiences with epidemics and restrictions [35].

3.4.7. Supply Shortages

Global suspension of vaccine companies and altered supply chains led to shortages in stock of vaccines and other supplies [31]. Addis Ababa, Ethiopia, experienced inadequate supplies of PPE [34], while Liberia and Malawi saw declines in vaccination due to shortages of vaccine stock [30]. The first dose of OPV was out of stock nationally from April to July 2020 in rural Gambia, causing major declines in the administration of the vaccine [36]. The Rural Western Area, Sierra Leone, reported experiencing no problems regarding vaccine supply [32].

3.4.8. Transportation Barriers

Travel restrictions and restricted movement were reported as factors influencing vaccination during the pandemic in Liberia and Malawi [30], Rwanda [33], and rural Gambia [36]. Kampala, Uganda, experienced closures of public transport and increased transport prices [38]. Additionally, a decrease in the use of motorcycle ambulances was reported in Nampula, Mozambique [41].

3.4.9. Workforce Changes

A redirected workforce toward COVID-19 care was experienced in Addis Ababa, Ethiopia [34]. The overall number of health professionals decreased in Nampula, Mozambique [41], while a lack of healthcare staff was reported in Kampala, Uganda [38].

3.5. Risk of Bias in Individual Studies

Using bias domains and scoring categories from the ROBINS-I tool, all studies had low or moderate risk of bias and were included in the synthesis of data. Most studies (92%) were categorized as having a moderate risk of bias due to missing data. However, a majority of the studies were categorized as low risk of bias due to confounding (92%), bias in the selection of participants into the study (92%), bias in the measurement of exposures or outcomes (85%), and bias in the selection of studies or reported outcomes (92%). We included a summary table of the risk of bias assessment in Supplementary Table S2.

4. Discussion

This comprehensive systematic review of 13 studies summarized the available data on changes in routine childhood vaccination in low-income countries during the COVID-19 pandemic. The review bridges gaps in the literature by addressing specific pandemic-driven impacts on children and summarizing the factors that influenced those impacts in low-income countries with residents that are vulnerable to poverty. Changes in vaccination practices, like vaccine coverage and clinic attendance, and influential factors were systematically examined using PRISMA 2020 guidelines and COSMOS-E recommendations. Furthermore, included studies were assessed for bias using a ROBINS-I tool that covered relevant domains of bias for our review. While vaccine types, vaccination changes, and influential factors varied across included studies, our results provide an account of how children in low-income countries weathered the pandemic. The results of this review reveal that most low-income countries experienced a reduction in routine childhood vaccination early in the COVID-19 pandemic. Several factors were reported as proposed influences on routine vaccination in children during the pandemic. Notable factors include fear of contracting COVID-19 in health facilities, changes in health system practices, and transportation barriers.

Declines in vaccination practices were reported for a majority of vaccines in most low-income countries studied. While some declines in vaccination were small or did not reach statistical significance, some declines were extreme. Sierra Leone and Afghanistan saw the largest declines in routine vaccination during the pandemic. The West Rural Area, Sierra Leone, experienced a substantial 84% decline in MCV 2 vaccination and over 50% decline in nine other vaccinations in March and April 2020. Laghman, Afghanistan, experienced large declines in overall vaccinations and nine individual vaccinations from April to July 2020. Declines were observed at least once for all individual vaccines studied and for overall vaccination coverage, fully vaccinated status, and vaccine clinic attendance. Increases reported during later months of the pandemic provide evidence of effective catch-up routines implemented to counteract downward trends. Given the extensive declines in vaccination rates observed in low-income countries during the pandemic, robust catch-up routines were imperative to restore progress from previous vaccination efforts.

Most of the included studies focused on the initial impact period of the pandemic and assessed the first few months after the pandemic was declared. All of the studies began their pandemic study period in March or April 2020, and most ended the study period by July 2020. Some studies chose not to include March 2020 in their study, while others included the month in the baseline study period. Most of the studies that did include March 2020 in the pandemic study period did not report results by month but instead reported totals for the entire study period. COVID-19 was declared a global pandemic by the World Health Organization (WHO) on March 11, 2020, and there was likely a delay in adverse outcomes, prompting studies to handle pandemic start times differently. Studies that divided the pandemic into phases found declines and increases in vaccination depending on the phase of the pandemic.

Changes in routine childhood vaccination practices are not a direct effect of the pandemic but are indirect results due to several influential factors. Low-income countries face distinctive factors influencing routine healthcare and vaccination. These populations often grapple with limited resources, inadequate healthcare infrastructure, and a higher prevalence of disease. Additionally, socioeconomic disparities contribute to challenges in delivering routine healthcare. Outside of the COVID-19 pandemic, factors that generally contribute to vaccine coverage inequality in low- and middle-income countries include maternal and paternal education, household wealth, ethnicity, caste, and area of residence. Urban–rural differences and distance to care influence the number of children who are vaccinated in these populations [19]. The COVID-19 pandemic revealed numerous factors that were reported as contributors to changes in routine vaccination practices during the pandemic in low-income countries. Routine childhood vaccination declines are more likely when there are more influential factors acting against it.

Vaccination rates during this period may have also been influenced by factors unrelated to COVID-19. Civil unrest and military activities from late 2019 to early 2023 likely impacted the well-being and health of people in certain low-income countries during this time. From 2020 to 2022, Ethiopia fought in the Tigray War between the Ethiopian government and the Tigray People's Liberation Front. It was one of the deadliest conflicts in recent history and set a record for the most people displaced in any country in a single year (2021) [42]. In May 2021, the United States began withdrawing from Afghanistan after two decades of military presence. With this came a subsequent change in government in Afghanistan. The Taliban took control of the capital city in August 2021, raising concerns about the rights and safety of Afghan citizens [43]. In addition to these conflicts, there was ongoing instability in the Democratic Republic of the Congo, Somalia, South Sudan, and Yemen.

There are some limitations that merit consideration when interpreting the results of this review. The primary limitation was the heterogeneity of vaccine types and analyses presented. A meta-analysis was considered but deemed inappropriate since we were unable to pool the effect estimates that were extracted. While we did not conduct a meta-analysis, we compiled and summarized the trends of both declines and increases in vaccination. Secondly, we did not present outcomes from all 28 low-income countries throughout the world due to a lack of available literature. We did include studies from 18 low-income countries that covered WHO African and Eastern Mediterranean Regions. The only region that included a low-income country that we were unable to obtain data from due to lack of papers is the South East Asian Region, which contains North Korea. We did not identify any drastic differences in social and economic facets and healthcare systems between the 18 countries included in this review and the 10 countries that were not included in this review apart from the distinct social and economic structures in North Korea. The countries we missed could have impacted our results, and the review may not be fully representative of what occurred in all low-income countries during the pandemic. Thirdly, there is the potential for selection bias since our study only included papers written in English. Because we studied routine childhood vaccinations throughout the world, it is possible that we failed to include literature written in languages other than English. However, a substantial portion of scientific literature is either in English or has been translated. Although not including studies that use other languages could introduce bias, only using English language studies allowed us to remain consistent throughout the review process. There is an additional potential source of selection bias that may have influenced our results, stemming from the process by which the identified papers were screened and selected. We significantly reduced the risk of bias by involving two reviewers in the screening and selection process. Using the ROBINS-I tool for risk of bias assessment, we found that a majority of studies included in the review had a low risk of bias in confounding, selection bias and measurement domains, suggesting the study findings are reliable. In several studies, we found a moderate risk of bias due to missing data collected from health facilities. No studies featured a high risk of bias for any of the bias domains, and all studies were included in the synthesis. Despite these limitations, we believe that this review successfully summarizes the current literature on routine childhood vaccination during the COVID-19 pandemic and identifies unique factors for changes in routine vaccination in low-income countries.

Although the next public health emergency may differ from COVID-19, we can use the lessons learned from this pandemic to guide practices for children in low-income settings. Compiling health outcomes during the pandemic and the reasons behind those outcomes helps inform preparedness efforts targeted at children who live in settings that put them at an increased risk of becoming infected or being exposed to poor outcomes. The COVID-19 pandemic has taught us to maintain strong communication with the community and try to mitigate fears, ensure transportation alternatives, and keep adequate stockpiles of essential supplies. It has also underscored the importance of maintaining routine health services such as vaccination and avoiding a complete shift of workers to emergency care, as it may result in the breakdown of other essential areas. If these factors are not effectively addressed during the next pandemic or public health emergency, we will likely again see declines in routine childhood vaccination, resulting in illness and mortality from preventable diseases.

5. Conclusions

Changes in routine childhood vaccination practices during the COVID-19 pandemic varied among low-income countries, but most saw declining vaccination trends, particularly during the initial months of the pandemic. Changes in routine childhood vaccination practices are indirect consequences due to multiple clinical, infrastructural, and social factors. Primary influential factors reported in low-income countries consisted of fear of contracting COVID-19 in health facilities, changes in health system practices like redirected care to patients with COVID-19, and transportation barriers. Although the COVID-19 public health emergency has been declared over, cataloging previous outcomes and lessons learned will help inform preparedness efforts for individuals vulnerable to poverty in the event of the next pandemic or public health emergency.

Supplementary Materials: The following supporting information can be downloaded at https://www.mdpi.com/article/10.3390/microorganisms12030573/s1, Table S1: Search strategy executed February 2023; Table S2: Risk of bias of included studies using ROBINS-I tool.

Author Contributions: Conceptualization, J.E.B. and K.G.K.; methodology, J.E.B., A.J., L.A.B., M.G., C.X. and K.G.K.; software, J.E.B., S.C. and K.G.K.; validation, J.E.B. and K.G.K.; formal analysis, J.E.B.; investigation, J.E.B. and K.G.K.; writing—original draft preparation, J.E.B. and K.G.K.; writing—review and editing, J.E.B., A.J., L.A.B., M.G., C.X., S.C. and K.G.K.; visualization, J.E.B.; supervision, K.G.K. All authors have read and agreed to the published version of the manuscript.

Funding: This research received no external funding.

Data Availability Statement: Data are contained within the articles and Supplementary Materials.

Conflicts of Interest: The authors declare no conflicts of interest.

References

1. World Health Organization. A Brief History of Vaccines. 2023. Available online: https://www.who.int/news-room/spotlight/history-of-vaccination/a-brief-history-of-vaccination#:~:text=Dr%20Edward%20Jenner%20created%20the,cowpox%20were%20immune%20to%20smallpox.&text=In%20May%201796,%20English%20physician,the%20hand%20of%20a%20milkmaid (accessed on 20 August 2023).
2. Mallory, M.L.; Lindesmith, L.C.; Baric, R.S. Vaccination-induced herd immunity: Successes and challenges. *J. Allergy Clin. Immunol.* **2018**, *142*, 64–66. [CrossRef] [PubMed]
3. GBD Vaccine Coverage Collaborators. Measuring routine childhood vaccination coverage in 204 countries and territories, 1980–2019: A systematic analysis for the Global Burden of Disease Study 2020, Release 1. *Lancet* **2021**, *398*, 503–521. [CrossRef] [PubMed]
4. UNICEF. Immunization. 2023. Available online: https://www.unicef.org/immunization (accessed on 20 August 2023).
5. Muhoza, P. Routine Vaccination Coverage—Worldwide, 2020. *MMWR Morb. Mortal. Wkly. Rep.* **2021**, *70*, 1495–1500. [CrossRef] [PubMed]
6. Rachlin, A. Routine Vaccination Coverage—Worldwide, 2021. *MMWR Morb. Mortal. Wkly. Rep.* **2022**, *71*, 1396–1400. [CrossRef] [PubMed]
7. Maltezou, H.C.; Medic, S.; Cassimos, D.C.; Effraimidou, E.; Poland, G.A. Decreasing routine vaccination rates in children in the COVID-19 era. *Vaccine* **2022**, *40*, 2525–2527. [CrossRef]
8. Cunniff, L.; Alyanak, E.; Fix, A.; Novak, M.; Peterson, M.; Mevis, K.; Eiden, A.L.; Bhatti, A. The impact of the COVID-19 pandemic on vaccination uptake in the United States and strategies to recover and improve vaccination rates: A review. *Hum. Vaccin. Immunother.* **2023**, *19*, 2246502. [CrossRef] [PubMed]
9. UNICEF. COVID-19 Pandemic Leads to Major Backsliding on Childhood Vaccinations, New WHO, UNICEF Data Shows. 2021. Available online: https://www.unicef.org/press-releases/covid-19-pandemic-leads-major-backsliding-childhood-vaccinations-new-who-unicef-data#:~:text=The%20data%20shows%20that%20middle,cent%20to%2085%20per%20cent. (accessed on 20 August 2023).

10. Vanderslott, S.; Dattani, S.; Spooner, F.; Roser, M. Vaccination. 2013. Available online: https://ourworldindata.org/vaccination (accessed on 1 September 2023).
11. Anderson, K.M.; Creanza, N. Internal and external factors affecting vaccination coverage: Modeling the interactions between vaccine hesitancy, accessibility, and mandates. *PLoS Global Public Health* **2023**, *3*, e0001186. [CrossRef]
12. Kaur, G. Routine Vaccination Coverage—Worldwide, 2022. *MMWR Morb. Mortal. Wkly. Rep.* **2023**, *72*, 1155–1161. [CrossRef]
13. World Health Organization. Childhood Immunization Begins Recovery after COVID-19 Backslide. 2023. Available online: https://www.who.int/news/item/18-07-2023-childhood-immunization-begins-recovery-after-covid-19-backslide (accessed on 1 September 2023).
14. World Health Organization. COVID-19 Pandemic Fuels Largest Continued Backslide in Vaccination in Three Decades. 2022. Available online: https://www.who.int/news/item/15-07-2022-covid-19-pandemic-fuels-largest-continued-backslide-in-vaccinations-in-three-decades#:~:text=Vaccine%20coverage%20dropped%20in%20every,points%20in%20just%20two%20years (accessed on 5 September 2023).
15. Yegros-Yegros, A.; van de Klippe, W.; Abad-Garcia, M.F.; Rafols, I. Exploring why global health needs are unmet by research efforts: The potential influences of geography, industry and publication incentives. *Health Res. Policy Syst.* **2020**, *18*, 47. [CrossRef]
16. Shet, A.; Carr, S.; Danovaro-Holiday, M.C.; Sodha, S.V.; Prosperi, C.; Wunderlich, J. Impact of the SARS-CoV-2 pandemic on routine immunization services: Evidence of disruption and recovery from 170 countries and territories. *The Lancet Global Health* **2022**, *10*, E186–E194. [CrossRef]
17. Lassi, Z.S.; Naseem, R.; Salam, R.A.; Siddiqui, F.; Das, J.K. The Impact of the COVID-19 Pandemic on Immunization Campaigns and Programs: A Systematic Review. *Int. J. Environ. Res. Public Health* **2021**, *18*, 988. [CrossRef] [PubMed]
18. Cardoso Pinto, A.M.; Ranasinghe, L.; Dodd, P.J.; Budhathoki, S.S.; Seddon, J.A.; Whittaker, E. Disruptions to routine childhood vaccinations in low- and middle-income countries during the COVID-19 pandemic: A systematic review. *Front. Pediatr.* **2022**, *10*, 979769. [CrossRef]
19. Ali, H.D.; Hartner, A.M.; Echeverria-Londono, S.; Roth, J.; Li, X.; Abbas, K.; Portnoy, A.; Vynnycky, E.; Woodruff, K.; Ferguson, N.M.; et al. Vaccine equity in low and middle income countries: A systematic review and meta-analysis. *Int. J. Equity Health* **2022**, *21*, 82. [CrossRef] [PubMed]
20. Hossain, M.M.; Abdulla, F.; Karimuzzaman; Rahman, A. Routine Vaccination Disruption in Low-Income Countries: An Impact of COVID-19 Pandemic. *Asia Pac. J. Public Health* **2020**, *32*, 509–510. [CrossRef] [PubMed]
21. Baciu, A.; Negussie, Y.; Geller, A.; Weinstein, J.N. (Eds.) *Communities in Action: Pathways to Health Equity. The Root Causes of Health Inequity*; National Academies Press (US): Washington, DC, USA, 2017.
22. Coalition, E.C.P.G. Child Poverty Facts. Available online: https://www.endchildhoodpoverty.org/facts-on-child-poverty#:~:text=Child%20poverty%20is%20not%20only,poor%20(as%20of%202018) (accessed on 22 January 2023).
23. Preferred Reporting Items for Systematic Reviews and Meta-Analyses. PRISMA 2020 Checklist. 2020. Available online: http://www.prisma-statement.org/ (accessed on 26 July 2023).
24. Dekkers, O.M.; Vandenbroucke, J.P.; Cevallos, M.; Renehan, A.G.; Altman, D.G.; Egger, M. COSMOS-E: Guidance on conducting systematic reviews and meta-analyses of observational studies of etiology. *PLoS Med.* **2019**, *16*, e1002742. [CrossRef] [PubMed]
25. World Bank. World Bank Country and Lending Groups. 2023. Available online: https://datahelpdesk.worldbank.org/knowledgebase/articles/906519-world-bank-country-and-lending-groups (accessed on 15 January 2023).
26. Cochrane. Covidence. 2022. Available online: https://community.cochrane.org/help/tools-and-software/covidence#:~:text=Covidence%20is%20the%20primary%20screening,and%20full%20text%20study%20reports (accessed on 10 February 2023).
27. Cochrane. ROBINS-I Tool 2022. Available online: https://methods.cochrane.org/methods-cochrane/robins-i-tool (accessed on 5 April 2023).
28. Thomas, J.; Harden, A. Methods for the thematic synthesis of qualitative research in systematic reviews. *BMC Med. Res. Methodol.* **2008**, *8*, 45. [CrossRef] [PubMed]
29. Kassie, A.; Wale, A.; Yismaw, W. Impact of Coronavirus Diseases-2019 (COVID-19) on Utilization and Outcome of Reproductive, Maternal, and Newborn Health Services at Governmental Health Facilities in South West Ethiopia, 2020: Comparative Cross-Sectional Study. *Int. J. Women's Health* **2021**, *13*, 479–488. [CrossRef]
30. Connolly, E.; Boley, E.; Fejfar, D.L.; Varney, P.; Aron, M.; Fulcher, I.; Lambert, W.; Ndayizigiye, M.; Law, M.; Mugunga, J.-C.; et al. Childhood immunization during the COVID-19 pandemic: Experiences in Haiti, Lesotho, Liberia and Malawi. *Bull. World Health Organ.* **2022**, *100*, 115–126C. [CrossRef]
31. Abid, Z.; Delgado, R.C.; Martinez, J.A.C.; González, P.A. The Impact of COVID-19 Pandemic Lockdown on Routine Immunization in the Province of Laghman, Afghanistan. *Risk Manag. Healthc. Policy* **2022**, *15*, 901–908. [CrossRef]
32. Buonsenso, D.; Cinicola, B.; Kallon, M.N.; Iodice, F. Child Healthcare and Immunizations in Sub-Saharan Africa During the COVID-19 Pandemic. *Front. Pediatr.* **2020**, *8*, 517. [CrossRef]
33. Wanyana, D.; Wong, R.; Hakizimana, D. Rapid assessment on the utilization of maternal and child health services during COVID-19 in Rwanda. *Public Health Action* **2021**, *11*, 12–21. [CrossRef]
34. Gebreegziabher, S.B.; Marrye, S.S.; Kumssa, T.H.; Merga, K.H.; Feleke, A.K.; Dare, D.J.; Hallström, I.K.; Yimer, S.A.; Shargie, M.B. Assessment of maternal and child health care services performance in the context of COVID-19 pandemic in Addis Ababa, Ethiopia: Evidence from routine service data. *Reprod. Health* **2022**, *19*, 42. [CrossRef]

35. Shapira, G.; Ahmed, T.; Drouard, S.H.P.; Fernandez, P.A.; Kandpal, E.; Nzelu, C.; Wesseh, C.S.; Mohamud, N.A.; Smart, F.; Mwansambo, C.; et al. Disruptions in maternal and child health service utilization during COVID-19: Analysis from eight sub-Saharan African countries. *Health Policy Plan.* **2021**, *36*, 1140–1151. [CrossRef]
36. Osei, I.; Sarwar, G.; Hossain, I.; Sonko, K.; Ceesay, L.; Baldeh, B.; Secka, E.; Mackenzie, G.A. Attendance and vaccination at immunization clinics in rural Gambia before and during the COVID-19 pandemic. *Vaccine* **2022**, *40*, 6367–6373. [CrossRef]
37. Masresha, B.G.; Luce, R., Jr.; Shibeshi, M.E.; Ntsama, B.; Ndiaye, A.; Chakauya, J.; Poy, A.; Mihigo, R. The performance of routine immunization in selected African countries during the first six months of the COVID-19 pandemic. *Pan Afr. Med. J.* **2020**, *37* (Suppl. S1), 12. [CrossRef]
38. Burt, J.F.; Ouma, J.; Lubyayi, L.; Amone, A.; Aol, L.; Sekikubo, M.; Nakimuli, A.; Nakabembe, E.; Mboizi, R.; Musoke, P.; et al. Indirect effects of COVID-19 on maternal, neonatal, child, sexual and reproductive health services in Kampala, Uganda. *BMJ Glob. Health* **2021**, *6*, e006102. [CrossRef]
39. Arsenault, C.; Gage, A.; Kim, M.K.; Kapoor, N.R.; Akweongo, P.; Amponsah, F.; Aryal, A.; Asai, D.; Awoonor-Williams, J.K.; Ayele, W.; et al. COVID-19 and resilience of healthcare systems in ten countries. *Nat. Med.* **2022**, *28*, 1314–1324. [CrossRef]
40. Kotiso, M.; Qirbi, N.; Al-Shabi, K.; Vuolo, E.; Al-Waleedi, A.; Naiene, J.; Senga, M.; Khalil, M.; Basaleem, H.; Alhidary, A. Impact of the COVID-19 pandemic on the utilisation of health services at public hospitals in Yemen: A retrospective comparative study. *BMJ Open* **2022**, *12*, e047868. [CrossRef]
41. das Neves Martins Pires, P.H.; Macaringue, C.; Abdirazak, A.; Mucufo, J.R.; Mupueleque, M.A.; Zakus, D.; Siemens, R.; Belo, C.F. Covid-19 pandemic impact on maternal and child health services access in Nampula, Mozambique: A mixed methods research. *BMC Health Serv. Res.* **2021**, *21*, 860. [CrossRef]
42. Centers for Preventive Action. Conflict in Ethiopia. Global Conflict Tracker 2023. Available online: https://www.cfr.org/global-conflict-tracker/conflict/conflict-ethiopia (accessed on 5 January 2024).
43. Centers for Preventive Action. Instability in Afghanistan. Global Conflict Tracker 2023. Available online: https://www.cfr.org/global-conflict-tracker/conflict/war-afghanistan (accessed on 5 January 2024).

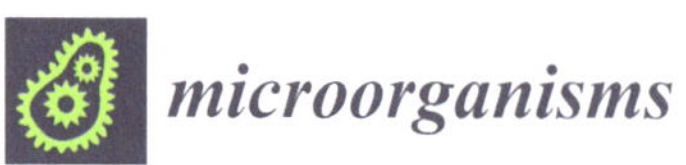 *microorganisms*

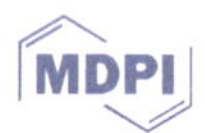

Brief Report

The Impact of the COVID-19 Pandemic on Cutaneous Drug Eruptions in a Swedish Health Region without Lockdown

Maria Pissa [1,2] and Sandra Jerkovic Gulin [2,3,*]

[1] Department of Dermatology and Venereology, Department of Dermatology and Sexual Health, Södersjukhuset, Karolinska University Hospital, 118 83 Stockholm, Sweden; maria.pissa@regionstockholm.se

[2] Department of Dermatology and Venereology, Ryhov County Hospital, 551 85 Jonkoping, Sweden

[3] Division of Cell Biology, Department of Biomedical and Clinical Sciences, Linkoping University, 581 83 Linkoping, Sweden

* Correspondence: sandra.jerkovicgulin@rjl.se or sandra.jerkovic.gulin@liu.se

Abstract: The incidence of severe cutaneous drug eruptions during the COVID-19 period in Sweden has not been studied previously. Our aim was to compare the incidence of these skin reactions in a Swedish health region during the COVID-19 pandemic period with that of the year after: we conducted a retrospective, observational cohort study using data from a national registry of patients diagnosed with cutaneous drug eruptions during the pandemic in Sweden. We included the number of patients diagnosed with severe cutaneous drug eruptions at the Department of Dermatology in the Jonkoping health region during the COVID-19 pandemic (1 April 2020 to 31 March 2021) and the reference period (1 April 2021 to 31 March 2022). We examined the monthly occurrences of cutaneous drug eruptions in three dermatology clinics within the Jonkoping health region. The frequency of these eruptions was determined for two distinct time periods: during the pandemic and post-pandemic. The study included 102 patients with cutaneous drug eruptions: 29 patients were diagnosed during the COVID-19 pandemic period and 73 were diagnosed during the reference period. The difference in the number of cutaneous drug eruptions cases (*p*-value = 0.0001, 95% CI 1.4995–3.5500, OR 2.3072) during the pandemic period compared to the post-pandemic period was significant. To our knowledge, the impact of the pandemic on cutaneous drug eruptions has not been investigated in EU countries. The increasing and differentiation of the number of diagnosed cutaneous drug eruptions cases after the pandemic could be explained by the removal of COVID-19 restrictions and the more frequent health-seeking behavior during the post-pandemic period.

Keywords: COVID-19; cutaneous drug eruptions; Stevens–Johnson syndrome; toxicoderma; toxic epidermal necrolysis

Citation: Pissa, M.; Jerkovic Gulin, S. The Impact of the COVID-19 Pandemic on Cutaneous Drug Eruptions in a Swedish Health Region without Lockdown. *Microorganisms* **2023**, *11*, 1913. https://doi.org/10.3390/microorganisms11081913

Academic Editor: Qibin Geng

Received: 25 June 2023
Revised: 20 July 2023
Accepted: 26 July 2023
Published: 27 July 2023

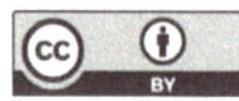

1. Introduction

In March 2020, the global healthcare system was confronted with an unprecedented crisis when the World Health Organization (WHO) declared the COVID-19 pandemic [1]. This declaration marked the beginning of a tumultuous period characterized by the rapid spread of the novel coronavirus and the subsequent collapse of healthcare infrastructures across multiple nations. The impact on specialist care services was particularly pronounced, as healthcare systems struggled to cope with the overwhelming burden of COVID-19 cases.

Sweden, like many other countries, experienced the profound effects of the pandemic; however, its approach to managing the pandemic differed from that of many other nations. On 24 January 2020, the first confirmed case of SARS-CoV-2 was identified at Ryhov County Hospital in Jonkoping, Sweden. Subsequently, the virus gained a foothold in the country, leading health authorities to implement various measures to mitigate its spread. In mid-March 2020, recommendations were issued, urging individuals aged 70 and above, as well as those belonging to high-risk groups, to adopt additional precautions such as practicing social distancing and adhering to strict hygiene protocols.

While the impact of COVID-19 on the healthcare system and general population has been extensively studied worldwide, there remains a dearth of research regarding the occurrence of drug eruptions during the pandemic in Sweden. Drug eruptions refer to adverse skin reactions or allergies triggered by different medicines. Understanding the occurrence and characteristics of drug eruptions during the COVID-19 pandemic is crucial for healthcare professionals to provide appropriate medical care and mitigate potential risks associated with drug-related adverse events. A spectrum of cutaneous reactions after mRNA COVID-19 vaccines has been reported, although mostly minor and self-limited [2–4].

Therefore, it is imperative to conduct a study to assess the occurrence and nature of drug eruptions during the COVID-19 pandemic in Sweden. Such research would provide valuable insights into the interplay between drug usage, immune responses, and viral infections, ultimately contributing to the development of enhanced therapeutic strategies and patient care protocols during times of healthcare crises. By identifying potential risk factors and patterns associated with drug eruptions in this unique context, healthcare professionals can better allocate resources and devise preventive measures, ultimately ensuring the well-being and safety of patients during this challenging time [4].

Through our retrospective analysis, we sought to elucidate any discernible variations in the frequency of cutaneous drug eruptions (CDEs) within the specified time periods. This investigation holds significant implications for understanding the interplay between drug usage, viral outbreaks, and the subsequent occurrence of adverse skin reactions. By acquiring a comprehensive understanding of the prevalence and characteristics of CDEs in the context of the COVID-19 pandemic, healthcare professionals can devise tailored strategies to mitigate risks and optimize patient care during similar healthcare crises in the future. This research holds significant value in shedding light on the impact of the pandemic on drug-induced skin reactions.

The primary aim was to assess and compare the incidence of CDE within Jonkoping County, a prominent health region in Sweden, during two distinct time periods: the 12-month span encompassing the COVID-19 pandemic (1 April 2020, to 31 March 2021), and the subsequent 12-month period following the pandemic (reference period). Investigating the incidence of CDEs during the COVID-19 pandemic in Sweden fills an existing knowledge gap in the literature. To our knowledge, no previous research has explored the impact of the pandemic on CDE occurrence in European Union (EU) countries, making our study unique in its contribution to the field of dermatology and drug safety. This study sought to provide critical insights into the prevalence and trends of CDEs in the context of the COVID-19 pandemic. Understanding the impact of the pandemic on CDE occurrence is vital for healthcare professionals to effectively manage these serious skin reactions and enhance patient safety.

2. Materials and Methods

This study was conducted as a retrospective, observational cohort study, focusing on three major hospitals: Ryhov County Hospital, Highland Hospital of Nassjo, and Varnamo Hospital. Jonkoping County, situated in the southeastern health region of Sweden, caters to a population of approximately 360,000 residents.

To gather comprehensive data, we analyzed the records of patients who received diagnoses of several systemic drug reactions including toxicoderma, toxic epidermal necrolysis (TEN), and Stevens–Johnson syndrome (SJS) at the Department of Dermatology within the Jonkoping health region. By identifying and analyzing cases of CDE, including severe and potentially life-threatening conditions such as TEN and SJS, we aimed to gauge the impact of the COVID-19 pandemic on the occurrence of drug-induced skin reactions.

The scope of our study extended over two distinct time periods, namely the COVID-19 pandemic period (1 April 2020 to 31 March 2021) and the subsequent post-pandemic period (1 April 2021 to 31 March 2022). This research endeavor was categorized as a quality review and underwent a thorough approval process from the Operations Manager and Head of the

Department of Dermatology at Ryhov County Hospital, located in the Jonkoping region of Sweden. The study was conducted in strict adherence to Section 31 of the Health and Medical Services Act, as outlined in the publication Lakartidningen 2015; 112: C9CL, ensuring compliance with the ethical and legal regulations governing healthcare research. To identify relevant cases for our analysis, we employed the ICD-10 codes (International Statistical Classification of Diseases, version 2019). All cases identified as L27.0 Generalized skin eruption due to drugs and medicaments/toxicoderma, L51.1 Bullous erythema multiforme/Stevens–Johnson syndrome (SJS), L51.2 Toxic epidermal necrolysis (TEN)/Syndrome Lyell during pandemic and post-pandemic period were included in the study. Cases coded with the following codes were excluded from the study: L27.1 Localized skin eruption due to drugs or medicaments, L56.0 Drug phototoxic response, L56.1 Drug photoallergic response, L51.8 Other erythema multiforme, L51.9 Erythema multiforme, unspecified.

By employing the standardized coding system, we aimed to ensure consistency and accuracy in case identification across the study. This approach allowed us the capture and analysis of a comprehensive dataset of patients who experienced cutaneous drug eruptions within the specified time periods. By utilizing this methodology, we sought to establish a comprehensive understanding of the occurrence and characteristics of cutaneous drug eruptions during the COVID-19 pandemic and the subsequent post-pandemic period.

In this study, we performed a comprehensive analysis to assess the monthly occurrences of different forms of CDE with a focus on toxicoderma, SJS, and TEN across the three dermatology clinics operating within the Jonkoping healthcare region. Our investigation aimed to examine the impact of the COVID-19 pandemic on the frequency of CDE cases by comparing the pandemic period (1 April 2020 to 31 March 2021) to the subsequent post-pandemic period (1 April 2021 to 31 March 2022).

3. Results

Our analysis yielded compelling results, revealing a notable disparity in the frequency of CDE cases between the two defined time periods, the pandemic period (1 April 2020 to 31 March 2021) and the subsequent post-pandemic period (1 April 2021 to 31 March 2022). We observed a substantial increase in the number of reported CDE cases during the post-pandemic period. During the pandemic period, a total of twenty-nine cases of CDE were documented across the three dermatology clinics. However, in the post-pandemic period, the number of reported cases surged significantly, reaching a total of seventy-three. The disparity in case numbers between the two periods was statistically significant ($p = 0.0001$, 95% CI 1.4995 to 3.5500, OR 2.3072). (Figure 1). To better understand the total number of consultations, in Figure 2, we provide data with a total number of patient consultations (digital referrals vs. physical visits) during the pandemic (1 April 2020 to 31 March 2021) and the after-pandemic periods (1 April 2021 to 31 March 2022).

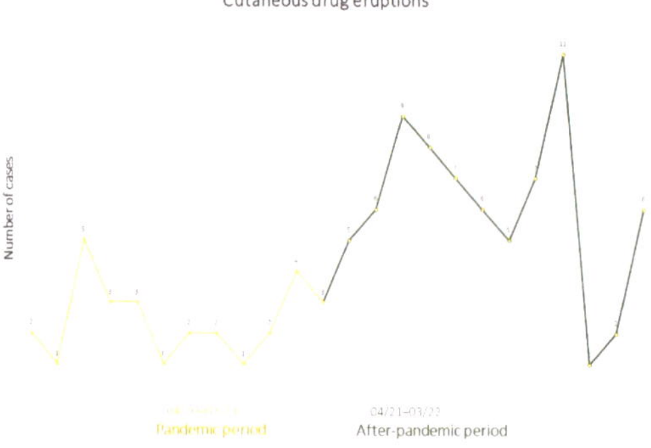

Figure 1. Number of cases of cutaneous drug eruptions during pandemic (1 April 2020 to 31 March 2021) and after-pandemic period (1 April 2021 to 31 March 2022).

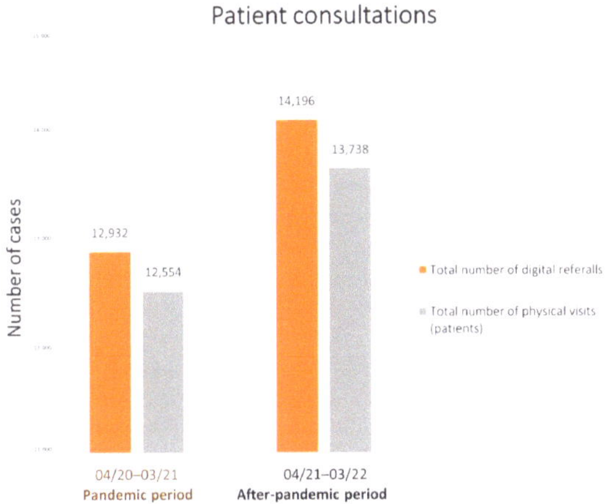

Figure 2. Total number of patient consultations (digital referrals vs. physical visits) during pandemic (1 April 2020 to 31 March 2021) and after-pandemic period (1 April 2021 to 31 March 2022).

4. Discussion

Within the current scientific landscape, there is a notable dearth of comprehensive research that specifically investigates the impact of the COVID-19 pandemic on the occurrences of CDE worldwide. Despite the increasing recognition of the pandemic's far-reaching effects, limited attention has been directed towards studying the association between the pandemic and the incidence of CDE cases worldwide. This research gap highlights a significant knowledge deficit that necessitates rigorous scientific inquiry to bridge the existing information void.

One intriguing observation that warrants investigation is the rise in the frequency of diagnosed CDE cases following the pandemic. Understanding the factors contributing to this trend poses a challenging task. One plausible contributing factor is the relaxation of COVID-19 restrictions that occurred as countries gradually emerged from the acute phase of the pandemic. The easing of lockdown measures, resulting in increased mobility and resumption of social interactions, may have inadvertently facilitated higher exposure to infective agents and, consequently, various drugs and medications. This increased exposure to potentially causative agents could have influenced the occurrence of CDE.

The relationship between the relaxation of COVID-19 restrictions and the subsequent rise in CDE cases is complex and probably multifactorial. The increased mobility and social interactions may have led to a greater utilization of medications, including prescription drugs, over-the-counter medications, and self-administered remedies. The diverse pharmacological profiles and potential side effects of these medications create an intricate web of interactions and reactions within the human body, including the skin. Consequently, the risk of developing CDE may have been elevated as a result of this increased medication usage and probably polypharmacy.

The study's main weakness lies in the absence of additional denominator data, such as CDE per consultation, CDE per cases, or CDE per patient-day. Without these data, it is difficult to draw definitive conclusions regarding the impact of the pandemic on medical care utilization and the true prevalence of CDEs during that period. As restrictions eased and vaccination rates increased, there might have been a release of pent-up demand for medical care, leading to an uptick in CDE diagnoses after the pandemic. To strengthen the study's findings and better understand the true effects of the pandemic on CDE prevalence, further research is needed, considering the factors mentioned above, and analyzing data from before, during and after the pandemic.

Another potential weakness of the study is the lack of analysis on sex, age, and ethnicity in relation to severe cutaneous drug eruptions during the COVID-19 pandemic. Understanding how these demographic factors may influence CDE occurrence could provide valuable insights into possible risk factors and tailored preventive measures. Future studies that consider these variables may further enhance the understanding of the impact of the pandemic on CDE prevalence.

Furthermore, the indirect consequences of the pandemic, such as psychological stressors and changes in healthcare-seeking behaviors, may also contribute to the observed rise in CDE cases. The psychological distress experienced during the pandemic period, including anxiety, fear, and social isolation, might have a profound impact on immune function and overall health. These psychosocial factors, in combination with the use of medications, may increase susceptibility to CDEs.

Is there a role of COVID-19 vaccination or COVID infection in the occurrence of CDE? Studies have reported a wide spectrum of cutaneous, mostly self-limited and minor, side effects [2,3]. Considering the impact of COVID-19 infection and vaccination on CDE prevalence is essential [4]. Some COVID-19 patients may require treatment with medications that have side effects, and the interplay between the infection and these drugs could lead to a higher incidence of serious CDEs. Additionally, the immune response triggered by COVID-19 could potentially influence the body's reactions to other drugs taken simultaneously, further impacting the occurrence of CDEs. Many questions are to be answered. The potential role of COVID-19 vaccination in the occurrence of CDE during the period after the COVID-19 pandemic is an important consideration. Currently, there is only limited scientific data available regarding the specific association between COVID-19 infection, COVID-19 vaccination and CDE. To provide concrete evidence and validate these hypotheses, additional studies should compare the rates of serious CDEs among individuals with the COVID-19 infection, vaccinated individuals, and those who have neither experienced infection nor received the vaccine.

However, the observed rise in CDE cases during the post-pandemic period is a complex phenomenon with potential interplay between multiple factors. Additional research is needed to delve deeper into the underlying mechanisms and risk factors associated with this trend. Epidemiological studies, encompassing diverse populations and different geographical regions, are needed to investigate the temporal trends and geographical variations in CDE occurrences during post-pandemic period.

Furthermore, the post-pandemic period might have influenced individual attitudes regarding seeking medical assistance resulting in drug prescription. It is plausible that the individuals who might have deferred non-urgent medical visits during the height of the pandemic due to fear of exposure or overwhelmed healthcare systems sought medical attention more promptly in the post-pandemic period. This shift in healthcare-seeking behavior could have contributed to the observed divergence in the frequency of diagnosed CDE cases.

Moreover, investigating the specific impact of COVID-19-related factors, such as the use of medications for COVID-19 treatment or prevention, immune dysregulation associated with the viral infection, or psychological stressors during the pandemic, may provide valuable insights into the etiology and pathogenesis of CDE in the context of the pandemic [4]. This knowledge will not only facilitate the development of preventive measures, early detection strategies, and optimal management protocols for CDE cases, but also contribute to the broader understanding of the interplay between pandemics, drug reactions, and health in general.

Moreover, comprehensive pharmacovigilance systems and post-marketing surveillance efforts should be strengthened to monitor and document CDE cases effectively. By collecting standardized and detailed data on medication use, drug reactions, and outcomes, researchers can gain valuable insights into the causative agents, risk factors, and clinical manifestations of CDE in the post-pandemic era. This information can help to guide clinical decision-making to minimize the occurrence and severity of CDE cases.

5. Conclusions

The scarcity of comprehensive research investigating the impact of the COVID-19 pandemic on the occurrences of CDE worldwide highlights a significant knowledge gap in the scientific community. The observed rise in the frequency of diagnosed CDE cases during post-pandemic period is probably the complex interplay between the relaxation of COVID-19 restrictions, increased medication usage, psychosocial factors and different immune reactions. By addressing this research gap, we can advance our understanding of the relationship between pandemics and cutaneous drug reactions, and ultimately enhance patient care, medication safety, and health measures.

Author Contributions: All authors have contributed significantly to this publication. Collection of data, study design, statistics and manuscript writing, S.J.G. and M.P. All authors have read and agreed to the published version of the manuscript.

Funding: This research was funded by FUTURUM-The Academy for Healthcare, Region Jönköping County.

Data Availability Statement: The data presented in this study are available on request from the corresponding author.

Conflicts of Interest: All authors declare no conflict of interest.

References

1. Huang, C.; Wang, Y.; Li, X.; Ren, L.; Zhao, J.; Hu, Y.; Zhang, L.; Fan, G.; Xu, J.; Gu, X.; et al. Clinical features of patients infected with 2019 novel coronavirus in Wuhan, China. *Lancet* **2020**, *395*, 497–506. [CrossRef] [PubMed]
2. McMahon, D.E.; Amerson, E.; Rosenbach, M.; Lipoff, J.B.; Moustafa, D.; Tyagi, A.; Desai, S.R.; French, L.E.; Lim, H.W.; Thiers, B.H.; et al. Cutaneous reactions reported after Moderna and Pfizer COVID-19 vaccination: A registry-based study of 414 cases. *J. Am. Acad. Dermatol.* **2021**, *85*, 46–55. [CrossRef] [PubMed]
3. Picone, V.; Martora, F.; Fabbrocini, G.; Marano, L. "Covid arm": Abnormal side effect after Moderna COVID-19 vaccine. *Dermatol. Ther.* **2022**, *35*, e15197. [CrossRef] [PubMed]
4. Wollina, U.; Karadağ, A.S.; Rowland-Payne, C.; Chiriac, A.; Lotti, T. Cutaneous signs in COVID-19 patients: A review. *Dermatol. Ther.* **2020**, *33*, e13549. [CrossRef] [PubMed]

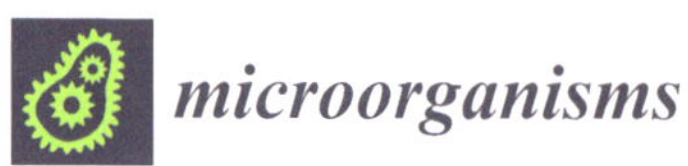

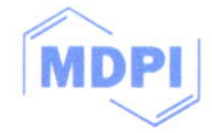

Review

The Renin–Angiotensin System (RAS) in COVID-19 Disease: Where We Are 3 Years after the Beginning of the Pandemic

Marco Prato [1], Natalia Tiberti [1], Cristina Mazzi [2], Federico Gobbi [1], Chiara Piubelli [1] and Silvia Stefania Longoni [1,*]

[1]   Department of Infectious, Tropical Diseases and Microbiology, IRCCS Sacro Cuore Don Calabria Hospital, Negrar di Valpolicella, 37024 Verona, Italy

[2]   Centre for Clinical Research, IRCCS Sacro Cuore Don Calabria Hospital, Negrar di Valpolicella, 37024 Verona, Italy

*   Correspondence: silvia.longoni@sacrocuore.it

Abstract: The RAS is a hormonal system playing a pivotal role in the control of blood pressure and electrolyte homeostasis, the alteration of which is associated with different pathologies, including acute respiratory distress syndrome (ARDS). As such, it is not surprising that a number of studies have attempted to elucidate the role and balance of the renin–angiotensin system (RAS) in COVID-19. In this review article, we will describe the evidence collected regarding the two main enzymes of the RAS (i.e., ACE and ACE2) and their principal molecular products (i.e., AngII and Ang1-7) in SARS-CoV-2 infection, with the overarching goal of drawing conclusions on their possible role as clinical markers in association with disease severity, progression, and outcome. Moreover, we will bring into the picture new experimental data regarding the systemic activity of ACE and ACE2 as well as the concentration of AngII and Ang1-7 in a cohort of 47 COVID-19 patients hospitalized at the IRCCS Sacro Cuore-Don Calabria Hospital (Negrar, Italy) between March and April 2020. Finally, we will discuss the possibility of considering this systemic pathway as a clinical marker for COVID-19.

Keywords: COVID-19; RAS pathway; ACE; ACE2; AngII; Ang1-7

Citation: Prato, M.; Tiberti, N.; Mazzi, C.; Gobbi, F.; Piubelli, C.; Longoni, S.S. The Renin–Angiotensin System (RAS) in COVID-19 Disease: Where We Are 3 Years after the Beginning of the Pandemic. *Microorganisms* **2024**, *12*, 583. https://doi.org/10.3390/microorganisms12030583

Academic Editor: Qibin Geng

Received: 30 January 2024
Revised: 4 March 2024
Accepted: 8 March 2024
Published: 14 March 2024

1. The Renin–Angiotensin System

Since the discovery of renin at the end of the 19th century, the renin–angiotensin system (RAS) has been largely studied for its important role in the regulation of blood pressure. The RAS is a hormonal system strictly involved in the control of blood pressure and electrolyte homeostasis [1]. Since it is present in several cells and tissues, the dysregulation of the RAS has been hypothesized to be involved in a number of different pathologies affecting multiple organs such as the liver, pancreas, skeletal muscle, kidney, lungs, blood vessels, heart, bone marrow, and nervous system [2,3].

The pathway comprises (i) a classic RAS, leading to the production of angiotensin II (AngII) through the ACE/AngII/AT1 axis; (ii) an alternative RAS, involving the production of angiotensin 1-7 (Ang1-7) through the ACE2/Ang1-7/MAS axis (Figure 1).

Renin and angiotensin-converting enzyme (ACE) are the two key enzymes of the classic RAS. The first is produced by the kidney and hydrolases the pro-hormone angiotensinogen, released by the liver, into angiotensin I (AngI) [3], while the second enzyme catalyzes the cleavage of AngII from AngI [3] (Figure 1). Depending on the target organ, AngII binding to its transmembrane AT1 receptor induces vasoconstriction (in vascular smooth muscles), sodium reabsorption (in the kidney), or aldosterone production (in the adrenal cortex) [3,4]. Indeed, AngII is a strong vasoconstrictor and pro-inflammatory hormone that acts both at renal and vascular levels to enhance the peripheral resistance of vessels, ultimately leading to high blood pressure (HBP) [5]. At the local level (i.e., heart, brain, and liver), it mediates local pathological events associated with inflammation, reactive oxygen species (ROS) production, and fibrosis, for instance [1].

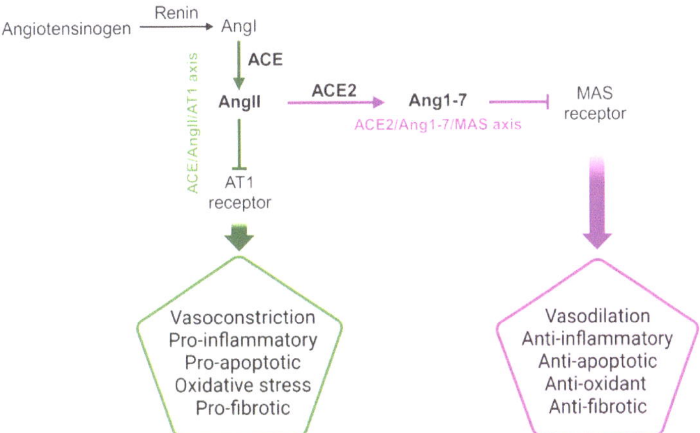

Figure 1. Schematic representation of the classical and alternative RAS. The main enzymes, hormones, and peptide products of the system are reported, together with the main systemic and local effects mediated by the RAS. The two enzymes and the two products described in this review manuscript are highlighted in bold. AngI: angiotensin I; AngII: angiotensin II; Ang1-7: angiotensin 1-7; ACE: angiotensin converting enzyme; ACE2: angiotensin converting enzyme 2. This figure was created using Biorender.com.

The alternative RAS was first described in the early 2000s following the discovery of angiotensin-converting enzyme 2 (ACE2) as an ACE counterpart. Indeed, ACE2 is responsible for the hydrolysis of AngII into Ang1-7 [6–9], which counteracts AngII effects by mediating anti-proliferative, anti-inflammatory, and anti-apoptotic responses [9,10], through binding to its natural transmembrane receptor MAS [2,3,11] (Figure 1).

Based on these premises, it is not surprising that the systemic or local activity of ACE and ACE2 and the concentration of AngII and Ang1-7 have been described in many human tissues and organs, and over the years, their involvement in cardiovascular diseases (CVD), hypertension, type 2 diabetes, and chronic kidney disease has been gradually elucidated [12–15]. Consequently, ACE inhibitors (e.g., Captopril) and angiotensin II type 1 (AT1) receptor blockers (ARBs) (e.g., Losartan) represent, nowadays, important therapeutic strategies against CVD, chronic kidney disease, and type 2 diabetes [16]. The RAS has also been proposed as an important player in the pathogenesis of acute respiratory distress syndrome (ARDS), the most severe form of acute lung injury [12,17]. In this particular context, it has been proposed that ACE2 activity could be necessary to counteract AngII, which is initially essential for an effective defense, but when chronically over-expressed could compromise the host immune defense, leading to potentially overwhelming bacterial infection [18]. Pathogens are among the major risk factors for ARDS, since pneumonia and non-pulmonary sepsis are, overall, responsible for 65–80% of all ARDS cases [19]. It might, thus, not be surprising that ACE2, which is highly expressed by oral cavity and lung epithelial cells [20], represents a molecular target for many respiratory pathogens. Consequently, the RAS, and particularly ACE2, have also been investigated in respiratory viral infections, including those caused by coronaviruses.

2. The RAS and Viral Respiratory Infections

Viral infections play an important role in ARDS onset, probably through the modulation and imbalance of the RAS [21]. It is known that the ACE2/Ang1-7/MAS axis is of particular importance in maintaining an equilibrium between an effective immune defense against microbial infections and in preventing immune-mediated tissue damage [17,18]. Different studies have attempted to elucidate the role of the RAS in lung pathologies associated with different viral infections in order to propose biomarkers of clinical utility. Indeed, an RAS imbalance has been described in patients with avian influenza (H5N1, H7N9), influenza A (H1N1), and hand, foot, and mouth disease (HFMD) caused by Coxsackie virus A16 (CA16) and enterovirus 71 (EV71). Significantly higher systemic concentrations of AngII have been reported in patients infected with H5N1 [22], H7N1, and H1N1 [23] when compared with uninfected control subjects. Interestingly, H7N1, which causes acute respiratory failures in humans, triggered higher and sustained circulating AngII levels than H1N1, while in both cases, plasma AngII concentrations were positively correlated with viral load [23]. These observations were also confirmed using a murine model since, in mice, H5N1 infection triggered a reduction in ACE2 expression in the lungs and an increase in AngII concentration in serum. During H7N1 and H5N1 infections, raised systemic AngII levels were associated with longer hospitalization and increased severity and mortality in both patients and mice [22,23]. These observations were corroborated by additional experimental data obtained using mice knock-out for ACE2 (ACE2-ko). Indeed, in agreement with increased circulating (c)AngII, ACE2-ko mice challenged with H5N1 presented a higher mortality rate and a more severe lung pathology, which was attenuated following treatment with recombinant ACE2 (rACE2) [22], suggesting a beneficial role of this enzyme in alleviating lung injuries during respiratory viral infections [22].

Serum concentrations of AngII were also found to be higher in pediatric patients with HFMD than in healthy controls, particularly in those with a severe clinical presentation [24], while local AngII (i.e., brain, skeletal muscle, and lungs) increased with disease progression in EV71-infected mice [24].

The systemic RAS balance was also investigated in severe acute respiratory syndrome (SARS) caused by a coronavirus (SARS-CoV) that appeared for the first time in 2002, causing potentially fatal lung injury and ARDS [25]. Interestingly, mACE2 (membrane ACE2) was identified as the virus receptor on many different types of host cells [25–27], mediating viral entry through the binding of the spike (S) protein of the viral envelope [26,28–30]. The same mechanism was also described for the human coronavirus NL63 (HCoV-NL63) discovered in the Netherlands in 2004 [31], even though it binds less efficiently to ACE2 [30].

Different studies have shown a reduction in ACE2 expression in the lungs following SARS-CoV infection in mice [30,32] and an association between this local ACE2 reduction and the development of severe acute respiratory failure [33]. This phenomenon was shown to be associated with the binding of the spike protein to ACE2 and with a subsequent shedding of ACE2 from the cell surface [30,32,34], suggesting that SARS-CoV could downregulate its own receptor.

A functional role for SARS-CoV S protein in worsening lung pathology, likely by deregulating the RAS, was also proposed [32] since mice treated with the Spike–Fc protein presented increased AngII in the lungs and worsened lung function, while blocking the RAS using a specific AT1 receptor inhibitor attenuated the development of acute lung failure [32]. This agrees with ACE2-ko mice presenting reduced pathologic alterations in the lungs following the injection of the Spike–Fc protein. Moreover, the treatment with rACE2 attenuated lung injury in both ACE2-ko and wild-type mice, suggesting the possibility of using rACE2 to modulate the RAS also during SARS-CoV infection [33].

Unfortunately, mainly as a consequence of SARS-CoV's high mortality rate and the relatively small number of registered cases, a more in-depth evaluation of RAS balance at the systemic level in clinical samples and the prognostic value of circulating RAS molecules in SARS-CoV patients has not been addressed.

2.1. RAS and COVID-19

Based on these observations, it is not surprising that when the entire world was exposed to the outbreak of a new coronavirus disease (COVID-19), caused by the previously unknown human coronavirus SARS-CoV-2, the attention of researchers was also drawn to the role and balance of the RAS during this novel viral infection [35–40].

Similarly to other coronaviruses, SARS-CoV-2 uses ACE2 expressed on host cells as the main receptor for cell invasion through the binding of the S protein of the viral envelope [41]. The cell surface expression of ACE2 is higher in alveolar pneumocytes, although a broad spectrum of human cells, including enterocytes and vascular endothelial cells, can express this receptor, offering multiple targets for viral entrance [42]. This wide distribution of ACE2 across cell types could, at least partly, explain the broad range of clinical manifestations of COVID-19, spanning from respiratory to gastrointestinal manifestations [35]. As already observed for SARS-CoV, SARS-CoV-2 binding to its receptor results in ACE2 downregulation at the transcriptional and protein expression level in vitro [43,44]. It was then hypothesized that this ACE2 downregulation could potentially lead to increased ACE, which, in turn, could promote the cytokine storm observed in patients with lung injury [36,45], although direct evidence is still missing.

Since the beginning of the pandemic, many authors have speculated about the modulation of the RAS by SARS-CoV-2 based on the following: (i) the important role of the RAS in the pathological mechanisms of acute lung injury and ARDS; (ii) the key role of ACE2 receptor in viral entrance; and (iii) the proposed ability of rACE2 to reduce lung injury in SARS-CoV infection. It has also been proposed that alterations in the RAS could predict the outcome of the disease [35–39], which is based on the hypothesis that, at the serum level, there would have been the same RAS imbalance [46,47] observed at the tissue level [48].

Many studies have tried to elucidate this putative link between systemic RAS imbalance and COVID-19 infection, with the main aim of finding prognostic markers of clinical utility as well as improving treatment strategies. Despite the huge efforts made by the scientific community, some limitations concerning the investigation of the RAS in COVID-19 arose, including the lack of a standardized strategy to determine circulating enzymatic activity and peptide concentration, and the lack of the systematic measurement of multiple RAS molecules. Moreover, most studies have been limited by a small sample size, by the lack of an in-depth clinical and demographic characterization of the study cohort, and by high heterogeneity in the timing of blood collection. Consequently, a straightforward comparison of the results obtained in the different studies can be found difficult.

In the following paragraphs, we will try to summarize the principal studies investigating circulating ACE, ACE2, AngII, and Ang1-7 in clinical samples from COVID-19 patients in order to highlight reproducible pieces of evidence across studies as well as potential inconsistencies that need to be further explored. Particular attention will be paid to patients' stratification based on disease severity and outcome to comprehensively evaluate the association of this metabolic pathway with the course of the disease.

2.1.1. Alterations in Circulating RAS Molecules in COVID-19 Patients Compared to Healthy Subjects

In the effort to evaluate a potential systemic imbalance in the RAS associated with COVID-19, a number of studies have measured and compared circulating RAS molecules between patients and control subjects (Table 1).

Table 1. Modulation of RAS molecules in COVID-19 patients during hospitalization compared to controls.

COVID-19	Controls	ACE (Act.)	ACE (Conc.)	ACE2 (Act.)	ACE2 (Conc.)	AngII (Conc.)	Ang1-7 (Conc.)	AngII/Ang1-7 (Ratio)	Ref.
Hospitalized, $n = 12$	Healthy, $n = 8$					↑			[49]
Hospitalized, $n = 74$	Healthy, $n = 55$			↑	↓	↑	↓	↑	[50]
Hospitalized, $n = 16$	Healthy, $n = 17$			↓	↑		↓		[51]
Hospitalized, $n = 519$	Healthy, $n = 201$				↓				[52]
Hospitalized, $n = 114$	Healthy, $n = 10$		≈		↑				[53]

Table 1. *Cont.*

COVID-19	Controls	ACE (Act.)	ACE (Conc.)	ACE2 (Act.)	ACE2 (Conc.)	AngII (Conc.)	Ang1-7 (Conc.)	AngII/Ang1-7 (Ratio)	Ref.
Hospitalized, $n = 10$	Healthy, $n = 5$			↑		↓	↑		[54]
Hospitalized, $n = 242$	Healthy, $n = 38$					↑			[55]
Hospitalized, $n = 30$	Healthy, $n = 14$					≈			[56]
Hospitalized, $n = 55$	Healthy, $n = 18$	≈							[57]
Hospitalized, $n = 84$	Healthy, $n = 18$		↓		↑	≈	↑		[58]
Hospitalized, $n = 81$	Healthy, $n = 316$	↓							[59]
Hospitalized, $n = 136$	Healthy, $n = 60$	↓							[60]
Hospitalized, $n = 112$	Healthy, $n = 27$					↓			[61]
Hospitalized, $n = 29$	Healthy, $n = 15$				↓	↑	≈		[42]
Hospitalized, $n = 19$	ARF non-COVID19, $n = 19$	↑							[62]
Hospitalized, $n = 82$	Critically ill non-COVID19 $n = 12$					↑			[63]
Hospitalized, $n = 52$	Sick non-COVID19 $n = 27$	≈	≈						[64]
Hospitalized, $n = 27$	Sick non-COVID19 $n = 14$						↓		[65]

Act.—activity; Conc.—concentration; Ref.—reference; ↓ represents lower values in COVID-19 patients compared to controls; ↑ represents higher values in COVID-19 patients compared to controls; ARF—acute respiratory failure; ≈ represents no statistically significant differences. Empty box means that no measurement was performed.

In an early report dating back to February 2020, Liu and co-workers reported increased levels of plasmatic AngII and decreased Ang1-7 in twelve SARS-CoV-2 patients presenting pneumonia compared with healthy subjects [49]. In agreement, raised AngII levels were also observed in critically ill patients with COVID-19 compared to critically ill patients without SARS-CoV-2 infection [63]. Similar results were obtained in an independent cohort of hospitalized patients [50], in which raised AngII concentrations were accompanied by decreased Ang1-7 and ACE2 concentrations but increased ACE2 activity in patients compared to controls [50].

Partly contrasting results were instead reported in severely ill hospitalized COVID-19 patients, who presented reduced cACE2 activity in both plasma and saliva when compared to negative controls [51]. In agreement with this reduced cACE2 activity, COVID-19 patients also displayed decreased Ang1-7 concentrations, indicating an overall downregulation of the alternative RAS pathway in this population. Interestingly, this reduction was accompanied by significantly increased concentrations of cACE2, suggesting that the reduction in ACE2 activity was not due to a reduced enzyme concentration. Moreover, treatment with convalescent plasma was reported to restore ACE2 activity after 60 days [51]. The systemic alteration in ACE2 concentration was not mirrored at the local level since no differences in ACE2 quantification in lung tissue from patients who died from COVID-19 or other pathological conditions were detected [51]. Unfortunately, disagreement among published data was also observed regarding cACE2 concentration, with two studies reporting lower [50,52] and four reporting higher cACE2 concentrations [51,53–55] in COVID-19 patients compared to healthy controls (Table 1). It might be worth reminding readers that enzyme concentration does not reflect activity. While the concentration of cACE2 could be of interest for speculation about the ability of the human body to capture the virus and avoid cell infection, it might only be of limited utility for the evaluation of the RAS balance since a high concentration of cACE2 or cACE does not directly reflect a high synthesis of their products in serum.

An overall potential downregulation of the RAS was reported by Henry and colleagues [65], who observed decreased AngI and Ang1-7 in COVID-19 patients upon hospital admission compared to healthy controls, even though the enzymatic activity and concentration of ACE were not significantly different, and the activity and concentration of ACE2 were not determined [65]. Avanoglu Guler et al. did not find any significant differences in ACE activity in infected subjects compared to healthy controls [57,64]. Lower cACE concentrations were instead observed in COVID-19 patients compared with healthy controls [58], even though this was accompanied by significantly high ACE2 and Ang1-7 concentrations in patients [58].

Contrasting results have, however, progressively been published. For instance, COVID-19 patients were reported to have the same [56] or even lower blood AngII concentrations than healthy controls [54]. In this latter study, COVID-19 patients, who were critically ill with respiratory failure and admitted to the intensive care unit (ICU), presented increased plasma ACE2 concentrations when compared to healthy controls. This increase was also associated with decreased AngII and, in contrast with what was reported by others [51], increased Ang1-7 formation, as determined by equilibration assay [54]. Lastly, increased activity of cACE has not been associated with COVID-19 [53,66]; rather, it has been shown to be lower in COVID-19 patients when compared to healthy controls [59].

2.1.2. Association between RAS Dysregulation and COVID-19 Severity or Outcome

When systemic AngII concentration was evaluated according to the severity of COVID-19, the reported data showed, again, a certain level of disagreement. An important bias in the early studies was the definition of severity itself. Indeed, especially at the beginning of the pandemic and before WHO guidelines were published [67], different criteria were used to classify hospitalized patients as mild, moderate, severe, or, in some cases, critical. It is, thus, not surprising that contrasting, or even opposite, results have been reported in the literature. It is also important to mention that, with respect to disease severity, cACE2 was the most investigated RAS molecule, while only a few studies also took into consideration cACE, AngII, and Ang1-7 activity or systemic concentration. A summary of the main results obtained for the evaluation of the RAS associated with disease severity is reported in Table 2.

Table 2. Modulation of RAS molecules in COVID-19 patients during hospitalization, stratified based on the severity of the disease.

COVID-19		ACE (Act.)	ACE (Conc.)	ACE2 (Act.)	ACE2 (Conc.)	AngII (Conc.)	Ang1-7 (Conc.)	AngII/Ang1-7 (Ratio)	Ref.
Severe, $n = 16$	Non-severe, $n = 120$	↓							[60]
Severe, $n = 59$	Non-severe, $n = 128$			↑					[68]
Severe, $n = 32$	Non-severe, $n = 94$					↑			[69]

Table 2. *Cont.*

COVID-19		ACE (Act.)	ACE (Conc.)	ACE2 (Act.)	ACE2 (Conc.)	AngII (Conc.)	Ang1-7 (Conc.)	AngII/Ang1-7 (Ratio)	Ref.
Severe, $n = 109$	Non-severe, $n = 196$				↑				[70]
Severe/critical, $n = 40$	Mild, $n = 42$					↑			[63]
Severe, $n = 11$	Mild, $n = 24$	≈							[57]
Severe, $n = 263$	Mild, $n = 82$				↓				[71]
Severe, $n = 11$	Critical, $n = 12$		≈		≈	↑	≈		[66]

Act.—activity; Conc.—concentration; Ref.—reference; ↓ represents lower values in COVID-19 patients compared to controls; ↑ represents higher values in COVID-19 patients compared to controls; ≈ represents no statistically significant differences. Empty box means that no measurement was performed.

In a small population of 12 patients, plasma AngII was shown to be associated with viral load and lung capacity since a significant negative correlation was reported with both the Ct (cycle threshold) value (Spearman rho $= -0.669$) and PaO_2/FiO_2 (correlation coefficient $= -0.545$) [49]. Such a relation was confirmed in a larger population encompassing 82 COVID-19 patients [63], in which significantly higher AngII concentrations, but not renin, were observed in severe and critically ill patients compared to those suffering from a mild infection [63,64]. Reindl-Schwaighofer and collaborators also reported higher AngII concentrations in severe COVID-19 patients than in non-severe patients [69]. Similarly, in critically ill COVID-19 patients, AngII levels upon admission were higher than those in severe patients and significantly decreased at discharge [66], while no differences were detected for ACE, ACE2, or Ang1-7 (Table 2). Interesting data are also available regarding cACE2 and COVID-19 severity since Akin and collaborators reported significantly higher cACE2 activity in severe patients than in non-severe ones [68] (Table 2). On the other hand, cACE activity has been reported to be lower in non-severe COVID-19 patients compared to severe patients [60] (Table 2).

A different trend was instead observed in patients suffering from hypertension [72]. In this particular population, severe cases presented higher ACE2 levels compared to both mild and moderate cases and decreased circulating AngII compared to mild subjects [72], suggesting that increased circulating ACE2 could be indicative of a more severe disease in patients under antihypertensive treatment. Indeed, a significant, although only moderate, positive correlation between plasmatic ACE2 and other indices of severity (i.e., D-dimer and length of hospitalization) was reported [72]. It is worth mentioning that different studies have reported that disease severity upon admission showed a stronger association with the presence of comorbidities, i.e., older age, hypertension, and body mass index (BMI), rather than with RAS circulating molecules [57,60,68,70]. Moreover, both ACE2 and AngII were partly influenced by the type of antihypertensive treatment since they were higher in patients under ARBs treatment compared to those taking ACEi [72]. In agreement with this, Files and colleagues did not observe differences between moderate and severe acute hypoxic respiratory failure (AHRF) COVID-19 patients for cACE2 activity and AngII and Ang1-7 concentrations [62]. Patients' stratification according to COVID-19 severity revealed lower cACE concentrations in mild compared to severe COVID-19 patients ($p = 0.054$), while among COVID-19 patients, those who developed cutaneous symptoms presented higher cACE2 concentrations than the rest of the patients (gastrointestinal and pulmonary) [73]. On the other hand, serum cACE and cACE2 concentrations did not show an association with the outcome of the diseases [53].

The association of soluble ACE activity and COVID-19 severity is also controversial since both unaltered and decreased activity were reported in severe patients in different studies [57,60]. Moreover, higher cACE2 activities and AngII/Ang1-7 ratios—a parameter frequently used as a surrogate for cACE2 activity—were observed in severe patients when compared with patients with influenza [69].

Interestingly, the contrasting data reported in the literature about the activity and the concentration of cACE2 could be explained by its time dependence. Reindl-Schwaighofer and collaborators reported lower cACE2 activities in blood taken early during hospitalization (i.e., days 0–3) compared with blood taken later (i.e., days 9–11) from the same COVID-19 patients, both severe and non-severe. Interestingly, when measured upon admission, they did not observe any significant differences in cACE2 activity between severe and non-severe patients, while they reported a 7-fold increase in severe patients during the course of the disease, with ACE2 being increased later during hospitalization [69].

These data suggest a pathophysiological role for cACE2, potentially inflammation-driven, aimed at counterbalancing an excess of AngII during the course of the infection. AngII and Ang1-7, in fact, were significantly higher and lower, respectively, in patients with severe COVID-19 upon admission and reverted a few days after hospitalization. This observation is reflected in the 4.5-fold higher Ang1-7/AngII ratio in severe COVID-19 patients 9–11 days after admission [69].

A trend, although not significant, toward increased levels of circulating AngII and decreased Ang1-7 was also observed in association with COVID-19 mortality in a cohort of 74 hospitalized patients suffering from mild or severe COVID-19 [50]. Interestingly, this trend translated into a significantly higher AngII/Ang1-7 ratio in patients who died compared to survivors, which also displayed a moderate potential as a predictor of mortality (AUC of 0.657). Indeed, patients with Ang II/Ang1-7 $\geq$ 3.45 had a 5-fold increased risk of mortality [50] (Table 3). Importantly, these observations were independent of the use of ACE inhibitors or ARBs [50].

Table 3. Modulation of RAS molecules in COVID-19 patients during hospitalization, stratified based on the outcome of the disease.

COVID-19		ACE (Act.)	ACE (Conc.)	ACE2 (Act.)	ACE2 (Conc.)	AngII (Conc.)	Ang1-7 (Conc.)	AngII/Ang1-7 (Ratio)	Ref.
Died, n = 25	Survived, n = 49			$\approx$	$\approx$	$\approx$	$\approx$	$\uparrow$	[50]
Died, n = 11	Survived, n = 17				$\uparrow$				[74]
ICU/died, n = 260	Transferred/ discharged, n = 331				$\downarrow$				[52]
Mechanical ventilation/died, n = 106	Non-ventilated survivors, n = 136				$\approx$				[55]
ICU, n = 8	Discharched, n = 22					$\approx$			[56]
Intubated, n = 79	Non-intubated, n = 225				$\uparrow$				[70]

Act.—activity; Conc.—concentration; Ref.—reference; $\downarrow$ represents lower values in COVID-19 patients compared to controls; $\uparrow$ represents higher values in COVID-19 patients compared to controls; $\approx$ represents no statistically significant differences. Empty box means that no measurement was performed.

Higher cACE2 levels were reported in COVID-19 patients with fatal outcomes compared to survivors [74] and in intubated patients compared with non-intubated COVID-19 patients [70]. Oppositely, Wuang and colleagues observed no significant differences in cACE2 concentrations between COVID-19 patients who survived compared to those who died from COVID-19 [55].

2.2. Systemic RAS during COVID-19: New Experimental Data

As already pointed out, an important limitation common to most of the published studies is the lack of measurement of the four main RAS players in the same cohort of patients. In our group, we tried to contribute to filling this gap by measuring cACE and cACE2 enzymatic activity, as well as AngII and Ang1-7 concentrations in the serum of SARS-CoV-2 patients ($n = 47$) and healthy controls ($n = 12$). COVID-19 patients were admitted to our hospital during the first COVID-19 wave from March to April 2020. The two groups—COVID-19 patients and controls—were matched for sex, with 55% males in the COVID-19 group and 50% in the control group, but not for age, with median ages of 75 (68–76) and 53.5 (52–57.25) (median and interquartile range), respectively. Additionally, 81% of COVID-19 patients presented comorbidities, while 37% were under ACEi/ARBs treatment. Data concerning the treatment and comorbidities for non-COVID-19 controls were not available. Based on a modified WHO score (WHO Working Group on the Clinical Characterization and Management of COVID-19 infection, 2020), COVID-19 patients were classified as mild (score 4, $n = 18$), moderate (score 5, $n = 23$), or severe (score ≥ 6, $n = 6$), as already reported elsewhere [75]. Patients were also stratified based on the clinical course during hospitalization (i.e., worsened ($n = 19$) or improved ($n = 28$)). The full demographic and clinical characteristics of the studied population as well as the laboratory findings are reported in the Supplementary Dataset and Supplementary S1. All subjects signed written informed consent, and the study was approved by the Ethical Committee of Verona and Rovigo provinces under protocol no. 63471/2020.

ACE2 activity was measured by an in-house method, while ACE activity was determined using the Angiotensin I Converting Enzyme (ACE) Activity Assay Kit (Fluorimetric) (Sigma-Aldrich, Merck KGaA, Darmstadt, Germany). The concentrations of AngII and Ang1-7 were measured using commercial ELISA kits (MybioSource, Inc., San Diego, CA, USA). A full description of the materials and methods used is reported in Supplementary Material S1.

Upon admission, we observed significantly lower ACE activities in COVID-19 patients compared with non-COVID-19 controls, while ACE2 activities and AngII and Ang1-7 concentrations did not differ between the two groups (Figure 2A).

In our population, the four molecules displayed different correlation profiles in COVID-19 patients and healthy controls. Indeed, in COVID-19, we observed a weak statistically significant negative correlation between Ang1-7 concentration and both cACE and cACE2, while in controls, Ang1-7 concentration was positively correlated with cACE2 (Figure 2B). COVID-19 patients were further stratified based on disease severity (i.e., severe $n = 6$, moderate $n = 23$, or mild $n = 18$), following a modified WHO score (Supplementary Material S1), or according to the clinical course during hospitalization (i.e., worsened $n = 19$ or improved $n = 28$) [75]. Despite these stratifications, we did not observe any significant differences between the subgroups for any of the measured enzymes or products. Similarly, we did not observe any significant difference in the AngII/Ang1-7 ratio.

Our COVID-19 population comprised 30% of subjects under ACE inhibitors (ACEi) or angiotensin receptor blockers (ARBs) treatment. As expected, we observed a significant difference in cACE2 activities and Ang1-7 concentrations in COVID-19 patients under ACEi or ARBs treatment. Specifically, we found higher cACE2 activities and lower Ang1-7 concentrations in those patients under ACEi/ARBs treatment (Figure 3A).

Our COVID-19 population comprised 38 patients (81%) presenting with comorbidities upon admission, mainly cardiovascular diseases (Table S1). Significantly higher ACE2 activities and lower AngII concentrations were observed in COVID-19 patients with comorbidities compared to those without, even though this last group had a small sample size (i.e., $n = 9$) (Figure 3B).

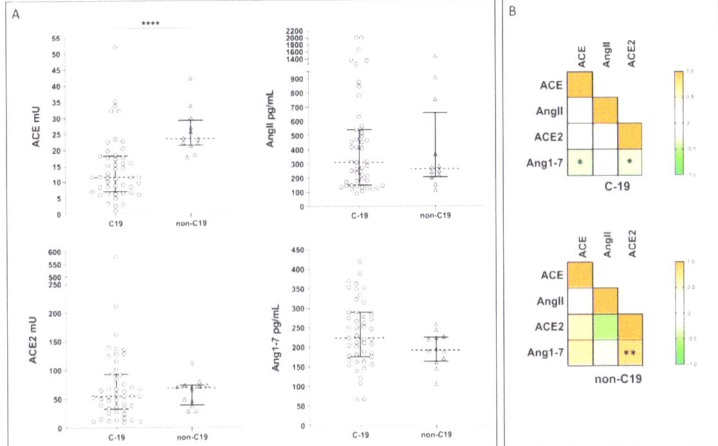

Figure 2. (**A**) Plots showing ACE and ACE2 activities and Ang1-7 and AngII concentrations in COVID-19 patients (C-19) and healthy controls (non-C19). Dotted line represents the median, and error bars represent the interquartile range. Statistical comparisons were computed using the Mann–Whitney test. **** = *p*-value < 0.0001. (**B**) Spearman correlation matrix for ACE and ACE2 activities, and Ang1-7 and AngII concentrations in COVID-19 patients (C-19) and healthy controls (non-C19). Color scale represents Spearman *rho* coefficient. Stars on plot indicate statistically significant correlations. * = *p*-value < 0.05; ** = *p*-value < 0.005.

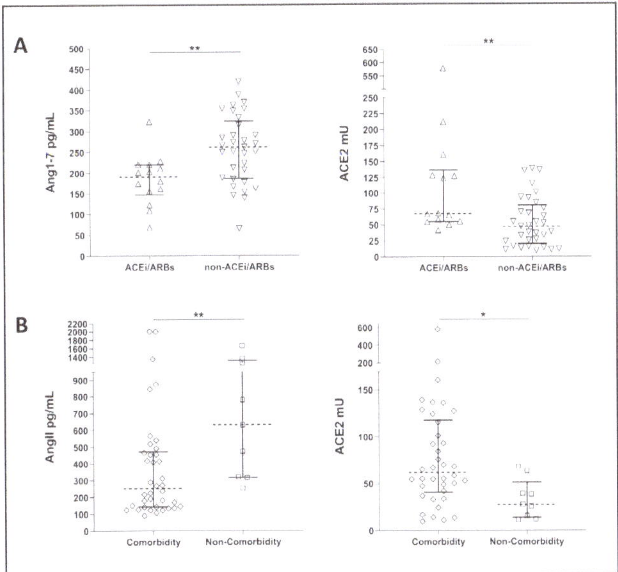

Figure 3. (**A**) Plots showing Ang1-7 concentrations and ACE2 activity in COVID-19 patients under ACEi/ARBs treatment (ACEi/ARBs) and COVID-19 patients not under ACEi/ARBs treatment (non-ACEi/ARBs). (**B**) Plots showing AngII concentrations and ACE2 activities in COVID-19 patients with comorbidities (comorbidity) and COVID-19 patients without comorbidities (non-comorbidity). Dotted line represents median, and error bars represent interquartile range. Statistical comparisons were computed using the Mann–Whitney test. * = *p*-value < 0.05; ** = *p*-value < 0.01.

In an attempt to establish whether some demographic or clinical factors could affect ACE and ACE2 activities or AngII and Agn1-7 concentrations in COVID-19 patients, we performed univariable and multivariable linear regression analyses (Tables S2 and S3). The univariable analysis showed a significant association of ACE2 and its product, Ang1-7, with ACE inhibitors, patients' age, and comorbidities, although only ACE inhibitors were still significant in the multivariable model. Among the assessed variables, only sex showed a weak association with ACE, while AngII was associated with sex and the presence of co-morbidities (Table S2), the latter was also significant in the multivariable analysis (Table S3). Our data suggest that during COVID-19, the RAS is much more likely to be modulated by the use of ACEi/ARBs or by the presence of co-morbidities (for AngII) than other factors (Table S3). Despite the fact that, in univariable analysis, sex seemed to influence the levels of AngII, we did not observe any significant influence in the multivariable model (Table S3).

Our study presents some limitations: (i) a low number of analyzed subjects; (ii) COVID-19 patients and control subjects were not matched by age, comorbidities, or treatments; (iii) there was a high prevalence of co-morbidities (80%) among COVID-19 patients; (iv) COVID-19 patients differed in their baseline medical therapy since 30% of them were on ACEi or angiotensin receptor blockers (ARBs); and (v) information about comorbidities or ACEi/ARBs treatment in the control subjects was not available. Despite these limitations, we showed that, overall, the RAS is not modulated during COVID-19 disease, except for the activity of ACE, which is reduced during SARS-CoV2 infection early during hospitalization.

3. Discussion and Concluding Remarks

Based on the current knowledge of the RAS in other diseases, it would be reasonable to think that higher ACE2 activity should lead to higher levels of Ang1-7, and likewise, higher ACE activity should correspond to higher levels of AngII. Moreover, high levels of AngII are known to lead to pro-inflammatory and pro-fibrotic effects, while Ang1-7 is associated with anti-inflammatory and anti-fibrotic effects [3,76–78]. Based on this knowledge, we expected COVID-19 to be associated with higher activity of ACE and, consequently, higher AngII levels, lower ACE2 activity, and lower Ang1-7 concentration. Additionally, we also expected this profile to be related to disease severity and outcomes. However, after a careful revision of the literature and some additional experimental data generated in our laboratory, it now seems evident that there is not a clear association between COVID-19 and a specific RAS dysregulation, as indicated by the contrasting results reported across studies (Tables 1–3). On the contrary, a number of studies investigating the RAS during either COVID-19 or other pathological conditions seem to suggest that co-morbidities or ACEi/ARBs treatment might exert a strong effect on the RAS balance [79–83]. To understand the role of co-morbidities in the regulation of the RAS, it is worth remembering that ACE2 is shed from the membrane surface and released into the blood stream following tissue damage [35,84]. It could be hypothesized that since SARS-CoV-2 uses ACE2 as a cellular entrance gate, the catalytic activity, at the tissue level, of this enzyme might be altered [85]. This could prevent the massive release of ACE2 into the blood stream, which is, instead, observed in other pathological conditions characterized by tissue damage [85], such as CVD, hypertension, type 2 diabetes, and chronic kidney disease, for which circulating ACE2 serves as a prognostic marker [86–89].

In fact, it has been reported that CVD patients present higher levels of cACE2 activity than healthy controls and that cACE2 activity correlates with the severity of the disease [90,91]. Most of the studies dealing with COVID-19 often did not fully describe the healthy control groups, especially with regard to the presence of comorbidities or treatment with RAS blockers. As reported in Table 1, a higher cACE2 activity was observed in COVID-19 patients when compared with healthy subjects with no history of CVD or previous treatment with ACEi/ARBs [50,54]. In our experimental data, instead, we did not observe differences in ACE2 activity in COVID-19 patients compared with healthy controls (Figure 2); however, we cannot exclude the presence of co-morbidities, such as CVD, in our control group since the information was not available.

Nonetheless, in our population of COVID-19 patients, we did observe significantly higher ACE2 activity in patients presenting at least one comorbidity compared to those presenting only with COVID-19 (Figure 3). cACE2 concentration was also reported to be higher in COVID-19 patients with pre-existing co-morbidities, such as CVD, hypertension, or kidney diseases, compared with patients without co-morbidities [70] as well as healthy controls with no history of comorbidities or RAS blocker treatment [53]. Opposite to what was believed at the beginning of the pandemic, scientific evidence has demonstrated the lack of association between the use of RAS blockers and susceptibility to SARS-CoV2 infection or disease severity [92–95]. Indeed, patients presenting CVD or kidney-related co-morbidities, which are often treated with RAS blockers such as ACEi/ARBs, calcium channel blockers, or beta-blockers, do not present less severe COVID-19 clinical presentation. No differences were recorded in cACE2 concentrations when comparing COVID-19 patients treated with ACEi/ARBs to COVID-19 patients without treatment [72].

It could be hypothesized that in order to counterbalance coronavirus's negative effects on the RAS, the kallikrein–kinin system (KKS) could be activated [85,96]. KKS is a system responsible for the production of bradykinin [85,97], a pro-inflammatory molecule and potent vasodilator [98], which has been found to be increased in COVID-19 patients [85,99]. Unfortunately, only a few studies have investigated the role of KKS and RAS during COVID-19, and further investigations should be performed.

It could, thus, be speculated that factors other than the SARS-CoV-2 infection might affect circulating ACE, ACE2, AngII, and Ang1-7 levels than COVID-19 itself, as also supported by our data.

This lack of association between a specific RAS imbalance and COVID-19 disease and the high disagreement between the results reported in the literature could be partly explained by a number of reasons. First, at the beginning of the pandemic, it was difficult to properly design and define the study cohorts, particularly for controls, which, most of the time, did not perfectly match COVID-19 patients in terms of age, comorbidities, and/or treatments. Second, until the release of the WHO's official guidelines in June 2020 [67], each study employed different classification criteria for the definition of severity. Third, the heterogeneity in the procedure for sample collection, such as the type of tubes, the use of protease inhibitors, the time delay between sample collection and analysis, the use of fresh or frozen samples, and the procedures for sample storage, might have influenced the results of the analyses.

In conclusion, based on our observations and a careful analysis of the literature, at the serum level, the RAS pathway does not present a clear imbalance in association with SARS-CoV-2 infection. From the studies reported in this review, it is not possible to exclude an RAS imbalance at the tissue level, which, however, would be of limited utility as a prognostic marker.

Thus, based on the pieces of evidence present in the literature, soluble ACE, ACE2, AngII, or Ang1-7 cannot currently be considered as markers for the diagnosis or prognosis of COVID-19. A number of additional factors (such as age, sex, co-morbidities, and treatments) are indeed likely to influence the RAS system during COVID-19 infection and deserve a more in-depth investigation. Moreover, research could also be extended to the KKS, as the natural counterbalance to the RAS, in order to build a more complete picture of the mechanisms leading to RAS alterations during COVID-19 infection.

Supplementary Materials: The following supporting information can be downloaded at: https://www.mdpi.com/article/10.3390/microorganisms12030583/s1, Supplementary Data Set; Supplemental-S1: MATERIAL AND METHODS: Bibliography research strategy, Study population [75,100], ACE2 Activity [101], ACE Activity, Angiotensin II and Angiotensin 1-7, List of reagent, Statistical analyses; Table S1: Demographic characteristics of the study population; Table S2: Results of univariable logistic regression models; Table S3: Multivariable logistic regression analysis to identify variables associated with ACE, ACE2, Ang 1-7, and AngII variability among COVID-19 patients. Only variables significant ($p < 0.2$) in the univariable analysis were included in the multivariable model.

Author Contributions: Conceptualization, M.P., F.G., C.P. and S.S.L.; methodology, M.P., N.T. and S.S.L.; formal analysis, C.M.; data curation, S.S.L.; writing—original draft preparation, N.T. and S.S.L.; writing—review and editing, M.P., N.T., C.M., F.G., C.P. and S.S.L. All authors have read and agreed to the published version of the manuscript.

Funding: This research was supported by EU funding within the MUR PNRR Extended Partnership initiative on Emerging Infectious Diseases (project no. PE00000007, INF-ACT), and by Italian Ministry of Health "Fondi Ricerca Corrente" project L1P6 to IRCCS Sacro Cuore Don Calabria Hospital.

Data Availability Statement: The datasets generated and analyzed during the current study are available in the Supplementary Materials.

Acknowledgments: The authors wish to thank the medical and nursing staff for their great effort during the pandemic in assisting the patients and for their support in sample collection. We also want to thank the colleagues involved in the diagnostic process of COVID-19.

Conflicts of Interest: The authors declare no conflicts of interest.

References

1. Eckenstaler, R.; Sandori, J.; Gekle, M.; Benndorf, R.A. Angiotensin II receptor type 1—An update on structure, expression and pathology. *Biochem. Pharmacol.* **2021**, *192*, 114673. [CrossRef] [PubMed]
2. Lavoie, J.L.; Sigmund, C.D. Minireview: Overview of the renin-angiotensin system—An endocrine and paracrine system. *Endocrinology* **2003**, *144*, 2179–2183. [CrossRef] [PubMed]
3. Vargas Vargas, R.A.; Varela Millan, J.M.; Fajardo Bonilla, E. Renin-angiotensin system: Basic and clinical aspects—A general perspective. *Endocrinol. Diabetes Nutr.* **2022**, *69*, 52–62. [CrossRef] [PubMed]
4. Lopez, D.L.; Casillas, O.E.; Jaramillo, H.J.; Romero-Garcia, T.; Vazquez-Jimenez, J.G. AT1 receptor downregulation: A mechanism for improving glucose homeostasis. *World J. Diabetes* **2023**, *14*, 170–178. [CrossRef] [PubMed]
5. Maranduca, M.A.; Vamesu, C.G.; Tanase, D.M.; Clim, A.; Drochioi, I.C.; Pinzariu, A.C.; Filip, N.; Dima, N.; Tudorancea, I.; Serban, D.N.; et al. The RAAS Axis and SARS-CoV-2: From Oral to Systemic Manifestations. *Medicina* **2022**, *58*, 1717. [CrossRef] [PubMed]
6. Donoghue, M.; Hsieh, F.; Baronas, E.; Godbout, K.; Gosselin, M.; Stagliano, N.; Donovan, M.; Woolf, B.; Robison, K.; Jeyaseelan, R.; et al. A novel angiotensin-converting enzyme-related carboxypeptidase (ACE2) converts angiotensin I to angiotensin 1-9. *Circ. Res.* **2000**, *87*, E1–E9. [CrossRef] [PubMed]
7. Ferrario, C.M. Angiotensin-converting enzyme 2 and angiotensin-(1-7): An evolving story in cardiovascular regulation. *Hypertension* **2006**, *47*, 515–521. [CrossRef]
8. Chappel, M.C.; Ferrario, C.M. ACE and ACE2: Their role to balance the expression of angiotensin II and angiotensin-(1-7). *Kidney Int.* **2006**, *70*, 8–10. [CrossRef]
9. Warner, F.J.; Guy, J.L.; Lambert, D.W.; Hooper, N.M.; Turner, A.J. Angiotensin converting enzyme-2 (ACE2) and its possible roles in hypertension, diabetes and cardiac function. *Lett. Pept. Sci.* **2003**, *10*, 377–385. [CrossRef]
10. Tamanna, S.; Clifton, V.L.; Rae, K.; van Helden, D.F.; Lumbers, E.R.; Pringle, K.G. Angiotensin Converting Enzyme 2 (ACE2) in Pregnancy: Preeclampsia and Small for Gestational Age. *Front. Physiol.* **2020**, *11*, 590787. [CrossRef]
11. Gomez, J.; Albaiceta, G.M.; Garcia-Clemente, M.; Lopez-Larrea, C.; Amado-Rodriguez, L.; Lopez-Alonso, I.; Hermida, T.; Enriquez, A.I.; Herrero, P.; Melon, S.; et al. Angiotensin-converting enzymes (ACE, ACE2) gene variants and COVID-19 outcome. *Gene* **2020**, *762*, 145102. [CrossRef] [PubMed]
12. Imai, Y.; Kuba, K.; Penninger, J.M. The renin-angiotensin system in acute respiratory distress syndrome. *Drug Discov. Today Dis. Mech.* **2006**, *3*, 225–229. [CrossRef] [PubMed]
13. Lew, R.A.; Warner, F.J.; Hanchapola, I.; Yarski, M.A.; Ramchand, J.; Burrell, L.M.; Smith, A.I. Angiotensin-converting enzyme 2 catalytic activity in human plasma is masked by an endogenous inhibitor. *Exp. Physiol.* **2008**, *93*, 685–693. [CrossRef] [PubMed]
14. Anguiano, L.; Riera, M.; Pascual, J.; Soler, M.J. Circulating ACE2 in Cardiovascular and Kidney Diseases. *Curr. Med. Chem.* **2017**, *24*, 3231–3241. [CrossRef] [PubMed]
15. Zisman, L.S.; Keller, R.S.; Weaver, B.; Lin, Q.; Speth, R.; Bristow, M.R.; Canver, C.C. Increased angiotensin-(1-7)-forming activity in failing human heart ventricles: Evidence for upregulation of the angiotensin-converting enzyme Homologue ACE2. *Circulation* **2003**, *108*, 1707–1712. [CrossRef] [PubMed]
16. Marx, N.; Federici, M.; Schutt, K.; Muller-Wieland, D.; Ajjan, R.A.; Antunes, M.J.; Christodorescu, R.M.; Crawford, C.; Di Angelantonio, E.; Eliasson, B.; et al. 2023 ESC Guidelines for the management of cardiovascular disease in patients with diabetes. *Eur. Heart J.* **2023**, *44*, 4043–4140. [CrossRef] [PubMed]
17. Hrenak, J.; Simko, F. Renin-Angiotensin System: An Important Player in the Pathogenesis of Acute Respiratory Distress Syndrome. *Int. J. Mol. Sci.* **2020**, *21*, 8038. [CrossRef] [PubMed]
18. Sodhi, C.P.; Nguyen, J.; Yamaguchi, Y.; Werts, A.D.; Lu, P.; Ladd, M.R.; Fulton, W.B.; Kovler, M.L.; Wang, S.; Prindle, T., Jr.; et al. A Dynamic Variation of Pulmonary ACE2 Is Required to Modulate Neutrophilic Inflammation in Response to Pseudomonas aeruginosa Lung Infection in Mice. *J. Immunol.* **2019**, *203*, 3000–3012. [CrossRef]

19. Pham, T.; Rubenfeld, G.D. Fifty Years of Research in ARDS. The Epidemiology of Acute Respiratory Distress Syndrome. A 50th Birthday Review. *Am. J. Respir. Crit. Care Med.* **2017**, *195*, 860–870. [CrossRef]

20. Salamanna, F.; Maglio, M.; Landini, M.P.; Fini, M. Body Localization of ACE-2: On the Trail of the Keyhole of SARS-CoV-2. *Front. Med.* **2020**, *7*, 594495. [CrossRef]

21. Gao, Y.L.; Du, Y.; Zhang, C.; Cheng, C.; Yang, H.Y.; Jin, Y.F.; Duan, G.C.; Chen, S.Y. Role of Renin-Angiotensin System in Acute Lung Injury Caused by Viral Infection. *Infect. Drug Resist.* **2020**, *13*, 3715–3725. [CrossRef]

22. Zou, Z.; Yan, Y.; Shu, Y.; Gao, R.; Sun, Y.; Li, X.; Ju, X.; Liang, Z.; Liu, Q.; Zhao, Y.; et al. Angiotensin-converting enzyme 2 protects from lethal avian influenza A H5N1 infections. *Nat. Commun.* **2014**, *5*, 3594. [CrossRef] [PubMed]

23. Huang, F.; Guo, J.; Zou, Z.; Liu, J.; Cao, B.; Zhang, S.; Li, H.; Wang, W.; Sheng, M.; Liu, S.; et al. Angiotensin II plasma levels are linked to disease severity and predict fatal outcomes in H7N9-infected patients. *Nat. Commun.* **2014**, *5*, 3595. [CrossRef]

24. Zhang, C.; Chen, S.; Zhou, G.; Jin, Y.; Zhang, R.; Yang, H.; Xi, Y.; Ren, J.; Duan, G. Involvement of the renin-angiotensin system in the progression of severe hand-foot-and-mouth disease. *PLoS ONE* **2018**, *13*, e0197861.

25. Imai, Y.; Kuba, K.; Penninger, J.M. The discovery of angiotensin-converting enzyme 2 and its role in acute lung injury in mice. *Exp. Physiol.* **2008**, *93*, 543–548. [CrossRef] [PubMed]

26. Li, W.; Moore, M.J.; Vasilieva, N.; Sui, J.; Wong, S.K.; Berne, M.A.; Somasundaran, M.; Sullivan, J.L.; Luzuriaga, K.; Greenough, T.C.; et al. Angiotensin-converting enzyme 2 is a functional receptor for the SARS coronavirus. *Nature* **2003**, *426*, 450–454. [CrossRef] [PubMed]

27. Ren, X.; Glende, J.; Al-Falah, M.; de Vries, V.; Schwegmann-Wessels, C.; Qu, X.; Tan, L.; Tschernig, T.; Deng, H.; Naim, H.Y.; et al. Analysis of ACE2 in polarized epithelial cells: Surface expression and function as receptor for severe acute respiratory syndrome-associated coronavirus. *J. Gen. Virol.* **2006**, *87 Pt 6*, 1691–1695. [CrossRef] [PubMed]

28. Wang, P.; Chen, J.; Zheng, A.; Nie, Y.; Shi, X.; Wang, W.; Wang, G.; Luo, M.; Liu, H.; Tan, L.; et al. Expression cloning of functional receptor used by SARS coronavirus. *Biochem. Biophys. Res. Commun.* **2004**, *315*, 439–444. [CrossRef]

29. Sha, A.; Chen, H. Infection routes, invasion mechanisms, and drug inhibition pathways of human coronaviruses on the nervous system. *Front. Neurosci.* **2023**, *17*, 1169740. [CrossRef]

30. Glowacka, I.; Bertram, S.; Herzog, P.; Pfefferle, S.; Steffen, I.; Muench, M.O.; Simmons, G.; Hofmann, H.; Kuri, T.; Weber, F.; et al. Differential downregulation of ACE2 by the spike proteins of severe acute respiratory syndrome coronavirus and human coronavirus NL63. *J. Virol.* **2010**, *84*, 1198–1205. [CrossRef]

31. Hofmann, H.; Pyrc, K.; van der Hoek, L.; Geier, M.; Berkhout, B.; Pohlmann, S. Human coronavirus NL63 employs the severe acute respiratory syndrome coronavirus receptor for cellular entry. *Proc. Natl. Acad. Sci. USA* **2005**, *102*, 7988–7993. [CrossRef] [PubMed]

32. Kuba, K.; Imai, Y.; Rao, S.; Gao, H.; Guo, F.; Guan, B.; Huan, Y.; Yang, P.; Zhang, Y.; Deng, W.; et al. A crucial role of angiotensin converting enzyme 2 (ACE2) in SARS coronavirus-induced lung injury. *Nat. Med.* **2005**, *11*, 875–879. [CrossRef] [PubMed]

33. Imai, Y.; Kuba, K.; Rao, S.; Huan, Y.; Guo, F.; Guan, B.; Yang, P.; Sarao, R.; Wada, T.; Leong-Poi, H.; et al. Angiotensin-converting enzyme 2 protects from severe acute lung failure. *Nature* **2005**, *436*, 112–116. [CrossRef]

34. Haga, S.; Yamamoto, N.; Nakai-Murakami, C.; Osawa, Y.; Tokunaga, K.; Sata, T.; Yamamoto, N.; Sasazuki, T.; Ishizaka, Y. Modulation of TNF-alpha-converting enzyme by the spike protein of SARS-CoV and ACE2 induces TNF-alpha production and facilitates viral entry. *Proc. Natl. Acad. Sci. USA* **2008**, *105*, 7809–7814. [CrossRef] [PubMed]

35. Beyerstedt, S.; Casaro, E.B.; Rangel, E.B. COVID-19: Angiotensin-converting enzyme 2 (ACE2) expression and tissue susceptibility to SARS-CoV-2 infection. *Eur. J. Clin. Microbiol. Infect. Dis.* **2021**, *40*, 905–919. [CrossRef] [PubMed]

36. Ngcobo, G.D. Measurement of serum ACE status may potentially improve the diagnosis of SARS-CoV-2 infection. *Sci. Afr.* **2021**, *14*, e01039. [CrossRef] [PubMed]

37. Bank, S.; De, S.K.; Bankura, B.; Maiti, S.; Das, M.; A Khan, G. ACE/ACE2 balance might be instrumental to explain the certain comorbidities leading to severe COVID-19 cases. *Biosci. Rep.* **2021**, *41*, BSR20202014. [CrossRef] [PubMed]

38. Ferrara, F.; Vitiello, A. Scientific Hypothesis for Treatment of COVID-19's Lung Lesions by Adjusting ACE/ACE2 Imbalance. *Cardiovasc. Toxicol.* **2021**, *21*, 498–503. [CrossRef]

39. Vidal-Petiot, E.; Gault, N. Renin-angiotensin system blockers and COVID-19. *BMC Med.* **2021**, *19*, 136. [CrossRef]

40. D'Ardes, D.; Boccatonda, A.; Rossi, I.; Guagnano, M.T.; Santilli, F.; Cipollone, F.; Bucci, M. COVID-19 and RAS: Unravelling an Unclear Relationship. *Int. J. Mol. Sci.* **2020**, *21*, 3003. [CrossRef]

41. Hoffmann, M.; Kleine-Weber, H.; Schroeder, S.; Kruger, N.; Herrler, T.; Erichsen, S.; Schiergens, T.S.; Herrler, G.; Wu, N.H.; Nitsche, A.; et al. SARS-CoV-2 Cell Entry Depends on ACE2 and TMPRSS2 and Is Blocked by a Clinically Proven Protease Inhibitor. *Cell* **2020**, *181*, 271–280.e8. [CrossRef] [PubMed]

42. Osman, I.O.; Melenotte, C.; Brouqui, P.; Million, M.; Lagier, J.C.; Parola, P.; Stein, A.; La Scola, B.; Meddeb, L.; Mege, J.L.; et al. Expression of ACE2, Soluble ACE2, Angiotensin I, Angiotensin II and Angiotensin-(1-7) Is Modulated in COVID-19 Patients. *Front. Immunol.* **2021**, *12*, 625732. [CrossRef]

43. Lu, Y.; Zhu, Q.; Fox, D.M.; Gao, C.; Stanley, S.A.; Luo, K. SARS-CoV-2 down-regulates ACE2 through lysosomal degradation. *Mol. Biol. Cell* **2022**, *33*, ar147. [CrossRef] [PubMed]

44. Triana, S.; Metz-Zumaran, C.; Ramirez, C.; Kee, C.; Doldan, P.; Shahraz, M.; Schraivogel, D.; Gschwind, A.R.; Sharma, A.K.; Steinmetz, L.M.; et al. Single-cell analyses reveal SARS-CoV-2 interference with intrinsic immune response in the human gut. *Mol. Syst. Biol.* **2021**, *17*, e10232. [CrossRef] [PubMed]

45. Ciulla, M.M. SARS-CoV-2 downregulation of ACE2 and pleiotropic effects of ACEIs/ARBs. *Hypertens. Res.* **2020**, *43*, 985–986. [CrossRef] [PubMed]
46. Kolberg, E.S.; Wickstrom, K.; Tonby, K.; Dyrhol-Riise, A.M.; Holten, A.R.; Amundsen, E.K. Serum ACE as a prognostic biomarker in COVID-19: A case series. *Acta Pathol. Microbiol. Immunol. Scand.* **2021**, *129*, 237–238. [CrossRef] [PubMed]
47. Kutz, A.; Conen, A.; Gregoriano, C.; Haubitz, S.; Koch, D.; Domenig, O.; Bernasconi, L.; Mueller, B.; Schuetz, P. Renin-angiotensin-aldosterone system peptide profiles in patients with COVID-19. *Eur. J. Endocrinol.* **2021**, *184*, 543–552. [CrossRef]
48. Saravi, B.; Li, Z.; Lang, C.N.; Schmid, B.; Lang, F.K.; Grad, S.; Alini, M.; Richards, R.G.; Schmal, H.; Sudkamp, N.; et al. The Tissue Renin-Angiotensin System and Its Role in the Pathogenesis of Major Human Diseases: Quo Vadis? *Cells* **2021**, *10*, 650. [CrossRef]
49. Liu, Y.; Yang, Y.; Zhang, C.; Huang, F.; Wang, F.; Yuan, J.; Wang, Z.; Li, J.; Li, J.; Feng, C.; et al. Clinical and biochemical indexes from 2019-nCoV infected patients linked to viral loads and lung injury. *Sci. China. Life Sci.* **2020**, *63*, 364–374. [CrossRef]
50. Amezcua-Guerra, L.M.; Del Valle, L.; Gonzalez-Pacheco, H.; Springall, R.; Marquez-Velasco, R.; Masso, F.; Brianza-Padilla, M.; Manzur-Sandoval, D.; Gonzalez-Flores, J.; Garcia-Avila, C.; et al. The prognostic importance of the angiotensin II/angiotensin-(1-7) ratio in patients with SARS-CoV-2 infection. *Ther. Adv. Respir. Dis.* **2022**, *16*, 17534666221122544. [CrossRef]
51. Daniell, H.; Nair, S.K.; Shi, Y.; Wang, P.; Montone, K.T.; Shaw, P.A.; Choi, G.H.; Ghani, D.; Weaver, J.; Rader, D.J.; et al. Decrease in Angiotensin-Converting Enzyme activity but not concentration in plasma/lungs in COVID-19 patients offers clues for diagnosis/treatment. *Mol. Therapy Methods Clin. Dev.* **2022**, *26*, 266–278. [CrossRef] [PubMed]
52. Diaz-Troyano, N.; Gabriel-Medina, P.; Weber, S.; Klammer, M.; Barquin-DelPino, R.; Castillo-Ribelles, L.; Esteban, A.; Hernandez-Gonzalez, M.; Ferrer-Costa, R.; Pumarola, T.; et al. Soluble Angiotensin-Converting Enzyme 2 as a Prognostic Biomarker for Disease Progression in Patients Infected with SARS-CoV-2. *Diagnostics* **2022**, *12*, 886. [CrossRef] [PubMed]
53. Lundstrom, A.; Ziegler, L.; Havervall, S.; Rudberg, A.S.; von Meijenfeldt, F.; Lisman, T.; Mackman, N.; Sanden, P.; Thalin, C. Soluble angiotensin-converting enzyme 2 is transiently elevated in COVID-19 and correlates with specific inflammatory and endothelial markers. *J. Med. Virol.* **2021**, *93*, 5908–5916. [CrossRef] [PubMed]
54. van Lier, D.; Kox, M.; Santos, K.; van der Hoeven, H.; Pillay, J.; Pickkers, P. Increased blood angiotensin converting enzyme 2 activity in critically ill COVID-19 patients. *ERJ Open Res.* **2021**, *7*, 00848–2020. [CrossRef] [PubMed]
55. Wang, K.; Gheblawi, M.; Nikhanj, A.; Munan, M.; MacIntyre, E.; O'Neil, C.; Poglitsch, M.; Colombo, D.; Del Nonno, F.; Kassiri, Z.; et al. Dysregulation of ACE (Angiotensin-Converting Enzyme)-2 and Renin-Angiotensin Peptides in SARS-CoV-2 Mediated Mortality and End-Organ Injuries. *Hypertension* **2022**, *79*, 365–378. [CrossRef] [PubMed]
56. Henry, B.M.; Benoit, S.; Lippi, G.; Benoit, J. Letter to the Editor—Circulating plasma levels of angiotensin II and aldosterone in patients with coronavirus disease 2019 (COVID-19): A preliminary report. *Prog. Cardiovasc. Dis.* **2020**, *63*, 702–703. [CrossRef] [PubMed]
57. Avanoglu Guler, A.; Tombul, N.; Aysert Yildiz, P.; Ozger, H.S.; Hizel, K.; Gulbahar, O.; Tufan, A.; Erbas, G.; Aygencel, G.; Guzel Tunccan, O.; et al. The assessment of serum ACE activity in COVID-19 and its association with clinical features and severity of the disease. *Scand. J. Clin. Lab. Investig.* **2021**, *81*, 160–165. [CrossRef]
58. Gerard, L.; Lecocq, M.; Bouzin, C.; Hoton, D.; Schmit, G.; Pereira, J.P.; Montiel, V.; Plante-Bordeneuve, T.; Laterre, P.F.; Pilette, C. Increased Angiotensin-Converting Enzyme 2 and Loss of Alveolar Type II Cells in COVID-19-related Acute Respiratory Distress Syndrome. *Am. J. Respir. Crit. Care Med.* **2021**, *204*, 1024–1034. [CrossRef]
59. Papadopoulou, A.; Fragkou, P.C.; Maratou, E.; Dimopoulou, D.; Kominakis, A.; Kokkinopoulou, I.; Kroupis, C.; Nikolaidou, A.; Antonakos, G.; Papaevangelou, V.; et al. Angiotensin-converting-enzyme insertion/deletion polymorphism, ACE activity, and COVID-19: A rather controversial hypothesis. A case-control study. *J. Med. Virol.* **2022**, *94*, 1050–1059. [CrossRef]
60. Zhu, Z.; Cai, T.; Fan, L.; Lou, K.; Hua, X.; Huang, Z.; Gao, G. The potential role of serum angiotensin-converting enzyme in coronavirus disease 2019. *BMC Infect. Dis.* **2020**, *20*, 883. [CrossRef]
61. Ozkan, S.; Cakmak, F.; Konukoglu, D.; Biberoglu, S.; Ipekci, A.; Akdeniz, Y.S.; Bolayirli, I.M.; Balkan, I.I.; Dumanli, G.Y.; Ikizceli, I. Efficacy of Serum Angiotensin II Levels in Prognosis of Patients With Coronavirus Disease 2019. *Crit. Care Med.* **2021**, *49*, e613–e623. [CrossRef] [PubMed]
62. Files, D.C.; Gibbs, K.W.; Schaich, C.L.; Collins, S.P.; Gwathmey, T.M.; Casey, J.D.; Self, W.H.; Chappell, M.C. A pilot study to assess the circulating renin-angiotensin system in COVID-19 acute respiratory failure. *Am. J. Physiol.-Lung Cell. Mol. Physiol.* **2021**, *321*, L213–L218. [CrossRef] [PubMed]
63. Wu, Z.; Hu, R.; Zhang, C.; Ren, W.; Yu, A.; Zhou, X. Elevation of plasma angiotensin II level is a potential pathogenesis for the critically ill COVID-19 patients. *Crit. Care* **2020**, *24*, 290. [CrossRef] [PubMed]
64. Henry, B.M.; Benoit, J.L.; Rose, J.; de Oliveira, M.H.S.; Lippi, G.; Benoit, S.W. Serum ACE activity and plasma ACE concentration in patients with SARS-CoV-2 infection. *Scand. J. Clin. Lab. Investig.* **2021**, *81*, 272–275. [CrossRef] [PubMed]
65. Henry, B.M.; Benoit, J.L.; Berger, B.A.; Pulvino, C.; Lavie, C.J.; Lippi, G.; Benoit, S.W. Coronavirus disease 2019 is associated with low circulating plasma levels of angiotensin 1 and angiotensin 1,7. *J. Med. Virol.* **2021**, *93*, 678–680. [CrossRef] [PubMed]
66. Camargo, R.L.; Bombassaro, B.; Monfort-Pires, M.; Mansour, E.; Palma, A.C.; Ribeiro, L.C.; Ulaf, R.G.; Bernardes, A.F.; Nunes, T.A.; Agrela, M.V.; et al. Plasma Angiotensin II Is Increased in Critical Coronavirus Disease 2019. *Front. Cardiovasc. Med.* **2022**, *9*, 847809. [CrossRef]
67. WHO Working Group on the Clinical Characterisation and Management of COVID-19 infection, A minimal common outcome measure set for COVID-19 clinical research. *Lancet Infect. Dis.* **2020**, *20*, e192–e197. [CrossRef]

68. Akin, S.; Schriek, P.; van Nieuwkoop, C.; Neuman, R.I.; Meynaar, I.; van Helden, E.J.; Bouazzaoui, H.E.; Baak, R.; Veuger, M.; Mairuhu, R.; et al. A low aldosterone/renin ratio and high soluble ACE2 associate with COVID-19 severity. *J. Hypertens.* **2022**, *40*, 606–614. [CrossRef]

69. Reindl-Schwaighofer, R.; Hodlmoser, S.; Eskandary, F.; Poglitsch, M.; Bonderman, D.; Strassl, R.; Aberle, J.H.; Oberbauer, R.; Zoufaly, A.; Hecking, M. ACE2 Elevation in Severe COVID-19. *Am. J. Respir. Crit. Care Med.* **2021**, *203*, 1191–1196. [CrossRef]

70. Kragstrup, T.W.; Singh, H.S.; Grundberg, I.; Nielsen, A.L.; Rivellese, F.; Mehta, A.; Goldberg, M.B.; Filbin, M.R.; Qvist, P.; Bibby, B.M. Plasma ACE2 predicts outcome of COVID-19 in hospitalized patients. *PLoS ONE* **2021**, *16*, e0252799. [CrossRef]

71. Shevchuk, O.; Pak, A.; Palii, S.; Ivankiv, Y.; Kozak, K.; Korda, M.; Vari, S.G. Blood ACE2 Protein Level Correlates with COVID-19 Severity. *Int. J. Mol. Sci.* **2023**, *24*, 13957. [CrossRef] [PubMed]

72. Elrayess, M.A.; Zedan, T.H.; Alattar, A.R.; Abusriwil, H.; Al-Ruweidi, M.; Almuraikhy, S.; Parengal, J.; Alhariri, B.; Yassine, H.M.; Hssain, A.A.; et al. Soluble ACE2 and angiotensin II levels are modulated in hypertensive COVID-19 patients treated with different antihypertension drugs. *Blood Press.* **2022**, *31*, 80–90. [CrossRef]

73. Maza, M.D.C.; Ubeda, M.; Delgado, P.; Horndler, L.; Llamas, M.A.; van Santen, H.M.; Alarcon, B.; Abia, D.; Garcia-Bermejo, L.; Serrano-Villar, S.; et al. ACE2 Serum Levels as Predictor of Infectability and Outcome in COVID-19. *Front. Immunol.* **2022**, *13*, 836516. [CrossRef] [PubMed]

74. Mohammadi, P.; Varpaei, H.A.; Seifi, A.; Zahak Miandoab, S.; Beiranvand, S.; Mobaraki, S.; Mohammadi, M.; Abdollahi, A. Soluble ACE2 as a Risk or Prognostic Factor in COVID-19 Patients: A Cross-sectional Study. *Med. J. Islam. Repub. Iran* **2022**, *36*, 135. [CrossRef] [PubMed]

75. Caldrer, S.; Mazzi, C.; Bernardi, M.; Prato, M.; Ronzoni, N.; Rodari, P.; Angheben, A.; Piubelli, C.; Tiberti, N. Regulatory T Cells as Predictors of Clinical Course in Hospitalised COVID-19 Patients. *Front. Immunol.* **2021**, *12*, 789735. [CrossRef] [PubMed]

76. Pucci, F.; Annoni, F.; Dos Santos, R.A.S.; Taccone, F.S.; Rooman, M. Quantifying Renin-Angiotensin-System Alterations in COVID-19. *Cells* **2021**, *10*, 2755. [CrossRef] [PubMed]

77. Gressens, S.B.; Leftheriotis, G.; Dussaule, J.C.; Flamant, M.; Levy, B.I.; Vidal-Petiot, E. Controversial Roles of the Renin Angiotensin System and Its Modulators During the COVID-19 Pandemic. *Front. Physiol.* **2021**, *12*, 624052. [CrossRef]

78. Oudit, G.Y.; Pfeffer, M.A. Plasma angiotensin-converting enzyme 2: Novel biomarker in heart failure with implications for COVID-19. *Eur. Heart J.* **2020**, *41*, 1818–1820. [CrossRef]

79. Chatterjee, S.; Nalla, L.V.; Sharma, M.; Sharma, N.; Singh, A.A.; Malim, F.M.; Ghatage, M.; Mukarram, M.; Pawar, A.; Parihar, N.; et al. Association of COVID-19 with Comorbidities: An Update. *ACS Pharmacol. Transl. Sci.* **2023**, *6*, 334–354. [CrossRef]

80. Fildes, J.E.; Walker, A.H.; Keevil, B.; Hutchinson, I.V.; Leonard, C.T.; Yonan, N. The effects of ACE inhibition on serum angiotensin II concentration following cardiac transplantation. *Transplantation* **2004**, *78*, 425. [CrossRef]

81. Emilsson, V.; Gudmundsson, E.F.; Aspelund, T.; Jonsson, B.G.; Gudjonsson, A.; Launer, L.J.; Jennings, L.L.; Gudmundsdottir, V.; Gudnason, V. Antihypertensive medication uses and serum ACE2 levels: ACEIs/ARBs treatment does not raise serum levels of ACE2. Preprint. *medRxiv* **2020**. [CrossRef]

82. Emilsson, V.; Gudmundsson, E.F.; Aspelund, T.; Jonsson, B.G.; Gudjonsson, A.; Launer, L.J.; Lamb, J.R.; Gudmundsdottir, V.; Jennings, L.L.; Gudnason, V. Serum levels of ACE2 are higher in patients with obesity and diabetes. *Obes. Sci. Pract.* **2020**, *7*, 239–243. [CrossRef] [PubMed]

83. Reindl-Schwaighofer, R.; Hödlmoser, S.; Domenig, O.; Krenn, K.; Eskandary, F.; Krenn, S.; Schörgenhofer, C.; Rumpf, B.; Karolyi, M.; Traugott, M.T.; et al. The systemic renin-angiotensin system in COVID-19. *Sci. Rep.* **2022**, *12*, 20117. [CrossRef] [PubMed]

84. Wang, K.; Gheblawi, M.; Oudit, G.Y.; Oudit, G.Y. Angiotensin Converting Enzyme 2: A Double-Edged Sword. *Circulation* **2020**, *142*, 426–428. [CrossRef] [PubMed]

85. Sohaei, D.; Hollenberg, M.; Janket, S.J.; Diamandis, E.P.; Poda, G.; Prassas, I. The therapeutic relevance of the Kallikrein-Kinin axis in SARS-cov-2-induced vascular pathology. *Crit. Rev. Clin. Lab. Sci.* **2023**, *60*, 25–40. [CrossRef] [PubMed]

86. Soro-Paavonen, A.; Gordin, D.; Forsblom, C.; Rosengard-Barlund, M.; Waden, J.; Thorn, L.; Sandholm, N.; Thomas, M.C.; Groop, P.H.; FinnDiane Study Group. Circulating ACE2 activity is increased in patients with type 1 diabetes and vascular complications. *J. Hypertens.* **2012**, *30*, 375–383. [CrossRef] [PubMed]

87. Yang, C.W.; Lu, L.C.; Chang, C.C.; Cho, C.C.; Hsieh, W.Y.; Tsai, C.H.; Lin, Y.C.; Lin, C.S. Imbalanced plasma ACE and ACE2 level in the uremic patients with cardiovascular diseases and its change during a single hemodialysis session. *Ren. Fail.* **2017**, *39*, 719–728. [CrossRef]

88. Ramchand, J.; Burrell, L.M. Circulating ACE2: A novel biomarker of cardiovascular risk. *Lancet* **2020**, *396*, 937–939. [CrossRef]

89. Fernández-Ruiz, I. ACE2 level as a marker of CVD. Nature reviews. *Cardiology* **2020**, *17*, 759.

90. Anguiano, L.; Riera, M.; Pascual, J.; Valdivielso, J.M.; Barrios, C.; Betriu, A.; Mojal, S.; Fernández, E.; Soler, M.J. NEFRONA study. Circulating angiotensin-converting enzyme 2 activity in patients with chronic kidney disease without previous history of cardiovascular disease. *Nephrol. Dial. Transplant.* **2015**, *30*, 1176–1185. [CrossRef]

91. Ramchand, J.; Patel, S.K.; Kearney, L.G.; Matalanis, G.; Farouque, O.; Srivastava, P.M.; Burrell, L.M. Plasma ACE2 Activity Predicts Mortality in Aortic Stenosis and Is Associated With Severe Myocardial Fibrosis. *Cardiovasc. Imaging* **2020**, *13*, 655–664. [CrossRef] [PubMed]

92. Fosbøl, E.L.; Butt, J.H.; Østergaard, L.; Andersson, C.; Selmer, C.; Kragholm, K.; Schou, M.; Phelps, M.; Gislason, G.H.; Gerds, T.A.; et al. Association of Angiotensin-Converting Enzyme Inhibitor or Angiotensin Receptor Blocker Use With COVID-19 Diagnosis and Mortality. *JAMA* **2020**, *324*, 168–177. [CrossRef] [PubMed]

93. Reynolds, H.R.; Adhikari, S.; Pulgarin, C.; Troxel, A.B.; Iturrate, E.; Johnson, S.B.; Hausvater, A.; Newman, J.D.; Berger, J.S.; Bangalore, S.; et al. Renin-Angiotensin-Aldosterone System Inhibitors and Risk of COVID-19. *N. Engl. J. Med.* **2020**, *382*, 2441–2448. [CrossRef] [PubMed]

94. Mancia, G.; Rea, F.; Ludergnani, M.; Apolone, G.; Corrao, G. Renin-Angiotensin-Aldosterone System Blockers and the Risk of COVID-19. *N. Engl. J. Med.* **2020**, *382*, 2431–2440. [CrossRef] [PubMed]

95. Dambha-Miller, H.; Hinton, W.; Wilcox, C.R.; Lemanska, A.; Joy, M.; Feher, M.; Stuart, B.; de Lusignan, S.; Hippisley-Cox, J.; Griffin, S. Mortality from angiotensin-converting enzyme-inhibitors and angiotensin receptor blockers in people infected with COVID-19: A cohort study of 3.7 million people. *Fam. Pract.* **2023**, *40*, 330–337. [CrossRef] [PubMed]

96. Schmaier, A.H. The plasma kallikrein-kinin system counterbalances the renin-angiotensin system. *J. Clin. Investig.* **2002**, *109*, 1007–1009. [CrossRef] [PubMed]

97. Garvin, M.R.; Alvarez, C.; Miller, J.I.; Prates, E.T.; Walker, A.M.; Amos, B.K.; Mast, A.E.; Justice, A.; Aronow, B.; Jacobson, D. A mechanistic model and therapeutic interventions for COVID-19 involving a RAS-mediated bradykinin storm. *eLife* **2020**, *9*, e59177. [CrossRef]

98. Bryant, J.W.; Shariat-Madar, Z. Human plasma kallikrein-kinin system: Physiological and biochemical parameters. *Cardiovasc. Hematol. Agents Med. Chem. (Former. Curr. Med. Chem. Cardiovasc. Hematol. Agents)* **2009**, *7*, 234–250. [CrossRef]

99. Ahiadu, B.K.; Ellis, T.; Graichen, A.; Kremer, R.B.; Rusling, J.F. Quantitative detection of RAS and KKS peptides in COVID-19 patient serum by stable isotope dimethyl labeling LC-MS. *Analyst* **2023**, *148*, 5926–5934. [CrossRef]

100. Marcolungo, L.; Beltrami, C.; Degli Esposti, C.; Lopatriello, G.; Piubelli, C.; Mori, A.; Pomari, E.; Deiana, M.; Scarso, S.; Bisoffi, Z.; et al. ACoRE: Accurate SARS-CoV-2 genome reconstruction for the characterization of intra-host and inter-host viral diversity in clinical samples and for the evaluation of re-infections. *Genomics* **2021**, *113*, 1628–1638. [CrossRef]

101. Xiao, F.; Burns, K.D. Measurement of Angiotensin Converting Enzyme 2 Activity in Biological Fluid (ACE2). *Methods Mol. Biol.* **2017**, *1527*, 101–115.

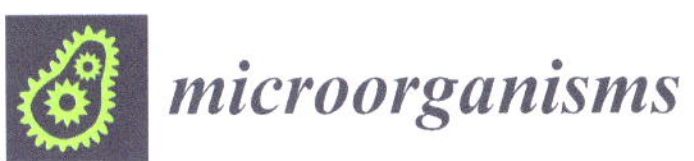

microorganisms

Review

SARS-CoV-2 and Other Respiratory Viruses in Human Olfactory Pathophysiology

Serigne Fallou Wade [1,*], Abou Abdallah Malick Diouara [2,*], Babacar Ngom [1], Fatou Thiam [2] and Ndongo Dia [3]

[1] École Supérieure des Sciences Agricoles et de l'Alimentation, Université Amadou Makhtar MBOW, Rue 21x20, 2ème Arrondissement, Pôle Urbain de Diamniadio, Dakar P.O. Box 45927, Senegal; babacar.ngom@uam.edu.sn

[2] Groupe de Recherche Biotechnologies Appliquées & Bioprocédés environnementaux (GRBA-BE), École Supérieure Polytechnique, Université Cheikh Anta Diop, Dakar P.O. Box 5085, Senegal; fatou54.thiam@ucad.edu.sn

[3] Virology Departement, Institut Pasteur de Dakar, 36, Avenue Pasteur, Dakar P.O. Box 220, Senegal; ndongo.dia@pasteur.sn

[*] Correspondence: serigne.wade@uam.edu.sn (S.F.W.); malick.diouara@ucad.edu.sn (A.A.M.D.)

Abstract: Acute respiratory viruses (ARVs) are the leading cause of diseases in humans worldwide. High-risk individuals, including children and the elderly, could potentially develop severe illnesses that could result in hospitalization or death in the worst case. The most common ARVs are the Human respiratory syncytial virus, Human Metapneumovirus, Human Parainfluenza Virus, rhinovirus, coronaviruses (including SARS and MERS CoV), adenoviruses, Human Bocavirus, enterovirus (-D68 and 71), and influenza viruses. The olfactory deficits due to ARV infection are a common symptom among patients. This review provides an overview of the role of SARS-CoV-2 and other common ARVs in the development of human olfactory pathophysiology. We highlight the critical need to understand the signaling underlying the olfactory dysfunction and the development of therapeutics for this wide-ranging category of AVRs to restore the altered or loss of smell in affected patients.

Keywords: respiratory viruses; anosmia; olfaction disorders; loss of smell; COVID-19

Citation: Wade, S.F.; Diouara, A.A.M.; Ngom, B.; Thiam, F.; Dia, N. SARS-CoV-2 and Other Respiratory Viruses in Human Olfactory Pathophysiology. *Microorganisms* **2024**, *12*, 540. https://doi.org/10.3390/microorganisms12030540

Academic Editor: Qibin Geng

Received: 13 October 2023
Revised: 7 November 2023
Accepted: 12 November 2023
Published: 7 March 2024

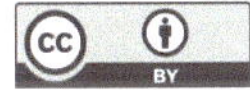

1. Introduction

Respiratory viral infections are very common and constitute a serious health concern around the world, with new infectious diseases continuing to emerge [1,2]. Such pathologies could lead to death, particularly in the elderly, and increase the expenses of the health care system worldwide. Respiratory viruses have the propensity to infect and trigger diseases through the human lower and upper respiratory tracts. We are more interested in viral upper respiratory infections (URI) as they are considered to be one of the most common causes of olfactory dysfunction, accounting for up to 45% of all cases [3,4]. Although the alteration of smell following viral URI is noticed in several cases, little treatment is currently available. The occurrence of this alteration is termed post-viral olfactory dysfunction (PVOD) [5–7]. The most common viruses implicated in PVOD include parainfluenza virus, rhinoviruses (RV), respiratory syncytial virus (RSV), and coronaviruses (CoV) [4,8–11]. In 1956, the RSV was found and isolated from chimpanzees and infants suffering severe lower respiratory tract illness a year later. In older children and healthy adults, the RSV causing repeated URI is common and can lead to symptomatic UR tract diseases [12]. According to Heikkinen and colleagues, 5% to 10% of URI are attributed to RSV. Studies performed in mice have shown that RSV infections are associated with damage to olfactory receptor neurons [13]. Despite these findings, the occurrence of olfactory loss associated with RSV infections seems low. It needs further investigations in broader regions of the world and during cold and warm periods to establish a clearer picture of this virus-induced olfactory dysfunction [11,14,15]. Like the RSV, the PIV was discovered in the 1950s and is associated with lower respiratory tract infections and URIs in children. Young children infected by this virus are often diagnosed with respiratory irritants, vitamin A deficiency, or malnutrition [16,17]. Although the PIV is found in respiratory secretions, the major diagnosis is observed from pulmonary secretions and confirmed by chest x-rays [18]. The RV that targets humans is considered among the most infectious agents worldwide and is associated with mild upper respiratory tract infections in people [19–21]. The CoV was identified in the 1960s. Little attention was given to this family of viruses until both outbreaks of the severe acute respiratory syndrome (SARS)-CoV and the Middle East respiratory syndrome (MERS)-CoV were identified in 2003 and 2012, respectively [22–24]. The novel coronavirus disease 2019 (COVID-19), caused by SARS-CoV-2, has spread fast all over the world [1,2]. Both MERS-CoV and SARS-CoV-2 are highly pathogenic coronaviruses and have a substantial spatial range of epidemics areas globally, but regarding MERS-CoV, the vast majority of cases are confined to the Middle East [23,24]. A key factor in the transmissibility of these viruses is the active virus replication in upper respiratory tract (URT) tissues and, therefore, its massive excretion [25,26]. Since the beginning of the pandemic, growing reports have shown the issues of partial to complete loss of smell in patients who contracted COVID-19 [27–30] and have brought new focus to PVOD. This review mainly focuses on understanding the molecular signaling underlying the olfactory pathophysiology in COVID-19-infected human patients and common viruses that induce URT infection. The importance of using such mechanisms in order to find potential targets to overcome the loss of smell will also be discussed.

2. Sources and Selection Criteria

The present study intends to synthesize the current knowledge regarding the relationship between the respiratory viral pathogenesis of the olfactory system and the mechanisms underlying the loss of smell in patients infected by respiratory viruses including COVID-19. We performed a literature search using mostly databases like PubMed Central (PMC), Google Scholar, and ScienceDirect to parse original articles, meta-analyses, and systematic reviews dealing with the animal and human respiratory viruses that have a negative impact on the olfactory system functionality. For our search, we used the combination of the following keywords: respiratory virus, coronavirus, rhinovirus, parainfluenza viruses and respiratory syncytial virus, anosmia, parosmia, hyposmia, olfactory epithelium, human, mouse, hamster, loss of smell, or olfactory dysfunction were considered in this review. Only the papers that met the keyword criteria listed above were considered in this work.

3. Olfactory Receptor and Odorant Detection

In most animals, the functional olfactory system detects and discriminates among diverse chemical stimuli. Odors are important for behaviors such as eating, mating, and avoiding dangerous smells, including smoke, leaking propane gas, and spoiled food [31–33]. The importance of the behaviors leads to a strong belief that the loss of olfactory function is indirectly life-threatening [34,35]. Two different olfactory systems have been developed in mammals such as rodents: the main olfactory epithelium (MOE), also called olfactory mucosa, connected to the main olfactory bulb, and the accessory system called the vomeronasal organ (VNO) connected to the accessory olfactory bulb [36–40]. Here, the VNO will not be discussed. The configuration of the olfactory epithelium (OE) presents unique cytological characteristics as it contains different cell types, such as the ciliated olfactory receptor neurons (ORNs), the sustentacular supporting cells, and the cells of Bowman's glands. The olfactory mucosa hosts many different types of cells, including ORNs in the intermediate layer, the sustentacular cells on the apical and basal sides, and the sensory cilia present at the apical pole where the dendrites of olfactory neurons are extended [41,42].

A deep understanding of the molecular signaling of smelling recognition is required to understand the basis of the olfactory system and, consequently, the loss of olfactory function. Starting from the beginning of the 1990s, pioneers have developed and studied the physiology of the olfactory system based on molecular biology, biochemistry, anatomy, and bioinformatics [31,43]. At first glance, getting insight into the molecular mechanisms of the perception of odors has emerged from several disciplines such as chemistry, biology, and professional odor detectors [31,43].

The detection occurs when the odorants penetrate into the nasal cavity and reach the olfactory mucosa. The odorants then interact with specific ORNs in the olfactory mucosa. Once an ORN is activated by an odorant, a nervous influx is sent to the cortex via the olfactory bulb. Readers interested in the mammalian olfactory epithelium and the perception of odor coding are invited to view an excellent review by Kurian and colleagues published in 2020 [44].

4. Viral Infection Causing Olfactory Dysfunction

The fact that the olfactory receptor neurons (ORNs) are found in the nasal cavity and expressed in the OE makes them directly exposed to all kinds of air-bound and airway pathogens that make the ORNs vulnerable. Whether the cause is physiological or pathological, the lifespan of ORNs is relatively short with a few weeks in the OE. Moreover, stem cell reprogramming ensures the continuous regeneration of new ORNs from OE basal cells either in a physiological turnover of ORNs or in response to inflammation and OE severe damage mediated by neural injury [45–47]. Several airway pathogens, such as viruses, are causing damage to OE, particularly through the sustentacular cells, triggering anosmia, hyposmia, phantosmia, or parmosmia in mammals [7,9,42,48,49]. Many respiratory tract infections due to viruses like RV, PIV, RSV, CoV, and Epstein-Barr viruses (EBV) [4,8–11] have been involved in the development of olfactory disorders such as partial or total loss of smell. Doty and others have termed this pathology as virus-induced olfactory dysfunction (PVOD) [3,5,6,50]. Viral infection destroys many cells within the apical layer of the OE, which could lead to ORN functional impairment in the nose. Interestingly, the OE basal cells can constantly replace damaged ORNs with new olfactory neurons, allowing patients to recover functional olfactory responses [46,47]. In the following sections, the common viral infection of the URT leading to olfactory dysfunction like anosmia, hyposmia, phantosmia, and parmosmia [4] in animal models and humans will be discussed.

5. Viruses Impacting Respiratory System

The respiratory system is exposed to the environment and is in permanent contact with air-way pathogens like viruses. A recent investigation in humans has identified 18 viruses in patients with PVOD. Several known viruses are associated with olfactory impairment, and it is crucial to investigate the mechanisms of infection as well as the specific receptors each virus targets (Table 1).

5.1. Case of the Parainfluenza Viruses

The presence of parainfluenza type 3 (PIV3) was observed in human nasal epithelial cells (HNECs) from 88% of patients with PVOD as compared to 9% of control patients [51]. This data suggests the potential involvement of PIV3 infection in the upper airway pathology. PIV3 in the turbinate epithelial cells of PVOD is responsible for 60% of hyposmia and 40% of anosmia in patients [51]. PIV3 has been shown to infect the HNECs and, therefore, exacerbate the production of IFN-γ and pro-inflammatory cytokines [52]. This data is in line with a previous study suggesting that PIV3 may cause olfactory dysfunction through mechanisms other than nasal obstruction in patients [9].

5.2. Case of the Sendai Virus (SeV) and Possible Interaction with PIV

The SeV, the murine counterpart of the human PIV, has been shown to directly infect the mouse brain via the olfactory neurons [53]. Another investigation demonstrated that SeV infection led to impairing mouse olfaction. Interestingly, the virus persists in OE and OB tissues for over two months and reduces the regenerative power and functionality of the ORNs [54]. Very recent findings have shown that the depletion of nasal cilia via the silencing of CEP83, a protein critical for motile cilia formation in all ciliated cells, would impede the PIV infection. Indeed, the PIV receptor CX3CR1 colocalizes to motile cilia and is a plausible viral entry mechanism into the cells [55]. An additional study showed that the intercellular adhesion molecule-1 (ICAM-1) and related cytokine molecules are induced by PIV3, and it is thought that this activation participates in the inflammation during infection by viruses [56,57] (Figure 1). Further research using the power of the transcriptomic analysis is necessary to help delineate the role of the PIV and implicated mechanisms in the development of the broad range of olfactory dysfunctions in patients and to find host-response transcript signatures for possible treatments. The study of the entire RNA transcripts in a biological sample is referred to as transcriptomics, technically available as microarrays and RNA sequencing (RNA-seq) [58]. Only recently, some precision medicine trials using transcriptome analysis have been applied in the field of cancer [59–63]. Data from the study of Rodon and colleagues suggest that clinical trials using transcriptomics analysis can increase the number of patients matched to drugs [62]. Recent findings on the molecular basis of neuroimmune responses revealed that the transcriptomic results are in line with a few previously reported studies of respiratory viral infections like Influenza A virus, RV, and RSV. Moreover, these data highlighted putative biomarkers of interest as a direct reflection of each virus infection and deserve further investigation for the evaluation/prediction of future innovative treatments [64–66].

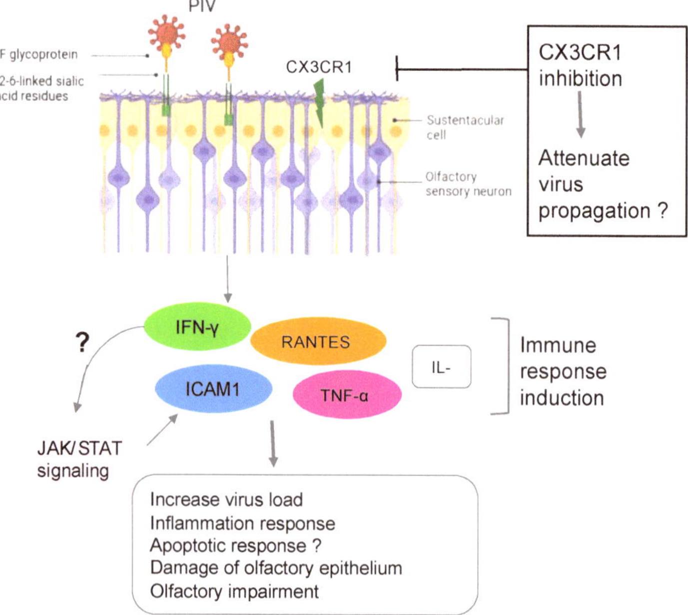

Figure 1. Action of PIV in the olfactory impairment. PIV induced the inflammation response with damage to olfactory epithelium and the impairment of olfactory response, leading to more virus susceptibility.

5.3. Case of the Respiratory Syncytial Virus (RSV)

Recent findings have demonstrated that the RSV can infect olfactory sensory neurons (OSNs) in the nasal cavity of the mouse before accessing the central nervous system of the animal [67]. As a PIV, the RSV targets the cilia of the epithelial cells in the airways by fusionning its F-glycoprotein to the cellular receptor human nucleolin (NCL). RSV also uses another mechanism that activates protein kinases like IGF1R to get into the cells [56,68,69]. Furthermore, recent studies have shown the essential role of the nucleolin

RNA binding domain RBD1,2 in allowing the infection of RSV [70]. Previous works have pointed out the importance of ORN progenitors in the turnover. They showed that RSV infection causes SOX2+ ORN progenitors damage prior to the manifestation of ORN impairment. Unfortunately, the airway allergy seems to amplify this damage induced by the RSV infection, leading to a possible loss of OMP+ ORNs [13]. Transcriptomic analysis demonstrated that olfactory signaling is among the altered pathways in patients suffering from RSV infection. This finding further supports previous work that described RSV as a causative agent of post-viral olfactory dysfunction. Interestingly, the authors highlighted that this molecular signaling could be a promising future route to investigate drug targets against RSV infection [3,34]. Sourimant et al. have recently shown that 4′-fluorouridine, a ribonucleoside analog, inhibits RSV in a selective manner in cells and human airway epithelia organoids. Although this oral therapeutic drug is efficient in small animal models, several years of investigations are needed before predicting/evaluating the outcome of applying such a type of molecule in humans [71] (Figure 2). Furthermore, many efforts are underway in the phase of clinical trials when mRNA vaccines are combined with antigens to fight multiple respiratory viruses, including the RSV [72,73].

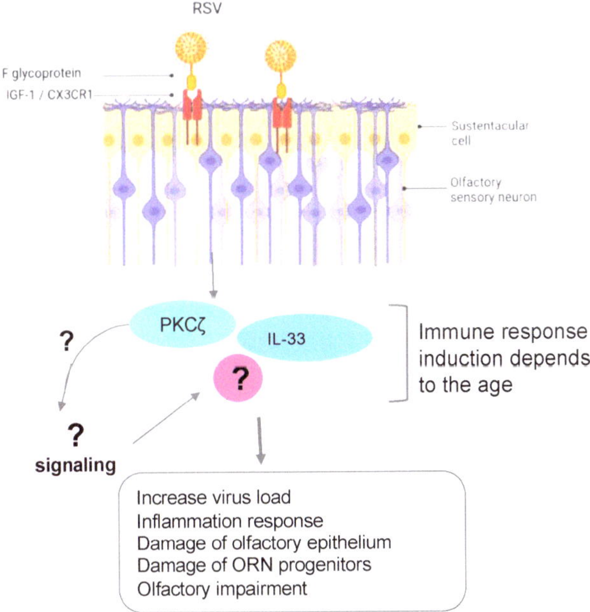

Figure 2. Role of RSV in olfactory impairment. RSV induced the inflammation response related to the age group with damage of olfactory epithelium and OSN progenitors and the impairment of olfactory response, leading to more virus susceptibility.

Table 1. Summary of virus-implication in PVOD.

Viruses	Animal or Cell Model	Effect of Respiratory Viruses on the Nasal Epithelial System	Comments	References
Parainfluenza virus	HNECs	PIV3 infection enhances the production of IFN-γ and generation of RANTES	• IFN-γ protein was observed in non-infected cells for up to 72 h. • 24 h post viral infection, were sufficient to notice significant increase of the IFN-γ but RANTES was detected only after 48 h. • Study using epithelial primary cells or animal model to help decipher the role of IFN-γ in PIV3 induced PVOD. • Data from Jun Tian et al. study provided some explanations on the later point.	[52]
	ALI-cultured NHE cells	Inhibition of cilia or microvilli may prevent airway entry and PIV spread throughout the viral-CX3CR1 receptor interactions in the ciliated HNEs	• Presence of nasal cilia enhances PIV infection. • Attenuation of virus trafficking might occur via CX3CR1 inhibition within the cilia as compared to TMPRSS2 inhibitor in SARS-CoV-2 propagation.	[55]
Sendai virus (SeV)	C57BL/6 mice and primary OSNs cultures	SeV prevents the primary cells from taking up the Ca^{2+} in the presence of odorants therefore altering directly the function of the OSN,	• SeV is the murine counterpart of the human PIV. • SeV triggers declination of the mouse olfactory function reaching a peak 15 days post-infection and persisting at least for 2 months in approximately 33% of animals • The virus decreases apoptosis and cell proliferation. • The normal cell turnover is lacking which may explain the inability of the olfactory epithelium to normally regenerate. • The inflammation after a virus infection may also be considered as an additional mechanism in driving the olfactory neuron impairment.	[54]
	HT1080 cells	ICAM-1 is activated by PIV3 throughout the induction of the JAK/STAT signaling pathways.	• The induction of ICAM-1 would trigger the inflammation during PIV3 infection. • This induction is IFN signaling-independent.	[57]
Respiratory syncytial virus (RSV)	Mice and airway organoid cultures	Prefusion RSV-F glycoprotein is required to bind with the IGF-1 receptor. Such association triggers the activation of PKCζ.	• Reduction of viral replication and pathology in RSV-infected mice after blunting PKCζ. • Nucleolin-specific antibodies decrease RSV infection as well as RNAi designed to cellular nucleolin expression • inhibition of RSV infections when a specific molecule targets the nucleolin RNA binding domain RBD1,2 of the virus. • Preventing the linkage between RSV-F glycoprotein and IGF-1 to occur could form the basis of new therapeutics to treat RSV infection.	[68–70]

Table 1. *Cont.*

Viruses	Animal or Cell Model	Effect of Respiratory Viruses on the Nasal Epithelial System	Comments	References
Respiratory syncytial virus (RSV)	Female BALB/c mice	Reduced SOX2$^+$ ORN progenitors was enhanced and prolonged in allergic mice infected by RSV.	• Expression of SOX2$^+$ ORN progenitors were affected in the nasal mucosa due to RSV transient infection. • Delayed RSV clearance and exacerbated progenitors damage observed in airway allergy mice.	[13]
Rhinoviruses	Sinus epithelial tissue, HeLa R-19, mouse L cells	The following three major types of cellular membrane glycoproteins ICAM-1, LDLR and CDHR3 are targeted by RV to gain entry into the host cell.	• Enhanced expression of these receptors increased RV interaction and enabled replication in nasal host cells. • Reduced virus adhesion throughout receptor-antibody would neutralize RV entry and attenuate cell inflammation leading to olfactory dysfunction.	[74–77]
	Sinonasal epithelial cells	H_2O_2 significantly reduced the production of (IFN-β) and type III (IFN- λ1 and λ2) interferons that was upregulated in cells infected with RV.	• Decrease expression of TLR3, RIG-1, MDA5, and IRF3 was observed in cells pretreated with H_2O_2. • Nrf2 siRNA showed decreased secretion of anti-viral interferons in transfected cells. • Oxidative stress inhibiting the anti-viral interferons in the sinonasal mucosa due to RV infection is a potential road to prevent inflammation-induced PVOD.	[78]
SARS-CoV-2	ciliated HNE cells	SARS-CoV-2 establishes a link with angiotensin-converting enzyme 2 (ACE2) receptor within the airway multicilia to traverse the mucus-mucin protective barrier.	• Depleting cilia prevents virus virus entry. • Inhibition of PAK1, PAK4 and SLK kinases activity reduces virus spread in mice. • Depleting cilia in nasal epithelial cells does not affect ACE2 and transmembrane serine protease 2 (TMPRSS2 levels). • More insight into cilia and microvilli reprogrammation for virus entry would identify marker candidates for treatment to block airway replication of SARS-CoV-2.	[55]
	K18-hACE2 mice, golden Syrian hamsters, cellular models	SARS-CoV-2 targets the sustentacular and Bowman gland cells by binding to their ACE2 and TMPRSS2 proteins.	• Exponential growth of the virus leading to the destruction of these supporting cells. • Significant reduced thickness of the mucus layer could be related to the Bowman's glands deterioration which are the precursor of the mucus. • Healthy mucus is crucial for odor detection as it enables odorants to diffuse to olfactory receptors. • Retraction of OSN cilia, although the mature OSN are free of SARS-CoV-2 viral load. • SARS-CoV-2 alterates throughout the supporting cells not only the structure of mucus but also the OSN cilia which contribute to the olfactory dysfunction.	[79–86]

Table 1. *Cont.*

Viruses	Animal or Cell Model	Effect of Respiratory Viruses on the Nasal Epithelial System	Comments	References
	K18-hACE2 mice, golden Syrian hamsters, cellular models	Supporting cells infected by SARS-CoV-2 affect the expression of the GLUT1/GLUT3 that interrupt the glucose trafficking to the cilia of the ORN in the mucus.	• Sustentacular cells and Bowman gland cells supply additional glucose to the cilia that is necessary for the ORN to respond to odorants. • SARS-CoV-2 uses the internal glucose as a fuel to maximize its replication thus preventing the cilia to undergo odorant-induced response of the ORN. • Loss of glucose normally supplied by sustentacular cells and Bowman gland cells. • SARS-CoV-2 exhibits supporting cell damage that consequently trigger the interruption of the supply of additional glucose to the cilia of the ORN via GLUT1/GLUT3.	[87–91]
	ALI and iALI cells	SARS-CoV-2 activates key molecular mechanisms after infecting ALI and iALI cellular models.	• SARS-CoV-2 infection in ALI and iALI cells activates inflammatory state and innate immune response. • The virus induces epithelial disruption, loss of mature ciliated cells. • miRNAs like MIR138 regulates ISG15 expression and plays a role in the virus-induced pro-inflammatory genes activation. • The option of miRNAs is promising for COVID-19 treatment and/or prevention.	[92]

Recently, RVs were shown to be among the more predominant causative agents of PVOD in patients. The study showed that patients with anosmia were higher than those with hyposmia (58.8% vs. 19.0%, $p = 0.018$) [8]. In line with these findings, it is tempting to suggest that the persistence of the virus could be one factor that governs a more severe injury to the olfactory system. In fact, RVs primarily invade the ciliated respiratory epithelial cells via the glycoprotein members such as the intercellular adhesion molecule 1 (ICAM-1), the low-density lipoprotein receptor (LDLR) family members, and the cadherin-related family member 3 (CDHR3) [74–77]. RV infection induces Toll-like receptor 7 (TLR7) and retinoic acid-inducible gene I (RIG-1) that trigger the activation of cytokine expression (type I and type III IFNs) [93–95]. Understanding the mechanisms of RV viral-induced asthma for new therapeutic directions has gained more attention in the recent past [96–98]. Papi et al. have investigated the role of reducing agents such as DMSO on RV infection in the nasal epithelium. They showed that rhinovirus-induced ICAM-1 mRNA expression was inhibited by reducing agents in a dose-dependent manner. Interestingly, NF-κB and TNF-α activation, which is necessary for the ICAM-1 promoter, was completely abolished in those treated epithelial cells [99]. Moreover, it has been shown that CDHR3 genetic variants impact on the severity of RV-related pediatric respiratory tract infections by upregulating the epithelial expression of RV receptors, thus helping clinicians predict the susceptibility and severity of RV infection [100]. Complementary recent studies have demonstrated that both vitamin D and hydrogen peroxide play a critical role in attenuating the RV, mediating the ICAM-1 activation and the production of type I (IFN-β) and type III (IFN-λ1 and λ2) interferons respectively [78,101] (Figure 3). To further support these collective findings, it would be interesting to document transcriptomic profiles from animal and cellular models infected by RVs and treated by those molecules. These works would shed light on the importance of genes, including the oxidant biomarkers to be considered for the future in the development of the treatment against RV infection.

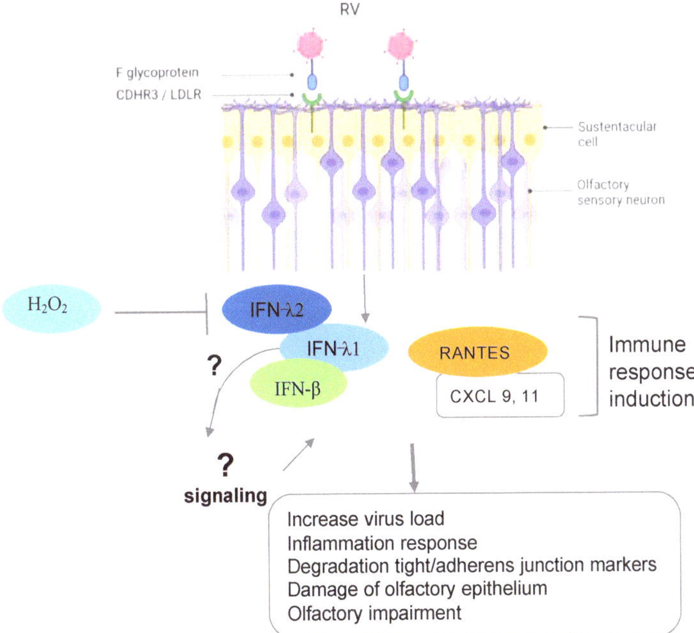

Figure 3. Implication of RV in olfactory impairment. RV induced the inflammation response with damage to the olfactory epithelium, the degradation of the tight junction and adherent junction markers, and the impairment of olfactory response leading to more virus susceptibility.

6. Mechanisms of SARS-CoV-2 Mediating the Loss of Smell

The post-COVID and the long-term-COVID have both tremendously triggered a lot of complications in different human systems. The loss or reduction of smell, among other complications of the nervous system, is an associated symptom for patients affected by different variants of COVID-19, including the omicron variant [102–106]. Moreover, studies reported that the prevalence of olfactory dysfunction differs greatly between populations and approaches [106–108]. Currently, many COVID-19 vaccines are authorized to help protect and eliminate the virus. The COVID-19 pathology and the cellular mechanism by which the olfactory dysfunction occurs have gained a lot of attention since the pandemic, and researchers are still investigating underlying signaling and complications (Table 1) [55,91,92,106,109–112]. Earlier in the pandemic, reports hypothesized that five potential mechanisms were considered to get insights into the olfactory dysfunction in COVID-19 patients: (1) obstruction/congestion and rhinorrhea of the nasal airway, (2) damage and loss of ORNs, (3) Olfactory center damage in the brain, (4) damage of the olfactory supporting cells in the OE, and (5) Inflammation-related olfactory epithelium dysfunction [107,113]. Butowt et al. have recently reviewed that at least the following hypotheses (1)–(3) turned out to be implausible in explaining the olfactory dysfunction in patients [113]. This allegation is further confirmed by very recent studies showing that SARS-CoV-2 infection significantly increased the expression of interferon-stimulated and inflammatory genes. Alteration of extracellular matrix genes was also observed in ALI and iALI-infected cells [92]. Here, we will particularly review the mechanisms related to the second, the fourth, and the fifth scenarios according to the available findings. Healthy sensory cilia of ORNs in the olfactory epithelium are crucial in perceiving odorant molecules before sending the information to the olfactory bulbs and then to the upper parts of the brain [45]. It has been reported in humans that SARS-CoV-2 may indirectly affect the olfactory cilia, hindering the smelling system's efficacy [114]. Reports suggested that ORNs lack the ability to express the entry proteins of SARS-CoV-2 in the OE. The virus seems to establish first contact in human nasal epithelia by binding its spike S protein to specific cells in the OE [115]. These reports are confirmed by a study based on in silico data, predicting that mature ORNs do not express the virus entry protein, the angiotensin-converting enzyme 2 (ACE2), and therefore are not likely to be infected by SARS-CoV-2 [81]. Furthermore, supporting data by Bryche et al. showed that SARS-CoV-2 was not detected in the ORNs of golden Siryan hamsters [85]. However, in a few cases, authors suggested that SARS-CoV-2 could infect ORNs in hamsters [111]. Based on the fact that COVID-19-related loss of smell disappeared within 1–2 weeks, while the regeneration of dead ORNs needs more than two weeks, many data tend to conclude that COVID-19-related olfactory dysfunction (OD) is not directly associated with the impairment of the ORNs [107,113,115–117]. Consequently, studying the entry protein expression within the cells in the OE will help to understand the sensitivity of the OE to SARS-CoV-2 infection related to the high prevalence of ODs in patients. Many groups are now interested in the organization of the sustentacular cells in the OE and thought that they might play a central role in leading to OD. A high level of expression of ACE2 and the transmembrane serine protease 2 (TMPRSS2) is particularly found on the sustentacular cells, suggesting a path to the neurotropism of SARS-CoV-2 in the OE. The ACE2 and TMPRSS2 are respectively known as the SARS-CoV-2 receptor and the SARS-CoV-2 cell entry-priming protease. ACE2 is found mainly on different parts of the sustentacular cells, both in humans and mice. The ACE2 and TMPRSS2 genes tend to be co-regulated [113,118–122]. Different approaches using tissues, cells, and organ systems in humans, golden Syrian hamsters, and hACE2 transgenic mice have been employed to study the pathological impact of the SARS-CoV-2. Here, we discussed findings related particularly to the OE in inducing ODs in humans. The spike protein (S protein) of SARS-CoV-2 mediates the passage of the virus into the host cell by fusing the viral and host cell membranes. In fact, via his spike S, SARS-CoV-2 employs ACE2 as the host functional receptor and TMPRSS2 as the cellular priming protease facilitating viral uptake, both signalings being confirmed by Single-cell RNA sequencing (scRNA-seq) datasets from the Human Cell Atlas consortium [123–125]. Another study showed that SARS-CoV-2 Nucleocapsid protein (NP) was observed in human OE through the neuronal marker Tuj1 9 h post-infection. This data further supported the enrichment of ACE2 in human olfactory sustentacular cells [119,126]. Earlier in the pandemic, the golden Syrian hamster was used as a model to document the pathology of SARS-CoV-2 in the OE post-infection. Reports showed that the sustentacular cells are rapidly infected by SARS-CoV-2. This viral neurotropism is associated with a massive recruitment of immune cells in the OE and lamina propria, which could drive the disorganization of the OE structure [85]. This study is consistent with a high level of Tumor Necrosis Factor α (TNF α) observed in OE samples from COVID-19-suffering patients and in ALI and iALI-infected cells [79,92]. Furthermore, the inflammation induced by SARS-CoV-2 infected supporting cells may play an important role in the onset and persistence of loss of smell in patients. This SARS-CoV-2-associated inflammation status was confirmed by the transcriptome of the in vitro human airway epithelium and by analyzing the expression of selected targets in the olfactory bulb using RNA-seq and RT-qPCR tools. Interestingly, this study showed that the proinflammatory markers, including NFKBIA, CSF1, FOSL1, Cxcl10, Il-1β, Ccl5, and Irf7 overexpression continued up to 14 dpi when animals had recovered from ageusia/anosmia [92,127]. These findings are in line with a very recent study showing the implication of immune cell infiltration and altered gene expression in OE in driving persistent smell loss in a subset of patients with SARS-CoV-2. Moreover, this study particularly demonstrates that T cell-mediated inflammation lasts longer in the OE after the acute SARS-CoV-2 infection has been eliminated from the tissue, suggesting a mechanistic insight into the long-term post-COVID-19 smell loss [105]. The OE disorganization is followed by a drastic deterioration of the cilia layer of the ORNs that leads to the impairment of the olfactory capacity of the animal [85]. Investigations in humans and hamsters using, respectively, Transmission Electron Microscopy (TEM) studies and Scanning Electron Microscopy (SEM) analysis showed various levels of cilia height that undergo regeneration in the course of patient recovery, including smell restoration. Data using the golden Syrian hamster showed that the regenerated cilia in the epithelium are accompanied by a decreased expression of FOXJ1+, highlighting the importance of this marker in respiratory ciliogenesis. This later finding by Schreiner et al., could in part shed light on the inquiry of how could we regenerate cilia during patient recovery, although a lot needs to be done in the roadmap of treating loss of smell related to nasal cilia deterioration by SARS-CoV-2 [55,104,128,129] (Figure 4; Table 1).

According to the literature, different variants of SARS-CoV-2 do not directly target the ORNs in the OE; instead, they are found in the majority expressed in the sustentacular cells [42]. A recent study by Seehusen et al. showed that K18-hACE2 transgenic mouse expressing the human ACE2 is highly sensitive to at least five variants of SARS-CoV-2 that infected not only the supportive cells in OE and the respiratory epithelium but invaded the CNS of the animal five days post-infection. Interestingly, the expression of hACE2 seems to convey higher binding affinity when compared to the wild-type mouse [130]. Using this transgenic mouse is revealed to be a serious option for therapy development against loss of smell as these animals exhibited low mortality when treated with COVID-19 convalescent antisera [80,130]. For instance, the miRNA is shown to play a crucial role in the regulation of immune genes deregulated, and the development of miRNA antagonists or mimics seems to be a promising new therapeutic strategy for the treatment of patients with COVID-19 on other respiratory viruses-induced PVOD [72,73,92,131–133].

It is now accepted that ACE2 is not the only obligate entry for SARS-CoV-2 as it has been suggested that molecules including PIKfyve or neuropilin-1 (NRP-1) may participate in SARS-CoV-2 entry [82–84]. Like ACE2, NRP-1 is highly expressed in the respiratory and olfactory epithelium, which further supports the infectivity and entry of SARS-CoV-2 in the human OE. NRP-1 is not only found in supportive cells but is expressed in nearly every cell type in the nasal passages, including the ORN, therefore giving SARS-CoV-2 a route to access those cells and impair the olfactory response. Interestingly, Daly et al.

demonstrated that the selective inhibition of the S1-NRP-1 interaction reduces SARS-CoV-2 infection [84,86,87].

Taken together, the high expression of ACE2, TMPRSS2, and NRP-1 in supportive and other olfactory cells and their impact on olfactory neurophysiology maintenance and in the development of human olfactory pathophysiology supports them as potential targets for signaling-based therapeutics of olfactory dysfunction.

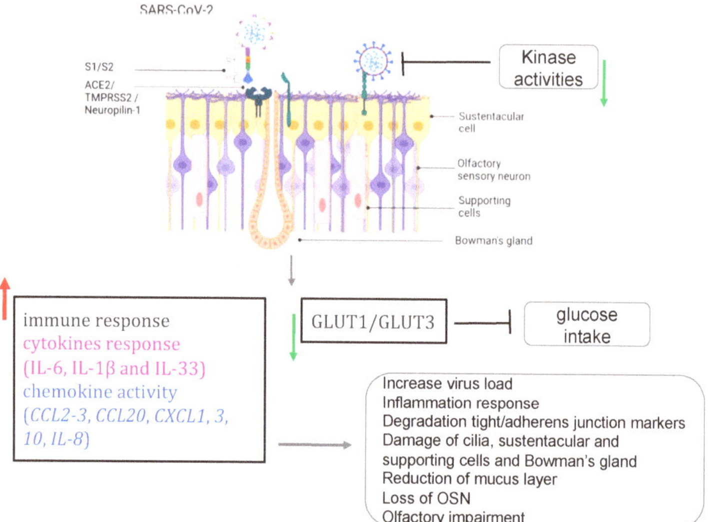

Figure 4. Role of SARS-CoV-2 in olfactory impairment. SARS-CoV-2 induced disruption of the nasal epithelium, with loss/damage of olfactory sensory neurons, sustentacular cells, Bowman's gland, and supporting cells. All figures were created with BioRender.com (accessed on 7 October 2023).

7. Pathological Implications of ARV Co-Infections

Coinfections with SARS CoV-2 and other ARVs may have tremendous pathological implications with potentially fatal outcomes [134–137]. The proportion of coinfections in SARS-CoV-2-infected patients and the types of viruses involved vary in different regions of the world depending on the sensitivity of the diagnostic tests used, population studied, climate, sampling period, and temporal variations in viral epidemiology. Some studies report proportions that vary from 1.7 to 20% [134,138–143]. Authors hypothesize that competitive advantage may play a role in SARS-CoV-2 interaction with other respiratory viruses during coinfection, and this is one reason why the coinfection rate in SARS-CoV-2 patients is much lower [142]. In many cases, the detection of RSV, influenza A, and other coinfections led to changes in clinical management in admitted patients to the medical intensive care unit [136,137].

Picornaviruses, influenza A and B, RSV, and parainfluenza are among the most detected viruses in COPD exacerbations [135]. Increased susceptibility to viral respiratory infections such as SARS-CoV-2 has been reported in chronic obstructive pulmonary disease (COPD), often worsened by bacterial co-infections and leading to serious clinical outcomes [137].

Trifonova et al. reported a more intensive replication of SARS CoV-2 and influenza viruses compared to that of other respiratory viruses involved in coinfections. The level of the viral load involved in mixed infections depends largely on the time of exposure to one virus relative to the other. These authors explain their findings by the fact of positive or negative interactions between SARS-CoV-2 and other respiratory viruses via interferon-mediated or other immunological mechanisms [134].

8. Clinical Trials for Respiratory Virus Infection

The protection against viral infection affecting human respiratory tracts constitutes a huge challenge and, therefore, forces clinicians and scientists to develop effective antivirals or vaccines to alleviate the death rate in patients [144]. Although mRNA COVID-19 vaccines are being authorized and administrated since 2020, for most of the respiratory viruses, there is no vaccine currently available. Moreover, in general, vaccination is efficient before the onset of the viral season infection. For example, the RSV seasonality was affected by the COVID-19 pandemic [145]. Currently, two molecules are being used against RSV: ribavirin for treatment and palivizumab for prevention. Many other antivirals to prevent RSV are in experimental stages as well as the use of anti-inflammatory drugs is to be considered, although the efficiency is to be verified [146]. To date, several recombinant RSV subunit vaccines are in different clinical phases 1 and 2 trials [147,148], which is in line with the undergoing clinical development of new vaccines for protecting the children and the elderly against RSV infection [149–153]. Very recently, the Food and Drug Administration (FDA) has approved the first vaccines for the prevention of RSV-associated low respiratory tract (LRT) in adults 60 years old and over. Both the GSK RSV vaccine and the Pfizer RSV vaccine were evaluated for their efficacy and safety. The efficacy of 1 dose of the GSK and Pfizer vaccine in preventing medically attended RSV-associated LRT was 77.5% and 81.0%, respectively, and both were safe according to the low severe reactogenicity events (group participants vs. control group participants) [145]. For instance, it is to be elucidated whether those new RSV vaccines will help to prevent the loss of smell within the URT in adults. The inhalation of ALX-0171 to prevent RSV infection in infants and toddlers is at Phase IIb clinical trial and is still under investigation for approval by the US FDA [154]. Regarding the PIV, the treatment is still for symptoms, although several investigations are being conducted to prepare a viable vaccine [155,156]. A study in 2019 has shown that DAS181, a sialidase fusion protein, may have clinical activity, particularly in immunocompromised patients with PIV, based on the data from the clinical phase 3 trials [157]. Karron and colleagues have recently conducted a phase I clinical trial of the live-attenuated recombinant human PIV2 in adults, as well as in children and seronegative children. In fact, rHPIV2-15C/948L/Δ1724 was appropriately restricted in replication in adults and HPIV2-seropositive children but was overattenuated for HPIV2 seronegative children. Their evaluation showed that the rHPIV2-15C/948L/Δ1724 represents less attenuated alternatives for pediatric vaccine development [158]. Further testing and clinical trials are required in the fight against the human PIV, especially PIV type 3, as it is considered to be the most virulent form of human PIV [159]. To our knowledge, there are no available vaccines or drugs against rhinovirus infections. Physical distancing seems to be not effective in reducing the transmission of this virus. But, it is essential to notice that rhinovirus infection is not associated with a significant rate of hospitalization or death [160]. Several researchers have demonstrated that daily dosing of 1 million IU of intranasal IFN-alpha gave 75–87% protection against rhinovirus infection [161,162]. The use of zinc gluconate lozenges has proven to be an effective treatment in reducing symptoms of rhinovirus infection [163]. For instance, if the vaccine against rhinovirus is not available, one may consider taking an antiviral with other antimediators for better protection from infection by the rhinovirus [164]. According to the WHO, COVID-19 treatment guidelines are evolving and fortunately several COVID-19 vaccines have been approved to actively immunize the general population. One can track the COVID-19 vaccines following this documentation [152].

9. Conclusions and Perspective

Our literature review further confirms the previous extended investigations showing that loss of smell and taste are among the key associated symptoms with most COVID-19 variants, including the omicron variant, which causes runny nose, headache, fatigue, sneezing, and sore throat [165]. The last three years have been an important rush towards deciphering the underlying mechanisms the SARS-CoV-2 deploys to impair the olfaction in infected patients. Furthermore, it is interesting to delineate the similarities and differences between the molecular mechanisms of SARS-CoV-2 and the other respiratory viruses induced olfactory dysfunction. Both SARS-CoV-2 and non-SARS-CoV-2 attach to the cilia during the initial stages of infection to later enter the nasal epithelium [55]. Interestingly, all these findings underline the importance of the immune-mediated inflammatory injury to the olfactory neuroepithelium that is now accepted as a consequence of those URT virus infections. However, the molecular signature related to the type of olfactory dysfunction, according to Table 1, seems particular for each respiratory virus. The animal or cellular models being used and the seasonal periods could add more complexity to the putative mechanisms for viral infection-induced olfactory dysfunction. Investigative literature on the COVID-19 mechanistic route has made clear that this virus seems to attach to ACE2-TMPRSS2 complex and/or NRP-1 on the host cell prior to infection and later triggers intrinsic immune responses. In the nasal mucosal microenvironment, those markers play a crucial role in inflammatory response mechanisms and are confirmed by several recent studies on understanding SARS-CoV-2 invasion [80,82–84,86,130,166]. Currently, the mechanism of how SARS-CoV-2 causes smell loss is widely documented, and more investigations are needed on the non-SARS-CoV-2 to complete the picture of comparing the particularity of each respiratory virus causing URT-related PVOD. For instance, this work emphasizes the urgency and necessity of finding an adequate therapeutic solution against COVID-19 and other respiratory viral pathogens-induced olfactory dysfunction. In addition, the mechanisms of taste dysfunction due to COVID-19 infection are not discussed in this review. But, it would be interesting to decipher the possible pathogenesis between ageusia and anosmia and other types of PVOD in COVID-19 and other non-COVID-19 patients in the future.

Author Contributions: Writing—original draft preparation, S.F.W. and A.A.M.D.; Writing—review and editing, S.F.W., A.A.M.D., B.N., F.T. and N.D.; Conceptualization and supervision, S.F.W. and A.A.M.D. All authors have read and agreed to the published version of the manuscript.

Funding: This research received no external funding.

Data Availability Statement: Data are contained within the article.

Conflicts of Interest: The authors declare no conflict of interest.

References

1. Wu, J.T.; Leung, K.; Leung, G.M. Nowcasting and forecasting the potential domestic and international spread of the 2019-nCoV outbreak originating in Wuhan, China: A modelling study. *Lancet* **2020**, *395*, 689–697. [CrossRef] [PubMed]
2. Hui, D.S.; Azhar, E.I.; Madani, T.A.; Ntoumi, F.; Kock, R.; Dar, O.; Ippolito, G.; McHugh, T.D.; Memish, Z.A.; Drosten, C.; et al. The continuing 2019-nCoV epidemic threat of novel coronaviruses to global health—The latest 2019 novel coronavirus outbreak in Wuhan, China. *Int. J. Infect. Dis.* **2020**, *91*, 264–266. [CrossRef] [PubMed]
3. Seiden, A.M. Postviral olfactory loss. *Otolaryngol. Clin. N. Am.* **2004**, *37*, 1159–1166. [CrossRef] [PubMed]
4. Zhen Yu, L.; Luigi Angelo, V.; Paolo, B.-R.; Abigail, W.; Claire, H. Post-viral olfactory loss and parosmia. *BMJ Med.* **2023**, *2*, e000382. [CrossRef]
5. Moran, D.T.; Jafek, B.W.; Eller, P.M.; Rowley, J.C., 3rd. Ultrastructural histopathology of human olfactory dysfunction. *Microsc. Res. Tech.* **1992**, *23*, 103–110. [CrossRef] [PubMed]
6. Welge-Lussen, A.; Wolfensberger, M. Olfactory disorders following upper respiratory tract infections. *Adv. Otorhinolaryngol.* **2006**, *63*, 125–132. [CrossRef]
7. Dicpinigaitis, P.V. Post-viral Anosmia (Loss of Sensation of Smell) Did Not Begin with COVID-19! *Lung* **2021**, *199*, 237–238. [CrossRef]
8. Tian, J.; Pinto, J.M.; Li, L.; Zhang, S.; Sun, Z.; Wei, Y. Identification of Viruses in Patients with Postviral Olfactory Dysfunction by Multiplex Reverse-Transcription Polymerase Chain Reaction. *Laryngoscope* **2021**, *131*, 158–164. [CrossRef]
9. Suzuki, M.; Saito, K.; Min, W.P.; Vladau, C.; Toida, K.; Itoh, H.; Murakami, S. Identification of viruses in patients with postviral olfactory dysfunction. *Laryngoscope* **2007**, *117*, 272–277. [CrossRef]
10. Imam, S.A.; Lao, W.P.; Reddy, P.; Nguyen, S.A.; Schlosser, R.J. Is SARS-CoV-2 (COVID-19) postviral olfactory dysfunction (PVOD) different from other PVOD? *World J. Otorhinolaryngol. Head. Neck Surg.* **2020**, *6* (Suppl. S1), S26–S32. [CrossRef]
11. Sugiura, M.; Aiba, T.; Mori, J.; Nakai, Y. An epidemiological study of postviral olfactory disorder. *Acta Otolaryngol. Suppl.* **1998**, *538*, 191–196. [CrossRef] [PubMed]

12. Diaz-Chiguer, D.L.; Tirado-Mendoza, R.; Marquez-Navarro, A.; Ambrosio-Hernandez, J.R.; Ruiz-Fraga, I.; Aguilar-Vargas, R.E.; Lira-Martinez, J.M.; Lopez-Valdes, J.C. Detection and molecular characterization of respiratory viruses that cause acute respiratory infection in the adult population. *Gac. Med. Mex.* **2019**, *155* (Suppl. S1), S7–S12. [CrossRef] [PubMed]
13. Ueha, R.; Mukherjee, S.; Ueha, S.; de Almeida Nagata, D.E.; Sakamoto, T.; Kondo, K.; Yamasoba, T.; Lukacs, N.W.; Kunkel, S.L. Viral disruption of olfactory progenitors is exacerbated in allergic mice. *Int. Immunopharmacol.* **2014**, *22*, 242–247. [CrossRef] [PubMed]
14. Heikkinen, T.; Jarvinen, A. The common cold. *Lancet* **2003**, *361*, 51–59. [CrossRef]
15. Potter, M.R.; Chen, J.H.; Lobban, N.S.; Doty, R.L. Olfactory dysfunction from acute upper respiratory infections: Relationship to season of onset. *Int. Forum Allergy Rhinol.* **2020**, *10*, 706–712. [CrossRef]
16. Henrickson, K.J. Parainfluenza viruses. *Clin. Microbiol. Rev.* **2003**, *16*, 242–264. [CrossRef]
17. Rafeek, R.A.M.; Divarathna, M.V.M.; Noordeen, F. A review on disease burden and epidemiology of childhood parainfluenza virus infections in Asian countries. *Rev. Med. Virol.* **2021**, *31*, e2164. [CrossRef]
18. Weston, S.; Frieman, M.B. Respiratory Viruses. In *Encyclopedia of Microbiology (Fourth Edition)*; Schmidt, T.M., Ed.; Academic Press: Oxford, UK, 2019; pp. 85–101. [CrossRef]
19. van Kempen, M.; Bachert, C.; Van Cauwenberge, P. An update on the pathophysiology of rhinovirus upper respiratory tract infections. *Rhinology* **1999**, *37*, 97–103.
20. Xatzipsalti, M.; Kyrana, S.; Tsolia, M.; Psarras, S.; Bossios, A.; Laza-Stanca, V.; Johnston, S.L.; Papadopoulos, N.G. Rhinovirus viremia in children with respiratory infections. *Am. J. Respir. Crit. Care Med.* **2005**, *172*, 1037–1040. [CrossRef]
21. Loeffelholz, M.J.; Trujillo, R.; Pyles, R.B.; Miller, A.L.; Alvarez-Fernandez, P.; Pong, D.L.; Chonmaitree, T. Duration of rhinovirus shedding in the upper respiratory tract in the first year of life. *Pediatrics* **2014**, *134*, 1144–1150. [CrossRef]
22. WHO. Severe Acute Respiratory Syndrome (SARS). Available online: https://www.who.int/health-topics/severe-acute-respiratory-syndrome#tab=tab_3 (accessed on 3 July 2023).
23. de Groot, R.J.; Baker, S.C.; Baric, R.S.; Brown, C.S.; Drosten, C.; Enjuanes, L.; Fouchier, R.A.; Galiano, M.; Gorbalenya, A.E.; Memish, Z.A.; et al. Middle East respiratory syndrome coronavirus (MERS-CoV): Announcement of the Coronavirus Study Group. *J. Virol.* **2013**, *87*, 7790–7792. [CrossRef] [PubMed]
24. Zaki, A.M.; van Boheemen, S.; Bestebroer, T.M.; Osterhaus, A.D.; Fouchier, R.A. Isolation of a novel coronavirus from a man with pneumonia in Saudi Arabia. *N. Engl. J. Med.* **2012**, *367*, 1814–1820. [CrossRef] [PubMed]
25. Khalafalla, A.I.; Lu, X.; Al-Mubarak, A.I.; Dalab, A.H.; Al-Busadah, K.A.; Erdman, D.D. MERS-CoV in Upper Respiratory Tract and Lungs of Dromedary Camels, Saudi Arabia, 2013–2014. *Emerg. Infect. Dis.* **2015**, *21*, 1153–1158. [CrossRef] [PubMed]
26. Wolfel, R.; Corman, V.M.; Guggemos, W.; Seilmaier, M.; Zange, S.; Muller, M.A.; Niemeyer, D.; Jones, T.C.; Vollmar, P.; Rothe, C.; et al. Virological assessment of hospitalized patients with COVID-2019. *Nature* **2020**, *581*, 465–469. [CrossRef]
27. de Melo, G.D.; Lazarini, F.; Levallois, S.; Hautefort, C.; Michel, V.; Larrous, F.; Verillaud, B.; Aparicio, C.; Wagner, S.; Gheusi, G.; et al. COVID-19-related anosmia is associated with viral persistence and inflammation in human olfactory epithelium and brain infection in hamsters. *Sci. Transl. Med.* **2021**, *13*, 596. [CrossRef] [PubMed]
28. Zazhytska, M.; Kodra, A.; Hoagland, D.A.; Frere, J.; Fullard, J.F.; Shayya, H.; McArthur, N.G.; Moeller, R.; Uhl, S.; Omer, A.D.; et al. Non-cell-autonomous disruption of nuclear architecture as a potential cause of COVID-19-induced anosmia. *Cell* **2022**, *185*, 1052–1064.e12. [CrossRef] [PubMed]
29. Bilinska, K.; Butowt, R. Anosmia in COVID-19: A Bumpy Road to Establishing a Cellular Mechanism. *ACS Chem. Neurosci.* **2020**, *11*, 2152–2155. [CrossRef]
30. Samaranayake, L.P.; Fakhruddin, K.S.; Panduwawala, C. Sudden onset, acute loss of taste and smell in coronavirus disease 2019 (COVID-19): A systematic review. *Acta Odontol. Scand.* **2020**, *78*, 467–473. [CrossRef]
31. Dammalli, M.; Dey, G.; Madugundu, A.K.; Kumar, M.; Rodrigues, B.; Gowda, H.; Siddaiah, B.G.; Mahadevan, A.; Shankar, S.K.; Prasad, T.S.K. Proteomic Analysis of the Human Olfactory Bulb. *OMICS* **2017**, *21*, 440–453. [CrossRef]
32. Dammalli, M.; Dey, G.; Kumar, M.; Madugundu, A.K.; Gopalakrishnan, L.; Gowrishankar, B.S.; Mahadevan, A.; Shankar, S.K.; Prasad, T.S.K. Proteomics of the Human Olfactory Tract. *OMICS* **2018**, *22*, 77–87. [CrossRef]
33. Oboti, L.; Peretto, P.; Marchis, S.D.; Fasolo, A. From chemical neuroanatomy to an understanding of the olfactory system. *Eur. J. Histochem.* **2011**, *55*, e35. [CrossRef] [PubMed]
34. Barral-Arca, R.; Gomez-Carballa, A.; Cebey-Lopez, M.; Bello, X.; Martinon-Torres, F.; Salas, A. A Meta-Analysis of Multiple Whole Blood Gene Expression Data Unveils a Diagnostic Host-Response Transcript Signature for Respiratory Syncytial Virus. *Int. J. Mol. Sci.* **2020**, *21*, 1831. [CrossRef] [PubMed]
35. Boesveldt, S.; Postma, E.M.; Boak, D.; Welge-Luessen, A.; Schopf, V.; Mainland, J.D.; Martens, J.; Ngai, J.; Duffy, V.B. Anosmia-A Clinical Review. *Chem. Senses* **2017**, *42*, 513–523. [CrossRef] [PubMed]
36. Firestein, S. How the olfactory system makes sense of scents. *Nature* **2001**, *413*, 211–218. [CrossRef]
37. Brennan, P.A.; Keverne, E.B. Something in the air? New insights into mammalian pheromones. *Curr. Biol.* **2004**, *14*, R81–R89. [CrossRef]
38. Buck, L.B. The molecular architecture of odor and pheromone sensing in mammals. *Cell* **2000**, *100*, 611–618. [CrossRef]
39. Mombaerts, P. Genes and ligands for odorant, vomeronasal and taste receptors. *Nat. Rev. Neurosci.* **2004**, *5*, 263–278. [CrossRef]
40. Restrepo, D.; Arellano, J.; Oliva, A.M.; Schaefer, M.L.; Lin, W. Emerging views on the distinct but related roles of the main and accessory olfactory systems in responsiveness to chemosensory signals in mice. *Horm. Behav.* **2004**, *46*, 247–256. [CrossRef]

41. Lavoie, J.; Gasso Astorga, P.; Segal-Gavish, H.; Wu, Y.C.; Chung, Y.; Cascella, N.G.; Sawa, A.; Ishizuka, K. The Olfactory Neural Epithelium As a Tool in Neuroscience. *Trends Mol. Med.* **2017**, *23*, 100–103. [CrossRef]
42. Liang, F.; Wang, Y. COVID-19 Anosmia: High Prevalence, Plural Neuropathogenic Mechanisms, and Scarce Neurotropism of SARS-CoV-2? *Viruses* **2021**, *13*, 2225. [CrossRef]
43. Olender, T.; Lancet, D.; Nebert, D.W. Update on the olfactory receptor (OR) gene superfamily. *Hum. Genom.* **2008**, *3*, 87–97. [CrossRef] [PubMed]
44. Kurian, S.M.; Gordon, S.; Barrick, B.; Dadlani, M.N.; Fanelli, B.; Cornell, J.B.; Head, S.R.; Marsh, C.L.; Case, J. Feasibility and Comparison Study of Fecal Sample Collection Methods in Healthy Volunteers and Solid Organ Transplant Recipients Using 16S rRNA and Metagenomics Approaches. *Biopreserv. Biobank.* **2020**, *18*, 425–440. [CrossRef] [PubMed]
45. Glezer, I.; Malnic, B. Olfactory receptor function. *Handb. Clin. Neurol.* **2019**, *164*, 67–78. [CrossRef] [PubMed]
46. Schwob, J.E. Neural regeneration and the peripheral olfactory system. *Anat. Rec.* **2002**, *269*, 33–49. [CrossRef] [PubMed]
47. Graziadei, P.P.; Graziadei, G.A. Neurogenesis and neuron regeneration in the olfactory system of mammals. I. Morphological aspects of differentiation and structural organization of the olfactory sensory neurons. *J. Neurocytol.* **1979**, *8*, 1–18. [CrossRef]
48. Urata, S.; Maruyama, J.; Kishimoto-Urata, M.; Sattler, R.A.; Cook, R.; Lin, N.; Yamasoba, T.; Makishima, T.; Paessler, S. Regeneration Profiles of Olfactory Epithelium after SARS-CoV-2 Infection in Golden Syrian Hamsters. *ACS Chem. Neurosci.* **2021**, *12*, 589–595. [CrossRef]
49. Lee, D.Y.; Lee, W.H.; Wee, J.H.; Kim, J.W. Prognosis of postviral olfactory loss: Follow-up study for longer than one year. *Am. J. Rhinol. Allergy* **2014**, *28*, 419–422. [CrossRef]
50. Doty, R.L.; Hawkes, C.H. Chemosensory dysfunction in neurodegenerative diseases. *Handb. Clin. Neurol.* **2019**, *164*, 325–360. [CrossRef]
51. Wang, J.H.; Kwon, H.J.; Jang, Y.J. Detection of parainfluenza virus 3 in turbinate epithelial cells of postviral olfactory dysfunction patients. *Laryngoscope* **2007**, *117*, 1445–1449. [CrossRef]
52. Lewandowska-Polak, A.; Brauncajs, M.; Paradowska, E.; Jarzebska, M.; Kurowski, M.; Moskwa, S.; Lesnikowski, Z.J.; Kowalski, M.L. Human parainfluenza virus type 3 (HPIV3) induces production of IFNgamma and RANTES in human nasal epithelial cells (HNECs). *J. Inflamm.* **2015**, *12*, 16. [CrossRef]
53. Mori, I.; Komatsu, T.; Takeuchi, K.; Nakakuki, K.; Sudo, M.; Kimura, Y. Parainfluenza virus type 1 infects olfactory neurons and establishes long-term persistence in the nerve tissue. *J. Gen. Virol.* **1995**, *76 Pt 5*, 1251–1254. [CrossRef] [PubMed]
54. Tian, J.; Pinto, J.M.; Cui, X.; Zhang, H.; Li, L.; Liu, Y.; Wu, C.; Wei, Y. Sendai Virus Induces Persistent Olfactory Dysfunction in a Murine Model of PVOD via Effects on Apoptosis, Cell Proliferation, and Response to Odorants. *PLoS ONE* **2016**, *11*, e0159033. [CrossRef]
55. Wu, C.T.; Lidsky, P.V.; Xiao, Y.; Cheng, R.; Lee, I.T.; Nakayama, T.; Jiang, S.; He, W.; Demeter, J.; Knight, M.G.; et al. SARS-CoV-2 replication in airway epithelia requires motile cilia and microvillar reprogramming. *Cell* **2023**, *186*, 112–130 e120. [CrossRef] [PubMed]
56. Lee, H.S.; Volpe, S.J.; Chang, E.H. The Role of Viruses in the Inception of Chronic Rhinosinusitis. *Clin. Exp. Otorhinolaryngol.* **2022**, *15*, 310–318. [CrossRef]
57. Gao, J.; Choudhary, S.; Banerjee, A.K.; De, B.P. Human parainfluenza virus type 3 upregulates ICAM-1 (CD54) expression in a cytokine-independent manner. *Gene Expr.* **2000**, *9*, 115–121. [CrossRef]
58. Cieslik, M.; Chinnaiyan, A.M. Cancer transcriptome profiling at the juncture of clinical translation. *Nat. Rev. Genet.* **2018**, *19*, 93–109. [CrossRef]
59. Worst, B.C.; van Tilburg, C.M.; Balasubramanian, G.P.; Fiesel, P.; Witt, R.; Freitag, A.; Boudalil, M.; Previti, C.; Wolf, S.; Schmidt, S.; et al. Next-generation personalised medicine for high-risk paediatric cancer patients—The INFORM pilot study. *Eur. J. Cancer* **2016**, *65*, 91–101. [CrossRef]
60. Weidenbusch, B.; Richter, G.H.S.; Kesper, M.S.; Guggemoos, M.; Gall, K.; Prexler, C.; Kazantsev, I.; Sipol, A.; Lindner, L.; Nathrath, M.; et al. Transcriptome based individualized therapy of refractory pediatric sarcomas: Feasibility, tolerability and efficacy. *Oncotarget* **2018**, *9*, 20747–20760. [CrossRef] [PubMed]
61. Tsimberidou, A.M.; Fountzilas, E.; Bleris, L.; Kurzrock, R. Transcriptomics and solid tumors: The next frontier in precision cancer medicine. *Semin. Cancer Biol.* **2022**, *84*, 50–59. [CrossRef]
62. Rodon, J.; Soria, J.C.; Berger, R.; Miller, W.H.; Rubin, E.; Kugel, A.; Tsimberidou, A.; Saintigny, P.; Ackerstein, A.; Brana, I.; et al. Genomic and transcriptomic profiling expands precision cancer medicine: The WINTHER trial. *Nat. Med.* **2019**, *25*, 751–758. [CrossRef]
63. Oberg, J.A.; Glade Bender, J.L.; Sulis, M.L.; Pendrick, D.; Sireci, A.N.; Hsiao, S.J.; Turk, A.T.; Dela Cruz, F.S.; Hibshoosh, H.; Remotti, H.; et al. Implementation of next generation sequencing into pediatric hematology-oncology practice: Moving beyond actionable alterations. *Genome Med.* **2016**, *8*, 133. [CrossRef]
64. Nicolas De Lamballerie, C.; Pizzorno, A.; Dubois, J.; Padey, B.; Julien, T.; Traversier, A.; Carbonneau, J.; Orcel, E.; Lina, B.; Hamelin, M.E.; et al. Human Respiratory Syncytial Virus-Induced Immune Signature of Infection Revealed by Transcriptome Analysis of Clinical Pediatric Nasopharyngeal Swab Samples. *J. Infect. Dis.* **2021**, *223*, 1052–1061. [CrossRef] [PubMed]
65. Dissanayake, T.K.; Schauble, S.; Mirhakkak, M.H.; Wu, W.L.; Ng, A.C.; Yip, C.C.Y.; Lopez, A.G.; Wolf, T.; Yeung, M.L.; Chan, K.H.; et al. Comparative Transcriptomic Analysis of Rhinovirus and Influenza Virus Infection. *Front. Microbiol.* **2020**, *11*, 1580. [CrossRef] [PubMed]

66. Al-Shalan, H.A.M.; Hu, D.; Wang, P.; Uddin, J.; Chopra, A.; Greene, W.K.; Ma, B. Transcriptomic Profiling of Influenza A Virus-Infected Mouse Lung at Recovery Stage Using RNA Sequencing. *Viruses* **2023**, *15*, 2198. [CrossRef]
67. Bryche, B.; Fretaud, M.; Saint-Albin Deliot, A.; Galloux, M.; Sedano, L.; Langevin, C.; Descamps, D.; Rameix-Welti, M.A.; Eleouet, J.F.; Le Goffic, R.; et al. Respiratory syncytial virus tropism for olfactory sensory neurons in mice. *J. Neurochem.* **2020**, *155*, 137–153. [CrossRef] [PubMed]
68. Griffiths, C.D.; Bilawchuk, L.M.; McDonough, J.E.; Jamieson, K.C.; Elawar, F.; Cen, Y.; Duan, W.; Lin, C.; Song, H.; Casanova, J.L.; et al. IGF1R is an entry receptor for respiratory syncytial virus. *Nature* **2020**, *583*, 615–619. [CrossRef]
69. Tayyari, F.; Marchant, D.; Moraes, T.J.; Duan, W.; Mastrangelo, P.; Hegele, R.G. Identification of nucleolin as a cellular receptor for human respiratory syncytial virus. *Nat. Med.* **2011**, *17*, 1132–1135. [CrossRef]
70. Mastrangelo, P.; Chin, A.A.; Tan, S.; Jeon, A.H.; Ackerley, C.A.; Siu, K.K.; Lee, J.E.; Hegele, R.G. Identification of RSV Fusion Protein Interaction Domains on the Virus Receptor, Nucleolin. *Viruses* **2021**, *13*, 261. [CrossRef]
71. Sourimant, J.; Lieber, C.M.; Aggarwal, M.; Cox, R.M.; Wolf, J.D.; Yoon, J.J.; Toots, M.; Ye, C.; Sticher, Z.; Kolykhalov, A.A.; et al. 4′-Fluorouridine is an oral antiviral that blocks respiratory syncytial virus and SARS-CoV-2 replication. *Science* **2022**, *375*, 161–167. [CrossRef]
72. Li, H.H.; Xu, J.; He, L.; Denny, L.I.; Rustandi, R.R.; Dornadula, G.; Fiorito, B.; Zhang, Z.Q. Development and qualification of cell-based relative potency assay for a human respiratory syncytial virus (RSV) mRNA vaccine. *J. Pharm. Biomed. Anal.* **2023**, *234*, 115523. [CrossRef]
73. Whitaker, J.A.; Sahly, H.M.E.; Healy, C.M. mRNA vaccines against respiratory viruses. *Curr. Opin. Infect. Dis.* **2023**, *36*, 385–393. [CrossRef] [PubMed]
74. Bochkov, Y.A.; Watters, K.; Ashraf, S.; Griggs, T.F.; Devries, M.K.; Jackson, D.J.; Palmenberg, A.C.; Gern, J.E. Cadherin-related family member 3, a childhood asthma susceptibility gene product, mediates rhinovirus C binding and replication. *Proc. Natl. Acad. Sci. USA* **2015**, *112*, 5485–5490. [CrossRef] [PubMed]
75. Staunton, D.E.; Merluzzi, V.J.; Rothlein, R.; Barton, R.; Marlin, S.D.; Springer, T.A. A cell adhesion molecule, ICAM-1, is the major surface receptor for rhinoviruses. *Cell* **1989**, *56*, 849–853. [CrossRef] [PubMed]
76. Hofer, F.; Gruenberger, M.; Kowalski, H.; Machat, H.; Huettinger, M.; Kuechler, E.; Blaas, D. Members of the low density lipoprotein receptor family mediate cell entry of a minor-group common cold virus. *Proc. Natl. Acad. Sci. USA* **1994**, *91*, 1839–1842. [CrossRef] [PubMed]
77. Bochkov, Y.A.; Gern, J.E. Rhinoviruses and Their Receptors: Implications for Allergic Disease. *Curr. Allergy Asthma Rep.* **2016**, *16*, 30. [CrossRef] [PubMed]
78. Lee, S.H.; Han, M.S.; Lee, T.H.; Lee, D.B.; Park, J.H.; Lee, S.H.; Kim, T.H. Hydrogen peroxide attenuates rhinovirus-induced anti-viral interferon secretion in sinonasal epithelial cells. *Front. Immunol.* **2023**, *14*, 1086381. [CrossRef]
79. Torabi, A.; Mohammadbagheri, E.; Akbari Dilmaghani, N.; Bayat, A.H.; Fathi, M.; Vakili, K.; Alizadeh, R.; Rezaeimirghaed, O.; Hajiesmaeili, M.; Ramezani, M.; et al. Proinflammatory Cytokines in the Olfactory Mucosa Result in COVID-19 Induced Anosmia. *ACS Chem. Neurosci.* **2020**, *11*, 1909–1913. [CrossRef]
80. Zheng, J.; Wong, L.R.; Li, K.; Verma, A.K.; Ortiz, M.E.; Wohlford-Lenane, C.; Leidinger, M.R.; Knudson, C.M.; Meyerholz, D.K.; McCray, P.B., Jr.; et al. COVID-19 treatments and pathogenesis including anosmia in K18-hACE2 mice. *Nature* **2021**, *589*, 603–607. [CrossRef]
81. Bilinska, K.; Jakubowska, P.; Von Bartheld, C.S.; Butowt, R. Expression of the SARS-CoV-2 Entry Proteins, ACE2 and TMPRSS2, in Cells of the Olfactory Epithelium: Identification of Cell Types and Trends with Age. *ACS Chem. Neurosci.* **2020**, *11*, 1555–1562. [CrossRef]
82. Davies, J.; Randeva, H.S.; Chatha, K.; Hall, M.; Spandidos, D.A.; Karteris, E.; Kyrou, I. Neuropilin-1 as a new potential SARS-CoV-2 infection mediator implicated in the neurologic features and central nervous system involvement of COVID-19. *Mol. Med. Rep.* **2020**, *22*, 4221–4226. [CrossRef]
83. Kang, Y.L.; Chou, Y.Y.; Rothlauf, P.W.; Liu, Z.; Soh, T.K.; Cureton, D.; Case, J.B.; Chen, R.E.; Diamond, M.S.; Whelan, S.P.J.; et al. Inhibition of PIKfyve kinase prevents infection by Zaire ebolavirus and SARS-CoV-2. *Proc. Natl. Acad. Sci. USA* **2020**, *117*, 20803–20813. [CrossRef] [PubMed]
84. Mayi, B.S.; Leibowitz, J.A.; Woods, A.T.; Ammon, K.A.; Liu, A.E.; Raja, A. The role of Neuropilin-1 in COVID-19. *PLoS Pathog.* **2021**, *17*, e1009153. [CrossRef] [PubMed]
85. Bryche, B.; St Albin, A.; Murri, S.; Lacote, S.; Pulido, C.; Ar Gouilh, M.; Lesellier, S.; Servat, A.; Wasniewski, M.; Picard-Meyer, E.; et al. Massive transient damage of the olfactory epithelium associated with infection of sustentacular cells by SARS-CoV-2 in golden Syrian hamsters. *Brain Behav. Immun.* **2020**, *89*, 579–586. [CrossRef] [PubMed]
86. Cantuti-Castelvetri, L.; Ojha, R.; Pedro, L.D.; Djannatian, M.; Franz, J.; Kuivanen, S.; van der Meer, F.; Kallio, K.; Kaya, T.; Anastasina, M.; et al. Neuropilin-1 facilitates SARS-CoV-2 cell entry and infectivity. *Science* **2020**, *370*, 856–860. [CrossRef] [PubMed]
87. Daly, J.L.; Simonetti, B.; Klein, K.; Chen, K.E.; Williamson, M.K.; Anton-Plagaro, C.; Shoemark, D.K.; Simon-Gracia, L.; Bauer, M.; Hollandi, R.; et al. Neuropilin-1 is a host factor for SARS-CoV-2 infection. *Science* **2020**, *370*, 861–865. [CrossRef]
88. Acevedo, C.; Blanchard, K.; Bacigalupo, J.; Vergara, C. Possible ATP trafficking by ATP-shuttles in the olfactory cilia and glucose transfer across the olfactory mucosa. *FEBS Lett.* **2019**, *593*, 601–610. [CrossRef]

89. Villar, P.S.; Vergara, C.; Bacigalupo, J. Energy sources that fuel metabolic processes in protruding finger-like organelles. *FEBS J.* **2021**, *288*, 3799–3812. [CrossRef]

90. Krishnan, S.; Nordqvist, H.; Ambikan, A.T.; Gupta, S.; Sperk, M.; Svensson-Akusjarvi, S.; Mikaeloff, F.; Benfeitas, R.; Saccon, E.; Ponnan, S.M.; et al. Metabolic Perturbation Associated With COVID-19 Disease Severity and SARS-CoV-2 Replication. *Mol. Cell Proteom.* **2021**, *20*, 100159. [CrossRef]

91. Khan, M.; Yoo, S.J.; Clijsters, M.; Backaert, W.; Vanstapel, A.; Speleman, K.; Lietaer, C.; Choi, S.; Hether, T.D.; Marcelis, L.; et al. Visualizing in deceased COVID-19 patients how SARS-CoV-2 attacks the respiratory and olfactory mucosae but spares the olfactory bulb. *Cell* **2021**, *184*, 5932–5949 e5915. [CrossRef]

92. Assou, S.; Ahmed, E.; Morichon, L.; Nasri, A.; Foisset, F.; Bourdais, C.; Gros, N.; Tieo, S.; Petit, A.; Vachier, I.; et al. The Transcriptome Landscape of the In Vitro Human Airway Epithelium Response to SARS-CoV-2. *Int. J. Mol. Sci.* **2023**, *24*, 12017. [CrossRef]

93. Lavoie, T.B.; Kalie, E.; Crisafulli-Cabatu, S.; Abramovich, R.; DiGioia, G.; Moolchan, K.; Pestka, S.; Schreiber, G. Binding and activity of all human alpha interferon subtypes. *Cytokine* **2011**, *56*, 282–289. [CrossRef]

94. Jaks, E.; Gavutis, M.; Uze, G.; Martal, J.; Piehler, J. Differential receptor subunit affinities of type I interferons govern differential signal activation. *J. Mol. Biol.* **2007**, *366*, 525–539. [CrossRef] [PubMed]

95. Donnelly, R.P.; Sheikh, F.; Kotenko, S.V.; Dickensheets, H. The expanded family of class II cytokines that share the IL-10 receptor-2 (IL-10R2) chain. *J. Leukoc. Biol.* **2004**, *76*, 314–321. [CrossRef] [PubMed]

96. Wang, Y.; Ninaber, D.K.; van Schadewijk, A.; Hiemstra, P.S. Tiotropium and Fluticasone Inhibit Rhinovirus-Induced Mucin Production via Multiple Mechanisms in Differentiated Airway Epithelial Cells. *Front. Cell Infect. Microbiol.* **2020**, *10*, 278. [CrossRef] [PubMed]

97. Lo, D.; Kennedy, J.L.; Kurten, R.C.; Panettieri, R.A., Jr.; Koziol-White, C.J. Modulation of airway hyperresponsiveness by rhinovirus exposure. *Respir. Res.* **2018**, *19*, 208. [CrossRef]

98. Loxham, M.; Smart, D.E.; Bedke, N.J.; Smithers, N.P.; Filippi, I.; Blume, C.; Swindle, E.J.; Tariq, K.; Howarth, P.H.; Holgate, S.T.; et al. Allergenic proteases cleave the chemokine CX3CL1 directly from the surface of airway epithelium and augment the effect of rhinovirus. *Mucosal Immunol.* **2018**, *11*, 404–414. [CrossRef]

99. Papi, A.; Papadopoulos, N.G.; Stanciu, L.A.; Bellettato, C.M.; Pinamonti, S.; Degitz, K.; Holgate, S.T.; Johnston, S.L. Reducing agents inhibit rhinovirus-induced up-regulation of the rhinovirus receptor intercellular adhesion molecule-1 (ICAM-1) in respiratory epithelial cells. *FASEB J.* **2002**, *16*, 1934–1936. [CrossRef]

100. Song, Y.P.; Tang, M.F.; Leung, A.S.Y.; Tao, K.P.; Chan, O.M.; Wong, G.W.K.; Chan, P.K.S.; Chan, R.W.Y.; Leung, T.F. Interactive effects between CDHR3 genotype and rhinovirus species for diagnosis and severity of respiratory tract infections in hospitalized children. *Microbiol. Spectr.* **2023**, *11*, e0118123. [CrossRef]

101. Greiller, C.L.; Suri, R.; Jolliffe, D.A.; Kebadze, T.; Hirsman, A.G.; Griffiths, C.J.; Johnston, S.L.; Martineau, A.R. Vitamin D attenuates rhinovirus-induced expression of intercellular adhesion molecule-1 (ICAM-1) and platelet-activating factor receptor (PAFR) in respiratory epithelial cells. *J. Steroid Biochem. Mol. Biol.* **2019**, *187*, 152–159. [CrossRef]

102. Khani, E.; Khiali, S.; Beheshtirouy, S.; Entezari-Maleki, T. Potential pharmacologic treatments for COVID-19 smell and taste loss: A comprehensive review. *Eur. J. Pharmacol.* **2021**, *912*, 174582. [CrossRef]

103. Silva Andrade, B.; Siqueira, S.; de Assis Soares, W.R.; de Souza Rangel, F.; Santos, N.O.; Dos Santos Freitas, A.; Ribeiro da Silveira, P.; Tiwari, S.; Alzahrani, K.J.; Goes-Neto, A.; et al. Long-COVID and Post-COVID Health Complications: An Up-to-Date Review on Clinical Conditions and Their Possible Molecular Mechanisms. *Viruses* **2021**, *13*, 700. [CrossRef] [PubMed]

104. Fernandez-de-Las-Penas, C.; Cancela-Cilleruelo, I.; Rodriguez-Jimenez, J.; Gomez-Mayordomo, V.; Pellicer-Valero, O.J.; Martin-Guerrero, J.D.; Hernandez-Barrera, V.; Arendt-Nielsen, L.; Torres-Macho, J. Associated-Onset Symptoms and Post-COVID-19 Symptoms in Hospitalized COVID-19 Survivors Infected with Wuhan, Alpha or Delta SARS-CoV-2 Variant. *Pathogens* **2022**, *11*, 725. [CrossRef] [PubMed]

105. Rodriguez-Sevilla, J.J.; Guerri-Fernandez, R.; Bertran Recasens, B. Is There Less Alteration of Smell Sensation in Patients with Omicron SARS-CoV-2 Variant Infection? *Front Med.* **2022**, *9*, 852998. [CrossRef] [PubMed]

106. Chee, J.; Chern, B.; Loh, W.S.; Mullol, J.; Wang, Y. Pathophysiology of SARS-CoV-2 Infection of Nasal Respiratory and Olfactory Epithelia and Its Clinical Impact. *Curr. Allergy Asthma Rep.* **2023**, *23*, 121–131. [CrossRef]

107. Mutiawati, E.; Fahriani, M.; Mamada, S.S.; Fajar, J.K.; Frediansyah, A.; Maliga, H.A.; Ilmawan, M.; Emran, T.B.; Ophinni, Y.; Ichsan, I.; et al. Anosmia and dysgeusia in SARS-CoV-2 infection: Incidence and effects on COVID-19 severity and mortality, and the possible pathobiology mechanisms—A systematic review and meta-analysis. *F1000Res* **2021**, *10*, 40. [CrossRef] [PubMed]

108. Butowt, R.; von Bartheld, C.S. Anosmia in COVID-19: Underlying Mechanisms and Assessment of an Olfactory Route to Brain Infection. *Neuroscientist* **2021**, *27*, 582–603. [CrossRef]

109. Kalra, R.S.; Dhanjal, J.K.; Meena, A.S.; Kalel, V.C.; Dahiya, S.; Singh, B.; Dewanjee, S.; Kandimalla, R. COVID-19, Neuropathology, and Aging: SARS-CoV-2 Neurological Infection, Mechanism, and Associated Complications. *Front. Aging Neurosci.* **2021**, *13*, 662786. [CrossRef]

110. Rebholz, H.; Braun, R.J.; Ladage, D.; Knoll, W.; Kleber, C.; Hassel, A.W. Loss of Olfactory Function-Early Indicator for COVID-19, Other Viral Infections and Neurodegenerative Disorders. *Front. Neurol.* **2020**, *11*, 569333. [CrossRef]

111. Reyna, R.A.; Kishimoto-Urata, M.; Urata, S.; Makishima, T.; Paessler, S.; Maruyama, J. Recovery of anosmia in hamsters infected with SARS-CoV-2 is correlated with repair of the olfactory epithelium. *Sci. Rep.* **2022**, *12*, 628. [CrossRef]

112. Tanzadehpanah, H.; Lotfian, E.; Avan, A.; Saki, S.; Nobari, S.; Mahmoodian, R.; Sheykhhasan, M.; Froutagh, M.H.S.; Ghotbani, F.; Jamshidi, R.; et al. Role of SARS-CoV-2 and ACE2 in the pathophysiology of peripheral vascular diseases. *Biomed. Pharmacother.* **2023**, *166*, 115321. [CrossRef]

113. Butowt, R.; Bilinska, K.; von Bartheld, C.S. Olfactory dysfunction in COVID-19: New insights into the underlying mechanisms. *Trends Neurosci.* **2023**, *46*, 75–90. [CrossRef]

114. Buqaileh, R.; Saternos, H.; Ley, S.; Aranda, A.; Forero, K.; AbouAlaiwi, W.A. Can cilia provide an entry gateway for SARS-CoV-2 to human ciliated cells? *Physiol. Genom.* **2021**, *53*, 249–258. [CrossRef] [PubMed]

115. Butowt, R.; Meunier, N.; Bryche, B.; von Bartheld, C.S. The olfactory nerve is not a likely route to brain infection in COVID-19: A critical review of data from humans and animal models. *Acta Neuropathol.* **2021**, *141*, 809–822. [CrossRef] [PubMed]

116. Lechien, J.R.; Chiesa-Estomba, C.M.; De Siati, D.R.; Horoi, M.; Le Bon, S.D.; Rodriguez, A.; Dequanter, D.; Blecic, S.; El Afia, F.; Distinguin, L.; et al. Olfactory and gustatory dysfunctions as a clinical presentation of mild-to-moderate forms of the coronavirus disease (COVID-19): A multicenter European study. *Eur. Arch. Otorhinolaryngol.* **2020**, *277*, 2251–2261. [CrossRef] [PubMed]

117. Lee, Y.; Min, P.; Lee, S.; Kim, S.W. Prevalence and Duration of Acute Loss of Smell or Taste in COVID-19 Patients. *J. Korean Med. Sci.* **2020**, *35*, e174. [CrossRef] [PubMed]

118. Fodoulian, L.; Tuberosa, J.; Rossier, D.; Boillat, M.; Kan, C.; Pauli, V.; Egervari, K.; Lobrinus, J.A.; Landis, B.N.; Carleton, A.; et al. SARS-CoV-2 Receptors and Entry Genes Are Expressed in the Human Olfactory Neuroepithelium and Brain. *iScience* **2020**, *23*, 101839. [CrossRef]

119. Chen, M.; Shen, W.; Rowan, N.R.; Kulaga, H.; Hillel, A.; Ramanathan, M., Jr.; Lane, A.P. Elevated ACE-2 expression in the olfactory neuroepithelium: Implications for anosmia and upper respiratory SARS-CoV-2 entry and replication. *Eur. Respir. J.* **2020**, *56*, 2001948. [CrossRef]

120. Hoffmann, M.; Kleine-Weber, H.; Schroeder, S.; Kruger, N.; Herrler, T.; Erichsen, S.; Schiergens, T.S.; Herrler, G.; Wu, N.H.; Nitsche, A.; et al. SARS-CoV-2 Cell Entry Depends on ACE2 and TMPRSS2 and Is Blocked by a Clinically Proven Protease Inhibitor. *Cell* **2020**, *181*, 271–280 e278. [CrossRef]

121. Ziegler, C.G.K.; Allon, S.J.; Nyquist, S.K.; Mbano, I.M.; Miao, V.N.; Tzouanas, C.N.; Cao, Y.; Yousif, A.S.; Bals, J.; Hauser, B.M.; et al. SARS-CoV-2 Receptor ACE2 Is an Interferon-Stimulated Gene in Human Airway Epithelial Cells and Is Detected in Specific Cell Subsets across Tissues. *Cell* **2020**, *181*, 1016–1035.e1019. [CrossRef]

122. Gkogkou, E.; Barnasas, G.; Vougas, K.; Trougakos, I.P. Expression profiling meta-analysis of ACE2 and TMPRSS2, the putative anti-inflammatory receptor and priming protease of SARS-CoV-2 in human cells, and identification of putative modulators. *Redox Biol.* **2020**, *36*, 101615. [CrossRef]

123. Sungnak, W.; Huang, N.; Becavin, C.; Berg, M.; Queen, R.; Litvinukova, M.; Talavera-Lopez, C.; Maatz, H.; Reichart, D.; Sampaziotis, F.; et al. SARS-CoV-2 entry factors are highly expressed in nasal epithelial cells together with innate immune genes. *Nat. Med.* **2020**, *26*, 681–687. [CrossRef]

124. Li, W.; Li, M.; Ou, G. COVID-19, cilia, and smell. *FEBS J.* **2020**, *287*, 3672–3676. [CrossRef]

125. Sternberg, A.; Naujokat, C. Structural features of coronavirus SARS CoV-2 spike protein: Targets for vaccination. *Life Sci.* **2020**, *257*, 118056. [CrossRef]

126. Chen, M.; Pekosz, A.; Villano, J.S.; Shen, W.; Zhou, R.; Kulaga, H.; Li, Z.; Beck, S.E.; Witwer, K.W.; Mankowski, J.L.; et al. Evolution of nasal and olfactory infection characteristics of SARS-CoV-2 variants. *bioRxiv* **2022**. [CrossRef]

127. von Bartheld, C.S.; Wang, L. Prevalence of Olfactory Dysfunction with the Omicron Variant of SARS-CoV-2: A Systematic Review and Meta-Analysis. *Cells* **2023**, *12*, 430. [CrossRef] [PubMed]

128. von Bartheld, C.S.; Hagen, M.M.; Butowt, R. The D614G Virus Mutation Enhances Anosmia in COVID-19 Patients: Evidence from a Systematic Review and Meta-analysis of Studies from South Asia. *ACS Chem. Neurosci.* **2021**, *12*, 3535–3549. [CrossRef]

129. Schreiner, T.; Allnoch, L.; Beythien, G.; Marek, K.; Becker, K.; Schaudien, D.; Stanelle-Bertram, S.; Schaumburg, B.; Mounogou Kouassi, N.; Beck, S.; et al. SARS-CoV-2 Infection Dysregulates Cilia and Basal Cell Homeostasis in the Respiratory Epithelium of Hamsters. *Int. J. Mol. Sci.* **2022**, *23*, 5124. [CrossRef]

130. Seehusen, F.; Clark, J.J.; Sharma, P.; Bentley, E.G.; Kirby, A.; Subramaniam, K.; Wunderlin-Giuliani, S.; Hughes, G.L.; Patterson, E.I.; Michael, B.D.; et al. Neuroinvasion and Neurotropism by SARS-CoV-2 Variants in the K18-hACE2 Mouse. *Viruses* **2022**, *14*, 1020. [CrossRef] [PubMed]

131. Trobaugh, D.W.; Klimstra, W.B. MicroRNA Regulation of RNA Virus Replication and Pathogenesis. *Trends Mol. Med.* **2017**, *23*, 80–93. [CrossRef] [PubMed]

132. Hanna, J.; Hossain, G.S.; Kocerha, J. The Potential for microRNA Therapeutics and Clinical Research. *Front. Genet.* **2019**, *10*, 478. [CrossRef]

133. Osan, J.K.; DeMontigny, B.A.; Mehedi, M. Immunohistochemistry for protein detection in PFA-fixed paraffin-embedded SARS-CoV-2-infected COPD airway epithelium. *STAR Protoc.* **2021**, *2*, 100663. [CrossRef]

134. Trifonova, I.; Christova, I.; Madzharova, I.; Angelova, S.; Voleva, S.; Yordanova, R.; Tcherveniakova, T.; Krumova, S.; Korsun, N. Clinical significance and role of coinfections with respiratory pathogens among individuals with confirmed severe acute respiratory syndrome coronavirus-2 infection. *Front. Public. Health* **2022**, *10*, 959319. [CrossRef] [PubMed]

135. Rohde, G.; Wiethege, A.; Borg, I.; Kauth, M.; Bauer, T.T.; Gillissen, A.; Bufe, A.; Schultze-Werninghaus, G. Respiratory viruses in exacerbations of chronic obstructive pulmonary disease requiring hospitalisation: A case-control study. *Thorax* **2003**, *58*, 37–42. [CrossRef] [PubMed]

136. Kim, H.J.; Choi, S.M.; Lee, J.; Park, Y.S.; Lee, C.H.; Yim, J.J.; Yoo, C.G.; Kim, Y.W.; Han, S.K.; Lee, S.M. Respiratory virus of severe pneumonia in South Korea: Prevalence and clinical implications. *PLoS ONE* **2018**, *13*, e0198902. [CrossRef] [PubMed]

137. Olloquequi, J. COVID-19 Susceptibility in chronic obstructive pulmonary disease. *Eur. J. Clin. Investig.* **2020**, *50*, e13382. [CrossRef]

138. Alhumaid, S.; Al Mutair, A.; Al Alawi, Z.; Alshawi, A.M.; Alomran, S.A.; Almuhanna, M.S.; Almuslim, A.A.; Bu Shafia, A.H.; Alotaibi, A.M.; Ahmed, G.Y.; et al. Coinfections with Bacteria, Fungi, and Respiratory Viruses in Patients with SARS-CoV-2: A Systematic Review and Meta-Analysis. *Pathogens* **2021**, *10*, 809. [CrossRef]

139. Cooksey, G.L.S.; Morales, C.; Linde, L.; Schildhauer, S.; Guevara, H.; Chan, E.; Gibb, K.; Wong, J.; Lin, W.; Bonin, B.J.; et al. Severe Acute Respiratory Syndrome Coronavirus 2 and Respiratory Virus Sentinel Surveillance, California, USA, May 10, 2020-June 12, 2021. *Emerg. Infect. Dis.* **2022**, *28*, 9–19. [CrossRef]

140. Jeong, S.; Lee, N.; Park, Y.; Kim, J.; Jeon, K.; Park, M.J.; Song, W. Prevalence and Clinical Impact of Coinfection in Patients with Coronavirus Disease 2019 in Korea. *Viruses* **2022**, *14*, 446. [CrossRef]

141. Kim, D.; Quinn, J.; Pinsky, B.; Shah, N.H.; Brown, I. Rates of Co-infection Between SARS-CoV-2 and Other Respiratory Pathogens. *JAMA* **2020**, *323*, 2085–2086. [CrossRef]

142. Nowak, M.D.; Sordillo, E.M.; Gitman, M.R.; Paniz Mondolfi, A.E. Coinfection in SARS-CoV-2 infected patients: Where are influenza virus and rhinovirus/enterovirus? *J. Med. Virol.* **2020**, *92*, 1699–1700. [CrossRef]

143. Burrel, S.; Hausfater, P.; Dres, M.; Pourcher, V.; Luyt, C.E.; Teyssou, E.; Soulie, C.; Calvez, V.; Marcelin, A.G.; Boutolleau, D. Co-infection of SARS-CoV-2 with other respiratory viruses and performance of lower respiratory tract samples for the diagnosis of COVID-19. *Int. J. Infect. Dis.* **2021**, *102*, 10–13. [CrossRef] [PubMed]

144. Nainwal, N. Treatment of respiratory viral infections through inhalation therapeutics: Challenges and opportunities. *Pulm. Pharmacol. Ther.* **2022**, *77*, 102170. [CrossRef] [PubMed]

145. Melgar, M.; Britton, A.; Roper, L.E.; Talbot, H.K.; Long, S.S.; Kotton, C.N.; Havers, F.P. Use of Respiratory Syncytial Virus Vaccines in Older Adults: Recommendations of the Advisory Committee on Immunization Practices—United States, 2023. *MMWR Morb. Mortal. Wkly. Rep.* **2023**, *72*, 793–801. [CrossRef] [PubMed]

146. Tregoning, J.S.; Schwarze, J. Respiratory viral infections in infants: Causes, clinical symptoms, virology, and immunology. *Clin. Microbiol. Rev.* **2010**, *23*, 74–98. [CrossRef] [PubMed]

147. Griffiths, C.; Drews, S.J.; Marchant, D.J. Respiratory Syncytial Virus: Infection, Detection, and New Options for Prevention and Treatment. *Clin. Microbiol. Rev.* **2017**, *30*, 277–319. [CrossRef]

148. Coultas, J.A.; Smyth, R.; Openshaw, P.J. Respiratory syncytial virus (RSV): A scourge from infancy to old age. *Thorax* **2019**, *74*, 986–993. [CrossRef]

149. Graham, B.S. Vaccine development for respiratory syncytial virus. *Curr. Opin. Virol.* **2017**, *23*, 107–112. [CrossRef]

150. Green, C.A.; Drysdale, S.B.; Pollard, A.J.; Sande, C.J. Vaccination against Respiratory Syncytial Virus. *Interdiscip. Top. Gerontol. Geriatr.* **2020**, *43*, 182–192. [CrossRef]

151. Ruckwardt, T.J.; Morabito, K.M.; Graham, B.S. Immunological Lessons from Respiratory Syncytial Virus Vaccine Development. *Immunity* **2019**, *51*, 429–442. [CrossRef]

152. COVID-19 Vaccine Tracker. Available online: https://www.raps.org/news-and-articles/news-articles/2020/3/covid-19-vaccine-tracker (accessed on 6 November 2023).

153. Clinical Trials. Available online: https://www.mayo.edu/research/clinical-trials/cls-20147700#moreinfo (accessed on 6 November 2023).

154. Dose Ranging Study of ALX-0171 in Infants Hospitalized for Respiratory Syncytial Virus Lower Respiratory Tract Infection (Respire). Available online: https://classic.clinicaltrials.gov/ct2/show/NCT02979431 (accessed on 6 November 2023).

155. Vainionpaa, R.; Hyypia, T. Biology of parainfluenza viruses. *Clin. Microbiol. Rev.* **1994**, *7*, 265–275. [CrossRef]

156. Sato, M.; Wright, P.F. Current status of vaccines for parainfluenza virus infections. *Pediatr. Infect. Dis. J.* **2008**, *27* (Suppl. 10), S123–S125. [CrossRef] [PubMed]

157. Chemaly, R.F.; Marty, F.M.; Wolfe, C.R.; Lawrence, S.J.; Dadwal, S.; Soave, R.; Farthing, J.; Hawley, S.; Montanez, P.; Hwang, J.; et al. DAS181 Treatment of Severe Lower Respiratory Tract Parainfluenza Virus Infection in Immunocompromised Patients: A Phase 2 Randomized, Placebo-Controlled Study. *Clin. Infect. Dis.* **2021**, *73*, e773–e781. [CrossRef] [PubMed]

158. Karron, R.A.; Herbert, K.; Wanionek, K.; Schmidt, A.C.; Schaap-Nutt, A.; Collins, P.L.; Buchholz, U.J. Evaluation of a Live-Attenuated Human Parainfluenza Virus Type 2 Vaccine in Adults and Children. *J. Pediatr. Infect. Dis. Soc.* **2023**, *12*, 173–176. [CrossRef]

159. Schmidt, A.C.; Schaap-Nutt, A.; Bartlett, E.J.; Schomacker, H.; Boonyaratanakornkit, J.; Karron, R.A.; Collins, P.L. Progress in the development of human parainfluenza virus vaccines. *Expert. Rev. Respir. Med.* **2011**, *5*, 515–526. [CrossRef] [PubMed]

160. Kasman, L.M. Engineering the common cold to be a live-attenuated SARS-CoV-2 vaccine. *Front. Immunol.* **2022**, *13*, 871463. [CrossRef]

161. Sung, R.Y.; Yin, J.; Oppenheimer, S.J.; Tam, J.S.; Lau, J. Treatment of respiratory syncytial virus infection with recombinant interferon alfa-2a. *Arch. Dis. Child.* **1993**, *69*, 440–442. [CrossRef] [PubMed]

162. Douglas, R.M.; Moore, B.; Miles, H.B.; Pinnock, C.B. Could preventive intranasal interferon lower the morbidity in children prone to respiratory illness? *Med. J. Aust.* **1990**, *152*, 524–528. [CrossRef]

163. Al-Nakib, W.; Higgins, P.G.; Barrow, I.; Batstone, G.; Tyrrell, D.A. Prophylaxis and treatment of rhinovirus colds with zinc gluconate lozenges. *J. Antimicrob. Chemother.* **1987**, *20*, 893–901. [CrossRef]

164. Gwaltney, J.M., Jr. Combined antiviral and antimediator treatment of rhinovirus colds. *J. Infect. Dis.* **1992**, *166*, 776–782. [CrossRef]
165. Iacobucci, G. COVID-19: Runny nose, headache, and fatigue are commonest symptoms of omicron, early data show. *BMJ* **2021**, *375*, n3103. [CrossRef]
166. Ohkubo, K.; Lee, C.H.; Baraniuk, J.N.; Merida, M.; Hausfeld, J.N.; Kaliner, M.A. Angiotensin-converting enzyme in the human nasal mucosa. *Am. J. Respir. Cell Mol. Biol.* **1994**, *11*, 173–180. [CrossRef] [PubMed]

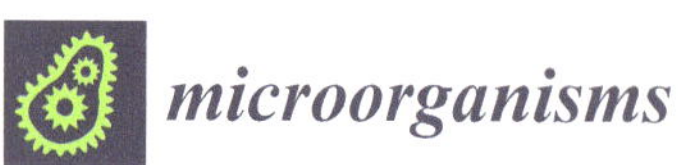

microorganisms

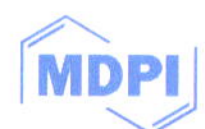

Article

SARS-CoV-2 Infection and Anemia—A Focus on RBC Deformability and Membrane Proteomics—Integrated Observational Prospective Study

Angelo D'Alessandro [1], Elena Krisnevskaya [2], Valentina Leguizamon [2], Ines Hernández [3], Carolina de la Torre [4], Joan-Josep Bech [4], Josep-Tomàs Navarro [3] and Joan-Lluis Vives-Corrons [2,*]

[1] Medical Campus, University of Colorado Anschutz, Aurora, CO 80045, USA; angelo.dalessandro@cuanschutz.edu
[2] Red Blood Cells and Haematopoietic Disorders, Josep Carreras Institute for Leukaemia Research (IJC), 08916 Badalona, Spain; ekrish6@gmail.com (E.K.); valen.velilla.vl@gmail.com (V.L.)
[3] Josep Carreras Leukaemia Research Institute, Haematology Department, ICO-Germans Trias i Pujol Hospital, Autonomous University of Barcelona, 08916 Badalona, Spain; ihernandez@iconcologia.net (I.H.); tnavarro@carrerasresearch.org (J.-T.N.)
[4] Proteomic Unit at Josep Carreras Leukaemia Research Institute IJC Building, Campus ICO-Germans Trias i Pujol, 08916 Badalona, Spain; cdelatorre@carrerasresearch.org (C.d.l.T.); jbech@carrerasresearch.org (J.-J.B.)
*   Correspondence: jlvives@clinic.cat

Abstract: Introduction: The multifaceted impact of COVID-19 extends beyond the respiratory system, encompassing intricate interactions with various physiological systems. This study elucidates the potential association between SARS-CoV-2 infection and anemia, with a particular emphasis on the deformability of red blood cells (RBCs), stability of hemoglobin, enzymatic activities, and proteomic profiles. Methods: The study encompasses a cohort of 74 individuals, including individuals positive for COVID-19, a control group, and patients with other viral infections to discern the specific effects attributable to COVID-19. The analysis of red blood cells was focused on deformability measured by osmotic gradient ektacytometry, hemoglobin stability, and glycolytic enzyme activity. Furthermore, membrane proteins were examined using advanced proteomics techniques to capture molecular-level changes. Results: Findings from the study suggest a correlation between anemia and exacerbated outcomes in COVID-19 patients, marked by significant elevations in d-dimer, serum procalcitonin, creatinine, and blood urea nitrogen (BUN) levels. These observations suggest that chronic kidney disease (CKD) may play a role in the development of anemia in COVID-19 patients, particularly those of advanced age with comorbidities. Furthermore, the proteomic analyses have highlighted a complex relationship between omics data and RBC parameters, enriching our understanding of the mechanisms underlying the disease. Conclusions: This research substantiates the complex interrelationship between COVID-19 and anemia, with a specific emphasis on the potential repercussions of SARS-CoV-2 infection on RBCs. The findings contribute to the growing body of evidence supporting the extensive impact of COVID-19 on RBCs.

Keywords: COVID-19; anemia; red blood cells; membranopathies; enzymopathies; ektacytometry; proteomics

Citation: D'Alessandro, A.; Krisnevskaya, E.; Leguizamon, V.; Hernández, I.; de la Torre, C.; Bech, J.-J.; Navarro, J.-T.; Vives-Corrons, J.-L. SARS-CoV-2 Infection and Anemia—A Focus on RBC Deformability and Membrane Proteomics—Integrated Observational Prospective Study. *Microorganisms* **2024**, *12*, 453. https://doi.org/10.3390/microorganisms12030453

Academic Editor: Qibin Geng

Received: 29 January 2024
Revised: 19 February 2024
Accepted: 22 February 2024
Published: 23 February 2024

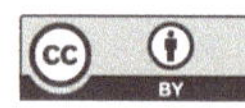

1. Introduction

The coronavirus infection (COVID-19) is caused by the SARS-CoV-2 virus and manifests primarily through symptoms such as shortness of breath, persistent cough, and fever. Given the critical role of red blood cells (RBCs) in oxygen transport and gas exchange, understanding the impact of COVID-19 on RBC properties is imperative. Previous studies have demonstrated alterations in the structural and functional proteins of RBCs in patients with COVID-19, correlated with disease severity and inflammatory markers such as interleukin-6 [1]. These alterations include the cleavage of the N-terminus cytosolic domain of band 3 (SLC4A1), attributable to oxidant stress or proteolytic activity [2] and changes in the band 3 interactome [3] involving key structural proteins such as ankyrin (ANK1) and spectrin (SPTA1 and SPTB). Subsequent research has further identified morphological changes in RBCs from COVID-19 patients and correlated these with proteome functional alterations [4,5]. While the mechanistic link to an increased hemolytic propensity of RBCs remains to be fully elucidated, a significant correlation has been established between altered red cell distribution widths (RDWs) and disease severity, indicating RDW as a potential marker for clinical outcomes in COVID-19 [6–8]. Additionally, Bergamaschi G et al. [9] have found in COVID-19-positive patients, the coexistence of anemia in 61% of cases compared to 45% of cases in a group of patients with clinical and laboratory findings suggestive of COVID-19, but with negative nasopharyngeal swab test. Recently, a comprehensive meta-analysis has highlighted a progressive decrease in hemoglobin levels as indicative of worse clinical progression in COVID-19 patients, pointing towards the potential role of SARS-CoV-2 RNA in contributing to anemia through effects on RBC structure [10].

It is well established that RBCs can be targeted by pathogens [11], leading to direct intravascular hemolysis or indirect clearance by reticuloendothelial systems. Given that RBCs cannot support viral replication, the possibility of SARS-CoV-2 RNA invasion into RBCs, similar to the behavior of flaviviruses like Zika, raises important questions regarding the unique or universal nature of RBC alterations in response to infections. In this context, it is worth mentioning that the activation of cGAS-STING-interferon-IDO1-kynurenine responses is a key determinant of prognosis in COVID-19 patients [12–14], yet these responses are universally triggered by almost any infective pathogen [15], especially when a background chronic inflammatory condition in aging is present.

Several years ago, an inhibition of liver pyruvate kinase (PKL) by physical interaction between the SARS-CoV-2 nucleocapsid protein and the enzymatic protein was described [16]. Since PKL and RBC PK (PKLR) share genetic encoding, a similar mechanism for reduced RBC lifespan and PKLR activity in COVID-19 in patients with COVID-19 infection was suggested. Unfortunately, this hypothesis could not be demonstrated in the present study.

Despite the frequent occurrence of anemia in COVID-19 patients, the direct link between the infection and anemia remains to be conclusively demonstrated, particularly once common causes related to iron metabolism and inflammatory conditions are excluded. This study aims to investigate the effects of COVID-19 on RBC (Hb), enzyme activities, and deformability in an effort to elucidate the mechanisms by which SARS-CoV-2 RNA may influence RBC dysfunction and contribute to anemia. Interestingly, a prevalence of anemia in COVID-19 patients has been documented, with a notable difference in incidence between patients testing positive for SARS-CoV-2 and those with similar symptoms but negative test results. The examination of proteomic biomarkers has contributed to enhancing the prediction of severe disease outcomes to improve the understanding of viral mechanisms and to explore more effective treatment strategies.

2. Materials and Methods

2.1. Patient Enrollment

The experimental design was based on an observational prospective study of a single cohort of 74 individuals (63 patients and 11 controls). Inclusion criteria were age >18 years and documented diagnosis of SARS-CoV-2 infection, confirmed by RT-PCR performed in at least one nasal/pharyngeal swab specimen. Viral infections with similar clinical COVID-19+ phenotype and negative RT-PCR in a nasal/pharyngeal swab specimen were also included. Exclusion criteria were age <18 years, not capable of signing the Informed Consent (IC), and a known history of a hereditary RBC defect. Accordingly, on the basis of anemia and the RT-PCR positivity, the patients were classified into four groups where patients negative for RT-PCR had viral infections not due to COVID-19 (Table 1). A fifth group with 11 healthy blood donors was included as the control group. Anemia was defined according to WHO (<120 g/L for women and <130 g/L for men). For the classification of the disease severity, the recommendations of the European Centre for Disease Prevention and Control [17] and the National Health Commission of the People's Republic of China and WHO [18] were used. Accordingly, patients with COVID-19 infection were classified into 4 categories: 1. Mild clinical symptoms without pneumonia at chest computed tomography; 2. Moderate fever and other respiratory symptoms with pneumonia seen at imaging; 3. Severe respiratory distress ($\geq$30 breaths per min), hypoxia (oxygen saturation: $\leq$93%), or abnormal results of blood gas analysis; and 4. Critical respiratory failure requiring mechanical ventilation, shock, or other organ(s) failure requiring intensive care unit monitoring and treatment. It should be mentioned that the study was performed during the pandemic and immediately after admission. For this reason, the main treatments received and the patient's clinical follow-up have not been considered here. The study with Ref. CEI PI-21-30-09 was approved by the Hospital Human Ethics Committee, and Informed Consent was signed by all the patients included in the study and performed in respect of the Declaration of Helsinki.

Table 1. Patients' clinical classification.

PATIENTS		GROUPS	NUMBER of CASES
COVID-19+	without ANEMIA	GROUP 1	13 (18%)
COVID-19+	with ANEMIA	GROUP 2	20 (27%)
VIRAL INFECTION	without ANEMIA	GROUP 3	10 (13%)
VIRAL INFECTION	with ANEMIA	GROUP 4	20 (27%)
HEALTHY CONTROLS		GROUP 5	11 (15%)

2.2. Hematological and Biochemical Parameters

Complete Blood Count (CBC) and basic biochemistry parameters were tested in all patients with SARS-CoV-2 positivity and other viral infections, as well as in the control group. In all patients with anemia, iron study, vitamin B12 and folate, C-reactive protein (CRP), and hepcidin were also tested. In all patients, hemoglobin stability was measured using the isopropanol test [19], and RBC enzyme activities were measured according to Beutler [20] with slight modifications [19].

2.3. RBC Deformability

RBC deformability was determined with a new-generation ektacytometer—a laser diffractometer that measures the deformability of an RBC population exposed to an increasing osmotic gradient under a constant shear stress [21]. The osmotic gradient ektacytometry (OGE) measures RBC geometry, cytoplasm viscosity, cell volume, and membrane fluidity by the RBCs' shift from discoid to elliptical shape, gauged by light scatters as the cell responds to shear forces over an osmotic gradient. In addition to rheological parameters, the ektacytometer allows for identification of eventual RBC structural abnormalities affecting membrane or hemoglobin content. The OGE profile obtained with the osmoscan module is a characteristic curve that shows the amount of deformability on the y-axis and the osmolality on the x-axis (Figure 1), as well as three main parameters: (a) EImax/Omax or the value of osmolality at maximum EI (deformability), (b) EImin/Omin, or the value at which RBCs have attained their critical hemolytic value due to osmotic shifting of water into the cell in a hypotonic environment (osmotic fragility), and (c) EIhyper/Ohyper, or the osmolality at which the index is midway between the maximal deformability and Omin (cellular hydration).

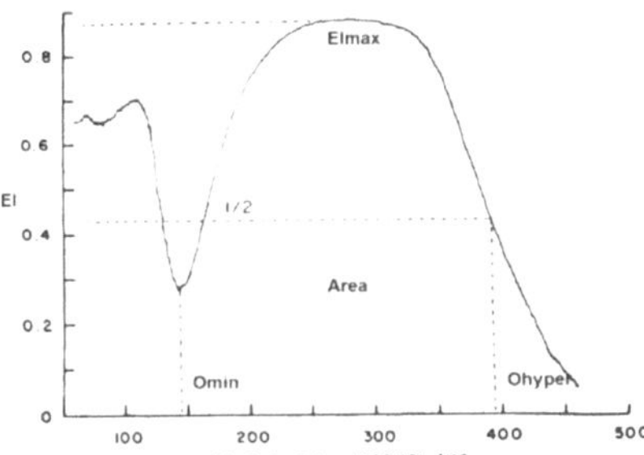

Figure 1. Graphic representation of the OGE profile obtained with the osmoscan module of the LoRRca ektacytometer. *y*-axis: elongation index (EI); *x*-axis: osmolality (mOsmol/Kg).

2.4. RBC Membrane Proteins (Proteomics)

Of the total cohort of 74 patients, RBC samples were available from 32 subjects for proteomic analyses. Specifically, proteomic analyses were performed on 11 healthy control subjects, patients with COVID-19 (with and without anemia), and patients with other viral infections (with and without anemia) (n = 6 for each one of these four groups). Patient samples were collected by centrifugation for 5 min at 150× g and were suspended in PBS containing 1 mM EDTA. Then, the slurry was passed through a leukocyte depletion filter. RBCs were washed four times with PBS and stored overnight on ice at 4 °C in PBS containing 10 mM glucose and EDTA-free protease inhibitor cocktail tablets (Roche, Mannheim, Germany). Proteomic analysis was performed on the day of collection, and the steps used for sample treatment are described below.

Sample preparation: RBCs were isolated according to Pesciotta et al. [22] and lysed in 0.1 M Tris-HCl containing 2% SDS and 0.05 M DTT at 100 °C for 5 min. RBC membranes were isolated by centrifugation at 21,000× g for 40 min and purified by 4–5 additional washes and centrifugations. Protein was quantified with the DC™ Protein Assay Kit II (Bio-Rad, Hercules, CA, USA).

Preparation of samples for protein digestion and peptide purification prior to mass spectrometry analysis was performed according to the conventional procedures for cell lysis, protein precipitation, and protein quantification. Prior to digestion, samples were reduced and alkylated with DTT and CAA; then, they were diluted with Tris 0.1 M to reach urea 2 mol/L. Lys-C was added at 1:100 (w/w) (enzyme-to-protein ratio), and protein digestion was carried out at 30 °C ON (overnight). The samples were diluted with Tris buffer (0.1 M) to achieve a final urea concentration of 0.8 mol/L. Trypsin was added to the diluted samples at a ratio of 1:100 (enzyme-to-protein ratio), and protein digestion was performed again at 30 °C for a duration of 8 h, allowing the trypsin enzyme to cleave the proteins into smaller peptides. The enzymatic reaction was stopped by adding formic acid (FA) to a final concentration of 10% (v/v). Digested peptides were cleared by centrifugation and purified using a reversed-phase C18 Microspin column according to the manufacturer's instructions. Elution of peptides was performed with 50% ACN in 0.1% TFA; then, peptides were dried by the speedVac at RT and stored at −80 °C until further processing.

LC-MS/MS Measurements: Tryptic peptide samples were reconstituted with 3% ACN and 0.1% FA aqueous solution at 100 ng/µL, and 8 µL (800 ng) was loaded into the Evotip. Peptides were separated using an Evosep EV1106 column (150 µm × 150 mm, 1.9 µm) (Evosep, Odense, Denmark) at a flow rate of 500 nL/min with an 88 min run. The column outlet was directly connected to an EASY-Spray source (Thermo Fisher Scientific, Waltham, MA, USA) fitted on an Orbitrap Eclipse™ Tribrid Mass Spectrometer (Thermo Fisher Scientific). The mass spectrometer was operated in a data-dependent acquisition (DDA) mode. In each data collection cycle, one full MS scan (375–1500 m/z) was acquired in the Orbitrap (1.2 × 105 resolution setting and automatic gain control (AGC) of 2 × 105). Ions were fragmented in the HCD with a collision energy of 28%, 0.25 activation Q, an AGC target of 5×10^4, an isolation window of 0.7 Da, a maximum ion accumulation time of 54 ms, and a turbo ion scan rate. Previously analyzed precursor ions were dynamically excluded for 15 s. MS2 were detected in the LC-MS Orbitrap (Thermo Fisher, Waltham, MA, USA) with a resolution of 30,000.

Data analysis and statistics for proteomic analyses: The .RAW files were processed using the MaxQuant 2.1.3.0 software. The peak lists were searched against a SwissProt Human Database (https://www.uniprot.org/ downloaded in 3 March 2021) with the help of the MaxQuant built-in Andromeda: a peptide search engine integrated into the MaxQuant environment. The false discovery rate (FDR) was assessed by using a decoy database. Trypsin was selected as the enzyme, and a maximum of two missed cleavages were allowed. Carbamidomethylating in cysteines was set as a fixed modification, whereas oxidation in methionine, acetylation at the protein N-terminal, and deamidation at asparagines and glutamines were used as variable modifications. Searches were performed using a peptide tolerance of 7 ppm and a product ion tolerance of 0.5 Da. The resulting data files were filtered for FDR. The quantification was performed using the iBAQ algorithm. The list of proteins was filtered to remove the 'potential contaminants', 'reverse', and 'only identified by site' proteins. The iBAQ-based intensity values were log2 transformed and analyzed to look for potential outliers, which were removed from the final data matrix. Additionally, we removed from the dataset the samples showing significant non-specific deformability alterations (ektacytometry). The samples present in the final data matrix were then normalized by median-centering the iBAQ intensity values. The statistical analysis was performed with the help of R (https://cran.r-project.org/) and Rstudio (https://www.rstudio.com) using the 'limma' package.

3. Results

3.1. General Hematological Data, Iron Metabolism and Inflammation Parameters

Table 2 summarizes the main demographic and laboratory parameters studied in the patients with laboratory-confirmed COVID-19+ compared to patients with viral infection but negative nasopharyngeal swab test and the control group. At hospital admission, the 20 patients of Group 2 (COVID-19+ with anemia) exhibited a more severe disease than the 13 patients of Group 1 (COVID-19+ without anemia). This difference was not observed between the 20 patients of Group 4 (viral infection with anemia) and the 10 patients of Group 3 (viral infection without anemia). WBC count was only slightly increased in patients COVID+ with anemia but moderately increased in patients with viral infection (with or without anemia). Platelet count was normal in all the patient groups. No association was found between hemoglobin concentration and the neutrophil-to-lymphocyte or the platelet-to-lymphocyte ratios. The d-dimer, serum procalcitonin, creatinine, and BUN were significantly increased in all the patients studied here, but especially in COVID-19+ patients with anemia (Group 2). Alkaline phosphatase, PCR, and hepcidin were also significantly increased in all groups, but especially in patients with viral infection and anemia (Group 4). Finally, iron metabolism parameters (serum iron, serum ferritin, and transferrin saturation index) were markedly abnormal in the same Group 4 when compared to the other groups.

3.2. Hemoglobin Stability

The isopropanol test was normal in all the patients included in this study, with the exception of five viral-infected patients—three with anemia and two without anemia. These patients were not the same as those with altered left-shifted curves. The study of these patients with high-performance liquid chromatography (HPLC) discarded unstable hemoglobinopathies.

3.3. RBC Enzyme Activities

RBC enzyme activities from the glycolytic pathway and the oxidative metabolism measured in all patients are summarized in Table 3. All enzyme activities were found to be within normal range, with the exception of pyruvate kinase (PK) and adenylate kinase

(AK). PK activity was significantly ($p < 0.05$) increased in COVID-19-positive patients with anemia (Group 2), and the AK activity was significantly ($p < 0.05$) increased in patients with anemia only (Groups 2 and 4). None of these increased enzyme activities were accompanied by an increased number of reticulocytes and/or circulating erythroblasts. No significant RBC morphological abnormalities were found.

Table 2. Hematological and biochemical parameters. Mean (SD).

		GROUP 1 COVID-19 Positive NO ANEMIA ($n = 13$)	GROUP 2 COVID-19 Positive ANEMIA ($n = 20$)	GROUP 3 VIRAL INFECTION NO ANEMIA ($n = 10$)	GROUP 4 VIRAL INFECTION ANEMIA ($n = 20$)	Normal Controls ($n = 11$)	p *
RBCs ($\times 10^{12}$/L)		4.61 (0.67)	3.86 (0.72)	4.53 (0.38)	3.80 (0.74)	4.51 (0.48)	
Hemoglobin (g/L)	M	142.7 (21.4)	121.4 (17.5)	131.1 (8.2)	108.1 (18.4)	139.0 (16.0)	
	F	136.0 (13.0)	107.5 (12.0)	124.5 [12.0]	101.5 (20.0)	131.0 (18.0)	
MCV (fl)		91.72 (4.68)	88.98 (6.63)	88.09 (5.28)	87.01 (7.51)	88.28 (3.10)	
MCH (pg)		30.85 (1.47)	29.20 (2.68)	29.04 (1.75)	29.03 (3.16)	30.24 (1.24)	
MCHC (g/L)		338.5 (8.00)	327.7 (8.90)	329.2 (5.30)	329.8 (8.80)	342.50 (7.20)	
RDW		13.52 (0.40)	15.7 (2.33)	14.88 (1.35)	15.58 (3.94)	13.25 (0.52)	
Reticulocytes (%)		0.87 (0.50)	1.47 (0.90)	1.15 (0.56)	1.51 (1.19)	1.15 (0.55)	0.125
Retis ($\times 10^9$/L)		40.45 (23.85)	53.61 (27.38)	52.23 (25.57)	55.32 (38.58)	51.98 (25.16)	0.537
WBCs ($\times 10^9$/L)		6.57 (4.44)	8.23 (4.62)	9.55 (3.88)	10.86 (5.68)	6.04 (1.61)	0.002
Platelets ($\times 10^9$/L)		170.77 (73.04)	241.05 (147.99)	225.2 (67.65)	259.6 (126.2)	251.91 (62.9)	0.121
MPV (fl)		8.39 (1.18)	8.41 (1.15)	8.41 (1.17)	8.51 (1.03)	8.74 (0.85)	0.703
Fibrinogen (g/L)		5.90 (1.32)	5.80 (1.42)	5.88 (5.61)	6.50 (0.97)	3.58 (1.58)	0.009
D-dimer (ng/L)		1469 (1653.07)	2858 (2548.69)	1375 (1438.96)	1074 (526.26)	294 (149.46)	0.046
Procalcitonin (ng/L)		2.80 (4.00)	58.20 (38.70)	5.30 (9.16)	16.70 (25.6)	5.00 (2.5)	0.001
Creatinine (mg/L)		8.70 (3.60)	16.9 (11.70)	10.10 (3.40)	12.20 (6.00)	6.90 (1.40)	0.003
BUN (mg/L)		403.60 (296.20)	824.70 (567.70)	536.70 (212.10)	505.2 (449.9)	220 (27.80)	0.001
PCR (mg/L)		627.50 (47.59)	767.10 (458.20)	586.10 (439.20)	1180 (775.60)	4.80 (2.10)	0.006
Hepcidin (nM/L)		44.71 (35.26)	70.93 (91.47)	194.77 (426.99)	212 (299.54)	9.55 (6.32)	0.009
Serum iron (mg/L)		664.02 (410.0)	544.40 (381.8)	465.7 (300.2)	213.0 (118.7)	1035(339.5)	0.002
Serum ferritin (ng/L)		1550 (522.50)	5375.3 (4052.2)	3681.40 (2839.80)	4520 (4611.4)	825 (741.7)	0.012
Serum transferrin (mg/L)		2136 (592.20)	1572 (561.20)	1747.10 (284.70)	2011 (468.20)	2650 (261.5)	0.002
Transferrin saturation Index (TSI)		24.00 (5.89)	26.67 (17.21)	21.29 (17.59)	7.80 (4.71)	28.5 (10.07)	0.003
Serum cobalamin (Vit B12) (pg/L)		577.0 (191.09)	908.63 (760.30)	640.29 (439.93)	614.60 (517.0)	486.43 (218.4)	0.971
Serum folate (ng/L)		66.00 (45.7)	59.40 (27.8)	69.90 (47.7)	74.7 (42.0)	55.0 (12.40)	0.809
Serum bilirubin (Total) (mg/L)		5.10 (1.1)	6.20 (4.5)	4.80 (0.19)	5.60 (2.50)	7.00 (2.90)	0.597
ALT (IU/L)		19.8 (12.1)	21.67 (10.32)	25.13 (19.14)	24.47 (13.89)	15.67 (7.23)	0.162
Alkaline phosphatase (IU/L)		86.25 (25.36)	72.5 (32.53)	69.86 (34.98)	118.69 (87.5)	50.80 (6.91)	0.085

Table 3. RBC enzyme activity (IU/gHb). Results are given as mean (SD). Since the majority of RBC enzymes do not follow a normal distribution, nonparametric statistical tests have been used (H of Krushal–Wallis).

	GROUP 1 COVID Positive NO ANEMIA ($n = 13$)	GROUP 2 COVID Positive ANEMIA ($n - 20$)	GROUP 3 COVID Negative NO ANEMIA ($n = 10$)	GROUP 4 COVID Negative ANEMIA ($n = 20$)	Reference Values ($n = 11$)	p *
Age	62.15 (21.5)	71.8 (14.23)	70.0 (19.50)	67.8 (18.72)	58.20 (15.50)	
Pyruvate kinase (PK)	13.1 (1.66)	14.40 (2.55)	13.10 (1.68)	12.55 (2.13)	11.23 (3.31)	0.047 *
Hexokinase (HK)	1.10 (0.34)	1.25 (0.36)	1.18 (0.16)	1.14 (0.36)	0.94 (0.34)	0.088
Glucose-6-phosphate dehydrogenase (G6PD)	7.48 (1.15)	7.62 (1.47)	8.53 (1.92)	7.29 (1.24)	7.53 (1.12)	0.517
Glucose phosphate isomerase (GPI)	53.22 (11.8)	55.28 (9.11)	52.13 (11.86)	50.81 (12.20)	53.05 (7.15)	0.729
Adenylate kinase (AK)	226.2 (23.7)	258.5 (38.25)	220.9 (37.50)	249.2 (38.24)	236.5 (33.32)	0.049 *
Phosphofructokinase (PFK)	10.45 (2.80)	11.28 (2.59)	9.73 (2.63)	10.53 (1.66)	9.42 (3.16)	0.412
Phosphoglycerate kinase (PGK)	31.57 (4.68)	32.30 (4.30)	31.67 (4.87)	31.62 (4.89)	30.74 (4.79)	0.765
Triosephosphate isomerase (TPI)	2032 (386)	2185 (435)	1975.4 (256)	2051.2 (246)	1897.1 (292)	0.291
Glutathione peroxidase (GPx)	16.3 (4.65)	18.88 (4.99)	17.17 (4.45)	16.66 (3.68)	16.04 (4.89)	0.403
Glutathione reductase (GR)	8.22 (1.82)	8.91 (2.57)	9.08 (2.61)	9.11 (2.74)	8.15 (1.97)	0.941
Reduced glutathione (GSH)	77.89 (14.7)	75.96 (14.27)	73.73 (7.20)	74.96 (18.79)	81.45 (13.04)	0.500
GSH Stability (+APH)	61.59 (17.3)	65.77 (12.50)	59.15 (18.54)	63.40 (25.26)	65.08 (20.24)	0.86 2

* Compared to normal controls.

3.4. RBC Deformability

All patients showed a normal OGE profile, with the exception of five patients with anemia—two COVID-19 positive and three COVID-19 negative—that exhibited a dehydrated RBC pattern of unknown origin. The genetic study of these patients by WES and a complete molecular panel for hemoglobinopathies (alpha and beta) discarded a hereditary RBC defect. The results of OGE parameters are summarized in Table 4. RBC deformability or maximum elongation index (EImax) was normal in all the patients, and only a significantly ($p < 0.05$) slight RBC overhydration (Ohyper and Area) was observed in Groups 2, 3, and 4. Usually, the normal range in Ohyper regions is rather wide, and the statistical significance obtained does not have great significance.

3.5. RBC Membrane Proteins (Proteomics)

An overview of the experimental design for the proteomic analyses performed herein is provided in Figure 2A. Significant proteomic alterations were observed across the four groups of patients, with the most significant alterations in Group 2 (COVID-19+ with anemia). Such differences are highlighted by unsupervised hierarchical clustering analysis (HCA—Figure 2B) and partially (PLS-DA—Figure 2C,D). A list of the protein variables with the largest loading weights from this analysis is provided in Figure 2C. Of note, this list includes levels of transferrin (TF), as measured by proteomics, and discriminating between anemic and non-anemic patients. The list also included a series of structural proteins (especially myosin heavy chains MYH10) and enzymes involved in immune functions, such as myeloperoxidase (MPO) and lysozyme (LYZ), suggesting elevated levels of these proteins in the residual plasma or cellular fraction enriched for the study of RBCs, despite buffy coat depletion. While Group 2 patients (COVID-19+ with anemia) showed the highest degree of separation from the other groups across principal component 1 (PC1), patients with infection other than SARS-CoV-2 showed the highest degree of separation across PC2 compared to the rest of the tested samples (Figure 2D).

Table 4. Osmoscan parameters. Statistical measurement by parametrical test (* $p < 0.05$).

	COVID	ANEMIA	VIRAL INFECTION	O Min (X ± SD)	EI Max (X ± SD)	O Max (X ±SD)	O Hyper (X ± SD)	Area (X ± SD)
Group 1	positive	NO		145 (5.7)	0.612 (0.01)	311 (8.9)	457 (16.7)	162 (7.45)
Group 2	positive	YES		137 (11.2)	0.607 (0.01)	300 (21.9)	464 (14.9) *	168 (7.5) *
Group 3	negative	NO	YES	136 (8.8) *	0.612 (0.01)	297 (22.6)	463 (13.2) *	172 (3.7) *
Group 4	negative	YES	YES	143 (11.1)	0.611 (0.01)	309 (21.1)	466 (13.7) *	168 (6.2) *
Normal Controls				146 (6.6)	0.613 (0.01)	309 (14.1)	449 (15.1)	160 (6.3)

O min: minimal osmolality (RBC osmotic fragility). EI max: maximum elongation index (RBC deformability). O max: osmolality at EI max (300 mOsm/kg). O hyper: at 50% of EI max (RBC hydration maximal osmolality).

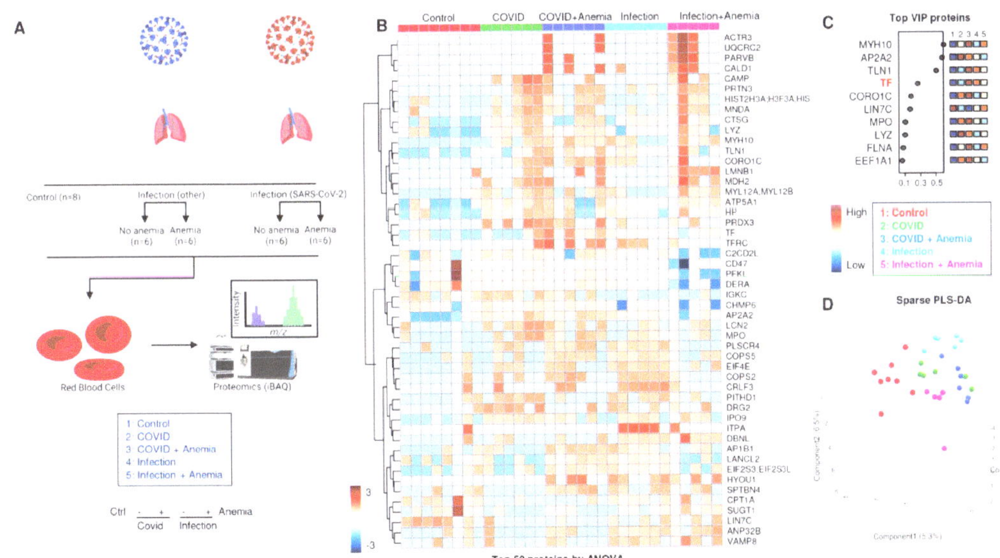

Figure 2. (**A**) Overview of the experimental design for the proteomic analyses performed here. (**B**) Proteomics alterations observed across the four groups of patients, with the differences highlighted by unsupervised hierarchical clustering analysis (HCA) and (**C**) with partially supervised partial least square-discriminant analysis (PLS-DA), including (**D**) a list of the protein variables with the largest loading weights.

The patients from Group 3 (viral infection without anemia) were characterized by a significant alteration in a subset of the proteome (Figure 3A), with significant depletion of several RBC membrane proteins (SLC4A1, ANK1, SPTA1, SPTB, stomatin (STOM), band 4.1 E4BP1, flotillin (FLOT2), glycolytic enzymes (fructose bisphosphate aldolase (ALD), glyceraldehyde-3-phosphate dehydrogenase (GAPDH)) and hemoglobin/heme metabolism enzymes (HBA, HBB, and biliverdin reductase B–BLVRB) (Figure 3B). This group was also characterized by an elevation in transcription factors and autophagy-related proteins, with a notable elevation in amyloid protein (APP) and mitochondrial malate dehydrogenase 2 (MDH2), suggesting an elevation in nucleated and mitochondria-containing blood cells in the RBC fraction tested herein (e.g., reticulocytes) (Figure 3C). This may be the result of stress erythropoiesis, resulting in incomplete mitochondrial clearance during the final phases of maturation, as reported by multiple groups, including ours, in the context of sickle cell disease.

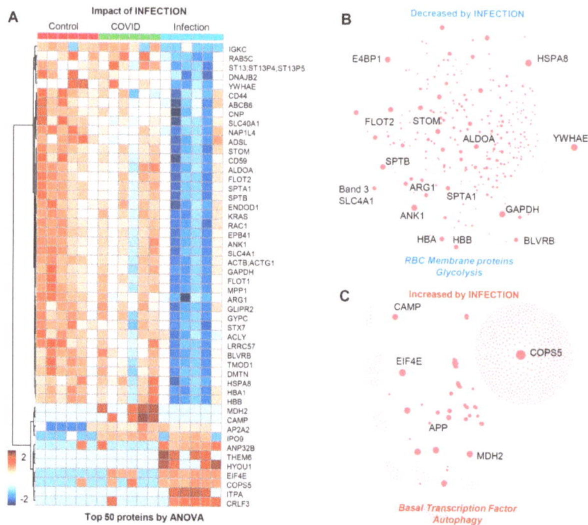

Figure 3. (Patients of Group 3) (**A**) Impact of infection on a subset of the proteome with: (**B**) significant depletion of several RBC membrane proteins and glycolytic enzymes and hemoglobin/heme metabolism and (**C**) elevation in transcription factors and autophagy-related proteins, especially amyloid protein (APP) and mitochondrial malate dehydrogenase 2 (MDH2).

The patients from Group 4 (viral infection with anemia) showed a significant decrease in several proteins (Figure 4A), mostly involved in infection responses (top enriched pathway suggests depression in components of the immune cascades activated by bacterial—*Staphylococcus aureus*—and viral—human papillomavirus—infections (Figure 4B)), suggesting that stronger immune responses are elicited by SARS-CoV-2 independently from anemia, while such responses are blunted in patients suffering from other viral infections in the context of anemia. The combination of anemia and viral infection was associated with elevated levels of components of the vesiculation machinery (Figure 4C).

In the patients from Group 2 (COVID-19+ with anemia), the anemia had a strong effect that can be appreciated at a glance from unsupervised hierarchical cluster analysis (HCA) and volcano plot analyses (Figure 5A,B). In particular, anemia was associated with elevation in protein components involved in necroptosis and AMPK signaling, with corresponding decreases in the levels of proteins involved in MAPK signaling and autophagy (Figure 5C,D). Pathway analyses of significantly increased and decreased proteins in anemic patients compared to non-anemic ones indicate an enrichment in cGMP-PKG signaling and mitochondrial components that participate in oxidative phosphorylation events, suggesting an association between anemia and the increase in young RBCs containing mitochondria. On the other hand, decreasing proteins in anemic RBC fractions included components of the autophagy and mTOR pathways.

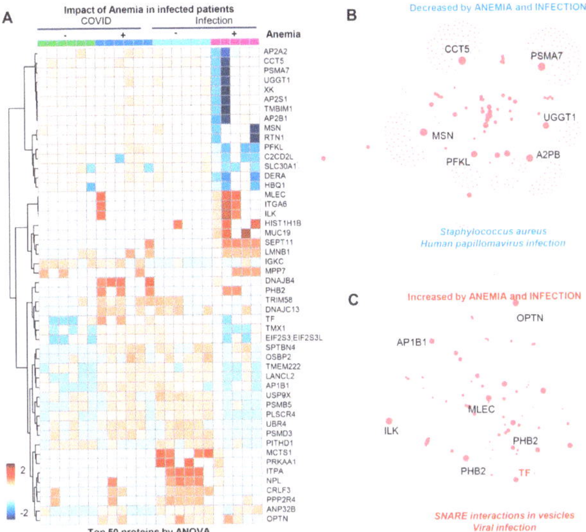

Figure 4. (Patients of Group 4) (**A**) Significant decrease in several proteins, mostly involved in infection responses. (**B**) Depression in components of the immune cascades activated by bacterial *Staphylococcus aureus* and viral infections. (**C**) Elevated levels of components of the vesiculation machinery.

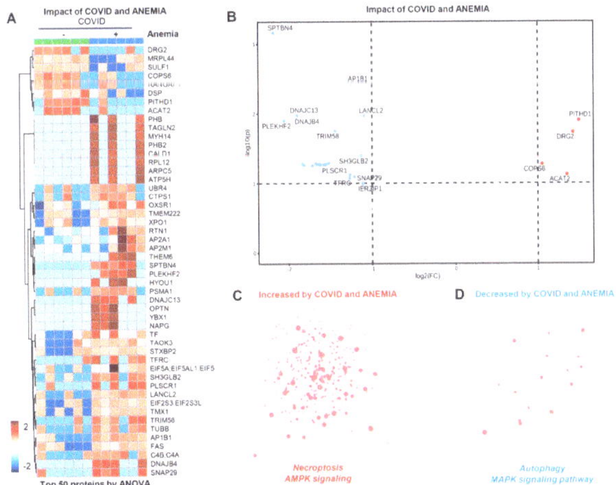

Figure 5. (Patients from Group 2) (**A,B**) Effect of anemia appreciated from unsupervised hierarchical cluster analysis (HCA) and volcano plot analyses. (**C**) Elevation in protein components involved in necroptosis and AMPK signaling. (**D**) Decreases in the levels of proteins involved in MAPK signaling and autophagy.

3.6. Omics Correlates to Clinical, Hematological, and Deformability Parameters

To determine the potential translational relevance of the proteomics observations, we correlated proteomics results to clinical, hematological, and biochemical parameters and RBC deformability measured by ektacytometry. Results showed four main clusters of highly connected variables. The largest cluster includes multiple hematological parameters (including RBC count, Hb concentration, and RDW), patient's age, markers of renal function (BUN and creatinine), a series of RBC structural and membrane proteins (E4BP2, SPTA1,

CD44, ANKFY1), hypoxia-upregulated 1 (HYOU1), and antioxidant capacity (reduced glutathione, glutathione peroxidase). A second cluster involved multiple markers of anemia (transferrin and serum iron), strongly associated with markers of one-carbon metabolism (B12, folate), liver metabolism (GGT, ALT, AST, LDH), ADP-ribosylation factors 1 and 3 (ARF1, ARF3), and the structural protein desmatin (DMTN). A third large cluster involved all parameters derived from the ektacytometric analysis, including the area of the osmoscan curve, and several proteins, including ACTBL2, 55kDa erythrocyte membrane protein (MPP1), and leucine-rich repeat-containing protein (LRRC57). Sub-networks included strongly connected hubs of transferrin and alfa-spectrin (SPTB), glycolytic and redox enzymes (HK, GSH), structural components (GYPC, FLOT2, ANK1), and RBC deformability (EImax). To further delve into these results, we plotted smile plots of Spearman correlates to patient age, RDW, PK activity, renal function (creatinine) and coagulability (d-dimer), common comorbidity factors in patients with severe COVID-19 infection (Figure 6). Top correlates to patient age indicate an age-dependent increase in renal dysfunction, which, in turn, is associated with markers of inflammation (e.g., RCP). Age and inflammation (IL-6, a marker of COVID-19 severity), as well as glycolytic enzymes (enolase–ENO1), also ranked amongst the top correlates to d-dimer measurements. As an internal validation of the quality of these correlative results, enzymatic assays of PK activity correlated significantly with the levels of RBC-PK isoforms (PKR) as detected via proteomics. The negative association between patient age and proteosome components (PSMD12, PSMA4) suggests a potential failure of protein degradation machinery in older subjects. Elevation in hemoglobin gamma chains (1 and 2) was negatively associated with PK activity and kidney function (elevated creatinine), suggestive of a linkage between anemia, kidney damage, and eventual subclinical hemolysis.

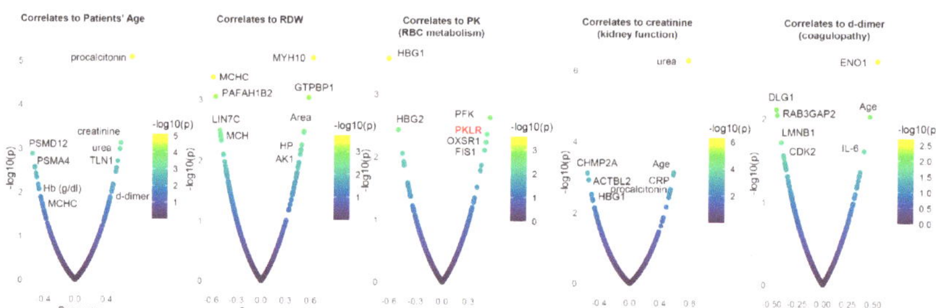

Figure 6. Spearman plot correlations with patient age, RDW, PK activity, kidney function (creatinine), and coagulability (d-dimer). As an internal validation of the quality of the observed correlative results, enzymatic assays of PK activity correlated significantly with the levels of RBC-PK isoforms (PKR) as detected via proteomics.

4. Discussion

The multifaceted etiology and prognosis of numerous clinical conditions, including those associated with respiratory complications such as COVID-19 infection, are significantly influenced by anemia [23,24]. Iron deficiency anemia (IDA) has been identified as a predisposing factor for lower respiratory tract infections in the pediatric demographic [25]. In adults, its presence upon hospital admission has been implicated as a potential determinant for adverse COVID-19 outcomes [26,27]. Recent investigations have linked anemia, particularly in the context of COVID-19, to increased mortality rates attributed to immune-mediated disruptions in iron homeostasis [28]. Furthermore, a reduction in hemoglobin levels has been observed in critically ill patients [29,30], underscoring the complex relationship between anemia and severe COVID-19 illness, which remains insufficiently elucidated. The pathogenesis of multifactorial anemia in SARS-CoV-2-infected individuals encompasses several mechanisms, including potential hemolysis induced by viral entry through erythrocyte membrane receptors [31], impaired erythropoiesis due to hematopoietic precursor invasion [32–34], and altered iron metabolism driven by pro-inflammatory cytokine-mediated upregulation of hepcidin [24,35]. However, since clinical and omics characterization of RBCs and plasma from COVID-19+ patients failed to document the increase in hemolysis, it can be assumed that the association of decreased iron availability, elevated levels of acute phase reactants, and a hindered erythropoiesis may explain the anemia of most COVID-19-infected patients [36].

This study introduces additional factors contributing to anemia in COVID-19 patients, emphasizing the comparative analysis of patients with other viral infections to enhance the understanding of this condition. Significantly, this research found elevated levels of d-dimer, procalcitonin (PCT), and markers of chronic kidney disease (CKD) in COVID-19 patients with anemia, suggesting a link between CKD and anemia in these patients. This association was further supported by a recent meta-analysis indicating a direct influence of aging and concurrent CKD on anemia in COVID-19 patients [37] in like fashion to patients suffering from CKD [38]. The study also highlights the role of elevated comorbidities, including renal dysfunction and alterations in erythrocyte structural membrane proteins, in the pathogenesis of anemia. Despite these findings, erythrocyte deformability was generally normal across the cohort, suggesting the complexity of anemia's impact on patient outcomes. Increased serum ferritin levels in anemic COVID-19 patients were noted, indicating inflammation. However, similar observations in patients with other viral infections suggest a broader context of anemia beyond COVID-19. Altogether, these observations may contribute to explaining the role of anemia and hypoxia [39]. The study underscores the importance of timely anemia management in hospitalized COVID-19 patients, suggesting that oxygen supplementation or steroids, in addition to standard care, may mitigate deterioration [40]. In this view, it is worth highlighting the reassuring evidence on the potential impact of COVID-19 on RBC oxygen kinetics [41] despite evidence of a potential disruption in the so-called oxygen-dependent metabolic modulation revolving around band 3 stability [1]. Furthermore, the analysis of hemoglobin stability and erythrocyte enzyme activities, including pyruvate kinase (PK) and adenylate kinase (AK), offers insights into the metabolic alterations associated with COVID-19 and anemia and its probable contribution to the prognostic role of anemia in COVID-19 Patients [42] Concerning hemoglobin, the coronavirus, similar to other viruses, is able to interact with protoporphyrin IX through the spike protein involving beta chains of Hb [43], causing eventual Hb denaturation and the inhibition of viral replication by blocking the SARS-CoV-2-cell fusion mediated by the spike protein [44]. Using the isopropanol test, we have analyzed the stability of the hemoglobin molecule in all the patients included in this study, and with the exception of five cases, all the patients exhibited a normal hemoglobin stability. Probably, in mature RBCs, the interaction between SARS-CoV-2 and hemoglobin can take place, but since the virus replication is prevented by the absence of a nucleus, the final effect on hemoglobin stability is not significant. The same may happen at the bone marrow level, where the virus enters the nascent erythroblasts through CD147 and CD26 [31]. Here, even though the virus can replicate, there may be no significant effect on hemoglobin stability. Concerning RBC enzyme activities, their measurement was performed in all the patients included in this study and showed normal values, with the exception of pyruvate kinase (PK) and adenylate kinase (AK), which exhibited a significant ($p < 0.05$) increase in activity in both COVID-19+ and virally infected patients with anemia. Previous studies on RBCs from COVID-19 patients have highlighted an increase in the glycolytic pathway manifested by a characteristic increase in glucose consumption accompanied by an accumulation of intermediates of glycolysis and higher levels of phosphofructokinase (PFK), the rate-limiting enzyme of glycolysis. Mammals have two pyruvate kinase genes, PK-LR and PK-M. PK-LR encodes for two PK isozymes: PKL (liver) and PKR (RBCs). The PK-M gene encodes for pyruvate kinase isozyme M1 (muscle and brain) and M2 (leukocytes and early fetal tissues). Only PKLR encodes for the RBC isozyme, which is affected in PK deficiency [45,46]. However, it has been shown that patients with severe COVID-19 disease exhibit a higher expression of leukocyte PKM2, suggesting that increased PKM2 is involved in the metabolic reprogramming process participating in the immune response induced by COVID-19 [47]. Adenylate kinase (AK) is the key enzyme of nucleotide metabolism and belongs to the nucleoside monophosphate kinase (NMPK) family [48]. The mechanism/s of the increased AK (AK1) activity in COVID-19+ patients with anemia is unknown, but increased AK, together with other biomarkers, can be helpful in assessing the risk of diseases where oxidative/inflammatory stress plays a crucial role in pathogenesis [49,50]. Of note, here, AK1 levels positively correlated with increases in RDW, a marker of disease severity and prognosis in COVID-19 patients [6,51]. This research sheds light on the direct effects of SARS-CoV-2 on erythrocyte structural proteins and metabolic pathways, potentially contributing to thromboembolic and coagulopathic complications [52]. Finally, the minimal changes observed through ektacytometry, despite proteomic evidence, pose a conundrum. It is plausible that, within our cohort, the protein modifications induced by viral interaction were not substantial enough to significantly alter red blood cell deformability.

In conclusion, this study highlights the complexity of RBC dynamics in the context of viral infections and enhances the understanding of anemia as a significant factor in the severity of outcomes in SARS-CoV-2-infected patients. Unfortunately, although these compelling findings are encouraging, the study's limitations, including a modest cohort size and geographical restrictions, suggest caution in generalizing the results, and we advocate for a deeper exploration of erythrocyte dynamics in viral infections.

Author Contributions: J.-L.V.-C. and E.K. conceived the original idea and performed the rheological studies. C.d.l.T. and J.-J.B. performed the numerical proteomic analysis. A.D. performed the calculation and interpretation of proteomic data and, with J.-L.V.-C., wrote the manuscript with strong input from J.-T.N.; I.H. and V.L. collected the samples from the hospital clinical departments. All authors have read and agreed to the published version of the manuscript.

Funding: This research was partially funded by a research grant number CEI PI-21-30 from Agios Pharmaceuticals, Inc.

Institutional Review Board Statement: This Project has been approved by the Hospital Human Ethics Committee (Ref: CEI PI-21-30).

Informed Consent Statement: Written informed consent has been obtained from the patient(s) to publish this paper.

Data Availability Statement: Data are contained within the article.

Acknowledgments: We are indebted to the support provided by the members of the clinical departments of the Hospital Germans Trias I Pujol (Campus ICO-HGTP) Cristina Tural Làcher from Internal Medicine Department, Roger Paredes Deirós, Lurdes Mateu Pruños and Bonaventura Clotet Capa from the Infectious Diseases Unit, Antoni Rosell Gratacos and Jorge Abad Capa from the Department of Pneumology.and Cristian Morales Indiano from the Clinical Laboratory of the Campus ICO-HGTP, Badalona (Barcelona), CATALONIA (Spain).

Conflicts of Interest: The authors declare no conflicts of interest, and the Company funder had no role in the design of the study; in the collection, analyses, or interpretation of data; in the writing of the manuscript; or in the decision to publish the results.

References

1. Thomas, T.; Stefanoni, D.; Dzieciatkowska, M.; Issaian, A.; Nemkov, T.; Hill, R.C.; Francis, R.O.; Hudson, K.E.; Buehler, P.W.; Zimring, J.C.; et al. Evidence of Structural Protein Damage and Membrane Lipid Remodeling in Red Blood Cells from COVID-19 Patients. *J. Proteome Res.* **2020**, *19*, 4455–4469. [CrossRef] [PubMed]
2. Rinalducci, S.; Ferru, E.; Blasi, B.; Turrini, F.; Zolla, L. Oxidative stress and caspase-mediated fragmentation of cytoplasmic domain of erythrocyte band 3 during blood storage. *Blood Transfus.* **2012**, *10* (Suppl. S2), S55–S62.
3. Issaian, A.; Hay, A.; Dzieciatkowska, M.; Roberti, D.; Perrotta, S.; Darula, Z.; Redzic, J.; Busch, M.P.; Page, G.P.; Rogers, S.C.; et al. The interactome of the N-terminus of band 3 regulates red blood cell metabolism and storage quality. *Haematologica* **2021**, *106*, 2971–2985. [CrossRef] [PubMed]
4. Recktenwald, S.M.; Simionato, G.; Lopes, M.G.M.; Gamboni, F.; Dzieciatkowska, M.; Meybohm, P.; Zacharowski, K.; von Knethen, A.; Wagner, C.; Kaestner, L.; et al. Cross-talk between red blood cells and plasma influences blood flow and omics phenotypes in severe COVID-19. *eLife* **2022**, *11*, e81316. [CrossRef]

5. Marchi, G.; Bozzini, C.; Bertolone, L.; Dima, F.; Busti, F.; Castagna, A.; Stranieri, C.; Fratta Pasini, A.M.; Friso, S.; Lippi, G.; et al. Red Blood Cell Morphologic Abnormalities in Patients Hospitalized for COVID-19. *Front. Physiol.* **2022**, *13*, 932013. [CrossRef]

6. Ramachandran, P.; Gajendran, M.; Perisetti, A.; Elkholy, K.O.; Chakraborti, A.; Lippi, G.; Goyal, H. Red Blood Cell Distribution Width in Hospitalized COVID-19 Patients. *Front. Med.* **2021**, *8*, 582403. [CrossRef] [PubMed]

7. Pouladzadeh, M.; Safdarian, M.; Choghakabodi, P.M.; Amini, F.; Sokooti, A. Validation of red cell distribution width as a COVID-19 severity screening tool. *Future Sci. OA* **2021**, *7*, FSO712. [CrossRef] [PubMed]

8. D'Alessandro, A.; Thomas, T.; Akpan, I.J.; Reisz, J.A.; Cendali, F.I.; Gamboni, F.; Nemkov, T.; Thangaraju, K.; Katneni, U.; Tanaka, K.; et al. Biological and Clinical Factors Contributing to the Metabolic Heterogeneity of Hospitalized Patients with and without COVID-19. *Cells* **2021**, *10*, 2293. [CrossRef]

9. Bergamaschi, G.; Borrelli de Andreis, F.; Aronico, N.; Lenti, M.V.; Barteselli, C.; Merli, S.; Pellegrino, I.; Coppola, L.; Cremonte, E.M.; Croce, G.; et al. Anemia in patients with COVID-19: Pathogenesis and clinical significance. *Clin. Exp. Med.* **2021**, *21*, 239–246. [CrossRef]

10. Lippi, G.; Mattiuzzi, C. Hemoglobin value may be decreased in patients with severe coronavirus disease 2019. *Hematol. Transfus. Cell Ther.* **2020**, *42*, 116–117. [CrossRef]

11. McCullough, J. RBCs as targets of infection. *Am. Soc. Hematol. Educ. Program* **2014**, *2014*, 404–409. [CrossRef]

12. Thomas, T.; Stefanoni, D.; Reisz, J.A.; Nemkov, T.; Bertolone, L.; Francis, R.O.; Hudson, K.E.; Zimring, J.C.; Hansen, K.C.; Hod, E.A.; et al. COVID-19 infection alters kynurenine and fatty acid metabolism, correlating with IL-6 levels and renal status. *JCI Insight* **2020**, *5*, e140327. [CrossRef]

13. Domizio, J.; Di Gulen, M.F.; Saidoune, F.; Thacker, V.V.; Yatim, A.; Sharma, K.; Nass, T.; Guenova, E.; Schaller, M.; Conrad, C.; et al. The cGAS–STING pathway drives type I IFN immunopathology in COVID-19. *Nature* **2022**, *603*, 145–151. [CrossRef] [PubMed]

14. Galbraith, M.D.; Kinning, K.T.; Sullivan, K.D.; Araya, P.; Smith, K.P.; Granrath, R.E.; Shaw, J.R.; Baxter, R.; Jordan, K.R.; Russell, S.; et al. Specialized interferon action in COVID-19. *Proc. Natl. Acad. Sci. USA* **2022**, *119*, e2116730119. [CrossRef]

15. Decout, A.; Katz, J.D.; Venkatraman, S.; Ablasser, A. The cGAS–STING pathway as a therapeutic target in inflammatory diseases. *Nat. Rev. Immunol.* **2021**, *21*, 548–569. [CrossRef]

16. Wei, W.-Y.; Li, H.-C.; Chen, C.-Y.; Yang, C.-H.; Lee, S.-K.; Wang, C.-W.; Ma, H.C.; Juang, Y.L.; Lo, S.Y. SARS-CoV nucleocapsid protein interacts with cellular pyruvate kinase protein and inhibits its activity. *Arch. Virol.* **2012**, *157*, 635–645. [CrossRef] [PubMed]

17. European Centre for Disease Prevention and Control. ECDC Assessment of the COVID-19 Situation in Europe as of 2 March 2020. Available online: https://www.ecdc.europa.eu/en/news-events/ecdc-assessment-covid-19-situationeurope-2-march-2020 (accessed on 28 January 2024).

18. *WHO-China Joint Mission on Coronavirus Disease 2019 (COVID-19)*; WHO: Geneva, Switzerland, 2020.

19. Vives-Corrons, J.L.; Aguilar Bascompte, J.L. *Manual of Hematology Laboratory Diagnostic Techniques*, 4th ed.; Elssevier-Masson: Paris, France, 2014. (In Spanish)

20. Weissman, S.M. Red Cell Metabolism. A Manual of Biochemical Methods. 2nd Edition. *Yale J. Biol. Med.* **1976**, *49*, 310–311.

21. Vives-Corrons, J.-L.; Krishnevskaya, E.; Rodriguez, I.H.; Ancochea, A. Characterization of hereditary red blood cell membranopathies using combined targeted next-generation sequencing and osmotic gradient ektacytometry. *Int. J. Hematol.* **2021**, *113*, 163–174. [CrossRef]

22. Pesciotta, E.N.; Lam, H.S.; Kossenkov, A.; Ge, J.; Showe, L.C.; Mason, P.J.; Bessler, M.; Speicher, D.W. In-Depth, Label-Free Analysis of the Erythrocyte Cytoplasmic Proteome in Diamond Blackfan Anemia Identifies a Unique Inflammatory Signature. *PLoS ONE* **2015**, *10*, e0140036. [CrossRef]

23. Hayden, S.J.; Albert, T.J.; Watkins, T.R.; Swenson, E.R. Anemia in critical illness: Insights into etiology, consequences, and management. *Am. J. Respir. Crit. Care Med.* **2012**, *185*, 1049–1057. [CrossRef]

24. Oh, S.M.; Skendelas, J.P.; Macdonald, E.; Bergamini, M.; Goel, S.; Choi, J.; Segal, K.R.; Vivek, K.; Nair, S.; Leff, J. On-admission anemia predicts mortality in COVID-19 patients: A single center, retrospective cohort study. *Am. J. Emerg. Med.* **2021**, *48*, 140–147. [CrossRef] [PubMed]

25. Mourad, S.; Rajab, M.; Alameddine, A.; Fares, M.; Ziade, F.; Merhi, B.A. Hemoglobin level as a risk factor for lower respiratory tract infections in Lebanese children. *N. Am. J. Med. Sci.* **2010**, *2*, 461–466. [CrossRef] [PubMed]

26. Taneri, P.E.; Gómez-Ochoa, S.A.; Llanaj, E.; Raguindin, P.F.; Rojas, L.Z.; Roa-Díaz, Z.M.; Salvador, D.; Groothof, D.; Minder, B.; Kopp-Heim, D.; et al. Anemia and iron metabolism in COVID-19: A systematic review and meta-analysis. *Eur. J. Epidemiol.* **2020**, *35*, 763–773. [CrossRef]

27. Fan, B.E.; Chong, V.C.L.; Chan, S.S.W.; Lim, G.H.; Lim, K.G.E.; Tan, G.B.; Mucheli, S.S.; Kuperan, P.; Ong, K.H. Hematologic parameters in patients with COVID-19 infection. *Am. J. Hematol.* **2020**, *95*, E131–E134. [PubMed]

28. Bellmann-Weiler, R.; Lanser, L.; Barket, R.; Rangger, L.; Schapfl, A.; Schaber, M.; Fritsche, G.; Wöll, E.; Weiss, G. Prevalence and Predictive Value of Anemia and Dysregulated Iron Homeostasis in Patients with COVID-19 Infection. *J. Clin. Med.* **2020**, *9*, 2429. [CrossRef] [PubMed]

29. Liu, X.; Zhang, R.; He, G. Hematological findings in coronavirus disease 2019: Indications of progression of disease. *Ann. Hematol.* **2020**, *99*, 1421–1428. [CrossRef]

30. Cavezzi, A.; Troiani, E.; Corrao, S. COVID-19: Hemoglobin, iron, and hypoxia beyond inflammation. A narrative review. *Clin. Pract.* **2020**, *10*, 1271. [CrossRef]

31. D'Alessandro, A.; Thomas, T.; Dzieciatkowska, M.; Hill, R.C.; Francis, R.O.; Hudson, K.E.; Zimring, J.C.; Hod, E.A.; Spitalnik, S.L.; Hansen, K.C. Serum Proteomics in COVID-19 Patients: Altered Coagulation and Complement Status as a Function of IL-6 Level. *J. Proteome Res.* **2020**, *19*, 4417–4427. [CrossRef]

32. Elahi, S. Hematopoietic responses to SARS-CoV-2 infection. *Cell. Mol. Life Sci.* **2022**, *79*, 187. [CrossRef]

33. Wang, X.; Wen, Y.; Xie, X.; Liu, Y.; Tan, X.; Cai, Q.; Zhang, Y.; Cheng, L.; Xu, G.; Zhang, S.; et al. Dysregulated hematopoiesis in bone marrow marks severe COVID-19. *Cell Discov.* **2021**, *7*, 60. [CrossRef]

34. Kucia, M.; Ratajczak, J.; Bujko, K.; Adamiak, M.; Ciechanowicz, A.; Chumak, V.; Brzezniakiewicz-Janus, K.; Ratajczak, M.Z. An evidence that SARS-CoV-2/COVID-19 spike protein (SP) damages hematopoietic stem/progenitor cells in the mechanism of pyroptosis in Nlrp3 inflammasome-dependent manner. *Leukemia* **2021**, *35*, 3026–3029. [CrossRef]

35. Camaschella, C.; Nai, A.; Silvestri, L. Iron metabolism and iron disorders revisited in the hepcidin era. *Haematologica* **2020**, *105*, 260–272. [CrossRef]

36. Drakesmith, H.; Prentice, A. Viral infection and iron metabolism. *Nat. Rev. Microbiol.* **2008**, *6*, 541–552. [CrossRef] [PubMed]

37. Bouchla, A.; Kriebardis, A.G.; Georgatzakou, H.T.; Fortis, S.P.; Thomopoulos, T.P.; Lekkakou, L.; Markakis, K.; Gkotzias, D.; Panagiotou, A.; Papageorgiou, E.G.; et al. Red Blood Cell Abnormalities as the Mirror of SARS-CoV-2 Disease Severity: A Pilot Study. *Front. Physiol.* **2021**, *12*, 825055. [CrossRef]

38. Bissinger, R.; Nemkov, T.; D'Alessandro, A.; Grau, M.; Dietz, T.; Bohnert, B.N.; Essigke, D.; Wörn, M.; Schaefer, L.; Xiao, M.; et al. Proteinuric chronic kidney disease is associated with altered red blood cell lifespan, deformability and metabolism. *Kidney Int.* **2021**, *100*, 1227–1239. [CrossRef] [PubMed]

39. Xu, P.; Chen, C.; Zhang, Y.; Dzieciatkowska, M.; Brown, B.C.; Zhang, W.; Xie, T.; Abdulmalik, O.; Song, A.; Tong, C.; et al. Erythrocyte transglutaminase-2 combats hypoxia and chronic kidney disease by promoting oxygen delivery and carnitine homeostasis. *Cell Metab.* **2022**, *34*, 299–316.e6. [CrossRef] [PubMed]

40. Aminianfar, M.; Soleiman-Meigooni, S.; Hamidi-Farahani, R.; Darvishi, M.; Hoseini-Shokouh, S.J.; Asgari, A.; Faraji-Hormozi, S.; Asli, M. Efficacy of Red Blood Cell Exchange as Adjunctive Treatment for Hypoxemia and Survival Rate of Patients with Severe Coronavirus-2 Disease: An Open-Labeled Phase 2 Randomized Clinical Trial. *Front. Med.* **2022**, *9*, 899593. [CrossRef]

41. Park, K.C.; Donovan, K.; McKechnie, S.; Ramamurthy, N.; Klenerman, P.; Swietach, P. Single-cell oxygen saturation imaging shows that gas exchange by red blood cells is not impaired in COVID-19 patients. *Br. J. Haematol.* **2020**, *190*, e229–e232. [CrossRef]

42. Zuin, M.; Rigatelli, G.; Quadretti, L.; Fogato, L.; Zuliani, G.; Roncon, L. Prognostic Role of Anemia in COVID-19 Patients: A Meta-Analysis. *Infect. Dis. Rep.* **2021**, *13*, 930–937. [CrossRef]

43. Liu, W.; Li, H. COVID-19:Attacks the 1-Beta Chain of Hemoglobin and Captures the Porphyrin to Inhibit Human Heme Metabolism. *ChemRxiv* **2020**. [CrossRef]

44. Lechuga, G.C.; Souza-Silva, F.; Sacramento, C.Q.; Trugilho, M.R.O.; Valente, R.H.; Napoleão-Pêgo, P.; Dias, S.S.; Fintelman-Rodrigues, N.; Temerozo, J.R.; Carels, N.; et al. SARS-CoV-2 Proteins Bind to Hemoglobin and Its Metabolites. *Int. J. Mol. Sci.* **2021**, *22*, 9035. [CrossRef] [PubMed]

45. Vives-Corrons, J.-L. The Rare Anaemias. In *Rare Diseases*; Zhan, H.W., Ed.; IntechOpen: Rijeka, Croatia, 2020.

46. Roy, M.K.; Cendali, F.; Ooyama, G.; Gamboni, F.; Morton, H.; D'Alessandro, A. Red Blood Cell Metabolism in Pyruvate Kinase Deficient Patients. *Front. Physiol.* **2021**, *12*, 735543. [CrossRef] [PubMed]

47. Allen, C.N.S.; Santerre, M.; Arjona, S.P.; Ghaleb, L.J.; Herzi, M.; Llewellyn, M.D.; Shcherbik, N.; Sawaya, B.E. SARS-CoV-2 Causes Lung Inflammation through Metabolic Reprogramming and RAGE. *Viruses* **2022**, *14*, 983. [CrossRef]

48. Chang, H.-Y.; Fu, C.-Y. Adenylate Kinase. In *Encyclopedia of Food Microbiology*, 2nd ed.; Batt, C.A., Tortorello, M.L., Eds.; Academic Press: Cambridge, MA, USA, 2014; pp. 18–23. ISBN 9780123847331.

49. McElvaney, O.J.; McEvoy, N.L.; McElvaney, O.F.; Carroll, T.P.; Murphy, M.P.; Dunlea, D.M.; Ní Choileáin, O.; Clarke, J.; O'Connor, E.; Hogan, G.; et al. Characterization of the Inflammatory Response to Severe COVID-19 Illness. *Am. J. Respir. Crit. Care Med.* **2020**, *202*, 812–821. [CrossRef] [PubMed]

50. Ionescu, M.I. Adenylate Kinase: A Ubiquitous Enzyme Correlated with Medical Conditions. *Protein J.* **2019**, *38*, 120–133. [CrossRef]

51. Foy, B.H.; Carlson, J.C.T.; Reinertsen, E.; Padros, I.; Valls, R.; Pallares Lopez, R.; Palanques-Tost, E.; Mow, C.; Westover, M.B.; Aguirre, A.D.; et al. Association of Red Blood Cell Distribution Width with Mortality Risk in Hospitalized Adults with SARS-CoV-2 Infection. *JAMA Netw. Open* **2020**, *3*, e2022058. [CrossRef]

52. Nappi, F.; Iervolino, A.; Avtaar Singh, S.S. Thromboembolic Complications of SARS-CoV-2 and Metabolic Derangements: Suggestions from Clinical Practice Evidence to Causative Agents. *Metabolites* **2021**, *11*, 341. [CrossRef]

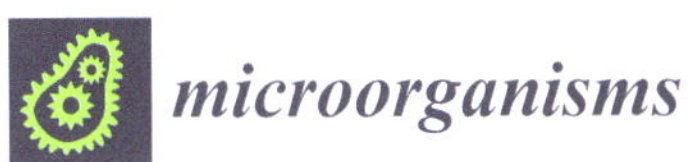
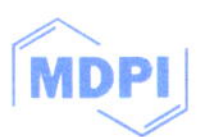

microorganisms

Article

P53-Independent G1-Cell Cycle Arrest Increases SARS-CoV-2 RNA Replication

Clara Husser [1], Hyesoo Kwon [2], Klara Andersson [3], Sofia Appelberg [4], Nuria Montserrat [5,6,7], Ali Mirazimi [1,2,4] and Vanessa M. Monteil [1,*]

[1] Department of Laboratory Medicine, Unit of Clinical Microbiology, Karolinska Institutet, 171 77 Stockholm, Sweden; clara.husser@hotmail.fr (C.H.); ali.mirazimi@ki.se (A.M.)
[2] National Veterinary Institute, 751 89 Uppsala, Sweden; hyesoo.kwon@sva.se
[3] Biomedrex Genetics, 141 52 Huddinge, Sweden; klara.andersson@biomedrex.com
[4] Department of Microbiology, Public Health Agency of Sweden, 171 65 Solna, Sweden; sofia.appelberg@folkhalsomyndigheten.se
[5] University of Barcelona, 08028 Barcelona, Spain 08028 Barcelona, Spain; nmontserrat@ibecbarcelona.eu
[6] Pluripotency for Organ Regeneration, Institute for Bioengineering of Catalonia (IBEC), The Barcelona Institute of Science and Technology (BIST), University of Barcelona, 08028 Barcelona, Spain
[7] Centro de Investigación Biomédica en Red en Bioingeniería, Biomateriales y Nanomedicina, Institució Catalana de Recerca i Estudis Avançats (ICREA), 08010 Barcelona, Spain
* Correspondence: vanessa.monteil@ki.se

Abstract: While having already killed more than 7 million of people worldwide in 4 years, SARS-CoV-2, the etiological agent of COVID-19, is still circulating and evolving. Understanding the pathogenesis of the virus is of capital importance. It was shown that in vitro and in vivo infection with SARS-CoV-2 can lead to cell cycle arrest but the effect of the cell cycle arrest on the virus infection and the associated mechanisms are still unclear. By stopping cells in the G1 phase as well as targeting several pathways involved using inhibitors and small interfering RNAs, we were able to determine that the cell cycle arrest in the late G1 is beneficial for SARS-CoV-2 replication. This cell cycle arrest is independent of p53 but is dependent on the CDC25A-CDK2/cyclin E pathway. These data give a new understanding in SARS-CoV-2 pathogenesis and highlight some possible targets for the development of novel therapeutic approaches.

Keywords: COVID-19; coronavirus; pathogenicity; replication; CDK2; cyclin E; CDC25A; treatments

Citation: Husser, C.; Kwon, H.; Andersson, K.; Appelberg, S.; Montserrat, N.; Mirazimi, A.; Monteil, V.M. P53-Independent G1-Cell Cycle Arrest Increases SARS-CoV-2 RNA Replication. *Microorganisms* **2024**, *12*, 443. https://doi.org/10.3390/ microorganisms12030443

Academic Editor: Qibin Geng

Received: 1 February 2024
Revised: 15 February 2024
Accepted: 17 February 2024
Published: 22 February 2024

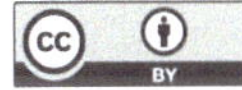

1. Introduction

Severe acute respiratory syndrome coronavirus 2 (SARS-CoV-2) is the etiological agent of Coronavirus disease 2019 (COVID-19). Patients develop flu-like symptoms that can evolve from mild to severe with lung damage but also injury to the kidneys, gastrointestinal tract, and cardiovascular system. More than 4 years after the beginning of the SARS-CoV-2-associated pandemic, the virus is still circulating at high levels worldwide and this high circulation rate favors the emergence of new variants. Despite the development of vaccines and some treatments, the virus is still causing mortality, highlighting the importance of better understanding its pathogenesis in order to develop novel antivirals.

The eukaryotic cell cycle is a meticulously coordinated and regulated series of events. It is divided into four stages: G1, during which cells prepare for DNA replication; S, during which DNA synthesis takes place; G2, during which cells prepare for division; and M, during which cells undergo mitosis. The transition between the different phases is carefully controlled by so-called cell cycle checkpoints [1]. A major cell cycle regulatory juncture is the G1 to S checkpoint, which ensures that the cell is ready to commit for cell division [2]. Hence, it is during the G1 phase that the cell integrates various signals to assess if the internal and external conditions are right for S-phase entry [3]. If those conditions are not met, the cell can exit the cell cycle into a stage called quiescence (G0).

The major driving force underlying cell cycle progression is the periodic synthesis and degradation of cyclins and their association with cyclin-dependent kinases (CDK) [1,4]. Each cyclin/CDK complex relates to a particular phase and transition of the cell cycle. To be activated, CDKs must be appropriately phosphorylated and must be in complex with the appropriate cyclin. When active, cyclin/CDK complexes phosphorylate key proteins of the cell cycle, including the retinoblastoma protein (pRb) [5]. Hypophosphorylated pRb exerts an inhibitory effect on the cell cycle by binding and regulating the transcription factor E2F [5]. In G1, active cyclin D/CDK4,6 and cyclin E/CDK2 complexes phosphorylate pRb. The resulting hyperphosphorylated form of pRb releases E2F and allows the expression of S-phase genes and the progression of the cell cycle [2,4,5]. Cyclin/CDK complexes are regulated by the cyclin-dependent kinase inhibitors (CDKi). CDKis can be divided into two families, the INK4 family (p15, p16, p18, p19), and the CIP/Kip family (p21, p27, p57) [2,6].

Viruses rely on host cell factors to replicate their genomes and generate new progeny viruses. Because of this dependence, viruses have evolved a myriad of mechanisms for exploiting host cell functions. Many viruses subvert the host cell cycle in order to increase their replication [7–9]. For example, severe acute respiratory syndrome coronavirus (SARS-CoV) and the mouse hepatitis virus (MHV) are known to induce a cell cycle arrest in infected host cells [10–13]. Given that SARS-CoV and SARS-CoV-2 are from the same species, it is reasonable to hypothesize that SARS-CoV-2 can also initiate cell cycle arrest. In vitro experiments using transfection of plasmid coding for SARS-CoV-2 viral proteins showed SARS-CoV-2 proteins N can induce a G0/G1 [14] or S-phase [15]. Infection experiments showed SARS-CoV-2 can causes cell cycle arrest in S [15,16] and G2/M stages [16]. All these studies suggest that SARS-CoV-2 could take advantage of the modulation of the cell cycle [15,17].

Understanding how different cell cycle phases are beneficial for SARS-CoV-2 pathogenesis could highlight some possible targets for the development of novel therapeutic approaches [18].

In this study, we show that the cell cycle arrest in late G1 is beneficial for SARS-CoV-2 replication. This cell cycle arrest is independent of p53 but is dependent on the cell division cycle 25 A (CDC25A)-CDK2/cyclin E pathway.

2. Materials and Methods

2.1. Cells and Virus

SARS-CoV-2 (GenBank accession number MT093571) was isolated and propagated on Vero-E6 cells (ATCC CRL-1586) as previously described [19]. A549 (ATCC CCL-185) were cultured on DMEM containing 10% FBS. Serum starvation to induce quiescence or synchronization of cells was performed by culturing cells in 0% FBS medium for 24 h.

Kidney organoids were prepared as previously described [19] and cultured in RPMI (ThermoFisher Scientific, Waltham, MA, USA).

Briefly, human embryonic stem cells (The National Bank of Stem Cells (ISCIII, Madrid, Spain)) were grown on vitronectin-coated plates (1001-015, Life Technologies, Carlsbad, CA, USA) and incubated with 0.5 mM EDTA (Merck, Darmstadt, Germany) at 37 °C for 3 min for disaggregation. In total, 100,000 cells/well were plated on a 24-well plate coated with 5 µL/mL vitronectin and further incubated with supplemented Essential 8 Basal medium at 37 °C overnight. The day after, named as day 0, the cells were treated for 3 days in Advanced RPMI 1640 basal medium (ThermoFisher Scientific) supplemented with 8 µM CHIR (Merck) and 1% penicillin-streptomycin and 1% of GlutaMAX (ThermoFisher Scientific). The medium was changed every day. From day 3 to 4, media were changed to Advanced RPMI supplemented with 200 ng/mL FGF9 (Peprotech, Cranbury, NJ, USA), 1 µg/mL heparin (Merck), and 10 ng/mL activin A (R&D System, Minneapolis, MN, USA). On day 4, the cultures were rinsed twice with PBS, and resuspended in Advanced RPMI supplemented with 5 µM CHIR, 200 ng/mL FGF9, and 1 µg/mL heparin. Cellular suspensions were seeded in a V-shape 96 multi-well plate at a final concentration of 100,000 cells/well and centrifuged at 2000 rpm for 3 min. The resulting spheroids were incubated during 1 h at 37 °C. Culture media was replaced by Advanced RPMI supplemented with 200 ng/mL FGF9 and 1 µg/mL heparin for 7 additional days. The media was changed every second day. From day 11 to 16, developing organoids were incubated only in the presence of Advanced RPMI, the media was changed every second day.

Lung organoids were kindly gifted by Prof. Haibo Zhang. The maturation media for lung organoids contained 75% IMDM, 25% Ham's F-12, 0.5% N2 supplement, 1% B27 supplement, 0.75% of BSA 7.5%, 1% PenStrep, 1% Glutamax and 3 µM CHIR99021, 10 ng/mL FGF10, 10 ng/mL FGF7, 50 nM Dexamethasone, 0.1 mM 8-Bromo-cAMP, 0.1 mM IBMX, 50 µg/mL ascorbic acid, and 0.4 µM monothioglycerol.

2.2. Treatment with EIPA

A549 cells were seeded at a density of 5×10^4 cells per well in a 48-well plate (Viability and infection assays) or at a density of 2×10^5 cells per well in a 6-well plate (Flow cytometry and Western blot assays). At 24 h post seeding, cells were treated with EIPA or mock-treated (DMSO 0.4%) at the indicated concentration for 24 h. Cells were then analyzed for cell cycle distribution by flow cytometry, for viability using a LIVE/DEAD cell imaging kit (#R37601, ThermoFisher Scientific), for Western blot or for infection as described below.

2.3. Viability/Cytotoxicity Assay

Mock and EIPA-treated cells were washed twice with PBS and 100 µL of fresh PBS was added per well. Reagents were thawed and mixed. In total, 100 µL of the reagent solution was added on top of the cells. The plate was incubated for 15 min at room temperature. Images of the cells were captured using confocal laser scanning microscope (Zeiss LSM 800) at 488/515 nm for live cells (green) and 570/602 nm for dead cells (red).

2.4. Western-Blot

Cells were washed once with PBS before being detached using 500 µL of trypsin. Cells were incubated for 5 min at 37 °C, allowing the cells to detach. A total of 500 µL of DMEM 10%FBS was added to stop the action of trypsin and the cells were transferred to 1.5 mL tube. Cells were pelleted by centrifugation at $400 \times g$ for 5 min. The supernatants were discarded and total proteins were extracted by lysing the cells with an in-house lysis buffer (pH 7.5) containing 10 mM Tris–HCl, 150 mM NaCl, 0.5% SDS, and 1% Triton X-100 supplemented with complete Protease Inhibitor Cocktail Tablets (Roche, Indianapolis, IN, USA) and NuPAGE LDS Sample Buffer (ThermoFisher Scientific) and β-Mercaptoethanol (Invitrogen, Waltham, MA, USA). The samples were boiled for 20 min at 98 °C. Total protein concentration was measured using Thermo Scientific Ionic Detergent Compatibility Reagent for Pierce 660 nm Protein Assay Reagent and Thermo Scientific Pierce Bovine Serum Albumin Standard Pre-Diluted Set as standard. For Western blot analyses, 20 µg of protein was separated in Criterion™ XT 4–12% Bis-Tris gels with XT MOPS running buffer and blotted onto PVDF membrane Trans-Blot Turbo Midi 0.2 µm (BioRad, Hercules, CA, USA). The membranes were blocked at room temperature for 1 h with 5% milk in PBST (PBS 0.01M + 0.1% Tween20). The membranes were then incubated with primary antibodies diluted in 5% milk/PBST for 1 h under rocking at room temperature. The membranes were then washed with PBST three times and then incubated with the secondary antibody diluted in 5% milk/PBST. After washing three times with PBST and once with PBS 1X, membrane-bound antibodies were detected by chemiluminescence using Amersham ECL Prime Western Blotting Detection Reagent (Cytiva, Marlborough, MA, USA).

Antibodies used: p-pRb (1/1000, #702097, ThermoFisher Scientific), p53 (1/1000, #MA5-12557, ThermoFisher Scientific), β-actin (1/2000, #MA5-15452, ThermoFisher Scientific), ACE2 (1/5000, #SAB3500346, Sigma), CDC25A (1/1000, PA5-77902, SAB3500346), Calnexin (1/10000, in-house), and cyclin E (1/1000, #11554-1-AP, ThermoFisher Scientific). Horseradish Peroxidase (HRP)-conjugate secondary antibody (AffiniPure Goat anti-rabbit (1/5000; #111-035-003) and/or AffiniPure goat anti-mouse (1/10,000; #115-035-174) (Jackson ImmunoResearch, West Grove, PA, USA) and Streptactine HRP-conjugate (#1610380, Bio-Rad) for ladder staining.

2.5. Flow Cytometry

The treated cells were detached using trypsin (ThermoFisher Scientific) (500 μL per well of a 6-well plate) for 5 min at 37 °C. A total of 500 μL of DMEM 10% FBS was added to each well and the cells were transferred to 15 mL tubes. The cells were centrifuged at $400 \times g$ for 5 min to pellet them The supernatant was carefully removed by pipetting. The cells were fixed in suspension by carefully adding chilled ethanol 70% and were vortexed before being incubated for 30 min at 4 °C. The cells were centrifuged at $400 \times g$ for 5 min. Ethanol was carefully discarded by pipetting. The cells were washed twice with PBS, being centrifuged at $400 \times g$ for 5 min after each washing and PBS carefully discarded. The cells were treated 50 mL of RNase A (100 μg/mL) and stained with 200 μL of propidium iodide (50 μg/mL, ThermoFisher Scientific) for 30 min at 4 °C in the dark. The cells were then analyzed on BD FACS CantoII (BD) and data were analyzed using ModFit LT 6.0 (Verity Software, Noida, Uttar Pradesh, India).

2.6. Treatments

A549 cells were seeded at a density of 5×10^4 cells per well in a 48-well plate in DMEM 5% FBS. At 24 h post-seeding, the supernatants were removed. The cells were washed once with PBS and the cells were treated with the respective concentration of compound:

Palbociclib 1 μM, Abemaciclib 1 μM, Gefitinib 25 μM, Cediranib 3 μM, Resveratrol 100 μM, Hesperidin 100 μM, AUZ-454 1 μM, 10 μM, and 20 μM in DMEM 5% FBS. All compounds were purchased from MedChem Express. After 24 h, supernatants were discarded. The cells were washed once with PBS and the cells were infected with SARS-CoV-2 as described below. EIPA treatment was used as a positive control and DMSO 0.4% as a negative (mock-treatment).

2.7. siRNA Transfection

In total, 5 pmol of negative control siRNA (Qiagen, Venlo, The Netherlands) or 5 pmol of human cyclin E1 siRNA (Horizon Discovery, Waterbeach, UK) were mixed in Opti-MEM (ThermoFisher Scientific) with lipofectamine RNAiMax (ThermoFisher Scientific) according to the company instructions. Briefly, 50 μL of the mix siRNA/lipofectamine were put in wells of a 48-well plate and 5×10^4 A549 cells were added on top (200 μL in DMEM 5%FBS). Cells were incubated at 37 °C for 48 h before being infected. The protocol was similar for the cells used for Western blot, using 25 pmol of siRNA in 250 μL of opti-MEM/lipofectamine RNAiMAX and adding 2×10^5 cells on top in 2 mL of DMEM 5% FBS and incubated for 48 h.

2.8. Infection

Cells were washed once with PBS. PBS was removed and all samples were infected for 1 h with SARS-CoV-2 (100 μL/well) at an MOI of 0.1 in 2% FBS medium containing the different compounds. At 1 hpi, the cells were then washed once with PBS and fresh medium 5%FBS containing the compounds. At 24 hpi, supernatant was removed. The cells were washed 3 times with PBS and all cells were lyzed using 100 μL per well of trizol (ThermoFisher Scientific).

Kidney organoids were infected with 10^3 PFU/organoids for 3 days or 10^6 PFU for 1 day in RPMI medium containing 50 μM of EIPA. Lung organoids were infected with 10^6 PFU for 3 days in maturation media containing EIPA under shaking.

2.9. RNA Extraction and RT-PCR Analysis

RNA was isolated from infected cells using Trizol (Invitrogen). Total RNA extraction from cells was performed using the Direct-zol RNA Miniprep kit (Zymo Research, Irvine, CA, USA). Equal amounts of Trizol and ethanol 100% were added to each sample and mixed.

The samples were then transferred on extraction columns and centrifuged at $12,000 \times g$ for 30 s. The flow-through were discarded in chemical waste for Trizol. A total of 400 µL of pre-wash buffer was added on top of each column and columns were centrifuged at $12,000 \times g$ for 30 s. The flow-through were discarded in chemical waste for alcohol and this step was repeated once. In total, 700 µL of washing buffer was added to each column and columns were centrifuged at $12,000 \times g$ for 2 min. Columns were transferred to 1.5 mL tubes and RNA was extracted by the addition of 30 µL of DNAse/RNase-free water on top of each column. The columns were centrifuged at $12,000 \times g$ for 30 s. The columns were discarded and the eluted RNA was stored at $-80\ ^{\circ}$C until qRT-PCR.

qRT-PCR mix was performed in 20 µL final volume in LightCycler Capillaries (Roche, Indianapolis, IN, USA) containing for SARS-CoV-2, 0.8 µL of forward primer (10 µM), 0.8 µL of reverse primer (10 µM), 0.4 µL of probe (10 µM), 5 µL of TaqMan Fast Virus 1-step master Mix (ThermoFisher Scientific), 5 µL of RNA and 8 µL of DNase/RNase-free water. For RNase P, 1 µL of forward primer (10 µM), 1µL of reverse primer (10 µM), 0.4 µL of probe (10 µM), 5 µL of TaqMan Fast Virus 1-step Master Mix (ThermoFisher Scientific), 5 µL of RNA, and 7.6 µL of DNase/RNase-free water.

qRT-PCR amplification was performed in a Roche LightCycler 4.0 Instrument under the following conditions: reverse transcription, 10 min at 50 $^{\circ}$C; denaturation, 2 min at 95 $^{\circ}$C; amplification 45 cycles of 10 s at 95 $^{\circ}$C for the denaturation and 40 s at 60 $^{\circ}$C for the annealing/extension step.

SARS-CoV-2 infection levels were calculated using E-gene SARS-CoV-2 primers/probe.

Forward primer: 5′-ACAGGTACGTTAATAGTTAATAGCGT-3′
Reverse primer: 5′-ATATTGCAGCAGTACGCACACA-3′
Probe: FAM-ACACTAGCCATCCTTACTGCGCTTCG-MGB

RNase P was used as an endogenous gene control to normalize the levels of intracellular viral RNA.

Forward primer: 5′-AGATTTGGACCTGCGAGCG-3′
Reverse primer: 5′-GAGCGGCTGTCTCCACAAGT-3′
Probe: FAM-TTCTGACCTGAAGGCTCTGCGCG-MGB

2.10. Statistical Analysis

All statistical analysis were performed using GraphPad Prism 10.

3. Results

3.1. Cell Cycle Arrest in G0/G1 P53-Independent Improves SARS-CoV-2 Infection

5-(N-Ethyl-N-isopropyl)amiloride (EIPA), an inhibitor of macropinocytosis, was used to treat A549 cells, an adenocarcinoma-derived human alveolar basal epithelial cell line. A549 cells were treated with 50 µM of EIPA or DMEM 0.4% (mock) in DMEM 5% for 24 h. These cells were then infected with SARS-CoV-2 (MOI 0.1) in medium containing EIPA. Surprisingly, 24 h post-infection (hpi), EIPA-treated cells showed a significant increase in SARS-CoV-2 infection compared to the mock-treated cells (Figure 1A). To determine if this effect was specific to SARS-CoV-2, the cells were treated and infected with another RNA virus, Hazara virus (HAZV), under the same conditions. As shown in Figure 1B, EIPA treatment was instead deleterious for HAZV infection. These data show that treatment with EIPA made A549 cells more susceptible to SARS-CoV-2 infection and this effect was specific to SARS-CoV-2.

Interestingly, EIPA treatment (50 µM, 24 h) of A549 cells visibly reduced the number of cells (Figure 2A, upper panel). According to the lack of dead cells in the EIPA-treated wells (Figure 2A lower panel), EIPA treatment was not cytotoxic. These data indicate that the reduced cell number seemed to be linked to a stop in cell growth. EIPA was previously shown to induce a cell cycle arrest in G0/G1 in MKN28 cells [20], as well as in A549 [21]. Cell cycle distribution in mock and EIPA-treated cells was assessed by flow cytometry. As shown in Figure 2B, EIPA treatment led to an increase in the cell number in G0/G1 and G2 stage compared to the S stage, with most of the cells being stopped in the G0/G1 phase. Western blot analysis of mock and EIPA-treated cells showed a dose-dependent low phosphorylation of the retinoblastoma protein (pRb), a marker of the G0/G1 stage, under treatment with EIPA, confirming that most of the cells were stopped in the G0/G1 stage (Figure 2C). Interestingly, when looking at the level of p53, a protein involved in the regulation of the cell proliferation, p53 did not show any variation under EIPA treatment, highlighting that the observed cell cycle arrest is p53-independent (Figure 2C).

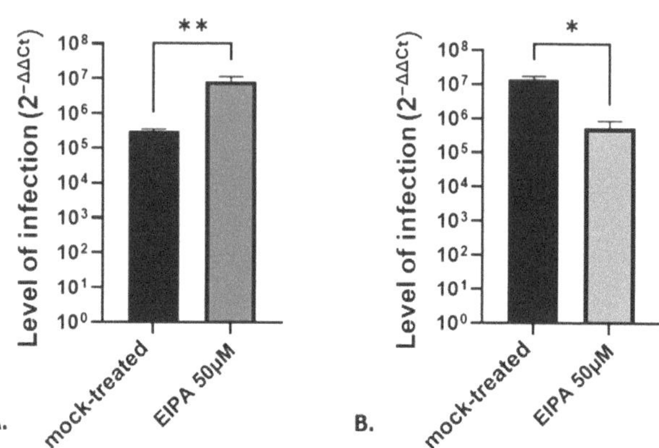

Figure 1. SARS-CoV-2 (**A**) and HAZV (**B**) infection level ($2^{-\Delta\Delta Ct}$) in mock-treated or EIPA-treated A549 cells. Student t-test * $p < 0.05$, ** $p < 0.01$.

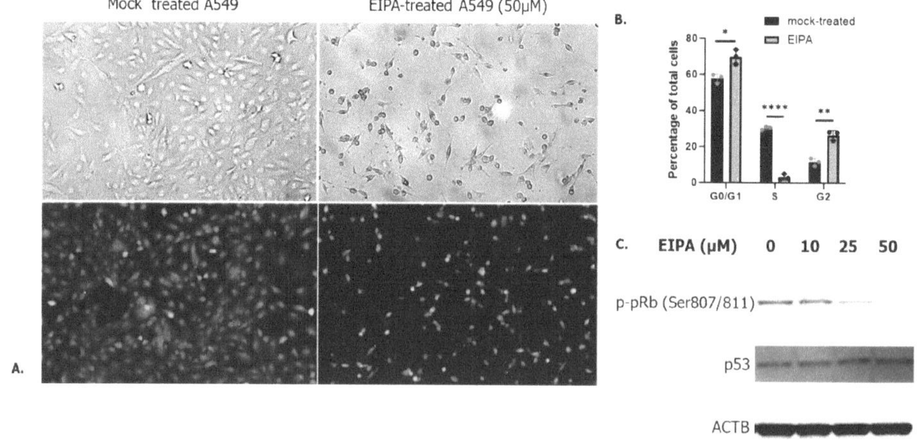

Figure 2. (**A**) Upper: Microscopy analysis of the mock-treated and EIPA-treated cells. Lower: A549 cells were stained for live (green) and dead (red) cells. Magnification $10\times$. (**B**) Cell cycle distribution of cells mock or EIPA-treated. Student t-test * $p < 0.05$, ** $p < 0.01$, **** $p < 0.0001$. (**C**) Staining of phosphorylated pRb and p53 by Western blot. Phosphorylation of pRb led to cell cycle progression from G1 to S. Lack of pRb phosphorylation is a marker of cell cycle arrest.

To confirm that the observed cell cycle arrest in G0/G1 is responsible for the increased SARS-CoV-2 infection, A549 cells were FBS starved for 24 h before being infected with SARS-CoV-2. Starvation, leading to a cell cycle arrest in G0/G1, led to an increase in SARS-CoV-2 infection (Figure 3), as previously observed in EIPA treated cells (Figure 1A).

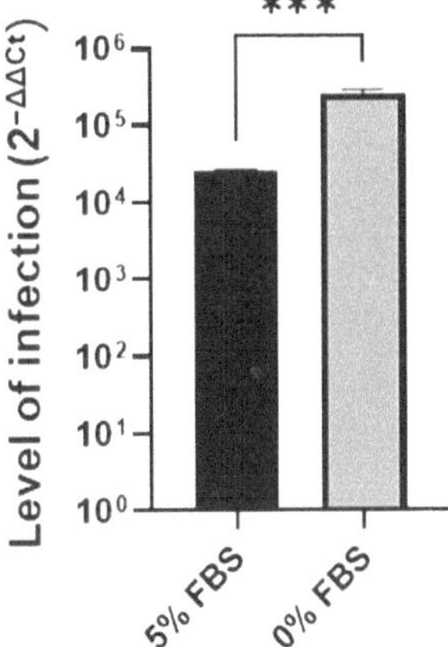

Figure 3. SARS-CoV-2 infection level in normal FBS (5%) or starved (0%) A549 cells. Student *t*-test *** $p < 0.001$.

3.2. SARS-CoV-2 Entry Step Is Not Affected by the Cell Cycle Arrest

The observed increase in SARS-CoV-2 infection in A549 cells treated with EIPA could be due to a higher infection at the attachment/entry step or higher RNA replication rate. To distinguish between these alternatives, EIPA and mock-treated cells were infected with SARS-CoV-2 (MOI 0.1) for 1h and the cells were recovered 1hpi. As shown in Figure 4A, EIPA treatment did not affect SARS-CoV-2 attachment/entry step. To complete these data, A549 cells starved/non starved and treated with several concentration of EIPA were tested for ACE2 expression, ACE2 being the main SARS-CoV-2 receptor [22–24] by Western blot. Figure 4B shows that A549 does not express ACE2 or at an undetectable level and this level of expression is not improved when the cells are treated with EIPA, confirming the absence of role for the entry step in the observed increased in SARS-CoV-2 infection.

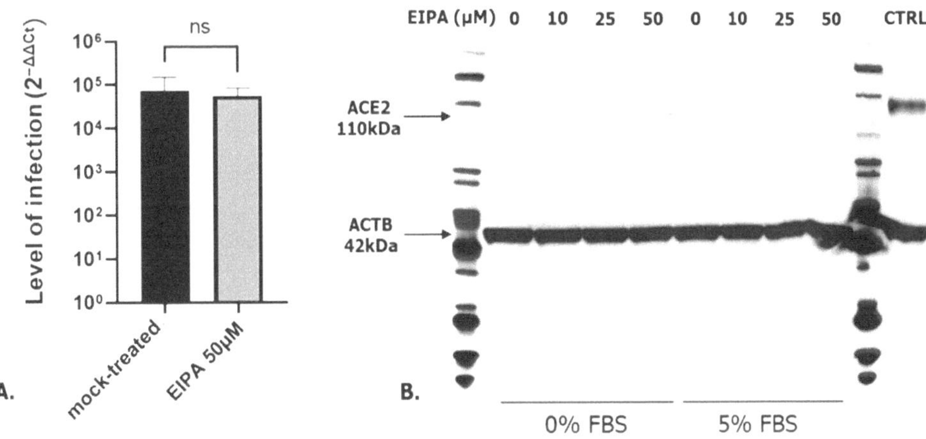

Figure 4. (**A**) Level of infection in mock or EIPA-treated A549 cells 1 hpi. Student *t*-test ns: non-significant. (**B**) Western blot analysis of ACE2 expression (CTRL: control, Vero E6 cell lysate).

3.3. Late G1 p53-Independent Cell Cycle Arrest Leads to an Increase in SARS-CoV-2 RNA Replication

Having found that G0/G1 cell cycle arrest was responsible for the increasing in SARS-CoV-2 RNA replication, we next focused on the cellular pathways involved in the G0/G1 stage (Figure 5A) in order to understand which pathways are important for SARS-CoV-2 replication. To do this, we used several compounds that are known to block the cell cycle in G0/G1 in A549 cells (Palbociclib [25], Abemaciclib [26,27], Gefitinib [28], Cediranib [29], Resveratrol [30], and Hesperidin [31]). These compounds target different pathways described in Figure 5B. Inhibitors of growth factor receptors (EGFR and VEGFR) tyrosine kinase (Gefitinib and Cediranib) led to an increase in SARS-CoV-2 infection (Figure 5C). Interestingly, Resveratrol, which blocks the cell cycle in a p53-independent manner, also positively affected SARS-CoV-2 infection while Hesperidin, blocking the cell cycle in a p53-dependent manner, did not affect SARS-CoV-2 infection (Figure 5C). These data are consistent with the non-variation in p53 expression in the EIPA-treated cells that was previously observed (Figure 2C), which was already suggestive of a p53-independent role of G0/G1 in SARS-CoV-2 infection. Interestingly, while Palbociclib, an inhibitor of CDK4/6, had no effect on SARS-CoV-2 infection, Abemaciclib, which is also an inhibitor of CDK4/6 but also of CDK2/cyclin E, increased SARS-CoV-2 infection (Figure 5C). These data show that the increased SARS-CoV-2 infection was not caused by blockade of the CDK4/6 pathway, i.e. early G1 stage, but was dependent on the blockade at the late G1 stage via the CDK2/cyclin E pathway.

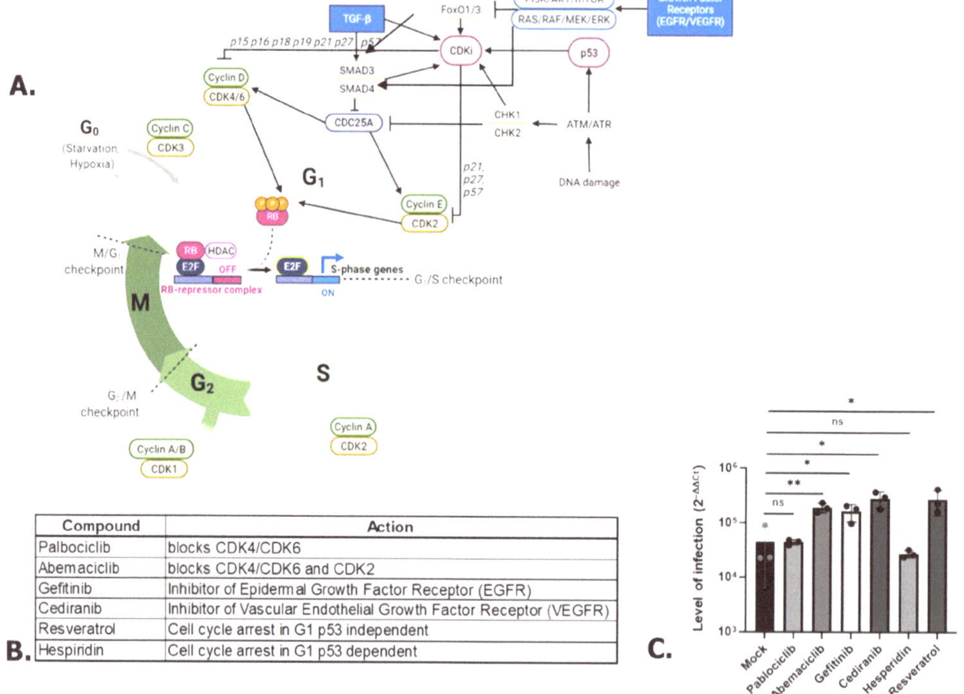

Compound	Action
Palbociclib	blocks CDK4/CDK6
Abemaciclib	blocks CDK4/CDK6 and CDK2
Gefitinib	Inhibitor of Epidermal Growth Factor Receptor (EGFR)
Cediranib	Inhibitor of Vascular Endothelial Growth Factor Receptor (VEGFR)
Resveratrol	Cell cycle arrest in G1 p53 independent
Hespiridin	Cell cycle arrest in G1 p53 dependent

Figure 5. (**A**) Scheme of some proteins involved in cell cycle regulation. Created with BioRender.com. (**B**) Compounds used in the study associated with their targets. (**C**) Effect of A549 treatments on SARS-CoV-2 replication. One-way ANOVA. * $p < 0.05$, ** $p < 0.01$, ns: non-significant.

3.4. Cell Cycle Arrest at the CDK2/Cyclin E Checkpoint via CDC25A Degradation Is Responsible for Higher Levels of SARS-CoV-2 Infection

Next, we wished to confirm the involvement of CDK2 in the enhancement of SARS-CoV-2 infection. Since the knock-down or knock-out of CDK2 does not affect cell proliferation [32], we instead treated cells with an inhibitor of CDK2 (AUZ 454) for 24 h before being infected with SARS-CoV-2. Treatment with the CDK2 inhibitor led to an increase in

SARS-CoV-2 infection, (Figure 6A). Since CDK2 and cyclin E are in complex and modulate the G1/S checkpoint, we also assessed the role of cyclin E in SARS-CoV-2 infection. Cyclin E was knocked down using siRNA (Figure 6B). The knock-down of cyclin E led to a significant increase in SARS-CoV-2 infection (Figure 6B). These data confirm the beneficial role of the inhibition of CDK2/cyclin E for SARS-CoV-2 replication.

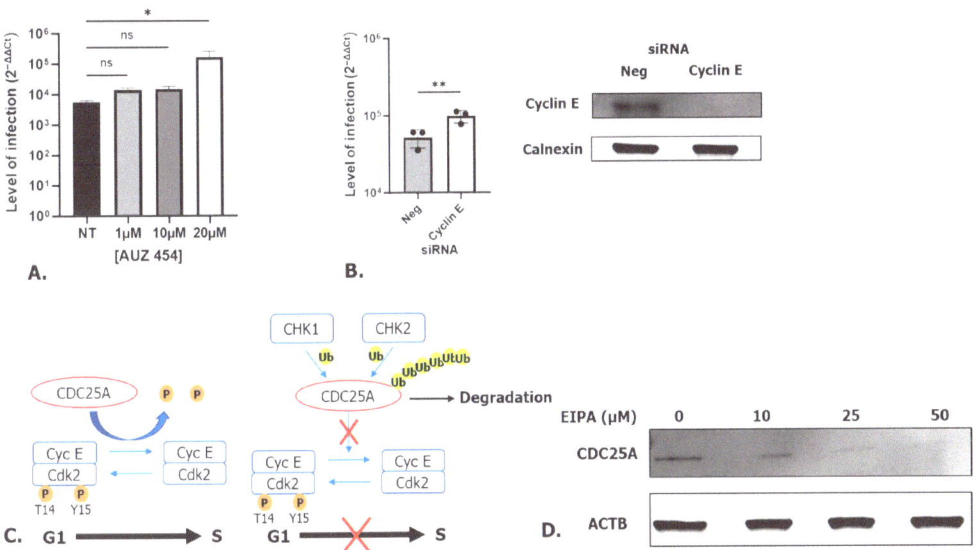

Figure 6. (**A**) Treatment of A549 cells with a specific inhibitor of CDK2. One-way ANOVA * $p < 0.05$ (**B**) A549 cells knocked down for cyclin E. One way ANOVA ** $p < 0.01$, ns: non-significant and Western blot analysis of cyclin E in siRNA-treated A549. (**C**) Scheme representing the role of CDC25A on cell cycle progression/arrest. (**D**) Western blot analysis of CDC25A in EIPA-treated A549 cells.

In order for the cells to pass from the G1 to the S phase, CDK2 has to be dephosphorylated by the cell division cycle 25A (CDC25A) phosphatase (Figure 6C). Under genotoxic insults, CDC25A is ubiquitinated by Checkpoint kinase 1 and 2 (CHK1 and CHK2) and is degraded by the proteasome. As a result, CDK2 is not dephosphorylated and cells stop in the G1 phase (Figure 6C). To determine if CDC25A is involved in the blocking of cells in the G1 stage while treated with EIPA, A549 cells were treated with different concentrations of EIPA for 24 h and the expression level of CDC25A was defined by Western blot. As shown in Figure 6D, CDC25A was degraded in a dose-dependent manner, confirming the role of the degradation of CDC25A in the blocking of the cell cycle in G1.

3.5. SARS-CoV-2 Infection Is Also Increased in Treated Human Kidney and Lung Organoids

Since A549 cells are a cancer-derived cell line, the validation of the findings in a more relevant model is essential. To achieve this, kidney as well as lung organoids were produced as previously described [19,33]. Kidney and lung organoids were treated with EIPA for 24 h before being infected with SARS-CoV-2 for 1 or 3 days. Consistent with our results in A549 cells, EIPA treatment led to a significant increase in SARS-CoV-2 infection in kidney (Figure 7A,B) and in lung (Figure 7C) organoids, suggesting EIPA treatment leads to a similar effect in organoids and in cancer cells.

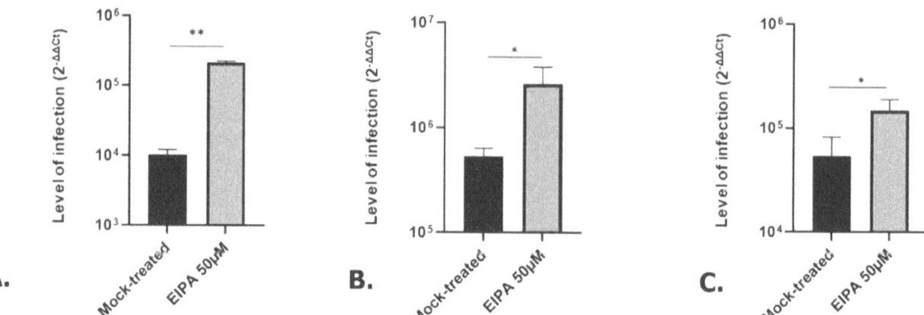

Figure 7. Level of infection in EIPA-treated kidney organoids ((A) 10^3 PFU/organoids, 3 dpi) and ((B) 10^6 PFU/organoids, 1 dpi) and lung organoids ((C) 10^6 PFU/organoids, 3 dpi). Student *t*-test. * $p < 0.05$, ** $p < 0.01$.

4. Discussion

On 31st of December 2023, SARS-CoV-2 was officially responsible for more than 770 million COVID-19 cases and 7 million deaths (WHO dashboard, https://data.who.int/dashboard/covid19/, accessed on 31 January 2024). The virus is still circulating and evolving, making the understanding of its pathogenesis essential.

Several studies have previously highlighted the role of p53 in SARS-CoV-2 infection [34,35], pointing out p53 as a potential target for the development of antivirals [36,37]. In contrast, our data show that the increase in SARS-CoV-2 replication observed when the cells are stopped in G1 is p53-independent, making the use of p53 targeting antivirals ineffective in this case. These data highlight the importance of finding several pathways used by SARS-CoV-2 in order to develop and use the appropriate antivirals to each situation.

Our data show that serum-starved cells and cells stopped in late G1 via CDK2/cyclin E inhibition leads to an increase in SARS-CoV-2 replication. It is possible to debate whether our experiments induce a G0 or G1 cell cycle arrest as it is commonly described that serum-starved cells are quiescent and stopped in an "out of cell cycle" stage named G0. However, G0 cells have the same amount of DNA as cells arrested in G1 and this cell cycle stage is commonly called G0/G1 as they cannot be distinguished. Some suggest that the G0 stage is not a bona fide cell cycle stage but instead a G1 stage where the cells are growing so slowly that they appear to be arrested. The aim of this study is not to debate the G0/G1 cell cycle definition, but a review discussing these terms is available [38].

We showed that blocking growth factor receptor (EGFR and VGFR) tyrosine kinases is beneficial for SARS-CoV-2 infection. Interestingly, a study using several inhibitors targeting several pathways downstream of growth factor receptor, PI3K, and MAPK pathways, showed an inhibition of SARS-CoV-2 replication [39]. None of the targets were in the cell cycle pathway we highlighted today (EGFR-(most probably Ras-Raf-MEK-ERK)-CDC25A-CDK2/cyclin E). This fact exemplifies the critical importance of studying in depth the mechanisms involved in SARS-CoV-2 (and any virus) pathogenesis to properly target the right pathway depending on the context of the infection.

Several studies have previously shown the ability of SARS-CoV-2 to drive cell cycle arrest in different phases [15,16]. We found that degradation of CDC25A, which inhibits CDK2 via the lack of its dephosphorylation, and treatment with a CDK2 inhibitor, both lead to an increase in SARS-CoV-2 replication. It was previously shown that the SARS-CoV-2 N protein is able to induce a Smad3-dependent cell cycle arrest in G1, via its interaction with Smad3, leading to acute kidney injury (AKI) [14]. Smad3 (Mothers against decapentaplegic homolog 3) protein, a transcription factor/tumor suppressor in the transforming growth factor–beta (TGF-β) signaling, triggers the cell death pathway in acute kidney injury [40] and induces a G1 cell cycle arrest in cells [41]. Smad3-/- mice exhibit metastatic colon cancer [42] and the loss of Smad3 expression increases susceptibility to tumorigenicity in human gastric cancer [43]. Importantly, Smad3 mediates degradation of CDC25A via the ubiquitination of CDC25A [44], blocking the cells in G1. All these data are consistent with our results and highlight the important role of the CDC25A/CDK2/cyclin E pathway-dependent G1 cell cycle arrest in SARS-CoV-2 infection. Further investigations will be conducted to understand how this CDC25A/CDK2/cyclin E pathway affects SARS-CoV-2 replication.

5. Conclusions

Studies have suggested that SARS-CoV-2 is able to stop the cell cycle of infected cells [14,16], but the effect of cell cycle arrest on SARS-CoV-2 infection is unknown. Our study showed that the late G1 cell cycle arrest dependent of the CDC25A/CDK2/cyclin E pathway and independent of P53, which is able to improve SARS-CoV-2 RNA replication.

Author Contributions: Conceptualization, V.M.M., C.H. and N.M.; data curation, C.H., H.K., K.A., S.A. and N.M.; formal analysis, V.M.M., C.H., H.K., K.A. and S.A.; funding acquisition, V.M.M., N.M. and A.M.; investigation, V.M.M. and C.H.; methodology, V.M.M. and C.H.; software, S.A.; validation, V.M.M. and A.M.; writing—original draft, V.M.M. and C.H.; writing—review and editing, V.M.M. and A.M. All authors have read and agreed to the published version of the manuscript.

Funding: This research was funded by Karolinska Institutet (FS-2022:0010). This work has received funding from the European Union's Horizon 2020 and Horizon Europe Research and Innovation Programme (European Research Council (ERC) ERC CoG-2020_101002478_ENGINORG to N.M. This project has received funding from the Innovative Medicines Initiative 2 Joint Undertaking (JU) under grant agreement no. 101005026. The JU receives support from the European Union's Horizon 2020 research and innovation program and EFPIA (A.M., and N.M.) and Fundació la Marató de TV3 201910-31 to N.M., and 202125-30 to N.M., and A.M. This study has been funded by Instituto de Salud Carlos III (ISCIII) through the Biobanks and Biomodels Platform and co-funded by the European Union (PTC20/00013, and 10 PTC20/00130 to N.M).

Data Availability Statement: All data are available upon request.

Acknowledgments: The authors would like to acknowledge Haibo Zhang (University of Toronto) for kindly gifted lung organoids.

Conflicts of Interest: The authors declare no conflicts of interest.

References

1. Barnum, K.J.; O'Connell, M.J. Cell cycle regulation by checkpoints. *Methods Mol. Biol.* **2014**, *1170*, 29–40. [CrossRef]
2. Donjerkovic, D.; Scott, D.W. Regulation of the G1 phase of the mammalian cell cycle. *Cell Res.* **2000**, *10*, 1–16. [CrossRef]
3. Hume, S.; Dianov, G.L.; Ramadan, K. A unified model for the G1/S cell cycle transition. *Nucleic Acids Res.* **2020**, *48*, 12483–12501. [CrossRef]
4. Bertoli, C.; Skotheim, J.M.; de Bruin, R.A. Control of cell cycle transcription during G1 and S phases. *Nat. Rev. Mol. Cell Biol.* **2013**, *14*, 518–528. [CrossRef]
5. Giacinti, C.; Giordano, A. RB and cell cycle progression. *Oncogene* **2006**, *25*, 5220–5227. [CrossRef]
6. Johnson, D.G.; Walker, C.L. Cyclins and cell cycle checkpoints. *Annu. Rev. Pharmacol. Toxicol.* **1999**, *39*, 295–312. [CrossRef]
7. Panda, M.; Kalita, E.; Rao, A.; Prajapati, V.K. Mechanism of cell cycle regulation and cell proliferation during human viral infection. *Adv. Protein Chem. Struct. Biol.* **2023**, *135*, 497–525. [CrossRef]
8. Bagga, S.; Bouchard, M.J. Cell cycle regulation during viral infection. *Methods Mol. Biol.* **2014**, *1170*, 165–227. [CrossRef]
9. Nascimento, R.; Costa, H.; Parkhouse, R.M. Virus manipulation of cell cycle. *Protoplasma* **2012**, *249*, 519–528. [CrossRef]
10. Chen, C.J.; Makino, S. Murine coronavirus replication induces cell cycle arrest in G0/G1 phase. *J. Virol.* **2004**, *78*, 5658–5669. [CrossRef]
11. Chen, C.J.; Sugiyama, K.; Kubo, H.; Huang, C.; Makino, S. Murine coronavirus nonstructural protein p28 arrests cell cycle in G0/G1 phase. *J. Virol.* **2004**, *78*, 10410–10419. [CrossRef]
12. Yuan, X.; Shan, Y.; Zhao, Z.; Chen, J.; Cong, Y. G0/G1 arrest and apoptosis induced by SARS-CoV 3b protein in transfected cells. *Virol. J.* **2005**, *2*, 66. [CrossRef]
13. Yuan, X.; Wu, J.; Shan, Y.; Yao, Z.; Dong, B.; Chen, B.; Zhao, Z.; Wang, S.; Chen, J.; Cong, Y. SARS coronavirus 7a protein blocks cell cycle progression at G0/G1 phase via the cyclin D3/pRb pathway. *Virology* **2006**, *346*, 74–85. [CrossRef]
14. Wang, W.; Chen, J.; Hu, D.; Pan, P.; Liang, L.; Wu, W.; Tang, Y.; Huang, X.R.; Yu, X.; Wu, J.; et al. SARS-CoV-2 N Protein Induces Acute Kidney Injury via Smad3-Dependent G1 Cell Cycle Arrest Mechanism. *Adv. Sci.* **2022**, *9*, e2103248. [CrossRef]

15. Quan, L.; Sun, X.; Xu, L.; Chen, R.A.; Liu, D.X. Coronavirus RNA-dependent RNA polymerase interacts with the p50 regulatory subunit of host DNA polymerase delta and plays a synergistic role with RNA helicase in the induction of DNA damage response and cell cycle arrest in the S phase. *Emerg. Microbes Infect.* **2023**, *12*, e2176008. [CrossRef]

16. Sui, L.; Li, L.; Zhao, Y.; Zhao, Y.; Hao, P.; Guo, X.; Wang, W.; Wang, G.; Li, C.; Liu, Q. Host cell cycle checkpoint as antiviral target for SARS-CoV-2 revealed by integrative transcriptome and proteome analyses. *Signal Transduct. Target. Ther.* **2023**, *8*, 21. [CrossRef]

17. Grand, R.J. SARS-CoV-2 and the DNA damage response. *J. Gen. Virol.* **2023**, *104*, 001918. [CrossRef]

18. Rizzo, R.; Caccuri, F.; Valacchi, G.; Zauli, G. Editorial: Cell cycle control as a new therapeutic approach for SARS-CoV-2 infection. *Front. Pharmacol.* **2023**, *14*, 1136277. [CrossRef]

19. Monteil, V.; Kwon, H.; Prado, P.; Hagelkrüys, A.; Wimmer, R.A.; Stahl, M.; Leopoldi, A.; Garreta, E.; Hurtado Del Pozo, C.; Prosper, F.; et al. Inhibition of SARS-CoV-2 Infections in Engineered Human Tissues Using Clinical-Grade Soluble Human ACE2. *Cell* **2020**, *181*, 905–913.e907. [CrossRef]

20. Hosogi, S.; Miyazaki, H.; Nakajima, K.; Ashihara, E.; Niisato, N.; Kusuzaki, K.; Marunaka, Y. An inhibitor of Na^+/H^+ exchanger (NHE), ethyl-isopropyl amiloride (EIPA), diminishes proliferation of MKN28 human gastric cancer cells by decreasing the cytosolic Cl^- concentration via DIDS-sensitive pathways. *Cell Physiol. Biochem.* **2012**, *30*, 1241–1253. [CrossRef]

21. Wang, B.Y.; Shen, H.T.; Lee, Y.L.; Chien, P.J.; Chang, W.W. Inhibition of Na+/H+ exchanger (NHE) 7 by 5-(N-ethyl-N-isopropyl)-Amiloride displays anti-cancer activity in non-small cell lung cancer by disrupting cancer stem cell activity and downregulating PD-L1 expression. *Am. J. Cancer Res.* **2023**, *13*, 4721–4733.

22. Shang, J.; Ye, G.; Shi, K.; Wan, Y.; Luo, C.; Aihara, H.; Geng, Q.; Auerbach, A.; Li, F. Structural basis of receptor recognition by SARS-CoV-2. *Nature* **2020**, *581*, 221–224. [CrossRef]

23. Lan, J.; Ge, J.; Yu, J.; Shan, S.; Zhou, H.; Fan, S.; Zhang, Q.; Shi, X.; Wang, Q.; Zhang, L.; et al. Structure of the SARS-CoV-2 spike receptor-binding domain bound to the ACE2 receptor. *Nature* **2020**, *581*, 215–220. [CrossRef]

24. Wang, Q.; Zhang, Y.; Wu, L.; Niu, S.; Song, C.; Zhang, Z.; Lu, G.; Qiao, C.; Hu, Y.; Yuen, K.Y.; et al. Structural and Functional Basis of SARS-CoV-2 Entry by Using Human ACE2. *Cell* **2020**, *181*, 894–904.e899. [CrossRef] [PubMed]

25. Liu, M.; Cui, L.; Li, X.; Xia, C.; Li, Y.; Wang, R.; Ren, F.; Liu, H.; Chen, J. PD-0332991 combined with cisplatin inhibits nonsmall cell lung cancer and reversal of cisplatin resistance. *Thorac. Cancer* **2021**, *12*, 924–931. [CrossRef]

26. Gelbert, L.M.; Cai, S.; Lin, X.; Sanchez-Martinez, C.; Del Prado, M.; Lallena, M.J.; Torres, R.; Ajamie, R.T.; Wishart, G.N.; Flack, R.S.; et al. Preclinical characterization of the CDK4/6 inhibitor LY2835219: In-vivo cell cycle-dependent/independent anti-tumor activities alone/in combination with gemcitabine. *Investig. New Drugs* **2014**, *32*, 825–837. [CrossRef]

27. Hino, H.; Iriyama, N.; Kokuba, H.; Kazama, H.; Moriya, S.; Takano, N.; Hiramoto, M.; Aizawa, S.; Miyazawa, K. Abemaciclib induces atypical cell death in cancer cells characterized by formation of cytoplasmic vacuoles derived from lysosomes. *Cancer Sci.* **2020**, *111*, 2132–2145. [CrossRef]

28. Hotta, K.; Tabata, M.; Kiura, K.; Kozuki, T.; Hisamoto, A.; Katayama, H.; Takigawa, N.; Fujimoto, N.; Fujiwara, K.; Ueoka, H.; et al. Gefitinib induces premature senescence in non-small cell lung cancer cells with or without EGFR gene mutation. *Oncol. Rep.* **2007**, *17*, 313–317. [CrossRef]

29. Guo, M.; Liu, Z.; Si, J.; Zhang, J.; Zhao, J.; Guo, Z.; Xie, Y.; Zhang, H.; Gan, L. Cediranib Induces Apoptosis, G1 Phase Cell Cycle Arrest, and Autophagy in Non-Small-Cell Lung Cancer Cell A549 In Vitro. *Biomed. Res. Int.* **2021**, *2021*, 5582648. [CrossRef]

30. Yuan, L.; Zhang, Y.; Xia, J.; Liu, B.; Zhang, Q.; Liu, J.; Luo, L.; Peng, Z.; Song, Z.; Zhu, R. Resveratrol induces cell cycle arrest via a p53-independent pathway in A549 cells. *Mol. Med. Rep.* **2015**, *11*, 2459–2464. [CrossRef]

31. Xia, R.; Sheng, X.; Xu, X.; Yu, C.; Lu, H. Hesperidin induces apoptosis and G0/G1 arrest in human non-small cell lung cancer A549 cells. *Int. J. Mol. Med.* **2018**, *41*, 464–472. [CrossRef]

32. Tetsu, O.; McCormick, F. Proliferation of cancer cells despite CDK2 inhibition. *Cancer Cell* **2003**, *3*, 233–245. [CrossRef]

33. Garreta, E.; Prado, P.; Stanifer, M.L.; Monteil, V.; Marco, A.; Ullate-Agote, A.; Moya-Rull, D.; Vilas-Zornoza, A.; Tarantino, C.; Romero, J.P.; et al. A diabetic milieu increases ACE2 expression and cellular susceptibility to SARS-CoV-2 infections in human kidney organoids and patient cells. *Cell Metab.* **2022**, *34*, 857–873.e859. [CrossRef]

34. Zhuang, Z.; Zhong, X.; Chen, Q.; Chen, H.; Liu, Z. Bioinformatics and System Biology Approach to Reveal the Interaction Network and the Therapeutic Implications for Non-Small Cell Lung Cancer Patients with COVID-19. *Front. Pharmacol.* **2022**, *13*, 857730. [CrossRef]

35. Lodi, G.; Gentili, V.; Casciano, F.; Romani, A.; Zauli, G.; Secchiero, P.; Zauli, E.; Simioni, C.; Beltrami, S.; Fernandez, M.; et al. Cell cycle block by p53 activation reduces SARS-CoV-2 release in infected alveolar basal epithelial A549-hACE2 cells. *Front. Pharmacol.* **2022**, *13*, 1018761. [CrossRef]

36. Milani, D.; Caruso, L.; Zauli, E.; Al Owaifeer, A.M.; Secchiero, P.; Zauli, G.; Gemmati, D.; Tisato, V. p53/NF-kB Balance in SARS-CoV-2 Infection: From OMICs, Genomics and Pharmacogenomics Insights to Tailored Therapeutic Perspectives (COVIDomics). *Front. Pharmacol.* **2022**, *13*, 871583. [CrossRef]

37. Bortot, B.; Romani, A.; Ricci, G.; Biffi, S. Exploiting Extracellular Vesicles Strategies to Modulate Cell Death and Inflammation in COVID-19. *Front. Pharmacol.* **2022**, *13*, 877422. [CrossRef]

38. Cooper, S. Reappraisal of serum starvation, the restriction point, G0, and G1 phase arrest points. *FASEB J.* **2003**, *17*, 333–340. [CrossRef]

39. Klann, K.; Bojkova, D.; Tascher, G.; Ciesek, S.; Münch, C.; Cinatl, J. Growth Factor Receptor Signaling Inhibition Prevents SARS-CoV-2 Replication. *Mol. Cell* **2020**, *80*, 164–174.e164. [CrossRef]
40. Wu, W.; Wang, X.; Yu, X.; Lan, H.Y. Smad3 Signatures in Renal Inflammation and Fibrosis. *Int. J. Biol. Sci.* **2022**, *18*, 2795–2806. [CrossRef]
41. Matsuura, I.; Denissova, N.G.; Wang, G.; He, D.; Long, J.; Liu, F. Cyclin-dependent kinases regulate the antiproliferative function of Smads. *Nature* **2004**, *430*, 226–231. [CrossRef]
42. Zhu, Y.; Richardson, J.A.; Parada, L.F.; Graff, J.M. Smad3 mutant mice develop metastatic colorectal cancer. *Cell* **1998**, *94*, 703–714. [CrossRef]
43. Han, S.U.; Kim, H.T.; Seong, D.H.; Kim, Y.S.; Park, Y.S.; Bang, Y.J.; Yang, H.K.; Kim, S.J. Loss of the Smad3 expression increases susceptibility to tumorigenicity in human gastric cancer. *Oncogene* **2004**, *23*, 1333–1341. [CrossRef]
44. Ray, D.; Terao, Y.; Nimbalkar, D.; Chu, L.H.; Donzelli, M.; Tsutsui, T.; Zou, X.; Ghosh, A.K.; Varga, J.; Draetta, G.F.; et al. Transforming growth factor beta facilitates beta-TrCP-mediated degradation of Cdc25A in a Smad3-dependent manner. *Mol. Cell Biol.* **2005**, *25*, 3338–3347. [CrossRef]

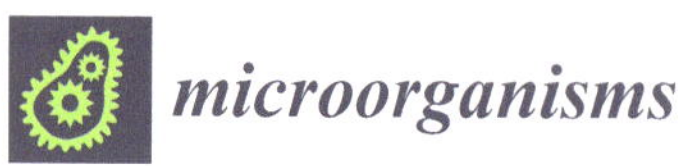 *microorganisms*

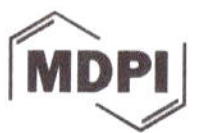

Article

DNA Methylation Levels of the ACE2 Promoter Are Not Associated with Post-COVID-19 Symptoms in Individuals Who Had Been Hospitalized Due to COVID-19

César Fernández-de-las-Peñas [1,2,*], Gema Díaz-Gil [3], Antonio Gil-Crujera [3], Stella M. Gómez-Sánchez [3], Silvia Ambite-Quesada [1], Juan Torres-Macho [4,5], Pablo Ryan-Murua [4], Anabel Franco-Moreno [4], Oscar J. Pellicer-Valero [6], Lars Arendt-Nielsen [2,7,8] and Rocco Giordano [2,9]

[1] Department of Physical Therapy, Occupational Therapy, Rehabilitation and Physical Medicine, Universidad Rey Juan Carlos, 28922 Alcorcón, Spain; silvia.ambite.quesada@urjc.es

[2] Center for Neuroplasticity and Pain (CNAP), Sensory Motor Interaction (SMI), Department of Health Science and Technology, Faculty of Medicine, Aalborg University, DK 9220 Aalborg, Denmark; lan@hst.aau.dk (L.A.-N.); rg@hst.aau.dk (R.G.)

[3] Research Group GAMDES, Department of Basic Health Sciences, Universidad Rey Juan Carlos (URJC), 28922 Alcorcón, Spain; gema.diaz@urjc.es (G.D.-G.); antonio.gil@urjc.es (A.G.-C.); stella.gomez@urjc.es (S.M.G.-S.)

[4] Department of Internal Medicine, Hospital Universitario Infanta Leonor-Virgen de la Torre, 28031 Madrid, Spain; juan.torresm@salud.madrid.org (J.T.-M.); pabloryan@gmail.com (P.R.-M.); anaisabel.franco@salud.madrid.org (A.F.-M.)

[5] Department of Medicine, School of Medicine, Universidad Complutense de Madrid, 28040 Madrid, Spain

[6] Image Processing Laboratory (IPL), Universitat de València, Parc Científic, 46980 Paterna, Spain; oscar.pellicer@uv.es

[7] Department of Gastroenterology & Hepatology, Mech-Sense, Aalborg University Hospital, DK 9100 Aalborg, Denmark

[8] Steno Diabetes Center North Denmark, Clinical Institute, Aalborg University Hospital, DK 9100 Aalborg, Denmark

[9] Department of Oral and Maxillofacial Surgery, Aalborg University Hospital, DK 9100 Aalborg, Denmark

* Correspondence: cesar.fernandez@urjc.es; Tel.: +34-91-488-88-84

Citation: Fernández-de-las-Peñas, C.; Díaz-Gil, G.; Gil-Crujera, A.; Gómez-Sánchez, S.M.; Ambite-Quesada, S.; Torres-Macho, J.; Ryan-Murua, P.; Franco-Moreno, A.; Pellicer-Valero, O.J.; Arendt-Nielsen, L.; et al. DNA Methylation Levels of the ACE2 Promoter Are Not Associated with Post-COVID-19 Symptoms in Individuals Who Had Been Hospitalized Due to COVID-19. *Microorganisms* **2024**, *12*, 1304. https://doi.org/10.3390/microorganisms12071304

Academic Editor: Qibin Geng

Received: 8 June 2024
Revised: 24 June 2024
Accepted: 26 June 2024
Published: 27 June 2024

Abstract: It is known that SARS-CoV-2 can translocate via membrane ACE2 exopeptidase into the host cells, and thus hypomethylation of ACE2 possibly upregulates its expression, enhancing the risk of SARS-CoV-2 infection. This study investigated if DNA methylation levels of the ACE2 promoter are associated with the development of post-COVID-19 symptomatology in a cohort of COVID-19 survivors who had been previously hospitalized. Non-stimulated saliva samples were obtained from 279 (51.5 male, mean age: 56.5 ± 13.0 years old) COVID-19 survivors who were hospitalized during the first wave of the pandemic. A face-to-face interview in which patients described the presence of post-COVID-19 symptoms (defined as a symptom that started no later than three months after SARS-CoV-2 infection) that they suffered from to an experienced healthcare trainer was conducted. Methylation of five CpG dinucleotides in the ACE2 promoter was quantified using bisulfite pyrosequencing. The percentage of methylation (%) was associated with the presence of the following reported post-COVID-19 symptoms: fatigue, dyspnea at rest, dyspnea at exertion, brain fog, memory loss, concentration loss, or gastrointestinal problems. Participants were assessed a mean of 17.8 (SD: 5.3) months after hospitalization. At that time, 88.1% of the patients experienced at least one post-COVID-19 symptom (mean number for each patient: 3.0; SD: 1.9 post-COVID-19 symptoms). Dyspnea at exertion (67.3%), fatigue (62.3%), and memory loss (31.2%) were the most frequent post-COVID-19 symptoms in the sample. Overall, the analysis did not reveal any difference in the methylation of the ACE2 promoter in any of the CpG locations according to the presence or absence of fatigue, dyspnea at rest, dyspnea at exertion, memory loss, brain fog, concentration loss, and gastrointestinal problems. This study did not find an association between methylation of ACE2 promoter and the presence of post-COVID-19 fatigue, dyspnea, cognitive or gastrointestinal problems in previously hospitalized COVID-19 survivors.

Keywords: methylation; ACE2; post-COVID-19; long COVID

1. Introduction

The coronavirus disease 2019 (COVID-19) pandemic, caused by the severe acute respiratory syndrome coronavirus 2 (SARS-CoV-2), challenged all healthcare systems around the world and a deeper understanding of the biological mechanisms behind individual responses to the virus was clearly needed. Building on this, the field of epigenetics might provide insights into how COVID-19 induces lasting changes in gene activity, potentially influencing long-term health outcomes. Epigenetics are those molecular processes regulating gene expression without modifying DNA sequence and phenotype and that are influenced by several factors, e.g., environmental exposures, stress, and nutrition [1]. Several epigenetic processes including methylation, histone protein modification, or the action of non-coding RNA (ncRNA) are described [2]. The effects of epigenetic changes induced by SARS-CoV-2 have been of interest from the beginning of the outbreak [3] but are still under investigation with research looking into possible systemic and cellular changes induced by COVID-19 [4]. DNA methylation is an epigenetic mark involved in gene expression regulation, catalyzed by a family of DNA methyltransferases that transfer a methyl group from S-adenyl methionine onto the DNA cytosine to form 5-methylcytosine [5]. In fact, some studies investigating methylation patterns in COVID-19 patients have revealed hypermethylation patterns in interferon-related genes and hypomethylation patterns in inflammatory-associated genes, supporting the presence of a dynamic epigenetic regulation (up or down) of genes in COVID-19 [6,7].

Several studies focusing on the viral mechanisms of SARS-CoV-2 infection have pointed to the importance of the surface receptor for the viral spike 1 protein (S1) of the angiotensin-converting enzyme 2 (ACE2) and transmembrane protease serine-2 (TMPRSS2) receptor in COVID-19 [8]. It is known that SARS-CoV-2 can translocate via membrane ACE2 exopeptidase into the host cells, and thus hypomethylation of ACE2 possibly upregulates its expression, enhancing the risk of SARS-CoV-2 infection [9]. Similar results were found in a previous study, where acute respiratory issues were associated with hypomethylation in the ACE2 promoter in blood [10]. Further, a study involving 500 COVID-19 patients showed that the involvement of the ACE2 gene depends on multiple individual variables such as sex, age, body mass index, smoking, and the presence of comorbidities, confirming hypomethylation in the ACE2 gene's promoter [11].

A growing healthcare problem associated with COVID-19 is the presence of long-lasting symptoms after the infection. The presence of a long-lasting symptomatology after COVID-19 has been called long COVID [12] or post-COVID-19 condition [13]. More than 100 long-lasting post-COVID-19 symptoms affecting respiratory, cardiovascular, immune, neurological, gastrointestinal, or musculoskeletal systems can be attributed to SARS-CoV-2 infection [14]. The Global Burden of Disease Long COVID study (which included 1.2 million of COVID-19 survivors) found that around 15% of individuals who had surpassed a SARS-CoV-2 infection experience post-COVID-19 symptoms up to one year after [15]. Thus, a recent meta-analysis found that up to 25–30% of patients reported post-COVID-19 symptoms two years after infection [16].

The underlying mechanisms explaining the development of post-COVID-19 symptomatology are still unknown and epigenetics have emerged as one potential crucial factor in elucidating them [17]. The fact that methylation changes identified during the acute COVID-19 phase persist one year after acute infection [18] can open a door for exploring an epigenetic relevance in the development of long-lasting post-COVID-19 symptoms. Thus, Nikesjö et al. described a specific DNA methylation signature in ten COVID-19 survivors suffering from post-COVID-19 symptoms lasting up to 10 months [19]. However, the processes by which epigenetics might fine tune the presence of long-lasting post-COVID-19 symptoms remain a major challenge, particularly in humans.

Therefore, the aim of this study was to investigate if DNA methylation pattern of the ACE2 promoter is associated with the presence of post-COVID-19 symptomatology in a cohort of individual who were hospitalized due to an acute SARS-CoV-2 infection.

2. Methods

2.1. Participants

A cohort of individuals who were hospitalized due to an acute SARS-CoV-2 infection during the first wave of the COVID-19 pandemic (March–May 2020) at four different urban hospitals in Madrid (Spain) were invited to participate in this study. To be included, a diagnosis of SARS-CoV-2 infection at hospital admission should have been confirmed by reverse transcription-polymerase chain reaction (RT-PCR) assay of nasopharyngeal and oral swab sample as well as clinical/radiological findings. The study was approved by the Ethics Committees of all involved institutions and hospitals (URJC0907202015920; HUFA 20/126; HCSC20/495E, HSO25112020; HUIL/092-20). All participants provided their written informed consent prior to the collection of any data.

2.2. Genome DNA Collection

Unstimulated whole saliva samples were collected into collection tubes according to standardized procedures: 1, patients were seated; 2, data collection was always conducted during the morning; and 3, patients were asked not to eat, drink, or chew gum for 1 h before sample collection. Saliva samples were centrifuged at 3000 rpm for 15 min to obtain the cell sediment and a self-collection procedure was carried out immediately afterwards and the samples were stored at $-20\ ^{\circ}$C until the analysis. Saliva was used instead of whole blood because it is non-invasive, stress-free, and ethically suitable assessment method.

Genomic DNA was extracted from 500 mL of saliva using a MagMAX™ DNA Multi-Sample Ultra 2.0 Kit (Thermo Fisher Scientific Inc., Hemel Hempstead, Hertfordshire, UK) according to the manufacturer's protocol. We automatically extracted DNA using the King Fisher Flex purification robot (Thermo Fisher). The resulting DNA was assessed for purity and concentration using Quant-iT™ PicoGreen™ dsDNA reagent" (Thermo Fisher, Waltham, MA, USA).

2.3. Differentially Methylation Profiling

Genomic DNA was bisulfite converted using the Epitech Fast 96 Bisulfite Kit (Cat n° 50959720, Werfen España, Barcelona) following the manufacturer's instructions. As a measure of successful conversion, the overall percentages of non-cytosine-phosphate-guanine (CpG) dinucleotides methylation varied from 0.03 to 0.06% among all loci and samples. Analyses of ACE2 promoter methylation were amplified using tailed oligos, i.e., a unique amplicon-specific part, fused to a $5'$-tail comprising sequences necessary for library preparation and sequencing reactions. A web-based program (http://www.urogene.org/methprimer, accessed on 1 February 2024) was used to identify CpG sites in the ACE2 promoter. Accordingly, five CpG sites of interest (CpG1, CpG2, CpG3, CpG4, CpG5) within the ACE2 promoter were selected according to the general rules and advice for primer design that were previously described [20,21] (Figure 1). The scores (percentage) were calculated by the PyroMark Assay Design, version 2.0.1.15 (Qiagen GmbH).

Analysis was performed using real time PCR with TB Green Premix Ex Taq II master-mix (Takara, France). Following ACE2-specific amplification, amplification products were purified from agarose gels, titrated, and diluted for further processing. NGS libraries were made using a collection of Illumina-compatible PCR primers including a 10 bp barcode identifier (MID) which was used to identify each sample within the pool. The products of this second amplification were evaluated using Bioanalyzer chips (Agilent, Santa Clara, CA, USA), titrated, and pooled, followed by additional bead-based purification and quantification. Finally, samples were subjected to Illumina sequencing in MiSeq (2 × 250 reads) (Illumina, Cambridge, UK).

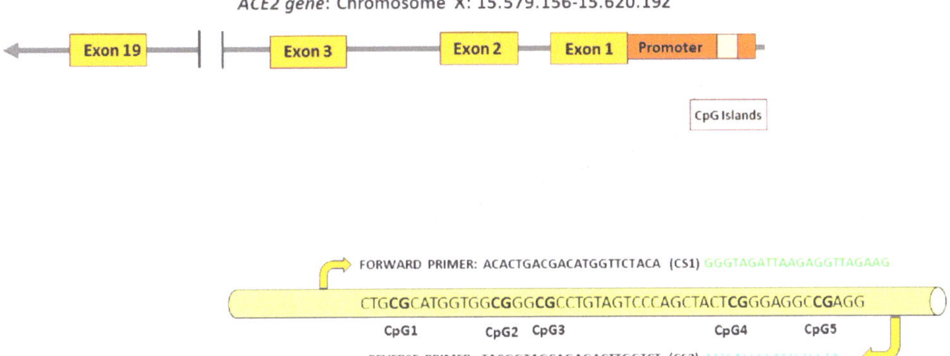

Figure 1. The CpG island sequence in the promoter region of human ACE2. A total of 5 CpG sites were analyzed. CpG sites are in bold. The primers used for DNA methylation sequencing are shown. Forward primer is shown in green color and reverse primer is shown in blue color. Both primers were fused to a 5′-tail comprising sequences (CS1 and CS2) necessary for library preparation and sequencing reactions.

The sequencing run yielded over 840,000 filtered, quality reads, an average of about 1800 reads per amplicon per sample (range 500 to 5000).

Bisulfite conversion, amplification of target sequences and sequencing were carried out at Fundación Parque Científico de Madrid (FPCM), c/Faraday 7, Madrid, Spain). Reads obtained were filtered and sorted according to their MID and the reference sequence. Alignments and calculation of the percentage methylation were subsequently performed using the freely available software Bismark (version 22.3). The percentage of methylation per sample within each CpG was calculated as the percentage C/C+T and used in the correlation analyses, the mean value of all CpG dinucleotides per amplicon was calculated to represent the methylation value of a particular locus. We analyzed the methylation percentage (%) of each position (CpG1, CpG2, CpG3, CpG4, CpG5) separately for the analysis

2.4. Collection Data

Data related to hospitalization due to COVID-19 were collected from hospital medical records: previous medical conditions, admission to intensive care unit (ICU), hospitalization stay (days).

Participants were scheduled for a face-to-face interview conducted by a healthcare professional. We used the definition proposed by Soriano et al. [13]: "post-COVID-19 condition occurs in people with a history of probable or confirmed SARS-CoV-2 infection, usually three months from the onset of infection, with symptoms that last for at least two months and cannot be explained by an alternative medical diagnosis. Common symptoms include, but are not limited to, fatigue, shortness of breath, and cognitive dysfunction, and generally have an impact on everyday functioning" [13]. Accordingly, patients were specifically asked to report the presence of any particular symptom that appeared in the following three months after their hospitalization due to SARS-CoV-2 infection and if that particular symptom still persisted at the time of the appointment. A predetermined list of symptoms (e.g., fatigue, dyspnea, brain fog, memory loss, anosmia, ageusia, hair loss, skin rashes, concentration loss, pain) was systematically used, although participants were free to report any symptom that they suffered from and attributed to the infection.

2.5. Statistical Analysis

Data were collected with STATA 16.1 and processed using Python's library pandas 0.25.3. Mean and standard deviation (SD) are presented for quantitative data and number of cases (percentages) are presented for categorical data. Differences in methylation percentages (%) according to the presence/absence of post-COVID-19 symptomatology were analyzed with one-way-ANOVA tests. The Shapiro–Wilk test was used to assess the assumption of normality. For all inferences, the level of significance was set at priori 0.05 with p-values from all tests being corrected (Holm–Bonferroni correction).

3. Results

From the 330 patients who were hospitalized due to COVID-19 in the four targeted hospitals during the first wave of the pandemic and who were invited to participate during the study period, 51 (15%) were excluded as follows: refused to attend the appointment (n = 30), saliva sample was compromised during methylation analyses (n = 14), and pregnancy (n = 7). Finally, 279 (48.7% female, mean age: 56.4 ± 12.8 years) patients were included in the study.

At the follow-up assessment (mean: 17.8; SD: 5.2 months after hospital discharge), 246 (88.1%) patients exhibited at least one post-COVID-19 symptom (mean number of symptoms per patient: 3.0; SD: 1.9). Dyspnea at exertion (67.3%), fatigue (62.3%), and memory loss (31.2%) were the most prevalent post-COVID-19 symptoms. Other prevalent post-COVID-19 symptoms were concentration loss (15%) and brain fog (14.6%).

For the main analyses, we considered the following post-COVID-19 symptoms: fatigue, dyspnea at rest, dyspnea at exertion, brain fog, memory loss, concentration loss, and gastrointestinal problems. Overall, the analysis did not reveal differences in the methylation of the ACE2 promoter in any of the CpG locations according to the presence or absence of fatigue (Table 1), dyspnea at rest (Table 2), dyspnea at exertion (Table 3), memory loss (Table 4), brain fog (Table 5), concentration loss (Table 6), and gastrointestinal problems (Table 7).

Table 1. Demographic, clinical, and methylation percentages in COVID-19 patients with or without post-COVID-19 fatigue.

	Post-COVID-19 Fatigue (n = 174)	No Post-COVID-19 Fatigue (n = 105)	p Value
Age, mean (SD), years	57.0 (12.5)	55.7 (13.1)	0.423
Gender, male/female (%) *	74 (42.5%)/100 (57.5%)	69 (65.7%)/36 (34.3%)	0.007 *
Weight, mean (SD), kg	81.5 (18.0)	80.5 (15.0)	0.675
Height, mean (SD), cm	166.5 (11.5)	169.0 (9.2)	0.679
Number of medical conditions	1.3 (1.0)	1.1 (1.0)	0.523
Pre-existing medical conditions, n (%)			
Hypertension	58 (33.3%)	37 (35.25%)	0.791
Diabetes	21 (12.1%)	8 (7.6%)	0.264
Cardiovascular Diseases	12 (6.9%)	8 (7.6%)	0.829
Asthma	20 (11.5%)	11 (10.5%)	0.805
Obesity	60 (34.5%)	25 (23.8%)	0.118
Chronic Obstructive Pulmonary Disease	3 (1.7%)	2 (1.9%)	0.913
Number of COVID-19-onset symptoms, mean (SD)	3.25 (1.0)	3.1 (1.0)	0.218
Days at hospital, mean (SD)	7.0 (5.8)	8.6 (10.0)	0.136
Intensive Care Unit (ICU) admission Yes/No, n (%)	8 (4.5%)/166 (95.5%)	2 (2%)/103 (98%)	0.326
CpG1 methylation (%)	93.3 (4.0)	93.7 (3.2)	0.335
CpG2 methylation (%)	40.4 (7.4)	39.4 (7.3)	0.259
CpG3 methylation (%)	43.6 (9.0)	42.8 (8.1)	0.437
CpG4 methylation (%)	45.5 (8.0)	45.6 (7.8)	0.937
CpG5 methylation (%)	0.6 (0.3)	0.6 (0.4)	0.804

n: number; SD: standard deviation; * Statistically significant differences between groups ($p < 0.05$).

Table 2. Demographic, clinical, and methylation percentages in COVID-19 patients with or without post-COVID-19 dyspnea at rest.

	Post-COVID-19 Dyspnea at Rest (n = 36)	No Post-COVID-19 Dyspnea at Rest (n = 243)	p Value
Age, mean (SD), years	55.0 (15.5)	57.7 (12.4)	0.421
Gender, male/female (%)	11 (30.5%)/25 (69.5%)	132 (64.3%)/111 (45.7%)	0.07
Weight, mean (SD), kg	81.0 (20.0)	81.9 (16.5)	0.933
Height, mean (SD), cm	165.5 (8.7)	168.0 (9.5)	0.501
Number of medical conditions	1.3 (1.0)	1.3 (1.0)	0.724
Pre-existing medical conditions, n (%)			
Hypertension	13 (36.1%)	82 (33.7%)	0.820
Diabetes	7 (19.4%)	22 (9.0%)	0.081
Cardiovascular Diseases	1 (2.8%)	19 (7.8%)	0.291
Asthma	4 (11.1%)	27 (11.1%)	0.636
Obesity	14 (38.9%)	71 (29.2%)	0.327
Chronic Obstructive Pulmonary Disease	1 (2.8%)	4 (1.7%)	0.636
Number of COVID-19-onset symptoms, mean (SD)	3.4 (1.0)	3.2 (1.0)	0.125
Days at hospital, mean (SD)	8.7 (5.8)	7.9 (9.0)	0.617
Intensive Care Unit (ICU) admission Yes/No, n (%)	1 (2.8%)/35 (97.2%)	9 (3.7%)/107 (96.3%)	0.623
CpG1 methylation (%)	93.0 (4.5)	93.5 (3.6)	0.350
CpG2 methylation (%)	37.9 (8.3)	40.3 (7.2)	0.061
CpG3 methylation (%)	40.7 (10.0)	43.7 (8.4)	0.054
CpG4 methylation (%)	44.3 (9.7)	45.7 (7.6)	0.322
CpG5 methylation (%)	0.6 (0.25)	0.6 (0.4)	0.623

n: number; SD: standard deviation.

Table 3. Demographic, clinical, and methylation pe percentages in COVID-19 patients with or without post-COVID-19 dyspnea on exertion.

	Post-COVID-19 Dyspnea on Exertion (n = 188)	No Post-COVID-19 Dyspnea Exertion (n = 91)	p Value
Age, mean (SD), years	56.5 (13.2)	56.5 (12.0)	0.997
Gender, male/female (%) *	82 (43.6%)/106 (56.4%)	61 (67.0%)/30 (33.0%)	0.008 *
Weight, mean (SD), kg	81.0 (17.5)	81.1 (15.0)	0.967
Height, mean (SD), cm	166.5 (9.5)	169.0 (9.6)	0.282
Number of medical conditions	1.3 (1.0)	1.1 (1.0)	0.205
Pre-existing medical conditions, n (%)			
Hypertension	62 (33.0%)	33 (36.25%)	0.659
Diabetes	20 (10.6%)	9 (9.9%)	0.855
Cardiovascular Diseases	14 (7.5%)	6 (6.6%)	0.802
Asthma	24 (12.8%)	7 (7.7%)	0.233
Obesity	64 (34.0%)	21 (23.1%)	0.120
Chronic Obstructive Pulmonary Disease	3 (1.6%)	2 (2.2%)	0.727
Number of COVID-19-onset symptoms, mean (SD)	3.2 (1.0)	3.25 (1.0)	0.637
Days at hospital, mean (SD)	8.2 (9.6)	7.6 (6.2)	0.608
Intensive Care Unit (ICU) admission Yes/No, n (%)	7 (3.7%)/181 (96.3%)	3 (3.3%)/88 (96.7%)	0.538
CpG1 methylation (%)	93.2 (4.2)	94.1 (2.5)	0.052

Table 3. *Cont.*

	Post-COVID-19 Dyspnea on Exertion (n = 188)	No Post-COVID-19 Dyspnea Exertion (n = 91)	*p* Value
CpG2 methylation (%)	40.2 (7.6)	39.7 (6.9)	0.578
CpG3 methylation (%)	43.4 (8.9)	43.0 (8.5)	0.681
CpG4 methylation (%)	45.7 (8.1)	45.4 (7.5)	0.742
CpG5 methylation (%)	0.6 (0.35)	0.6 (0.35)	0.517

n: number; SD: standard deviation; * Statistically significant differences between groups ($p < 0.05$).

Table 4. Demographic, clinical, and methylation percentages in COVID-19 patients with or without post-COVID-19 memory loss.

	Post-COVID-19 Memory Loss (n = 87)	No Post-COVID-19 Memory Loss (n = 192)	*p* Value
Age, mean (SD), years	57.9 (12.3)	55.8 (13.0)	0.204
Gender, male/female (%)	8 (44.7%)/49 (56.3%)	107 (54.7%)/87 (45.3%)	0.222
Weight, mean (SD), kg	81.2 (16.9)	81.0 (16.8)	0.867
Height, mean (SD), cm	166.7 (9.5)	168.0 (9.5)	0.469
Number of medical conditions	1.45 (1.0)	1.2 (1.0)	0.07
Pre-existing medical conditions, n (%)			
Hypertension	35 (40.2%)	60 (31.25%)	0.233
Diabetes *	14 (16.1%)	15 (7.8%)	0.046 *
Cardiovascular Diseases	6 (6.9%)	14 (7.3%)	0.909
Asthma *	16 (18.4%)	15 (7.8%)	0.014 *
Obesity	24 (27.6%)	61 (31.8%)	0.557
Chronic Obstructive Pulmonary Disease	0 (0.0%)	5 (2.6%)	0.132
Number of COVID-19-onset symptoms, mean (SD) *	3.4 (0.8)	3.1 (1.1)	0.04 *
Days at hospital, mean (SD)	9.1 (12.3)	7.5 (6.4)	0.159
Intensive Care Unit (ICU) admission Yes/No, n (%)	4 (4.6%)/83 (95.4%)	6 (3.1%)/186 (96.9%)	0.09
CpG1 methylation (%)	93.1 (4.9)	93.6 (3.1)	0.263
CpG2 methylation (%)	41.1 (7.1)	39.5 (7.4)	0.096
CpG3 methylation (%)	44.6 (8.3)	42.7 (8.7)	0.087
CpG4 methylation (%)	46.5 (7.8)	45.1 (7.9)	0.177
CpG5 methylation (%)	0.6 (0.25)	0.6 (0.4)	0.086

n: number; SD: standard deviation; * Statistically significant differences between groups ($p < 0.05$).

Table 5. Demographic, clinical, and methylation percentages in COVID-19 patients with or without post-COVID-19 brain fog.

	Post-COVID-19 Brain Fog (n = 41)	No Post-COVID-19 Brain Fog (n = 238)	*p* Value
Age, mean (SD), years	55.1 (12.8)	56.7 (12.8)	0.459
Gender, male/female (%)	17 (41.5%)/24 (58.5%)	126 (52.9%)/112 (47.1%)	0.331
Weight, mean (SD), kg	81.6 (19.0)	81.0 (16.3)	0.805
Height, mean (SD), cm	166.5 (9.9)	167.5 (9.5)	0.580
Number of medical conditions	1.35 (1.0)	1.3 (1.0)	0.331

Table 5. *Cont.*

	Post-COVID-19 Brain Fog (n = 41)	No Post-COVID-19 Brain Fog (n = 238)	p Value
Pre-existing medical conditions, n (%)			
Hypertension	11 (26.83%)	84 (35.3%)	0.390
Diabetes	6 (14.6%)	23 (9.7%)	0.361
Cardiovascular Diseases	1 (2.5%)	19 (8.0%)	0.221
Asthma	7 (17.1%)	24 (10.1%)	0.215
Obesity	14 (34.1%)	71 (29.8%)	0.643
Chronic Obstructive Pulmonary Disease	0 (0.0%)	5 (2.1%)	0.353
Number of COVID-19-onset symptoms, mean (SD)	3.4 (0.9)	3.15 (1.0)	0.142
Days at hospital, mean (SD)	7.5 (7.0)	8.1 (9.0)	0.673
Intensive Care Unit (ICU) admission Yes/No, n (%)	2 (4.9%)/39 (95.1%)	8 (3.3%)/230 (96.7%)	0.657
CpG1 methylation (%)	93.7 (4.4)	93.4 (3.7)	0.748
CpG2 methylation (%)	41.4 (6.6)	39.8 (7.5)	0.197
CpG3 methylation (%)	44.6 (8.1)	43.1 (8.8)	0.306
CpG4 methylation (%)	46.7 (7.5)	45.4 (8.0)	0.319
CpG5 methylation (%)	0.6 (0.4)	0.65 (0.35)	0.612

n: number; SD: standard deviation.

Table 6. Demographic, clinical, and methylation percentages in COVID-19 patients with or without post-COVID-19 concentration loss.

	Post-COVID-19 Concentration Loss (n = 42)	No Post-COVID-19 Concentration Loss (n = 237)	p Value
Age, mean (SD), years	54.5 (12.4)	57.0 (12.9)	0.311
Gender, male/female (%) *	16 (28.1%)/26 (61.9%)	127 (54.6%)/110 (46.4%)	0.007 *
Weight, mean (SD), kg	80.7 (16.4)	81.0 (16.9)	0.898
Height, mean (SD), cm	165.5 (9.75)	167.0 (9.5)	0.202
Number of medical conditions	1.3 (1.0)	1.3 (1.0)	0.989
Pre-existing medical conditions, n (%)			
Hypertension	14 (33.3%)	81 (34.2%)	0.931
Diabetes	2 (4.8%)	27 (11.4%)	0.219
Cardiovascular Diseases	2 (4.8%)	18 (7.6%)	0.525
Asthma	4 (9.5%)	27 (11.4%)	0.737
Obesity	19 (45.2%)	66 (27.8%)	0.06
Chronic Obstructive Pulmonary Disease	0 (0.0%)	5 (2.1%)	0.346
Number of COVID-19-onset symptoms, mean (SD)	3.3 (1.1)	3.2 (1.0)	0.554
Days at hospital, mean (SD)	8.5 (7.7)	7.9 (8.8)	0.708
Intensive Care Unit (ICU) admission Yes/No, n (%)	2 (4.7%)/40 (95.3%)	8 (3.4%)/229 (94.6%)	0.657
CpG1 methylation (%)	93.1 (4.5)	93.5 (3.6)	0.497
CpG2 methylation (%)	38.9 (7.6)	40.1 (7.3)	0.292
CpG3 methylation (%)	42.2 (8.6)	43.5 (8.7)	0.368
CpG4 methylation (%)	43.5 (7.6)	45.9 (8.0)	0.066
CpG5 methylation (%)	0.6 (0.3)	0.6 (0.4)	0.506

n: number; SD: standard deviation; * Statistically significant differences between groups ($p < 0.05$).

Table 7. Demographic, clinical, and methylation percentages in COVID-19 patients with or without post-COVID-19 gastrointestinal symptomatology.

	Post-COVID-19 Gastrointestinal Symptoms (n = 25)	No Post-COVID-19 Gastrointestinal Symptoms (n = 254)	*p* Value
Age, mean (SD), years	55.0 (14.1)	56.6 (12.7)	0.536
Gender, male/female (%)	11 (44.0%)/14 (56.0%)	132 (52.0%)/122 (48.0%)	0.586
Weight, mean (SD), kg	81.2 (21.2)	81.0 (16.4)	0.947
Height, mean (SD), cm	168.5 (12.7)	167.5 (9.2)	0.475
Number of medical conditions	1.2 (1.0)	1.3 (1.0)	0.523
Pre-existing medical conditions, n (%)			
Hypertension	10 (40.0%)	85 (33.5%)	0.593
Diabetes	1 (4.0%)	28 (11.0%)	0.299
Cardiovascular Diseases	1 (4.0%)	19 (7.5%)	0.535
Asthma	3 (12.0%)	28 (11.0%)	0.889
Obesity	50 (20.0%)	80 (31.5%)	0.320
Chronic Obstructive Pulmonary Disease	1 (4.0%)	4 (1.6%)	0.387
Number of COVID-19-onset symptoms, mean (SD)	3.35 (0.8)	3.2 (1.0)	0.408
Days at hospital, mean (SD)	5.7 (2.5)	8.2 (9.0)	0.168
Intensive Care Unit (ICU) admission Yes/No, n (%)	0 (0.0%)/25 (100%)	10 (3.9%)/244 (96.1%)	0.412
CpG1 methylation (%)	91.3 (6.0)	93.7 (3.4)	0.002
CpG2 methylation (%)	40.5 (8.0)	40.0 (7.3)	0.711
CpG3 methylation (%)	42.2 (9.2)	43.4 (8.6)	0.527
CpG4 methylation (%)	44.3 (9.5)	45.7 (7.7)	0.411
CpG5 methylation (%)	0.55 (0.45)	0.6 (0.35)	0.295

n: number; SD: standard deviation.

Small differences were identified depending on the presence/absence of some post-COVID-19 symptoms. The most significant difference was that the presence of post-COVID-19 fatigue ($p = 0.007$, Table 1), dyspnea on exertion ($p = 0.008$, Table 3), or concentration loss ($p = 0.007$, Table 6) was more prevalent in females than in males. In addition, a significantly higher proportion of patients reporting post-COVID-19 memory loss suffered from diabetes ($p = 0.046$) or asthma ($p = 0.014$) before the infection.

4. Discussion

This study did not find an association between the methylation of the ACE2 promoter and the presence of post-COVID-19 fatigue, dyspnea, cognitive or gastrointestinal problems up to one year and a half after the infection in previously hospitalized COVID-19 survivors.

We observed that up of 90% of our cohort of COVID-19 survivors who were hospitalized during the first wave of the pandemic reported post-COVID-19 symptomatology up to 18 months after hospital discharge because SARS-CoV-2. Previous meta-analyses have reported that 25–30% of COVID-19 survivors exhibit post-COVID-19 symptoms one or two years after an acute SARS-CoV-2 infection [15,16]; thus, our prevalence rate was much higher than that in the published literature. Different features of our cohort of COVID-19 survivors could explain the differences in prevalence rates of post-COVID-19 symptoms. First, the sample included in our study were patients infected with the historical strain (i.e., during the first wave of the pandemic). Current data suggest that the prevalence rate of post-COVID-19 symptoms is higher in patients infected with the historical strain than in those individuals infected with the Alpha, Delta, or Omicron variants [22,23]. Second, all participants in our study had been infected and developed post-COVID-19 symptoms before vaccination. Evidence supports that vaccination is able to decrease the risk of post-COVID-19 symptomatology if administered before SARS-CoV-2 infection and before the development of post-COVID-19 symptoms, but its effects on those with ongoing symptomatology is still not clear [24]. Third, the current study included a cohort of previously hospitalized patients with, therefore, moderate to severe COVID-19. Although it has been suggested that hospitalized and non-hospitalized patients develop post-COVID-19 symptoms, a meta-analysis has found that COVID-19 survivors who had been hospitalized are at a higher risk of suffering from some post-COVID-19 symptoms such as dyspnea or pain than COVID-19 survivors who are not hospitalized [25].

It seems that the post-COVID-19 condition has multifactorial and multiple mechanisms, e.g., viral persistence, long-lasting inflammation, endothelial dysfunction, reactivation latent infections, immune system dysregulation, and alteration in gut microbiota have been proposed [17]. Our study did not find an association between methylation of ACE2 promoter and the presence of long-lasting post-COVID-19 fatigue, dyspnea, cognitive or gastrointestinal problems. The present results are contrary to those found by Nikesjö et al. who described a specific DNA methylation signature in ten COVID-19 survivors with post-COVID-19 symptomatology 10 months after the acute infection [19]. Similarly, Balnis et al. identified a hypermethylation pattern in interferon-related genes and a hypomethylation pattern in inflammatory-related genes not only at the acute COVID-19 phase [7] but also one year after the infection [18] in a sample of 15 patients. Differences in DNA methylation techniques and specific gene promoters could explain discrepancies among the studies. It is possible that DNA methylation of gene promoters related to the pro-inflammatory response associated with SARS-CoV-2 could be revealed to have some associations with post-COVID-19 symptomatology. In addition, the small sample size and the lack of a comparative group of COVID-19 survivors without post-COVID-19 symptoms in previously published studies also limit their comparability with the current one.

An important topic to consider is that no timeframe can currently be made for DNA methylation, since this is variable [26]. In fact, no longitudinal studies have investigated the possible variations of DNA methylation throughout time. It is possible that SARS-CoV-2 can lead to DNA methylation changes in some genes at the acute phase of the infection but these changes reverse with time. The fact that DNA methylation alterations are reversible opens the possibility of using DNA methylation or demethylation as targets for therapeutic treatments [27].

Finally, the results of the current study should be analyzed considering its potential limitations. First, we included a cohort of patients who were hospitalized due to COVID-19 during the first wave of the pandemic, when the historical SARS-CoV-2 strain was predominant; hence, an extrapolation of our results should be performed with caution. Second, the cross-sectional design did not permit to identify the longitudinal evolution of DNA methylation alterations and the fluctuating nature of these changes. Third, the current study focused solely on DNA methylation changes in the ACE2 promoter. Population-based studies that include whole DNA methylation analyses could help to identify epigenetic changes associated with post-COVID-19 symptomatology.

5. Conclusions

This study did not find an association between methylation of ACE2 promoter and the presence of post-COVID-19 fatigue, dyspnea, cognitive or gastrointestinal problems up to one and a half years after an acute SARS-CoV-2 infection in a cohort of COVID-19 survivors who required hospitalization during the first wave of the outbreak.

Author Contributions: All the authors cited in the manuscript had substantial contributions to the concept and design, the execution of the work, or the analysis and interpretation of data; drafting or revising the manuscript and have read and approved the final version of the paper. C.F.-d.-l.-P.: conceptualization, visualization, methodology, validation, data curation, writing—original draft, writing—review, editing. G.D.-G.: methodology, validation, data curation, writing—original draft, writing—review, editing. A.G.-C.: methodology, validation, data curation, writing—original draft, writing—review and editing. S.M.G.-S.: validation, data curation, writing—original draft, writing—review and editing. S.A.-Q.: validation, writing—original draft, writing—review and editing. J.T.-M.: validation, writing—original draft writing—review, and editing. P.R.-M.: validation, writing—original draft, writing—review, and editing. A.F.-M.: validation, writing—original draft writing—review, editing. O.J.P.-V.: validation, data curation, writing—original draft, writing—review, and editing. L.A.-N.: methodology, validation, data curation, writing—original draft, writing—review and editing. R.G.: methodology, validation, supervision, writing—original draft writing—review, and editing. All authors have read and agreed to the published version of the manuscript.

Funding: The project was supported by a grant from the Novo Nordisk Foundation NNF 21OC0067235 (Denmark) and by a grant associated with the Fondo Europeo De Desarrollo Regional—Recursos REACT-UE del Programa Operativo de Madrid 2014–2020, en la línea de actuación de proyectos de I+D+i en materia de respuesta a COVID 19 (LONG-COVID-EXP-CM).

Institutional Review Board Statement: The study was approved by the Ethics Comittees of all institutions/hospitals (URJC0907202015920 15 July 2020; HUFA 20/126 6 July 2020; HCSC20/495E 10 July 2020, HSO25112020 4 December 2020; HUIL/092-20 6 November 2020).

Informed Consent Statement: All participants provided their written informed consent prior to collecting any data.

Data Availability Statement: All data are presented in the text of the paper and are available on appropriate requirement from the corresponding author.

Conflicts of Interest: The authors declare no conflicts of interest. The funders had no role in the design of the study; in the collection, analyses, or interpretation of data; in the writing of the manuscript, or in the decision to publish the results.

References

1.   Deans, C.; Maggert, K.A. What do you mean, "epigenetic"? *Genetics* **2015**, *199*, 887–896. [CrossRef] [PubMed]
2.   Capp, J.P. Interplay between genetic, epigenetic, and gene expression variability: Considering complexity in evolvability. *Evol. Appl.* **2021**, *14*, 893–901. [CrossRef] [PubMed]
3.   Mantovani, A.; Netea, M.G. Trained innate immunity, epigenetics, and COVID-19. *N. Engl. J. Med.* **2020**, *383*, 1078–1080. [CrossRef] [PubMed]
4.   Behura, A.; Naik, L.; Patel, S.; Das, M.; Kumar, A.; Mishra, A.; Nayak, D.K.; Manna, D.; Mishra, A.; Dhiman, R. Involvement of epigenetics in affecting host immunity during SARS-CoV-2 infection. *Biochim. Biophys. Acta Mol. Basis Dis.* **2023**, *1869*, 166634. [CrossRef] [PubMed]
5.   Moore, L.D.; Le, T.; Fan, G. DNA methylation and its basic function. *Neuropsychopharmacology* **2013**, *38*, 23–38. [CrossRef] [PubMed]
6.   Dey, A.; Vaishak, K.; Deka, D.; Radhakrishnan, A.K.; Paul, S.; Shanmugam, P.; Daniel, A.P.; Pathak, S.; Duttaroy, A.K.; Banerjee, A. Epigenetic perspectives associated with COVID-19 infection and related cytokine storm: An updated review. *Infection* **2023**, *51*, 1603–1618. [CrossRef] [PubMed]
7.   Balnis, J.; Madrid, A.; Hogan, K.J.; Drake, L.A.; Chieng, H.C.; Tiwari, A.; Vincent, C.E.; Chopra, A.; Vincent, P.A.; Robek, M.D.; et al. Blood DNA Methylation and COVID-19 outcomes. *Clin. Epigenet.* **2021**, *13*, 118. [CrossRef] [PubMed]
8.   Singh, H.O.; Choudhari, R.; Nema, V.; Khan, A.A. ACE2 and TMPRSS2 polymorphisms in various diseases with special reference to its impact on COVID-19 disease. *Microb. Pathog.* **2021**, *150*, 104621. [CrossRef] [PubMed]
9.   Faramarzi, A.; Safaralizadeh, R.; Dastmalchi, N.; Teimourian, S. Epigenetic-related effects of COVID-19 on human cells. *Infect. Disord. Drug Targets* **2022**, *22*, 21–26. [CrossRef] [PubMed]
10. Najafipour, R.; Mohammadi, D.; Momeni, M.; Moghbelinejad, S. ACE-2 Expression and methylation pattern in bronchoalveolar lavage fluid and bloods of Iranian ARDS COVID-19 patients. *Int. J. Mol. Cell Med.* **2022**, *11*, 55–63. [PubMed]
11. Daniel, G.; Paola, A.R.; Nancy, G.; Fernando, S.O.; Beatriz, A.; Zulema, R.; Julieth, A.; Claudia, C.; Adriana, R. Epigenetic mechanisms and host factors impact ACE2 gene expression: Implications in COVID-19 susceptibility. *Infect. Genet. Evol.* **2022**, *104*, 105357. [CrossRef] [PubMed]
12. Fernández-de-las-Peñas, C. Long COVID: Current definition. *Infection* **2022**, *50*, 285–286. [CrossRef] [PubMed]
13. Soriano, J.B.; Murthy, S.; Marshall, J.C.; Relan, P.; Diaz, J.V.; WHO Clinical Case Definition Working Group on Post-COVID-19 Condition. A clinical case definition of post-COVID-19 condition by a Delphi consensus. *Lancet Infect. Dis.* **2022**, *22*, e102–e107. [CrossRef] [PubMed]
14. Hayes, L.D.; Ingram, J.; Sculthorpe, N.F. More Than 100 Persistent Symptoms of SARS-CoV-2 (Long COVID): A scoping review. *Front. Med.* **2021**, *8*, 750378. [CrossRef] [PubMed]

15. Global Burden of Disease Long COVID Collaborators; Wulf Hanson, S.; Abbafati, C.; Aerts, J.G.; Al-Aly, Z.; Ashbaugh, C.; Ballouz, T.; Blyuss, O.; Bobkova, P.; Bonsel, G.; et al. Estimated global proportions of individuals with persistent fatigue, cognitive, and respiratory symptom clusters following symptomatic COVID-19 in 2020 and 2021. *JAMA* **2022**, *328*, 1604–1615. [PubMed]

16. Fernández-de-las-Peñas, C.; Notarte, K.I.; Macasaet, R.; Velasco, J.V.; Catahay, J.A.; Therese Ver, A.; Chung, W.; Valera-Calero, J.A.; Navarro-Santana, M. Persistence of post-COVID symptoms in the general population two years after SARS-CoV-2 infection: A systematic review and meta-analysis. *J. Infect.* **2024**, *88*, 77–88. [CrossRef] [PubMed]

17. Fernández-de-las-Peñas, C.; Raveendran, A.V.; Giordano, R.; Arendt-Nielsen, L. Long COVID or post-COVID-19 condition: Past, present and future research directions. *Microorganisms* **2023**, *11*, 2959. [CrossRef] [PubMed]

18. Balnis, J.; Madrid, A.; Hogan, K.J.; Drake, L.A.; Adhikari, A.; Vancavage, R.; Singer, H.A.; Alisch, R.S.; Jaitovich, A. Whole-Genome methylation sequencing reveals that COVID-19-induced epigenetic dysregulation remains 1 year after hospital discharge. *Am. J. Respir. Cell Mol. Biol.* **2023**, *68*, 594–597. [CrossRef] [PubMed]

19. Nikesjö, F.; Sayyab, S.; Karlsson, L.; Apostolou, E.; Rosén, A.; Hedman, K.; Lerm, M. Defining post-acute COVID-19 syndrome (PACS) by an epigenetic biosignature in peripheral blood mononuclear cells. *Clin. Epigenet.* **2022**, *14*, 172. [CrossRef] [PubMed]

20. Mikeska, T.; Felsberg, J.; Hewitt, C.A.; Dobrovic, A. Analysing DNA methylation using bisulphite pyrosequencing. *Methods Mol. Biol.* **2011**, *791*, 33–53.

21. Fan, R.; Mao, S.Q.; Gu, T.L.; Zhong, F.D.; Gong, M.L.; Hao, L.M.; Yin, F.Y.; Dong, C.Z.; Zhang, L.N. Preliminary analysis of the association between methylation of the ACE2 promoter and essential hypertension. *Mol. Med. Rep.* **2017**, *15*, 3905–3911. [CrossRef] [PubMed]

22. Fernández-de-las-Peñas, C.; Notarte, K.I.; Peligro, P.J.; Velasco, J.V.; Ocampo, M.J.; Henry, B.M.; Arendt-Nielsen, L.; Torres-Macho, J.; Plaza-Manzano, G. Long-COVID symptoms in individuals infected with different SARS-CoV-2 variants of concern: A systematic review of the literature. *Viruses* **2022**, *14*, 2629. [CrossRef] [PubMed]

23. Du, M.; Ma, Y.; Deng, J.; Liu, M.; Liu, J. Comparison of long COVID-19 caused by different SARS-CoV-2 strains: A systematic review and meta-analysis. *Int. J. Environ. Res. Public Health* **2022**, *19*, 16010. [CrossRef] [PubMed]

24. Watanabe, A.; Iwagami, M.; Yasuhara, J.; Takagi, H.; Kuno, T. Protective effect of COVID-19 vaccination against long COVID syndrome: A systematic review and meta-analysis. *Vaccine* **2023**, *41*, 1783–1790. [CrossRef] [PubMed]

25. Yuan, N.; Lv, Z.H.; Sun, C.R.; Wen, Y.Y.; Tao, T.Y.; Qian, D.; Tao, F.P.; Yu, J.H. Post-acute COVID-19 symptom risk in hospitalized and non-hospitalized COVID-19 survivors: A systematic review and meta-analysis. *Front. Public Health* **2023**, *11*, 1112383. [CrossRef] [PubMed]

26. Møller Johansen, L.; Gerra, M.C.; Arendt-Nielsen, L. Time course of DNA methylation in pain conditions: From experimental models to humans. *Eur. J. Pain* **2021**, *25*, 296–312. [CrossRef] [PubMed]

27. Tajerian, M.; Alvarado, S.; Millecamps, M.; Vachon, P.; Crosby, C.; Bushnell, M.C.; Szyf, M.; Stone, L.S. Peripheral nerve injury is associated with chronic, reversible changes in global DNA methylation in the mouse prefrontal cortex. *PLoS ONE* **2013**, *8*, e55259. [CrossRef] [PubMed]

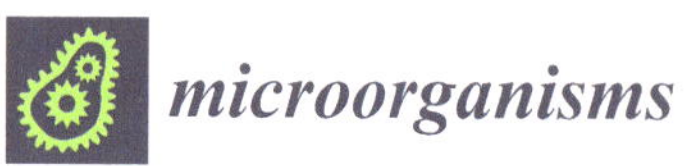 *microorganisms*

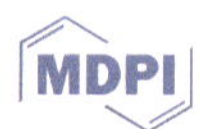

Brief Report

CD147 rs8259T>A Variant Confers Susceptibility to COVID-19 Infection within the Mexican Population

Luis M. Amezcua-Guerra [1], Carlos A. Guzmán-Martín [2], Isela Montúfar-Robles [3], Rashidi Springall [1], Adrián Hernández-Díazcouder [4], Rosa Elda Barbosa-Cobos [5,6], Fausto Sánchez-Muñoz [1,*] and Julián Ramírez-Bello [7,*]

[1] Immunology Department, Instituto Nacional de Cardiología Ignacio Chávez, Mexico City 14080, Mexico; lmamezcuag@gmail.com (L.M.A.-G.); raspringall@yahoo.com (R.S.)
[2] Postgraduate Doctoral Program in Biological and Health Sciences, Universidad Autónoma Metropolitana, Mexico City 14387, Mexico; mcarlos93@gmail.com
[3] Research Unit, Hospital Juárez de México, Mexico City 07760, Mexico; ismontufar@gmail.com
[4] Obesity and Asthma Research Laboratory, Hospital Infantil de México Federico Gómez, Mexico City 06720, Mexico; adrian.hernandez.diazc@hotmail.com
[5] Rheumatology Department, Hospital Juárez de México, Mexico City 07760, Mexico; rebcob@yahoo.com
[6] The American British Cowdray Medical Center, Mexico City 05348, Mexico
[7] Endocrinology Department, Instituto Nacional de Cardiología Ignacio Chávez, Mexico City 14080, Mexico
[*] Correspondence: fausto22@yahoo.com (F.S.-M.); dr.julian.ramirez.inc@gmail.com (J.R.-B.); Tel.: +(52)-1-5523328417 (F.S.-M.); +(52)-1-7777910155 (J.R.-B.)

Abstract: Background: Coronavirus disease 2019 (COVID-19) is caused by the severe acute respiratory syndrome coronavirus 2 (SARS-CoV-2). Clinical manifestations of COVID-19 range from mild flu-like symptoms to severe respiratory failure. Nowadays, extracellular matrix metalloproteinase inducer (EMMPRIN), also known as cluster of differentiation 147 (CD147) or BASIGIN, has been studied as enabling viral entry and replication within host cells. However, the impact of the *CD147* rs8259T>A single nucleotide variant (SNV) on SARS-CoV-2 susceptibility remains poorly investigated. Objective: To investigate the impact of rs8259T>A on the *CD147* gene in individuals from Mexico with COVID-19 disease. Methods: We genotyped the *CD147* rs8359T>A SNV in 195 patients with COVID-19 and 185 healthy controls from Mexico. In addition, we also measured the expression levels of CD147 and TNF mRNA and miR-492 from whole blood of patients with COVID-19 through RT-q-PCR. Results: We observed a significant association between the *CD147* rs8259T>A SNV and susceptibility to COVID-19: T vs. A; OR 1.36, 95% CI 1.02–1.81; $p = 0.037$; and TT vs. AA; OR 1.77, 95% CI 1.01–3.09; $p = 0.046$. On the other hand, we did not find differences in CD147, TNF or miR-492 expression levels when considering the genotypes of the *CD147* rs8259T>A SNV. Conclusions: Our results suggest that the *CD147* rs8259T>A variant is a risk factor for COVID-19.

Keywords: CD147; Basigin; single nucleotide polymorphism; rs8259; COVID-19

Citation: Amezcua-Guerra, L.M.; Guzmán-Martín, C.A.; Montúfar-Robles, I.; Springall, R.; Hernández-Díazcouder, A.; Barbosa-Cobos, R.E.; Sánchez-Muñoz, F.; Ramírez-Bello, J. *CD147* rs8259T>A Variant Confers Susceptibility to COVID-19 Infection within the Mexican Population. *Microorganisms* **2023**, *11*, 1919. https://doi.org/10.3390/microorganisms11081919

Academic Editor: Qibin Geng

Received: 5 June 2023
Revised: 21 July 2023
Accepted: 25 July 2023
Published: 28 July 2023

1. Introduction

Coronavirus disease 2019 (COVID-19), caused by the severe acute respiratory syndrome coronavirus 2 (SARS-CoV-2), has resulted in over 6.8 million deaths worldwide [1,2]. The clinical manifestations of COVID-19 range from mild flu-like symptoms to severe respiratory failure [3]. The ability of SARS-CoV-2 to infect host cells is primarily governed by the interactions between the viral spike (S) protein and its human receptor angiotensin-converting enzyme-2 (ACE2). These interactions initiate a cascade of events that enable viral entry and replication within the host cells [4]. Initially, the human ACE2 receptor was identified as the primary host cell receptor for the S protein [5]. Nevertheless, further investigations revealed additional molecules involved in mediating viral infection, such as extracellular matrix metalloproteinase inducer (EMMPRIN), also known as cluster of differentiation 147 (CD147) or BASIGIN [6]. Although the impact of CD147 on SARS-CoV-2 infection remains poorly investigated, its significance should not be underestimated.

CD147, a highly glycosylated transmembrane glycoprotein belonging to the immunoglobulin superfamily, is expressed in diverse immune cells and plays a role in triggering inflammation with the release of cytokines such as interleukin (IL)-6 and tumor necrosis factor (TNF), induction of matrix metalloproteinase 2 (MMP)-2, IL-9, interferon (IFN)-gamma, and immune cell activation [7]. In recent years, genetic research has been focused on understanding how single nucleotide variants (SNVs) can influence infectious disease susceptibility. SNVs are among the most common genetic variations, occurring approximately every 1200 base pairs (bp) when comparing a pair of human chromosomes [8]. This information is often used to uncover why some people are more likely to have a certain disease or condition than others, including COVID-19.

For instance, a meta-analysis conducted by Li and colleagues assessed the association between interferon-induced transmembrane protein 3 (*IFITM3*) variants and susceptibility to COVID-19. Notably, they identified an association between the *IFITM3* rs12252A>G SNV and COVID-19 infection [9]. On the other hand, some studies on SNVs in COVID-19 have been focused on genes encoding SARS-CoV-2 receptors or on proteases that prime the S protein, such as ACE2 and TMPRSS2, respectively [10,11]. In addition, a recent study evaluated the *CD147* rs8259T>A SNV in patients with COVID-19 [12]. CD147 is another receptor of the S protein [13]. Izmailova and colleagues aimed to investigate potential associations between the *CD147* rs8259T>A, *ACE2* rs4240157T>C, *TMPRSS2* rs12329760C>T, and *TMPRSS11A* rs353163C/T variants and COVID-19 severity in the Ukrainian population. They analyzed these variants among cases divided into three groups: without oxygen therapy, non-invasive oxygen therapy, and invasive oxygen therapy. Interestingly, they only found frequency differences for the *TMPRSS2* rs12329760C>T variant in the group receiving invasive oxygen therapy, but they did not identify an association between *CD147* rs8259T>A and COVID-19 susceptibility or severity [12]. However, given the sample size reported in that study, it is necessary to evaluate whether this same variant is a risk factor in populations with a different genetic background. The *CD147* rs8259T>A variant is in the 3′-untranslated region (3′ UTR) of *CD147* on chromosome 19:582927 and has been evolutionarily conserved in several eutherian mammals (Figure 1a–c).

Despite several studies investigating different SNVs in genes such as *TMPRSS2*, *ACE1*, *ACE2*, and others with COVID-19 susceptibility, it remains unclear whether the *CD147* rs8259T>A variant confers susceptibility to this infectious disease in the Mexican population. Therefore, our objective was to investigate the impact of the *CD147* rs8259T>A variant in individuals from Mexico who have contracted COVID-19. In addition, we evaluated whether the genotypes of the *CD147* variant are associated with CD147, TNF, and miR-492 expression levels. Thus, we aim to contribute to the understanding of the genetic factors influencing COVID-19 susceptibility.

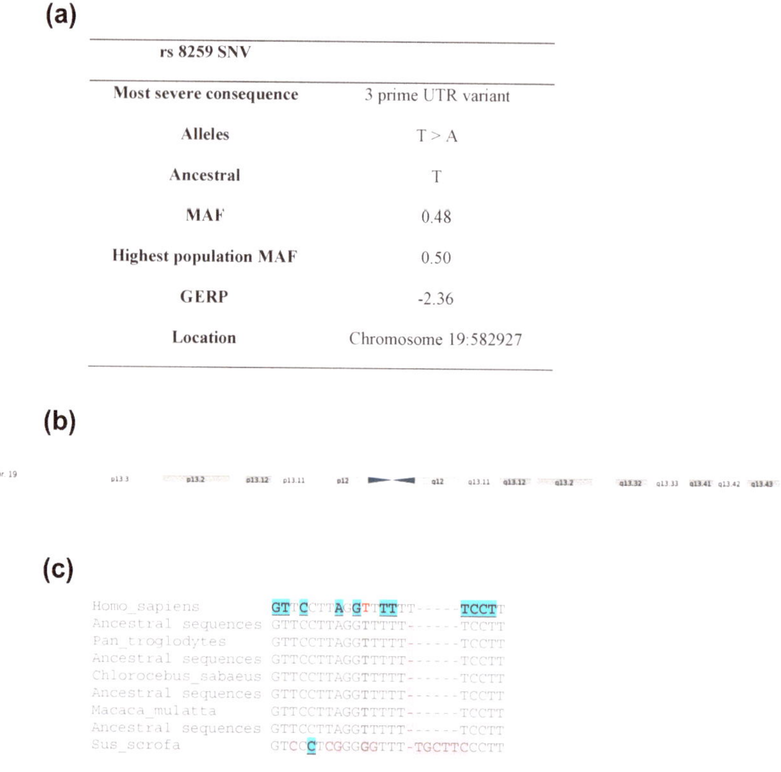

Figure 1. Information on *CD147* rs8259 SNV. (**a**) Some features of CD147 rs8259T>A, (**b**) 19:582927 chromosomic localization (enclosed in the red box), and (**c**) conservation through eutherian mammals. Blue color denotes variants in the 3′ UTR (untranslated region), red indicates the focus variant, and pink represents those that differ from the primary species.

2. Materials and Methods

2.1. Study Population

In this study, a total of 195 symptomatic patients with COVID-19 confirmed by RT-qPCR test were enrolled from the Hospital Juárez de México. The recruitment period spanned from October 2020 and January 2021, during which the original strain of SARS-CoV-2 was observed. The diagnosis of COVID-19 was made based on clinical characteristics, such as loss of taste, dry cough, fatigue, fever, diarrhea, nasal congestion, sore throat, conjunctivitis, headache, musculoskeletal pain, skin rashes, dizziness, heart rate, and oxygen saturation, together with a positive PCR test for SARS-CoV-2. Laboratory parameters were collected from medical records on the same day as the study sampling. For the control group, we included 195 individuals who were not infected with SARS-CoV-2, and their samples were collected during the period of 2016 to 2018. Participants in the control group had no history of chronic-inflammatory, autoimmune, or cancer diseases (conditions where CD147 is widely expressed), and they were free from respiratory diseases. Additionally, individuals in the control group tested negative for COVID-19 infection based on RT-qPCR. Our study was conducted in accordance with the principles outlined in the Declaration of Helsinki and received approval from the Ethics, Biosecurity, and Research Committees of the Hospital Juárez de México (project number HJM 024/22-I). All patients or their relatives provided informed consent by signing the institutional consent letter.

2.2. Genetic Analysis

Whole blood samples (5 mL) were collected in EDTA tubes following WHO recommendations for sampling and processing biological samples from COVID-19 cases [14]. Genomic DNA was extracted using the QIAamp DNA Blood Mini kit (QIAGEN, Hilden, Germany). DNA integrity was evaluated by agarose gel electrophoresis (1% agarose gel stained with ethidium bromide). The purity and concentration of the extracted DNA were measured using a NanoDrop 2000 spectrophotometer (Thermo Fisher's Scientific, Wilmington, DE, USA). Genotyping of the rs8259T>A variant was performed using Applied Biosystems TaqMan Genotyping Assays (Foster City, CA, USA), according to the manufacturer's instructions.

2.3. CD147, miR-492, and TNF mRNA Expression

K-EDTA whole blood samples (400 µL) were isolated using Tripure reagent and subsequently treated with DNAse I (Roche, Penzberg, Germany). For CD147, TNF, and GAPDH mRNA levels, 50 ng of total RNA was amplified by one-step RT-qPCR with the QuantiNova Probe RT-PCR Kit (Qiagen, Hilden, Germany).

For miR-492 and U6 (used as endogenous control) levels, 20 ng of total RNA was retrotranscribed using the TaqMan miRNA RT kit (Applied Biosystems, Foster City, CA, USA). For qPCR, 1 µL of cDNA was used along with the QuantiNova Probe PCR Master Mix (Qiagen), following the manufacturer's instructions.

CD147 mRNA levels were compared with whole blood from 25 patients and 25 controls. In addition, we evaluated the levels of miR-492, CD147, and TNF mRNA considering the three genotypes of *CD147* rs8259T>A from 25 randomized samples of patients with COVID-19, maintaining the same percentages of genotypes identified in all patients with this infectious disease.

The qPCR was performed using the Oppus CFX96 system (BioRad, Hercules, CA, USA). The cycling conditions consisted of an initial denaturation at 95 °C for 10 min, followed by 45 cycles at 95 °C for 15 s, 60 °C for 60 s, and 72 °C for 1 s. Expression levels were measured in duplicate and normalized using glyceraldehyde-3-phosphate dehydrogenase (GAPDH) sequence 5′-AGCCACATCGCTCAGACAC-3′ and 5′-GCCCAATACGACCAAATCC-3′ as the reference. The following NCBI assay genes and TaqMan catalog numbers were used: CD147: Hs00936295_m1, Catalog #4331182; TNF: Hs00174128_m1, Catalog #4331182; hsa-miR-492: 001039, U6: Catalog #4427975 (Thermo Fisher, Foster City, California). Relative quantification was performed using the 2 −delta Ct ($2^{-\Delta Ct}$) method.

2.4. Statistical Analysis

Hardy-Weinberg equilibrium analysis was conducted using the web software https://ihg.helmholtz-muenchen.de accessed on 17 January 2023. Alleles and genotype frequencies were calculated using GraphPad Prism software v8. To evaluate susceptibility between *CD147* variants and COVID-19, we compared allelic and genotypic frequencies between SARS-CoV-2-infected patients and controls. Additional statistical analyses were carried out in SPSS v26. A comparison of expression levels of TNF, miR-492, and CD147 mRNAs between different genotype groups was carried out using the Kruskal–Wallis test. The association between genotypes and susceptibility to COVID-19 infection was evaluated using the chi-square test. Correlation analysis was performed using the Pearson test. A p-value less than 0.05 was considered statistically significant.

3. Results

Among the 195 COVID-19 patients included in our study, a median age of 55 years (IQR 46 to 66) was observed, and 122 (62.6%) patients were male. Mechanical ventilation was required for 60 (30.8%) patients during hospitalization. Clinical improvement was observed in 68.2% of the cases, while 31.8% ultimately died. The main clinical and laboratory data are summarized in Table 1.

Table 1. Demographic and clinical data of COVID-19 participants.

	COVID-19 Patients (n = 195)
Age in years, median (IQR)	55 (46–66)
Male sex, n (%)	122 (62.6)
Outcome	
• Clinical improvement, n (%)	133 (68.2)
• Death, n (%)	62 (31.8)
Mechanical Ventilation, n (%)	60 (30.8)
Diabetes Mellitus, n (%)	69 (35.4)
Systemic Hypertension, n (%)	82 (42.1)
Obesity, n (%)	82 (42.1)
Serum creatinine, median (IQR)	0.87 (0.66–1.35)
Ferritin, median (IQR)	686 (386–1028.7)
Lactic Dehydrogenase, median (IQR)	363.7 (268–471)
C-reactive protein, median (IQR)	8.9 (3.8–23.4)
Total bilirubin, median (IQR)	0.6 (0.43–0.80)
ALT, median (IQR)	47.5 (28–72)
AST, median (IQR)	40 (27–67)

Main clinical characteristics of COVID-19 patients; quantitative variables are represented with median and interquartile range, and qualitative variables are shown with frequencies and percentages. ALT—alanine aminotransferase, AST—aspartate aminotransferase.

Regarding the allele and genotypic frequencies in controls, we identified a normal distribution of genotypes of the *CD147* rs8259T>A variant in controls. The distribution of allele and genotype frequencies of the *CD147* rs8259T>A variant in cases and controls is presented in Figure 2. Our analyses revealed, after adjusting for age, gender, comorbidities, etc., an association between the *CD147* rs8259T>A SNV and COVID-19 infection; T vs. A (OR 1.36, 95% CI 1.02 to 1.81, and p = 0.037) and TT vs. AA (OR 1.77, 95% CI 1.01 to 3.09 and p = 0.046) (Figure 2). However, no significant differences were found in the quantitative laboratory variables or clinical traits associated with COVID-19 among the genotype groups of *CD147* rs8259T>A (Table 2). Our data suggest that this variant is a risk factor for COVID-19, but it is not associated with severity.

Table 2. Comparison of quantitative and qualitative variables in different genotype groups in patients with COVID-19.

	TT (n = 62)	TA (n = 85)	AA (n = 48)	p
Mechanical Ventilation (n, %)	18 (29.0)	27 (31.8)	15 (31.3)	0.787
Diabetes mellitus (n, %)	24 (38.7)	27 (31.8)	18 (37.5)	0.644
Systemic Hypertension (n, %)	25 (40.3)	37 (43.5)	19 (39.6)	0.882
Male (n, %)	39 (62.9)	54 (63.5)	29 (60.4)	0.936
Obesity (n, %)	29 (46.8)	34 (40)	19 (35.6)	0.659
Creatinine (mg/dL)	0.84 (0.69–1.28)	0.88 (0.62–1.32)	0.96 (0.73–1.42)	0.31
Ferritin (ng/mL)	681 (348–1074)	686 (377–1295)	693 (396–992)	0.78
LDH (IU/L)	366 (256–489)	362 (275–460)	350 (269–558)	0.84
CRP (mg/dL)	6.38 (3.3–21.1)	10.20 (4.0–22.2)	8.32 (4.3–65.2)	0.60

(a)

SNP	Population	Allele		Genotype		
		T	A	TT	TA	AA
rs8259	Controls (n=185)	0.61 (226)	0.39 (144)	0.40 (73)	0.43 (80)	0.17 (32)
	Cases (n=195)	0.54 (209)	0.46 (181)	0.32 (62)	0.44 (85)	0.24 (48)

(b)

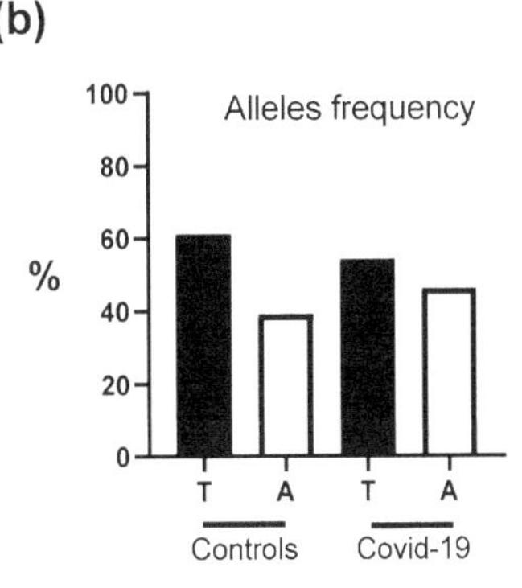

(c)

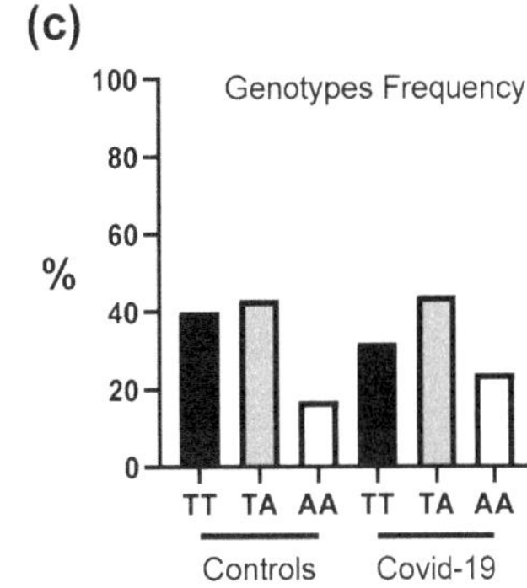

(d)

Risk allele 2	T vs A	TT vs TA	TT vs AA	TT vs TA+AA
OR	1.359	1.251	1.766	1.398
(95% CI)	(1.018 – 1.814)	(0.793 – 1.973)	(1.008 – 3.095)	(0.917 – 2.131)
Chi2	4.35	0.93	3.98	2.43
P value	**P=0.0369**	P=0.3353	**P=0.0459**	P=0.1186

Figure 2. (**a–c**) Allele and genotype frequencies of *CD147* rs8259T>A observed on both controls and COVID-19 patients. (**d**) Association analysis of the *CD147* rs8259T>A variant in cases vs. controls CI—Confidence interval, OR—Odds ratio; significant *p*-values are in bold.

Additionally, we compared the expression levels of CD147 mRNA levels in 25 COVID-19 patients and 25 controls, and we found a higher expression in COVID-19 patients compared with controls (COVID-19 median: 2.01, IQR 0.63 to 3.97; controls median 0.96, IQR 0.69 to 1.52, $p = 0.04$) (Figure 3a). Next, we conducted an analysis of the expression of the CD147 (Figure 3b), miR-492 (Figure 3c), and TNF mRNAs (Figure 3d) considering the genotypes of rs8259T/A. After analysis, we did not identify any statistically significant difference between the genotypes of the aforementioned molecules in patients with COVID-19: CD147 (TT genotype median 1.93, IQR 0.697 to 3.32 vs. TA genotype median 2.13, IQR 1.142 to 5.863 vs. AA genotype median 3.02, IQR 0.85 to 11.93; $p > 0.05$; Figure 3b), miR-492 (TT genotype median 0.034, IQR 0.019 to 0.086 vs. TA genotype median 0.028, IQR 0.014 to 0.052 vs. AA genotype median 0.019, IQR 0.007 to 0.076; $p > 0.05$; Figure 3c), and TNF (TT genotype median 4.30, IQR 0.50 to 12.43 vs. TA genotype median 1.87, IQR 0.57 to 3.04 vs. AA genotype median 1.92, IQR 0.70 to 3.32; $p > 0.05$; Figure 3d).

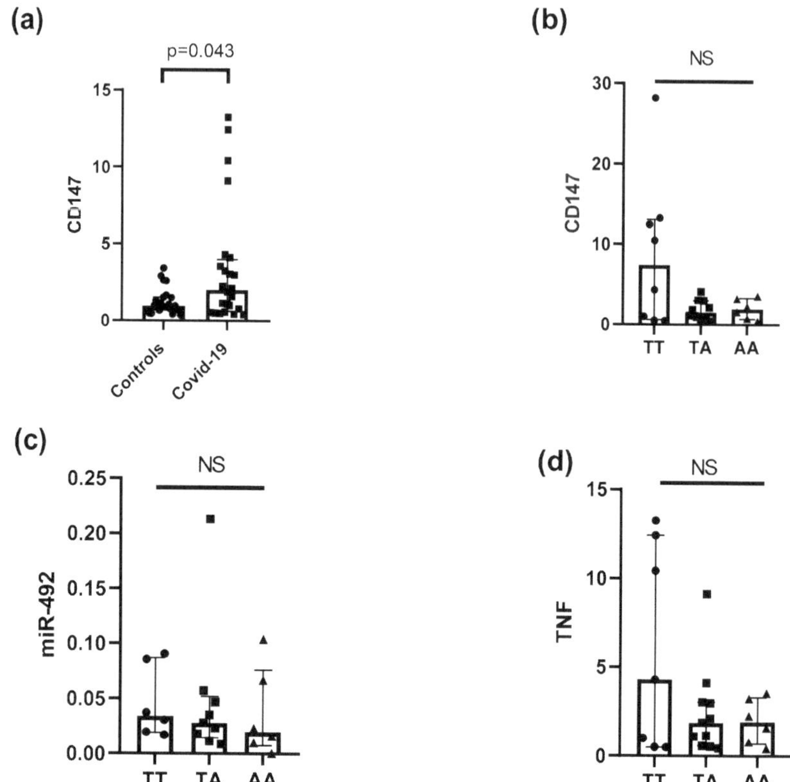

Figure 3. CD147, TNF, and miR-492 mRNA levels in patients with COVID-19. (**a**) CD147 mRNA levels in 25 COVID-19 patients and 25 controls. (**b**) CD147, (**c**) miR-492, and (**d**) TNF mRNA levels considering the three genotypes (TT, TA, and AA) of the *CD147* rs8259T>A in 25 patients with COVID-19. NS: Not Significative.

4. Discussion

CD147, a transmembrane glycoprotein belonging to the immunoglobulin superfamily, has been implicated in viral infections. Like the human ACE2 receptor, CD147 has been reported to be another human receptor for the S protein of SARS-CoV-2 and to be involved in viral entry [10,15]. In addition, previous studies have demonstrated the functional role of CD147 in facilitating SARS-CoV-2 infection [16]. Indeed, CD147 interacts with the S protein of SARS-CoV-2, thereby participating in the entry route of SARS-CoV-2 into infected human cells [15].

Some authors have suggested that certain variants in the *CD147* gene could be important to the susceptibility and/or severity of COVID-19 [6,17,18], given the significance of CD147 in the entry of SARS-CoV-2 into human host cells [17,18]. Thus, in this study, we investigated whether the *CD147* rs8259T>A variant is associated with COVID-19 infection in the Mexican population. To the best of our knowledge, only one study has previously reported on the role of the rs8259T>A variant in COVID-19 susceptibility and severity in the Ukrainian population; however, they did not find any association [12]. In contrast, our study revealed a significant association with COVID-19 susceptibility. These discrepant findings between the two studies may be attributed to several factors. Firstly, the difference in the number of control samples could have influenced the results. Our study had a larger control group, consisting of 185 Mexican mestizos, compared to their study's 92 controls. A larger control group provides more statistical power to detect associations accurately.

Additionally, the genetic ancestry of the study populations might have played a crucial role. Our study included participants from Central Mexico, where the genetic background is characterized by approximately 52% European, 44% Amerindian, and 4% African ancestry [19]. Indeed, the genotype frequencies of the CD147 rs8259T>A variant in our Mexican controls are different from those identified in the Ukrainian controls [12]. These differences could lead to the fact that in Mexicans it is a risk factor, while in Ukrainians it is not. Given the lack of association reported in the European population and the association we identified in a Latin American population, other studies should be conducted in other populations with different genetic backgrounds to determine whether this CD147 variant is indeed a risk factor for SARS-CoV-2 infection and COVID-19. On the other hand, in our study, we assessed whether the rs8259T>A variant is associated with specific laboratory parameters or clinical features related to COVID-19. However, after analysis, we did not observe any significant associations, indicating that it is not associated with disease severity in our study population.

It is worth noting that the A allele or AA genotype of the *CD147* rs8259T>A variant, which we identified as a risk factor for COVID-19, has previously been reported as a risk factor for chronic heart failure (CHF) in Chinese patients [20]. Moreover, a study by Yingzhen Weng et al. explored the role of SNVs in *CD147* and matrix metalloproteinase-9 (MMP-9) in the susceptibility and severity of coronary artery disease (CAD). They genotyped the rs8259T>A, rs28915400G>T, rs4919859G>C, rs6758G>A, and rs8637G>A *CD147* variants and rs3918242C>T *MMP-9* variant in 812 patients and 258 controls and found associations between rs8259T>A and rs3918242C>T variants and CAD, suggesting their involvement in the pathological process of the disease [21].

Finally, we investigated the expression levels of CD147 mRNA between patients with COVID-19 and controls, as well as whether the three genotypes of rs8259T>A were associated with abnormal levels of CD147, miR-492, and TNF mRNA expression in patients with COVID-19. We observed significantly higher expression levels of CD147 mRNA in patients with COVID-19 compared to controls. This finding suggests that CD147 may play a role in the pathogenesis or progression of COVID-19. The elevated expression of CD147 in patients with COVID-19 is in line with previous studies that have reported an increase of CD147 mRNA in some inflammatory and autoimmune diseases [13,22,23]. These results highlight the potential of CD147 as a biomarker or therapeutic target for COVID-19. The CD147 mRNA or protein is expressed in high levels in whole blood and in PBMCs of controls, as previously reported [6,24,25] and as we also identified in our study. Our analysis did not reveal any statistically significant difference in CD147, miR-492, and TNF expression levels among the three genotypes of rs8259T>A in patients with COVID-19. We did not carry out any study of the expression of CD147, miR-492, and TNF considering the genotypes of the *CD147* rs8259T>A variant in controls, this being one of the limitations of our study.

On the other hand, the A/A and T/A genotypes of the *CD147* rs8259T>A variant have been associated with higher expression levels of CD147 mRNA or protein in PBMCs from patients with ACS but not in patients with stable angina [24]. Thus, the effect of genotypes of the CD147 rs8259T>A variant on the expression of its mRNA appears to depend on the cell type, tissue, or disease. As far as we know, the expression of miR-492 had not been evaluated in patients with COVID-19, but a study showed that this miRNA is expressed in PBMCs from healthy controls [25]. In this sense, we also found an expression of this miRNA in whole blood cells of our controls. miR-492 has been reported to bind to the T allele of the *CD147* rs8259T>A variant; meanwhile, the A allele destroys the binding site for this miRNA, which generates an increase in CD147 protein expression [24]. In this same study, it was reported that the AA genotype of rs8259T>A is associated with an increased production of CD147 protein (but not mRNA) in PBMCs from patients with psoriasis versus the TT genotype [25]. Therefore, the effect of the three genotypes (T/T, T/A, and A/A) of this variant on its protein or mRNA expression levels appears to depend on the cell type, tissue, or disease [24,25]. In line with the information reported by Wu et al., we do not observe statistically significant differences in CD147 mRNA levels considering the genotypes of this variant in patients with psoriasis and stable angina [24,25]. Although we did not identify differences in TNF mRNA expression considering the three rs8259T>A genotypes, we know that TNF is a cytokine that mediates inflammation and can cause detrimental tissue damage, that it promotes lung fibrosis, which later results in pneumonia, pulmonary edema, and acute respiratory distress syndrome, that it promotes inflammation and that it is associated with morbidity and mortality in patients with COVID-19 [26].

It is important to acknowledge the limitations of our study. Although we conducted a comprehensive analysis of the *CD147* rs8259T>A variant in relation to COVID-19, laboratory parameters, and gene expression, our findings are based on a specific population and may not be generalizable to other ethnicities or regions.

5. Conclusions

Our data suggest that this *CD147* rs8259T>A variant is a risk factor for COVID-19 in the Mexican population. These findings highlight the potential involvement of CD147 in the pathogenesis of COVID-19 and suggest the importance of genetic factors in disease susceptibility. Understanding the role of CD147 and its variants in COVID-19 may contribute to the development of personalized medicine and targeted therapeutic interventions.

Author Contributions: Conceptualization: F.S.-M., L.M.A.-G. and J.R.-B.; Methodology, formal analysis, and investigation: F.S.-M., L.M.A.-G., C.A.G.-M. and J.R.-B.; Writing original draft preparation: L.M.A.-G., C.A.G.-M., I.M.-R. and R.S.; Funding acquisition:, J.R.-B., R.E.B.-C., F.S.-M. and A.H.-D.; Supervision L.M.A.-G., C.A.G.-M., I.M.-R., R.S., A.H.-D., R.E.B.-C., F.S.-M. and J.R.-B.; Review and Editing: A.H.-D., R.E.B.-C., I.M.-R. and R.S. All authors have read and agreed to the published version of the manuscript.

Funding: Open Access funding for this article was supported by Instituto Nacional de Cardiología Ignacio Chávez.

Data Availability Statement: Raw data are available directly from the corresponding authors with a reasonable request.

Conflicts of Interest: The authors declare no conflict of interest.

References

1. Wang, H.; Paulson, K.R.; Pease, S.A.; Watson, S.; Comfort, H.; Zheng, P.; Aravkin, A.Y.; Bisignano, C.; Barber, R.M.; Alam, T.; et al. Estimating excess mortality due to the COVID-19 pandemic: A systematic analysis of COVID-19-related mortality, 2020–2021. *Lancet* **2022**, *399*, 1513–1536. [CrossRef]
2. WHO Coronavirus (COVID-19) Dashboard | WHO Coronavirus (COVID-19) Dashboard with Vaccination Data. Available online: https://covid19.who.int/ (accessed on 5 March 2023).
3. Fricke-Galindo, I.; Falfán-Valencia, R. Genetics Insight for COVID-19 Susceptibility and Severity: A Review. *Front. Immunol.* **2021**, *12*, 622176. [CrossRef]
4. Zhang, J.; Xiao, T.; Cai, Y.; Chen, B. Structure of SARS-CoV-2 spike protein. *Curr. Opin. Virol.* **2021**, *50*, 173–182. Available online: https://pubmed.ncbi.nlm.nih.gov/34534731/ (accessed on 1 May 2023). [CrossRef]
5. Scialo, F.; Daniele, A.; Amato, F.; Pastore, L.; Matera, M.G.; Cazzola, M.; Castaldo, G.; Bianco, A. ACE2: The Major Cell Entry Receptor for SARS-CoV-2. *Lung* **2020**, *198*, 867–877. Available online: https://pubmed.ncbi.nlm.nih.gov/33170317/ (accessed on 1 May 2023). [CrossRef]
6. Radzikowska, U.; Ding, M.; Tan, G.; Zhakparov, D.; Peng, Y.; Wawrzyniak, P.; Wang, M.; Li, S.; Morita, H.; Altunbulakli, C.; et al. Distribution of ACE2, CD147, CD26, and other SARS-CoV-2 associated molecules in tissues and immune cells in health and in asthma, COPD, obesity, hypertension, and COVID-19 risk factors. *Allergy* **2020**, *75*, 2829. [CrossRef]
7. Asgari, R.; Vaisi-Raygani, A.; Aleagha, M.S.E.; Mohammadi, P.; Bakhtiari, M.; Arghiani, N. CD147 and MMPs as key factors in physiological and pathological processes. *Biomed. Pharmacother.* **2023**, *157*, 113983. [CrossRef]
8. Fridley, B.L.; Biernacka, J.M. Gene set analysis of SNP data: Benefits, challenges, and future directions. *Eur. J. Hum. Genet.* **2011**, *19*, 837. [CrossRef]
9. Li, Y.; Wei, L.; He, L.; Sun, J.; Liu, N. Interferon-induced transmembrane protein 3 gene polymorphisms are associated with COVID-19 susceptibility and severity: A meta-analysis. *J. Infect.* **2022**, *84*, 825–833. [CrossRef]
10. Martínez-Gómez, L.E.; Herrera-López, B.; Martinez-Armenta, C.; Ortega-Peña, S.; Camacho-Rea, M.d.C.; Suarez-Ahedo, C.; Vázquez-Cárdenas, P.; Vargas-Alarcón, G.; Rojas-Velasco, G.; Fragoso, J.M.; et al. ACE and ACE2 Gene Variants Are Associated With Severe Outcomes of COVID-19 in Men. *Front. Immunol.* **2022**, *13*, 812940. [CrossRef]

11. Posadas-Sánchez, R.; Fragoso, J.M.; Sánchez-Muñoz, F.; Rojas-Velasco, G.; Ramírez-Bello, J.; López-Reyes, A.; Martínez-Gómez, L.E.; Sierra-Fernández, C.; Rodríguez-Reyna, T.; Regino-Zamarripa, N.E.; et al. Association of the Transmembrane Serine Protease-2 (TMPRSS2) Polymorphisms with COVID-19. *Viruses* **2022**, *14*, 1976. [CrossRef]

12. Kaidashev, I.; Izmailova, O.; Shlykova, O.; Kabaliei, A.; Vatsenko, A.; Ivashchenko, D.; Dudchenko, M.; Volianskyi, A.; Zelinskyy, G.; Koval, T.; et al. Polymorphism of tmprss2 (rs12329760) but not ace2 (rs4240157), tmprss11a (rs353163) and cd147 (rs8259) is associated with the severity of COVID-19 in the Ukrainian population. *Acta Bio. Medica. Atenei Parm.* **2023**, *94*, e2023030. [CrossRef]

13. Behl, T.; Kaur, I.; Aleya, L.; Sehgal, A.; Singh, S.; Sharma, N.; Bhatia, S.; Al-Harrasi, A.; Bungau, S. CD147-spike protein interaction in COVID-19: Get the ball rolling with a novel receptor and therapeutic target. *Sci. Total Environ.* **2022**, *808*, 152072–152072. [CrossRef] [PubMed]

14. Laboratory Testing for Coronavirus Disease (COVID-19) in Suspected Human Cases. Available online: https://apps.who.int/iris/handle/10665/331501 (accessed on 18 May 2023).

15. Wang, K.; Chen, W.; Zhang, Z.; Deng, Y.; Lian, J.Q.; Du, P.; Wei, D.; Zhang, Y.; Sun, X.-X.; Gong, L.; et al. CD147-spike protein is a novel route for SARS-CoV-2 infection to host cells. *Signal Transduct. Target. Ther.* **2020**, *5*, 283. [CrossRef] [PubMed]

16. Chen, Z.; Mi, L.; Xu, J.; Yu, J.; Wang, X.; Jiang, J.; Xing, J.; Shang, P.; Qian, A.; Li, Y.; et al. Function of HAb18G/CD147 in Invasion of Host Cells by Severe Acute Respiratory Syndrome Coronavirus. *J. Infect. Dis.* **2005**, *191*, 755–760. [CrossRef] [PubMed]

17. Adimulam, T.; Arumugam, T.; Gokul, A.; Ramsuran, V. Genetic Variants within SARS-CoV-2 Human Receptor Genes May Contribute to Variable Disease Outcomes in Different Ethnicities. *Int. J. Mol. Sci.* **2023**, *24*, 8711. Available online: https://www.mdpi.com/1422-0067/24/10/8711/htm (accessed on 18 May 2023). [CrossRef]

18. Hashemi, S.M.A.; Thijssen, M.; Hosseini, S.Y.; Tabarraei, A.; Pourkarim, M.R.; Sarvari, J. Human gene polymorphisms and their possible impact on the clinical outcome of SARS-CoV-2 infection. *Arch. Virol.* **2021**, *166*, 2089.

19. Price, A.L.; Patterson, N.; Yu, F.; Cox, D.R.; Waliszewska, A.; McDonald, G.J.; Tandon, A.; Schirmer, C.; Neubauer, J.; Bedoya, G.; et al. A Genomewide Admixture Map for Latino Populations. *Am. J. Hum. Genet.* **2007**, *80*, 1024–1036. [CrossRef]

20. Li, M.-P.; Hu, X.-L.; Yang, Y.-L.; Zhang, Y.-J.; Zhou, J.-P.; Peng, L.-M.; Tang, J.; Chen, X.-P. Basigin rs8259 Polymorphism Confers Decreased Risk of Chronic Heart Failure in a Chinese Population. *Int. J. Environ. Res. Public Health* **2017**, *14*, 211. [CrossRef]

21. Weng, Y.; Chen, T.; Ren, J.; Lu, D.; Liu, X.; Lin, S.; Xu, C.; Lou, J.; Chen, X.; Tang, L. The Association Between Extracellular Matrix Metalloproteinase Inducer Polymorphisms and Coronary Heart Disease: A Potential Way to Predict Disease. *DNA Cell Biol.* **2020**, *39*, 244–254. [CrossRef]

22. Geng, J.; Chen, L.; Yuan, Y.; Wang, K.; Wang, Y.; Qin, C.; Wu, G.; Chen, R.; Zhang, Z.; Wei, D.; et al. CD147 antibody specifically and effectively inhibits infection and cytokine storm of SARS-CoV-2 and its variants delta, alpha, beta, and gamma. *Signal Transduct. Target. Ther.* **2021**, *6*, 347. [CrossRef]

23. Springall, R.; González-Flores, J.; García-Ávila, C.; Juárez-Vicuña, Y.; Hernández-Diazcouder, A.; Márquez-Velasco, R.; Cásares-Alvarado, S.; Sánchez-Muñoz, F.; Basilio-Gálvez, E.; Castillo-Salazar, M.; et al. Elevated Levels of Soluble CD147 are Associated with Hyperinflammation and Disease Severity in COVID-19: A Proof-of-Concept Clinical Study. *Arch. Immunol. Ther. Exp.* **2022**, *70*, 18. [CrossRef]

24. Yan, J.; Mao, Y.; Wang, C.; Wang, Z. Association Study between an SNP in CD147 and Its Expression with Acute Coronary Syndrome in a Jiangsu Chinese Population. *Medicine* **2015**, *94*, e1537. [CrossRef]

25. Wu, L.-S.; Li, F.-F.; Sun, L.-D.; Li, D.; Su, J.; Kuang, Y.-H.; Chen, G.; Chen, X.-P.; Chen, X. A miRNA-492 binding-site polymorphism in BSG (basigin) confers risk to psoriasis in Central South Chinese population. *Hum. Genet.* **2011**, *130*, 749–757. [CrossRef]

26. Mohd Zawawi, Z.; Kalyanasundram, J.; Mohd Zain, R.; Thayan, R.; Basri, D.F.; Yap, W.B. Prospective Roles of Tumor Necrosis Factor-Alpha (TNF-α) in COVID-19: Prognosis, Therapeutic and Management. *Int. J. Mol. Sci.* **2023**, *24*, 6142. [CrossRef]

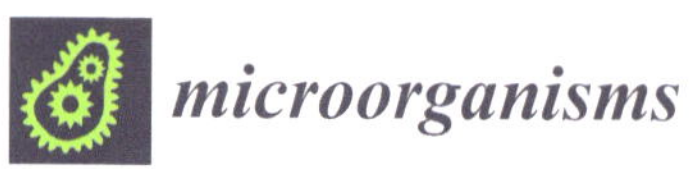 *microorganisms*

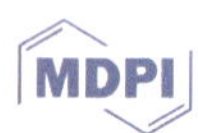

Brief Report

Increased Expression of lncRNA AC000120.7 and SENP3-EIF4A1 in Patients with Acute Respiratory Distress Syndrome Induced by SARS-CoV-2 Infection: A Pilot Study

Javier González-Ramírez [1,2,†], Ana Gabriela Leija-Montoya [3,†], Nicolás Serafín-Higuera [4], Carlos A. Guzmán-Martín [5], Luis M. Amezcua-Guerra [5], Carlos Olvera-Sandoval [3], Jesús René Machado-Contreras [3], Armando Ruiz-Hernández [3], Adrián Hernández-Díazcouder [5,6], Julia Dolores Estrada-Guzmán [3] and Fausto Sánchez-Muñoz [5,*]

[1] Facultad de Enfermería, Universidad Autónoma de Baja California, Av. Álvaro Obregón y Calle "G" S/N, Col. Nueva, Mexicali 21100, Baja California, Mexico; javier.gonzalez.ramirez@uabc.edu.mx
[2] Laboratorio de Biología Celular, Unidad de Ciencias de la Salud Campus Mexicali, Universidad Autónoma de Baja California, Calle de la Claridad S/N, Col. Plutarco Elías Calles, Mexicali 21376, Baja California, Mexico
[3] Facultad de Medicina Mexicali, Universidad Autónoma de Baja California, Dr. Humberto Torres Sanginés S/N, Centro Cívico, Mexicali 21000, Baja California, Mexico; gabriela.leija@uabc.edu.mx (A.G.L.-M.); olvera.carlos@uabc.edu.mx (C.O.-S.); rene.machado@uabc.edu.mx (J.R.M.-C.); armando.ruiz.hernandez@uabc.edu.mx (A.R.-H.); juliaestrada@uabc.edu.mx (J.D.E.-G.)
[4] Facultad de Odontología, Universidad Autónoma de Baja California, Zotoluca S/N, Fracc. Calafia, Mexicali 21040, Baja California, Mexico; nserafin@uabc.edu.mx
[5] Departamento de Inmunología, Instituto Nacional de Cardiología Ignacio Chávez, Juan Badiano No. 1, Col. Sección XVI, Tlalpan, Mexico City 14080, Mexico; gmcarlos93@gmail.com (C.A.G.-M.); lmamezcuag@gmail.com (L.M.A.-G.); adrian.hernandez.diazc@hotmail.com (A.H.-D.)
[6] Laboratorio de Investigación en Obesidad y Asma, Hospital Infantil de México Federico Gómez, Calle Doctor Márquez 162, Cuauhtémoc, Mexico City 06720, Mexico
[*] Correspondence: fausto22@yahoo.com; Tel.: +52-5523328417
[†] These authors contributed equally to this work.

Citation: González-Ramírez, J.; Leija-Montoya, A.G.; Serafín-Higuera, N.; Guzmán-Martín, C.A.; Amezcua-Guerra, L.M.; Olvera-Sandoval, C.; Machado-Contreras, J.R.; Ruiz-Hernández, A.; Hernández-Díazcouder, A.; Estrada-Guzmán, J.D.; et al. Increased Expression of lncRNA AC000120.7 and SENP3-EIF4A1 in Patients with Acute Respiratory Distress Syndrome Induced by SARS-CoV-2 Infection: A Pilot Study. *Microorganisms* 2023, 11, 2342. https://doi.org/10.3390/microorganisms11092342

Academic Editor: Qibin Geng

Received: 9 August 2023
Revised: 16 September 2023
Accepted: 17 September 2023
Published: 19 September 2023

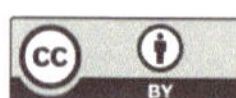

Abstract: COVID-19, a disease caused by the SARS-CoV-2 virus, poses significant threats to the respiratory system and other vital organs. Long non-coding RNAs have emerged as influential epigenetic regulators and promising biomarkers in respiratory ailments. The objective of this study was to identify candidate lncRNAs in SARS-CoV-2-positive individuals compared to SARS-CoV-2-negative individuals and investigate their potential association with ARDS-CoV-2 (acute respiratory distress syndrome). Employing qRT-PCR, we meticulously examined the expression profiles of a panel comprising 84 inflammation-related lncRNAs in individuals presenting upper respiratory infection symptoms, categorizing them into those testing negative or positive for SARS-CoV-2. Notably, first-phase PSD individuals exhibited significantly elevated levels of AC000120.7 and SENP3-EIF4A1. In addition, we measured the expression of two lncRNAs, AC000120.7 and SENP3-EIF4A1, in patients with ARDS unrelated to SARS-CoV-2 ($n = 5$) and patients with ARDS induced by SARS-CoV-2 (ARDS-CoV-2, $n = 10$), and interestingly, expression was also higher among patients with ARDS. Intriguingly, our interaction pathway analysis unveiled potential interactions between lncRNA AC000120.7, various microRNAs, and genes associated with inflammation. This study found higher expression levels of lncRNAs AC000120.7 and SENP3-EIF4A1 in the context of infection-positive COVID-19, particularly within the complex landscape of ARDS.

Keywords: COVID-19; SARS-CoV-2; long non-coding RNA; acute respiratory distress syndrome

1. Introduction

In December 2019, an outbreak of severe pneumonia caused by a novel coronavirus was identified, leading to the recognition of severe acute respiratory syndrome coronavirus 2 (SARS-CoV-2) as the causative agent of coronavirus disease 2019 (COVID-19) [1]. While most patients with COVID-19 experience mild symptoms, many patients may develop severe disease. Diagnostic considerations of COVID-19 include recent-onset fever and upper or lower respiratory infection symptoms [2,3]. To confirm the diagnosis, testing for SARS-CoV-2 in samples from the upper respiratory tract using PCR is essential [4]. Early onset of dyspnea and hypoxemia may lead to severe forms of COVID-19, which are associated with the development of acute respiratory distress syndrome (ARDS). These patients face a high mortality rate due to shock, thrombosis, and multiple organ dysfunction [5,6].

Long non-coding RNAs (lncRNAs) are transcripts that exceed 200 nucleotides in length and lack protein-coding capacity [7]. LncRNAs exhibit significant heterogeneity and possess remarkable functional adaptability. They can adapt to different molecular structures and establish distinct molecular interactions [8]. LncRNAs are involved in transcriptional regulation and RNA processing, functioning as "molecular decoys" for microRNAs (miRNAs), serving as "scaffolds" for proteins, and even as precursors for miRNAs [9]. These lncRNAs have emerged as promising targets for clinical and therapeutic research [10]. SARS-CoV-2 studies have shown an association between lncRNA expression patterns and the severity of infection [11]. However, the number of studies exploring this relationship remains low, highlighting a knowledge gap that needs to be addressed [12]. Therefore, the aim of this study was to identify potential candidate lncRNAs in individuals with a confirmed SARS-CoV-2 diagnosis in comparison to those who tested negative for the virus. Additionally, we sought to explore the potential associations between the expression of these lncRNAs and the development of ARDS.

2. Materials and Methods

2.1. Ethics Statement

The study protocol received approval from the Ethics Committee of the Faculty of Medicine of Mexicali, with registration number FMM/CEI-FMM/003/2021-1. Prior to their inclusion in the study, all participants provided written informed consent. For the second phase of the study, the patients were required to sign an informed consent form upon their hospital admission. This phase was conducted at the Ignacio Chávez National Institute of Cardiology, located in Mexico City, Mexico. The study was approved by the local ethics committee, under project number 20-1186. All procedures were carried out in accordance with the 2013 Declaration of Helsinki, its addenda, and local regulations.

2.2. Subjects

We conducted a two-phase investigation: In the initial phase, we recruited a total of six patients with upper respiratory infection symptoms from the COVID-19 Diagnosis Center of the Faculty of Medicine Mexicali UABC. Among them, three patients tested negative for SARS-CoV-2 diagnosis (NSD), and three tested positive for SARS-CoV-2 diagnosis (PSD), through RT-PCR. Inclusion criteria: The participants enrolled in this study were individuals seeking evaluation at the COVID-19 Diagnostic Center of the Mexicali School of Medicine, presenting with at least one characteristic symptom of SARS-CoV-2 infection, including but not limited to cough, fever, headache, myalgia, and arthralgia. Eligible participants fell within the age range of 20 to 60 years, with no gender restrictions. Exclusion criteria: Excluded from the study were individuals who were pregnant, asymptomatic individuals, those currently undergoing antiviral treatment, or samples that were deemed to be in suboptimal condition or poorly preserved. Elimination criteria: Samples with insufficient volume, low leukocyte recovery, evidence of RNA degradation, improper storage conditions, or sample contamination were subject to elimination from the study.

Biological specimens were collected from unvaccinated individuals. Nasopharyngeal samples were obtained using swabs, while peripheral blood samples were collected and stored in EDTA tubes. The samples were promptly refrigerated between 4 and 8 °C until use.

The second phase of the study was conducted at the Ignacio Chávez National Institute of Cardiology in Mexico City, Mexico. In this phase, we recruited a total of 15 patients from the intensive care unit, all of whom had been diagnosed with ARDS. Among these patients, five had ARDS unrelated to SARS-CoV-2 (ARDS), while the remaining ten were diagnosed with ARDS caused by SARS-CoV-2 (ARDSCoV-2). The inclusion criteria were as follows: confirmed diagnosis of COVID-19 based on a positive PCR test for SARS-CoV-2 for the ARDS-CoV-2 group and at least 2 negative PCR tests for SARS-CoV-2 for the ARDS group without COVID-19; patients over 18 years old admitted to the intensive care unit (ICU) at Ignacio Chávez National Institute of Cardiology for the treatment of severe acute respiratory distress syndrome. Exclusion criteria: if patients or their legally authorized representatives refused to provide informed consent for participation in the study.

2.3. SARS-CoV-2 Detection in the NSD and PSD Groups

The extraction of viral RNA in nasopharyngeal swab samples was performed using the Quick RNA MiniPrep Kit (Zymo Research, Irvine, CA, USA), following the supplier's instructions. RT-qPCR was performed using the protocol published by the US Centers for Disease Control and Prevention (CDC), Atlanta (CDC 2019-nCoV Real-Time RT-PCR Diagnostic Panel), which detects SARS-CoV-2-specific gene fragments, and the human RNase P housekeeping gene was determined as an extraction control.

The qRT-PCR reaction was performed on a CFX96 (Bio-Rad, Hercules, CA, USA) with the SuperScript™ III One-Step RT-PCR System and Platinum™ Taq DNA Polymerase kits (Thermo Fisher, Waltham, MA, USA), along with specific primers and probes for SARS-CoV-2 as described above. The thermocycling conditions were RT at 55 °C for 10 min, inactivation at 95 °C for 2 min, denaturation at 95 °C for 5 s, amplification at 60 °C for 30 s, and the last two steps were repeated for 45 cycles.

2.4. Isolation of Leukocytes in the NSD and PSD Groups

Samples of blood were collected and dispensed in KEDTA tubes (Becton Dickinson, Franklin Lakes, NJ, USA). Erythrocytes from blood were lysed using an ACK (ammonium–chloride–potassium) lysing buffer. The tubes were mixed (8 inversions) and incubated for 3–5 h at 4 °C until processing. Then, 0.8 mL of whole blood was mixed with 14 mL of ACK lysing buffer at room temperature and incubated for 8 min. After centrifugation at $300 \times g$ for 5 min at room temperature, the supernatant was collected. The pellet was washed twice with 5 mL of phosphate-buffered saline and centrifuged at 4 °C. White blood cell samples were mixed with 1 mL of TRIzol reagent (Invitrogen, Waltham, MA, USA), followed by storage at −20 °C until processing.

2.5. Total RNA Isolation and cDNA Synthesis in the NSD and PSD Groups

Total RNA was extracted from leukocytes by the Tripure method, following the manufacturer's protocol (Roche; Basel, Switzerland). The RNA obtained from each sample was quantified using a nanophotometer to ensure accurate measurements. The quality of the RNA was assessed by determining the 260/280 nm absorbance ratio for each RNA sample, which was consistently recorded as 1.9 ± 0.2. The RNA isolated from leukocytes was immediately converted to cDNA, as described below.

2.6. cDNA Synthesis and qRT-PCR Analysis in the NSD and PSD Groups

The synthesis of cDNA was performed using 1 μg of total RNA with an RT2 First Strand Kit (QIAGEN, Hilden, Germany). The cDNA manufacturing protocol included a treatment to avoid DNA carryover (DNase I for 30 min at 42 °C), and it was performed according to the manufacturer's instructions. The qRT-PCR was performed using RT2 SYBR® Green qPCR Master Mix (Qiagen; Hilden, Germany). The reaction (25 μL) was placed into the wells of the QIAGEN Inflammatory Responses RT2 lncRNA PCR array kit (Qiagen; Hilden, Germany), which contains the pairs of specific, predesigned, and laboratory-verified oligonucleotides. The lncRNA expression levels were normalized to those of the internal control RN7SK. Values are the means $\pm$ SE. The relative expression values were tested with an unpaired *t*-test (* $p < 0.05$).

2.7. Total RNA Isolation in the ARDS and ARDS-CoV-2 Groups

Total RNA was extracted from total blood by the Tripure method, following the manufacturer's protocol (Roche; Basel, Switzerland). To remove any DNA contamination, the isolated RNA was treated with DNase (Thermo Fisher Scientific, Waltham, MA, USA). The quality and purity of the RNA were assessed by determining the 260/280 nm absorbance ratio for each RNA sample, using a nanophotometer. The isolated RNA was immediately used for RT-qPCR.

2.8. RT-qPCR Analysis in the ARDS and ARDS-CoV-2 Groups

LncRNAs were determined using one-step RT-qPCR with the RT 2 lncRNA qPCR assay for AC000120.7 (Qiagen catalog number: LPH15155A-200, NCBI Entrez Gene: ENST00000414227) and SENP3-EIF4A1 (Qiagen catalog number: LPH24757A-200, NCBI Entrez Gene: ENST00000579777) (Qiagen; Hilden, Germany). Each one-step RT-qPCR reaction used 90 ng of total RNA that had been isolated following the manufacturer's protocol (Qiagen; Hilden, Germany). The one-step RT-qPCR reaction program consisted of 10 min at 50 °C for reverse transcription and 2 min at 95 °C for initial PCR activation, followed by 40 cycles at 95 °C for 5 s and 60 °C at 10 s. PCR was performed using a CFX96 system (Bio-Rad; CA, USA). The lncRNAs' relative concentrations were normalized with Ct values of GAPDH (primer L: AGCCACATCGCTCAGACAC, primer R: GCCCAATAC-GACCAAATCC), and the values were calculated using the $2^{-\Delta Ct}$ formula.

2.9. Statistical Analysis

Statistical analyses were performed using SPSS v26.0 software (SPSS Inc., Chicago, IL, USA) for all quantitative data, while GraphPad Prism v9 software was employed for data visualization. Quantitative variables were presented as either medians with interquartile ranges (IQRs) or means with standard deviations, depending on the nature of the data, while qualitative data were expressed as frequencies and percentages. In the first phase, differences in lncRNA expression were assessed using Welch's test. In the second phase, the Mann–Whitney U test was utilized. A *p*-value of less than 0.05 was considered statistically significant.

2.10. Pathway Network Interaction Analysis

We constructed an interaction map of the lncRNA pathways, focusing on the predicted interactions of lncRNAs AC000120.7 and SENP3-EIF4A1 with various microRNAs and genes. These interactions were established through base-pairing interactions sourced from reputable databases: miRnet.ca (https://www.mirnet.ca/. Accessed on: 5 July 2023), the RNA interactome Database (https://www.rna-society.org/rnainter/, Accessed on: 5 July 2023), RNAcentral (https://rnacentral.org/ Accessed on: 5 July 2023; https://diana.e-ce.uth.gr/lncbasev3. Accessed on: 5 July 2023), LNCipedia (https://lncipedia.org/. Accessed on: 5 July 2023), and LncRRIsearch (http://rtools.cbrc.jp/LncRRIsearch/. Accessed on: 5 July 2023). Network analysis was performed by integrating all of the information with Cytoscape 3.9.1. These interactions can be seen in Figure 1a. Furthermore, we conducted enrichment analysis using the bioinformatics tool DAVID Bioinformatics Resources (https://david.ncifcrf.gov/. Accessed on: 6 July 2023) to identify and explore the implicated pathways.

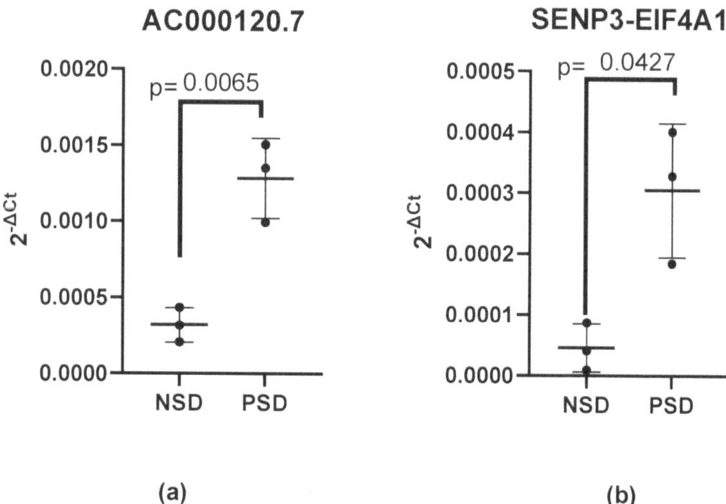

Figure 1. (**a**) AC000120.7 and (**b**) SENP3-EIF4A1 expression levels in leukocytes of patients: NSD (negative for SARS-CoV-2) and PSD (positive for SARS-CoV-2). The lncRNAs' expression levels were normalized to those of the internal control RNA component of 7SK nuclear ribonucleoprotein (RN7SK). Values are the means ± SE. The relative expression values were tested with unpaired *t*-tests.

3. Results

A two-phase pilot study was conducted; in the first phase, three NSD and three PSD patients with flu-like symptoms participated. Their characterization and main symptomatology are shown in Table 1.

Table 1. Clinical characteristics of patients with upper respiratory infection symptoms who were negative (NSD) or positive (PSD) for SARS-CoV-2 infection according to RT-PCR.

RT-PCR Positive or Negative Cases		NSD			PSD		
General	Female	x	x	x		x	x
	Male				x		
	Age	54	25	29	45	54	23
Symptoms	Sudden onset of symptoms						
	Fever	x		x			
	Cough	x	x	x	x	x	
	Headache	x		x	x	x	x
	Dyspnea	x				x	
	Irritability		x	x		x	x
	Diarrhea		x	x			
	Chest pain		x			x	
	Chills			x		x	
	Odynophagia	x		x			
	Myalgia	x		x	x	x	
	Arthralgia	x		x		x	x
	Malaise	x		x	x	x	
	Rhinorrhea	x		x			x
	Abdominal pain	x		x			
	Anosmia						x
Comorbidities	Hypertension	x					
	Smoking						x
Treatment	Antipyretics			x	x	x	x
Epidemiological history	Contact with influenza or COVID-19 cases in the last 2 weeks		x				x

NSD (negative for SARS-CoV-2 diagnosis) and PSD (positive for SARS-CoV-2 diagnosis).

In first phase, a comprehensive analysis was conducted on a set of 84 genes associated with the human inflammatory response. The results revealed elevated expression levels of lncRNA AC000120.7 (means: 0.001284 vs. 0.0003186, 95% CI: 0.0004081 to 0.001523, effect size: 4.764, actual statistical power: 0.987, p = 0.0130) and SENP3-EIF4A1 (means: 0.0003047 vs. 4.546×10^{-5}, 95% CI: 1.787×10^{-5} to 0.0005007, effect size: 3.133, actual statistical power: 0.814, p = 0.0427) in patients with PSD as compared to those with NSD, respectively (Figure 1a,b).

In the second phase of the study, it was observed that higher expression of AC000120.7 (median: 0.02860, 95% CI: 0.01911 to 0.03533 vs. 0.01097, 95% CI: 0.003105 to 0.02078, effect size: 1.6139, actual power: 0.9636142, p = 0.0280) and SENP3-EIF4A1 (median: 0.01065, 95% CI: 0.006911 to 0.01781 vs. 0.003380, 95% CI: −0.001671 to 0.01220, effect size: 1.062352, actual power: 0.9506665, p = 0.0400) remained in patients diagnosed with ARDS-CoV-2 compared to patients with ARDS (Figure 2a,b). The main features of the patients are presented in Table 2.

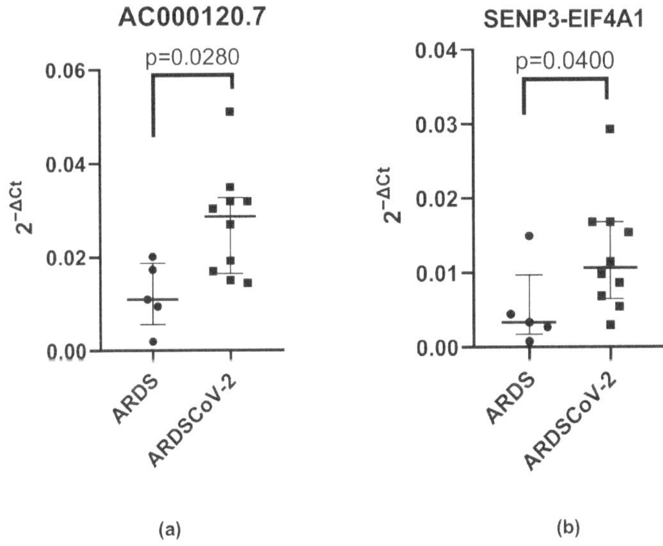

Figure 2. (**a**) AC000120.7 and (**b**) SENP3-EIF4A1 expression levels in the blood of patients with ARDS (acute respiratory distress syndrome not caused by SARS-CoV-2) and ARDS-CoV-2 (patients with acute respiratory distress syndrome caused by SARS-CoV-2). The relative expression values were tested with the Mann–Whitney test.

Table 2. Main clinical and demographic data of patients with acute respiratory distress syndrome, either positive or negative for SARS-CoV-2 infection.

	Negative for COVID-19 (n = 5)	Positive for COVID-19 (n = 10)
Age, years	64 (53.5–67)	64 (52.5–72.7)
Female, n (%)	2 (40)	4 (40)
Male, n (%)	3 (60)	6 (60)
Invasive mechanical ventilation	3 (60)	3 (30)
Death (%)	2 (40)	2 (20)
Diabetes (%)	1 (20)	3 (30)
Systemic hypertension	3 (60)	5 (50)

Data are expressed as medians with interquartile ranges for quantitative variables, and as frequencies and percentages for qualitative variables.

Finally, utilizing the bioinformatics tool miRNet 2.0 (available at https://www.mirnet. ca/. Accessed on: 5 July 2023), we constructed an interaction pathway that unveiled predicted interactions involving lncRNA AC000120.7 (also called KRIT1) with various miRNAs and genes. Notably, within this pathway, we observed the presence of several genes associated with inflammation and COVID-19 that have been previously identified by other researchers, including IL-6, basigin, and MMP9 (Figure 3).

(a)

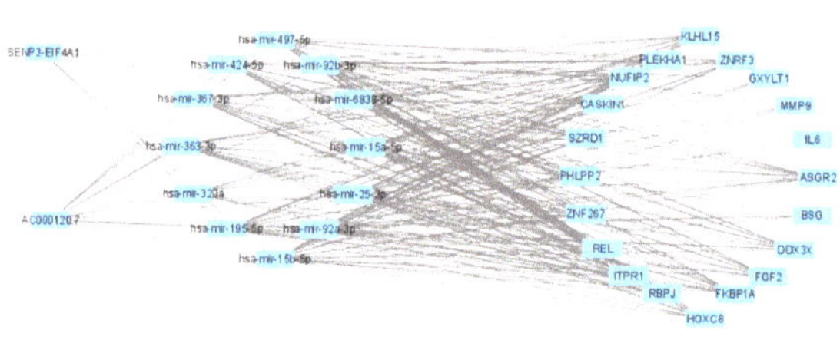

(b)

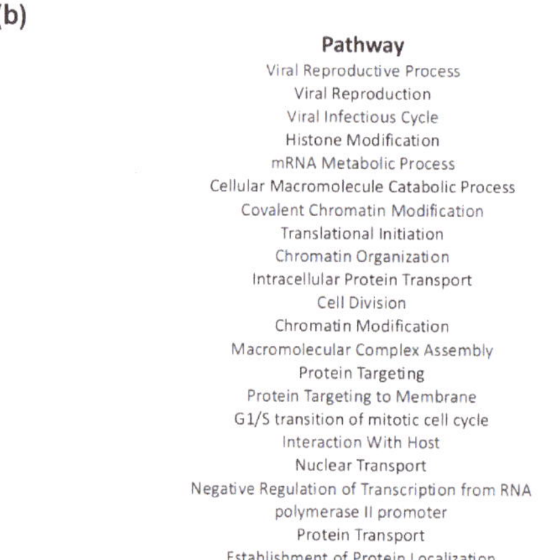

Figure 3. Bioinformatics analysis: (**a**) Interaction pathway with the predicted interactions of lncRNAs AC000120.7 and SENP-EIF4A1 with diverse microRNAs and genes; interestingly, we can appreciate some inflammation-related COVID-19 genes previously described by other authors, such as IL-6, basigin, and MMP9. (**b**) Enrichment analysis of the interaction network, in which several viral pathways are implicated.

4. Discussion

In this pilot study, our aim was to assess the expression levels of inflammation-related lncRNAs in leukocyte samples obtained from both SARS-CoV-2-positive and SARS-CoV-2-negative patients, especially in those with acute respiratory distress syndrome, through qRT-PCR. Interestingly, we observed elevated expression levels of lncRNAs AC000120.7 and SENP3-EIF4A1 in PSD patients compared to NSD patients. Likewise, we observed that association with SARS-CoV-2 infection persisted in the subsequent study involving patients with ARDS. Additionally, a bioinformatics analysis identified the interaction of these lncRNAs with various miRNAs and genes, including inflammation- and COVID-19-associated genes like IL-6, basigin, and MMP9.

To the best of our knowledge, this is the first study examining the expression profile of inflammatory lncRNAs in leukocytes of SARS-CoV-2 patients Prior investigations have primarily centered on the analysis of lncRNAs within peripheral blood mononuclear cells (PBMCs) and whole blood. Notably, two of these prior studies utilized in silico methodologies, employing bioinformatics approaches to explore lncRNAs as potential candidates involved in various adverse reactions associated with COVID-19 [13,14]. In contrast, another study conducted a comprehensive transcriptional analysis of lncRNAs using RNA-Seq on PBMC samples from COVID-19 patients, albeit without subsequent qRT-PCR validation [15]. It is intriguing to note that significant differences in the expression levels of lncRNAs AC000120.7 and SENP3-EIF4A1, as observed in our study, were not reported in these prior investigations. Possible contributors to this discrepancy may encompass methodological disparities, including variations in PBMC acquisition techniques [16,17].

Due to the lack of information in the literature about long non-coding RNAs AC000120.7 and SENP3-EIF4A1, we searched a variety of databases, such as NCBI (https://www.ncbi.nlm.nih.gov/. Accessed on: 5 July 2023), the RNA Interactome Database (https://www.rna-society.org/rnainter/. Accessed on: 5 July 2023), RNA Central (https://rnacentral.org/ Accessed on: 5 July 2023; https://diana.e-ce.uth.gr/lncbasev3. Accessed on: 5 July 2023), LNCipedia (https://lncipedia.org/. Accessed on: 5 July 2023), and LncRRIsearch (http://rtools.cbrc.jp/LncRRIsearch/. Accessed on: 5 July 2023), looking for diverse aliases for those long non-coding RNAs. Consequently, through the bioinformatics tool miRNet 2.0 (https://www.mirnet.ca/. Accessed on: 5 July 2023), we created an interaction pathway with the predicted interactions of lncRNAs AC000120.7 (KRIT1) and SENP3-EIF4A1 with diverse microRNAs and genes. Notably, our observations unveiled the presence of a range of genes linked to inflammation and COVID-19, such as IL-6, basigin, and MMP9. This discovery aligns with the extensive exploration by various researchers into the role of cytokines in the pathophysiology of COVID-19 infection [18,19]. Furthermore, a study conducted by Springall and collaborators revealed an intriguing association of IL-6, MMP9, and other cytokines with CD147, a molecule proposed as a potential entry point for the host receptor in COVID-19 [20].

AC000120.7 is an lncRNA that exhibits increased expression in PSD patients compared to NSD patients. Upon investigating its potential functionality, we observed that AC000120.7 overlaps with the sense strand of the gene encoding the KRIT1 protein [21]. However, since this strand is in the sense orientation, it is unlikely to harm mRNA or protein production. Notably, this lncRNA has also been reported in another inflammatory condition, periodontitis, although the specific molecular mechanisms underlying its involvement in periodontitis have yet to be described [22].

SENP3-EIF4A1 is an lncRNA located on chromosome 17's p-arm at position 13.1 [20]. Previous studies have linked this lncRNA to hepatocellular carcinoma, suggesting its potential as a diagnostic biomarker for this disease [23]. In addition, it has been described that SENP3-EIF4A1 inhibits the activity of miR-195-5p, as a negative correlation has been observed between miR-195-5p and SENP3-EIF4A1 [24]. Interestingly, this interaction can be observed in our interaction pathway image (Figure 1). The significance of its interaction with miR-195-5p in our results stems from the fact that this miRNA negatively regulates the expression of inflammatory factors, such as vascular endothelial growth factor A (VEGFA) [25]. VEGFA contributes to increased vascular permeability during various stages of inflammation [26], and its presence has been associated with the development of neurological symptoms in COVID-19 patients. VEGF also facilitates the recruitment of inflammatory cells and has been identified as a promising therapeutic target for suppressing inflammation during SARS-CoV-2 infection with neurological symptoms [27]. On the other hand, miR-195 has been implicated in macrophage polarization within the cardiovascular system. It inhibits the mediators of the TLR2 inflammatory pathway and affects the recruitment capacity and migration profile of smooth muscle cells [28]. Notably, COVID-19 is associated with cardiovascular manifestations, such as myocardial injury and arrhythmias. Some patients, especially those without the typical symptoms of fever or cough, may present with cardiac symptoms as the initial clinical manifestation of COVID-19. However, the etiology of heart failure in COVID-19 can arise from factors such as hypoxia, cytokine release, volume overload, renal failure, stress, or critical illness. Furthermore, underlying subclinical heart failure may be uncovered or exacerbated by SARS-CoV-2 infection [29]. Another important aspect to consider is the potential impact of SENP3-EIF4A1 blocking the activity of miR-195-5p. Rat models have demonstrated that when miR-195-5p is overexpressed in vitro and in vivo, there is a significant reduction in the production of pro-inflammatory cytokines in pulmonary macrophages in rats with obstructive pulmonary disease [30]. Finally, the impact of SENP3-EIF4A1 in inhibiting miR-195-5p, along with its subsequent effects on the inhibition of inflammatory factors such as VEGFA, the modulation of the TLR2 inflammatory pathway, and the potential attenuation of pro-inflammatory cytokine production in COVID-19, remain areas that require further investigation.

In the context of COVID-19 infection, our results add to the knowledge that has shown lncRNAs to exhibit potential roles in immune evasion, modulation of cytokine storms, and the regulation of both innate and adaptive immune responses [31]. They may contribute to immune evasion by interfering with crucial immune pathways, possibly binding to the viral genome and, thus, affecting viral replication [17,32]. Moreover, certain lncRNAs enhance innate immune activation and inflammatory responses, such as lnc02384, which promotes IFN-γ synthesis. Additionally, lncRNAs like NORAD, RAD51-AS1, GAS5, NEAT1, and MALAT1 appear to regulate cytokine and chemokine expression, contributing to cytokine storms [11]. While these findings offer insights into lncRNAs' roles in SARS-CoV-2 infection, further research is required to uncover precise mechanisms. Understanding these mechanisms could have vital implications for antiviral therapies and managing immune responses in COVID-19 patients.

This study presents some limitations that need to be acknowledged. Firstly, the sample size in this research was relatively small, which may limit the generalizability of the results. Although we aimed to compensate for this limitation by conducting a comprehensive analysis of a panel of inflammation-related lncRNAs, the small sample size remained a constraint. Secondly, in this pilot study, our primary objective was to investigate the differences in lncRNA expression between these two specific patient groups, but the absence of a control group consisting of healthy individuals was a limitation. The inclusion of healthy controls would have provided valuable baseline data for the expression levels of the studied lncRNAs and enabled a clearer distinction between individuals with SARS-CoV-2 infection and those without. However, we consider that our data are important because this is the first time that the expression of lncRNAs has been compared between two entities where similarities and differences are both recognized.

We hold the belief that our discoveries possess a provocative essence and will act as a catalyst for forthcoming research initiatives. These studies should primarily focus on validating our results across diverse population groups, utilizing a combination of qRT-PCR, RNA-Seq, and/or in situ hybridization techniques. Furthermore, these investigations should delve more profoundly into unraveling the intricate molecular mechanisms governed by these lncRNAs within the context of SARS-CoV-2 infection. Specifically, the study of lncRNAs holds promise for advancing our future understanding of coronaviruses.

5. Conclusions

In conclusion, this study sheds light on the potential roles of lncRNAs AC000120.7 and SENP3-EIF4A1 as candidate biomarkers of COVID-19, particularly in the context of ARDS. We observed elevated expression levels of these lncRNAs in SARS-CoV-2-positive individuals, indicating their potential relevance in the pathogenesis of the disease. However, further functional studies are needed to elucidate their precise roles in COVID-19 and ARDS. Additionally, our findings underscore the importance of considering lncRNAs as potential diagnostic and therapeutic targets in respiratory diseases. Furthermore, validating these lncRNAs' roles and exploring their clinical applications could have significant implications for the management and treatment of COVID-19 and related respiratory conditions.

Author Contributions: Conceptualization: J.G.-R., A.G.L.-M., F.S.-M., C.A.G.-M., N.S.-H., L.M.A.-G., C.O.-S. and J.R.M.-C.; methodology, formal analysis, and investigation: J.G.-R., A.G.L.-M., F.S.-M., N.S.-H., C.A.G.-M., L.M.A.-G., A.R.-H., C.O.-S., A.H.-D., J.R.M.-C. and J.D.E.-G.; writing—original draft preparation: J.G.-R., A.G.L.-M., F.S.-M., C.A.G.-M., L.M.A.-G. and N.S.-H.; funding acquisition: J.G.-R., A.G.L.-M., F.S.-M., N.S.-H., C.O.-S., J.R.M.-C. and J.D.E.-G.; supervision: F.S.-M., J.G.-R., A.G.L.-M., N.S.-H., C.O.-S. and J.R.M.-C.; review and editing: A.R.-H., A.H.-D., C.O.-S., J.R.M.-C. and J.D.E.-G. All authors have read and agreed to the published version of the manuscript.

Funding: We thank to Consejo Nacional de Humanidades, Ciencias y Tecnologías (CONAHCYT) for the support (Grant CF-2023-I-1400 to NSH).

Data Availability Statement: All data generated or analyzed during this study are included in this article. Further inquiries can be directed to the corresponding author.

Acknowledgments: We thank Gustavo Martínez-Coronilla for their critical review of the document.

Conflicts of Interest: The authors declare that they have no conflict of interest.

References

1. Ganesh, B.; Rajakumar, T.; Malathi, M.; Manikandan, N.; Nagaraj, J.; Santhakumar, A.; Elangovan, A.; Malik, Y.S. Epidemiology and Pathobiology of SARS-CoV-2 (COVID-19) in Comparison with SARS, MERS: An Updated Overview of Current Knowledge and Future Perspectives. *Clin. Epidemiol. Glob. Health* **2021**, *10*, 100694. [CrossRef]
2. Wiersinga, W.J.; Rhodes, A.; Cheng, A.C.; Peacock, S.J.; Prescott, H.C. Pathophysiology, Transmission, Diagnosis, and Treatment of Coronavirus Disease 2019 (COVID-19): A Review. *JAMA* **2020**, *324*, 782–793. [CrossRef]
3. Alkhathami, M.G.; Advani, S.; Al Shehri, M.K.; Abalkhail, A.; Alkhathami, F.; Al Salamah, J.A.; Albeashy, E. Prevalence and Mortality of Lung Comorbidities Among Patients with COVID-19: A Systematic Review and Meta-Analysis. *Lung India* **2021**, *38*, S31–S40. [CrossRef]
4. Mohamadian, M.; Chiti, H.; Shoghli, A.; Biglari, S.; Parsamanesh, N.; Esmaeilzadeh, A. COVID-19: Virology, Biology and Novel Laboratory Diagnosis. *J. Gene Med.* **2021**, *23*, e3303. [CrossRef]
5. Krynytska, I.; Marushchak, M.; Birchenko, I.; Dovgalyuk, A.; Tokarskyy, O. COVID-19-Associated Acute Respiratory Distress Syndrome versus Classical Acute Respiratory Distress Syndrome (a Narrative Review). *Iran. J. Microbiol.* **2021**, *13*, 737–747. [CrossRef]
6. Li, X.; Xu, S.; Yu, M.; Wang, K.; Tao, Y.; Zhou, Y.; Shi, J.; Zhou, M.; Wu, B.; Yang, Z.; et al. Risk Factors for Severity and Mortality in Adult COVID-19 Inpatients in Wuhan. *J. Allergy Clin. Immunol.* **2020**, *146*, 110–118. [CrossRef] [PubMed]
7. Chillón, I.; Marcia, M. The Molecular Structure of Long Non-Coding RNAs: Emerging Patterns and Functional Implications. *Crit. Rev. Biochem. Mol. Biol.* **2020**, *55*, 662–690. [CrossRef] [PubMed]
8. Montoya, G.L.; Ramírez, J.G.; Basilio, J.S.; Higuera, I.S.; Espinoza, M.I.; González, R.G.; Higuera, N.S. Long Non-Coding RNAs: Regulators of the Activity of Myeloid-Derived Suppressor Cells. *Front. Immunol.* **2019**, *10*, 1734. [CrossRef]
9. Mercer, T.R.; Dinger, M.E.; Mattick, J.S. Long Non-Coding RNAs: Insights into Functions. *Nat. Rev. Genet.* **2009**, *10*, 155–159. [CrossRef]
10. Guzmán-Martín, C.A.; Juárez-Vicuña, Y.; Domínguez-López, A.; González-Ramírez, J.; Amezcua-Guerra, L.M.; Martínez-Martínez, L.A.; Sánchez-Muñoz, F. LncRNAs Dysregulation in Monocytes from Primary Antiphospholipid Syndrome Patients: A Bioinformatic and an Experimental Proof-of-Concept Approach. *Mol. Biol. Rep.* **2022**, *50*, 937–941. [CrossRef] [PubMed]
11. Lin, Y.; Sun, Q.; Zhang, B.; Zhao, W.; Shen, C. The Regulation of LncRNAs and MiRNAs in SARS-CoV-2 Infection. *Front. Cell Dev. Biol.* **2023**, *11*, 1229393. [CrossRef] [PubMed]
12. Zhong, Y.; Ashley, C.L.; Steain, M.; Ataide, S.F. Assessing the Suitability of Long Non-Coding RNAs as Therapeutic Targets and Biomarkers in SARS-CoV-2 Infection. *Front. Mol. Biosci.* **2022**, *9*, 975322. [CrossRef] [PubMed]
13. Moazzam-Jazi, M.; Lanjanian, H.; Maleknia, S.; Hedayati, M.; Daneshpour, M.S. Interplay between SARS-CoV-2 and Human Long Non-Coding RNAs. *J. Cell. Mol. Med.* **2021**, *25*, 5823–5827. [CrossRef]
14. Huang, K.; Wang, C.; Vagts, C.; Raguveer, V.; Finn, P.W.; Perkins, D.L. Long Non-Coding RNAs (LncRNAs) NEAT1 and MALAT1 Are Differentially Expressed in Severe COVID-19 Patients: An Integrated Single-Cell Analysis. *PLoS ONE* **2022**, *17*, e0261242. [CrossRef] [PubMed]
15. Cheng, J.; Zhou, X.; Feng, W.; Jia, M.; Zhang, X.; An, T.; Luan, M.; Pan, Y.; Zhang, S.; Zhou, Z.; et al. Risk Stratification by Long Non-Coding RNAs Profiling in COVID-19 Patients. *J. Cell. Mol. Med.* **2021**, *25*, 4753–4764. [CrossRef]
16. Zampetaki, A.; Albrecht, A.; Steinhofel, K. Long Non-Coding RNA Structure and Function: Is There a Link? *Front. Physiol.* **2018**, *9*, 1201. [CrossRef]
17. Ouyang, J.; Hu, J.; Chen, J.L. LncRNAs Regulate the Innate Immune Response to Viral Infection. *Wiley Interdiscip. Rev. RNA* **2016**, *7*, 129–143. [CrossRef]
18. Aghamohamadi, N.; Shahba, F.; Zarezadeh Mehrabadi, A.; Khorramdelazad, H.; Karimi, M.; Falak, R.; Emameh, R.Z. Age-Dependent Immune Responses in COVID-19-Mediated Liver Injury: Focus on Cytokines. *Front. Endocrinol.* **2023**, *14*, 1139692. [CrossRef]

19. Zaira, B.; Yulianti, T.; Levita, J. Correlation between Hepatocyte Growth Factor (HGF) with D-Dimer and Interleukin-6 as Prognostic Markers of Coagulation and Inflammation in Long COVID-19 Survivors. *Curr. Issues Mol. Biol.* **2023**, *45*, 5725–5740. [CrossRef]

20. Springall, R.; González-Flores, J.; García-Ávila, C.; Juárez-Vicuña, Y.; Hernández-Diazcouder, A.; Márquez-Velasco, R.; Cásares-Alvarado, S.; Sánchez-Muñoz, F.; Basilio-Gálvez, E.; Castillo-Salazar, M.; et al. Elevated Levels of Soluble CD147 Are Associated with Hyperinflammation and Disease Severity in COVID-19: A Proof-of-Concept Clinical Study. *Arch. Immunol. Ther. Exp.* **2022**, *70*, 18. [CrossRef]

21. Zhou, M.; Wang, X.; Shi, H.; Cheng, L.; Wang, Z.; Zhao, H.; Yang, L.; Sun, J. Characterization of Long Non-Coding RNA-Associated CeRNA Network to Reveal Potential Prognostic LncRNA Biomarkers in Human Ovarian Cancer. *Oncotarget* **2016**, *7*, 12598–12611. [CrossRef] [PubMed]

22. Sánchez-Muñoz, F.; Martínez-Coronilla, G.; Leija-Montoya, A.G.; Rieke-Campoy, U.; Angelina Lopez-Carrasco, R.; de Lourdes Montaño-Pérez, M.; Beltrán-Partida, E.; Bojórquez-Anaya, Y.; Serafin-Higuera, N.; González-Ramírez, J. Periodontitis May Modulate Long-Non Coding RNA Expression. *Arch. Oral Biol.* **2018**, *95*, 95–99. [CrossRef] [PubMed]

23. Wang, K.; Chen, W.; Zhang, Z.; Deng, Y.; Lian, J.Q.; Du, P.; Wei, D.; Zhang, Y.; Sun, X.X.; Gong, L.; et al. CD147-Spike Protein Is a Novel Route for SARS-CoV-2 Infection to Host Cells. *Signal Transduct. Target. Ther.* **2020**, *5*, 283. [CrossRef] [PubMed]

24. Chen, L.; Miao, X.; Si, C.; Qin, A.; Zhang, Y.; Chu, C.; Li, Z.; Wang, T.; Liu, X. Long Non-Coding RNA SENP3-EIF4A1 Functions as a Sponge of MiR-195-5p to Drive Triple-Negative Breast Cancer Progress by Overexpressing CCNE1. *Front. Cell Dev. Biol.* **2021**, *9*, 647527. [CrossRef]

25. Xu, Y.; Jiang, W.; Zhong, L.; Li, H.; Bai, L.; Chen, X.; Lin, Y.; Zheng, D. miR-195-5p alleviates acute kidney injury through repression of inflammation and oxidative stress by targeting vascular endothelial growth factor A. *Aging* **2020**, *12*, 10235–10245. [CrossRef]

26. Lee, Y.C. The Involvement of VEGF in Endothelial Permeability: A Target for Anti-Inflammatory Therapy. *Curr. Opin. Investig. Drugs* **2005**, *6*, 1124–1130.

27. Yin, X.X.; Zheng, X.R.; Peng, W.; Wu, M.L.; Mao, X.Y.; Mao, X.Y.; Mao, X.Y.; Mao, X.Y. Vascular Endothelial Growth Factor (VEGF) as a Vital Target for Brain Inflammation during the COVID-19 Outbreak. *ACS Chem. Neurosci.* **2020**, *11*, 1704–1705. [CrossRef]

28. Bras, J.P.; Silva, A.M.; Calin, G.A.; Barbosa, M.A.; Santos, S.G.; Almeida, M.I. MiR-195 Inhibits Macrophages pro-Inflammatory Profile and Impacts the Crosstalk with Smooth Muscle Cells. *PLoS ONE* **2017**, *12*, e0188530. [CrossRef]

29. Nishiga, M.; Wang, D.W.; Han, Y.; Lewis, D.B.; Wu, J.C. COVID-19 and Cardiovascular Disease: From Basic Mechanisms to Clinical Perspectives. *Nat. Rev. Cardiol.* **2020**, *17*, 543–558. [CrossRef]

30. Li, S.; Jiang, L.; Yang, Y.; Cao, J.; Zhang, Q.; Zhang, J.; Wang, R.; Deng, X.; Li, Y. MiR-195-5p Inhibits the Development of Chronic Obstructive Pulmonary Disease via Targeting Siglec1. *Hum. Exp. Toxicol.* **2020**, *39*, 1333–1344. [CrossRef]

31. Ding, J.; Chen, J.; Yin, X.; Zhou, J. Current Understanding on Long Non-Coding RNAs in Immune Response to COVID-19. *Virus Res.* **2023**, *323*, 198956. [CrossRef] [PubMed]

32. Enguita, F.J.; Leitão, A.L.; McDonald, J.T.; Zaksas, V.; Das, S.; Galeano, D.; Taylor, D.; Wurtele, E.S.; Saravia-Butler, A.; Baylin, S.B.; et al. The Interplay between LncRNAs, RNA-Binding Proteins and Viral Genome during SARS-CoV-2 Infection Reveals Strong Connections with Regulatory Events Involved in RNA Metabolism and Immune Response. *Theranostics* **2022**, *12*, 3946–3962. [CrossRef] [PubMed]

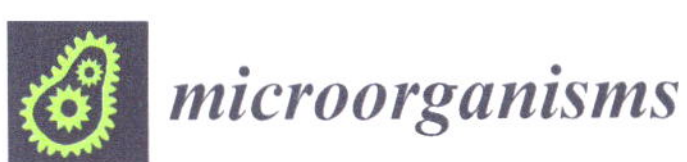

microorganisms

MDPI

Article

Type I Interferon Pathway-Related Hub Genes as a Potential Therapeutic Target for SARS-CoV-2 Omicron Variant-Induced Symptoms

Zhiwei Lin [1,†], Mingshan Xue [1,2,†], Ziman Wu [1], Ze Liu [1], Qianyue Yang [1], Jiaqing Hu [1], Jiacong Peng [1], Lin Yu [1,*] and Baoqing Sun [1,2,*]

[1] Department of Clinical Laboratory, National Center for Respiratory Medicine, National Clinical Research Center for Respiratory Disease, State Key Laboratory of Respiratory Disease, Guangzhou Institute of Respiratory Health, The First Affiliated Hospital of Guangzhou Medical University, Guangzhou 510120, China; veelin0419@stu.gzhmu.edu.cn (Z.L.)

[2] Guangzhou Laboratory, Guangzhou 510005, China

* Correspondence: yulin@gzhmu.edu.cn (L.Y.); sunbaoqing@vip.163.com (B.S.)

† Zhiwei Lin and Mingshan Xue should be regarded as co-first authors.

Abstract: Background: The global pandemic of COVID-19 is caused by the rapidly evolving severe acute respiratory syndrome coronavirus 2 (SARS-CoV-2). The clinical presentation of SARS-CoV-2 Omicron variant infection varies from asymptomatic to severe disease with diverse symptoms. However, the underlying mechanisms responsible for these symptoms remain incompletely understood. Methods: Transcriptome datasets from peripheral blood mononuclear cells (PBMCs) of COVID-19 patients infected with the Omicron variant and healthy volunteers were obtained from public databases. A comprehensive bioinformatics analysis was performed to identify hub genes associated with the Omicron variant. Hub genes were validated using quantitative RT-qPCR and clinical data. DSigDB database predicted potential therapeutic agents. Results: Seven hub genes (IFI44, IFI44L, MX1, OAS3, USP18, IFI27, and ISG15) were potential biomarkers for Omicron infection's symptomatic diagnosis and treatment. Type I interferon-related hub genes regulated Omicron-induced symptoms, which is supported by independent datasets and RT-qPCR validation. Immune cell analysis showed elevated monocytes and reduced lymphocytes in COVID-19 patients, which is consistent with retrospective clinical data. Additionally, ten potential therapeutic agents were screened for COVID-19 treatment, targeting the hub genes. Conclusions: This study provides insights into the mechanisms underlying type I interferon-related pathways in the development and recovery of COVID-19 symptoms during Omicron infection. Seven hub genes were identified as promising biological biomarkers for diagnosing and treating Omicron infection. The identified biomarkers and potential therapeutic agent offer valuable implications for Omicron's clinical manifestations and treatment strategies.

Keywords: COVID-19; SARS-CoV-2; Omicron; biomarker; type I interferon

Citation: Lin, Z.; Xue, M.; Wu, Z.; Liu, Z.; Yang, Q.; Hu, J.; Peng, J.; Yu, L.; Sun, B. Type I Interferon Pathway-Related Hub Genes as a Potential Therapeutic Target for SARS-CoV-2 Omicron Variant-Induced Symptoms. *Microorganisms* **2023**, *11*, 2101. https://doi.org/10.3390/microorganisms11082101

Academic Editors: Vittorio Sambri and Qibin Geng

Received: 14 July 2023
Revised: 2 August 2023
Accepted: 15 August 2023
Published: 17 August 2023

1. Introduction

The COVID-19 pandemic, caused by the severe acute respiratory syndrome coronavirus 2 (SARS-CoV-2), has presented an unparalleled global public health challenge. SARS-CoV-2 infection leads to a spectrum of clinical outcomes, ranging from asymptomatic cases to severe illness characterized by symptoms such as high fever, cough, fatigue, and dyspnea, ultimately leading to respiratory failure [1,2]. Since 2019, there have been more than 755 million cumulative cases of COVID-19 globally and more than 6.83 million deaths [3]. No specific antiviral therapy for the pandemic COVID-19 exists yet, particularly for the milder-seeming Omicron variant. Numerous vaccines are under development, and several previously FDA-approved drugs have been repurposed to slow the progression of COVID-19 [4].

Recent real-world studies indicate that the Omicron variant, which is currently predominant, may exhibit milder clinical manifestations compared to earlier variants, with lower hospitalization rates and shorter lengths of stay observed in certain regions [5–8]. The formation of multinucleated syncytia, reflecting cell–cell fusion during viral infection, represents a crucial pathological step in SARS-CoV-2 infection [9,10]. In vitro, assays have demonstrated the reduced formation of multinucleated syncytia by the Omicron variant compared to previous variants, along with higher cell viability [11–13]. This evidence supports the notion that the Omicron variant manifests with reduced severity compared to its predecessors. However, it is crucial to recognize that thousands of deaths continue to occur worldwide, particularly in developing countries where underreporting is common due to factors like limited testing capacity [14]. Furthermore, the highly transmissible Omicron variant continues to strain healthcare systems significantly [15,16]. Therefore, gaining a comprehensive understanding of the underlying pathogenesis of the SARS-CoV-2 Omicron variant and its association with symptomatic presentation remains a paramount research priority.

Type I interferons (IFN-I), including IFN-α and IFN-β, play a pivotal role in the pathogenesis of COVID-19, acting as crucial antiviral factors [17]. Upon activation of the JAK-STAT pathway by the IFN-I receptor complex, the inhibitory effect of type I interferon on SARS-CoV replication suggests its potential for viral clearance [18]. The timing of the IFN-I response varies, with an early response observed in mild cases and a delayed response in severe cases of COVID-19 [19,20]. Single-cell RNA analysis of peripheral blood mononuclear cells from severe COVID-19 patients has revealed up-regulation of IFN-I and other inflammatory cytokines [21]. Thus, the IFN-I pathway may contribute to symptom development, and early administration of IFN-I could potentially enhance viral clearance. A meta-analysis has supported the potential of JAK inhibitor baricitinib as a candidate drug against COVID-19 [22]. The current research on COVID-19 has extensively covered various variants' clinical manifestations and transmission dynamics, including the Omicron strain [23,24]. However, despite the prevalence of symptomatic infections caused by the Omicron variant, there still exists a gap in understanding the specific molecular mechanisms driving symptom development and potential therapeutic interventions. Unraveling this association could unveil potential therapeutic targets for Omicron-dominant COVID-19 cases [25–27].

Addressing existing gaps in the literature, this study employed various methods to investigate the uniqueness of COVID-19 infection with the Omicron variant. These methods included the analysis of gene expression datasets [28], functional annotation using bioinformatics tools, pathway analysis, and construction of protein–protein interaction networks [29–32]. The obtained results were validated using clinical samples. By applying a bioinformatics approach, this study is the first to identify differences in hub genes and pathways associated with COVID-19 symptoms. Given the heterogeneity of COVID-19 symptoms and the ongoing uncertainty regarding its pathogenesis, our findings hold significant value in contributing to the diagnosis and prognosis of COVID-19.

2. Materials and Methods

2.1. Data Collection and Differential Expression Analysis of Genes

Microarray gene expression datasets were acquired from the GEO database (accessible at https://www.ncbi.nlm.nih.gov/gds, accessed on 10 January 2023) for COVID-19 patients and their matched controls. The search in the GEO database utilized the keywords "COVID-19", "symptoms", "SARS-CoV-2", and "Omicron". The selection of the COVID-19 microarray dataset followed specific criteria, including human PBMC samples, mRNA gene expression profiles, a minimum of three samples per group, and array-based expression profiling as the study type. Three datasets, namely GSE201530, GSE179627, and GSE167930, were identified and included in this study.

The GSE201530 dataset, consisting of 39 COVID-19 patients infected with the SARS-CoV-2 Omicron variant and 8 healthy controls, was utilized for the analysis and identification of hub genes. To validate the diagnostic efficacy of the hub genes, the GSE179627 dataset was used as an independent validation set. Furthermore, the GSE167930 dataset, comprising 21 healthy controls, 7 asymptomatic infected patients, 13 symptomatic infected patients, and 15 recovering patients, was utilized to identify central genes associated with COVID-19 symptoms. A schematic representation of the study design can be found in Figure 1.

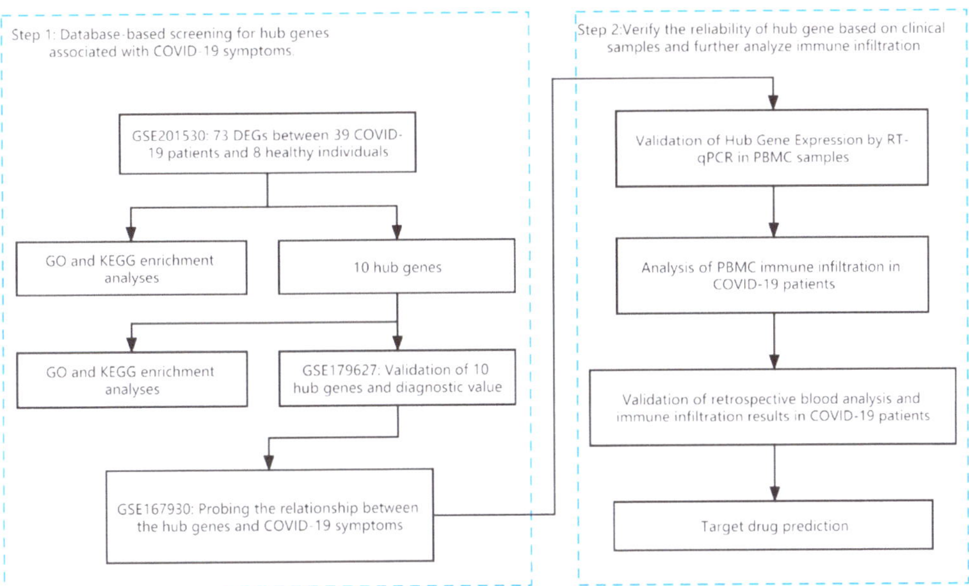

Figure 1. A visual representation of the study design.

To ensure the quality of the dataset samples, we utilized the R package "arrayQualityMetrics". Data standardization was performed using the "affy" or "limma" packages, renowned for their application in linear models for microarray data. The identification of statistically significant differentially expressed genes (DEGs) between COVID-19 and control samples in each dataset was performed using the "limma (version 3.40.6)" package in R. DEGs with adjusted p-values < 0.05 and | log2 Fold change (logFC) | > 2 were considered statistically significant. To visualize the results, volcanic and thermal maps were generated using the R packages "ggplot2 (version 3.3.6)" and "heatmap", respectively.

2.2. Functional Enrichment Analysis

Gene ontology (GO) is widely used for gene annotation, including molecular functions (MF), biological pathways (BP), and cellular components (CC). Kyoto Encyclopedia of Genes and Genomes (KEGG) enrichment analysis provides valuable insights into gene functions and high-level genomic functional information. To gain a comprehensive understanding of the role of target genes, we utilized the "clusterProfiler (version 4.4.4)" package in R for analyzing GO functions and performing KEGG pathway enrichment analysis. The results of the enrichment analysis were visualized using the "ggplot2 (version 3.3.6)" package. Visualizations such as string and bubble plots were generated to depict the joint logFC enrichment analysis of GO and KEGG, utilizing the "ggplot2 (version 3.3.6)" package.

2.3. Protein–Protein Interaction (PPI) Analysis of Differentially Expressed Genes and Identification of Hub Genes

The protein–protein interaction (PPI) network of differentially expressed genes was examined using the STRING database (accessible at https://string-db.org/, accessed on

5 March 2023). Hub genes, which exert a significant influence on other genes within the network, were identified based on their centrality scores. The analysis data from STRING were imported into Cytoscape software (version 3.8.1). We designated the top 10 scoring genes as hub genes using the MCC algorithm from Cytoscape's cytoHubba plugin. Additionally, the co-expression network of DEGs was analyzed using Cytoscape's MCODE plugin, and the most significant clusters containing hub genes were visualized. Further analysis involved a Venn diagram to determine the intersection of hub genes obtained from these two methods, resulting in the final set of identified hub genes.

2.4. Construction of the miRNA-Target Regulatory Network

To predict the miRNAs and TFs associated with the hub genes, we utilized the miRNet database (accessible at https://www.miRNet.ca/, accessed on 22 Apirl 2023). Subsequently, we constructed and visualized regulatory networks involving mRNA–miRNA and mRNA–TF interactions using Cytoscape software (version 3.8.1).

2.5. Validation of the Diagnostic Value of Hub Genes

To assess the sensitivity and specificity of the target genes, we conducted ROC curve analysis using HiPlot software (version 0.1.0). Multigene ROC analysis was performed by calculating the predicted probability of multiple genes contributing to the results in each sample based on a binary Logit model. This analysis was conducted using SPSS 25.0 software. The results were quantified as the area under the ROC curve (AUC), considering genes with an AUC > 0.6 as diagnostically significant.

2.6. Immune Infiltration Analysis

The proportion of 22 immune cell types in the samples was estimated using "CIBER-SORTx" (accessible at https://cibersortx.stanford.edu/, accessed on 20 May 2023). CIBER-SORTx is an analytical tool that utilizes gene expression data to provide mixed estimates of the abundance of different immune cell types within a cell population.

2.7. Retrospective Analysis of Blood Counts in COVID-19 Patients

Demographic and clinical information of COVID-19 patients, including gender, age, and symptoms, were collected using an electronic case system. Each isolate was cultured and verified. Continuous variables were presented as median (interquartile range [IQR]). Differences in continuous variables between two groups were assessed using the Mann–Whitney Wilcoxon rank-sum test. A *p*-value < 0.05 was considered statistically significant.

2.8. Real-Time Quantitative Polymerase Chain Reaction (RT-qPCR) Verification

To validate the findings obtained from the bioinformatics analysis, peripheral blood mononuclear cell (PBMC) samples were collected from 20 COVID-19 patients infected with the Omicron variant and 20 healthy individuals as controls. Total RNA was extracted using TRIzol reagent (Invitrogen, Carlsbad, CA, USA), and approximately 2 µg of total RNA was reverse transcribed using the iScript cDNA Synthesis Kit (Bio-Rad, Hercules, CA, USA). RT-qPCR was performed on a CFX Connect Real-Time PCR detection system (Bio-Rad) using ChamQ SYBR Color qPCR Master Mix (Vazyme, Nanjing, China). The relative mRNA expression was calculated using the $2^{-\Delta\Delta Ct}$ method. The primer sequences used in the experiment are provided in Table 1. Statistical analysis was performed using one-way analysis of variance with SPSS 25.0 software (IBM, Armonk, NY, USA), and statistical significance was defined as a *p*-value < 0.05.

Table 1. Primer sequences used for RT-qPCR.

Gene		Sequence (5′ -> 3′)	Length	Tm	Location
IFI27	Forward Primer	TGCTCTCACCTCATCAGCAGT	21	62.9	12–32
	Reverse Primer	CACAACTCCTCCAATCACAACT	22	60.2	126–105
IFI44	Forward Primer	ATGGCAGTGACAACTCGTTTG	21	61.1	1–21
	Reverse Primer	TCCTGGTAACTCTCTTCTGCATA	23	60	212–190
IFI44L	Forward Primer	AGCCGTCAGGGATGTACTATAAC	23	61	133–155
	Reverse Primer	AGGGAATCATTTGGCTCTGTAGA	23	60.8	248–226
ISG15	Forward Primer	CGCAGATCACCCAGAAGATCG	21	62.6	89–109
	Reverse Primer	TTCGTCGCATTTGTCCACCA	20	62.4	240–221
MX1	Forward Primer	GTTTCCGAAGTGGACATCGCA	21	62.9	7–27
	Reverse Primer	CTGCACAGGTTGTTCTCAGC	20	61.2	128–109
OAS3	Forward Primer	GAAGGAGTTCGTAGAGAAGGCG	22	62.1	66–87
	Reverse Primer	CCCTTGACAGTTTTCAGCACC	21	61.4	179–159
USP18	Forward Primer	CCTGAGGCAAATCTGTCAGTC	21	60.4	21–41
	Reverse Primer	CGAACACCTGAATCAAGGAGTTA	23	60	220–198
GAPDH	Forward Primer	GGAGCGAGATCCCTCCAAAAT	21	61.6	108–128
	Reverse Primer	GGCTGTTGTCATACTTCTCATGG	23	60.9	304–282

2.9. Prediction of Potential Therapeutic Agents

The DSigDB database (available at http://tanlab.ucdenver.edu/DSigDB, accessed on 30 May 2023) was utilized to predict potential therapeutic agents for COVID-19 based on protein–drug interaction data. The thresholds set for selection were FDR < 0.05 and composite score > 5000.

2.10. Statistical Analysis

Statistical analyses were performed using GraphPad Prism 9 and R software (version 4.2.2). The data were presented as mean ± standard deviation, and a comparison between groups was conducted using an unpaired Student's *t*-test. A *p*-value less than 0.05 was considered statistically significant.

3. Results

3.1. Screening and Functional Enrichment Analysis of Differentially Expressed Genes in PBMC of Omicron Infection

The differential gene analysis of the GSE201530 dataset was conducted using the "limma" package in R, resulting in the identification of 73 differentially expressed genes (33 up-regulated and 40 down-regulated), as shown in Figure 2A (Supplementary Table S1). The screening criteria applied were | log2(FC) | > 2 and adj. *p*-value < 0.05.

To evaluate the reproducibility of the data within the group, UMAP analysis was performed, demonstrating satisfactory reproducibility, as depicted in Figure 2B. Volcano plots illustrating the differentially expressed genes were generated using the "ggplot2 [3.3.6]" package in R, with the parameters Log2FC > 2 and adj. *p*-value < 0.05, as shown in Figure 2C.

GO and KEGG enrichment analyses were conducted on the differentially expressed genes (Supplementary Table S2). The results revealed significant GO enrichments related to virus response, defense response to symbiont, defense response to virus, response to type I interferon, regulation of viral life cycle, cellular response to type I interferon, and the type I interferon signaling pathway. In the KEGG enrichment analysis, the differentially expressed genes were primarily associated with diseases such as COVID-19, Influenza A, and Chagas disease, as depicted in Figure 2E–H.

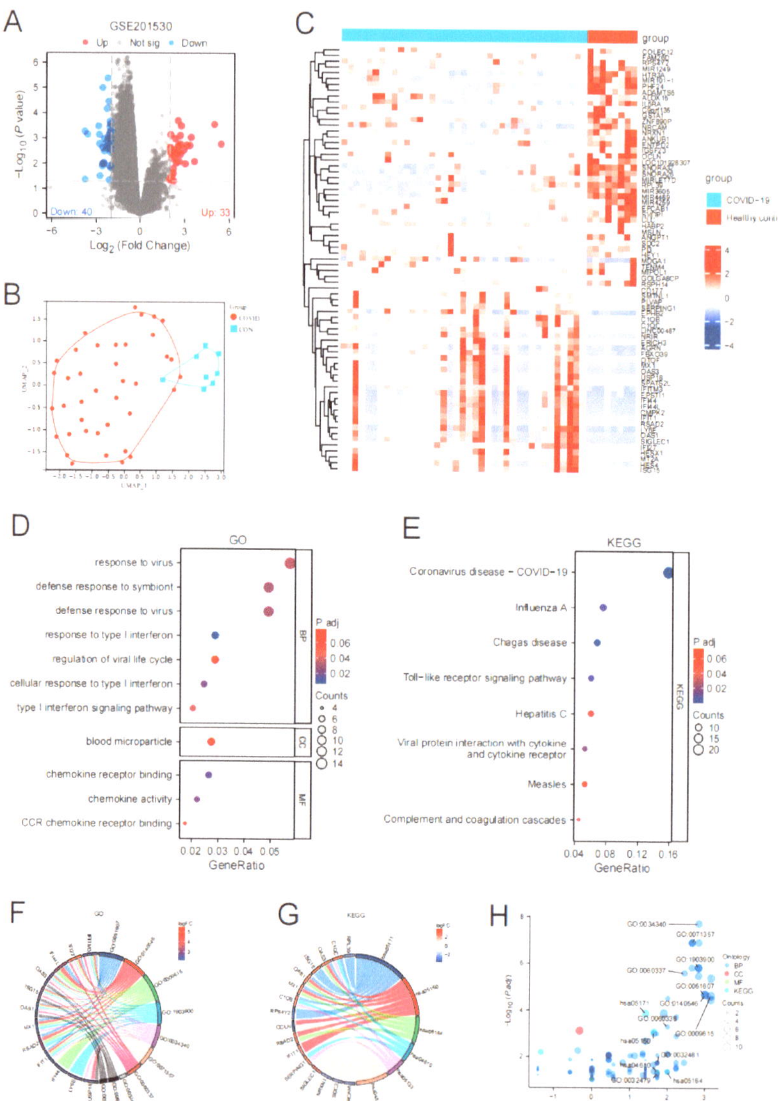

Figure 2. Comprehensive analysis of gene expression and functional annotation in COVID-19. volcano plot (**A**); GSE201530UMAP plot (**B**); heat map of DEGs (**C**); GO/KEGG categories and pathways (**D,E**); chord diagram describing the relationship between GO/KEGG terms of genes and biological processes (**F–H**).

3.2. Gene Screening and Functional Enrichment Analysis of PBMC Hub Genes in Omicron Infection

The differentially expressed genes obtained earlier were used to construct a protein-protein interaction network using the STRING database (accessible at https://string-db. org/, accessed on 5 March 2023) (Figure 3A). The data from STRING were imported into Cytoscape software (version 3.8.1), and the MCODE plugin was utilized to analyze the co-expression network of the differentially expressed genes. The visualization of the most significant clusters revealed the hub genes: IFI44L, RSAD2, IFI27, MX1, OAS1, LY6E,

IFIT1, OAS3, EPSTI1, IFITM3, CMPK2, IFI44, ISG15, and USP18 (Figure 3B). Furthermore, the cytohubba plugin in Cytoscape, employing the MCC algorithm, identified the top 10 scoring genes as hub genes: OAS1, IFI44, IFI44L, MX1, OAS3, USP18, IFIT1, RSAD2, IFI27, and ISG15 (Figure 3C). VENN plots confirmed that these 10 genes exhibited common differential expression in the gene set, thus confirming their status as the final identified hub genes: OAS1, IFI44, IFI44L, MX1, OAS3, USP18, IFIT1, RSAD2, IFI27, and ISG15 (Figure 3D). The visualization of the hub genes was presented in a volcano plot generated using the "ggplot2" package in R software (version 4.2.2) (Figure 3E).

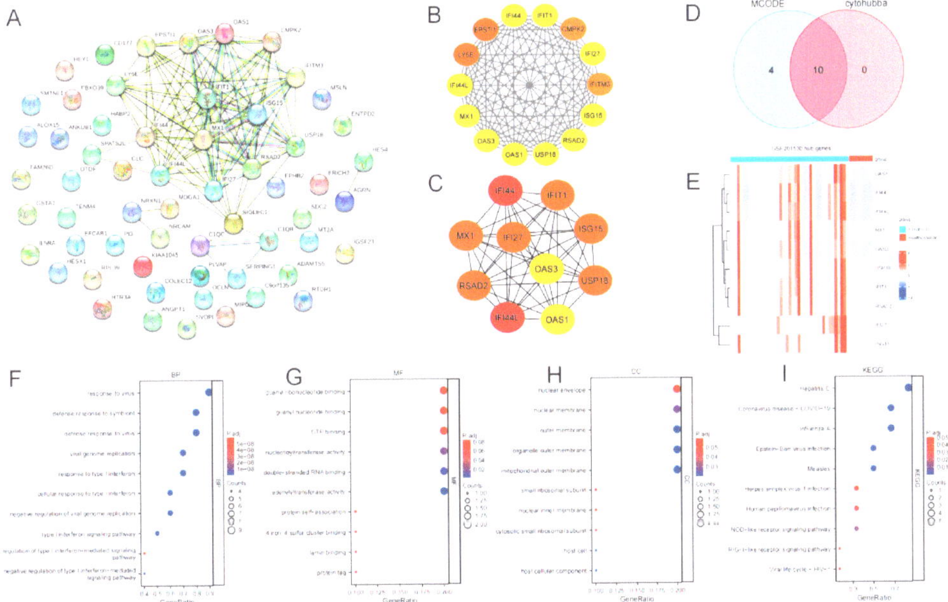

Figure 3. Identification and validation of hub genes. STRING (**A**); MCODE hub genes (**B**); cytohubba-MCC hub genes (**C**); VENN of MCODE hub genes and cytohubba-MCC hub genes (**D**); heatmap of 10 hub genes (**E**); GO/KEGG categories and pathways (**F–I**).

Following the hub genes analysis, GO and KEGG enrichment analyses were performed (Supplementary Table S3). The results demonstrated significant enrichment in GO terms associated with the response to virus, response to type I interferon, cellular response to type I interferon, type I interferon signaling pathway, and regulation of type I interferon-mediated signaling. The KEGG analysis revealed the involvement of multiple viral infectious diseases, including COVID-19 (Figure 3F–I).

3.3. Confirmation of Hub Genes Expression and Diagnostic Value in GSE179627

GSE179627 was utilized to verify the expression levels of the selected target genes. The results demonstrated consistent expression patterns between COVID-19 patients with Omicron infection and healthy individuals for the 10 hub genes (OAS1, IFI44, IFI44L, MX1, OAS3, USP18, IFIT1, RSAD2, IFI27, and ISG15) (Figure 4A–J).

ROC curves were generated using the data from COVID-19 patients with Omicron infection and healthy individuals to assess the diagnostic value of these 10 genes. The results indicated that these genes hold significant diagnostic value for COVID-19 patients. The AUC values were as follows: OAS1, 0.8352 (95% CI: 0.6697 to 1.000); IFI44, 0.8409 (95% CI: 0.6974 to 0.9844); IFI44L, 0.8561 (95% CI: 0.7306 to 0.9815); MX1, 0.9091 (95% CI: 0.8048 to 1.000); OAS3, 0.8371 (95% CI: 0.6585 to 1.000); USP18, 0.9375 (95% CI: 0.8576 to 1.000);

IFIT1, 0.7424 (95% CI: 0.5451 to 0.9397); RSAD2, 0.8864 (95% CI: 0.7744 to 0.9984); IFI27, 0.9867 (95% CI: 0.9591 to 1.000); and ISG15, 0.8504 (95% CI: 0.6896 to 1.000) (Figure 4K–T).

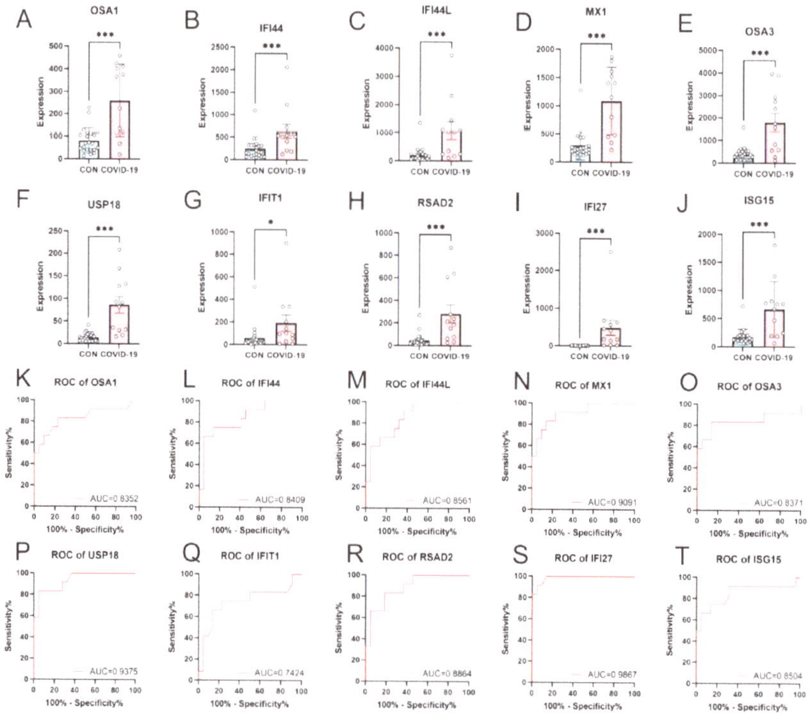

Figure 4. Confirmation of hub genes expression and diagnostic value. Comparison of hub genes expression in the GSE179627 dataset (**A–J**); diagnostic ROC curves of COVID-19 versus 10 hub genes in healthy samples (**K–T**). *, $p < 0.05$; ***, $p < 0.001$.

3.4. Investigation of the Relationship between Hub Genes and Omicron Infection

To examine the impact of hub genes on the symptoms manifested after SARS-CoV-2 infection in humans, we utilized GSE167930, which included healthy individuals, asymptomatic infected individuals, symptomatic infected individuals, and recovering patients. The analysis revealed no statistically significant difference in the expression of the 10 hub genes between asymptomatic infected individuals and healthy individuals. However, a notable statistically significant difference or a trend towards elevated expression was observed for all 10 hub genes in symptomatic infected individuals compared to both healthy and asymptomatic infected individuals (although the difference was not statistically significant in the latter case). Importantly, during the recovery period of COVID-19, 7 out of the 10 hub genes (IFI44, IFI44L, MX1, OAS3, USP18, IFI27, and ISG15) exhibited a significant decrease, reaching levels comparable to those of healthy individuals (Figure 5A–J).

Furthermore, we conducted GO and KEGG enrichment analyses for the seven hub genes related to COVID-19 symptoms (Supplementary Table S4). The results indicated that the most significant GO enrichment was observed for multiple type I interferon-related categories, including response to virus, response to type I interferon, cellular response to type I interferon, and type I interferon signaling pathway. The KEGG analysis demonstrated the involvement of various viral infectious diseases, including COVID-19. Based on the identified DEGs and the enrichment analyses of the hub genes, the results highlighted the involvement of seven potential biomarkers in abnormal signaling pathways associated with COVID-19 symptom production and recovery, primarily related to type I interferon signaling pathways (Figure 5K,L).

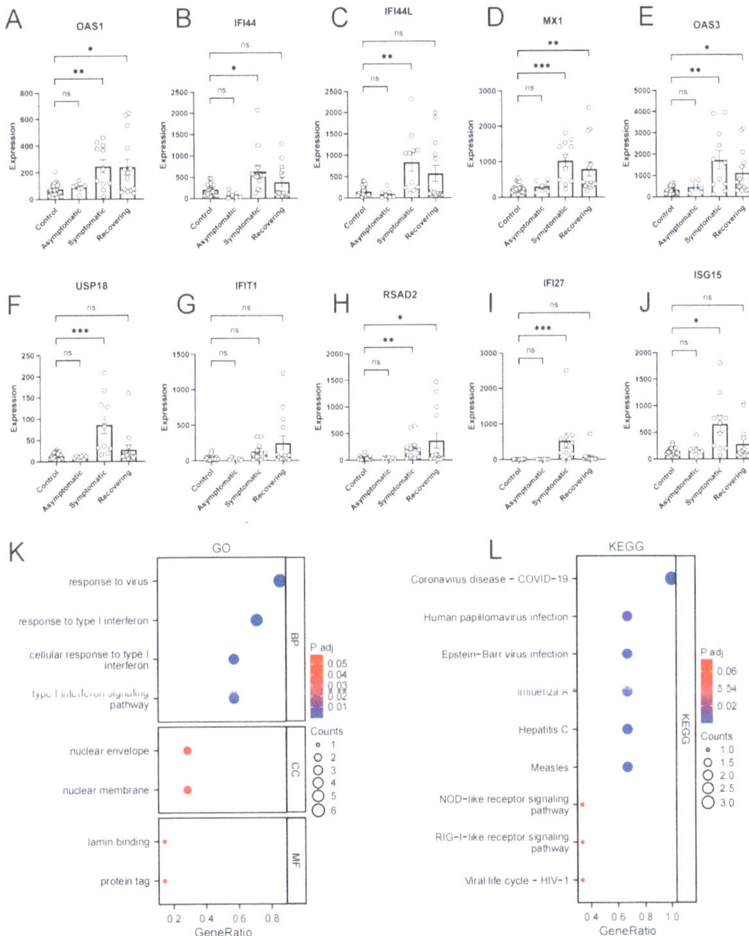

Figure 5. Association of hub genes with COVID-19 symptoms and signaling pathways. Comparison of hub genes expression in different groups (**A–J**); GO/KEGG categories and pathways (**K,L**). *, $p < 0.05$; **, $p < 0.01$; ***, $p < 0.001$.

3.5. Validation of Hub Genes Expression by RT-qPCR

To validate the findings derived from the bioinformatics analysis, PBMC samples were collected from 20 COVID-19 patients infected with the Omicron variant and 20 healthy individuals as controls. The expression levels of the hub genes, namely IFI44, IFI44L, MX1, OAS3, USP18, IFI27, and ISG15, were examined using RT-qPCR. The results revealed a significant upregulation of these genes in the COVID-19 group compared to the control group, which aligns with the patterns observed in the microarray analysis (Figure 6). This validation provides strong support for the reliability of the bioinformatics analysis and reinforces the evidence suggesting the dysregulation of these hub genes in COVID-19.

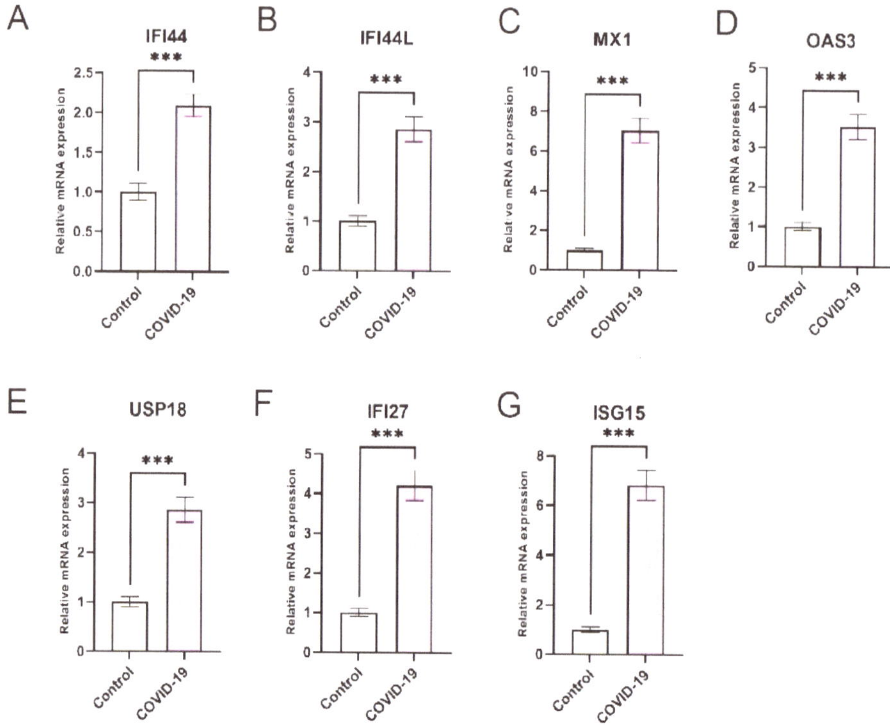

Figure 6. Validation of hub genes expression in COVID-19 patients. RT-PCR analysis of PBMC IFI44, IFI44L, MX1, OAS3, USP18, IFI27, and ISG15 expression from control and COVID-19 (n = 20) (**A–G**). ***, $p < 0.001$.

3.6. Construction of mRNA-miRNA and mRNA-TF Regulatory Networks

The miRNet tool was utilized to integrate the results of the seven COVID-19 symptom-related hub genes with the miRNA interaction network, resulting in the identification of 150 miRNAs and 305 mRNA-miRNA pairs. Subsequently, Cytoscape was employed to construct co-expression networks of mRNA and miRNAs (Figure 7A). Notably, there were 63 miRNAs found to regulate IFI27 (e.g., hsa-mir-146a-5p), 36 miRNAs regulating IFI44 (e.g., hsa-mir-26b-5p), 79 miRNAs regulating IFI44L (e.g., hsa-mir-124-3p), 29 miRNAs regulating ISG15 (e.g., hsa-mir-1-3p), 46 miRNAs regulating MX1 (e.g., hsa-mir-204-5p), 57 miRNAs regulating OAS3 (e.g., hsa-mir-143-3p), and 23 miRNAs regulating USP18 (e.g., hsa-mir-26b-5p) (Supplementary Table S5).

Furthermore, the results of the seven COVID-19 symptom-related hub genes were integrated with the transcription factor (TF) interaction network to identify 89 TFs and 179 mRNA-TF pairs. Cytoscape was then employed to construct co-expression networks of mRNA and TFs. The analysis revealed that 3 TFs were involved in regulating IFI27 (e.g., NR2C2), 36 miRNAs regulated IFI44 (e.g., ZNF143) (Figure 7B), 3 TFs regulated IFI44L (e.g., EED), 80 TFs regulated ISG15 (e.g., ZKSCAN1), 1 TF regulated MX1 (WRNIP1), 4 TFs regulated OAS3 (e.g., TRIM22), and 9 TFs regulated USP18 (e.g., MBD1) (Supplementary Table S6).

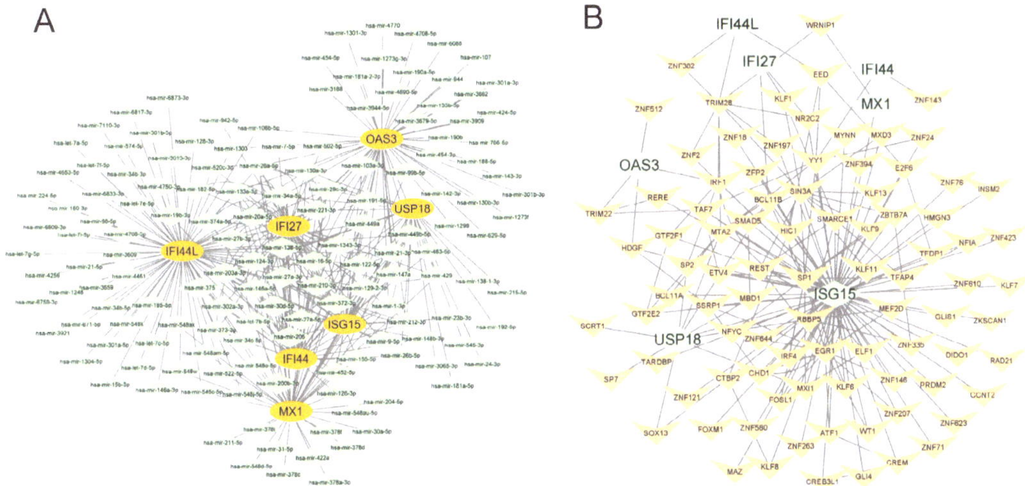

Figure 7. mRNA-miRNA and mRNA-TF interaction networks in COVID-19 symptom-related hub genes. mRNA and miRNAs co-expression network. The network depicts the interaction between the seven hub genes (IFI27, IFI44, IFI44L, ISG15, MX1, OAS3, and USP18) and their corresponding miRNAs. Various miRNAs, such as hsa-mir-146a-5p and hsa-mir-26b-5p, regulate the expression of these hub genes (**A**); mRNA and TF co-expression network. The network shows the interaction between the seven hub genes and transcription factors (TFs). TFs, including NR2C2 and ZNF143, are involved in regulating the expression of these hub genes (**B**).

3.7. Analysis of PMBC Immune Infiltration in Omicron Infection

Based on the GSE201530 dataset, "CIBERSORTx" (https://cibersortx.stanford.edu/, accessed on 20 May 2023) compared the different immune infiltration patterns of COVID-19 patients and normal controls. The results showed that the proportion of monocytes, T cells CD4 memory activated, and Mast cells resting was significantly increased in COVID-19 patients with Omicron infection, while T cells CD4 memory resting was significantly decreased (Figure 8A). Cell types with an expression of 0 that were not present in the sample were further excluded. The PBMC-associated immune cells were selected and the results of correlation analysis between immune cells are shown in Figure 8B.

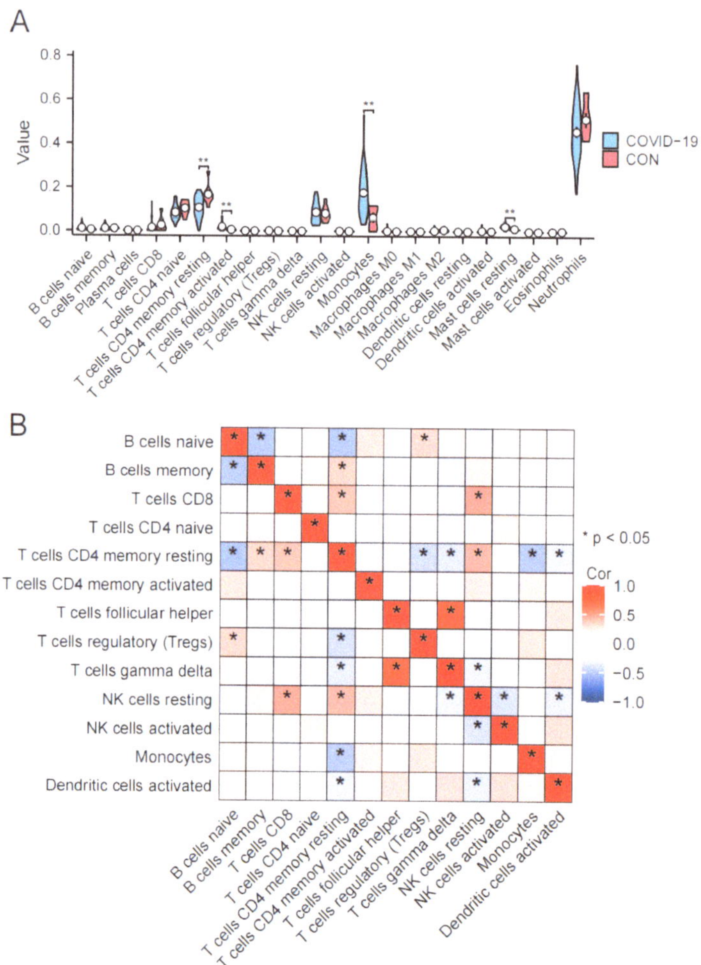

Figure 8. The immune cell infiltration patterns in COVID-19 patients with Omicron infection. Pattern of immune cell infiltration in COVID-19, monocytes, T cells CD4 memory activated, and Mast cells resting ratios were significantly increased, while T cells CD4 memory resting was significantly decreased (**A**). The correlation analysis between immune cells (**B**). *, $p < 0.05$; **, $p < 0.01$.

3.8. Validation of Retrospective Blood Analysis and Immune Infiltration Results in Omicron Infection

Neutrophil (NEU%), monocyte (MONO% and MONO), mean corpuscular volume (MCV), mean platelet volume (MPV), platelet large cell ratio (PLCR) and C-reactive protein (CRP) were significantly increased in COVID-19 patients than that in healthy controls ($p < 0.05$) (Table 2). Lymphocytes (LYM and LYM%), eosinophils (EOS and EOS%), basophils (BASO and BASO%), red blood cell (RBC), hemoglobin (HGB), hematocrit (HCT), mean corpuscular hemoglobin concentration (MCHC), blood platelet (PLT), platelet distribution width (PDW), plateletcrit (PCT) and platelet large cell ratio (PLCR) were lower in COVID-19 patients ($p < 0.05$). The elevated monocytes in the COVID-19 group were consistent with the results of the immune infiltration fraction in clinical blood tests.

Table 2. Basic information of healthy controls and COVID-19 patients.

	Healthy Controls	COVID-19	p
N	20	20	
Age	47.5, (32.75, 60.25)	49.45, (29.5, 69)	0.736
WBC, 10^9/L	5.98, (5.3, 6.75)	5.53, (4.15, 7.05)	0.304
NEU%	57.64, (53.08, 62.3)	64.29, (56.83, 73.28)	0.012
LYM%	32.08, (27.58, 37.4)	22.08, (13.05, 32.1)	0.001
MONO%	6.86, (6.23, 7.6)	11.93, (8.73, 14.63)	<0.001
EOS%	2.86, (1.53, 4)	1.22, (0.23, 1.38)	<0.001
BASO%	0.71, (0.5, 0.98)	0.49, (0.33, 0.6)	0.010
NEU, 10^9/L	3.56, (3.05, 3.7)	3.64, (2.6, 4.67)	0.790
LYM, 10^9/L	2.06, (1.65, 2.48)	1.16, (0.69, 1.54)	<0.001
MONO, 10^9/L	0.44, (0.33, 0.5)	0.65, (0.42, 0.87)	0.006
EOS, 10^9/L	0.18, (0.15, 0.22)	0.06, (0.01, 0.1)	<0.001
BASO, 10^9/L	0.09, (0.06, 0.12)	0.03, (0.02, 0.03)	<0.001
RBC, 10^{12}/L	4.78, (4.6, 4.9)	4.38, (3.98, 4.67)	0.001
HGB, g/L	139.35, (124.25, 149)	125.35, (118.25, 136.75)	0.012
HCT%	0.42, (0.4, 0.44)	0.4, (0.37, 0.43)	0.025
MCV, fL	87.3, (85.23, 90.68)	91.46, (89.85, 94.9)	<0.001
MCH, Pg	29.93, (28.03, 31.58)	29.4, (28.7, 31)	0.838
MCHC, g/L	341.55, (332.25, 349.75)	321.08, (315.25, 327)	<0.001
RDW-SD, fL	42.55, (39, 45.75)	43.65, (41.1, 46)	0.293
RDW-CV	12.92, (12.53, 13.35)	13.16, (12.23, 13.68)	0.621
PLT, 10^9/L	244.2, (132, 358.75)	171.8, (123.25, 219.25)	0.010
MPV, fL	8.56, (7.6, 9.5)	11.25, (10, 12.6)	<0.001
PDW	20.6, (18, 24.25)	14.12, (10.58, 16.8)	<0.001
PCT	0.26, (0.2, 0.32)	0.19, (0.15, 0.22)	<0.001
P-LCR	24.25, (16.25, 29)	34.57, (22.93, 46.13)	0.006
CRP	0.27(0.1, 0.4)	17.1, (1.97, 14.16)	<0.001

WBC: White blood cell; NEU: Neutrophil; LYM: Lymphocyte; MONO: Monocyte; BASO: Basophil; EOS: Eosinophils; NRBC: Nucleated red blood cell; HGB: Hemoglobin; HCT: Hematocrit; MCV: Erythrocyte mean corpuscular volume; MCH: Mean corpuscular hemoglobin; MCHC: Mean corpuscular hemoglobin concentration; RDW-SD: Red blood cell distribution width-standard deviation; RDW-CV: Red blood cell distribution width-coefficient of variance; PLT: Blood platelet; MPV: Mean platelet volume; PCT: Plateletcrit; PLCR: Platelet large cell ratio; CRP: C-reactive protein; PDW: Platelet distribution width.

3.9. Target Drug Prediction

The DSigDB database was used to predict potential target drugs associated with seve target hub genes that may treat Omicron infection by modulating the hub genes. A total of 123 target drugs were finally predicted; the composite scores and corresponding target genes are listed in Supplementary Table S7. The top 10 predicted target drugs according to the composite scores are shown in Figure 9 The top 10 predicted targets according to the composite score are shown in Figure 9. Among them, acetohexamide is expected to be a potential drug for the treatment of Omicron infection.

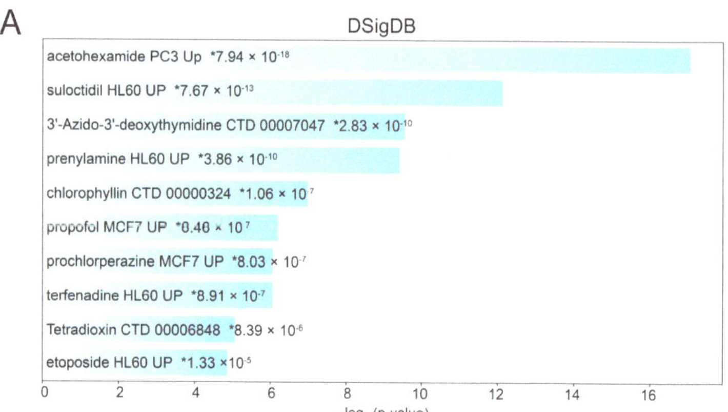

B

Index	Name	P-value	Adjusted p-value	Odds Ratio	Combined score
1	acetohexamide PC3 UP	7.94×10^{-18}	9.77×10^{-16}	7,050.35	277,601.52
2	suloctidil HL60 UP	7.67×10^{-13}	4.72×10^{-11}	882.58	24,620.10
3	3-Azido-3'-deoxythymidine CTD 00007047	2.83×10^{-10}	1.16×10^{-8}	319.97	7,034.66
4	prenylamine HL60 UP	3.86×10^{-10}	1.19×10^{-8}	782.71	1,6965.34
5	chlorophyllin CTD 00000324	1.06×10^{-7}	2.61×10^{-6}	554.61	8,906.19
6	propofol MCF7 UP	6.46×10^{-7}	1.33×10^{-5}	293.26	4,179.67
7	prochlorperazine MCF7 UP	8.03×10^{-7}	1.37×10^{-5}	271.88	3,815.72
8	terfenadine HL60 UP	8.91×10^{-7}	1.37×10^{-5}	262.32	3,654.40
9	Tetradioxin CTD 00006848	8.39×10^{-6}	1.15×10^{-4}	113,624.00	1,328,140.36
10	etoposide HL60 UP	1.33×10^{-5}	1.64×10^{-4}	103.38	1160.54

Figure 9. Predicted target drugs for Omicron infection modulating the hub genes. Bar graph of DSigDB (**A**); Table of DSigDB (**B**). The top 10 predicted target drugs, based on composite scores, are presented. Notably, acetohexamide emerges as a promising candidate for the treatment of COVID-19. *, *p*-value.

4. Discussion

The emergence of novel coronaviruses and their potential global impact on public health have become a major concern in recent years [3]. With the ongoing challenges posed by the SARS-CoV-2 Omicron variant, it is crucial to identify potential biomarkers and explore associated mechanisms using bioinformatics approaches to enhance the diagnosis and treatment of this variant.

In this study, we analyzed the PBMC microarray dataset (GSE201530) from the GEO database to identify differentially expressed genes (DEGs) associated with SARS-CoV-2 Omicron variant infection. Through this analysis, we identified 10 hub genes through the construction of a protein–protein interaction (PPI) network. These findings were validated using an independent PBMC dataset of COVID-19 patients (GSE179627), which consistently demonstrated the expected expression patterns of these 10 genes and their diagnostic value. Additionally, we analyzed a dataset comprising healthy individuals, asymptomatic infected individuals, symptomatic infected individuals, and recovered infected individuals (GSE167930) to identify seven target hub genes (IFI44, IFI44L, MX1, OAS3, USP18, IFI27, and ISG15) that showed correlations with symptom onset and recovery from COVID-19. Further GO and KEGG pathway analyses at different stages of genetic screening revealed significant enrichment in pathways related to virus response, defense response to virus, response to type I interferon, cellular response to type I interferon, and the type I interferon signaling pathway. Moreover, we analyzed the miRNAs corresponding to these seven target hub genes and constructed interaction networks with transcription factors (TFs) using the miRNet tool.

In the analysis of the GSE201530 dataset with the "CIBERSORTx" tool, we observed a significant increase in the proportion of monocytes, activated memory CD4 T cells and resting mast cells in COVID-19 patients. Conversely, we observed a notable decrease in the proportion of resting memory T cells CD4. Furthermore, we identified a correlation between elevated monocyte levels and decreased proportions of resting memory T cells CD4. To support these findings, we reviewed blood counts recorded in hospital medical records of symptomatic COVID-19 patients with Omicron infection, which demonstrated that abnormally elevated monocyte ratios and higher monocyte counts were associated with an increased risk of developing symptomatic COVID-19 compared to normal subjects, aligning with the results obtained from immune infiltration analysis.

Moreover, we conducted RT-qPCR to validate the up-regulated expression levels of these seven genes in PBMCs of COVID-19 patients infected with the Omicron variant. The consistent up-regulation of these genes supports their potential crucial role in the progression of COVID-19. The expression trends of many key DEGs found in this study align with previously reported results, further validating the reliability of the database and our data analysis.

Among the seven target hub genes, MX1, OAS3, USP18, IFI27, and ISG15 are characterized as type I interferon-related genes [33]. MX1 acts as an effector protein of the IFN system and plays a crucial role in responding to SARS-CoV-2 infection, with its expression significantly increasing with viral load escalation [34]. Importantly, MX1 directly impacts the viral ribonucleoprotein complex, and its antiviral function relies on the essentiality of its gTPase activity [35]. The interferon-induced antiviral enzyme known as $2'$-$5'$-oligoadenylate synthase (OAS) encompasses OAS1, OAS2, OAS3, and OASL [36]. OAS3 serves as a key player in antiviral action and signal transduction [37]. Additionally, IFI27 (also referred to as ISG12 or p27), an interferon α-inducible gene (and to a lesser extent, interferon γ), exhibits nuclear membrane localization and contributes to diverse biological processes [37]. Notably, a cohort study demonstrated that IFI27 expression was observed in the blood of COVID-19 patients and positively correlated with elevated viral load [38].

IFI44L, an IFN-inducible protein with similarities to IFN-I, is induced by various viruses [39]. As an IFN-I negative regulator, IFI44L mitigates antimicrobial inflammatory factors by negatively regulating the NF-κB pathway and inhibiting STAT1 activation, thereby inhibiting IFN-I and ISG production [40]. Acting as a feedback regulator of the IFN response, IFI44L potentially promotes viral replication by modulating the innate immune response following viral infection [41]. Interestingly, our study reveals a significant overlap between these seven target hub genes and the results obtained from bioinformatics analyses of diseases such as dengue fever [42]. Previous studies have demonstrated shared pathophysiological pathways between dengue fever and COVID-19, including fever, plasma leakage, low platelet count, and coagulation disorders [43]. Therefore, further discussions are warranted to explore potential therapeutic approaches to symptomatic COVID-19 by referencing strategies employed against dengue fever.

The initial defense against viral infection is the interferon I (IFN-I) response, which induces the activation of hundreds of interferon-stimulated genes (ISGs) through the JAK/STAT signaling pathway [44]. Severe lung inflammation leading to respiratory failure in SARS coronavirus type 2-infected patients is primarily attributed to cytokine dysregulation. Severe cases of COVID-19 exhibit impaired production of both IFN-I and interferon II (IFN-II) and downregulation of ISGs [45,46]. The hub genes identified in this study have the potential to counteract COVID-19 development by modulating interferon activity. To identify potential compounds, we conducted a screening process based on the DSigDB database. Among the ranked *p*-values, acetohexamide emerged as a promising candidate for COVID-19 patients with Omicron infection treatment. A study utilizing three molecular docking programs aimed to repurpose FDA-approved drugs targeting the functional structural domain of csBiP, specifically the BiP functional domain, as antivirals against COVID-19, and acetohexamide was among the selected ligands [47]. The potential therapeutic role of acetohexamide in the treatment of COVID-19, particularly in the context of Omicron infection, warrants further investigation and validation through in vitro and clinical studies. Such studies will help elucidate its mechanism of action and assess its safety and efficacy in combating the virus. This research direction represents a promising avenue for the development of targeted therapies to mitigate the impact of COVID-19, especially in the context of emerging variants like the Omicron variant.

Compared to previous studies on Omicron variants, this study brings innovation by specifically focusing on targets associated with symptom development and outcomes. The identification of hub genes related to the Type I interferon pathway highlights their critical role as key therapeutic targets. The validation of our results using patient samples in a clinical setting enhances the accuracy and scientific validity of our findings. However, this study has several limitations that should be acknowledged and taken into consideration. Firstly, there is still a lack of sufficient transcriptomic research related to Omicron variant infection, particularly concerning the differential expression of genes in individuals with different symptoms, leading to a scarcity of available datasets. Secondly, the diagnostic value of research findings such as hub genes and predicted drugs needs to be further verified by additional experimental exploration and clinical trials to establish their potential clinical relevance and utility, which is the direction of future research.

Despite these limitations, this study provides valuable insights into the molecular mechanisms underlying the pathogenesis of the SARS-CoV-2 Omicron variant and its association with the symptomatic presentation. The identified hub genes and enriched pathways offer potential targets for further investigation and the development of therapeutic interventions for Omicron-dominant COVID-19 cases. Further research in this area will be crucial for advancing our understanding of the virus and improving the management of COVID-19 patients.

5. Conclusions

In this study, our investigation successfully identified seven hub genes (IFI44, IFI44L, MX1, OAS3, USP18, IFI27, and ISG15) associated with antiviral activity and the type I interferon response as potential biomarkers for the diagnosis and treatment of COVID-19 in individuals infected with the Omicron variant. Through the construction of a comprehensive network of mRNA–miRNA and mRNA–TF interactions, we gained valuable insights into the regulatory mechanisms underlying Omicron infection. Our immune infiltration analysis and retrospective clinical data analysis provided compelling evidence of a correlation between elevated monocytes and the development of Omicron infection. We also identified ten agents as promising drug candidates that specifically target these hub genes for treating Omicron infection. These findings significantly advance our understanding of COVID-19 symptom development and recovery and highlight the potential of further investigating type I interferon-related pathways to identify therapeutic targets and biomarkers for COVID-19 patients, particularly those infected with the Omicron variant.

Supplementary Materials: The following supporting information can be downloaded at: https://www.mdpi.com/article/10.3390/microorganisms11082101/s1.

Author Contributions: Conceptualization, Z.L. (Zhiwei Lin), L.Y. and B.S.; Data curation, M.X. and Z.W.; Formal analysis, Z.L. (Zhiwei Lin) and Z.W.; Funding acquisition, B.S.; Investigation, M.X. and J.P.; Methodology, Z.L. (Zhiwei Lin); Project administration, B.S.; Resources, J.H.; Software, M.X., Z.L. (Ze Liu) and J.P.; Supervision, L.Y. and B.S.; Validation, J.H.; Writing—original draft, Z.L. (Zhiwei Lin), Z.L. (Ze Liu) and Q.Y.; Writing—review & editing, Z.L. (Zhiwei Lin). All authors have read and agreed to the published version of the manuscript.

Funding: The study was supported by the Chinese National Natural Science Foundation (81960023), State Key Laboratory Project (SKLRD-Z-202305), Zhongnanshan Medical Foundation of Guangdong Province (ZNSXS-20220080), Guangdong-Hong Kong-Macao Joint Laboratory for Respiratory Infectious Diseases Project (GHMJLRID-Z-202102), Precision Medicine Joint Foundation of Guangdong Basic and Applied Basic Research Foundation (2021B1515230008).

Institutional Review Board Statement: The studies involving human participants were reviewed and approved by The First Affiliated Hospital of Guangzhou Medical University Scientific Research Project Reviews Ethics Committee, clinical research approval 2021 No.31. The patients/participants provided their written informed consent to participate in this study.

Data Availability Statement: The original contributions presented in the study are included in the article/Supplementary Material, further inquiries can be directed to the corresponding authors.

Acknowledgments: The authors would like to express their gratitude to Yaqin Li (Guangdong University of Foreign Studies) for the expert linguistic services provided.

Conflicts of Interest: The authors declare that the research was conducted in the absence of any commercial or financial relationships that could be construed as a potential conflict of interest.

References

1. Carlos, W.G.; Dela Cruz, C.S.; Cao, B.; Pasnick, S.; Jamil, S. Novel Wuhan (2019-nCoV) coronavirus. *Am. J. Respir. Crit. Care Med.* **2020**, *201*, P7–P8. [CrossRef]
2. Song, F.; Shi, N.; Shan, F.; Zhang, Z.; Shen, J.; Lu, H.; Ling, Y.; Jiang, Y.; Shi, Y. Emerging 2019 novel coronavirus (2019-nCoV) pneumonia. *Radiology* **2020**, *295*, 210–217. [CrossRef]
3. Weekly Epidemiological Update on COVID-19. 2021. Available online: https://covid19.who.int/ (accessed on 4 June 2023).
4. Al-Karmalawy, A.A.; Soltane, R.; Abo Elmaaty, A.; Tantawy, M.A.; Antar, S.A.; Yahya, G.; Chrouda, A.; Pashameah, R.A.; Mustafa, M.; Abu Mraheil, M.; et al. Coronavirus Disease (COVID-19) Control between Drug Repurposing and Vaccination: A Comprehensive Overview. *Vaccines* **2021**, *9*, 1317. [CrossRef] [PubMed]
5. UK Health Security Agency. SARS-CoV-2 Variants of Concern and Variants under Investigation in England-Technical Briefing: Update on Hospitalisation and Vaccine Effectiveness for Omicron VOC-21NOV-01 (B.1.1.529). Available online: https://assets.publishing.service.gov.uk/government/uploads/system/uploads/attachment_data/file/1045619/Technical-Briefing-31-Dec-2021-Omicron_severity_update.pdf (accessed on 9 June 2023).
6. Ulloa, A.C.; Buchan, S.A.; Daneman, N.; Brown, K.A. Estimates of SARS-CoV-2 Omicron variant severity in Ontario, Canada. *J. Am. Med. Assoc.* **2022**, *327*, 1286–1288. [CrossRef] [PubMed]
7. Iuliano, A.D.; Brunkard, J.M.; Boehmer, T.K.; Peterson, E., Adjei, S., Binder, A.M.; Cobb, S.; Graff, P.; Hidalgo, P.; Panaggio, M.J. Trends in disease severity and health care utilization during the early Omicron variant period compared with previous SARS-CoV-2 high transmission periods—United States, December 2020–January 2022. *Morb. Mortal. Wkly. Rep.* **2022**, *71*, 146–152. [CrossRef]
8. Lewnard, J.A.; Hong, V.X.; Patel, M.M.; Kahn, R.; Lipsitch, M.; Tartof, S.Y. Clinical outcomes among patients infected with Omicron (B.1.1.529) SARS-CoV-2 variant in southern California. *medRxiv* **2022**. [CrossRef]
9. Bussani, R.; Schneider, E.; Zentilin, L.; Collesi, C.; Ali, H.; Braga, L.; Volpe, M.C.; Colliva, A.; Zanconati, F.; Berlot, G.; et al. Persistence of viral RNA, pneumocyte syncytia and thrombosis are hallmarks of advanced COVID-19 pathology. *EBioMedicine* **2020**, *61*, 103104. [CrossRef] [PubMed]
10. Sanders, D.W.; Jumper, C.C.; Ackerman, P.J.; Bracha, D.; Donlic, A.; Kim, H.; Kenney, D.; Castello-Serrano, I.; Suzuki, S.; Tamura, T.; et al. SARS-CoV-2 requires cholesterol for viral entry and pathological syncytia formation. *eLife* **2021**, *10*, e65962. [CrossRef]
11. Meng, B.; Abdullahi, A.; Ferreira, I.A.; Goonawardane, N.; Saito, A.; Kimura, I.; Yamasoba, D.; Gerber, P.P.; Fatihi, S.; Rathore, S.; et al. Altered TMPRSS2 usage by SARS-CoV-2 Omicron impacts tropism and fusogenicity. *Nature* **2022**, *603*, 706–714. [CrossRef]
12. Suzuki, R.; Yamasoba, D.; Kimura, I.; Wang, L.; Kishimoto, M.; Ito, J.; Morioka, Y.; Nao, N.; Nasser, H.; Uriu, K.; et al. Attenuated fusogenicity and pathogenicity of SARS-CoV-2 Omicron variant. *Nature* **2022**, *603*, 700–705. [CrossRef]
13. Shuai, H.; Chan, J.F.W.; Hu, B.; Chai, Y.; Yuen, T.T.T.; Yin, F.; Huang, X.; Yoon, C.; Hu, J.C.; Liu, H.; et al. Attenuated replication and pathogenicity of SARS-CoV-2 B.1.1.529 Omicron. *Nature* **2022**, *603*, 693–699. [CrossRef] [PubMed]
14. Fan, Y.; Li, X.; Zhang, L.; Wan, S.; Zhang, L.; Zhou, F. SARS-CoV-2 Omicron variant: Recent progress and future perspectives. *Signal Transduct. Target. Ther.* **2022**, *7*, 141. [CrossRef] [PubMed]
15. Jassat, W.; Karim, S.; Mudara, C. Clinical severity of COVID-19 patients admitted to hospitals in Gauteng, South Africa during the omicron-dominant fourth wave. *SSRN Electron. J.* **2021**. [CrossRef]
16. Mahase, E. COVID-19: Hospital admission 50–70% less likely with omicron than delta, but transmission a major concern. *BMJ* **2021**, *375*, n3151. [CrossRef] [PubMed]
17. Ramasamy, S.; Subbian, S. Critical Determinants of Cytokine Storm and Type I Interferon Response in COVID-19 Pathogenesis. *Clin. Microbiol. Rev.* **2021**, *34*, e00299-20. [CrossRef]
18. Zheng, B.; He, M.-L.; Wong, K.-L.; Lum, C.T.; Poon, L.L.M.; Peng, Y.; Guan, Y.; Lin, M.C.M.; Kung, H.-F. Potent Inhibition of SARS-associated coronavirus (SCoV) infection and replication by type I interferons (IFN-α/β) but not by type II interferon (IFN-γ). *J. Interferon Cytokine Res.* **2004**, *24*, 388–390. [CrossRef]

19. Jamilloux, Y.; Henry, T.; Belot, A.; Viel, S.; Fauter, M.; El Jammal, T.; Walzer, T.; François, B.; Sève, P. Should we stimulate or suppress immune responses in COVID-19? Cytokine and anti-cytokine interventions. *Autoimmun. Rev.* **2020**, *19*, 102567. [CrossRef]

20. Channappanavar, R.; Fehr, A.R.; Vijay, R.; Mack, M.; Zhao, J.; Meyerholz, D.K.; Perlman, S. Dysregulated type I interferon and inflammatory monocyte-macrophage responses cause lethal pneumonia in SARS-CoV-infected mice. *Cell Host Microbe* **2016**, *19*, 181–193. [CrossRef]

21. Lee, J.S.; Park, S.; Jeong, H.W.; Ahn, J.Y.; Choi, S.J.; Lee, H.; Choi, B.; Nam, S.K.; Sa, M.; Kwon, J.-S.; et al. Immunophenotyping of COVID-19 and influenza highlights the role of type I interferons in development of severe COVID-19. *Sci. Immunol.* **2020**, *5*, eabd1554. [CrossRef]

22. Lin, Z.; Niu, J.; Xu, Y.; Qin, L.; Ding, J.; Zhou, L. Clinical efficacy and adverse events of baricitinib treatment for coronavirus disease-2019 (COVID-19): A systematic review and meta-analysis. *J. Med. Virol.* **2022**, *94*, 1523–1534. [CrossRef] [PubMed]

23. Asante, I.A.; Hsu, S.N.; Boatemaa, L.; Kwasah, L.; Adusei-Poku, M.; Odoom, J.K.; Awuku-Larbi, Y.; Foulkes, B.H.; Oliver-Commey, J.; Asiedu, E.K.; et al. Repurposing an integrated national influenza platform for genomic surveillance of SARS-CoV-2 in Ghana: A molecular epidemiological analysis. *Lancet Glob. Health.* **2023**, *11*, e1075–e1085. [CrossRef] [PubMed]

24. Ma, K.C.; Shirk, P.; Lambrou, A.S.; Hassell, N.; Zheng, X.Y.; Payne, A.B.; Ali, A.R.; Batra, D.; Caravas, J.; Chau, R.; et al. Genomic Surveillance for SARS-CoV-2 Variants: Circulation of Omicron Lineages—United States, January 2022–May 2023, MMWR. *Morb. Mortal. Wkly. Rep.* **2023**, *72*, 651–656. [CrossRef] [PubMed]

25. Newman, A.M.; Liu, C.L.; Green, M.R.; Gentles, A.J.; Feng, W.; Xu, Y.; Hoang, C.D.; Diehn, M.; Alizadeh, A.A. Robust enumeration of cell subsets from tissue expression profiles. *Nat. Methods* **2015**, *12*, 453–457. [CrossRef] [PubMed]

26. Gentles, A.J.; Newman, A.M.; Liu, C.L.; Bratman, S.V.; Feng, W.; Kim, D.; Nair, V.S.; Xu, Y.; Khuong, A.; Hoang, C.D.; et al. The prognostic landscape of genes and infiltrating immune cells across human cancers. *Nat. Med.* **2015**, *21*, 938–945. [CrossRef] [PubMed]

27. Kawada, J.I.; Takeuchi, S.; Imai, H.; Okumura, T.; Horiba, K.; Suzuki, T.; Torii, Y.; Yasuda, K.; Imanaka-Yoshida, K.; Ito, Y. Immune cell infiltration landscapes in pediatric acute myocarditis analyzed by CIBERSORT. *J. Cardiol.* **2021**, *77*, 174–178. [CrossRef]

28. Lee, H.K.; Knabl, L.; Walter, M.; Furth, P.A.; Hennighausen, L. Limited cross-variant immune response from SARS-CoV-2 Omicron BA.2 in naïve but not previously infected outpatients. *iScience* **2022**, *25*, 105369. [CrossRef]

29. Szklarczyk, D.; Franceschini, A.; Kuhn, M.; Simonovic, M.; Roth, A.; Minguez, P.; Doerks, T.; Stark, M.; Muller, J.; Bork, P.; et al. The STRING database in 2011: Functional interaction networks of proteins, globally integrated and scored. *Nucleic Acids Res.* **2011**, *39*, D561–D568. [CrossRef]

30. Shannon, P.; Markiel, A.; Ozier, O.; Baliga, N.S.; Wang, J.T.; Ramage, D.; Amin, N.; Schwikowski, B.; Ideker, T. Cytoscape: A software environment for integrated models of biomolecular interaction networks. *Genome Res.* **2003**, *13*, 2498–2504. [CrossRef]

31. Zhang, J.; Lin, D.; Li, K.; Ding, X.; Li, L.; Liu, Y.; Liu, D.; Lin, J.; Teng, X.; Li, Y.; et al. Transcriptome Analysis of Peripheral Blood Mononuclear Cells Reveals Distinct Immune Response in Asymptomatic and Re-Detectable Positive COVID-19 Patients. *Front. Immunol.* **2021**, *12*, 716075. [CrossRef]

32. Zhou, Z.; Zhou, X.; Cheng, L.; Wen, L.; An, T.; Gao, H.; Deng, H.; Yan, Q.; Zhang, X.; Li, Y.; et al. Machine learning algorithms utilizing blood parameters enable early detection of immunethrombotic dysregulation in COVID-19. *Clin. Transl. Med.* **2021**, *11*, e523. [CrossRef]

33. Zhang, C.; Feng, Y.G.; Tam, C.; Wang, N.; Feng, Y. Transcriptional Profiling and Machine Learning Unveil a Concordant Biosignature of Type I Interferon-Inducible Host Response Across Nasal Swab and Pulmonary Tissue for COVID-19 Diagnosis. *Front. Immunol.* **2021**, *12*, 733171. [CrossRef] [PubMed]

34. Bizzotto, J.; Sanchis, P.; Abbate, M.; Lage-Vickers, S.; Lavignolle, R.; Toro, A.; Olszevicki, S.; Sabater, A.; Cascardo, F.; Vazquez, E.; et al. SARS-CoV-2 Infection Boosts MX1 Antiviral Effector in COVID-19 Patients. *iScience* **2020**, *23*, 101585. [CrossRef] [PubMed]

35. Verhelst, J.; Parthoens, E.; Schepens, B.; Fiers, W.; Saelens, X. Interferon-inducible protein Mx1 inhibits influenza virus by interfering with functional viral ribonucleoprotein complex assembly. *J. Virol.* **2012**, *86*, 13445–13455. [CrossRef]

36. Zhang, Y.; Yu, C. Prognostic Characterization of OAS1/OAS2/OAS3/OASL in Breast Cancer. *BMC Cancer* **2020**, *20*, 575.

37. Papac-Milicevic, N.; Breuss, J.M.; Zaujec, J.; Ryban, L.; Plyushch, T.; Wagner, G.A.; Fenzl, S.; Dremsek, P.; Cabaravdic, M.; Steiner, M.; et al. The interferon stimulated gene 12 inactivates vasculoprotective functions of NR4A nuclear receptors. *Circ. Res.* **2012**, *110*, e50–e63. [CrossRef]

38. Shojaei, M.; Shamshirian, A.; Monkman, J.; Grice, L.; Tran, M.; Tan, C.W.; Teo, S.M.; Rodrigues Rossi, G.; McCulloch, T.R.; Nalos, M.; et al. IFI27 transcription is an early predictor for COVID-19 outcomes, a multi-cohort observational study. *Front. Immunol.* **2023**, *13*, 1060438. [CrossRef]

39. Zhao, M.; Zhou, Y.; Zhu, B.; Wan, M.; Jiang, T.; Tan, Q.; Liu, Y.; Jiang, J.; Luo, S.; Tan, Y.; et al. Ifi44l promoter methylation as a blood biomarker for systemic lupus erythematosus. *Ann. Rheum. Dis.* **2016**, *75*, 1998–2006. [CrossRef]

40. DeDiego, M.L.; Nogales, A.; Martinez-Sobrido, L.; Topham, D.J. Interferon-induced protein 44 interacts with cellular FK506-binding protein 5, negatively regulates host antiviral responses, and supports virus replication. *mBio* **2019**, *10*, e01839-19. [CrossRef] [PubMed]

41. DeDiego, M.L.; Martinez-Sobrido, L.; Topham, D.J. Novel functions of Ifi44l as a feedback regulator of host antiviral responses. *J. Virol.* **2019**, *93*, e01159-19. [CrossRef]

42. Xie, L.M.; Yin, X.; Bi, J.; Luo, H.M.; Cao, X.J.; Ma, Y.W.; Liu, Y.L.; Su, J.W.; Lin, G.L.; Guo, X.G. Identification of potential biomarkers in dengue via integrated bioinformatic analysis. *PLoS Negl. Trop. Dis.* **2021**, *15*, e0009633. [CrossRef]
43. Harapan, H.; Ryan, M.; Yohan, B.; Abidin, R.S.; Nainu, F.; Rakib, A.; Jahan, I.; Emran, T.B.; Ullah, I.; Panta, K.; et al. COVID-19 and dengue: Double punches for dengue-endemic countries in Asia. *Rev. Med. Virol.* **2021**, *31*, e2161. [CrossRef] [PubMed]
44. Stark, G.R.; Darnell, J.E., Jr. The jak-stat pathway at twenty. *Immunity* **2012**, *36*, 503–514. [CrossRef] [PubMed]
45. Hadjadj, J.; Yatim, N.; Barnabei, L.; Corneau, A.; Boussier, J.; Pere, H.; Charbit, B.; Bondet, V.; Chenevier-Gobeaux, C.; Breillat, P.; et al. Impaired type I interferon activity and exacerbated inflammatory responses in severe COVID-19 patients. *Science* **2020**, *369*, 718–724. [CrossRef] [PubMed]
46. Blanco-Melo, D.; Nilsson-Payant, B.E.; Liu, W.-C.; Uhl, S.; Hoagland, D.; Møller, R.; Jordan, T.X.; Oishi, K.; Panis, M.; Sachs, D.; et al. Imbalanced host response to SARS-CoV-2 drives development of COVID-19. *Cell* **2020**, *181*, 1036–1045.e9. [CrossRef]
47. Zhang, Y.; Greer, R.A.; Song, Y.; Praveen, H.; Song, Y. In silico identification of available drugs targeting cell surface BiP to disrupt SARS-CoV-2 binding and replication: Drug repurposing approach. *Eur. J. Pharm. Sci.* **2021**, *160*, 105771. [CrossRef] [PubMed]

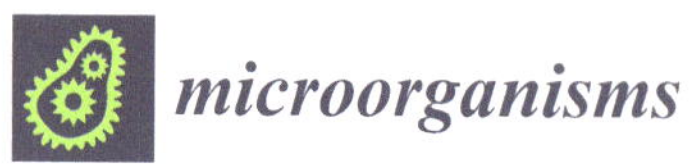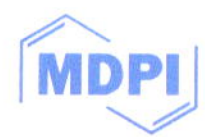

Review

Back to the Future: Immune Protection or Enhancement of Future Coronaviruses

Merit Bartels, Eric Sala Solé , Lotte M. Sauerschnig and Ger T. Rijkers *

Science and Engineering Department, University College Roosevelt, 4331 CB Middelburg, The Netherlands; m.bartels@ucr.nl (M.B.); e.salasole@ucr.nl (E.S.S.); l.sauerschnig@ucr.nl (L.M.S.)
* Correspondence: g.rijkers@ucr.nl; Tel.: +31-118-655-500

Abstract: Before the emergence of SARS-CoV-1, MERS-CoV, and most recently, SARS-CoV-2, four other coronaviruses (the alpha coronaviruses NL63 and 229E and the beta coronaviruses OC43 and HKU1) had already been circulating in the human population. These circulating coronaviruses all cause mild respiratory illness during the winter seasons, and most people are already infected in early life. Could antibodies and/or T cells, especially against the beta coronaviruses, have offered some form of protection against (severe) COVID-19 caused by infection with SARS-CoV-2? Related is the question of whether survivors of SARS-CoV-1 or MERS-CoV would be relatively protected against SARS-CoV-2. More importantly, would humoral and cellular immunological memory generated during the SARS-CoV-2 pandemic, either by infection or vaccination, offer protection against future coronaviruses? Or rather than protection, could antibody-dependent enhancement have taken place, a mechanism by which circulating corona antibodies enhance the severity of COVID-19? Another related phenomenon, the original antigenic sin, would also predict that the effectiveness of the immune response to future coronaviruses would be impaired because of the reactivation of memory against irrelevant epitopes. The currently available evidence indicates that latter scenarios are highly unlikely and that especially cytotoxic memory T cells directed against conserved epitopes of human coronaviruses could at least offer partial protection against future coronaviruses.

Keywords: SARS-CoV-2; COVID-19; human coronaviruses; conserved T-cell epitopes; antibody-dependent enhancement; original antigenic sin

Citation: Bartels, M.; Sala Solé, E.; Sauerschnig, L.M.; Rijkers, G.T. Back to the Future: Immune Protection or Enhancement of Future Coronaviruses. *Microorganisms* **2024**, *12*, 617. https://doi.org/10.3390/microorganisms12030617

Academic Editor: Qibin Geng

Received: 5 February 2024
Revised: 14 March 2024
Accepted: 16 March 2024
Published: 19 March 2024

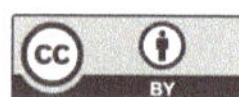

1. Introduction

The COVID-19 pandemic outbreak has brought attention to a critical global public health issue that has affected billions of people. The virus that causes COVID-19 is SARS-CoV-2, which displays a high degree of similarity to the SARS-CoV species that caused the 2003 coronavirus outbreak. This has greatly aided the identification and full genetic characterization of SARS-CoV-2 [1]. The rapid spread of the illness necessitated the development of preventative and therapeutic measures for the care of SARS-CoV-2-infected individuals. Thanks to the development and implementation of effective vaccines, and probably also the emergence of the omicron variant, the pandemic could be brought under control. On 17 March 2023, the Director-General of the WHO indicated that he was confident that in 2023, COVID-19 would be over as a public health emergency of international concern [2] and, indeed, in May 2023, the WHO declared that COVID-19 is now an established and ongoing health issue which no longer constitutes a public health emergency of international concern [3]. SARS-CoV-2, however, has not disappeared from the world and still causes severe disease in the most vulnerable. In an optimistic scenario, it can be envisioned that within time, SARS-CoV-2 can be added to the so-called cold cousins, i.e., the circulating coronaviruses that cause the common cold during winter seasons (229E, OC43, NL63, and HKU1 [4]). The human population then would be relatively protected against future variants of SARS-CoV-2. It has to be emphasized that the timeline of the evolutionary conversion of a severe acute respiratory coronavirus to a common cold coronavirus is difficult to predict and could potentially take tens to hundreds of years. In a pessimistic scenario where novel coronaviruses adapt to humans, immunological memory would not protect against novel coronaviruses but instead, due to antibody-dependent and related mechanisms, could enhance the severity of the disease. In this paper, currently available evidence will be discussed, which suggests that T-cell memory, directed against conserved epitopes on the spike protein and nucleocapsid protein, could protect against future coronaviruses.

Coronaviruses (CoVs) are positive-sense, single-stranded RNA viruses; they are members of the family Coronaviridae, subfamily Coronavirinae, and order Nidovirales. CoVs possess one of the largest genomes among all RNA viruses. Four species of coronaviruses, including alpha, beta, gamma, and delta, can be distinguished. SARS-CoV-2 belongs to the species severe acute respiratory syndrome-related coronavirus [5]. Originally, they were categorized based on serology; however, the categories named above are based on phylogenetic clustering [6].

The spike, envelope, membrane, and nucleocapsid are the four main structural proteins that make up the coronavirus virion structure (Figure 1). Although the number and location of accessory ORFs present in different coronavirus species vary, distinct coronavirus strains share a common genetic organization for the coding region, encoding for a canonical set of genes in the order 5′ end–ORF1a/b replicase, spike, envelope, membrane, nucleocapsid–3′ end. The subgenomic mRNAs that carry out gene translation combine with the viral genome to form a 5′ and 3′ co-terminal nested set. Subgenomic mRNAs are present along with a common 5′ leader sequence and a 3′ terminal sequence. The genome contains small untranslated regions at both the 3′ and 5′ ends. In addition, the viral genome encodes a number of nonstructural proteins (NSPs), such as the papain-like protease (PLpro), the coronavirus main protease (3CLpro), and the RNA-dependent RNA polymerase (RdRp) [7].

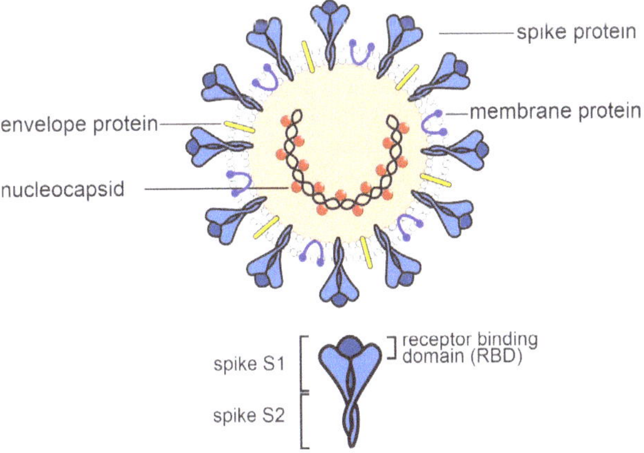

Figure 1. Structure of SARS-CoV-2 with major structural proteins. The immunologically relevant domains of the spike protein (S1, S2, and RBD) are indicated.

Before the emergence of SARS-CoV-1, Middle Eastern respiratory syndrome coronavirus (MERS-CoV), and most recently, SARS-CoV-2, four other coronaviruses had already been circulating in the human population: the alpha coronaviruses NL63 and 229E and the beta coronaviruses OC34 and HKU1 (SARS-CoV-1, MERS-CoV, and SARS-CoV-2 are also beta coronaviruses) [8]. The circulating coronaviruses all cause mild respiratory illness during the winter seasons (which is the reason why they are sometimes called the "cold cousins" of SARS-CoV-2), and most people are already infected in early life [9,10]. Could antibodies or T cells (especially against the beta coronaviruses), which have originally been generated after exposure to a circulating coronavirus, have offered some form of protection against (severe) COVID-19 caused by SARS-CoV-2 infection? Related is the question of whether survivors of SARS-CoV-1 or MERS-CoV would be relatively protected against SARS-CoV-2.

2. The Immune Response to SARS-CoV-2 Infection and Vaccination

Upon infection with SARS-CoV-2, an innate immune response is initiated in the respiratory tract. This involves massive activation of mainly proinflammatory cytokines [11,12]. The size of the initial viral load and the effectiveness of the innate immune response—especially the type I interferon-mediated response—appears to be crucial in determining the course of the subsequent adaptive response and the final clinical outcome [13]. Effective interferon signaling plays a critical role in acute infection, as demonstrated by both acquired and genetic factors. The indicators of severe clinical outcomes include early and persistent inflammation with elevated interferon (IFN)-α, TNF, and IFN-γ, as well as a slow decline in the viral load [14].

Like other viral respiratory infections, SARS-CoV-2 infection promotes the fast production of IgM, IgG, and IgA antibodies. These antibodies, including those that bind to the spike protein and nucleocapsid, are detectable in the sera as early as one-week post-infection. The speed at which these reactions occur suggests that the antibodies originate from extrafollicular differentiation of naive B cells into short-lived antibody-secreting cells, independent of the traditional germinal center reaction [15]. These antibodies also show neutralizing activity against live or pseudotyped SARS-CoV-2; the latter activity can be readily detected in convalescent sera, though the degree of neutralization that can be achieved varies widely between people. The inconsistent outcomes of plasma therapy, which was tried early in the pandemic, could be partially explained by this variability [16].

2.1. The Humoral Immune Response to SARS-CoV-2 Infection

Hashem et al. studied the relationship between the severity of disease and the antibody titers in COVID-19 patients [17]. It was found that COVID-19 patients who experienced severe or moderate infections exhibited noticeably higher total neutralizing antibody (nAbs) levels. Furthermore, compared to mild cases, severe cases had significantly higher levels of IgG antibodies directed against the S1 subunit of the spike protein (S1). Notably, anti-N IgG and IgM levels were induced at higher levels in moderate and severe cases compared to mild infections, and these levels were significantly correlated with the severity of the disease [18]. Anti-S1 and N antibodies (IgG and IgM), as well as nAbs, were found to be significantly higher in patients who required ICU admission or had fatal outcomes when patients were stratified based on their need for ICU admission or infection outcome. Similar findings were also published by Liu et al. and Rijkers et al., who reported that nAbs were higher in hospitalized COVID-19 patients as compared to healthcare workers with mild clinical symptoms, not requiring hospitalization [19,20]. These findings unequivocally demonstrate the relationship between the severity of the COVID-19 infection and the activation state of the humoral immune system as a whole.

Neutralizing antibodies are mostly directed against the receptor-binding domain (RBD) of the SARS-CoV-2 spike protein (indicated in Figure 2) but can also be directed against the N-terminal domain or the stem helix region or the fusion peptide region in the S2 subunit of the spike protein [21]. Evolutionary variability of the virus, reflected in the successive appearance of alpha, delta, and omicron variants, caused changes in an increasing number of amino acids within the RBD and a concomitant loss of the neutralizing capacity of existing antibodies.

COVID-19 and Response to Vaccination in Patients with Humoral Immunodeficiency or B-Cell-Depletion Therapy

The importance of the role played by humoral immunity in COVID-19, as well as a correlation of protection against COVID-19 after vaccination, remains uncertain because

SARS-CoV-2 infection or vaccination induces both a humoral and cellular immune response. Patients with agammaglobulinemia lack (functional) B cells but have an intact cellular immune system. The immune response of agammaglobulinemia patients during SARS-CoV-2 infection and the outcome of COVID-19 could serve as a model to further investigate the relative role of humoral and cellular immunity.

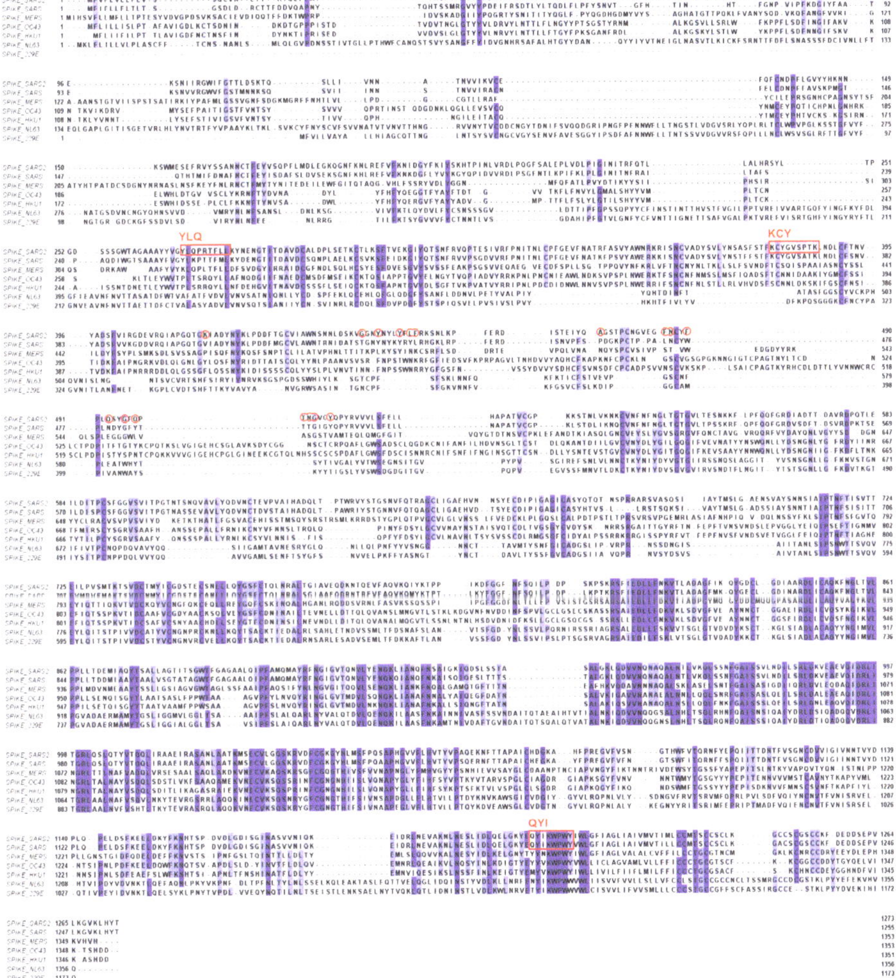

Figure 2. Homology between spike proteins of the human coronaviruses. The amino acids constituting the ACE2-receptor-binding domain of SARS-CoV-2 are encircled in red. Major CD8+ T-cell epitopes are indicated by red rectangles and their first three amino acids according to the SARS-CoV-2 sequence. YLQ = YLQPRTFLL (269–277); KCY = KCYGVSPTKL (378–386); QYI = QYIKWPWYI (1208–1216) [22]. Shades of blue indicate different degrees of identity between the compared protein sequences. Figures 2 and 3 were created using Clustal Omega version 1.2.2 (http://www.clustal.org/omega/ (accessed on 30 January 2024)) and Jalview sequence alignment software version 2.11.2.0 (https://www.jalview.org/ (accessed on 30 January 2024)). All viral peptide sequences were retrieved from the UniProt database (https://www.uniprot.org/ (accessed on 30 January 2024)).

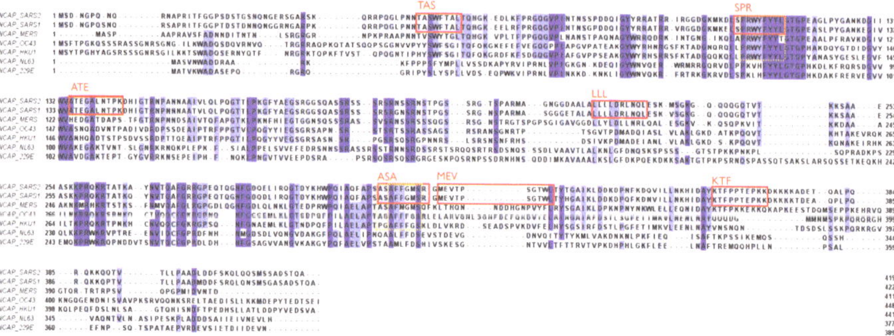

Figure 3. Major T-cell epitopes within the nucleocapsid protein. All epitopes are indicated by their first three letters. TAS = TASWFTAL (49–56); SPR = SPRWYFYYL (105–113); ATE = ATEGALNTPK (134–143); LLL = LLLDRLNQL (222–230); ASA = ASAFFGMSR (311–319); KTF = KTFPPTEPKK (361–369); MEV = MEVTPSGTWL (322–331). Further details are provided in the legend of Figure 2. Based on data from [22–24].

Soresina et al. described the cases of two X-linked agammaglobulinemia (XLA) patients who developed pneumonia as a clinical manifestation of SARS-CoV-2 infection but did recover without requiring oxygen ventilation or intensive care treatment [25]. The cases of two adolescent male XLA patients were discussed by Devassikutty et al., where, except for delayed recovery, both patients had successful outcomes [26]. In a paper on seven patients (two with agammaglobulinemia and five with common variable immunodeficiency (CVID)), it was noted that a milder course of COVID-19 was observed in agammaglobulinemia as compared to the CVID patients. Furthermore, their COVID-19 course had a shorter duration and required no need for anti-inflammatory treatment with an IL-6-blocking drug [27]. These data, on an admittedly low number of patients, indicate that in the complete absence of B cells, such as in the case of XLA, COVID-19 does not necessarily take a severe course. It could be argued that XLA patients are substituted with intravenous immunoglobulins (IVIG) and that antibodies contained within the preparation confer protection against COVID-19. The above-mentioned studies, however, were all published in the first year of the pandemic, and at that time, IVIG preparations did not (yet) contain SARS-CoV-2 IgG antibodies.

From these findings in patients with B-cell deficiencies, it can be speculated that B-cell depletion may not have a major detrimental effect on COVID-19 recovery. In B-cell lymphoma patients treated with rituximab and bendamustine, the humoral immune response (but not the T-cell response) to SARS-CoV-2 vaccination is impaired, as would be expected from a B-cell-depleting treatment [28]. Similar results were published by Candon et al. and Ishio et al. [29,30]. Patients with B-cell lymphoma who were successfully treated with rituximab and recovered show normal antibody responses after (mRNA) SARS-CoV-2 vaccines [31]. Finally, in a group of patients with childhood-onset nephrotic syndrome who received rituximab for its steroid/calcineurin-inhibitor sparing effect, SARS-CoV-2 antibodies largely persisted. This indicates that long-lived plasma cells play a major role in maintaining antibody levels [32].

Most of the patients with multiple sclerosis who were treated with rituximab had a mild course of COVID-19 [33]. In a French cohort study on COVID-19 in patients with inflammatory rheumatic and musculoskeletal diseases treated with rituximab, severe disease occurred more frequently than in non-rituximab-treated patients [34]. For other rituximab indications, variable effects on the incidence and severity of COVID-19 have been reported, but an extensive discussion of these data is beyond the scope of this paper.

2.2. T-Cell-Mediated Immunity against Coronaviruses

Probably fueled by the massive reports in the popular press on vaccination and immunity, the general conception is that mainly antibodies directed against the SARS-CoV-2 spike protein offer protection against disease. Furthermore, antibody levels should remain high in order to stay protected. The role of T-cell-mediated immunity against SARS-CoV-2, and viruses in general, has received relatively little attention. Of the papers dealing with SARS-CoV-2 immunity, 87% concern humoral immunity, and only 13% address T-cell immunity.

Importance of T-Cell Immunity

T cells, in principle, can respond to any viral peptides, including those of more conserved regions. SARS-CoV-2, as well as SARS-CoV-1, for that matter, can enter the host cells through binding to the ACE2 receptor. Upon entry, viral capsid proteins are broken down by enzymatic degradation, setting free the genetic material and exploiting the host cellular machinery for viral replication purposes [35]. Simultaneously, viral proteins are further processed by the proteasome, after which any peptide that fits can be bound in the groove of an MHC class I molecule (HLA-A, -B, -C) and, upon cell surface expression, be presented to CD8$^+$ T cells or bind to MHC class II (HLA-DR, -DP, DQ) [36] molecules on antigen-presenting cells (APCs) to CD4$^+$ T-helper cells. The selective interaction with the TCR elicits either a cytotoxic response by CD8$^+$ T cells or the activation of CD4$^+$ T-helper cells that are necessary for proper stimulation of B-lymphocytes and antibody production [37]. Because all viral peptides, including those derived from non-structural regions, have the potential to elicit a T-cell response, they play a determining role in adaptive cellular immunity. Tarke et al., by using overlapping peptides spanning all structural and non-structural viral proteins, identified several hundred T-cell epitopes for CD4$^+$ T cells and CD8$^+$ T cells, highlighting the diverse T-cell response to the virus [38]. Additionally, abortive infections can exist where T-cell responses may clear the virus before sufficient viral replication or antibody production has taken place. This process is explored in a study by Swadling et al., who found that the T cells involved in this process are mainly directed against non-structural proteins of the replication-transcription complex [22]. It should be kept in mind that most studies on T-cell epitope mapping are performed with peripheral blood T cells. The T cells that have infiltrated infected tissue, such as the lung, may have a different specificity pattern [39].

The receptor-binding domain of the spike protein of SARS-CoV-2 is localized in the N-terminal region of the protein and contains 17 amino acids that directly interact with the ACE2 receptor in human host cells (Figure 2). Within the conserved regions of the spike proteins of the other hCoVs, there is little sequence homology. Homologies are more prominent in the C-terminal regions of the spike proteins, which is also the part where most CD8$^+$ T-cell epitopes are found (Figure 2) [40].

As indicated above, the spike protein contains many T-cell epitopes, of which three can be considered major epitopes, as defined by Ferretti et al., termed YLQ, KCY, and QYI [40]. All three epitopes are located outside the RBD of SARS-CoV-2. The QYI epitope is highly conserved in SARS-CoV-1 and MERS-CoV, as well as in the other hCoVs. Furthermore, in the variants of SARS-CoV-2, from alpha to omicron, including the omicron subvariants, the QYI epitope remains unchanged. However, the epitope closest to the RBD (KCY) has been mutated in the omicron variants [23].

The nucleocapsid (N) protein is well conserved and has been shown to display a high degree of homology between different coronavirus strains [24]. N proteins are associated with the viral RNA (see Figure 1) and are not accessible for antibodies in an intact virus particle. Therefore, anti-N antibodies, which are produced in large quantities following infection, cannot prevent the spread of the virus within the body. N proteins can, however, serve as important T-cell epitopes [41]. Six major epitopes have been identified in SARS-CoV-2, as indicated in Figure 3. Furthermore, all six epitopes are identical in SARS-CoV-1 and SARS-CoV-2 (including the delta and omicron variants of SARS-CoV-2), plus they are located within conserved regions of the different beta coronavirus strains. More specifically, the ASA epitope is conserved in all known human beta coronaviruses and SPR to a lesser degree (Figure 3). The MEV epitope is identical in SARS-CoV-1 and SARS-CoV-2 but not found in other human beta coronaviruses [42]. SARS-CoV-1 survivors showed a robust T-cell response when activated in vitro with N-protein epitopes, including ASA and SPR [42]. This is evidence supporting the suggestion that memory T-cells from previous infections with circulating coronaviruses could have been reactive to SARS-CoV-2 and thus have aided in the cellular protection against severe disease. Any possible existing cross-reactive T-cell immunity or cross-reactive antibodies against SARS-CoV-2 could therefore have resulted from prior infection with another coronavirus, i.e., SARS-CoV-1 or MERS-CoV [18,43], and this would have had a much bigger impact than one of the common cold viruses, OC43, HKU1, NL63, or 229E10 [10,44–46]. In a similar scenario, long-lasting cellular immunity could be provided through cross-reactivity against homologous epitopes for new coronaviruses in the future.

When targeting cellular immunity, the focus should be on MHC class I epitopes, which are present on all nucleated cells [47], including those with ACE2 receptors. Displaying viral peptides via MHC I elicits a direct response of cytotoxic CD8$^+$ T cells, leading to programmed cell death of the virally infected cell [48]. This immediately halts viral replication as the host cell is necessary for the production of the virus. In COVID-19, an early cytotoxic T-cell response has been observed to correlate with efficient viral clearance and a mild disease course [14,39,45,46]. In addition, CD8$^+$ memory T cells generated by previous infection with coronaviruses facilitate a quick response to reinfection by the same strain and might aid in fighting infection by a new strain or entirely new virus [48], provided there would be sufficient sequence homology between relevant epitopes. Therefore, T-cell immunity and especially MHC class I epitopes should receive careful consideration when designing vaccines in the future [45,49].

Furthermore, Verma et al. found that peptides of the N protein can bind with high affinity to TLR4, expressed on monocytes and macrophages [41]. Triggering of TLR4 could be beneficial as this improves antigen uptake and presentation to both CD4$^+$ T cells, stimulating the B-cell response and antibody production as well as to CD8$^+$ T cells [50]. Hence, identifying and utilizing epitopes that are recognized by APCs additionally to providing binding sites for MHC I could thus promote both cellular and humoral immunity. As indicated above, apart from the spike and N proteins, many T-cell epitopes in SARS-CoV-2 are also found in non-structural parts (NSPs) like ORF1ab or ORF3a [38,51]. However, immunodominant are epitopes of the N protein, giving rise to the highest frequency of specific T-cells [14,52]. Overall, the indicated (immuno-)dominant HLA alleles in response to SARS-CoV-2 are HLA-A*01:01, HLA-A*02:01, HLA-A*03:01, HLA-A*11:01, HLA-A*26:01, HLA-A*68:01, HLA-B*07:02, HLA-B*08:01, and HLA-B*35:01 [38,40]. These HLA alleles specifically have been shown to interact with a wide variety of different structural and non-structural SARS-CoV-2 peptides, and at least one of these prominent HLA class I alleles is present in about 85% of the world's population [40]. All SARS-CoV-2 T-cell epitopes discussed in this paper can interact with at least one of these aforementioned alleles.

3. Potential Negative Impact of Existing Antibodies and Memory B Cells on Future Viruses

When, as discussed above, a novel emerging coronavirus would have considerable antigenic differences with circulating coronaviruses, existing antibodies and memory B cells would offer no protection. It is even possible that existing antibodies and memory B cells would have a negative effect and cause more severe clinical expression of the infection. Two different but partly overlapping mechanisms could be involved. The first one is antibody-dependent enhancement, and the second is the original antigenic sin.

3.1. Antibody-Dependent Enhancement (ADE)

Antibody-dependent enhancement (ADE) refers to the enhancement of disease due to the presence of antibodies to the pathogen that has caused the disease. These antibodies could have been induced by previous exposure to the given pathogen, which caused a primary immune response, or previous vaccination, which has induced the production of antibodies. Also, passively administered antibodies (either prophylactic or therapeutic) could potentially lead to ADE. As far as coronaviruses are concerned, there has been a precedent of ADE after vaccination. Cats vaccinated against feline infectious peritonitis virus, a coronavirus, did produce anti-viral antibodies, but after being challenged with the live virus, they were more susceptible than the non-vaccinated control animals [53,54]. While ADE is of concern to vaccine development in general, it was especially relevant for coronavirus vaccines (see above). Thus, the interest in ADE rose during the SARS-CoV-2 pandemic (Figure 4).

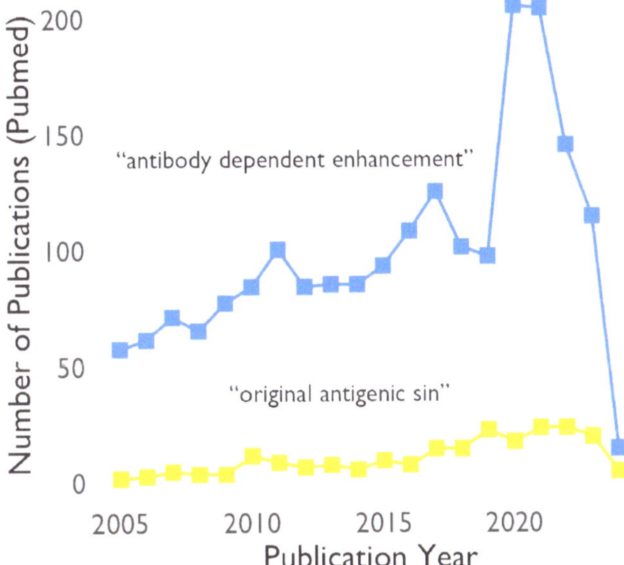

Figure 4. Number of publications per year retrieved from PubMed (https://pubmed.ncbi.nlm.nih.gov/ (accessed on 14 January 2024)) using the search terms "antibody dependent enhancement" or "original antigenic sin" during the past 20 years.

3.1.1. In Vitro Studies on Antibody-Dependent Enhancement

Wan et al. mentioned the mechanism by which previous coronaviruses have undergone ADE, specifically MERS-CoV and SARS-CoV [55]. Using monoclonal antibodies specifically targeted to the receptor-binding domain (RBD) of SARS-CoV, Wan et al. found that entry into CD32A-expressing cells was mediated by this monoclonal antibody; however, it blocked entry into cells that expressed the ACE2 receptor [55]. This inhibitory effect serves as a possible mechanism by which ADE could occur with blood lymphocytes since they show poor ACE2 expression as compared to tissue-resident macrophages.

3.1.2. In Vivo Indications for Antibody-Dependent Enhancement

In vivo evidence of ADE has been observed and studied in dengue virus infections. The proposed mechanism for the ADE of dengue virus entails a primary infection of a specific serotype during which antibodies are produced that neutralize the serotype of the primary infection [56]. ADE then occurs during a secondary dengue infection of a different serotype, and the same antibodies no longer function to the original extent. Instead of neutralizing the viral particles, they potentiate the entry into leukocytes [56]. This is achieved as the Fab part of these antibodies will bind to the viral particles, leaving the Fc part open to interact with Fcγ receptors on cells of the immune system. This will then allow leukocytes to recognize and neutralize the virus in normal function; however, in ADE, the Fc part of the antibody will mediate the entry of the viral particles into leukocytes, particularly the macrophages, which will lead to viral replication inside of the leukocytes and ultimately enhancement of the disease. This mechanism of disease enhancement is similar to that discussed in the case of coronaviruses (see above) [57]. The specific glycosylation states of IgG antibodies generated during a SARS-CoV-2 infection have been linked to how the course of the disease will progress ultimately. Afucosylation of the IgG antibodies leads to an increase in the affinity to FcγRIIIA (CD16a) and, thus, an increase in antibody-dependent cellular cytotoxicity (ADCC) [58,59]. Other modifications to antibodies and different antibody classes need to be researched to elucidate the roles that galactosylation and sialylation have on complement activation and disease progression, which could play a role in ADE through the aforementioned mechanism.

When ADE occurs in cases of SARS-CoV-2 infection, it is expected that after vaccination, COVID-19 will take a more severe course. However, studies on breakthrough infections [60,61] as well as case–control studies [62] have shown that vaccinated individuals with breakthrough COVID-19 infections experience milder symptoms, with fewer hospital and ICU admission and lower mortality rates as compared to unvaccinated individuals [63].

3.1.3. Proposed Mechanisms of Antibody-Dependent Enhancement

Fc gamma receptors (FcγRs) are involved in the specific signaling pathways that purportedly cause ADE and are primarily expressed on the surface of leukocytes. If the binding of the Fc part of IgG would mediate viral entry into the leukocytes, on top of the capacity of the virus to enter target cells expressing ACE2 receptors, this could lead to ADE (Figure 5).

Upon engagement with immune complexes formed by antibodies and their corresponding antigens, FcγRs initiate intracellular signaling cascades, leading to various cellular responses, including phagocytosis: antibody-dependent cellular phagocytosis, ADCP [64], production of pro-inflammatory cytokines and cellular activation [65]. In the context of ADE, these signaling pathways may inadvertently contribute to increased infection by promoting the uptake of virus-containing immune complexes. Therefore, in ADE, the phagocytic cells could serve as a (additional) host for the virus.

Also, the complement system may play a critical role in ADE. There are two main mechanisms involving complement that have been exploited by viruses, namely a C1q-mediated mechanism [66,67] and a C3-mediated mechanism [68,69] (Figure 5c,d).

3.2. The Original Antigenic Sin

Apart from ADE, another potential negative effect of immunological memory for future coronaviruses would be the so-called original antigenic sin [70]. This phenomenon was first described by Thomas Francis Jr. in 1960 and states that a new strain of an existing virus (in his case, influenza virus) could activate memory B cells specific for a previous strain. Those antibodies could bind to the new strain but not neutralize the virus [71]. This phenomenon needs to be considered when designing and evaluating current and future coronavirus vaccines [72]. Current data do not point toward a role for "original antigenic sin" in the immune response to SARS-CoV-2 infection or vaccination [73,74].

Within the T-cell system, an equivalent of ADE or original antigenic sin has not been described. Any negative effect of existing T-cell memory on protection against disease caused by future coronavirus infections, therefore, is not to be expected.

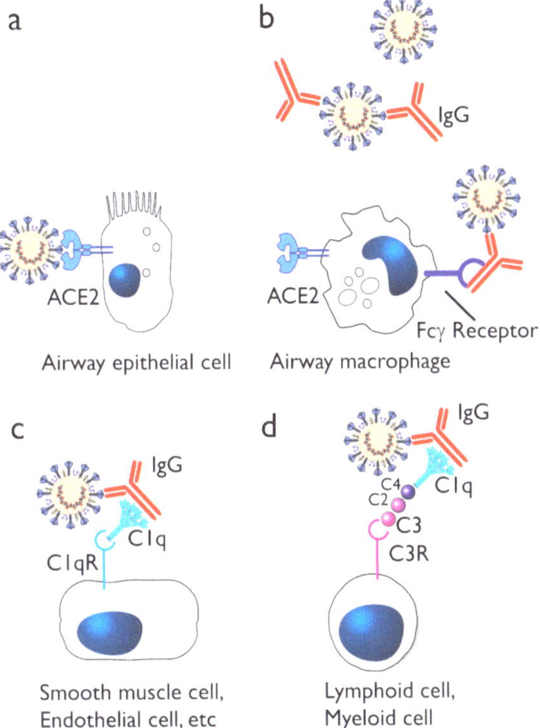

Figure 5. Cellular tropism of SARS-CoV-2 and the potential mechanism of antibody-dependent enhancement. Human cells expressing the angiotensin-converting enzyme 2 (ACE2), such as airway epithelial cells (panel (**a**)) and airway macrophages (panel (**b**)), can be infected by SARS-CoV-2. When IgG antibodies (against viral surface proteins such as the spike protein) are generated, these can form immune complexes with the virus. The Fc part of the IgG can be bound by cellular Fcγ receptors, which enables the virus to enter the cell via this route (panel (**b**)). When the complement system is activated, C1q binds to the IgG, and the complex can be captured by C1q receptors (C1qR) (panel (**c**)). Ongoing complement activation leads to binding and activation of C4, C2, and C3 (C1r and C1s are not shown). C3 receptors (C3Rs), which include complement receptor 1 (CR1), CR2, and CR3, can also bind the complex of virus, antibody, and complement proteins (panel (**d**)).

4. Concluding Remarks and Outlook for the Future

The best model to assess the protective effect of existing immunological memory for future coronaviruses is to compare COVID-19 incidence and severity in survivors of SARS-CoV-1 or MERS-CoV infection. In SARS-CoV-1 survivors, cross-reactive SARS-CoV-2 IgG antibodies can be detected, and these SARS survivors also generate a much stronger antibody response after SARS-CoV-2 vaccination [75]. In a retrospective cohort study, it was found that symptomatic MERS-CoV patients were at a lower risk for COVID-19 [76]. Care must be taken when interpreting these data because SARS-CoV-1 and MERS-CoV patients survived without being vaccinated or specifically treated. Therefore, they can have an immune system that was and remained a priori better equipped to combat coronaviruses.

Our analysis of the literature shows and confirms that cytotoxic T cells against conserved epitopes on the SARS-CoV-2 spike protein and nucleocapsid protein are expanded during infection and do limit the severity of COVID-19 [14,77]. Based on these findings, it is possible that existing memory T cells, generated during exposure to circulating hCoVs, including SARS-CoV-1 and MERS, have offered partial protection against COVID-19 caused by SARS-CoV-2 infection and thus could have contributed to a lower case-fatality rate of

SARS-CoV-2 as compared to SARS and MERS. Therefore, it should be considered to include conserved epitopes of both the spike protein and nucleocapsid protein in future vaccines in order to induce a robust and lasting T-cell response against these relevant epitopes [77]. Appelberg et al. have shown that in their prototype universal SARS-CoV-2 vaccine, the inclusion of only the relevant nucleoprotein T-cell epitopes provided 60% protection against lethal infection in mice [78]. Future coronavirus vaccines ideally would be pancoronavirus vaccines [79]. Such a vaccine cannot be solely based on spike proteins or epitopes thereof because not all coronaviruses use ACE2 as a cellular receptor. T-cell epitopes of the nucleocapsid protein are conserved among the current hCoVs, and indeed, those epitopes are included in a number of pancoronavirus vaccines currently under development [80].

Regarding the outlook for the future, it should be noted that this review is restricted to an analysis of the immunological factors that may protect against future coronaviruses or enhance disease severity. Other factors, such as virological, societal, and environmental, can be as important or even more important than immune memory and cross-reactivity as such.

Infection with SARS-CoV-2, or vaccination for that matter, induces a strong response of both the humoral and cellular immune systems. In the assessment of the immune status of patients with COVID-19, as well as in the analysis of the immune response to vaccination, emphasis is mostly placed on the quantitation of (neutralizing) antibodies. Although no protective antibody titers have been established, the magnitude of the antibody response is taken as a correlate of protection. T-cell immunity appears to be more important and is directed to epitopes of viral proteins, which are largely conserved among the hCoVs, including the variants of SARS-CoV-2. It, therefore, would be appropriate to (also) implement T-cell-based diagnostic assays. Development and implementation of these assays will be part of preparing for the future.

In their search for the origin of SARS-CoV-2, Temmam et al. have sampled Rhinolophus bats in northern Laos [81]. Many previously unknown coronaviruses were found, including five sarbecoviruses. Three of those (BANAL-52, BANAL-103, and BANAL-236) are close relatives of SARS-CoV-2 and can bind to human ACE2 [82]. These data show that bats, as well as many other animal species for that matter, are a large reservoir from which new coronaviruses can emerge with the potential to set off a new pandemic.

Thanks to the advancement of medical sciences, the original Darwinian principles of struggle for life and survival of the fittest no longer hold completely true. Yet, despite vaccines, diagnostics, and advanced treatment, the burden of infectious diseases, including SARS-CoV-2, weighs on those with an impaired immune system. The "fitness" of the immune system, however, is not as easy to determine as, for instance, that of the cardiac or respiratory system. Unfortunately, there is no simple litmus test for the immune system.

The research team of Amy Huei-Yi Lee has developed a multiomic data integration tool that has the potential to create a kind of immune signature that could predict response to vaccination [82]. On a much larger scale, an initiative has been taken to collect thousands of immune parameters (cells, proteins, genes) of hundreds of thousands of people across the globe in a project called the Human Immunome Project (https://www.humanimmunomeproject.org/ (accessed on 8 January 2024)) [83]. Advancements like these will make it possible to predict whether or not a new virus, or any other microorganism, would have the potential to give rise to endemic or pandemic outgrowth.

Author Contributions: Conceptualization, G.T.R., M.B., E.S.S. and L.M.S.; methodology, M.B. and G.T.R.; formal analysis, M.B.; writing—original draft preparation, G.T.R., M.B., E.S.S. and L.M.S.; writing—review and editing, G.T.R.; visualization, M.B., E.S.S., L.M.S. and G.T.R.; supervision, G.T.R. All authors have read and agreed to the published version of the manuscript.

Funding: Article Processing Charges of this manuscript were covered by a grant (2024-025) from the Research Fund of the University College Roosevelt.

Acknowledgments: We apologize to all colleagues who have contributed immensely to our current understanding of the immunobiology of SARS-CoV-2 and other coronaviruses but whose work we could not include or cite due to space restrictions. We gratefully acknowledge the assistance of Theresa Dinse for language editing.

Conflicts of Interest: The authors declare no conflicts of interest.

References

1. Zhu, N.; Zhang, D.; Wang, W.; Li, X.; Yang, B.; Song, J.; Zhao, X.; Huang, B.; Shi, W.; Lu, R.; et al. China Novel Coronavirus Investigating Research Team ANovel Coronavirus from Patients with Pneumonia in China 2019. *N. Engl. J. Med.* **2020**, *382*, 727–733. [CrossRef]
2. World Health Organization. Virtual Press Conference on COVID-19 & Other Global Health Emergencies. Available online: https://www.who.int/publications/m/item/virtual-press-conference-on-covid-19---other-global-health-emergencies (accessed on 14 January 2024).
3. Harris, E. WHO Declares End of COVID-19 Global Health Emergency. *JAMA* **2023**, *329*, 1817. [CrossRef]
4. Cohen, J. COVID's cold cousins. Four largely ignored coronaviruses circulate in humans without causing great harm and may portend the future for SARS-CoV-2. *Science* **2024**, *383*, 141–145. [CrossRef]
5. Coronaviridae Study Group of the International Committee on Taxonomy of Viruses. The species Severe acute respiratory syndrome-related coronavirus: Classifying 2019-nCoV and naming it SARS-CoV-2. *Nat. Microbiol.* **2020**, *5*, 536–544. [CrossRef]
6. Al-Qahtani, W.S.; Alneghery, L.M.; Alqahtani, A.Q.S.; Al-Kahtani, M.D.; Alkahtani, S. A review of comparison study between corona viruses (SARS-CoV, mers-cov) and novel corona virus (COVID-19). *Rev. Mex. Ing. Química* **2020**, *19* (Suppl. 1), 201–212. [CrossRef]
7. Yang, H.; Rao, Z. Structural biology of SARS-CoV-2 and implications for therapeutic development. *Nat. Rev. Microbiol.* **2021**, *19*, 685–700. [CrossRef]
8. Tang, G.; Liu, Z.; Chen, D. Human coronaviruses: Origin, host and receptor. *J. Clin. Virol.* **2022**, *155*, 105246. [CrossRef]
9. Rajapakse, N.; Dixit, D. Human and novel coronavirus infections in children: A review. *Paediatr. Int. Child Health* **2021**, *41*, 36–55. [CrossRef] [PubMed]
10. van der Hoek, L.; Pyrc, K.; Jebbink, M.F.; Vermeulen-Oost, W.; Berkhout, R.J.; Wolthers, K.C.; Wertheim-van Dillen, P.M.; Kaandorp, J.; Spaargaren, J.; Berkhout, B. Identification of a new human coronavirus. *Nat. Med.* **2004**, *10*, 368–373. [CrossRef] [PubMed]
11. Hu, B.; Huang, S.; Yin, L. The cytokine storm and COVID-19. *J. Med. Virol.* **2021**, *93*, 250–256. [CrossRef] [PubMed]
12. Fajgenbaum, D.C.; June, C.H. Cytokine Storm. *N. Engl. J. Med.* **2020**, *383*, 2255–2273. [CrossRef]
13. Lei, X.; Dong, X.; Ma, R.; Wang, W.; Xiao, X.; Tian, Z.; Wang, C.; Wang, Y.; Li, L.; Ren, L.; et al. Activation and evasion of type I interferon responses by SARS-CoV-2. *Nat. Commun.* **2020**, *11*, 3810. [CrossRef]
14. Moss, P. The T cell immune response against SARS-CoV-2. *Nat Immunol.* **2022**, *23*, 186–193. [CrossRef]
15. Woodruff, M.C.; Ramonell, R.P.; Nguyen, D.C.; Cashman, K.S.; Saini, A.S.; Haddad, N.S.; Ley, A.M.; Kyu, S.; Howell, J.C.; Ozturk, T.; et al. Extrafollicular B cell responses correlate with neutralizing antibodies and morbidity in COVID-19. *Nat Immunol.* **2020**, *21*, 1506–1516. [CrossRef] [PubMed]
16. Zhang, Q.; Wang, Y.; Qi, C.; Shen, L.; Li, J. Clinical trial analysis of 2019-nCoV therapy registered in China. *J. Med. Virol.* **2020**, *92*, 540–545. [CrossRef]
17. Hashem, A.M.; Algaissi, A.; Almahboub, S.A.; Alfaleh, M.A.; Abujamel, T.S.; Alamri, S.S.; Alluhaybi, K.A.; Hobani, H.I.; AlHarbi, R.H.; Alsulaiman, R.M.; et al. Early Humoral Response Correlates with Disease Severity and Outcomes in COVID-19 Patients. *Viruses* **2020**, *12*, 1390. [CrossRef] [PubMed]
18. Ng, K.W.; Faulkner, N.; Cornish, G.H.; Rosa, A.; Harvey, R.; Hussain, S.; Ulferts, R.; Earl, C.; Wrobel, A.G.; Benton, D.J.; et al. Preexisting and de novo humoral immunity to SARS-CoV-2 in humans. *Science* **2020**, *370*, 1339–1343. [CrossRef]
19. Liu, X.; Wang, J.; Xu, X.; Liao, G.; Chen, Y.; Hu, C.H. Patterns of IgG and IgM antibody response in COVID-19 patients. *Emerg. Microbes Infect.* **2020**, *9*, 1269–1274. [CrossRef] [PubMed]
20. Rijkers, G.; Murk, J.L.; Wintermans, B.; van Looy, B.; van den Berge, M.; Veenemans, J.; Stohr, J.; Reusken, C.; van der Pol, P.; Reimerink, J. Differences in Antibody Kinetics and Functionality Between Severe and Mild Severe Acute Respiratory Syndrome Coronavirus 2 Infections. *J. Infect. Dis.* **2020**, *222*, 1265–1269. [CrossRef]
21. Chen, Y.; Zhao, X.; Zhou, H.; Zhu, H.; Jiang, S.; Wang, P. Broadly neutralizing antibodies to SARS-CoV-2 and other human coronaviruses. *Nat. Rev. Immunol.* **2023**, *23*, 189–199. [CrossRef]
22. Swadling, L.; Maini, M.K. Can T cells abort SARS-CoV-2 and other viral infections? *Int. J. Mol. Sci.* **2023**, *24*, 4371. [CrossRef] [PubMed]
23. Suardana, I.B.K.; Mahardika, B.K.; Pharmawati, M.; Sudipa, P.H.; Sari, T.K.; Mahendra, N.B.; Mahardika, G.N. Whole-Genome Comparison of Representatives of All Variants of SARS-CoV-2, Including Subvariant BA.2 and the GKA Clade. *Adv. Virol.* **2023**, *2023*, 6476626. [CrossRef] [PubMed]
24. Bai, Z.; Cao, Y.; Liu, W.; Li, J. The SARS-CoV-2 Nucleocapsid Protein and Its Role in Viral Structure, Biological Functions, and a Potential Target for Drug or Vaccine Mitigation. *Viruses* **2021**, *13*, 1115. [CrossRef] [PubMed]

25. Soresina, A.; Moratto, D.; Chiarini, M.; Paolillo, C.; Baresi, G.; Focà, E.; Bezzi, M.; Baronio, B.; Giacomelli, M.; Badolato, R. Two X-linked agammaglobulinemia patients develop pneumonia as COVID-19 manifestation but recover. *Pediatr. Allergy Immunol.* **2020**, *31*, 565–569. [CrossRef] [PubMed]

26. Devassikutty, F.M.; Jain, A.; Edavazhippurath, A.; Joseph, M.C.; Peedikayil, M.M.T.; Scaria, V.; Sandhya, P.; Govindaraj, G.M. X-Linked Agammaglobulinemia and COVID-19: Two Case Reports and Review of Literature. *Pediatr. Allergy Immunol. Pulmonol.* **2021**, *34*, 115–118. [CrossRef] [PubMed]

27. Quinti, I.; Locatelli, F.; Carsetti, R. The Immune Response to SARS-CoV-2 Vaccination: Insights Learned from Adult Patients with Common Variable Immune Deficiency. *Front. Immunol.* **2022**, *12*, 815404. [CrossRef] [PubMed]

28. Vanni, A.; Salvati, L.; Mazzoni, A.; Lamacchia, G., Capone, M., Francalanci, S., Kiros, S.T.; Cosmi, L.; Puccini, B.; Ciceri, M.; et al. Bendamustine impairs humoral but not cellular immunity to SARS-CoV-2 vaccination in rituximab-treated B-cell lymphoma-affected patients. *Front. Immunol.* **2023**, *14*, 1322594. [CrossRef]

29. Candon, S.; Lemee, V.; Leveque, E.; Etancelin, P.; Paquin, C.; Carette, M.; Contentin, N.; Bobee, V.; Alani, M.; Cardinael, N.; et al. Dissociated humoral and cellular immune responses after a three-dose schema of BNT162b2 vaccine in patients receiving anti-CD20 monoclonal antibody maintenance treatment for B-cell lymphomas. *Haematologica* **2022**, *107*, 755–758. [CrossRef]

30. Ishio, T.; Tsukamoto, S.; Yokoyama, E.; Izumiyama, K.; Saito, M.; Muraki, H.; Kobayashi, M.; Mori, A.; Morioka, M.; Kondo, T. Anti-CD20 antibodies and bendamustine attenuate humoral immunity to COVID-19 vaccination in patients with B-cell non-Hodgkin lymphoma. *Ann. Hematol.* **2023**, *12*, 1421–1431. [CrossRef]

31. Perry, C.; Luttwak, E.; Balaban, R.; Shefer, G.; Morales, M.M.; Aharon, A.; Tabib, Y.; Cohen, Y.C.; Benyamini, N.; Beyar-Katz, O.; et al. Efficacy of the BNT162b2 mRNA COVID-19 vaccine in patients with B-cell non-Hodgkin lymphoma. *Blood Adv.* **2021**, *5*, 3053–3061. [CrossRef]

32. Lu, L.; Chan, C.Y.; Lim, Y.Y.; Than, M.; Teo, S.; Lau, P.Y.W.; Ng, K.H.; Yap, H.K. SARS-CoV-2 Humoral Immunity Persists Following Rituximab Therapy. *Vaccines* **2023**, *11*, 1864. [CrossRef]

33. Bsteh, G.; Assar, H.; Hegen, H.; Heschl, B.; Leutmezer, F.; Di Pauli, F.; Gradl, C.; Traxler, G.; Zulehner, G. AUT-MuSC investigators. COVID-19 severity and mortality in multiple sclerosis are not associated with immunotherapy: Insights from a nation-wide Austrian registry. *PLoS ONE* **2021**, *16*, e0255316. [CrossRef]

34. Avouac, J.; Drumez, E.; Hachulla, E.; Seror, R.; Georgin-Lavialle, S.; El Mahou, S.; Pertuiset, E.; Pham, T.; Marotte, H. FAIR/SFR/SNFMI/SOFREMIP/CRI/IMIDIATE consortium and contributors. COVID-19 outcomes in patients with inflammatory rheumatic and musculoskeletal diseases treated with rituximab: A cohort study. *Lancet Rheumatol.* **2021**, *3*, e419–e426. [CrossRef]

35. Anand, P.; Puranik, A.; Aravamudan, M.; Venkatakrishnan, A.J. Soundararajan VSARS-CoV-2 strategically mimics proteolytic activation of human ENaC. *Elife* **2020**, *9*, e58603. [CrossRef]

36. Kotsias, F.; Cebrian, I.; Alloatti, A. Antigen processing and presentation. *Int. Rev. Cell Mol. Biol.* **2019**, *348*, 69–121. [CrossRef]

37. Nagler, A.; Kalaora, S.; Barbolin, C.; Gangaev, A.; Ketelaars, S.L.C.; Alon, M.; Pai, J.; Benedek, G.; Yahalom-Ronen, Y.; Erez, N.; et al. Identification of presented SARS-CoV-2 HLA class I and HLA class II peptides using HLA peptidomics. *Cell Rep.* **2021**, *35*, 109305. [CrossRef]

38. Tarke, A.; Sidney, J.; Kidd, C.K.; Dan, J.M.; Ramirez, S.I.; Yu, E.D.; Mateus, J.; da Silva Antunes, R.; Moore, E.; Rubiro, P.; et al. Comprehensive analysis of T cell immunodominance and immunoprevalence of SARS-CoV-2 epitopes in COVID-19 cases. *Cell Rep. Med.* **2021**, *2*, 100204. [CrossRef] [PubMed]

39. Bertoletti, A.; Tan, A.T.; Le Bert, N. The T-cell response to SARS-CoV-2: Kinetic and quantitative aspects and the case for their protective role. *Oxf. Open Immunol.* **2021**, *2*, iqab006. [CrossRef]

40. Ferretti, A.P.; Kula, T.; Wang, Y.; Nguyen, D.M.V.; Weinheimer, A.; Dunlap, G.S.; Xu, Q.; Nabilsi, N.; Perullo, C.R.; Cristofaro, A.W.; et al. Unbiased Screens Show CD8+ T Cells of COVID-19 Patients Recognize Shared Epitopes in SARS-CoV-2 that Largely Reside outside the Spike Protein. *Immunity* **2020**, *53*, 1095–1107. [CrossRef] [PubMed]

41. Verma, J.; Kaushal, N.; Manish, M.; Subbarao, N.; Shakirova, V.; Martynova, E.; Liu, R.; Hamza, S.; Rizvanov, A.A.; Khaiboullina, S.F.; et al. Identification of conserved immunogenic peptides of SARS-CoV-2 nucleocapsid protein. *J. Biomol. Struct. Dyn.* **2023**, 1–17. [CrossRef] [PubMed]

42. Le Bert, N.; Tan, A.T.; Kunasegaran, K.; Tham, C.Y.L.; Hafezi, M.; Chia, A.; Chng, M.H.Y.; Lin, M.; Tan, N.; Linster, M.; et al. SARS-CoV-2-specific T cell immunity in cases of COVID-19 and SARS, and uninfected controls. *Nature* **2020**, *584*, 457–462. [CrossRef] [PubMed]

43. AlKhalifah, J.M.; Seddiq, W.; Alshehri, M.A.; Alhetheel, A.; Albarrag, A.; Meo, S.A.; Al-Tawfiq, J.A.; Barry, M. Impact of MERS-CoV and SARS-CoV-2 Viral Infection on Immunoglobulin-IgG Cross-Reactivity. *Vaccines* **2023**, *11*, 552. [CrossRef] [PubMed]

44. Kesheh, M.M.; Hosseini, P.; Soltani, S.; Zandi, M. An overview on the seven pathogenic human coronaviruses. *Rev. Med. Virol.* **2022**, *32*, e2282. [CrossRef]

45. Kundu, R.; Narean, J.S.; Wang, L.; Fenn, J.; Pillay, T.; Fernandez, N.D.; Conibear, E.; Koycheva, A.; Davies, M.; Tolosa-Wright, M.; et al. Cross-reactive memory T cells associate with protection against SARS-CoV-2 infection in COVID-19 contacts. *Nat. Commun.* **2022**, *13*, 80. [CrossRef]

46. Loyal, L.; Braun, J.; Henze, L.; Kruse, B.; Dingeldey, M.; Reimer, U.; Kern, F.; Schwarz, T.; Mangold, M.; Unger, C.; et al. Cross-reactive CD4+ T cells enhance SARS-CoV-2 immune responses upon infection and vaccination. *Science* **2021**, *374*, eabh1823. [CrossRef] [PubMed]

47. Hewitt, E.W. The MHC class I antigen presentation pathway: Strategies for viral immune evasion. *Immunology* **2003**, *110*, 163–169. [CrossRef]

48. Cassioli, C.; Baldari, C.T. The Expanding Arsenal of Cytotoxic T Cells. *Front. Immunol.* **2022**, *13*, 883010. [CrossRef]

49. Niessl, J.; Sekine, T.; Buggert, M. T cell immunity to SARS-CoV-2. *Semin. Immunol.* **2021**, *55*, 101505. [CrossRef]

50. Tay, C.; Kanellakis, P.; Hosseini, H.; Cao, A.; Toh, B.H.; Bobik, A.; Kyaw, T. B Cell and CD4 T Cell Interactions Promote Development of Atherosclerosis. *Front. Immunol.* **2020**, *10*, 3046. [CrossRef]

51. Kared, H.; Redd, A.D.; Bloch, E.M.; Bonny, T.S.; Sumatoh, H.; Kairi, F.; Carbajo, D.; Abel, B.; Newell, E.W.; Bettinotti, M.P.; et al. SARS-CoV-2-specific CD8+ T cell responses in convalescent COVID-19 individuals. *J. Clin. Investig.* **2021**, *131*, e145476. [CrossRef]

52. Song, G.; He, W.T.; Callaghan, S.; Anzanello, F.; Huang, D.; Ricketts, J.; Torres, J.L.; Beutler, N.; Peng, L.; Vargas, S.; et al. Cross-reactive serum and memory B-cell responses to spike protein in SARS-CoV-2 and endemic coronavirus infection. *Nat. Commun.* **2021**, *12*, 2938. [CrossRef]

53. Vennema, H.; de Groot, R.J.; Harbour, D.A.; Dalderup, M.; Gruffydd-Jones, T.; Horzinek, M.C.; Spaan, W.J. Early death after feline infectious peritonitis virus challenge due to recombinant vaccinia virus immunization. *J. Virol.* **1990**, *64*, 1407–1409. [CrossRef]

54. Olsen, C.W.; Corapi, W.V.; Ngichabe, C.K.; Baines, J.D.; Scott, F.W. Monoclonal antibodies to the spike protein of feline infectious peritonitis virus mediate antibody-dependent enhancement of infection of feline macrophages. *J. Virol.* **1992**, *66*, 956–965. [CrossRef] [PubMed]

55. Wan, Y.; Shang, J.; Sun, S.; Tai, W.; Chen, J.; Geng, Q.; He, L.; Chen, Y.; Wu, J.; Shi, Z.; et al. Molecular Mechanism for Antibody-Dependent Enhancement of Coronavirus Entry. *J. Virol.* **2020**, *94*, e02015-19. [CrossRef]

56. Takada, A.; Kawaoka, Y. Antibody-dependent enhancement of viral infection: Molecular mechanisms and in vivo implications. *Rev. Med. Virol.* **2003**, *13*, 387–398. [CrossRef]

57. Arvin, A.M.; Fink, K.; Schmid, M.A.; Cathcart, A.; Spreafico, R.; Havenar-Daughton, C.; Lanzavecchia, A.; Corti, D.; Virgin, H.W. A perspective on potential antibody-dependent enhancement of SARS-CoV-2. *Nature* **2020**, *584*, 353–363. [CrossRef]

58. Pongracz, T.; Vidarsson, G.; Wuhrer, M. Antibody glycosylation in COVID-19. *Glycoconj. J.* **2022**, *39*, 335–344. [CrossRef] [PubMed]

59. van Osch, T.L.J.; Nouta, J.; Derksen, N.I.L.; van Mierlo, G.; van der Schoot, C.E.; Wuhrer, M.; Rispens, T.; Vidarsson, G. Fc galactosylation promotes hexamerization of human IgG1, leading to enhanced classical complement activation. *J. Immunol.* **2021**, *207*, 1545–1554. [CrossRef] [PubMed]

60. Bergwerk, M.; Gonen, T.; Lustig, Y.; Amit, S.; Lipsitch, M.; Cohen, C.; Mandelboim, M.; Levin, E.G.; Rubin, C.; Indenbaum, V.; et al. COVID-19 Breakthrough Infections in Vaccinated Health Care Workers. *N. Engl. J. Med.* **2021**, *385*, 1474–1484. [CrossRef]

61. Chandan, S.; Khan, S.R.; Deliwala, S.; Mohan, B.P.; Ramai, D.; Chandan, O.C.; Facciorusso, A. Postvaccination SARS-CoV-2 infection among healthcare workers: A systematic review and meta-analysis. *J. Med. Virol.* **2022**, *94*, 1428–1441. [CrossRef]

62. Tenforde, M.W.; Self, W.H.; Adams, K.; Gaglani, M.; Ginde, A.A.; McNeal, T.; Ghamande, S.; Douin, D.J.; Talbot, H.K.; Casey, J.D.; et al. Association Between mRNA Vaccination and COVID-19 Hospitalization and Disease Severity. *JAMA* **2021**, *326*, 2043–2054. [CrossRef]

63. Nakayama, E.E.; Shioda, T. SARS-CoV-2 Related Antibody-Dependent Enhancement Phenomena In Vitro and In Vivo. *Microorganisms* **2023**, *11*, 1015. [CrossRef] [PubMed]

64. Weiskopf, K.; Weissman, I.L. Macrophages are critical effectors of antibody therapies for cancer. *MAbs* **2015**, *7*, 303–310. [CrossRef] [PubMed]

65. Junker, F.; Gordon, J.; Qureshi, O. Fc Gamma Receptors and Their Role in Antigen Uptake, Presentation, and T Cell Activation. *Front. Immunol.* **2020**, *11*, 1393. [CrossRef] [PubMed]

66. von Kietzell, K.; Pozzuto, T.; Heilbronn, R.; Grössl, T.; Fechner, H.; Weger, S. Antibody-mediated enhancement of parvovirus B19 uptake into endothelial cells mediated by a receptor for complement factor C1q. *J. Virol.* **2014**, *88*, 8102–8115. [CrossRef] [PubMed]

67. Eggleton, P.; Tenner, A.J.; Reid, K.B. C1q receptors. *Clin. Exp. Immunol.* **2000**, *120*, 406–412. [CrossRef] [PubMed]

68. Wen, J.; Cheng, Y.; Ling, R.; Dai, Y.; Huang, B.; Huang, W.; Zhang, S.; Jiang, Y. Antibody-dependent enhancement of coronavirus. *Int. J. Infect. Dis.* **2020**, *100*, 483–489. [CrossRef]

69. Thomas, S.; Smatti, M.K.; Ouhtit, A.; Cyprian, F.S.; Almaslamani, M.A.; Thani, A.A.; Yassine, H.M. Antibody-Dependent Enhancement (ADE) and the role of complement system in disease pathogenesis. *Mol. Immunol.* **2022**, *152*, 172–182. [CrossRef] [PubMed]

70. Monto, A.S.; Malosh, R.E.; Petrie, J.G.; Martin, E.T. The Doctrine of Original Antigenic Sin: Separating Good from Evil. *J. Infect. Dis.* **2017**, *215*, 1782–1788. [CrossRef]

71. Francis, T. On the doctrine of original antigenic sin. *Proc. Am. Philos. Soc.* **1960**, *104*, 572–578.

72. Petráš, M.; Králová Lesná, I. SARS-CoV-2 vaccination in the context of original antigenic sin. *Hum. Vaccines Immunother.* **2022**, *18*, 1949953. [CrossRef]

73. Pillai, S. SARS-CoV-2 vaccination washes away original antigenic sin. *Trends Immunol.* **2022**, *43*, 271–273. [CrossRef]

74. Rijkers, G.T.; van Overveld, F.J. The "original antigenic sin" and its relevance for SARS-CoV-2 (COVID-19) vaccination. *Clin. Immunol. Commun.* **2021**, *1*, 13–16. [CrossRef]

75. Xia, C.S.; Zhan, M.; Liu, Y.; Yue, Z.H.; Song, Y.; Zhang, F.; Wang, H. SARS-CoV-2 antibody response in SARS survivors with and without the COVID-19 vaccine. *Int. J. Antimicrob. Agent* **2023**, *62*, 106947. [CrossRef] [PubMed]
76. El-Saed, A.; Othman, F.; Baffoe-Bonnie, H.; Almulhem, R.; Matalqah, M.; Alshammari, L.; Alshamrani, M.M. Symptomatic MERS-CoV infection reduces the risk of future COVID-19 disease; A retrospective cohort study. *BMC Infect. Dis.* **2023**, *23*, 757. [CrossRef]
77. Sette, A.; Sidney, J.; Crotty, S. T Cell Responses to SARS-CoV-2. *Annu. Rev. Immunol.* **2023**, *41*, 343–373. [CrossRef] [PubMed]
78. Appelberg, S.; Ahlén, G.; Yan, J.; Nikouyan, N.; Weber, S.; Larsson, O.; Höglund, U.; Aleman, S.; Weber, F.; Perlhamre, E.; et al. A universal SARS-CoV DNA vaccine inducing highly cross-reactive neutralizing antibodies and T cells. *EMBO Mol. Med.* **2022**, *14*, c15821. [CrossRef]
79. Altmann, D.M.; Boyton, R.J. COVID-19 vaccination: The road ahead. *Science* **2022**, *375*, 1127–1132. [CrossRef]
80. Dolgin, E. Pan-coronavirus vaccine pipeline takes form. *Nat. Rev. Drug Discov.* **2022**, *21*, 324–326. [CrossRef]
81. Temmam, S.; Vongphayloth, K.; Baquero, E.; Munier, S.; Bonomi, M.; Regnault, B.; Douangboubpha, B.; Karami, Y.; Chrétien, D.; Sanamxay, D.; et al. Bat coronaviruses related to SARS-CoV-2 and infectious for human cells. *Nature* **2022**, *604*, 330–336. [CrossRef]
82. Shannon, C.P.; Blimkie, T.M.; Ben-Othman, R.; Gladish, N.; Amenyogbe, N.; Drissler, S.; Edgar, R.D.; Chan, Q.; Krajden, M.; Foster, L.J.; et al. Multi-Omic Data Integration Allows Baseline Immune Signatures to Predict Hepatitis B Vaccine Response in a Small Cohort. *Front. Immunol.* **2020**, *11*, 578801. [CrossRef] [PubMed]
83. Leslie, M. Giant project will chart human immune diversity to improve drugs and vaccines. *Science* **2024**, *383y*, 13–14. [CrossRef] [PubMed]

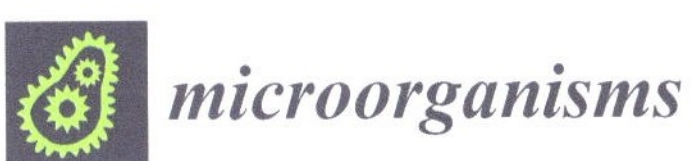 *microorganisms*

Article

Development of a Melting-Curve-Based Multiplex Real-Time PCR Assay for the Simultaneous Detection of Viruses Causing Respiratory Infection

Eliandro Reis Tavares [1,†], Thiago Ferreira de Lima [2,†], Guilherme Bartolomeu-Gonçalves [3], Isabela Madeira de Castro [2], Daniel Gaiotto de Lima [1], Paulo Henrique Guilherme Borges [2], Gerson Nakazato [2], Renata Katsuko Takayama Kobayashi [2], Emerson José Venancio [3], César Ricardo Teixeira Tarley [4], Elaine Regina Delicato de Almeida [5], Marsileni Pelisson [3], Eliana Carolina Vespero [3], Andrea Name Colado Simão [3], Márcia Regina Eches Perugini [3], Gilselena Kerbauy [6], Marco Aurélio Fornazieri [7], Maria Cristina Bronharo Tognim [8], Viviane Monteiro Góes [9], Tatiana de Arruda Campos Brasil de Souza [10], Danielle Bruna Leal Oliveira [11,12], Edison Luiz Durigon [12], Lígia Carla Faccin-Galhardi [2], Lucy Megumi Yamauchi [1,2,*] and Sueli Fumie Yamada-Ogatta [1,2,*]

[1] Laboratory of Molecular Biology of Microorganisms, Department of Microbiology, State University of Londrina, Londrina 86057-970, Brazil; tavares.eliandro@uel.br (E.R.T.); dgaiotto2@gmail.com (D.G.d.L.)

[2] Graduate Program in Microbiology, Department of Microbiology, State University of Londrina, Londrina 86057-970, Brazil; ferreira.thiagodelima@gmail.com (T.F.d.L.); isabela.mcastro@uel.br (I.M.d.C.); pauloguilhermeph@gmail.com (P.H.G.B.); gnakazato@uel.br (G.N.); kobayashirkt@uel.br (R.K.T.K.); lgalhardi@uel.br (L.C.F.-G.)

[3] Graduate Program in Clinical and Laboratory Pathophysiology, Department of Pathology, Clinical and Toxicological Analysis, State University of Londrina, Londrina 86038-350, Brazil; guilherme.bartolomeu@uel.br (G.B.-G.); emersonj@uel.br (E.J.V.); marsileni@uel.br (M.P.); elianacv@uel.br (E.C.V.); deianame@uel.br (A.N.C.S.); marciaperugini@uel.br (M.R.E.P.)

[4] Graduate Program in Chemistry, Department of Chemistry, State University of Londrina, Londrina 86057-970, Brazil; tarley@uel.br

[5] Department of Pathology, Clinical and Toxicological Analysis, State University of Londrina, Londrina 86038-350, Brazil; elainedelicato@hotmail.com

[6] Graduate Program in Nursing, Department of Nursing, State University of Londrina, Londrina 86038-350, Brazil; gilselena@uel.br

[7] Graduate Program in Health Sciences, Department of Clinical Surgery, State University of Londrina, Londrina 86038-350, Brazil; marcofornazieri@gmail.com

[8] Department of Basic Health Sciences, State University of Maringá, Maringá 87020-900, Brazil; mcbtognim@uem.br

[9] Institute of Molecular Biology of Paraná, Curitiba 81350-010, Brazil; viviane@ibmp.org.br

[10] Carlos Chagas Institute, Oswaldo Cruz Foundation (FIOCRUZ-Pr), Curitiba 81350-010, Brazil; tatiana.brasil@fiocruz.br

[11] Albert Einstein Hospital, São Paulo 05652-900, Brazil; danielle.durigon@einstein.br

[12] Laboratory of Clinical and Molecular Virology, University of São Paulo, São Paulo 05508-000, Brazil; eldurigo@usp.br

* Correspondence: lionilmy@uel.br (L.M.Y.); ogatta@uel.br (S.F.Y.-O.)

† These authors contributed equally to this work.

Citation: Tavares, E.R.; de Lima, T.F.; Bartolomeu-Gonçalves, G.; de Castro, I.M.; de Lima, D.G.; Borges, P.H.G.; Nakazato, G.; Kobayashi, R.K.T.; Venancio, E.J.; Tarley, C.R.T.; et al. Development of a Melting-Curve-Based Multiplex Real-Time PCR Assay for the Simultaneous Detection of Viruses Causing Respiratory Infection. *Microorganisms* **2023**, *11*, 2692. https://doi.org/10.3390/microorganisms11112692

Academic Editor: Qibin Geng

Received: 25 September 2023
Revised: 19 October 2023
Accepted: 30 October 2023
Published: 2 November 2023

Abstract: The prompt and accurate identification of the etiological agents of viral respiratory infections is a critical measure in mitigating outbreaks. In this study, we developed and clinically evaluated a novel melting-curve-based multiplex real-time PCR (M-m-qPCR) assay targeting the RNA-dependent RNA polymerase (RdRp) and nucleocapsid phosphoprotein N of SARS-CoV-2, the Matrix protein 2 of the Influenza A virus, the RdRp domain of the L protein from the Human Respiratory Syncytial Virus, and the polyprotein from Rhinovirus B genes. The analytical performance of the M-m-qPCR underwent assessment using in silico analysis and a panel of reference and clinical strains, encompassing viral, bacterial, and fungal pathogens, exhibiting 100% specificity. Moreover, the assay showed a detection limit of 10 copies per reaction for all targeted pathogens using the positive controls. To validate its applicability, the assay was further tested in simulated nasal fluid spiked with the viruses mentioned above, followed by validation on nasopharyngeal swabs collected from 811 individuals. Among them, 13.4% (109/811) tested positive for SARS-CoV-2, and 1.1% (9/811) tested positive for Influenza A. Notably, these results showed 100% concordance with those obtained using a commercial kit. Therefore, the M-m-qPCR exhibits great potential for the routine screening of these respiratory viral pathogens.

Keywords: COVID-19; SARS-CoV-2; Influenza A virus; Human Respiratory Syncytial Virus; Human Rhinovirus B; nucleic acid amplification test

1. Introduction

Historically, mankind has witnessed the emergence of infectious agents, some of which have unleashed devastating effects on the human population, such as those responsible for the smallpox and influenza pandemics [1]. Given their ease of transmission via aerosol, respiratory viral pathogens have been implicated as potential catalysts of pandemics, as exemplified in the past two decades by the emergence of severe acute respiratory syndrome coronavirus (SARS-CoV) in 2002; H1N1 Influenza A in 2009; Middle East respiratory syndrome coronavirus (MERS-CoV) in 2012; and most recently, SARS-CoV-2 in 2020 [2,3]. In addition to the route of transmission, respiratory viruses share several common characteristics: (i) their capacity to affect healthy and immunocompromised individuals of all ages; (ii) the substantial global burden of epidemics caused by these viruses, amounting to millions of cases annually; (iii) the propensity of viral RNA polymerases to exhibit a low fidelity rate, leading to point mutations in each replication cycles [4] and the subsequent emergence of variants; (iv) the ability to cause infections that can manifest as either symptomatic or asymptomatic cases; (v) their potential to induce elevated rates of hospitalization, morbidity, and mortality, especially among young children, the elderly, and adults with underlying chronic diseases; (vi) the significant economic impact they impose, encompassing treatment costs, absenteeism from work/school, and productivity losses [5–9].

SARS-CoV-2, an enveloped single-stranded positive-sense RNA virus belonging to the *Coronaviridae* family [3], is the causative agent of COVID-19 (Coronavirus Disease-19), a potentially fatal severe acute respiratory syndrome characterized by high rates of transmission and infection. Since its initial identification in 2019 in Wuhan, this disease has affected more than 771 million individuals worldwide, with cumulative deaths surpassing 6.9 million [2]. Both symptomatic and asymptomatic patients exhibit a high viral load in the nostrils shortly after infection onset, highlighting their crucial role in the virus transmission chain and the importance of detecting SARS-CoV-2 within the population [10,11]. The success in containing the spread of COVID-19 has been attributed to a set of non-pharmacological measures such as social distancing, mask-wearing, rigorous hand hygiene, travel restrictions, and temporary school closures. Furthermore, extensive diagnostic testing to detect SARS-CoV-2 within the population and subsequent vaccination campaigns have played pivotal roles in managing the pandemic. However, along with the intrinsic characteristics of viral RNA polymerases, the viral genome can undergo recombination and reassortment, contributing to high diversity and the emergence of new variants. Thus, the availability of assays for diagnosing/monitoring the infectious agent remains an essential component of infection control strategies [12].

Generally, the most common symptoms of COVID-19 are indistinguishable from those associated with other viral agents causing respiratory infections. These symptoms include fever, headache, cough, muscle ache, fatigue, dyspnea, and loss of smell and taste [3,13]. Therefore, syndromic diagnosis cannot identify specific viral pathogens responsible for respiratory tract infections. In fact, epidemics of viral respiratory tract infections caused by non-coronaviruses remain highly prevalent worldwide and can lead to severe consequences in susceptible individuals. Notable examples of such viral agents include the influenza (FLU) virus, Human Respiratory Syncytial Virus (HRSV), and Human Rhinovirus B (HRV-B).

Epidemiological studies have shown that most viruses responsible for respiratory tract infections exhibit seasonal patterns. Specifically, FLU and HRSV tend to be more prevalent during winter, while HRV-B can be detected throughout the year [8]. Nevertheless, the COVID-19 pandemic has impacted the epidemiology of viral infections, including the genetic diversity of these non-SARS-CoV-2 viral agents during the pandemic. A significant decrease in respiratory infections and hospitalizations caused by non-SARS-CoV-2 viruses has been observed globally [14–16]. Despite this decrease, cases of co-infection involving SARS-CoV-2 and these viral agents have also been reported during the COVID-19 pandemic [17–19].

Seasonal influenza is primarily caused by the influenza virus, mainly of type A (FLU-A), which circulates worldwide. This enveloped virus consists of a single strand of RNA divided into eight negative-sense RNA segments and belongs to the *Orthomyxoviridae* family. The severity of the disease ranges from mild to severe, with specific populations at a higher risk of developing severe illness. These include pregnant women, younger children, the elderly, and individuals with underlying chronic conditions such as pulmonary, cardiac, renal, metabolic, liver, or hematologic diseases. Additionally, individuals with immuno-suppressive conditions, including those undergoing chemotherapy or steroid treatment or with malignancies, are also more susceptible to severe outcomes [6]. According to the World Health Organization (WHO), the annual epidemic burden of severe influenza illnesses is estimated to be around 3 to 5 million cases, resulting in approximately 290,000 to 650,000 deaths [20]. Control measures for FLU-A infections include vaccines and antiviral drugs [21]. However, akin to SARS-CoV-2, new subtypes and variants of FLU-A emerge frequently, and occasionally, a new human strain may arise from an animal source, thereby posing a potential threat to human populations [6,22].

Human Respiratory Syncytial Virus (HRSV), an enveloped single-strand, negative-sense RNA virus belonging to the *Pneumoviridae* family, can cause the common cold in individuals of all ages. However, it is particularly notorious as a leading cause of lower respiratory tract infection in young children [5,23]. In this vulnerable population, HRSV infection may progress to potentially fatal conditions such as bronchiolitis and community-acquired pneumonia [5]. Furthermore, adults with underlying diseases (including chronic pulmonary or circulatory diseases and functional disability) and the elderly also face a heightened risk of experiencing severe HRSV infections [24]. Currently, only two HRSV vaccines have been approved by the U.S. Food and Drug Administration for use in adults over 60 years [5,25]. Moreover, the first monoclonal antibody was recently approved to prevent HRSV infections in children [5].

Rhinovirus (HRV), a non-enveloped single-strand, positive-sense RNA virus of the *Picornaviridae* family, has been identified as the primary causative agent of the common cold, particularly affecting children [7,26,27]. Typically, infections caused by this virus exhibit a mild and self-limiting course; however, they can also progress to severe manifestations, including community-acquired pneumonia [26], with a high risk of death [5]. Moreover, HRV is important in asthma exacerbation [28]. Unfortunately, despite medical advancements, no approved vaccines or other preventive therapies are available for HRV infection [5].

The early and accurate identification of viral pathogens causing respiratory infections is crucial to control their spread and provide specific and immediate treatment, thus avoiding outbreaks and complications for patients [29]. While isolation and identification of the infectious agent are considered standards for clinical laboratory diagnosis, it is essential to acknowledge that these techniques are labor-intensive, time-consuming, and possess limited sensitivity [30]. Conversely, nucleic acid amplification tests (NAATs) have demonstrated remarkable specificity and sensitivity in detecting the etiological agents of infections, surpassing conventional culture-based testing methods [12,31]. Multiplex polymerase chain reaction (PCR)-based tests, for instance, enable the simultaneous detection of several molecular markers using distinct pairs of oligonucleotide primers. Amplicons can be detected either through agarose gel electrophoresis or in real-time (m-qPCR) using DNA-intercalating fluorophores during PCR or specific probes complementary to the target gene.

Real-time PCR (qPCR) remains the gold standard for the detection of SARS-CoV-2 and other respiratory viruses in clinical and environmental samples, and most in-house and commercial tests rely on the use of fluorescent probes [31–35]. This study aimed to develop a melting-curve-based multiplex real-time PCR assay (M-m-qPCR) for the simultaneous detection of four respiratory viral pathogens: SARS-CoV-2, FLU-A, HRSV, and HRV-B. This assay targets specific genes, including the RNA-dependent RNA polymerase (RdRp) and the nucleocapsid phosphoprotein N of SARS-CoV-2, the Matrix protein 2 of FLU-A, the RdRp domain of the L protein from HRSV, and the polyprotein from HRV-B. The potential usefulness of this assay was evaluated using nasopharyngeal swab specimens.

2. Materials and Methods

2.1. Oligonucleotide Primers and Positive Controls

The nucleotide sequences of the genes encoding RdRp (gene: ORF1ab) and nucleocapsid phosphoprotein N (gene: N) of SARS-CoV-2, Matrix protein 2 (gene: M2) of FLU-A, the RdRp domain of the L protein (gene: L) of HRSV, and the polyprotein (gene: 5′ untranslated region-UTR) of HRV-B were obtained from the GenBank/EMBL databases (available on the website http://www.ncbi.nlm.nih.gov accessed on 24 August 2020). These sequences were analyzed using the BioEdit v.7.2.0 software. Specific primers were designed based on the consensus sequence of each gene, employing the OligoAnalyzer™ tool (http://www.idtdna.com, accessed on 28 August 2020). Additionally, primers targeting the human tRNA-processing ribonuclease P (RNase P) gene [34,36] were also included in this study. Detailed information on the primer sequences and the expected size of the amplicons can be found in Table 1. To create positive controls, the consensus sequences of each viral target were inserted into plasmid pUC57 (Figure S1, FastBio Ltd.a, Ribeirão Preto, Brazil).

Table 1. Characteristics of oligonucleotide primers of melting-curve-based multiplex real-time PCR.

Virus	Gene	Primers		Amplicon Size (pb)	Annealing Temperature (°C)
SARS-CoV-2	ORF1ab	RdRp-SARS-CoV-2-F RdRp-SARS-CoV-2-R	AGCTTGTCACACCGTTTCT AGTCTGTGTCAACATCTCTATTTCT	282	61
	N	NC-SARS-CoV-2-F NC-SARS-CoV-2-R	ACACCAATAGCAGTCCAGATG ATTCAAGGCTCCCTCAGTTG	197	61
FLU-A	M2	M-IAV-F M-IAV-R	TCTAACCGAGGTCGAAACGTA TGGTCTTGTCTTTAGCCATTCC	142	61
HRSV	L	RdRp-HRSV- F RdRp-HRSV-R	AGAGAGGACCCACTAAACCA ATGCATACACCCAATCCAAT	138	61
HRV-B	5′-UTR	pp-HRV-F pp-HRV-R	GTGTTCGATCAGGTGAGTTT CGAGTCTTCACACCATGTC	143	61

RNA-dependent RNA polymerase (RdRp) (ORF1ab gene) and the nucleocapsid phosphoprotein N (gene N) of SARS-CoV-2, the Matrix protein 2 (gene M2) of the Influenza A virus (FLU-A), the RdRp domain of the L protein (gene L) from Human Respiratory Syncytial Virus (HRSV), and the polyprotein (5′-UTR) from Human Rhinovirus B (HRV-B).

2.2. Viral and Microbial Strains

A panel comprising 47 viral strains, 12 bacteria, and 10 fungi (Table 2) was used to develop the assays. This panel encompassed various microbial and viral species components of the respiratory tract microbiota or pathogens associated with this anatomical site. Three colony-forming units (CFUs) of each bacterial and fungal species were cultivated at 37 °C for 24 h in tryptic soy broth (TSB, Oxoid, São Paulo, Brazil) and Sabouraud dextrose broth (SDB, Himedia, Thane, India), respectively. Following cultivation, the microbial cells were harvested via centrifugation (10,000× *g* for 5 min), washed twice with sterile PBS, and processed for DNA purification. Bacterial and fungal cultures were kept at −80 °C in TSB containing 20% glycerol and SDB containing 20% glycerol, respectively. Viruses were obtained from the viral collection of the Laboratory of Virology (LAVIR) of the State University of Londrina (UEL) and the Laboratory of Clinical and Molecular Virology of the University of São Paulo.

Table 2. Panel of positive controls, viruses, and microorganisms used to evaluate the melting curve-based multiplex real-time PCR specificity.

	Targets				
	RdRp-SARS-CoV-2	N-SARS-CoV-2	M2-FLU-A	L-HRSV	5′-UTR-HRV-B
Positive Control	+	+	+	+	+
SARS-CoV-2 LMM 38135	+	+	−	−	−
SARS-CoV-2 MAM 87209	+	+	−	−	−
SARS-CoV-2 HM11-20	+	+	−	−	−
SARS-CoV-2 LFL11-20	+	+	−	−	−
SARS-CoV-2 AGBCS11-20	+	+	−	−	−
SARS-CoV-2 PQB12-20	+	+	−	−	−
SARS-CoV-2 AOC12-20	+	+	−	−	−
SARS-CoV-2 CNPB11-20	+	+	−	−	−
SARS-CoV-2 MPC12-20	+	+	−	−	−
SARS-CoV-2 MKA01-21	+	+	−	−	−
SARS-CoV-2 BWS02-21	+	+	−	−	−
SARS-CoV-2 VCS02-21	+	+	−	−	−
SARS-CoV-2 EOC02-21	+	+	−	−	−
SARS-CoV-2 SMGC02-21	+	+	−	−	−
SARS-CoV-2 VRS02-21	+	+	−	−	−
SARS-CoV-2 SS09-21	+	+	−	−	−
SARS-CoV-2 ARM09-21	+	+	−	−	−
SARS-CoV-2 CHB09-21	+	+	−	−	−
SARS-CoV-2 ALMO12-21	+	+	−	−	−
SARS-CoV-2 MPV10-21	+	+	−	−	−
SARS-CoV-2 DIBM12-21	+	+	−	−	−
SARS-CoV-2 PLCSC01-22	+	+	−	−	−
Human Rhinovirus HRV 3760	−	−	−	−	+
Human Rhinovirus HRV HRV01	−	−	−	−	+
Human Rhinovirus HRV HRV02	−	−	−	−	+
Human Respiratory Syncytial Virus HRSV 3760	−	−	−	+	−
Human Respiratory Syncytial Virus HRSV 4226	−	−	−	+	−
Human Respiratory Syncytial Virus HRSV 4122	−	−	−	+	−
Human Respiratory Syncytial Virus HRSV IVC1	−	−	−	+	−
Human Respiratory Syncytial Virus HRSV IVC2	−	−	−	+	−
Human Respiratory Syncytial Virus HRSV IVC3	−	−	−	+	−
Influenza Virus A FLU-A/H1N1 FLU	−	−	+	−	−
Influenza Virus A FLU-A/H3N2	−	−	+	−	−
Influenza Virus A FLU-A CS1	−	−	+	−	−
Influenza Virus A FLU-A CS2	−	−	+	−	−
Influenza Virus A FLU-A CS3	−	−	+	−	−
Influenza Virus A FLU-A CS4	−	−	+	−	−
Influenza Virus A FLU-A CS5	−	−	+	−	−
Influenza Virus B	−	−	−	−	−
Human Enterovirus (HEV)	−	−	−	−	−
Seasonal Coronavirus (HCoVs)	−	−	−	−	−
Parainfluenza Virus 1 (HPIV1)	−	−	−	−	−
Parainfluenza Virus 2 (HPIV2)	−	−	−	−	−
Parainfluenza Virus 3 (HPIV3)	−	−	−	−	−
Parainfluenza Virus 4 (HPIV4)	−	−	−	−	−
Human Adenovirus ADV 3226	−	−	−	−	−
Human Adenovirus ADH 4122	−	−	−	−	−
Staphylococcus aureus ATCC 25923	−	−	−	−	−
Staphylococcus epidermidis ATCC 35984	−	−	−	−	−
Staphylococcus haemolyticus ATCC 29968	−	−	−	−	−
Staphylococcus saprophyticus ATCC 15305	−	−	−	−	−
Staphylococcus pseudintermedius SIG34	−	−	−	−	−
Staphylococcus schleiferi	−	−	−	−	−
Pseudomonas aeruginosa ATCC 27858	−	−	−	−	−
Klebsiella pneumonia ATCC 10031	−	−	−	−	−
Klebsiella pneumoniae kp39	−	−	−	−	−
Enterococcus faecalis ATCC 51299	−	−	−	−	−
Enterococcus faecium ATCC 6569	−	−	−	−	−
Escherichia coli ATCC 25922	−	−	−	−	−
Candida albicans ATCC 25923	−	−	−	−	−
Candida glabrata ATCC 2001	−	−	−	−	−
Candida krusei ATCC 34135	−	−	−	−	−
Candida parapsilosis ATCC 22019	−	−	−	−	−
Candida tropicalis ATCC 28707	−	−	−	−	−
Candida auris 10913	−	−	−	−	−
Cryptococcus neoformans ATCC 34872	−	−	−	−	−
Cryptococcus gattii ATCC 32269	−	−	−	−	−
Paracoccidioides brasiliensis Pb1 8	−	−	−	−	−
Histoplasma capsulatum I	−	−	−	−	−

2.3. Nucleic Acid Purification

The QIAamp® DNA Mini kit (QIAGEN, São Paulo, Brazil) and QIAamp® Viral RNA Mini kit (QIAGEN, São Paulo, Brazil) were used for DNA and RNA purification, respectively, according to manufacturer's recommendations.

2.4. PCR Design

The amplification reaction conditions were determined through a two-step process. First, the annealing temperatures and primer concentrations were established via conventional PCR. Subsequently, the established conditions were tested in qPCR assays. Therefore, each primer pair, at concentrations ranging from 0.5 to 2 μM, was used in conventional PCRs with a final volume of 20 μL. The reaction mix contained 20 mM of Tris-HCl (pH 8.4), 5 mM of KCl, 1.5 mM of $MgCl_2$, 100 μM of each dNTP, 2.5 U of *Taq* DNA polymerase (Invitrogen, São Paulo, Brazil), and 1×10^6 copies of the positive control. The amplification reactions were performed in a Veriti 96-well Thermal Cycler (Applied Biosystems, São Paulo, Brazil) with an initial denaturation at 95 °C for 1 min, followed by 35 cycles of 95 °C for 30 s, an annealing temperature gradient ranging from 60 °C to 70 °C for 1 min, and an extension step at 72 °C for 45 s. Negative template control (NTC) reactions without template nucleic acid were carried out simultaneously. Subsequently, amplicons were analyzed via 3% agarose gel electrophoresis after staining with GelRed® (Biotium-Uniscience, Osasco, Brazil).

An annealing temperature of 61 °C and a primer concentration of 1 μM were selected to validate the optimized conditions in the qPCR assays, using the positive controls and nucleic acid purified of each viral strain as templates. Thus, all qPCRs were performed using a Rotor-Gene Q 5PlexHRM (QIAGEN, Hilden, Germany) in a final volume of 20 μL, which contained 1 μM of each viral primer pair, 1 μM of human RNase P primers, and QuantiNova SYBR® Green RT-PCR mix (QIAGEN, São Paulo, Brazil), following the manufacturer's recommendations. The cycling conditions were as follows: an initial denaturation at 95 °C for 2 min, followed by 40 cycles of 95 °C for 30 s, 61 °C for 30 s, and 72 °C for 30 s. Melting curves were acquired using 0.5 °C steps with a hold of 60 s at each step, ranging from 60 to 99 °C. NTC reactions were carried out simultaneously. Data were analyzed using the Rotor-Gene Q series software version 2.1.0.9.

2.5. Analytical Specificity, Sensitivity, and Performance in Virus-Spiked Swabs

The specificity of the M-m-qPCR was assessed using 100 ng of nucleic acid obtained from cultures or clinical samples of a panel of bacteria, fungi, and viruses (Table 2). All amplification reactions were performed in duplicate in three independent experiments. Moreover, the primer sequences targeting the selected genes were compared with nucleotide sequences available in the GenBank databases of the National Center for Biotechnology Information (NCBI, http://www.ncbi.nlm.nih.gov accessed on 28 August 2020) using the Blast algorithm (blastn).

The sensitivity of the M-m-qPCR was empirically determined using positive controls ranging from 10^0 to 10^6 copies per reaction. Each strain was processed in triplicate on five consecutive days. For each primer pair, a standard curve was generated from the C_T values as a function of the positive plasmid copy number, and the R^2 was calculated to evaluate the efficiency of the reaction. The slope of this line was used to determine the efficiency (E) according to the following equation: $E = 10^{-1/slope} - 1$. The sensitivity of the M-m-qPCR was also determined using SARS-CoV-2 RNA. Therefore, Vero ATCC CCL81 (Merck, São Paulo, Brazil) cells were cultured in Dulbecco's modified Eagle's medium (DMEM, Invitrogen-Gibco, Waltham, MA, USA), supplemented with 10% fetal bovine serum (Invitrogen-Gibco), glutamine (2 mM, Sigma-Aldrich, St. Louis, MI, USA), streptomycin (100 μg/mL, Gibco BRL, Waltham, MA, USA), and penicillin (100 IU/mL, Novafarma Ind. Farm., Anápolis, Brazil). SARS-CoV-2/human/BRA/SP02cc/2020 stock was obtained via inoculation in Vero cells until a cytopathic effect was achieved (CPE ~90%) and stored at −80 °C. The virus titration was performed using a median tissue culture infectious dose ($TCID_{50}$/mL) assay [37]. Cells were seeded into 96-well plates (5×10^4 cells/mL) 24 h before the experiment. Viruses were 10-fold serially diluted in DMEM (10^{-1} to 10^{-12}). The medium was removed from the cell culture plates, and then, virus dilutions were added in sextuplicate and incubated at 37 °C. Visualizations were performed daily in an inverted light microscope (Axiovert 100, Carl Zeiss, Oberkochen, Germany) to observe the CPE over 72 h. The viral titer was calculated using the Spearman and Kärber algorithm [38] and expressed in $TCID_{50}$/mL. The viral titer was determined as 1.44×10^7 $TCID_{50}$/mL. The limit of detection (LoD) was established using the SARS-CoV-2 viral concentration (Genomic Copy Equivalents—GCEs) ranging from 5 to 10,000 GCEs.

The performance of the M-m-qPCR was analyzed using simulated swabs spiked with the viruses. Initially, swabs were soaked in a 2% polyethylene oxide (*w/v*) solution that mimics mucus [39]. Afterward, 100 μL aliquots of each supernatant from virus-infected cells with cytopathic effects were used to spike the swabs, which were further processed for RNA extraction as described above.

2.6. Performance of the Multiplex Real-Time PCR Assay in Clinical Samples

The performance of the M-m-qPCR was initially evaluated using nasopharyngeal samples collected from 20 patients who sought care for respiratory syndromes at reference centers in Londrina, Paraná, Brazil, and tested positive for COVID-19. Nasopharyngeal secretions were collected using Rayon swabs (Inlab, São Paulo, Brazil) and maintained in viral transport medium (DMEM containing 1000 IU/mL penicillin, 1000 μg/mL streptomycin, and 25 μg/mL amphotericin B). Patients were randomly selected according to a C_T value < 21 detected using the TaqPath™ COVID-19 CE-IVD RT-PCR kit and the 7500 Real-Time PCR System (ThermoFisher Scientific, Waltham, MA, USA) for SARS-CoV-2 detection. The viral species were further confirmed through genome or Spike protein-encoding gene (gene S) sequencing. The sequencing library preparation for the Illumina platform was performed using the Nextera XT Kit (Illumina, San Diego, CA, USA), according to the manufacturer's instructions. Libraries were quantified using the Qubit fluorimetric method (ThermoFisher Scientific, Waltham, MA, USA) and sequenced on the NextSeq 550 instrument with 300 paired-end cycle kits (Illumina, San Diego, CA, USA) at the Hospital Israelita Albert Einstein, São Paulo, Brazil. The data underwent filtering and trimming to achieve a Phred score of <20. The genome was assembled using an "ab initio" strategy with reference genome NC_045512.2 (SAR-CoV-2) and the SPADES software, v.3.13.1. Whole-genome consensus sequences were classified using the Phylogenetic Assignment of Named Global Outbreak Lineages (PANGOLIN) software, v3.1.18 (pangolearn 2022-01-20, constellations v0.1.2, scorpio v0.3.16, and pango-designation release v1.2.123) [40]. The whole-genome sequences of the viral strains were submitted to DDBJ/ENA/GenBank under the submission number SUB12140327.

Next, the performance of the M-m-qPCR for SARS-CoV-2 in clinical samples was compared with the results obtained from the Molecular SARS-CoV-2 (E)—Bio-Manguinhos kit (FIOCRUZ, Curitiba, Brazil). This comparison involved 811 individuals who exhibited symptoms of respiratory infection and/or had contact with people diagnosed with COVID-19 between November 2020 and May 2023. The study protocol was approved by the Ethics Committee of the UEL (Document 47784621.2.0000.5231, Opinion Number 4.862.243—CEP/UEL). Written informed consent was obtained from all participants, including their agreement with the publication of this report and any accompanying images. Nasopharyngeal swabs from each participant were collected using Rayon swabs (Inlab, São Paulo, Brazil). The swabs were transferred to a tube containing 560 μL of lysis buffer from the QIAamp® Viral RNA Mini kit (QIAGEN, São Paulo, Brazil) and incubated at room temperature for 30 min before undergoing nucleic acid purification, as recommended by the manufacturer.

3. Results and Discussion

3.1. Melting-Curve-Based Multiplex Real-Time PCR Assay

NAATs have been used in many clinical laboratories to diagnose different infectious diseases because of their high specificity and sensitivity, as well as their ability to provide rapid results. However, culture-based tests to identify viral agents, along with many microorganisms, are known for their time-consuming and labor-intensive nature, in addition to their limited sensitivity [30]. Moreover, several clinically relevant viruses are challenging to cultivate in vitro [30] or require a high biosafety level (BSL) laboratory for handling, such as SARS-CoV-2 (requiring BSL-3 for viral culture versus BSL-2 for NAATs) [34].

The main outcome of our study is methodological. We developed a melting-curve-based real-time multiplex-PCR assay using SYBR green dye, allowing for the simultaneous detection of SARS-CoV-2, FLU-A, HRSV, and HRV-B (Figure 1). To enhance the specificity and accuracy of the assays, our selection of target nucleotide sequences was based on the following criteria: (i) essential gene status; (ii) conserved sequences within the species to avoid false-negative results due to genetic variations; (iii) non-overlapping melting temperature (Tm) ranges for the different amplicons within the assay; (iv) the presence of secondary structures and dimerization (self- and heterodimerization) not exceeding 10% of the Tm and total ΔG values, respectively, of the primers.

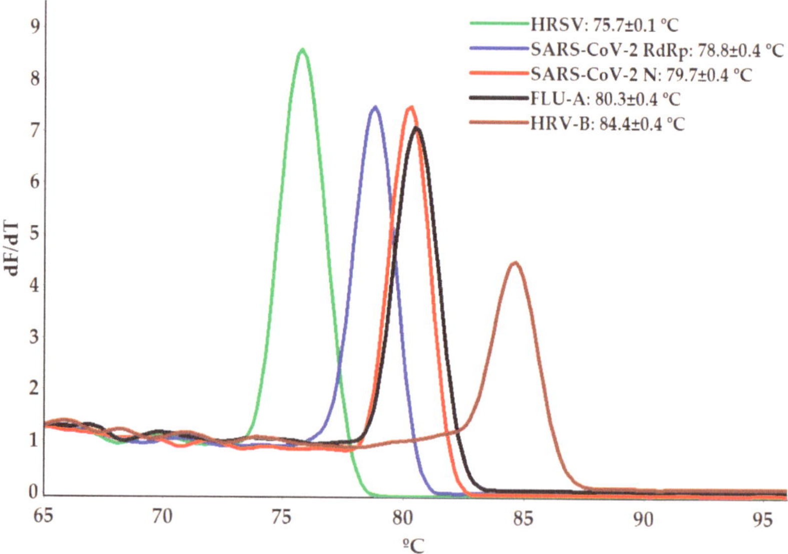

Figure 1. Melting curve analyses showing the melting temperature (Tm) peaks of RNA-dependent RNA polymerase (RdRp) and the nucleocapsid phosphoprotein N of SARS-CoV-2, the Matrix protein 2 of the Influenza A virus (FLU-A), the RdRp domain of the L protein from Human Respiratory Syncytial Virus (HRSV), and the 5′-UTR polyprotein from Human Rhinovirus B (HRV-B) amplicons using the positive (plasmid) controls.

These genes have been studied as potential therapeutic targets for the development of antiviral agents [4,41–44], reinforcing their crucial role in viral life cycles. For SARS-CoV-2, genes encoding RdRp (ORF1ab) and N (gene: N) proteins were selected for primer design in this study. These genes have been recognized as reliable targets for NAATs [45–47]. Indeed, most available NAATs for detecting SARS-CoV-2 contain redundancies to avoid targeting failures resulting from viral genomic mutations [45]. Notably, a high degree of structural conservation has been observed among viral RdRps [48]. Nonetheless, variations in RNA binding, polymerization, and the presence of accessory domains have also been noted among these enzymes [4]. The N gene, conversely, is highly conserved, sharing over

98% similarity across various SARS-CoV-2 variants, including Wuhan (China), Alpha (UK), Beta (South Africa), Gamma (Brazil), Delta (India), Epsilon (USA), and Omicron (South Africa) [43]. The N protein is the most abundant in virions and plays several essential roles in the SARS-CoV-2 life cycle, including transcription, the replication of the viral genome, the encapsidation of the viral genome into a ribonucleotide complex, and assembly into viral particles [47].

The L protein of HRSV contains an RdRp domain (RNA transcription/replication), a polyribonucleotidyltransferase (cap addition) domain, and a methyltransferase (cap methylation) domain, all of which are indispensable for the viral replicative cycle. Notably, the C-terminal region of the L protein is the most variable domain among non-segmented negative-strand viruses [44].

Regarding HRV-B, its genome consists of a positive-sense single-strand RNA of approximately 7200 bp that encodes a single open reading frame (ORF). The $5'$-terminal sequence (80 to 84 bases) exhibits minimal structural variation across species and displays a cloverleaf-like (CL) motif, which interacts with viral and cellular proteins to initiate RNA synthesis. Immediately following the CL motif, all Rhinoviruses share unique sequences consisting of a pyrimidine-rich spacer segment with short oligo C (Cytosine) and oligo U (Uracil) units interspersed with Adenines [49]. In our study, the specific primers for HRV-B detection target the $5'$-UTR polyprotein, a region commonly employed for the detection of this virus in clinical samples [7].

Finally, the M2 protein of FLU-A, an integral membrane protein that forms a pH-regulated ion channel, plays an essential role in viral replication and can contribute to host pathogenicity by interfering with cellular homeostasis or interacting with and modulating the host proteome [42].

To establish the amplification conditions for detecting these genes, we initially conducted conventional monoplex PCRs using synthetic viral controls (positive plasmid controls). Each specific primer pair (1 µM) successfully generated amplicons of the expected sizes, as shown in Table 1, with an annealing temperature of 61 °C. The identity of each amplicon was further confirmed via sequencing and searching for nucleotide sequence homology in the GenBank/EMBL databases.

Afterward, we used the positive controls to determine the equivalent Tms of each primer in the monoplex qPCR assays. All primer pairs successfully amplified the corresponding genes, generating dissociation curves with a single peak (Figure S2). The Tm values of all amplicons are presented in Figure 1 and Figure S2. These Tm values were further confirmed in monoplex qPCR using RNA purified from viral cultures. To evaluate the quality of the nucleic acid purification and the presence of potential PCR-interfering substances, primers targeting the human tRNA processing ribonuclease P (RNase P) gene were also included [34,50], resulting in a Tm value of 82.1 ± 0.50 °C (Figure S2).

3.2. Analytical Performance of the Assay

The specificity of each primer pair targeting the selected genes was initially analyzed in silico using the GenBank/EMBL database on the NCBI homepage. No matches were found other than those with the corresponding genes of specific viral species and the human genome, indicating that amplification signal of non-target sequences that result in cross-reactivity is not likely to occur. Subsequently, the specificity of the M-m-qPCR was confirmed using nucleic acid from the panel of bacteria, fungi, and viruses (Table 2). Amplification signals were detected only for the specific viral agents, demonstrating no cross-reactivity among non-target species.

To assess the linearity and limit of detection (LoD) of the M-m-qPCR for the target genes, tenfold serial dilutions ranging from 10^0 to 10^6 copies per reaction of each positive control from specific viral species were prepared. Each concentration was analyzed in six replicates every day for five days ($n = 30$). The LoD of the m-qPCR for the target genes was 10 copies per reaction, and the reaction efficiencies, calculated from the slope of the standard curves, ranged from 98 to 100% (Figure 2). The mean C_T values of the target genes, using the LoD, were 29.8 (Orf1a/b) and 28.7 (N) for SARS-CoV-2, 29.7 (5′-UTR-polyprotein) for HRV-B, 28.1 (L) for HRSV, and 27.3 (M2) for FLU-A.

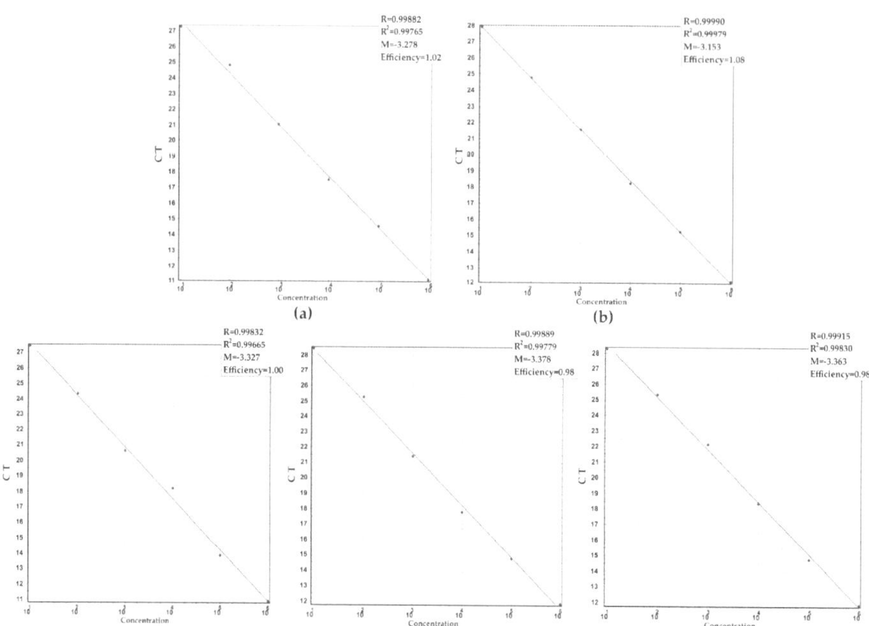

Figure 2. Sensitivity of multiplex real-time PCR assays. (**a**) RNA-dependent RNA polymerase (ORF1a/b) of SARS-CoV-2; (**b**) nucleocapsid phosphoprotein N (gene N) of SARS-CoV-2; (**c**) Matrix protein 2 (gene M2) of Influenza A virus; (**d**) RdRp domain of L protein (gene L) from Human Respiratory Syncytial Virus; (**e**) polyprotein (5′-UTR-polyprotein) from Human Rhinovirus B. Amplification plot of tenfold serial dilution corresponding to 10^1 to 10^6 copies of the positive controls. Standard curve represented by linear regression line for threshold cycle (C_T) versus copy numbers. Slope (M), regression coefficient (R), and efficiency of the real-time PCR method are shown (**a–e**).

The sensitivity of M-m-qPCR was also evaluated using SARS-CoV-2 (SARS-CoV-2/human/BRA/SP02cc/2020 strain) RNA. The LoD of the assay for the RdRp- and N-encoding genes of SARS-CoV-2 was 5 GCEs, displaying C_T values of 22.6 (RdRp) and 23.6 (N) (Figure S3). These slight differences can be explained by the viral titration method used. The median $TCID_{50}$ is defined as the dilution of a virus required to infect 50% of a given cell culture and is widely used for determining viral infectivity [51]. Therefore, it is possible that a higher load of viral particles was assessed in this assay.

According to these results, the M-m-qPCR is considered positive for all viruses when amplification signals for each specific gene target, as well as the control, are detected with C_T values ≤ 30 using the Rotor-Gene Q 5PlexHRM System. The performance of the M-m-qPCR is comparable to that exhibited by the two commercial kits that were used in this study. The TaqPath™ COVID-19 CE-IVD RT-PCR kit targets the genes encoding the ORF1ab, N protein, and S protein of SARS-CoV-2. According to the technical note, the LoD of the assay is 10 GCEs, with C_T cut-off values of ≤ 37 for all viral targets. The valid C_T values for the internal control (MS2 phage) are ≤ 32 using the 7500 Real-Time PCR System. On the other hand, the Molecular SARS-CoV-2 (E)—Bio-Manguinhos kit targets the genes encoding the ORF1ab and the envelope protein (E), and the LoD of the assay is 304 GCEs. The test is considered positive for SARS-CoV-2 when amplification signals for E and RdRp targets, as well as the internal control (RNase P), are detected with C_T values of ≤ 40, ≤ 35, or ≤ 37, respectively, also using the 7500 Real-Time PCR System. In addition to the primers, both kits use fluorescent probes as an amplification detection system.

Next, the performance of the M-m-qPCR assay was analyzed using a swab saturated with synthetic nasal mucus and spiked with the target viruses. Amplification signals were detected for all viruses, and the dissociation curves generated melting peaks corresponding to each specific target, as generated for the positive controls.

Based on these data, the optimized M-m-qPCR assay consists of a reaction mixture with a final volume of 20 µL. Tube 1 contains 1 µM of forward and reverse primers targeting the genes encoding the SARS-CoV-2 RdRp and N proteins, 2×10^3 copies of the positive control, and a QuantiNova SYBR® Green RT-PCR mix. Tube 2 includes 1 µM of forward and reverse primers targeting the HRV-B 5′-UTR-polyprotein, the HRSV RdRp domain of the L protein, the FLU-A Matrix protein 2 encoded genes, 2×10^3 copies of the positive control, and a QuantiNova SYBR® Green RT-PCR mix. In Tube 3, the reagents include 1 µM of forward and reverse primers targeting the human RNase P-encoded gene and a QuantiNova SYBR® Green RT-PCR mix. In all tubes, 5 µL of template nucleic acid is added, and the final volume is adjusted with deionized water. NTC reactions, which lack any template nucleic acid, are carried out simultaneously.

3.3. Performance of the Assay in Clinical Samples

To assess the performance of the M-m-qPCR for SARS-CoV-2 detection in clinical samples, genomic RNAs extracted from nasopharyngeal specimens collected from 20 COVID-19-positive patients ($C_T < 21$) diagnosed with the TaqPath™ COVID-19 CE-IVD RT-PCR kit were tested with the M-m-qPCR. The developed assay was capable of detecting all SARS-CoV-2 strains (Table 3). In addition, viral genome sequencing conducted as part of the study showed that the standardized M-m-qPCR assay could detect several SARS-CoV-2 variants, including variants of concern (VOCs) (Table 3).

Table 3. Panel of different variants of SARS-CoV-2 used to validate the performance of the melting-curve based multiplex real time PCR specificity.

Date	Viral Strain	Pango Lineage
2020-11	SARS CoV 2 LAVIR HM UEL	B.1.1.33
2020-11	SARS-CoV-2 LAVIR-AB-UEL	B.1.1.143
2020-11	SARS-CoV-2 LAVIR-PB-UEL	B.1.1.28
2020-11	SARS-CoV-2 LAVIR-LL-UEL	B.1.1.33
2020-11	SARS-CoV-2 LAVIR-CB-UEL	P.2
2020-12	SARS-CoV-2 LAVIR-AC-UEL	B.1.1.28
2020-12	SARS-CoV-2 LAVIR-MC-UEL	P.2
2021-01	SARS-CoV-2 LAVIR-MA-UEL	P.2
2021-02	SARS-CoV-2 LAVIR-BS-UEL	B.1.1.7
2021-02	SARS-CoV-2 LAVIR-VCS-UEL	B.1.1.7
2021-02	SARS-CoV-2 LAVIR-SC-UEL	B.1.1.7
2021-02	SARS-CoV-2 LAVIR-VRS-UEL	B.1.1.7
2021-02	SARS-CoV-2 LAVIR-EC-UEL	B.1.1.7
2021-09	SS09-21	Delta (B.1.617.2-like)
2021-09	ARM09-21	Delta (B.1.617.2-like)
2021-09	CHB09-21	Delta (B.1.617.2-like)
2021-12	ALMO12-21	Omicron (BA.1-like)
2021-10	MPV10-21	Delta (B.1.617.2-like)
2021-12	DIBM12-21	Omicron (BA.1-like)
2022-01	PLCSC01-22	Delta (B.1.617.2-like)

Date: Clinical sample collection period. Viral strain: Nasopharyngeal specimens collected from COVID-19-positive patients (CT < 21) diagnosed with TaqPath™ COVID-19 CE-IVD RT-PCR kit. Pango lineage: Defined according to the Spike protein-encoding gene sequence analysis.

Furthermore, the performance of the M-m-qPCR was analyzed in nasopharyngeal swabs obtained from 811 individuals with respiratory infection symptoms and/or who had contact with individuals diagnosed with COVID-19. The results of the M-m-qPCR were compared with those obtained using the Molecular SARS-CoV-2 (E)—Bio-Manguinhos kit. Among the 811 participants in the survey, 502 (61.9%) were females, and 309 (38.1%) were males, with ages ranging from 5 to 85 years. Among them, 109 (13.4%) were positive for SARS-CoV-2, and 9 (1.1%) were positive for FLU-A. Notably, there was a 100% agreement between all positive and negative results obtained using the M-m-qPCR and those obtained with the commercial kit for SARS-CoV-2.

Some studies have used the melting curve strategy to detect the etiological agents of infections. Tavares et al. [52] described real-time PCR assays targeting the intergenic spacer 1 (IGS1) region from an rDNA locus to differentiate *Cryptococcus gattii sensu lato* and *Cryptococcus neoformans sensu lato*. Otaguiri et al. [31] reported a good agreement between a culture-based and a melting curve-based multiplex real-time PCR assay targeting the *cfb* gene for the detection of *Streptococcus agalactiae* in the rectal–vaginal swabs of pregnant women. Lastly, Sun et al. [53] described a high-resolution melting (HRM) multiplex assay for the direct detection of SARS-CoV-2 variants, and good agreement was observed with standard Sanger sequencing.

Our study has some limitations. (i) None of the clinical samples generated amplification signals for HRSV or HRV-B genetic markers. However, in simulated swabs saturated with synthetic mucus and spiked with the viruses, amplification signals were detected for all specific genetic markers. This result may be attributed to a reported reduction in positive cases and hospitalizations due to other respiratory viruses during the COVID-19 pandemic, as indicated in previous studies [14–16]. Moreover, as mentioned before, these viral agents are common causes of respiratory infections, mainly among children [23]. Thus, the lower percentage of children tested in our study may have contributed to these results. Further assays conducted during the post-COVID pandemic period will provide valuable insights into the performance of M-m-qPCR during the circulation of seasonal respiratory viruses. (ii) The LoD of the assay was determined using the synthetic plasmid (positive control), which may not fully reflect the assay sensitivity when applied to clinical samples, as the RNA purification procedure may interfere with the result. Particularly for SARS-CoV-2, assay sensitivity was similar using RNA extracted from viral cultures in Vero ATCC CCL81 cells. (iii) The probability of developing a false positive on the M-m-qPCR was not assessed with biological samples proven negative for respiratory infections. However, some precautions were taken to reduce the likelihood of false positives, including the following: (a) all primers were analyzed in silico to assess similarity with nucleotide sequences from humans and other infectious agents of respiratory infections and to identify secondary structures and dimerization potential; (b) all biological samples from the 811 individuals were processed immediately after nasopharyngeal swab collection; (c) all samples collected from the 811 individuals were simultaneously tested with the Molecular SARS-CoV-2 (E)—Bio-Manguinhos kit; (d) inconclusive tests—that is, when no amplification signal from the internal control (RNase P) was detected, the assay was repeated with a new biological sample. (iv) Only two commercial kits for detecting SARS-CoV-2 were used in our study. Therefore, we cannot generalize our findings to all real-time PCR systems. (v) The method still requires thermal cycling equipment.

Despite these limitations, our results demonstrated the following advantages: (i) the entire test, including RNA purification, sample preparation, and M-m-qPCR analysis, can be performed in about 4 h—this rapid turnaround time is crucial for ensuring timely diagnosis and patient management; (ii) the test exhibits comparable sensitivity and specificity to fluorescent probe-based NAATs; (iii) we estimated the labor costs (equipment and personal were not included) associated with nasopharyngeal swab collection and the processing of M-m-qPCR, providing insights into the economic feasibility of this method, and the value was estimated at USD 6.50; (iv) the assay can be readily adapted to a multiplex-standard PCR format, making it suitable for use in settings lacking real-time PCR equipment; and

(v) as the methodology is based on a melting curve, new genetic markers for the detection of other viral agents causing respiratory infections can be incorporated into the assay.

The recent literature data report a transition from the pandemic phase of COVID-19 to an endemic state. Although mortality rates have reduced significantly, severe disease cases can occur, particularly among individuals with risk factors [54,55]. This highlights the enduring presence of SARS-CoV-2, which may co-circulate with other respiratory viral agents, and, therefore, the continuous surveillance of these viral agents remains imperative.

4. Patents

This study resulted in a patent application to the Brazilian National Institute of Intellectual Property (INPI-https://www.gov.br/inpi/pt-br—number BR 10 2023 017320 9) (accessed on 20 September 2023).

Supplementary Materials: The following supporting information can be downloaded at https://www.mdpi.com/article/10.3390/microorganisms11112692/s1: Figure S1: Construction of pUC57 (positive controls) carrying the consensus sequences of target genes used in melting-curve-based multiplex real-time PCR. (**a**) RNA-dependent RNA polymerase (RdRp) and the nucleocapsid phosphoprotein N of SARS-CoV-2; (**b**) Matrix protein 2 of Influenza A virus (FLU-A); (**c**) and the RdRp domain of the L protein from Human Respiratory Syncytial Virus (HRSV) and the 5′-UTR polyprotein from Human Rhinovirus B (HRV-B). Figure S2: Monoplex real-time PCR for determining melting temperature peaks (Tms) of RNA-dependent RNA polymerase (RdRp) and the nucleocapsid phosphoprotein (N) of SARS-CoV-2, Matrix protein 2 (M2) of the Influenza A virus (FLU-A), the RdRp domain of the L protein (L) from Human Respiratory Syncytial Virus (HRSV), and the 5′-UTR polyprotein from Human Rhinovirus B (HRV-B) amplicons using positive (plasmid) controls. RNase P amplicon Tm peak was determined using human nasopharyngeal swab samples. Figure S3: Performance of real-time PCR assay for SARS-CoV-2. Melting temperature peaks (Tms) of (**a**) RNA-dependent RNA polymerase (RdRp) and (**c**) nucleocapsid phosphoprotein N of SARS-CoV-2 (**c**) using SARS-CoV-2/human/BRA/SP02cc/2020 culture in Vero ATCC CCL81 cells. Sensitivity of real-time PCR assays: Amplification pattern of serial dilution corresponding to 10,000, 1000, 100, 10, and 5 viral particles. The virus titration was determined using a tissue culture infectious dose (TCID$_{50}$/mL) assay [37]. (**b**) RNA-dependent RNA polymerase (RdRp) and (**d**) nucleocapsid phosphoprotein N.

Author Contributions: Conceptualization, E.R.T., L.M.Y. and S.F.Y.-O.; methodology, E.R.T., T.F.d.L., G.B.-G., I.M.d.C., D.G.d.L., P.H.G.B., E.R.D.d.A., M.P., E.C.V., A.N.C.S., M.R.E.P. and G.K.; validation, V.M.G., T.d.A.C.B.d.S. and L.C.F.-G.; resources, M.C.B.T., D.B.L.O. and E.L.D.; writing—original draft preparation, E.R.T. and S.F.Y.-O.; writing—review and editing, E.R.T., G.B.-G., L.M.Y. and S.F.Y.-O.; funding acquisition, G.N., R.K.T.K., E.J.V., C.R.T.T., M.A.F. and S.F.Y.-O. All authors have read and agreed to the published version of the manuscript.

Funding: The present study was supported by grants from the Conselho Nacional de Desenvolvimento Científico e Tecnológico (CNPq, Process 402387/2020-1), the Coordenação de Aperfeiçoamento de Pessoal de Nível Superior (CAPES, Financial Code 01) and Fundação Araucária (FA/PR, Agreement 219/2023 PDI).

Institutional Review Board Statement: The study protocol was approved by the Ethics Committee of the Universidade Estadual de Londrina (Document 47784621.2.0000.5231, Opinion Number 4.862.243-CEP/UEL).

Informed Consent Statement: Written informed consent was obtained from all participants agreeing with the publication of this report and any accompanying images.

Data Availability Statement: Data are contained within the article and Supplementary Materials.

Acknowledgments: T.F.d.L., G.B.-G., I.M.d.C. and P.H.G.B. were funded by a graduate scholarship from CAPES. D.G.d.L. was funded by an undergraduate scholarship from Fundação Araucária. G.N., R.K.T.K., C.R.T.T., M.A.F., T.d.A.C.B.d.S., L.C.F.-G. and S.F.Y.-O. (CNPq, Process 309260/2022-1) were funded by a research fellowship from CNPq. We thank the Instituto Nacional de Controle de Qualidade em Saúde (INCQS), Fundação Oswaldo Cruz-Rio de Janeiro, Brazil, for kindly donating the bacterial and fungal reference strains.

Conflicts of Interest: The authors declare no conflict of interest.

References

1. Cunha, B.A. Influenza: Historical aspects of epidemics and pandemics. *Infect. Dis. Clin. N. Am.* **2004**, *18*, 141–155. [CrossRef] [PubMed]
2. WHO Coronavirus Disease (COVID-19). Available online: https://www.who.int/health-topics/coronavirus#tab=tab_1 (accessed on 19 October 2023).
3. Guest, P.C.; Hawkins, S.F.C.; Rahmoune, H. Rapid Detection of SARS-CoV-2 Variants of Concern by Genomic Surveillance Techniques. *Adv. Exp. Med. Biol.* **2023**, *1412*, 491–509. [PubMed]
4. Ramaswamy, K.; Rashid, M.; Ramasamy, S.; Jayavelu, T.; Venkataraman, S. Revisiting Viral RNA-Dependent RNA Polymerases: Insights from Recent Structural Studies. *Viruses* **2022**, *14*, 2200. [CrossRef] [PubMed]
5. Langedijk, A.C.; Bont, L.J. Respiratory syncytial virus infection and novel interventions. *Nat. Rev. Microbiol.* **2023**, *21*, 734–749. [CrossRef] [PubMed]
6. Liang, Y. Pathogenicity and virulence of influenza. *Virulence* **2023**, *14*, 2223057. [CrossRef] [PubMed]
7. Ljubin-Sternak, S.; Meštrović, T. Rhinovirus-A True Respiratory Threat or a Common Inconvenience of Childhood? *Viruses* **2023**, *15*, 825. [CrossRef]
8. Moriyama, M.; Hugentobler, W.J.; Iwasaki, A. Seasonality of Respiratory Viral Infections. *Annu. Rev. Virol.* **2020**, *7*, 83–101. [CrossRef]
9. Nikolai, L.A.; Meyer, C.G.; Kremsner, P.G.; Velavan, T.P. Asymptomatic SARS Coronavirus 2 infection: Invisible yet invincible. *Int. J. Infect. Dis.* **2020**, *100*, 112–116. [CrossRef]
10. Zou, L.; Ruan, F.; Huang, M.; Liang, L.; Huang, H.; Hong, Z.; Yu, J.; Kang, M.; Song, Y.; Xia, J.; et al. SARS-CoV-2 Viral Load in Upper Respiratory Specimens of Infected Patients. *N. Engl. J. Med.* **2020**, *382*, 1177–1179. [CrossRef]
11. Costa, R.; Bueno, F.; Albert, E.; Torres, I.; Carbonell-Sahuquillo, S.; Barrés-Fernández, A.; Sánchez, D.; Padrón, C.; Colomina, J.; Lázaro Carreño, M.I.; et al. Upper respiratory tract SARS-CoV-2 RNA loads in symptomatic and asymptomatic children and adults. *Clin. Microbiol. Infect.* **2021**, *27*, 1858.e1–1858.e7. [CrossRef]
12. Dorta-Gorrín, A.; Navas-Méndez, J.; Gozalo-Margüello, M.; Miralles, L.; García-Hevia, L. Detection of SARS-CoV-2 Based on Nucleic Acid Amplification Tests (NAATs) and Its Integration into Nanomedicine and Microfluidic Devices as Point-of-Care Testing (POCT). *Int. J. Mol. Sci.* **2023**, *24*, 10233. [CrossRef] [PubMed]
13. Huang, C.; Wang, Y.; Li, X.; Ren, L.; Zhao, J.; Hu, Y.; Zhang, L.; Fan, G.; Xu, J.; Gu, X.; et al. Clinical features of patients infected with 2019 novel coronavirus in Wuhan, China. *Lancet* **2020**, *395*, 497–506. [CrossRef] [PubMed]
14. Varela, F.H.; Scotta, M.C.; Polese-Bonatto, M.; Sartor, I.T.S.; Ferreira, C.F.; Fernandes, I.R.; Zavaglia, G.O.; de Almeida, W.A.F.; Arakaki-Sanchez, D.; Pinto, L.A.; et al. Absence of detection of RSV and influenza during the COVID-19 pandemic in a Brazilian cohort: Likely role of lower transmission in the community. *J. Glob. Health* **2021**, *11*, 05007. [CrossRef] [PubMed]
15. Habbous, S.; Hota, S.; Allen, V.G.; Henry, M.; Hellsten, E. Changes in hospitalizations and emergency department respiratory viral diagnosis trends before and during the COVID-19 pandemic in Ontario, Canada. *PLoS ONE* **2023**, *18*, e0287395. [CrossRef] [PubMed]
16. Principi, N.; Autore, G.; Ramundo, G.; Esposito, S. Epidemiology of Respiratory Infections during the COVID-19 Pandemic. *Viruses* **2023**, *15*, 1160. [CrossRef] [PubMed]
17. Guido, G.; Lalle, E.; Mosti, S.; Mencarini, P.; Lapa, D.; Libertone, R.; Ianniello, S.; Ricciuto, G.M.; Vaia, F.; Maggi, F.; et al. Recovery from Triple Infection with SARS-CoV-2, RSV and Influenza virus: A case report. *J. Infect. Public Health* **2023**, *16*, 1045–1047. [CrossRef]
18. Malveste Ito, C.R.; Moreira, A.L.E.; Silva, P.A.N.D.; Santos, M.O.; Santos, A.P.D.; Rézio, G.S.; Brito, P.N.; Rezende, A.P.C.; Fonseca, J.G.; Peixoto, F.A.O.; et al. Viral Coinfection of Children Hospitalized with Severe Acute Respiratory Infections during COVID-19 Pandemic. *Biomedicines* **2023**, *11*, 1402. [CrossRef]
19. Maltezou, H.C.; Papanikolopoulou, A.; Vassiliu, S.; Theodoridou, K.; Nikolopoulou, G.; Sipsas, N.V. COVID-19 and Respiratory Virus Co-Infections: A Systematic Review of the Literature. *Viruses* **2023**, *15*, 865. [CrossRef]
20. WHO Influenza (Seasonal). Available online: https://www.who.int/news-room/fact-sheets/detail/influenza-(seasonal) (accessed on 20 September 2023).
21. Luo, J.; Zhang, Z.; Zhao, S.; Gao, R. A Comparison of Etiology, Pathogenesis, Vaccinal and Antiviral Drug Development between Influenza and COVID-19. *Int. J. Mol. Sci.* **2023**, *24*, 6369. [CrossRef]
22. Pillai, T.K.; Johnson, K.E.; Song, T.; Gregianini, T.S.; Tatiana, G.; Wang, G.; Medina, R.A.; Van Bakel, H.; García-Sastre, A.; Nelson, M.I.; et al. Tracking the emergence of antigenic variants in influenza A virus epidemics in Brazil. *Virus Evol.* **2023**, *9*, vead027. [CrossRef]
23. Fontes, V.; Ferreira, H.; Ribeiro, M.; Pinheiro, A.; Maramaldo, C.; Pereira, E.; Batista, L.; Júnior, A.; Lobato, L.; Silva, F.; et al. High Incidence of Respiratory Syncytial Virus in Children with Community-Acquired Pneumonia from a City in the Brazilian Pre-Amazon Region. *Viruses* **2023**, *15*, 1306. [CrossRef] [PubMed]
24. Nguyen-Van-Tam, J.S.; O'Leary, M.; Martin, E.T.; Heijnen, E.; Callendret, B.; Fleischhackl, R.; Comeaux, C.; Tran, T.M.P.; Weber, K. Burden of respiratory syncytial virus infection in older and high-risk adults: A systematic review and meta-analysis of the evidence from developed countries. *Eur. Respir. Rev.* **2022**, *31*, 220105. [CrossRef] [PubMed]
25. Altman, J.D.; Rouse, B.T. The Long-Awaited Respiratory Syncytial Virus Vaccine. *J. Interferon Cytokine Res.* **2023**, *43*, 285–286. [CrossRef] [PubMed]

26. Ferreira, H.L.D.S.; Costa, K.L.P.; Cariolano, M.S.; Oliveira, G.S.; Felipe, K.K.P.; Silva, E.S.A.; Alves, M.S.; Maramaldo, C.E.C.; de Sousa, E.M.; Rego, J.S.; et al. High incidence of rhinovirus infection in children with community-acquired pneumonia from a city in the Brazilian pre-Amazon region. *J. Med. Virol.* **2019**, *91*, 1751–1758. [CrossRef] [PubMed]
27. Moreira, A.L.E.; da Silva, P.A.N.; Assunção, L.D.P.; Santos, M.O.; Ito, C.R.M.; de Araújo, K.M.; Cunha, M.O.; Rabelo, V.D.C.; de Souza, P.P.; Maia, S.B.S.; et al. Profile analysis of emerging respiratory virus in children. *Eur. J. Clin. Microbiol. Infect. Dis.* **2023**, *42*, 873–882. [CrossRef]
28. Nakagome, K.; Nagata, M. Innate Immune Responses by Respiratory Viruses, Including Rhinovirus, During Asthma Exacerbation. *Front. Immunol.* **2022**, *13*, 865973. [CrossRef] [PubMed]
29. Brendish, N.J.; Malachira, A.K.; Beard, K.R.; Ewings, S.; Clark, T.W. Impact of turnaround time on outcome with point-of-care testing for respiratory viruses: A post hoc analysis from a randomised controlled trial. *Eur. Respir. J.* **2018**, *52*, 1800555. [CrossRef]
30. Hodinka, R.L. Point: Is the era of viral culture over in the clinical microbiology laboratory? *J. Clin. Microbiol.* **2013**, *51*, 2–4. [CrossRef]
31. Otaguiri, E.S.; Morguette, A.E.B.; Morey, A.T.; Tavares, E.R.; Kerbauy, G.; de Almeida Torres, R.S.L.; Chaves Júnior, M.; Tognim, M.C.B.; Góes, V.M.; Krieger, M.A.; et al. Development of a melting-curve based multiplex real-time PCR assay for simultaneous detection of *Streptococcus agalactiae* and genes encoding resistance to macrolides and lincosamides. *BMC Pregnancy Childbirth* **2018**, *18*, 126. [CrossRef]
32. Gunson, R.N.; Collins, T.C.; Carman, W.F. Real-time RT-PCR detection of 12 respiratory viral infections in four triplex reactions. *J. Clin. Virol.* **2005**, *33*, 341–344. [CrossRef]
33. Paulino, R.D.S.; Benega, M.A.; Santos, K.C.; Silva, D.B.; Pereira, J.C.; Sasaki, N.A.; Silva, P.E.; Curti, S.P.; Oliveira, M.I.; Carvalhanas, T.R.; et al. Differential diagnosis of respiratory viruses by using real time RT-PCR methodology. *Rev. Inst. Med. Trop. Sao Paulo* **2013**, *55*, 432. [CrossRef] [PubMed]
34. WHO Information for the Molecular Detection of Influenza Viruses. Available online: https://cdn.who.int/media/docs/default-source/influenza/molecular-detention-of-influenza-viruses/protocols_influenza_virus_detection_feb_2021.pdf?sfvrsn=df7d2 68a_5 (accessed on 20 September 2023).
35. Hayes, E.K.; Gouthro, M.T.; LeBlanc, J.J.; Gagnon, G.A. Simultaneous detection of SARS-CoV-2, influenza A, respiratory syncytial virus, and measles in wastewater by multiplex RT-qPCR. *Sci. Total Environ.* **2023**, *889*, 164261. [CrossRef] [PubMed]
36. Altman, S. The road to RNase P. *Nat. Struct. Biol.* **2000**, *7*, 827–828. [CrossRef]
37. Reed, L.J.; Muench, H. A simple method of estimating fifty per cent endpoints. *Am. J. Epidemiol.* **1938**, *27*, 493–497. [CrossRef]
38. Hierholzer, J.C.; Killington, R.A. *Virology Methods Manual*; Mahy, B., Kangro, H., Eds.; Academic Press: Amsterdam, The Netherlands, 1996; Chapter 2; pp. 25–46.
39. Ghezzi, C.E.; Hartigan, D.R.; Hardick, J.P.; Gore, R.; Adelfio, M.; Diaz, A.R.; McGuinness, P.D.; Robinson, M.L.; Buchholz, B.O.; Manabe, Y.C. Preclinical Validation of a Novel Injection-Molded Swab for the Molecular Assay Detection of SARS-CoV-2. *Diagnostics* **2022**, *12*, 206. [CrossRef]
40. O'Toole, Á.; Scher, E.; Underwood, A.; Jackson, B.; Hill, V.; McCrone, J.T.; Colquhoun, R.; Ruis, C.; Abu-Dahab, K.; Taylor, B.; et al. Assignment of epidemiological lineages in an emerging pandemic using the pangolin tool. *Virus Evol.* **2021**, *7*, veab064. [CrossRef]
41. Bauer, L.; Lyoo, H.; van der Schaar, H.M.; Strating, J.R.; van Kuppeveld, F.J. Direct-acting antivirals and host-targeting strategies to combat enterovirus infections. *Curr. Opin. Virol.* **2017**, *24*, 1–8. [CrossRef]
42. Manzoor, R.; Igarashi, M.; Takada, A. Influenza A Virus M2 Protein: Roles from Ingress to Egress. *Int. J. Mol. Sci.* **2017**, *18*, 2649. [CrossRef]
43. Royster, A.; Ren, S.; Ma, Y.; Pintado, M.; Kahng, E.; Rowan, S.; Mir, S.; Mir, M. SARS-CoV-2 Nucleocapsid Protein Is a Potential Therapeutic Target for Anticoronavirus Drug Discovery. *Microbiol. Spectr.* **2023**, *11*, e0118623. [CrossRef]
44. Sutto-Ortiz, P.; Eléouët, J.F.; Ferron, F.; Decroly, E. Biochemistry of the Respiratory Syncytial Virus L Protein Embedding RNA Polymerase and Capping Activities. *Viruses* **2023**, *15*, 341. [CrossRef]
45. Burns, B.L.; Moody, D.; Tu, Z.J.; Nakitandwe, J.; Brock, J.E.; Bosler, D.; Mitchell, S.L.; Loeffelholz, M.J.; Rhoads, D.D. Design and Implementation of Improved SARS-CoV-2 Diagnostic Assays to Mitigate the Impact of Genomic Mutations on Target Failure: The Xpert Xpress SARS-CoV-2 Experience. *Microbiol. Spectr.* **2022**, *10*, e0135522. [CrossRef] [PubMed]
46. Cheng, L.; Lan, L.; Ramalingam, M.; He, J.; Yang, Y.; Gao, M.; Shi, Z. A review of current effective COVID-19 testing methods and quality control. *Arch. Microbiol.* **2023**, *205*, 239. [CrossRef] [PubMed]
47. Wu, W.; Cheng, Y.; Zhou, H.; Sun, C.; Zhang, S. The SARS-CoV-2 nucleocapsid protein: Its role in the viral life cycle, structure and functions, and use as a potential target in the development of vaccines and diagnostics. *Virol. J.* **2023**, *20*, 6. [CrossRef] [PubMed]
48. Mönttinen, H.A.M.; Ravantti, J.J.; Poranen, M.M. Structure Unveils Relationships between RNA Virus Polymerases. *Viruses* **2021**, *13*, 313. [CrossRef] [PubMed]
49. Palmenberg, A.C.; Spiro, D.; Kuzmickas, R.; Wang, S.; Djikeng, A.; Rathe, J.A.; Fraser-Liggett, C.M.; Liggett, S.B. Sequencing and analyses of all known human rhinovirus genomes reveal structure and evolution. *Science* **2009**, *324*, 55–59. [CrossRef]
50. Pasqualotto, A.C.; Seus, A.L. COVID-19 PCR: Frequency of internal control inhibition in clinical practice. *Access Microbiol.* **2023**, *5*, acmi000478.v3. [CrossRef]
51. Lei, C.; Yang, J.; Hu, J.; Sun, X. On the calculation of $TCID_{50}$ for quantitation of virus infectivity. *Virol. Sin.* **2021**, *36*, 141–144. [CrossRef]

52. Tavares, E.R.; Azevedo, C.S.; Panagio, L.A.; Pelisson, M.; Pinge-Filho, P.; Venancio, E.J.; Barros, T.F.; Yamada-Ogatta, S.F.; Yamauchi, L.M. Accurate and sensitive real-time PCR assays using intergenic spacer 1 region to differentiate *Cryptococcus gattii sensu lato* and *Cryptococcus neoformans sensu lato*. *Med. Mycol.* **2016**, *54*, 89–96.
53. Sun, L.; Wang, L.; Zhang, C.; Xiao, Y.; Zhang, L.; Zhao, Z.; Ren, L.; Peng, J. Rapid Detection of Predominant SARS-CoV-2 Variants Using Multiplex High-Resolution Melting Analysis. *Microbiol. Spectr.* **2023**, *11*, e0005523. [CrossRef]
54. Biancolella, M.; Colona, V.L.; Mehrian-Shai, R.; Watt, J.L.; Luzzatto, L.; Novelli, G.; Reichardt, J.K.V. COVID-19 2022 update: Transition of the pandemic to the endemic phase. *Hum. Genom.* **2022**, *16*, 19. [CrossRef]
55. Biancolella, M.; Colona, V.L.; Luzzatto, L.; Watt, J.L.; Mattiuz, G.; Conticello, S.G.; Kaminski, N.; Mehrian-Shai, R.; Ko, A.I.; Gonsalves, G.S.; et al. COVID-19 annual update. A narrative review. *Hum. Genom.* **2023**, *17*, 68. [CrossRef] [PubMed]

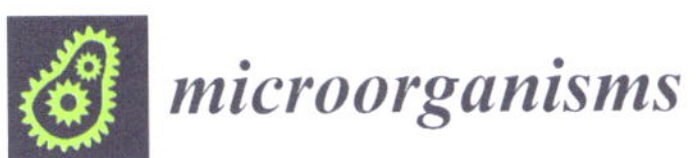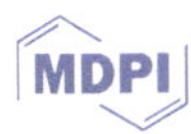

Article

SARS-CoV-2 Rapid Antigen Test Based on a New Anti-Nucleocapsid Protein Monoclonal Antibody: Development and Real-Time Validation

Fabiana Fioravante Coelho [1,2,3], Miriam Aparecida da Silva [4], Thiciany Blener Lopes [3], Juliana Moutinho Polatto [4], Natália Salazar de Castro [3], Luis Adan Flores Andrade [3], Karine Lima Lourenço [3], Hugo Itaru Sato [3], Alex Fiorini de Carvalho [3], Helena Perez Coelho [3], Flávia Fonseca Bagno [3], Daniela Luz [4], Vincent Louis Viala [4], Pedro Queiroz Cattony [4], Bruna de Sousa Melo [4], Ana Maria Moro [4], Wagner Quintilio [4], Ana Paula Barbosa [4], Camila Gasque Bomfim [5], Camila Pereira Soares [5], Cristiane Rodrigues Guzzo [5], Flavio Guimarães Fonseca [3], Edison Luiz Durigon [5], Ricardo Tostes Gazzinelli [3], Santuza M. Ribeiro Teixeira [3], Roxane Maria Fontes Piazza [4] and Ana Paula Fernandes [1,3,*]

1   Faculdade de Farmácia, Universidade Federal de Minas Gerais, Belo Horizonte 31270-901, Brazil; ffioravante23@gmail.com
2   Hospital da Polícia Militar de Minas Gerais, Polícia Militar de Minas Gerais, Belo Horizonte 30110-013, Brazil
3   Centro de Tecnologia em Vacinas, Universidade Federal de Minas Gerais, Belo Horizonte 31310-260, Brazil; thicy_lopes@hotmail.com (T.B.L.); natsalazar@gmail.com (N.S.d.C.); luisadanflores@gmail.com (L.A.F.A.); karine_lourenco@hotmail.com (K.L.L.); hugo_itaru@hotmail.com (H.I.S.); alexficar@gmail.com (A.F.d.C.); helenaperezcoelho@gmail.com (H.P.C.); flavia.bagno@gmail.com (F.F.B.); fdafonseca@icb.ufmg.br (F.G.F.); ricardo.gazzinelli@fiocruz.br (R.T.G.); santuzat@ufmg.br (S.M.R.T.)
4   Instituto Butantan, São Paulo 05503-900, Brazil; miriam.silva@butantan.gov.br (M.A.d.S.); juliana.yassuda@butantan.gov.br (J.M.P.); daniela.luz@butantan.gov.br (D.L.); vincent.viala@butantan.gov.br (V.L.V.); pedro.cattony@butantan.gov.br (P.Q.C.); brn.smelo@gmail.com (B.d.S.M.); ana.moro@butantan.gov.br (A.M.M.); wagner.quintilio@butantan.gov.br (W.Q.); ana2.barbosa@usp.br (A.P.B.); roxane.piazza@butantan.gov.br (R.M.F.P.)
5   Department of Microbiology, Institute of Biomedical Sciences, University of São Paulo, São Paulo 05508-900, Brazil; camila.bomfim@usp.br (C.G.B.); camilasoares350@gmail.com (C.P.S.); crisguzzo@usp.br (C.R.G.); elduri go@usp.br (E.L.D.)
*   Correspondence: apfernandes.ufmg@gmail.com; Tel.: +55-31-3401-1226

Citation: Coelho, F.F.; da Silva, M.A.; Lopes, T.B.; Polatto, J.M.; de Castro, N.S.; Andrade, L.A.F.; Lourenço, K.L.; Sato, H.I.; de Carvalho, A.F.; Coelho, H.P.; et al. SARS-CoV-2 Rapid Antigen Test Based on a New Anti-Nucleocapsid Protein Monoclonal Antibody: Development and Real-Time Validation. *Microorganisms* **2023**, *11*, 2422. https://doi.org/10.3390/microorganisms11102422

Academic Editors: Qibin Geng and Simone Peletto

Received: 12 July 2023
Revised: 27 August 2023
Accepted: 1 September 2023
Published: 28 September 2023

Abstract: SARS-CoV-2 diagnostic tests have become an important tool for pandemic control. Among the alternatives for COVID-19 diagnosis, antigen rapid diagnostic tests (Ag-RDT) are very convenient and widely used. However, as SARS-CoV-2 variants may continuously emerge, the replacement of tests and reagents may be required to maintain the sensitivity of Ag-RDTs. Here, we describe the development and validation of an Ag-RDT during an outbreak of the Omicron variant, including the characterization of a new monoclonal antibody (anti-DTC-N 1B3 mAb) that recognizes the Nucleocapsid protein (N). The anti-DTC-N 1B3 mAb recognized the sequence TFPPTEPKKDKKK located at the C-terminus of the N protein of main SARS-CoV-2 variants of concern. Accordingly, the Ag-RDT prototypes using the anti-DTC-N 1B3 mAB detected all the SARS-CoV-2 variants—Wuhan, Alpha, Gamma, Delta, P2 and Omicron. The performance of the best prototype (sensitivity of 95.2% for samples with Ct ≤ 25; specificity of 98.3% and overall accuracy of 85.0%) met the WHO recommendations. Moreover, results from a patients' follow-up study indicated that, if performed within the first three days after onset of symptoms, the Ag-RDT displayed 100% sensitivity. Thus, the new mAb and the Ag-RDT developed herein may constitute alternative tools for COVID-19 point-of-care diagnosis and epidemiological surveillance.

Keywords: SARS-CoV-2; diagnosis; nucleocapsid (N) antigen; IgG2b monoclonal antibody; Ag-RDT development; validation; follow-up study

1. Introduction

The CoronaVirus Disease 2019 (COVID-19), caused by the new coronavirus named Severe Acute Respiratory Syndrome CoronaVirus 2 (SARS-CoV-2), has caused more than 770 million infections and more than 6.9 million deaths worldwide since it was declared a pandemic [1]. COVID-19 vaccination campaigns were essential for pandemic control, but vaccination has progressed slowly worldwide, and it is estimated that only 5 billion people are fully vaccinated. Although vaccines greatly reduced the incidence of severe COVID-19 and death cases, they do not fully prevent transmission and infection by SARS CoV 2 [2].

A combination of high infection rates, low vaccine coverage, especially in developing countries, and high virus mutation rates contributed to the appearance of SARS-CoV-2 variants, classified either as variants of concern (VOC) or variants of interest (VOI) [3,4]. VOCs and VOIs accumulated mutations, mainly in the Spike protein, leading to an escape from neutralizing antibodies induced by previous infections or vaccination. The SARS-CoV-2 VOCs Delta and Omicron spread worldwide at a speed never seen before for any other variant. The Gamma variant was detected in Brazil in April 2021 [3] and was replaced by the Delta variant, which circulated in Brazil until December 2021 [4]. The Delta variant accumulated a total of nine mutations at the Spike protein [5]. On 26 November 2021, the Omicron BA.1 variant, which displayed 62 nonsynonymous mutations in its genome, 36 of them in the Spike gene, was described in South Africa. In December 2021, the Omicron BA.1 variant was detected in Brazil [6], quickly replacing the Delta variant.

In the current context, while efficient COVID-19 treatments are not widely available, the world population is not fully vaccinated and pre-existing antibodies induced either by previous infections or vaccination may not be sufficient to protect against the continuous emergence of new VOCs, one of the mainstay measures for COVID-19 control remains the prompt identification of SARS-CoV-2 infection in symptomatic individuals and contact cases. As fast as infected individuals are identified, countermeasures including isolation and case notification should be adopted to reduce transmission. In this scenario, antigen rapid diagnostic tests (Ag-RDTs) have become a highly cost-effective alternative compared to the real-time quantitative polymerase chain reaction (RTq-PCR), the gold standard for COVID-19 diagnosis. If correctly performed and interpreted, Ag-RDT can play a significant role in the continuous efforts for disease control, including its use in primary health attention rooms and self-testing [7–9]. It has also proved to be a valuable tool for epidemiologic surveys in field conditions. Consequently, during the pandemic, its use spread worldwide and was incorporated into routine tests for the diagnosis of respiratory virus infections. However, the continuous improvements in Ag-RDT, the target study population, and the continuous emergence of new SARS-CoV-2 variants may influence the performance of Ag-RDT [10].

In contrast to the Spike protein, which is the hotspot for mutations on the SARS-CoV-2 genome due to intense evolutionary pressure to escape host antibody responses, the Nucleocapsid protein (N) is not only more conserved among variants, but is also more abundantly expressed during infection [11]. Therefore, the N protein has become one of the main targets for Ag-RDTs development, and some of them are commercially available. Despite the appearance of SARS-CoV-2 variants, the sensitivity of N-based Ag-RDT remains high, so far [12].

Herein, we describe the engineering process to develop an Ag-RDT based on N protein detection, including a new anti-N monoclonal antibody production and characterization, as well as its validation during an Omicron BA.1 variant outbreak in Brazil under field conditions.

2. Materials and Methods

2.1. Ethical Approval

This study was conducted in agreement with the Ethical Principles in Human Research, approved by the Research Ethics Committee/UFMG (CAAE: 1686320.0.0000.5149). For animal use, this study was carried out following the recommendations of Ethical Principles in Animal Research, adopted by the Brazilian Council of Animal Experimentation. The Ethical Committee for Animal Research from Butantan Institute approved the research protocol (2715140420).

2.2. Populational Study

The nasopharyngeal samples were collected from patients attending the public health system in the city of Guaranésia, a small Brazilian town with 19 k habitants [13], in the state of Minas Gerais, at the border with São Paulo State. Sample collection and testing were performed for citizens with suggestive COVID-19 symptoms. The samples were obtained from 1 December 2022 to 8 February 2022, during the outbreak of the Omicron BA.1 variant in the southeast region of Brazil. All samples (n = 939) were submitted to RT-qPCR for the diagnosis of SARS-CoV-2 infection.

According to the epidemiological report released by the public health authorities of Minas Gerais State Health Department (SES/MG), by 8 February 2022, 14,350 citizens of Guaranésia had already been immunized with two doses of the vaccines against COVID-19 [14]. This number corresponds to approximately 75.5% of the total city population. In addition, 16,504 inhabitants had already received at least the first dose of the vaccine (approximately 86.8% of the total population).

2.3. Follow-Up Study

Patients (n = 38) from Belo Horizonte-Minas Gerais (Brazil) with a diagnosis of COVID-19 by RT-qPCR were monitored for 17 days, since the day of symptoms onset (day 0), from 23 December 2021 to 15 February 2022, to assess the sensitivity of the Ag-RDT in parallel with the RT-qPCR test, according to the reported number of days of symptoms of the patient. At least two samples from the 38 patients were collected throughout the infection. The follow-up study totaled 112 positive samples collected. Of the 38 individuals included in this cohort, 84.4% received two vaccine doses against COVID-19, 9.4% received three doses and 3.0% received only one dose. The administration of RNA vaccines was predominant (52%) among these patients, followed by viral vector vaccines (29%) and inactivated vaccines (19%). Samples were assayed with prototype 2.

2.3.1. Sampling

For each patient, two nasopharyngeal swabs were collected, one for Ag-RDT and the other for RT-qPCR, from each nostril. Samples for Ag-RDT were collected with nylon swabs in 0.3 mL of inactivation buffer and kept at $-20\,^{\circ}$C until testing. Samples for RT-qPCR were collected with rayon swabs in 1 mL of virus transport media and kept in 4–8 $^{\circ}$C until RNA extraction, as previously described [15].

2.3.2. RT-qPCR and RNA Sequencing

The RNA extraction from the samples was performed using the NucleoSpin® RNA Virus (Nagel, Germany), according to manufacturing protocols. Briefly, from 1 mL of the Virus Transport Media with the sample, 150 µL was used for RNA extraction and the remainder was stored at $-80\,^{\circ}$C for eventual repetitions or RNA sequencing. The RT-qPCR was performed using two different protocols on QuantStudio™ 3 and 5 Real-time PCR System (Applied Biosystems™, Waltham, MA, USA) and 5 Real-time PCR System (Applied Biosystems™). The main protocol followed the Charité/Berlin [16] recommendations, targeting the viral gene coding for the E protein with a reported sensibility to detect the 3.9 copies of SARS-CoV-2 genome per reaction [16]. Our internal validation disclosed 2.0 genome copies per reaction. When the result was inconclusive, we used the Center for Disease Control and Prevention (CDC) protocol [17], which targets the viral genes N1 and N2, with the sensibility to detect at least 5 copies/reaction [17]. Both protocols used the human RNAse P as the endogenous reaction control.

Thirty-five samples with Ct < 29 were selected for gene amplification, with PCR primers targeting the Spike gene, and the 1569 bp amplicons were sequenced using primers selected following the ARTIC protocol [18]. Sequences of all oligonucleotides can be found in Supplementary Table S1. The 1569 bp amplified region encodes amino acids S371, S373, S375, T376, D405, R408, K417, N440, G446, L452, S477, T478, E484, F486, Q493, G496, Q498, N501, Y505, F486, T547, A570, D614, H655, N679, P681, and S704, which have been associated with the characterization of several VOIs and the VOCs. Reverse transcription reactions and PCR amplifications were performed as previously described [19]. The assembling of Sanger contigs was performed with the GeneStudio software [Geneious Prime version 2022.0.1]. The Benchling platform [https://www.benchling.com/ (accessed on 24 August 2023)] was used for the visualization of alignments and the samples were manually genotyped via the evaluation of the modifications of interest in the sequences.

2.4. Expression and Purification of Nucleocapsid Recombinant Proteins DTC-N, N-Terminal Domain (Residues 47–177), and C-terminal Domain (Residues 210–419)

The codon-optimized, full-length (rDTC-N) coding region of the nucleocapsid (N) gene of SARS-CoV-2 (Genebank accession number: MT126808.1) was inserted into the pET-24a-(+) expression vector. The DNA fragments coding for the N-terminal domain (N_NTD47-177, residues 47 to 177) and C-terminal domain (N_CTD210-419, residues 210 to 419) were amplified with PCR using SARS-CoV-2 cDNA transcribed from the RNA isolated from the second Brazilian patient [20]. The primers used for PCR amplification were as follows: N_NTD47-177: 5′ AGCATAGCTAGCAATAA-TACTGCGTCTTGGTTCACCG 3′ and 5′ ATTATCGGATCCTTATCTGCTCCCTTCTGCG-TAGAAG 3′. N_CTD210-419: 5′ AG-CATAGCTAGCATGGCTGGCAATGGCGG 3′ and 5′ AT-TATCGGATCCTTAGGCCTGAGT TGAGTCAGC 3′, cloned into the expression vector pET-28a. All three proteins were expressed in *Escherichia coli* strain BL21(DE3). The recombinant antigens were purified with affinity chromatography using nickel columns in an AKTA Prime plus system following the manufacturer's instructions (GE Healthcare, Chicago, IL, USA) [21]. The eluted fractions containing the purified proteins were analyzed using SDS-PAGE, Western blot with Anti-His Tag antibody (Supplementary Figure S1). The full-length N recombinant protein was used for the mouse immunization and production of the new monoclonal antibody anti-DTC-N 1B3 (anti-DTC-N 1B3 mAb), and was applied at Ag-RDT's control line. The proteins containing the N-terminal (N_NTD47-177) and C-terminal domains (N_CTD210-419) were used to determine the epitope localization recognized by the anti-DTC-N 1B3 mAb.

2.5. SARS-CoV-2 Nucleocapsid Monoclonal Antibody (mAb) Production and Characterization

The immunization protocol was followed as described before [22,23]. Briefly, 10 μg of recombinant full-length N protein (rDTC-N) was used as the antigen. The mouse with the highest antibody titer was boosted with 10 μg of rDTC-N five days prior to cell fusion. Cells from the popliteal lymph node were fused to SP2/O-Ag14 mouse myeloma cells as previously described [24]. The supernatant fluids were screened for specific antibodies via indirect ELISA, in which 100 μL of hybridoma supernatant was added to a 96-well MaxiSorp microplate (Nunc®, Rochester, NY, USA) previously coated with 10 μg/mL of purified rDTC-N. mAb isotyping and purification of the mAb present in the supernatant were performed as described previously [22]. The anti-DTC-N 1B3 mAb binding kinetics to recombinant DTC-N was evaluated via surface plasmon resonance (SPR) in a Cytiva Biacore T-200 system. The NTA sensor (Cytiva, Uppsala, Sweden) was equilibrated in HBS-N buffer (0.01 M Hepes pH 7.4 and 0.15 M NaCl, 25 °C) and sensitized with 50 mM $NiCl_2$ for 60 s at 10 μL/min. The DTC-N protein at 1 μg/mL was captured in an NTA sensor chip (300 s, 10 μL/min). Three different sample concentrations ranging from 100 to 11.1 μg/mL (three-fold dilution) were injected sequentially (180 s association, 420 s dissociation, 30 μL/min). Between cycles, the sensor surface was regenerated with a 30 μL pulse of 0.25 M EDTA disodium. Kinetics parameters were calculated using a Langmuir 1:1 fitting model with BiaEvalutation Software 3.0. The experiment was performed in duplicate and the result was expressed as the average from the two independent assays.

2.5.1. mAb Sequencing

Total RNA was extracted from 6×10^5 cells producing the mAb with the RNeasy Mini Kit (QIA-GEN, Hilden, Germany), following the manufacturer's recommendations. Reverse transcription was obtained using random hexamer primers supplied by First-Strand cDNA Synthesis (GE Healthcare, USA). The heavy and light chain variable domains' amplification was carried out using degenerate primers [25], and the amplicons were sequenced with the SANGER method [26] to confirm the sequences as variable chains. The NGS sequencing library was prepared using 50 ng of cDNA (quantified with Qubit dsDNA BR Assay Kit–Thermo Fisher Scientific, Waltham, MA, USA) and the Nextera XT DNA Library preparation kit (Illumina, San Diego, CA, USA) using dual-index tagging, according to manufacturer's instructions. The library's size distribution was measured using the automated capillary electrophoresis system GelBot (Loccus, Cotia, Brazil) and the average size was used to normalize the library for the final loading concentration of 600 pM. The library was sequenced on a NextSeq 2000 P2 2 × 100 bp flow cell (Illumina, San Diego, CA, USA). The raw data were automatically converted and trimmed online at the Basespace web-based cloud (Illumina, USA). To ensure mAb had no clonal diversity, we mapped the NGS reads to the variable chains reference sequence of the cloning expression cassette, previously sequenced with SANGER using the Map to Reference tool with default parameters on Geneious Prime 2022.1.1. The alignment of the reads was manually inspected for nucleotide variation.

2.5.2. Epitope Characterization and Structure Analysis

Peptide mapping was performed using PEPperPRINT (Heidelberg, Germany), according to their protocols. The N-protein sequences of SARS-CoV-2 (UniProt ID: P0DTC9), SARS-CoV (P59595), MERS-CoV (K9N4V7), HCoV-OC43 (P33469), HCoV-NL63 (Q6Q1R8), HCoV-229E (P15130), and HCoV-HKU1 (isolate 1: Q5MQC6; isolate 2: Q14EA6; isolate 5: Q0ZME3) were elongated with neutral GSGSGSG linkers at the C- and N-terminus to avoid truncated peptides. Briefly, an N-protein peptide microarray was incubated with anti-DTC-N 1B3 mAb at concentrations of 1 µg/mL, 10 µg/mL, and 100 µg/mL, followed by staining with secondary and control antibodies as well as being read out with an Innopsys InnoScan 710-IR Microarray Scanner at scanning gains of 50/10 (red/green). Microarray image analysis was undertaken with a PepSlide® analyzer and summarized in the Excel file Microarray Data Mouse mAb 1B3 (PEP20225052421).xlsx.

For structure analysis, we determined the recognition pattern of anti-DTC-N 1B3 mAb between non-treated rDTC-N and treated rDTC-N (heated at 100 °C or 50 mM DTT also heated at 100 °C, both for 10 min). The mAb was also evaluated using indirect ELISA, in which MaxiSorp microplates (Thermo Fisher Scientific, Waltham, MA, USA) were coated with 10 µg/mL of rDTC-N, treated or non-treated. Phosphate-buffered saline (PBS) with bovine serum albumin (BSA) 1% was added as a blocking agent and incubated for 1 h at 37 °C. Next, the anti-DTC-N 1B3 mAb was diluted (log2) in an initial concentration of 7.15 µg/mL, followed by incubation with goat anti-mouse IgG conjugated with horseradish peroxidase (Sigma-Aldrich, St. Louis, MO, USA) diluted 1:5000 in PBS-BSA 0.1% solution. Reactions were developed with 0.5 mg/mL O-phenylenediamine (OPD; Sigma Aldrich Co., St. Louis, MO, USA) plus 0.5-µL/mL hydrogen peroxide in 0.05 M citrate-phosphate buffer, pH 5.0, in the dark, at room temperature. The reactions were interrupted after 15 min by the addition of 50 µL of 1 M HCl. The absorbance was measured at 492 nm in a Multiskan EX ELISA reader (Labsystems, Milford, MA, USA). At each step, the volume added was 100 µL/well, except in the washing and blocking steps, when the volume used was 200 µL/well. Between incubation periods, the plates were washed three times with PBS-Tween 0.05%. All experiments were carried out in technical duplicates, and the results corresponded to three independent experiments (biological replicates). The nitrocellulose membranes (GE-Healthcare, Freiburg, Germany) containing the transferred proteins DTC-N (SARS-CoV-2), N-terminus protein N (SARS-CoV-2), C-terminus protein N (SARS-CoV-2), DENV-2 NS1 recombinant protein and full protein N (SARS-CoV-2) from

12% polyacrylamide gel electrophoresis containing sodium dodecyl sulfate (SDS-PAGE) were blocked with BSA 1% for 1 h at 37 °C and then they were tested with an anti-DTC-N 1B3 mAb (1:100) at a concentration of 870 µg/mL. Next, the membranes were incubated with goat anti-mouse IgG conjugated with peroxidase (1:5000). The reactive protein bands were identified with 10 mg DAB in 15 mL Tris-buffered saline plus 12 µL H_2O_2 (30%).

2.6. SARS-CoV-2 Samples

The SARS-CoV-2 viral strains used in this study were from the lineage B (isolate BRA/SP02/2020), Delta (EPI_ISL_2965577), and Omicron (EPI_ISL_7699344) variants. Viral stocks were propagated in Vero E6 cells (ATCC CRL-1586) at 37 °C with 5% CO_2 and observed for cytopathic effects (CPE) daily up to 72 h. Viruses were titrated in Vero E6 cells using a plaque forming units (PFU) assay [20]. Viral aliquots were kept at -80 °C until further use. The identity of all samples was confirmed by genome sequencing. Before use, samples were heated at 60 °C for 1 h to inactivate the virus. Parallel analyses of the diluted stock viruses were performed using RT-qPCR and the developed Ag-RDT. The results obtained were compared with the purpose of certifying the ability of the Ag-RDT to specifically detect the original SARS-CoV-2 virus, as well as its variants.

2.7. Antigen Rapid Diagnostic Test (Ag-RDT)

The Ag-RDT developed was based on the lateral flow immunochromatographic principle. Several membranes were superposed, each one containing a specific reagent. The test and control lines were sprayed and immobilized on the nitrocellulose membrane using the Continuous Dispenser HGS101 (Autokun®, Hangzhou, China). The antibodies were conjugated to colloidal gold nanoparticles [27] and dispensed onto a glass fiber. The glass fiber was also used on the sample pad. A cellulose fiber was used to absorb all the reagents at the opposite end of the test membranes. The superposed membranes' strips were placed on a plastic cassette, which was the dispositive where the test was performed. In the presence of SARS-CoV-2, the virus N protein reacted with the monoclonal antibody in the conjugate pad and as the complex flowed through the nitrocellulose membrane, it was captured by a second monoclonal antibody dispensed on the test line. The results were visually read 20 min after sample application, and any color intensity formed in the test line was considered positive. In the absence of SARS-CoV-2, no reactivity was presented at the test line. The remaining conjugate, bound to the control line, resulted in a color change that was required to validate the test.

2.7.1. Inactivation Buffer

The inactivation buffer used to collect the sample for the Ag-RDT was designed to lyse the cells and expose the viral antigens, as well as to maintain the structure of the viral protein. It contained Tris-NaCl buffer (pH 8.5) and Tergitol® NP-40 as a lysis agent. Nasal swab samples were collected in vials containing 0.3 mL of buffer.

2.7.2. Prototype 1

Initially, we used a pair of commercial monoclonal antibodies anti-N (mAb A and mAb B) from Fapon Biotech® (Dongguan, China), to prototype an Ag-RDT (prototype 1). By using this pair of mAb previously tested in the prototype, we were able to set up all the other components and variables that may interfere with an Ag-RDT performance. Prototype 1 was then used as a proof of concept for the correct assembly of all test components and reagents. The mAb A was immobilized on the nitrocellulose membrane as the test line in a concentration varying between 0.2 and 4.0 mg/mL. The recombinant protein N was dispensed as the control line in the same concentration range as the test line. The mAb B was used as the conjugate. In this way, the mAb B was mixed with colloidal gold nanoparticles of 20 nm, incubated at room temperature for 5 min, and blocked with BSA (Sigma-Aldrich®) for the same time. After this process, the solution was centrifuged at 8 °C, the supernatant was discarded, and the pellet was resuspended in a storage buffer, dispensed on glass fiber, and dried at room temperature and <40% humidity. The strips were superposed, cut, and placed in plastic cassettes.

2.7.3. Prototype 2

After prototype 1 had been set up and tested, we gradually replaced one of the commercial mAb with the newly developed anti-DTC-N 1B3 mAb (mAb C), generating prototype 2. A mixture of mAb A and mAb C was immobilized on the nitrocellulose membrane as the test line in a concentration varying between 0.2 and 4.0 mg/mL. All the remaining conditions used for prototype 1 were maintained for this second prototype.

2.7.4. Prototype 3

In prototype 3, the commercial mAb B was completely replaced with mAb C, as the conjugate, using colloidal gold nanoparticles of 40 nm. All other remaining conditions of prototype 1 were maintained.

2.8. Assaying Ag-RDT Prototypes with SARS-CoV-2 Virus

Before starting the tests, all reagents and samples were brought to room temperature. The samples were homogenized, and 120 µL of samples were applied to the sample cavity of the cassette. All three prototypes were initially evaluated using dilutions of the SARS-CoV-2 virus collected in DMEM medium and inactivated by heat, as described above. Virus stocks' dilutions (1:2 up to 1:1024) were prepared using the inactivation buffer, which was used as negative control.

2.9. Assaying Ag-RDT Prototypes with Patients' Samples for Validation

As previously mentioned, prototype 1 was used as a proof of concept for the correct assembly of all test components and reagents and was assayed using 17 swab samples of patients, 10 of which were negative and 7 positive in RT-qPCR. For the validation of prototypes 2 and 3, 2 different sets of 120 positive and 60 negative samples of patients from the Guaranésia cohort were assayed on each prototype, and the results were compared to the results of RT-qPCR. Two sets of samples were required for the evaluation of each prototype, due to the limitation of the sample's volume. For each test, 120 µL of samples were added and the results were read after 20 min.

2.10. Stability Assay

The stability assay was performed by the aggression of prototypes at 45 °C, to estimate the real-time stability of the Ag-RDT [28]. The tests were packed in sachets containing silica gel and sealed before being placed at 45 °C. They were evaluated at day 0 (before being placed in the incubator) and every 7 days after that. For the evaluation, 4 cassettes were removed from the stove and evaluated with serial dilutions of heat-inactivated SARS-CoV-2 virus stocks and with an inactivation buffer (negative control). For each test, 120 µL of samples were added and the results were read after 20 min. For the determination of real-time stability, samples of Ag-RDT prototype 3 were maintained under standard storage conditions, at room temperature and under humidity control. The evaluation procedure was performed as described above for over 14 months.

2.11. Statistical Analysis

Descriptive statistics were used to analyze the data. Sensitivity was defined as the proportion of SARS-CoV-2 positive patients correctly identified by the Ag-RDT that was also positive by RT-qPCR. Specificity was defined as the proportion of samples correctly identified as negative by Ag-RDT and also categorized as negative by RT-qPCR. Sensitivity was evaluated globally and according to the Ct value for the E gene or the N gene using different cutoffs (Ct $\leq$ 25; 25 $\leq$ Ct $\leq$ 30 and Ct > 30) and the days post onset of symptoms (0–3 days; 4–7 days; >7 days). Accuracy was calculated by dividing the sum of the true positives and true negatives by the total number of samples analyzed. The concordance between RT-qPCR and Ag-RDT was calculated using the Kappa (k) index, according to Cohen [29]. Statistical analysis was carried out using MedCalc version 20.118 (MedCalc Software) and the GraphPad Prism 8.0.1 software. The 95% confidence intervals (CI) for sensitivity, specificity, and accuracy were calculated using the Clopper–Pearson method. The Mann–Whitney test was used to estimate statistical differences between pairs of tests. Differences were considered statistically significant with the p-value < 0.05.

Statistical analyses of data obtained for the characterization of anti-DTC-N 1B3 mAb were performed with two-way variance analysis followed by the ANOVA post-test. (** $p = 0.0018$). Differences between means of the ELISA optical density of reactivity with the intact protein and treated fractions were analyzed using an unpaired Student's t-test; *** $p = 0.0009$ compared to DTT-treated protein and * $p = 0.01$ compared to heat-treated protein.

3. Results

3.1. Population Characteristics

From 1 December 2021 to 8 February 2022, 939 samples were collected in the city of Guaranésia, Minas Gerais, for simultaneous analysis using RT-qPCR and Ag-RDT. The distribution of positive and negative samples and their corresponding Ct values are shown in Supplementary Figure S3. Among the 939 samples evaluated, 22.68% (213/939) were negative for SARS-CoV-2 on RT-qPCR analysis, 76.25% (716/939) were positive, based on the detection of the gene E sequence, and 1.06% (10/939) showed an inconclusive result. From the positive samples, 64.4% (461/716) showed Ct values ≤ 25; 11.59% (83/716) showed Ct values between 25 and 30; and 24.0% (172/716) had a Ct value > 30. For the evaluation of the Ag-RDT prototype 2, 180 samples characterized with RT-qPCR were selected: 60 (33.3%) negative samples and 120 (66.7%) positive samples (65.8% with Ct values ≤ 25; 15.0% with $25 <$ Ct value ≤ 30 and 19.2% with Ct value > 30). For the evaluation of the Ag-RDT prototype 3, an additional 180 samples also characterized with RT-qPCR were selected: 60 (33.3%) negative samples and 120 (66.7%) positive samples (70.0% with Ct values ≤ 25; 12.5% with Ct value between 25 and 30 and 17.5% with Ct value > 30). The positive samples were selected in a way to approximate the proportion of Ct values detected in the population.

For the follow-up study, 112 positive samples detected using RT-qPCR were collected sequentially after the onset of symptoms from 38 patients living in the city of Belo Horizonte, from 23 December 2021 to 15 February 2022. According to the day of onset of symptoms, 22.3% (25/112) of the samples were collected between 0 and 3 days, 40.2% (45/112) between 4 and 7 days, and 37.5% (42/112) were collected from the 8th until the 17th day of the symptom onset. The Ct means found in the RT-qPCR for each group were 21.5, 25.2, and 30.8, respectively.

DNA sequencing, performed in 35 samples from Guaranésia and Belo Horizonte cities, indicated the predominance of the Omicron BA.1 variant of SARS-CoV-2, which was detected in 100% of the samples analyzed.

3.2. SARS-CoV-2 Nucleocapsid mAb (Anti-DTC-N 1B3 mAb) Functional Characterization

After fusion, only one secretory hybridoma was generated, named 1B3. The clone was expanded, supernatants were collected and the mAb was purified (Figure 1A). The mAb-protein interaction association and dissociation rates (mean $\pm$ SD, $n = 2$) were measured using surface plasmon resonance (SPR); rates of $(7.2 \pm 0.5) \times 10^3$ M^{-1} s^{-1} and $(3.27 \pm 0.01) \times 10^{-4}$ s^{-1}, respectively, were found with a corresponding binding affinity K_D of $(4.5 \pm 0.3) \times 10^{-8}$ M. To determine the anti-DTC-N 1B3 isotype, antibodies that recognized specifically IgG1, 2a, 2b, IgG3 ($p \leq 0.0001$), and IgA and IgM subclasses were used in ELISA. Significant reactivity ($p \leq 0.0001$) with the N protein was observed only for IgG2b, when compared to all the other isotypes (Figure 1B). The location of the epitope recognized by the anti-DTC-N 1B3 on the N protein was confirmed via immunoblotting (Figure 1C). This analysis revealed that the anti-DTC-N 1B3 mAb recognizes not only the full-length

N recombinant protein, but also its C-terminal domain. No reactivity was detected in the N-terminus region. The recognition pattern of the anti-DTC-N 1B3 mAb was then evaluated with ELISA using either non-treated rDTC-N or treated rDTC-N (heated at 100 °C or 50 mM DTT also heated at 100 °C, both for 10 min). The results indicated that the recognized epitope was at least partially represented by conformational structures, since reactivity was affected by treatments that may affect the N protein structure (Figure 1D). The epitope mapping resulted in the recognition of peptides with the consensus motif TFPPTEPKKDKKK of SARS-CoV-2, and SARS-CoV (Figure 1E), which aligned with the C-terminus sequence of the protein and was not mutated in the Omicron variant (Supplementary Figure S2). Anti-DTC-N 1B3 mAb CDRs domains were confirmed using the SANGER method after random primers' detection and the NGS sequencing library (Supplementary Figure S1).

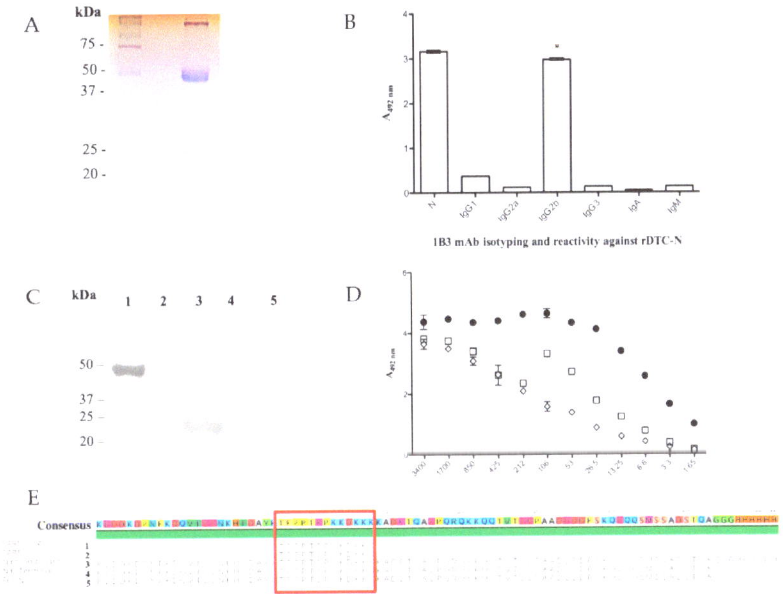

Figure 1. Anti-DTC-N 1B3 mAb purification and characterization. (**A**) The 12% SDS/PAGE anti-DTC-N 1B3 mAb profile stained with Coomassie Blue after the G protein affinity column purification. (**B**) Anti-DTC-N 1B3 mAb isotyping analysis. C96 MaxiSorp ELISA microtiter plates coated with 10 µg/mL of recombinant rDTC-N or 1 µg/mL of IgG1, 2a, 2b, IgG3, IgA, and IgM, incubated with 100 µL supernatants of anti-DTC-N 1B3 mAb and with rat anti-mouse kappa conjugated with horseradish (1:1000). The asterisk (*) indicates statistically significant differences as compared to all the other isotypes of IgG, and IgA and IgM subclasses ($p \leq 0.0001$). (**C**) Immunoblotting analysis. Nitrocellulose membrane containing 10 µg of (1) DTC-N (SARS-CoV-2); (2) N-terminus protein N (SARS-CoV-2); (3) C-terminus protein N (SARS-CoV-2); (4) DENV-2 NS1 recombinant protein; (5) full-length control protein N (SARS-CoV-2). Membrane was probed with the anti-DTC-N 1B3 mAb (1:100) at a concentration of 870 µg/mL and goat anti-mouse IgG conjugated with peroxidase (1:5000). (**D**) Anti-DTC-N 1B3 recognition patter. The 10 µg/mL rDTC-N, heated-treated [100 °C for 10 min (□), DTT-treated (◇), or intact (●) were used as solid phase-bound antigens. The anti-DTC-N 1B3 mAb was serially diluted (log2) from an initial concentration of 0.007 µg/mL. (**E**) Alignments of the anti-DTC-N 1B3 mAb epitope with N protein sequences. The epitope sequence recognized by anti-DTC-N 1B3 mAb was aligned with protein N partial sequences, comprised between amino acids 352 and 434 from SARS-CoV-2, SARS, and with sequences obtained for the full-length N and N-terminal recombinant proteins.

3.3. Ag-RDT Validation

3.3.1. Prototype 1 Performance

Prototype 1, used only as a proof of concept, was initially tested against the SARS-CoV2 variants' culture stocks (Wuhan, Alpha, Gamma, Delta, P2, and Omicron). Positive results were detected in samples from all tested SARS-CoV-2 cultured stocks in dilutions of up to 1:1024, with high signal intensity, regardless of the variant. This prototype detected five out of seven positive patient samples with Ct values between 19.1 and 26.4, whereas the two undetected samples had Ct values of 29.5 and 32.7. Nonspecific reactions were not observed in any of the 10 negative samples evaluated. Color intensities of the reactions for this prototype are shown in Figure 2A.

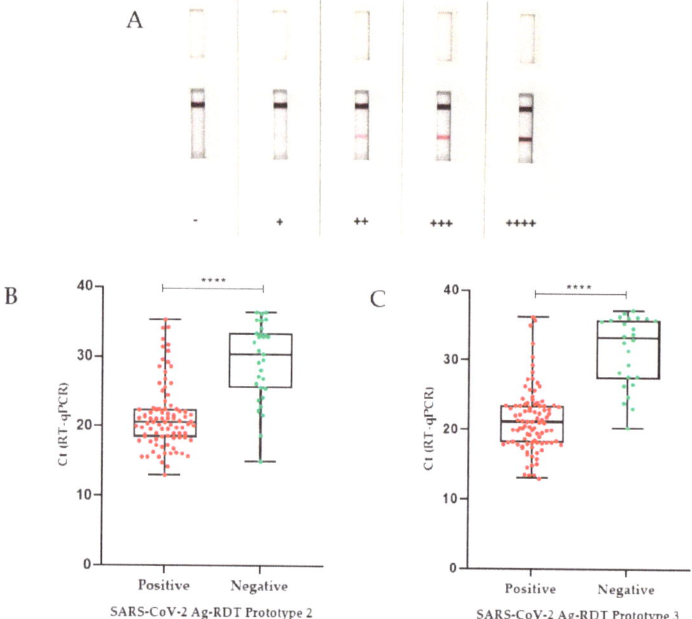

Figure 2. Validation of Ag-RDT prototypes based on RT-qPCR. (**A**) Illustrative figures of Ag-RDT results. Figures show tests with different intensities of reaction as detected by the Ag-RDT. According to the signal strength of the positive samples on the test line (T), the results were classified as + (low intensity), ++ (moderate to low intensity), +++ (moderate to high intensity), and ++++ (high intensity). In the absence of the appearance of a test line (T), the sample was considered negative ($-$). (**B**) Box plot analysis of RT-qPCR and Ag-RDT prototype 2. RT-qPCR Ct values (for positive samples only) as compared with positive and negative results obtained with prototype 2 Ag-RDT. The median Ct value found for the false-negative samples on SARS-CoV-2 Ag-RDT (30.4) was significantly different from the median Ct value found for the positive samples on SARS-CoV-2 Ag-RDT (20.6). (**C**) Box plot analysis of RT-qPCR Ct value (positive only) compared with prototype 3 Ag-RDT results. The median Ct value found for the false-negative samples on SARS-CoV-2 Ag-RDT (33.2) was significantly different from the median Ct value found for the positive samples on SARS-CoV-2 Ag-RDT (21.1) ($p < 0.0001$ was indicated by ****). Boxplot analysis (2B and 2D) was performed by applying the Mann–Whitney test, using the GraphPad Prism 8.0.1 software. The line across the box is the median. The whiskers represent all points showing minimum to maximum quartiles.

3.3.2. Prototype 2 Performance

Sensitivity results (95% CI) for prototype 2 were extracted according to the Ct of the samples obtained using the RT-qPCR technique. The sensitivity values obtained for samples with Ct $\leq$ 25 was 91.1% (CI 82.6–96.4%); for samples with Ct between 25 and 30 it was 55.6% (CI 30.8–78.5%); and for samples with Ct > 30 it was 30.4% (CI 13.2–52.9%). The overall sensitivity of this Ag-RDT prototype was 74.2% (CI 65.4–81.7%). The specificity of the test was 90% (CI 79.5–96.2%) and the overall accuracy found was 79.4% (CI 72.8–85.1%) (Table 1). The median Ct found for the false-negative samples (30.4) was significantly different ($p < 0.0001$) from the median value determined for the positive ones (20.6), according to the Mann–Whitney test (Figure 2B).

Table 1. Prototype 2 and 3's performances according to RT-qPCR results.

Prototype 2						
RT-qPCR Positive Samples	Ct	Ag-RDT Positive	Ag-RDT Negative	Sensitivity (95% CI)	Specificity (95% CI)	Accuracy (95% CI)
79	Ct $\leq$ 25	72	7	91.1% (82.6–96.4%)		90.6% (83.5–94.9%)
18	25 < Ct $\leq$ 30	10	8	55.6% (30.8–78.5%)	90% (79.5–96.2%) 54/60	82.1% (71.7–89.8%)
23	Ct > 30	7	16	30.4% (13.2–52.9%)		71.2% (62.7–82.6%)
120	Total	89	31	74.2% (65.4–81.7%)		79.4% (72.8–85.1%)

Prototype 3						
RT-qPCR positive sample	Ct	Ag-RDT positive	Ag-RDT negative	Sensitivity (95% CI)	Specificity (95% CI)	Accuracy (95% CI)
84	Ct $\leq$ 25	80	4	95.2% (88.2–98.7%)		96.5% (92.1–98.8%)
15	25 < Ct $\leq$ 30	9	6	60.0% (32.3–83.6%)	98.3% (91.1–99.9%) 59/60	90.7% (81.7–96.2%)
21	Ct > 30	5	16	23.8% (8.2–47.2%)		79.0% (68.5–87.3%)
120	Total	94	26	78.3% (69.9–85.3%)		85.0% (78.9–89.9%)

95% CI: calculated with the Clopper–Pearson method using MedCalc Software.

The agreement between Ag-RDT and RT-qPCR results for all samples corresponded to a moderate Kappa index (agreement = 79.4%, k = 0.579). When considering only samples with high viral loads (Ct $\leq$ 25), an excellent concordance was obtained (agreement = 90.6%, k = 0.811).

Prototype 2 was stable for 45 days at 45 °C, which corresponded to approximately 12 months at room temperature.

3.3.3. Prototype 3 Performance

To improve Ag-RDT specificity and to reduce the dependency on commercial antibodies, we developed prototype 3 by replacing mAb B with mAb C (anti-DTC-N 1B3 mAb). As shown for prototype 2, prototype 3 was also able to detect all analyzed SARS-CoV-2 variants—Wuhan, Alpha, Gamma, Delta, P2, and Omicron. The sensitivity (95% CI) for prototype 3 was also categorized according to the Ct of the samples obtained with the RT-qPCR. The sensitivity obtained for samples with Ct $\leq$ 25 was 95.2% (CI 88.2–98.7%); it was 60.0% (CI 32.3–83.6%) for samples with Ct between 25 and 30, and 23.8% (CI 8.2–47.2%) for samples with Ct > 30. The specificity of the test was 98.3% (CI 91.1–99.9%) and the overall accuracy found was 85.0% (CI 78.9–89.9%) (Table 1). The median Ct found in the false-negative samples (33.2) was significantly different ($p < 0.0001$) from the median value of the positive ones (21.1), as detected using the Mann–Whitney test (Figure 2C). Prototype 3 has displayed a real-time stability of 14 months, so far.

3.4. Ag-RDT Follow-Up Study

The sensitivity of Ag-RDT tests may vary during the progress of the SARS-CoV-2 infection, after the onset of symptoms [30]. Therefore, we performed sequential sampling for patients from the Belo Horizonte cohort, starting from the day of PCR diagnosis and symptoms onset. This follow-up study indicated that whenperformed within the first three days after the onset of symptoms, when patients displayed a mean Ct of 21.5, the Ag-RDT displayed a 100% (CI 86.3–100.0%) sensitivity. Between 4 and 7 days after symptom onset, the sensitivity of the Ag-RDT was reduced to 64.4% (CI 48.8–78.1%), whereas the percentage of positive results obtained from the eighth day post symptoms onset was further reduced to 42.8% (CI 27.7–59.0%) (Table 2). As noted before, the sensitivity observed between the days after symptoms onset correlated with the viral load, i.e., it decreased with the increase in the mean Ct of the samples.

Table 2. Diagnostic performance of the developed Ag-RDT (prototype 2), according to the day of symptoms onset.

Days of Symptoms Onset	RT-qPCR Positive Samples	Mean Ct	Ag-RDT Positive Samples	Sensitivity (95% CI)
0 to 3	25	21.5	25	100.0% (86.3–100.0%)
4 to 7	45	25.2	29	64.4% (48.9–78.1%)
>7	42	30.8	18	42.8% (27.7–59.0%)

95% CI: calculated with the Clopper–Pearson method using MedCalc Software.

A summary of the prototypes' performances compared to some commercial kits is presented in Table 3. The reported sensitivity of commercial kits varies from 92.9% to 100% for samples with Ct ≤ 25, while specificity varies from 83.3% to 100%.

Table 3. Summary of the prototypes' performances compared to commercial kits.

Author	Country	Samples (*n*) +	Samples (*n*) −	Commercial Kit	Sensitivity Ct ≤ 25	Sensitivity Overall	Specificity
Rastawicki, 2021 [31]	Poland	95	46	PCL COVID-19 Ag Rapid FIA (ROK)	92.9%	38.9%	83.3%
Pérez-García, 2021 [32]	Spain	186	170	Panbio COVID-19 Ag Rapid Test Abbott (USA)	98.9%	60.0%	100%
				SD Biosensor Ag (ROK)	97.4%	66.5%	97.3%
Blairon, 2021 [33]	Belgium	150	49	Coronavirus Ag Rapid Test Cassette Bio-Rad (USA)	97.1%	60.0%	100%
				GSD NovaGen SARS-CoV-2 Antigen Rapid Test (China)	95.7%	59.3%	85.7%
				Aegle Coronavirus Ag Rapid Test Cassette LumiraDx (UK)	97.1%	61.1%	100%
Sood, 2021 [34]	USA	226	548	BinaxNOW™ Abbott (USA)	93.8%	56.2%	98.4%
Choudhary, 2022 [35]	India	129	627	SD Biosensor, Inc. (ROK)	NR	55.0%	99.2%
Nóra, 2022 [36]	Hungary	40	58	GenBody COVID-19 Ag (ROK)	93.8%	62.0%	86.4%
Wegrzynska, 2023 [37]	Poland	103	301	GenBody COVID-19 Ag (ROK)	100%	97.1%	100%
Prototypes	Brazil	120	60	SARS-CoV-2 Ag RDT Prototype 2 (Brazil)	92.0%	74.1%	90.0%
		120	60	SARS-CoV-2 Ag RDT Prototype 3 (Brazil)	95.2%	78.3%	98.3%

NR: Not reported; +: Positive; −: Negative.

4. Discussion

After more than 3 years of the COVID-19 pandemic, SARS-CoV-2 Ag-RDT has become an important alternative for diagnosis, patient follow-up and to improve the efficacy of disease control. While the effective implementation of Ag-RDTs requires constant surveillance of their analytical performance, as new SARS-CoV-2 variants may emerge, new reagents and test availability may ensure that a loss of sensitivity of Ag-RDTs will be specifically overcome.

Here, we report a complete engineering process for developing a SARS-CoV-2 Ag-RDT, including the production of N recombinant protein as well as the production and characterization of a new mAb (anti-DTC-N 1B3 mAb) that is specific for this protein. So far, more than 30 mutations, some of them very frequent, have been reported among the variants of SARS-CoV-2. In contrast, only four main mutations are present in N protein [38,39]. Therefore, the use of mAbs directed to different and conserved epitopes of the N protein may improve sensitivity, overcoming losses caused by the high mutation rates of Spike as a target antigen. Indeed, anti-N mAbs have been successfully used for the development of commercially available Ag-RDT tests [10,12,40], as well as in other sensitive assays [41]. In addition to the high mutation rate, the Spike protein has several sites of post-transcriptional modifications and usually requires eukaryotic expression systems for its expression as a recombinant protein in a correct conformation [42]. In contrast, the N protein was easily expressed in prokaryotic cells, which is convenient for the generation of monoclonal antibodies and its use as a reagent in RDT.

To prototype the Ag-RDT, initially we used a pair of antibodies for the detection of the virus N antigen, which were commercially available. Using these mAbs, all the reagents, membranes and detection conditions were tested. Then, the commercial mAb was replaced with the new mAb anti-DTC-N 1B3. The epitope mapping of the anti-DTC-N 1B3 mAb revealed a sequence present in the C-terminus of the N protein that was conserved in all main VOCs of SARS-CoV-2 analyzed. To address this question experimentally, we tested the performance of the Ag-RDT prototypes with viral culture stocks corresponding to the main VOCs that circulated globally. In agreement, the Ag-RDT prototypes were able to detect all tested variants of SARS-CoV-2 and showed a performance similar to commercial tests [43].

The performance of the Ag-RDT prototypes was also challenged in a real-time validation test with samples collected from patients during an outbreak of the Omicron variant in Brazil. According to WHO, Ag-RDTs should meet a minimum performance requirements of $\geq$80% sensitivity and $\geq$97% specificity [7]. Since the specificity of prototype 2 was 90% and, therefore, beneath the value recommended by WHO, an improved prototype was developed by replacing the commercial mAb B with the anti-DTC-N 1B3 mAb. Prototype 3 showed 98.3% specificity and 95.2% sensitivity when tested with samples with Ct $\leq$ 25, meeting WHO's criteria. This performance was also similar to those found for tests currently available on the market. The distribution of the Ct values of true positive and false negative samples and the concordance index of Ag-RDT with RT-qPCR were also comparable to those reported for commercial SARS-CoV-2 antigen tests [30,32], indicating the potential of the Ag-RDT developed here as a tool for COVID-19 diagnosis. Although a sensitivity of 100% has been reported for some commercial tests, direct comparisons of their performance with our data may be compromised given the differences in VOCs prevalence, the vaccination status of the populations and the assay conditions for comparison with RT-qPCR [44]. In agreement, Nora et al. (2022) reported the evaluation of 10 commercial kits' on-field conditions and found, for some of them, important differences on their performance when compared to previously reported data [36,37].

The follow-up study aimed at evaluating the correlation between the dynamics of viral loads, after symptoms onset and the sensitivity of the Ag-RDT, since this may provide additional information on the performance of the Ag-RDT in patients with confirmed diagnosis at different time points, either with high or low viral loads. As observed in other studies [30,44], and following the dynamics of viral infection, the Ct of the samples increased after the symptoms onset, reaching the detection limit of the assay, evidencing a constant decrease in the viral loads. In our study, this decrease was more pronounced after 4 days past symptoms onset, when patients presented a mean Ct > 25.

RT-qPCR is considered the gold standard for COVID-19 diagnosis, and thus used to evaluate the performance of Ag-RDTs. Nonetheless, some aspects may be considered for results' interpretations when comparing these tests, given that targets and conditions for these assays are quite different. In the present study, samples for Ag-RDT and RT-qPCR were collected concomitantly for each patient, but from different nostrils and maintained in different buffers. These different conditions may have introduced a bias in the viral load between the two samples. Another aspect is the fact that it is still unclear whether the persistent detection of SARS-CoV-2 RNA in routine nasopharyngeal swabs of COVID-19 patients represents replicating virus or simply viral nucleic acid in cell debris [45]. There is no clear evidence for a correlation between RNA viral load and infectivity and transmissibility, i.e., whether RT-qPCR results in patients with Ct > 25 indicate the presence of intact viral particles or reminiscent sub-genomic fragments [46]. This correlation is even more complicated when extrapolated for Ag-RDT, since the targets for RT-qPCR and Ag-RDT are different. Despite the lower sensitivity when compared to molecular testing, it has been argued that antigen tests may be a better indicator of viral infectivity. Nevertheless, there is a significant consensus that, in the presence of symptoms, a negative Ag-RDT test should be validated by a RT-qPCR test [47].

It has been reported that vaccination affects the duration of symptoms and the viral loads measured with RT-qPCR [48]. There is also evidence that SARS-CoV-2 T cell responses, besides neutralizing antibodies induced by either natural infection or vaccines, limit the disease severity by providing a rapid viral clearance [49–52]. The developed prototypes were validated during the outbreak of the Omicron variant in the city of Guaranésia, Minas Gerais, Brazil, after this population had already reached a significant level of vaccination coverage. The sensitivity of prototypes dropped among patients from this population with Ct values higher than 25. Therefore, the high rate of vaccination in Guaranésia's population may explain the decrease in the sensitivity values for the Ag-RDT prototypes tested in patients with Ct > 25.

Whilst our study aimed at contributing with new reagents and valuable insights into the detection and characterization of SARS-CoV-2 and its variants, some limitations are noteworthy, including testing on a limited sample size and the evaluation of a specific population, from a single region, in a specific period of time. Further independent validation studies could enhance the robustness of our findings and confirm the diagnostic accuracy of the Ag-RDT in more diverse settings. Whereas our assay exhibited high sensitivity, it is important to acknowledge that false negatives might occur, especially in cases of low viral loads. Optimizing sensitivity for varying viral loads could enhance its effectiveness. The potential for bias in sample collection, even with rigorous protocols, could impact the representativeness of our study population. Strategies to minimize selection bias during sample collection would boost the validity of our results. While the developed prototypes showed specificity for SARS-CoV-2, potential cross-reactivity with other related pathogens was not exhaustively investigated. Moreover, the potential for detecting emerging variants, such as those associated with VOCs, warrants the continuous surveillance and adaptation of the diagnostic test. In addition, further studies evaluating the stability of our assay components over extended periods would provide confidence in its reliability. Finally, some of these limitations may be related to the fact that the prototypes were produced in a laboratory setting. Industrial prototypes may be further optimized, allowing adjustments to improve the performance and additional validation assays.

5. Conclusions

Results of this study indicated that, using a new anti-N mAb, the Ag-RDT developed displayed high sensitivity and specificity, regardless of the most significant VOCs circulating worldwide and the immune status of the population, and may, therefore, constitute an alternative tool for improving point-of-care diagnosis and for epidemiological and follow-up studies of COVID-19.

Supplementary Materials: The following supporting information can be downloaded at: https://www.mdpi.com/article/10.3390/microorganisms11102422/s1, Table S1. Primers used for PCR amplification and Sanger sequencing. In the table are present the identifiers and sequences of the primers (Primer ID, Sequence (5′–3′). The nCoV-2019_75_LEFT, nCoV-2019_77_RIGHT and CTR1 primers were used for the obtention of 1569 bp. Figure S1. Anti-HisTag immunoblotting of purified Nucleocapsid fragments. A. Full-length (N_Full1-419); B. N-terminal domain (N_NTD47-177); C. C-terminal domain (N_CTD210-419); D. Precision Plus Protein Kaleidoscope Standards (Bio-Rad). Figure S2. Protein N sequence across SARS-CoV-2 variants of concern (VOC) Alpha (B.1.1.7), Beta (B.1.351), Gamma (P.1), Delta (B.1.617.2) and Omicron (B.1.1.529) compared with Wuhan (Hu) sequence as reference. Yellow squares represent most mutagenic sites. The red region represents the conservate epitope among SARS-CoV-2 lineages, which is recognized by monoclonal antibody in ag-RDT. Sequences aligned by multalin (http://multalin.toulouse.inra.fr/multalin/ accessed on 27 September 2022). Image adapted from Biorender (http://biorender.com). Figure S3. Cohort samples' characterization using RT-qPCR. [A] Samples collected from patients of the cohort of Guaranésia City were categorized according to the Cycle threshold (Ct) values detected in positive samples and arranged in a sectorized percentage graph. Samples from this cohort were selected to evaluate the performance of prototype 1, as proof of concept, and to validate prototypes 2 and 3, aiming to maintain the Cts distribution in the same or as close as possible to the Cts proportions of the original population. [B] The follow-up study samples were longitudinally grouped as 0–3 days, 4–7 days, or more than 7 days after symptoms onset, respectively, and characterized using RT-qPCR and Ag-RDT.

Author Contributions: Antigen Rapid Diagnostic Tests (Ag-RDT) development and validation: Conceptualization: F.F.C. and A.P.F.; Data curation: F.F.C., T.B.L., L.A.F.A., K.L.L., H.I.S., A.F.d.C., C.P.S. and A.P.F.; Formal analysis: F.F.C. and A.P.F.; Investigation: F.F.C., T.B.L., L.A.F.A., K.L.L., H.I.S., A.F.d.C., H.P.C. and C.P.S.; Methodology: F.F.C., T.B.L. and A.P.F.; Project administration: F.F.C. and A.P.F.; Resources: F.G.F., R.T.G., S.M.R.T., E.L.D. and A.P.F.; Validation: F.F.C.; Visualization: F.F.C. and A.P.F.; Writing—original draft: F.F.C., L.A.F.A., K.L.L. and A.P.F.; Writing—review and editing: F.F.C., T.B.L., L.A.F.A., H.I.S. and A.P.F.; Supervision: F.G.F., R.T.G., S.M.R.T. and A.P.F.; Funding acquisition: A.P.F. and R.T.G. Expression and Purification of Nucleocapsid Recombinant Proteins DTC-N, N-terminal domain and C-terminal domain: Data curation: N.S.d.C., F.F.B. and C.R.G.; Formal analysis: C.R.G.; Investigation: N.S.d.C. and F.F.B.; Methodology: N.S.d.C., F.F.B. and C.R.G.; Resources: F.G.F., R.T.G., S.M.R.T. and A.P.F.; Validation: N.S.d.C. and C.R.G.; Writing—original draft: C.R.G.; Writing—review and editing: C.R.G.; Supervision: C.R.G., F.G.F., R.T.G., S.M.R.T. and A.P.F. SARS-CoV-2 Nucleocapsid Monoclonal Antibody (mAb) production and characterization: Conceptualization: M.A.d.S., D.L. and R.M.F.P.; Data curation: M.A.d.S., D.L., V.L.V. and R.M.F.P.; Formal analysis: M.A.d.S., J.M.P., D.L., V.L.V., P.Q.C., B.d.S.M., A.M.M., W.Q., A.P.B., C.G.B. and R.M.F.P.; Investigation: M.A.d.S., J.M.P., D.L., V.L.V., P.Q.C., B.d.S.M., W.Q., A.P.B. and C.G.B.; Methodology: M.A.d.S., J.M.P., D.L., V.L.V., P.Q.C., B.d.S.M., W.Q., A.P.B., C.G.B. and R.M.F.P.; Resources: V.L.V. and R.M.F.P.; Validation: M.A.d.S., J.M.P., D.L., V.L.V., P.Q.C., B.d.S.M., W.Q., A.P.B., C.G.B. and R.M.F.P.; Visualization: M.A.d.S., J.M.P., B.d.S.M., A.M.M. and W.Q.; Writing—original draft: M.A.d.S., D.L., W.Q. and R.M.F.P.; Writing—review and editing: M.A.d.S., D.L. and R.M.F.P.; Supervision: R.M.F.P. All authors have read and agreed to the published version of the manuscript.

Funding: This study received funding from the Brazilian Ministry of Science, Technology and Innovation (MCTI) through the "Rede Virus initiative", grants FINEP 01.20.0005.00 and 01.20.0039.00, CAPES and CNPq 403549/2020-5.

Institutional Review Board Statement: The study was conducted in agreement with the Ethical Principles in Human Research, approved by the Research Ethics Committee/UFMG (CAAE: 1686320.0.0000.5149). For animal use, this study was carried out following the recommendations of Ethical Principles in Animal Research, adopted by the Brazilian Council of Animal Experimentation. The Ethical Committee for Animal Research from Butantan Institute approved the research protocol (2715140420).

Informed Consent Statement: Informed consent was obtained from all subjects involved in the study.

Data Availability Statement: Not applicable.

Acknowledgments: We thank all the patients, the Health System of the City of Guaranésia for patients' recruitment and sample transportation to the CTVACINAS lab, the Transportation Department at the Federal University of Minas Gerais (UFMG) for helping with the follow-up logistics, and the Brazilian Mail Agency (Correios do Brasil) for logistics regarding RedeVirus materials, and finally we thank the teams of CTVACINAS/UFMG, Butantan Institute and the Microbiology Department of the University of São Paulo.

Conflicts of Interest: The authors declare no conflict of interest.

References

1. WHO Coronavirus (COVID-19) Dashboard. Available online: https://covid19.who.int/ (accessed on 4 September 2023).
2. Rahman, S.; Rahman, M.M.; Miah, M.; Begum, M.N.; Sarmin, M.; Mahfuz, M.; Hossain, M.E.; Rahman, M.Z.; Chisti, M.J.; Ahmed, T. COVID-19 Reinfections among Naturally Infected and Vaccinated Individuals. *Sci. Rep.* **2022**, *12*, 1438. [CrossRef]
3. Giovanetti, M.; Fonseca, V.; Wilkinson, E.; Tegally, H.; San, E.J.; Althaus, C.L.; Xavier, J.; Nanev Slavov, S.; Viala, V.L.; Ranieri Jerônimo Lima, A. Replacement of the Gamma by the Delta Variant in Brazil: Impact of Lineage Displacement on the Ongoing Pandemic. *Virus Evol.* **2022**, *8*, veac024. [CrossRef]
4. Naveca, F.G.; Nascimento, V.; Souza, V.; Corado, A.L.; Nascimento, F.; Silva, G.; Mejía, M.C.; Brandão, M.J.; Costa, Á.; Duarte, D. Spread of Gamma (P. 1) Sub-Lineages Carrying Spike Mutations Close to the Furin Cleavage Site and Deletions in the N-Terminal Domain Drives Ongoing Transmission of SARS-CoV-2 in Amazonas, Brazil. *medRxiv* **2021**, *10*, e02366-21. [CrossRef]
5. Baral, P.; Bhattarai, N.; Hossen, M.L.; Stebliankin, V.; Gerstman, B.S.; Narasimhan, G.; Chapagain, P.P. Mutation-Induced Changes in the Receptor-Binding Interface of the SARS-CoV-2 Delta Variant B. 1.617. 2 and Implications for Immune Evasion. *Biochem. Biophys. Res. Commun.* **2021**, *574*, 14–19. [CrossRef]
6. Adamoski, D.; Baura, V.A.D.; Rodrigues, A.C.; Royer, C.A.; Aoki, M.N.; Tschá, M.K.; Bonatto, A.C.; Wassem, R.; Nogueira, M.B.; Raboni, S.M. SARS-CoV-2 Delta and Omicron Variants Surge in Curitiba, Southern Brazil, and Its Impact on Overall COVID-19 Lethality. *Viruses* **2022**, *14*, 809. [CrossRef] [PubMed]
7. World Health Organization. *Antigen-Detection in the Diagnosis of SARS-CoV-2 Infection: Interim Guidance, 6 October 2021*; World Health Organization: Geneva, Switzerland, 2021.
8. Ricks, S.; Kendall, E.A.; Dowdy, D.W.; Sacks, J.A.; Schumacher, S.G.; Arinaminpathy, N. Quantifying the Potential Value of Antigen-Detection Rapid Diagnostic Tests for COVID-19: A Modelling Analysis. *BMC Med.* **2021**, *19*, 75. [CrossRef]
9. Peacock, W.F.; Soto-Ruiz, K.M.; House, S.L.; Cannon, C.M.; Headden, G.; Tiffany, B.; Motov, S.; Merchant-Borna, K.; Chang, A.M.; Pearson, C. Utility of COVID-19 Antigen Testing in the Emergency Department. *J. Am. Coll. Emerg. Physicians Open* **2022**, *3*, e12605. [CrossRef]
10. Kim, J.; Sung, H.; Lee, H.; Kim, J.-S.; Shin, S.; Jeong, S.; Choi, M.; Lee, H.-J. Development Committee and Clinical Evidence Research Team in National Evidence-Based Healthcare Collaborating Agency. Clinical Performance of Rapid and Point-of-Care Antigen Tests for SARS-CoV-2 Variants of Concern: A Living Systematic Review and Meta-Analysis. *Viruses* **2022**, *14*, 1479. [CrossRef]
11. Woo, P.C.; Lau, S.K.; Tsoi, H.; Chan, K.; Wong, B.H.; Che, X.; Tam, V.K.; Tam, S.C.; Cheng, V.C.; Hung, I.F. Relative Rates of Non-Pneumonic SARS Coronavirus Infection and SARS Coronavirus Pneumonia. *Lancet* **2004**, *363*, 841–845. [CrossRef]
12. Weishampel, Z.A.; Young, J.; Fischl, M.; Fischer, R.J.; Donkor, I.O.; Riopelle, J.C.; Schulz, J.E.; Port, J.R.; Saturday, T.A.; van Doremalen, N. OraSure InteliSwab™ Rapid Antigen Test Performance with the SARS-CoV-2 Variants of Concern—Alpha, Beta, Gamma, Delta, and Omicron. *Viruses* **2022**, *14*, 543. [CrossRef]
13. Prefeitura de Guaranésia. Available online: https://www.prefguaranesia.mg.gov.br/adm2017/ (accessed on 1 September 2022).
14. Secretaria de Estado de Minas Gerais, S. Boletim Epidemiológico Coronavírus. Available online: https://coronavirus.saude.mg.gov.br/boletim (accessed on 1 September 2022).
15. Carvalho, A.F.; Rocha, R.P.; Gonçalves, A.P.; Silva, T.; Sato, H.I.; Vuitika, L.; Bagno, F.F.; Sérgio, S.A.; Figueiredo, M.M.; Martins, R.B. The Use of Denaturing Solution as Collection and Transport Media to Improve SARS-CoV-2 RNA Detection and Reduce Infection of Laboratory Personnel. *Braz. J. Microbiol.* **2021**, *52*, 531–539. [CrossRef] [PubMed]
16. Corman, V.M.; Landt, O.; Kaiser, M.; Molenkamp, R.; Meijer, A.; Chu, D.K.; Bleicker, T.; Brünink, S.; Schneider, J.; Schmidt, M.L. Detection of 2019 Novel Coronavirus (2019-NCoV) by Real-Time RT-PCR. *Eurosurveillance* **2020**, *25*, 2000045. [CrossRef]
17. Lu, X.; Wang, L.; Sakthivel, S.K.; Whitaker, B.; Murray, J.; Kamili, S.; Lynch, B.; Malapati, L.; Burke, S.A.; Harcourt, J. US CDC Real-Time Reverse Transcription PCR Panel for Detection of Severe Acute Respiratory Syndrome Coronavirus 2. *Emerg. Infect. Dis.* **2020**, *26*, 1654. [CrossRef]
18. Tyson, J.R.; James, P.; Stoddart, D.; Sparks, N.; Wickenhagen, A.; Hall, G.; Choi, J.H.; Lapointe, H.; Kamelian, K.; Smith, A.D. Improvements to the ARTIC Multiplex PCR Method for SARS-CoV-2 Genome Sequencing Using Nanopore. *BioRxiv* **2020**. [CrossRef]
19. Dorlass, E.G.; Lourenço, K.L.; Magalhaes, R.D.M.; Sato, H.; Fiorini, A.; Peixoto, R.; Coelho, H.P.; Telezynski, B.L.; Scagion, G.P.; Ometto, T. Survey of SARS-CoV-2 Genetic Diversity in Two Major Brazilian Cities Using a Fast and Affordable Sanger Sequencing Strategy. *Genomics* **2021**, *113*, 4109–4115. [CrossRef]

20. Araujo, D.B.; Machado, R.R.G.; Amgarten, D.E.; Malta, F.D.M.; de Araujo, G.G.; Monteiro, C.O.; Candido, E.D.; Soares, C.P.; de Menezes, F.G.; Pires, A.C.C.; et al. SARS-CoV-2 Isolation from the First Reported Patients in Brazil and Establishment of a Coordinated Task Network. *Mem. Inst. Oswaldo Cruz* **2020**, *115*, e200342. [CrossRef]

21. Bagno, F.F.; Sérgio, S.A.R.; Figueiredo, M.M.; Godoi, L.C.; Andrade, L.A.F.; Salazar, N.C.; Soares, C.P.; Aguiar, A.; Almeida, F.J.; da Silva, E.D.; et al. Development and validation of an enzyme-linked immunoassay kit for diagnosis and surveillance of COVID-19. *J. Clin. Virol. Plus* **2022**, *2*, 100101. [CrossRef]

22. Rocha, L.B.; Luz, D.E.; Moraes, C.T.; Caravelli, A.; Fernandes, I.; Guth, B.E.; Horton, D.S.; Piazza, R.M. Interaction between Shiga Toxin and Monoclonal Antibodies: Binding Characteristics and in Vitro Neutralizing Abilities. *Toxins* **2012**, *4*, 729–747. [CrossRef] [PubMed]

23. Rocha, L.B.; Alves, R.P.D.S.; Caetano, B.A.; Pereira, L.R.; Mitsunari, T.; Amorim, J.H.; Polatto, J.M.; Botosso, V.F.; Gallina, N.M.F.; Palacios, R. Epitope Sequences in Dengue Virus NS1 Protein Identified by Monoclonal Antibodies. *Antibodies* **2017**, *6*, 14. [CrossRef]

24. Köhler, G.; Milstein, C. Continuous Cultures of Fused Cells Secreting Antibody of Predefined Specificity. *Nature* **1975**, *256*, 495–497. [CrossRef] [PubMed]

25. Caldas, C.; Coelho, V.P.; Rigden, D.J.; Neschich, G.; Moro, A.M.; Brígido, M.M. Design and Synthesis of Germline-Based Hemi-Humanized Single-Chain Fv against the CD18 Surface Antigen. *Protein Eng.* **2000**, *13*, 353–360. [CrossRef]

26. Sanger, F.; Nicklen, S.; Coulson, A.R. DNA Sequencing with Chain-Terminating Inhibitors. *Proc. Natl. Acad. Sci. USA* **1977**, *74*, 5463–5467. [CrossRef] [PubMed]

27. Frens, G. Controlled Nucleation for the Regulation of the Particle Size in Monodisperse Gold Suspensions. *Nat. Phys. Sci.* **1973**, *241*, 20–22. [CrossRef]

28. Matejtschuk, P.; Phillips, P. Product Stability and Accelerated Degradation Studies. *Med. Anim. Cell Cult.* **2007**, 503–522.

29. Cohen, J. A Coefficient of Agreement for Nominal Scales. *Educ. Psychol. Meas.* **1960**, *20*, 37–46. [CrossRef]

30. Begum, M.N.; Jubair, M.; Nahar, K.; Rahman, S.; Talha, M.; Sarker, M.S.; Uddin, A.N.; Khaled, S.; Uddin, M.S.; Li, Z. Factors Influencing the Performance of Rapid SARS-CoV-2 Antigen Tests under Field Condition. *J. Clin. Lab. Anal.* **2022**, *36*, e24203. [CrossRef]

31. Rastawicki, W.; Gierczyński, R.; Juszczyk, G.; Mitura, K.; Henry, B.M. Evaluation of PCL Rapid Point of Care Antigen Test for Detection of SARS-CoV-2 in Nasopharyngeal Swabs. *J. Med. Virol.* **2021**, *93*, 1920–1922. [CrossRef]

32. Pérez-García, F.; Romanyk, J.; Moya Gutiérrez, H.; Labrador Ballestero, A.; Pérez Ranz, I.; González Arroyo, J.; González Ventosa, V.; Pérez-Tanoira, R.; Domingo Cruz, C.; Cuadros-González, J. Comparative Evaluation of Panbio and SD Biosensor Antigen Rapid Diagnostic Tests for COVID-19 Diagnosis. *J. Med. Virol.* **2021**, *93*, 5650–5654. [CrossRef]

33. Blairon, L.; Cupaiolo, R.; Thomas, I.; Piteüs, S.; Wilmet, A.; Beukinga, I.; Tré-Hardy, M. Efficacy Comparison of Three Rapid Antigen Tests for SARS-CoV-2 and How Viral Load Impact Their Performance. *J. Med. Virol.* **2021**, *93*, 5783–5788. [CrossRef]

34. Sood, N.; Shetgiri, R.; Rodriguez, A.; Jimenez, D.; Treminino, S.; Daflos, A.; Simon, P. Evaluation of the Abbott BinaxNOW Rapid Antigen Test for SARS-CoV-2 Infection in Children: Implications for Screening in a School Setting. *PLoS ONE* **2021**, *16*, e0249710. [CrossRef]

35. Choudhary, S.; Ishrat, A. Validation of Rapid SARS-COV-2 Antigen Detection Test as a Screening Tool for Detection of Covid-19 Infection at District Hospital in Northern India. *Asian J. Med. Sci.* **2022**, *13*, 7–10. [CrossRef]

36. Nóra, M.; Déri, D.; Veres, D.S.; Kis, Z.; Barcsay, E.; Pályi, B. Evaluating the Field Performance of Multiple SARS-Cov-2 Antigen Rapid Tests Using Nasopharyngeal Swab Samples. *PLoS ONE* **2022**, *17*, e0262399. [CrossRef] [PubMed]

37. Wegrzynska, K.; Walory, J.; Charkiewicz, R.; Lewandowska, M.A.; Wasko, I.; Kozinska, A.; Majewski, P.; Baraniak, A. Clinical Validation of GenBody COVID-19 Ag, Nasal and Nasopharyngeal Rapid Antigen Tests for Detection of SARS-CoV-2 in European Adult Population. *Biomedicines* **2023**, *11*, 493. [CrossRef]

38. SARS-CoV-2 Variants of Concern as of 24 August 2023. Available online: https://www.ecdc.europa.eu/en/covid-19/variants-concern (accessed on 25 August 2023).

39. Abavisani, M.; Rahimian, K.; Mahdavi, B.; Tokhanbigli, S.; Mollapour Siasakht, M.; Farhadi, A.; Kodori, M.; Mahmanzar, M.; Meshkat, Z. Mutations in SARS-CoV-2 Structural Proteins: A Global Analysis. *Virol. J.* **2022**, *19*, 220. [CrossRef]

40. Liotti, F.M.; Menchinelli, G.; Lalle, E.; Palucci, I.; Marchetti, S.; Colavita, F.; La Sorda, M.; Sberna, G.; Bordi, L.; Sanguinetti, M. Performance of a Novel Diagnostic Assay for Rapid SARS-CoV-2 Antigen Detection in Nasopharynx Samples. *Clin. Microbiol. Infect.* **2021**, *27*, 487–488. [CrossRef]

41. Diao, B.; Wen, K.; Zhang, J.; Chen, J.; Han, C.; Chen, Y.; Wang, S.; Deng, G.; Zhou, H.; Wu, Y. Accuracy of a Nucleocapsid Protein Antigen Rapid Test in the Diagnosis of SARS-CoV-2 Infection. *Clin. Microbiol. Infect.* **2021**, *27*, 289.e1–289.e4. [CrossRef]

42. Jackson, C.B.; Farzan, M.; Chen, B.; Choe, H. Mechanisms of SARS-CoV-2 Entry into Cells. *Nat. Rev. Mol. Cell Biol.* **2022**, *23*, 3–20. [CrossRef]

43. Deerain, J.; Druce, J.; Tran, T.; Batty, M.; Yoga, Y.; Fennell, M.; Dwyer, D.E.; Kok, J.; Williamson, D.A. Assessment of the Analytical Sensitivity of 10 Lateral Flow Devices against the SARS-CoV-2 Omicron Variant. *J. Clin. Microbiol.* **2022**, *60*, e02479-21. [CrossRef] [PubMed]

44. Rohde, J.; Himmel, W.; Hofinger, C.; Lâm, T.-T.; Schrader, H.; Wallstabe, J.; Kurzai, O.; Gágyor, I. Diagnostic Accuracy and Feasibility of a Rapid SARS-CoV-2 Antigen Test in General Practice–a Prospective Multicenter Validation and Implementation Study. *BMC Prim. Care* **2022**, *23*, 149. [CrossRef]

45. Batra, A.; Clark, J.R.; Kang, A.K.; Ali, S.; Patel, T.R.; Shlobin, N.A.; Hoffman, S.C.; Lim, P.H.; Orban, Z.S.; Visvabharathy, L. Persistent Viral RNA Shedding of SARS-CoV-2 Is Associated with Delirium Incidence and Six-Month Mortality in Hospitalized COVID-19 Patients. *GeroScience* **2022**, *44*, 1241–1254. [CrossRef]

46. Badu, K.; Oyebola, K.; Zahouli, J.Z.; Fagbamigbe, A.F.; de Souza, D.K.; Dukhi, N.; Amankwaa, E.F.; Tolba, M.F.; Sylverken, A.A.; Mosi, L. SARS-CoV-2 Viral Shedding and Transmission Dynamics: Implications of WHO COVID-19 Discharge Guidelines. *Front. Med.* **2021**, *8*, 648660. [CrossRef] [PubMed]

47. Binnicker, M.J. Can Testing Predict SARS-CoV-2 Infectivity? The Potential for Certain Methods to Be Surrogates for Replication-Competent Virus. *J. Clin. Microbiol.* **2021**, *59*, e00469-21. [CrossRef] [PubMed]

48. Ronchini, C.; Gandini, S.; Pasqualato, S.; Mazzarella, L.; Facciotti, F.; Mapelli, M.; IEO Covid Team, Frige', G.; Passerini, R.; Pase, L.; et al. Lower Probability and Shorter Duration of Infections after COVID-19 Vaccine Correlate with Anti-SARS-CoV-2 Circulating IgGs. *PLoS ONE* **2022**, *17*, e0263014. [CrossRef] [PubMed]

49. Moderbacher, C.R.; Ramirez, S.I.; Dan, J.M.; Grifoni, A.; Hastie, K.M.; Weiskopf, D.; Belanger, S.; Abbott, R.K.; Kim, C.; Choi, J. Antigen-Specific Adaptive Immunity to SARS-CoV-2 in Acute COVID-19 and Associations with Age and Disease Severity. *Cell* **2020**, *183*, 996–1012.e19. [CrossRef]

50. Kalimuddin, S.; Tham, C.Y.; Qui, M.; de Alwis, R.; Sim, J.X.; Lim, J.M.; Tan, H.-C.; Syenina, A.; Zhang, S.L.; Le Bert, N. Early T Cell and Binding Antibody Responses Are Associated with COVID-19 RNA Vaccine Efficacy Onset. *Med* **2021**, *2*, 682–688.e4. [CrossRef]

51. Mazzoni, A.; Vanni, A.; Spinicci, M.; Lamacchia, G.; Kiros, S.T.; Rocca, A.; Capone, M.; Di Lauria, N.; Salvati, L.; Carnasciali, A.; et al. SARS-CoV-2 Infection and Vaccination Trigger Long-Lived B and CD4+ T Lymphocytes with Implications for Booster Strategies. *J. Clin. Investig.* **2022**, *132*, e157990. [CrossRef]

52. Azevedo, P.O.; Hojo-Souza, N.S.; Faustino, L.P.; Fumagalli, M.J.; Hirako, I.C.; Oliveira, E.R.; Figueiredo, M.M.; Carvalho, A.F.; Doro, D.; Benevides, L. Differential Requirement of Neutralizing Antibodies and T Cells on Protective Immunity to SARS-CoV-2 Variants of Concern. *NPJ Vaccines* **2023**, *8*, 15. [CrossRef]

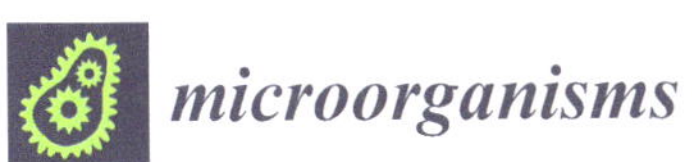

microorganisms

MDPI

Article

Utilizing Protein–Peptide Hybrid Microarray for Time-Resolved Diagnosis and Prognosis of COVID-19

Peiyan Zheng [1,†], Baolin Liao [2,†], Jiao Yang [3], Hu Cheng [3,4], Zhangkai J. Cheng [1], Huimin Huang [1], Wenting Luo [1], Yiyue Sun [3,4], Qiang Zhu [5], Yi Deng [3,4], Lan Yang [3], Yuxi Zhou [3], Wenya Wu [3,4], Shanhui Wu [1], Weiping Cai [2], Yueping Li [2], Xiaoneng Mo [2], Xinghua Tan [2], Linghua Li [2], Hongwei Ma [3,*] and Baoqing Sun [1,*]

[1] Department of Clinical Laboratory, National Center for Respiratory Medicine, National Clinical Research Center for Respiratory Disease, State Key Laboratory of Respiratory Disease, Guangzhou Institute of Respiratory Health, The First Affiliated Hospital of Guangzhou Medical University, Guangzhou 510120, China; gdmcslxx@126.com (P.Z.); jasontable@gmail.com (Z.J.C.); huanghuimin311@126.com (H.H.); xveyin@163.com (W.L.); wushanhui2020@126.com (S.W.)

[2] Guangzhou Institute of Clinical Medicine of Infectious Diseases, Guangzhou Eighth People's Hospital, Guangzhou Medical University, Guangzhou 510440, China; polinlbl@163.com (B.L.); gz8hcwp@126.com (W.C.); gz8hlypicu@126.com (Y.L.); moxiaoneng@126.com (X.M.); gz8htxh@126.com (X.T.); llheliza@126.com (L.L.)

[3] Division of Nanobiomedicine, Suzhou Institute of Nano-Tech and Nano-Bionics, Chinese Academy of Sciences, Suzhou 215123, China; jyang2018@sinano.ac.cn (J.Y.); chh22@mail.ustc.edu.cn (H.C.); ustcsyy@163.com (Y.S.); wanx@mail.ustc.edu.cn (Y.D.); yanglbio@foxmail.com (L.Y.); zyx1997@mail.ustc.edu.cn (Y.Z.); wuwenya4925@163.com (W.W.)

[4] Nano Science and Technology Institute, University of Science and Technology of China, Suzhou 215123, China

[5] State Key Laboratory of Respiratory Disease, Guangzhou Institutes of Biomedicine and Health Chinese Academy of Sciences, Guangzhou 510530, China; zhu_qiang@gibh.ac.cn

* Correspondence: hwma2008@sinano.ac.cn (H.M.); sunbaoqing@vip.163.com (B.S.)

† These authors contributed equally to this work.

Citation: Zheng, P.; Liao, B.; Yang, J.; Cheng, H.; Cheng, Z.J.; Huang, H.; Luo, W.; Sun, Y.; Zhu, Q.; Deng, Y.; et al. Utilizing Protein–Peptide Hybrid Microarray for Time-Resolved Diagnosis and Prognosis of COVID-19. *Microorganisms* **2023**, *11*, 2436. https://doi.org/10.3390/microorganisms11102436

Academic Editor: Qibin Geng

Received: 29 August 2023
Revised: 21 September 2023
Accepted: 23 September 2023
Published: 28 September 2023

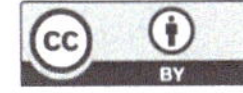

Abstract: The COVID-19 pandemic has highlighted the urgent need for accurate, rapid, and cost-effective diagnostic methods to identify and track the disease. Traditional diagnostic methods, such as PCR and serological assays, have limitations in terms of sensitivity, specificity, and timeliness. To investigate the potential of using protein–peptide hybrid microarray (PPHM) technology to track the dynamic changes of antibodies in the serum of COVID-19 patients and evaluate the prognosis of patients over time. A discovery cohort of 20 patients with COVID-19 was assembled, and PPHM technology was used to track the dynamic changes of antibodies in the serum of these patients. The results were analyzed to classify the patients into different disease severity groups, and to predict the disease progression and prognosis of the patients. PPHM technology was found to be highly effective in detecting the dynamic changes of antibodies in the serum of COVID-19 patients. Four polypeptide antibodies were found to be particularly useful for reflecting the actual status of the patient's recovery process and for accurately predicting the disease progression and prognosis of the patients. The findings of this study emphasize the multi-dimensional space of peptides to analyze the high-volume signals in the serum samples of COVID-19 patients and monitor the prognosis of patients over time. PPHM technology has the potential to be a powerful tool for tracking the dynamic changes of antibodies in the serum of COVID-19 patients and for improving the diagnosis and prognosis of the disease.

Keywords: receptor binding domain (RBD) probe; sero-IgG dynamic (IsD) events; PPHM assay; serological assays; SARS-CoV-2

1. Introduction

The sudden outbreak of SARS-CoV-2 has been declared a public health emergency of international concern by the World Health Organization [1–4]. SARS-CoV-2 mainly infects the human lower respiratory tract (lungs) and causes various clinical symptoms such as cough, fever, fatigue, and tachypnea [5–7]. According to the different manifestations of pulmonary imaging and clinical symptoms, COVID-19 infections can be classified into four groups (mild, moderate, severe, and critical) [6]. The method of adopting specific strategies to treat patients based on the severity of their condition is currently highly efficient, and most "mild" or "moderate" patients can recover quickly [8]. However, in the case of misclassification of the severity level or insufficient medical care, moderate patients may develop severe or critical conditions, and the risk of death for critical patients increases sharply [6,9]. Thus, a time-resolved diagnosis to accurately estimate the disease status, progression, and prognosis is key to reducing mortality rates of COVID-19 patients.

Lower sensitivity for diagnosis and limited information for prognosis are two well-known shortcomings of traditional receptor-binding domain (RBD)-based serological assays [10]. Although they are mature technologies, RBD-based serological assays typically achieve a sensitivity of approximately 85% [4] owing to the so-called window periods for IgM and IgG production. Recent studies demonstrated that anti-RBD IgG sero-dynamic curves provide limited information on the prognosis, as anti-RBD IgG levels plateau within 14 days post-onset (d.p.o.) and remain at that level even when the severity of the COVID-19 case changes [11].

The humoral immune response can produce functional antibodies (e.g., neutralizing antibodies) to effectively clear the viruses and plays a pivotal role in blocking viral infections [12–14]. Previous studies on human immunodeficiency virus, influenza virus, and other viruses have reported that the differences in antibody dynamics during the viral acute infection period in the humoral immune response are linked to differential disease outcomes [15–18]. Few studies have successfully shown the differences in antibody dynamics against viral proteins in the humoral immune response among different types of COVID-19 patients. SARS-CoV-2 has an abundant number of B-cell linear epitopes [19–23], warranting further studies on the differences in antibody dynamics among different groups of COVID-19 patients from the viewpoint of B-cell linear epitopes.

Upon infection with the SARS-CoV-2 virus, the cellular microenvironment consequently undergoes an acute change [20,24,25]. Significant differences in cytokine levels (e.g., IL-6) and plasma protein levels (e.g., C-reactive protein, CRP) were reported among different groups of COVID-19 patients [26], and both indices were considered potential biomarkers for the diagnosis, progression, and prognosis of COVID-19. Therefore, the identification of biomarkers for diagnostic measures and the development of antigenic targets for vaccines are highly important. Peptide microarrays have been shown to display large numbers of putative target proteins translated into overlapping linear (and cyclic) peptides for multiplexed, high-throughput antibody analysis [9].

In this study, we aim to investigate the opportunities for harnessing B-cell linear epitopes to support COVID-19 diagnosis and prognosis using a discovery cohort and a quarantine cohort, both comprising longitudinal serum samples (i.e., sequential serum samples from a single patient). We introduce a novel diagnostic approach based on protein–peptide hybrid microarray (PPHM) high-throughput screening. This method uses multiple phases of sero-antibody dynamics to capture the changes in the antibody dynamics in serum against different polypeptide epitopes or protein antigens at high resolution. The PPHM platform was used to identify a SARS-CoV-2 epitope containing short peptides (ECSP). Our findings demonstrate that PPHM can provide earlier diagnosis and more accurate prognosis of COVID-19 compared to traditional methods. We also show that PPHM can be used to classify patients into different disease-severity groups and monitor disease progression over time. We hope that our findings will contribute to the ongoing efforts to combat the COVID-19 pandemic and provide a useful tool for clinicians and researchers working in this field.

2. Materials and Methods

2.1. Ethics Approval

This study was approved by the Medical Ethics Committee of the First Affiliated Hospital of Guangzhou Medical University (ethics approval no. gyfyy-2020-76). All study participants provided written informed consent.

2.2. Patients and Serum Sample Collection

This study included two cohorts (discovery and quarantine) and followed the experimental design shown in Figure S1A,B. The discovery cohort (Figure S1A, left) comprised 20 COVID-19 patients (patient #1 to patient #20, a total of 323 serum samples) who were confirmed to have SARS-CoV-2 infection using reverse transcript quantitative polymerase chain reaction (RT-qPCR) and were admitted or transferred to the First Affiliated Hospital of Guangzhou Medical University in February 2020. These patients were initially diagnosed with different disease severity levels based on the classification guidelines of the COVID-19 Diagnosis Program (5th edition) [27]. Respiratory swabs, sputum, and serum samples were collected at different time periods after the symptom onset. Clinical data were retrieved from the medical records of the patients. Among these patients, four with moderate COVID-19 were cured and discharged from the hospital; we labeled these four patients the "moderate-cured" group. Thirteen patients with severe/critical COVID-19 who survived and were discharged from the hospital by the time we started our study (end of June 2020) were labeled the "severe/critical-cured" group. The remaining three patients who were in critical condition and still in the intensive care unit (ICU) at the end of June 2020 owing to other comorbidities were labeled the "critical" group (Figure S1A, left). The gender distribution was different among the patient groups in the discovery cohort, with a higher proportion of males among the critical group, a finding similar to those of previous reports [28,29] (Figure S1C). There were no differences in the median age of the patient groups in the discovery cohort (Figure S1D).

Among 60 patients in the quarantine cohort (individuals who were diagnosed with COVID-19 during mandatory quarantine upon their entry to China), male patients accounted for 53.3% of the total, and their median age was 45. The majority of the patients had moderate cases of COVID-19 (33/60, 55%). The average d.p.o. for the quarantine cohort was 5.8; this cohort supplied the early-stage samples, which were lacking in the discovery cohort.

We had access to many longitudinal serum samples collected at multiple time points throughout the course of the disease for each patient (Figure S1A,E); thus, we were able to develop an informative serological screening strategy to detect the responsive antibodies against B-cell epitopes over time. As illustrated in Figure S1B, we used PPHM technology to perform the serological screening and the array that contains the probes based on whole SARS-CoV-2 proteins (i.e., containing both conformational and linear B-cell epitopes) and the peptides derived from SARS-CoV-2 proteins (i.e., containing linear B-cell epitopes). We were thus able to examine the antibody levels against both types of probes over time during the progression of the disease. Ultimately, we were able to capture informative data trends, which could not have been acquired using other strategies (e.g., solely whole-protein-based serological assays) [30,31].

2.3. Peptides and Proteins

By analyzing the amino acid sequence of the SARS-CoV-2 strain (MN908947), 20-mer peptides with an overlap of 10 aa residues, partially covering four structural proteins (S, N, M, E) of SARS-CoV-2, were chemically synthesized by GenScript (Jiangsu, China), and ultimately yielded 136 peptides. We also purchased the RBD protein (GenScript, Jiangsu, China) and N protein (VACURE Biotechnology, Sichuan, China) of SARS-CoV-2 and set them as protein probes in the experiments.

2.4. Real-Time PCR Detection of SARS-CoV-2 Infection

Nucleic acid was extracted from the samples collected via nasopharyngeal swabbing following the instructions of a commercial viral RNA extraction kit (DaAn Gene Co., Ltd. of Sun Yat-sen University, Guangzhou, China). A real-time PCR assay kit targeting SARS-CoV-2 ORF1ab and N gene regions was also purchased from DaAn Gene Co., Ltd. Initially confirmed patients or those with negative nucleic acid test results were evaluated by combining two consecutive and consistent test results, with an interval of at least 24 h between the two tests.

2.5. Fabrication of PPHM-1 Microarray

PPHM-1, with the entire panel of 136 peptides and 2 SARS-CoV-2 proteins, was fabricated as described in Figure S2A–C. Briefly, approximately 0.6 NL of each peptide (0.1 mg/ML) or protein (1 Mm) was printed onto the Ipdms substrate membrane using the non-contact printer sciFLEXARRAYER S1 (Capital Bio, Beijing, China) to form a 4 × 4 array (12 arrays with different probes produced for initial serum screening). In each array, three positive controls were printed with human IgG at a concentration of 10 μg/ML, and one negative control was printed with buffer.

2.6. Determination of Peptide Composition for PPHM-2 Microarray

Two batches of peptides were enrolled for the fabrication of PPHM-2: ① 27 peptides (from PPHM-1) that specifically interact with the initial serum samples; ② 18 peptides with low detection-signal values for IgG when screened against PPHM-1 by optimizing the following serum-screening conditions: (i) increasing the concentration of serum samples, (ii) increasing the incubation time of serum samples with the microarray, or (iii) increasing both.

The initial screening of four COVID-19 serum samples (Figure S2D) was Serum-(Patient #19)-8 d.p.o. (Serum-(Patient ID)-d.p.o.), Serum-(Patient #20)-18 d.p.o., Serum-(Patient #1)-23 d.p.o., and Serum-(Patient #19)-39 d.p.o. Fifty archived anonymous serum samples were enrolled as a negative control, which included 12 SARS-convalescent samples, 5 samples from prostatitis, 6 samples from patients who were infected with EV71, and 27 samples from healthy donors. One randomly selected serum sample from healthy donors was enrolled for initial screening (Figure S2D). The selection of the samples was based on a combination of factors designed to screen specific short peptide antibody combinations for the PPHM-2 and give representative antibody responses in SARS-CoV-2

Forty-five peptides (potential ECSPs) and two proteins (Figure S2E) were finally selected and printed in a 4 × 4 array using the same approach as that used for producing PPHM-1. The printing concentration was 0.1 mg/ML for each peptide and 1 Mm for each protein. A total of four arrays were produced for COVID-19 cohort screening.

2.7. Serum Screening against PPHM Microarrays

Serum was first diluted 100-fold (40-fold for optimized conditions) with serum-dilution buffer (1% bovine serum albumin, 1% casein, 0.5% sucrose, 0.2% polyvinylpyrrolidone, 0.5% Tween20 in 0.01 M phosphate-buffered saline, Ph 7.4). Thereafter, 100 ML of the diluted sample was added to each microarray well and incubated for 30 min (or 2 h) on a shaker (500 rpm, 37 °C); the well incubated with serum-dilution buffer only was set as an experimental control. Thereafter, the microarray was rinsed three times with washing buffer (0.01 M PBST) and incubated with 100 ML of horseradish peroxidase (HRP) conjugated goat anti-human IgG (ZSGB-BIO, Beijing, China) for another 30 min on a shaker (500 rpm, 37 °C). Human HRP-IgG was diluted 10,000-fold with peroxidase conjugate stabilizer/diluent (Thermo Scientific, Waltham, MA, USA) for experimental use. Finally, 100 ML of one-step Ultra TMB-Blotting Solution (Thermo Scientific) was used to detect the informative signal of IgGs against probes using a microarray imager (Suzhou Epitope, Suzhou, China). The data were processed using IBT software, which was also developed by Suzhou Epitope (Suzhou, China). The signal for each dot was calculated using the following equation: Signal dot = Signal readout − Signal background.

2.8. Detection of Dynamic Changes in IL-6 and CRP Tests for COVID-19 Patients

Owing to the medical treatment context for each patient, some standard clinical parameters were not tracked throughout the course of the disease. Overall, the COVID-19 patients enrolled in our study had complete clinical records of routine blood examinations and serological assays. The frequency of these examinations and assays was determined by physicians, and the results of the serological assays were associated with the data mainly covering the serum levels of cytokines (IL-2, IL-4, IL-6, IL-10, TNF-α, and IFN-γ) and CRP.

3. Results
3.1. Identification and Characterization of ECSPs for COVID-19 Diagnosis
3.1.1. Identification of ECSPs Using Protein–Peptide Hybrid Microarray

A two-level PPHM screening strategy was employed in this study [25,32,33]. In the first-level screening, 136 peptides extracted from four structural proteins of SARS-CoV-2 (Figure S2A–C and Table S2) were used to screen one negative sample and four positive samples. A heat map was generated to exclude non-responsive peptides (Figure S2D). Approximately 20% of the immunogen-derived peptides were responsive to the four positive samples (Table S3). Subsequently, 18 potential ECSPs were identified and used for the second-level screening [25]. This involved 45 peptides (potential ECSPs) and 2 proteins (N protein and RBD), comprising PPHM-2 (Figure S2E). PPHM-2 was then used to screen 323 serum samples of 20 COVID-19 patients (discovery cohort) (Table S3). Thus, IgG levels against both protein and peptide probes were monitored throughout the course of the disease to obtain the IsD curves of the peptide probes.

3.1.2. Characterization of ECSPs Using Serological Assays

At different detection time points, a positive IgG signal value (signal value $\geq$ 10) against a potential ECSP at one time point was regarded as an ECSP IsD curve. Counts for the ECSP IsD curves in the moderate-cured group were lower than those in the severe/critical-cured or critical group (Figures S2G and S3), suggesting weaker humoral immune responses. Unlike the protein IsD curves, which display simple, similar dynamic changes [34], the ECSP IsD curves intertwine in patient #1 (Figure S2F). Dissection identified six different types of ECSP IsD curves in patient #1, which provided more detailed information than the protein IsD curves (Figure S2H).

The accepted model for the IgG lifecycle, which includes three distinct stages [10] and corresponds to ① rising, ② plateau, and ③ decreasing levels of IgG production (Figure S2I), could explain the observed ECSP IsD curves. These curves reflected a single stage of IgG production, the lifecycle of IgG production, or multiple cycle combinations (Figure S2H(i–vi)).

The humoral immune system produces IgGs which recognize various antigens [35], including whole proteins and peptides, some of which recognize only whole proteins and conformational epitopes, while others recognize only peptides (e.g., internal linear epitopes, Figure S4B,C). The limited number of interacting epitopes with peptide probes in PPHM diminish compensation of IgG signals from different interacting epitopes, enabling the observation of detailed stages of the epitope-specific IgG lifecycle, i.e., the ESCP IsD curves (Figure S2H).

Analysis of the IgG signals against different ECSPs at various time points revealed different-looking curves in the same period and indicated multiple distinct wave phases. Placing three randomly selected ECSP IsD curves together (Figure S2J) demonstrated an example of a "distinct wave phase" scenario. Thus, we used the term "multiple phases of antibody sero-dynamics" (MPAD) to refer to the collections of IsD curves (both proteins and ECSPs) for each patient. MPAD was evident in the PPHM screening results of the discovery cohort (Figures S2F and S5).

3.2. Comparison of ECSP IsD Curves with RBD IsD Curves for COVID-19 Diagnosis

3.2.1. Results of PPHMCOVID-19 Assay

To compare IgG dynamics against different antigens, eight ECSPs and one protein (RBD) were selected from the PPHMCOVID-19 assay for high-efficiency COVID-19 diagnosis (referred to as PPHMCOVID-19 afterward). DMI is the sum of the assigned values of the eight peptide probes and one protein probe (RBD). We proposed four types of results according to antibody development upon SARS-CoV-2 infection:

- Type #1 is negative (DMI < 2 and anti-RBD IgG negative);
- Type #2 is positive (DMI ≥ 2 but anti-RBD IgG negative);
- Type #3 is positive (DMI ≥ 2 and anti-RBD IgG positive);
- Type #4 is negative (DMI < 2 and anti-RBD IgG positive).

3.2.2. Early Diagnosis by Type #2 Results

Among the 60 patients in the quarantine cohort, 42 were symptomatic and positive for serological assays. These were divided into three groups based on the number of types of PPHMCOVID-19 identified along their IsD curves (Figure S6A–C). Group 1 (14/40, 35%) sequentially showed type #1, type #2 and type #3 results (Figures S6A,G and 1A). This enabled earlier COVID-19 diagnosis as two or more anti-ECSP IgGs entered the seropositive period earlier than the anti-RBD IgG (first identification of type #1 results was 3–14 days post-onset, average 7.5 days; type #2 results 8–20 days post-onset, average 12.8 days; seroconversion lag between anti-ECSP IgGs and anti-RBD IgGs 3–13 days post-onset, average 5.2 days). Group 2 (17/40, 42.5%) showed type #1 results initially, followed by type #3 results (Figures S6B and 2B). Type #2 results were absent due to rapid development of anti-RBD IgGs. Group 3 (9/40, 22.5%) showed type #3 results from the first sampling point (Figures S6C and 1C). Unusually long incubation periods could explain the missing values for type #2 and type #3 results in this group.

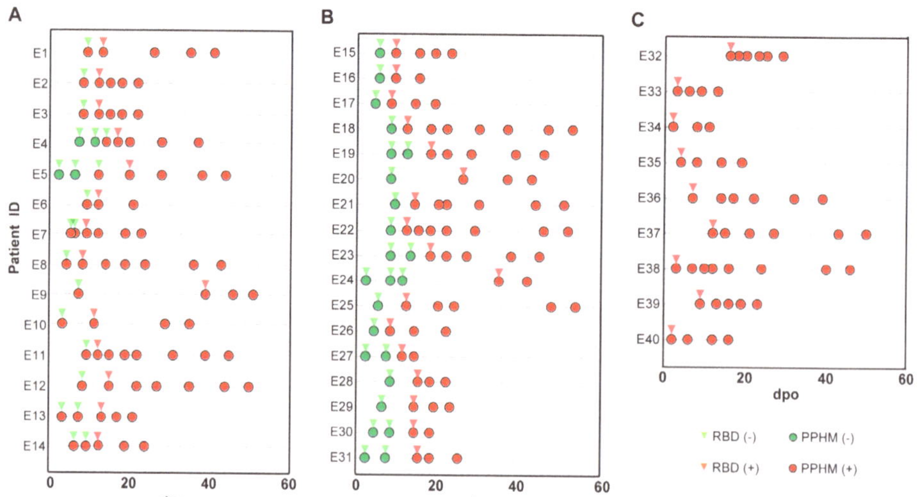

Figure 1. The representative patient information of the three groups, as well as the detection time and results of PPHM COVID−19. (**A**) A total of 14 patients of group 1 obtained an earlier diagnosis because of a situation in which two or more anti-ECSP IgGs entered the sero-positive period earlier than the anti-RBD IgG; (**B**) 17 patients were categorized into Group 2; (**C**) 9 patients were categorized into Group 3.

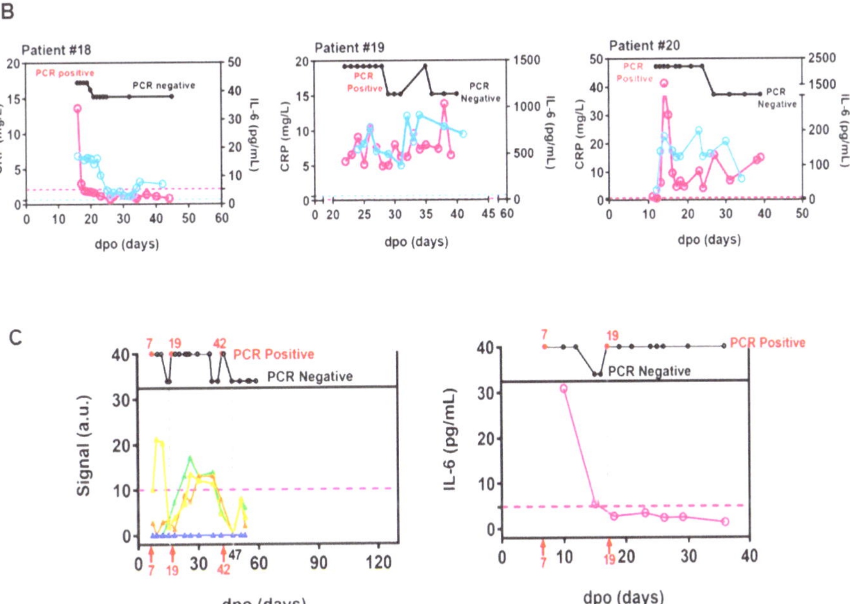

Figure 2. ECSP IsD curves outperformed infection-related biomarkers in predicting COVID-19 prognosis. (**A**) The predictive ability of ECSP IsD curves in patients with different severity levels at different periods. (**B**) The dynamic changes in both IL-6 levels (purple) and CRP levels (blue) for three COVID-19 patients from the Critical patient group. The threshold for normal levels of IL-6 and CRP are presented with dashed lines of the corresponding color. High levels of IL-6 and CRP indicate poor disease prognosis. (**C**) The ECSP IsD curves of P-N37~P-N40 (bottom) and the dynamic changes of PCR results detected at different time points (top) for Patient #4 (left). the color design used for these four ECSP IsD curves is the same as in Figure 3D, and the threshold for a valid IgG signal is presented as a dashed line. The dynamic changes in the IL-6 level for Patient #4 (right); a normal IL-6 level is presented as a dashed line.

The combination of multiple IsD curves enabled excellent diagnostic performance. Different patients had different anti-ECSP IgG-positive combinations, enabling early diagnosis by type #2 results (Figure S6). Although type #4 result was not obtained due to the limited observation period, some ECSP IsD curves showed a trend of decline (Figure S6E,F). One subgroup of COVID-19 patients showed unusually early sero-reversion, with a frequency of 5% in the discovery and validation cohorts.

3.2.3. PPHMCOVID-19 Compared to PCR and RBD-Based Serological Assays

Out of the 60 patients in quarantine, 42 were symptomatic and 18 asymptomatic COVID-19 patients. Among the 42 symptomatic patients, 28 had multiple positive PCR results (Figure S6A). Of these 28, 11 (39.3%) had PCR, PPHMCOVID-19, and RBD-based serological assays sequentially indicating positive results. For example, patient #E5 had seven paired PCR and serum samples 1–44 days post-onset (d.p.o.); three were positive, while the subsequent five negatives were due to viral clearance by 12 d.p.o. Their PPHMCOVID-19 and RBD-based assays had positive results at 12 and 20 d.p.o., respectively, closing the "blind zone" (Figure S6G). We plotted the d.p.o.s of the first positive results of these three assays (Figure S6H). PCR, PPHMCOVID-19, and RBD-based serological assays had positive results 1–7 (median 4), 3–14 (median 7), and 8–20 d.p.o. (median 12), respectively. Of the 14 patients with one positive PCR result (Figure S6I), only three (21.4%) had positive PCR, PPHMCOVID-19, and RBD-based serological assays. Of the 18 asymptomatic patients, only one (patient #E44; Figure S6J) had sequential positive results from all three tests. Nine asymptomatic patients had positive PPHMCOVID-19 and RBD-based serological assay results (50%; median 8 d.p.h.), the other nine negative results. Overall, 25 (41.7%) patients had negative PCR from the first day of hospitalization. PPHMCOVID-19 fills the "blind zone" between PCR and RBD-based tests and offers additional clinically actionable information.

3.2.4. ECSP IsD Curves Revealing Differential IgG Dynamics in Humoral Immune Responses among Patient Groups

To assess whether ECSP IsD curves can be used for prognosis, we performed a high-throughput analysis of the whole MPAD data of the discovery cohort. We identified an area where the ECSPs exhibited moderate response rates (~50%) to all serum samples but an extremely low response rate to samples from a certain patient group (Figure 3A, in the yellow box). Except for P-N25, other ECSPs (P-N37–P-N40) revealed varying response rates among the three patient groups (Figure 3B), implying differences in IsD against them.

We then determined the IgG signals against ECSPs (P-N37–P-N40) at various time points, resulting in ECSP IsD curves for each patient group (Figure 3C). These curves showed distinct patterns for different patient groups, suggesting differential humoral immune responses (Figure 3C,D). Protein IsD curves among the three groups showed similar trends with almost equivalent IgG levels throughout the disease progression [34,36].

ECSP IsD curves of P-N37–P-N40 were mostly consistent with the patterns depicted in earlier analyses (Figure S2H). The only exception here was type ii, which was present in the IsD curves of the N protein (Figure 3C). The ECSP IsD curves of the moderate-cured patients showed a simple curve pattern (Figure S2H(iv,v)) four or eight weeks after the symptom onset, reflecting a "short-term" lifecycle of IgG production (Figure 3C,D). The P-N37–P-N40 ECSP IsD curves among the severe/critical-cured patients indicated a long-lasting humoral immune response stronger than that of the moderate-cured patients (Figure 3C).

The ECSP IsD curve patterns of the critical patients were different from the other groups, with varying signals for P-N38 (Figure 3C). This detected response among the critical patients can be used as an indicator of poor prognosis.

ECSP IsD curves of P-N37–P-N40 enable time-resolved monitoring of humoral immune responses of COVID-19 patients with distinct disease statuses. The dynamics of IgG production vary in the early stage of the disease (within four to eight weeks of symptom onset). Further divergence in the IgG dynamics is evident after eight weeks between the severe/critical-cured and critical patient groups. These results suggest that ECSP IsD curves of P-N37–P-N40 can be used to monitor severity, diagnose disease progression, and assess prognosis.

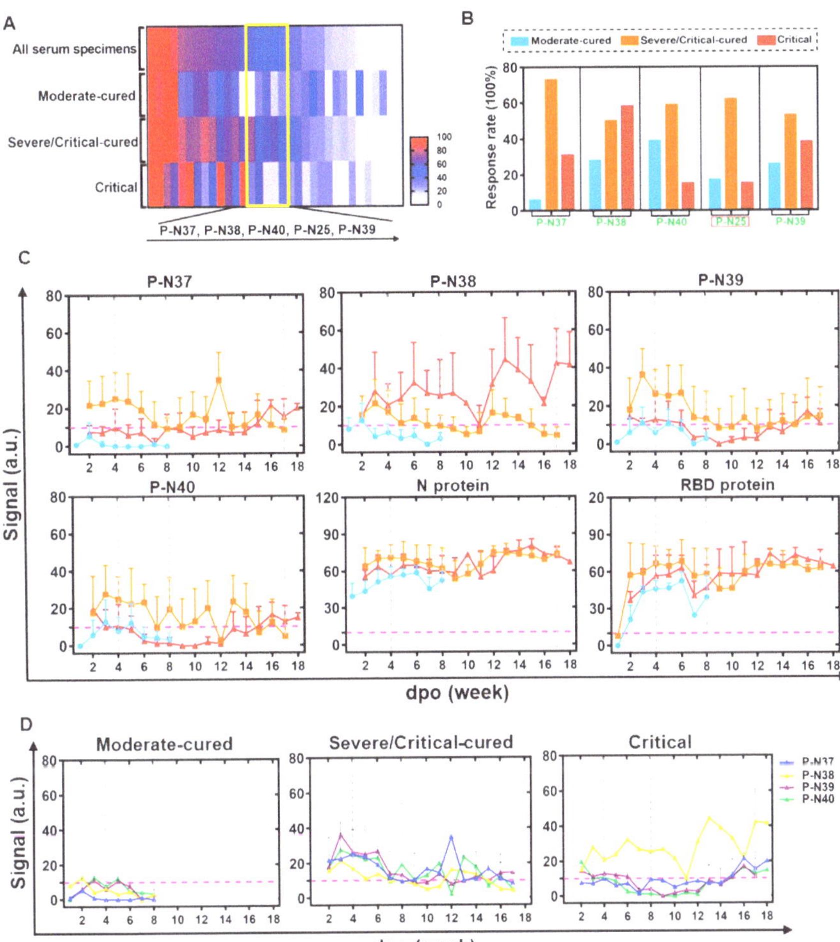

Figure 3. ECSP IsD curves reveal differential IgG dynamics in humoral immune responses among three patient groups. (**A**) A heat map was produced according to the response rates for ECSPs among the three indicated patient groups, based on PPHM-2 screening within the discovery cohort. The yellow box indicates ECSPs which yield moderate response rates (~50%) among patients generally, but which exhibit a low response rate among a single patient group. The ECSPs from the yellow box are detailed at the bottom of the panel. (**B**) Calculation of the response rate for the identified ECSPs in each patient group. (**C**) The IsD curves detected using P-N37~P-N30, N protein, and RBD probes in each of the three patient groups. Data for each time point are shown as the mean + SEM (the average of data for at least three samples). The differential IsD curve patterns were observed in different patient groups during different stages of disease course (defined with the dashed grey line). The color design for the ECSP IsD curves for the patient groups is the same as in Figure 3B. (**D**) The overlaps of ECSP IsD curves of P-N37~P-N40 in the three patient groups. The characteristics of the ECSP IsD curve of P-N38 in the Critical patient group can be used as an index to indicate poor prognosis.

3.3. Automatic Severity Classification Based on PPHM Data

Twenty patients were classified into three groups based on their ECSP IsD curves of P-N37–P-N40, which were examined at 0–30, 30–60, and 60–120 d.p.o. (Figure S7). The terms 'declining' and 'rising' refer to synchronous changes in IgG signals, while 'irregular' denotes asynchronous fluctuations. The classification outcome supports the inference that ECSP IsD curves are suitable for predicting COVID-19 prognosis and identifying patients with comorbidities, such as serious inflammatory responses. When combined with PCR testing, ECSP IsD curves improve the time-resolved diagnosis of the disease.

We developed a software program for the automatic processing of PPHM data from longitudinal sera to help clinicians determine disease severity and prognosis. The response trends are automatically determined as declining, oscillating, or persistent. Patients with at least 50% declining response in the first cycle and 100% declining response in the second were classified as "moderate-cured". Those with 100% persistent or oscillating responses in the third cycle were considered "severe/critical". Of the discovery cohort of 20 patients, 19 (95%) had their cured status correctly predicted.

3.4. ECSP IsD Curves for Predicting COVID-19 Prognosis

Infection-related biomarkers such as IL-6 and CRP are widely used to predict disease progression and prognosis. However, they are known to be sensitive to antibiotics and drugs that are commonly used to treat inflammatory responses, which are frequent comorbidities with infectious diseases [5,37–39]. On the other hand, antibody production levels are less influenced by antibiotics [40].

We investigated whether ECSP IsD curves of P-N37–P-N40 provide more clinically accurate and actionable information than IL-6 and CRP as biomarkers for prognosis. Recent studies have indicated that IL-6 and CRP can be used to assess COVID-19 disease progression and prognosis [26]. Generally, a return of IL-6 or CRP to normal levels indicates a good prognosis (Figures S7 and 1B). However, irregularities in the P-N37–P-N40 IsD curves can indicate a patient with comorbidities such as serious inflammatory responses (Figure S8). It is evident that the first two patients in Section A show a clear decline in antibody levels before day 60 (D60). However, a similar trend is observed for patient #7 in Group B. Additionally, when examining the kinetics for patient #3 in Group A, there is a modest yet significant increase in antibody levels at D90, a pattern also observed for patient #12 in Group B.

The data of patient #4 revealed the potential for PPHM COVID-19 data to be more informative than IL-6 or CRP data. This patient was placed in the moderate-cured patient group, and test results indicated viral presence at 7–17 d.p.o./19–42 d.p.o. and viral clearance at 17–19 d.p.o./after 47 d.p.o. (Figure 2C). Two distinct P-N37–P-N40 IsD curves reflected the virus status change. Anti-ECSP IgG production after 19 d.p.o. was characteristic of critical patient group patterns (Figure 3D). This oscillating biomarker data explained the patient's initial misclassification as a critical patient, and also captured the viral clearance process that IL-6 trends may have missed (Figure 2C). These results suggest caution should be taken when using IL-6 levels as biomarkers for COVID-19 treatment.

3.5. Differentiating COVID-19 Severity Levels through ECSP IsD Curves

Three checking cycles for PMI model were defined as "0–30 dpo" (first checking cycle), "30–60 dpo" (second checking cycle), and "60–120 dpo" (third checking cycle), respectively (Figure 4). The disease severities of the confirmed COVID-19 patients can be initially distinguished according to the ECSP IsD curves of P-N37~P-N40 during the first checking cycle. The patients with P-N37~P-N40 IsD curves similar to Image ① can be confidently diagnosed as moderate patients who should recover soon with standard treatments; these patients will not require further assessment in the second or third checking cycles. In contrast, patients with P-N37~P-N40 IsD curves similar to Image ② or ③ should be understood as severe or critical patients; these patients will require further assessment during the second checking cycle. If, during the second checking cycle, the ECSP IsDs appear similar to Image ④, these patients are recovering well and will likely become moderate patients. One of two alternatives at this point is patients with ECSP IsD curves that appear similar to Image ⑤; such patients should be given continuous examination throughout the third checking cycle, and if their ECSP IsD curves (or at least three ECSP IsD curves) appear similar to Image ⑤/⑦ during the third checking cycle, such patients are recovering from the disease with a curable outcome. The second alternative is when the second checking cycle ECSP IsD curves appear similar to Image ⑥; these critical patients show irregular anti-(P-N37~P-N40) IgG production that may reflect serious comorbidities (inflammatory responses), and they should be treated with intensive care as soon as possible. Such patients may have third checking cycle ECSP IsD curves that appear similar to Image ⑧, which indicates a very poor prognosis.

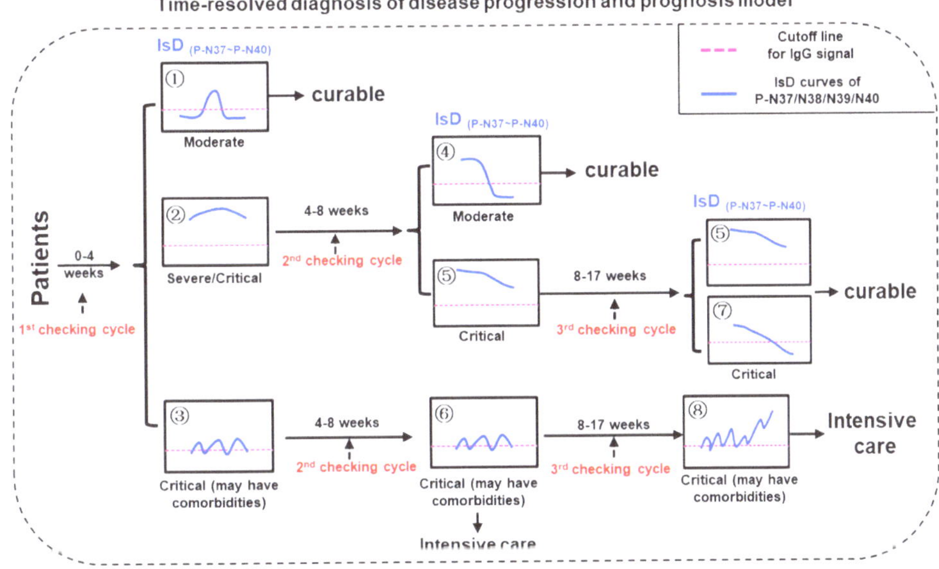

Figure 4. The model for time-resolved diagnosis of COVID-19 disease progression and prognosis (PPHM-MPAD-IsD "PMI" model).

4. Discussion

For traditional whole-protein-based serological assays, the detection of an antibody in a single serum sample may reflect either a previous infection/vaccination or an ongoing infection. To overcome this ambiguity, the currently promulgated practice guideline to confirm an ongoing infection is to require evidence for either (i) a seroconversion or (ii) a greater than fourfold increase in the "specific" IgG level. Our analysis of IsD curves emphasized that meeting these two requirements is exceedingly difficult in practice [10].

We previously conducted a PPHM-based study, which detected a short-lived characteristic for anti-ECSP IgGs in peste des petits ruminants virus (PPRV) vaccination [25]. We successfully used this feature to differentiate between infected and vaccinated animals for a live attenuated PPR vaccine. Specifically, by 40 days post-vaccination (d.p.v.), anti-ECSP IgGs were no longer detectable, and the detection of anti-(F protein) IgGs indicated the effectiveness of the vaccine. If anti-ECSP IgGs were detected after 40 d.p.v.—regardless of the level of anti-(F protein) IgGs—then we could infer that PPRV infection must have occurred. In the present study, we found the same short-lived characteristic for anti-ECSP IgGs in SARS-CoV-2 infection, and hypothesized that a positive anti-ECSP IgG signal from PPHMCOVID-19 can confirm ongoing infection based on a single serum sample.

Our analyses of longitudinal serum samples from the two cohorts supported the following conclusions: (1) anti-ECSP IgGs are short-lived relative to anti-RBD IgGs; (2) ECSP IsD curves from PPHM data support an earlier diagnosis than traditional whole-protein based serological assays; and (3) PPHMCOVID-19 can cover the blind zone of COVID-19 diagnosis created by PCR- and RBD-based chemiluminescent immunoassay (CLIA) assays.

The practical utility of these conclusions is evident considering that latitudinal serum samples are typically the only available samples in common clinical practice. In the study conducted in parallel using a large latitudinal sera cohort, PPHMCOVID-19 was applied to latitudinal serum samples and achieved earlier diagnosis and higher sensitivity than traditional whole-protein-based serological assays. Thus, the longitudinal serum analysis suggests that some anti-ECSP IgGs have earlier seroconversion than anti-RBD IgG, and thus PPHM has the capacity for an earlier diagnosis than traditional whole-protein-based serological assays.

Current strategies for predicting COVID-19 disease progression and prognosis are based on the diagnostic results obtained from a few time points at a very early stage of the disease course [26,41]. In this study, we used the information that MPAD data from PPHM testing can provide to accurately predict the disease status and progression in real time. This time-resolved diagnosis and prognosis can support improved clinical care. Continuous monitoring can prevent the misevaluation of the disease progression or final disease outcome. A cytokine storm is known to be a manifestation of the severity of virus-linked diseases, and can occur in COVID-19 patients [42,43]. Both antibiotics and hormone drugs are commonly used to manage the inflammatory responses of associated comorbidities in COVID-19 patients. Although these medications can quickly return the levels of infection-related biomarkers (e.g., IL-6 and CRP) to normal levels, patients treated with these drugs are at risk of virus recurrence (such as Patient # 4) [44–46]. The lifecycle of antibody production is less sensitive to antibiotics and hormone drugs than the monitoring of inflammatory responses [37,39]. These results indicate how IL-6 trends can be affected by the administration of antibiotics and hormonal drugs, and that caution should be exercised when using IL-6 levels as biomarkers for COVID-19 treatment. While several treatments have emerged for COVID-19, novel cell-based approaches have shown significant potential in managing the disease [47]. Accordingly, using ECSP IsD curves to monitor antibody production is more reliable and safer for prognosis and clinical applications.

The main limitation of this study is the lack of a validation group for the prognosis test. That is, the prognosis potential of P-N37–P-N40 was only explored in a small discovery cohort. Although we did assemble a training group (Figures S9 and S10), retrospective studies that included samples representing the highly informative "third checking cycle" (Figure 3) for these patients were not available due to the limited sampling duration. An ideal validation group for assessing the prognosis performance of P-N37–P-N40 would comprise data from a larger cohort that specifically includes serum samples taken during the third checking cycle.

Despite this limitation, the context of the ongoing COVID-19 pandemic supports our reporting of the potential of using P-N37–P-N40 IsD curves for prognosis. This study highlights the unique application potential of MPAD based on PPHM data and will be of interest to researchers and clinicians who work in this field. Using the data provided by MPAD, we are planning to develop an algorithm for mining neutralization- and indicator-related ECSPs, involving heuristic inputs as well as machine learning methods to accommodate the full scope of available information. Equally important are carefully planned clinical cohort studies that include systematic serological sampling across the full disease course. ECSP IgG sero dynamic (IsD) curves enable substantially earlier COVID-19 diagnosis than RBD IsD curves (e.g., 6 days earlier). We performed a retrospective study to analyze the PPHM data collected from the discovery cohort: (i) at different time points after symptom onset, (ii) in multiple individual patients, with (iii) different disease severities, and (iv) differential disease outcomes. Four ECSPs showed prognosis potential, and the severity classification of COVID-19 patients was completed using an automated software program that supports the automatic processing of PPHM data from longitudinal sera. Even if the lack of data on immunocompromised people may limit the generalizability of our results, we believe that this methodology could be adapted to study these special populations and could offer valuable insights into their antibody responses. The noteworthy implication of this study lies in its application of machine learning to accelerate the detection and classification computational processes for the large datasets generated by the microarray. Therefore, a deep collaboration with data scientists to explore how to integrate machine learning into the PPHM platform will be a direction for the future development of this technology.

5. Conclusions

In conclusion, our study demonstrates that PPHM provides a more comprehensive and high-resolution view of sero-antibody dynamics in COVID-19 patients than traditional single-protein methods. While PCR remains the diagnostic gold standard, PPHM contributes valuable supplementary data on the host's immune response. The method is particularly useful in monitoring post-infection immunity in patients at risk of reinfection, evaluating disease progression in hospitalized patients, and assessing vaccine efficacy. Our preliminary findings also indicate that the early convalescent phase (2–3 weeks post symptom onset) is the optimal time for blood-sample collection to obtain a robust antibody profile. Furthermore, the validation of our proposed prognostic algorithm in a larger cohort with longitudinal sera samples from different stages of the COVID-19 disease course is warranted to further establish its clinical utility and accuracy.

Supplementary Materials: The following supporting information can be downloaded at: https://www.mdpi.com/article/10.3390/microorganisms11102436/s1, Figure S1: Study strategy and basic information about the COVID-19 patients; Figure S2: Multiple phases of sero-antibody dynamics (MPAD) are evident in PPHM screening results; Figure S3: The counts for the ECSP IsD curves in ECAH COVID-19 patient from the discovery cohort; Figure S4: N protein blocking experiment; Figure S5: The "multiple phases of antibody sero-dynamics" (MPAD) in two representative COVID-19 patients; Figure S6: Some anti-ECSP IgGs showed earlier sero-conversion than anti-RBD IgG and some anti-ECSP IgGs are short lived compared with anti-RBD IgGs; Figure S7: The dynamic curves of CRP and IL-6 in individual patients; Figure S8: The ECSP IsD curves of P-N37~P-N40 in individual patient; Figure S9: The basic information for patients in training group; Figure S10: The ECSP IsD curves of P-N37~P-N40 in individual patient from the training group; Table S1: Demographic characteristics of the quarantine cohort; Table S2: Peptide information of PPHM-1; Table S3: Peptide information of PPHM-2 (partial peptides from PPHM-1).

Author Contributions: H.M. and B.S. conceived the study; P.Z., B.L., H.H., W.L., Q.Z., S.W., W.C., L.Y., X.M. and X.T. performed all the experiments; Y.S., Y.L., Y.D., W.W. and Y.Z. analyzed the results; J.Y., H.C., P.Z., Z.J.C., L.L. and H.M. wrote the manuscript. All authors have read and agreed to the published version of the manuscript.

Funding: This study was supported by the National Natural Science Foundation of China (82302607, 31901065); Science and Technology Innovation Committee Project of Guangzhou (202201020524); Cultivation Project of the First Affiliated Hospital of Guangzhou Medical University (ZH202105); Guangzhou Basic Research Program on People's Livelihood Science and Technology (2020020200050); Jiangsu Natural Science Foundation (BK20190230); National Natural Science Foundation of China (31901065); Guangdong Basic and Applied Basic Research Foundation (2022A1515110555, 2023A1515010932); the Emergency Key Project of Guangzhou Laboratory (EKPG21-30-2); Municipal and University (Hospital) joint funding project of Guangzhou Municipal Science and Technology Bureau (202201020250), and Emergency Grants for SARS-CoV-2 drug development (2022YFC0869400).

Institutional Review Board Statement: This study was conducted in accordance with the ethical principles with the Declaration of Helsinkiand was approved by the Medical Ethics Committee of the First Affiliated Hospital of Guangzhou Medical University (ethics approval no. gyfyy-2021-31) and Guangzhou Eighth People's Hospital (202002135). Written informed consent was obtained from all participants prior to the study in strict adherence to the ethical standards outlined in the Declaration of Helsinki.

Informed Consent Statement: Informed consent was obtained from all subjects involved in the study.

Data Availability Statement: The data that support the findings of this study are partially available in the supplementary materials of this article. The full dataset generated and/or analyzed during the current study are not publicly available due to ethical considerations, but are available from the corresponding author upon reasonable request.

Acknowledgments: We would like to extend our deepest gratitude to ZHONGNANSHAN MEDICAL FOUNDATION OF GUANGDONG PROVINCE (Grant No. ZNSA-20220009) for funding this research. We also appreciate all those who offered assistance during the research and writing process.

Conflicts of Interest: The authors declare no conflict of interest. The funders had no role in the design of the study; in the collection, analyses, or interpretation of data; in the writing of the manuscript; or in the decision to publish the results.

References

1. Wu, F.; Zhao, S.; Yu, B.; Chen, Y.M.; Wang, W.; Song, Z.G.; Hu, Y.; Tao, Z.W.; Tian, J.H.; Pei, Y.Y.; et al. A new coronavirus associated with human respiratory disease in China. *Nature* **2020**, *579*, 265–269. [CrossRef] [PubMed]

2. Zhou, P.; Yang, X.L.; Wang, X.G.; Hu, B.; Zhang, L.; Zhang, W.; Si, H.R.; Zhu, Y.; Li, B.; Huang, C.L.; et al. A pneumonia outbreak associated with a new coronavirus of probable bat origin. *Nature* **2020**, *579*, 270–273. [CrossRef] [PubMed]

3. Zhu, N.; Zhang, D.; Wang, W.; Li, X.; Yang, B.; Song, J.; Zhao, X.; Huang, B.; Shi, W.; Lu, R.; et al. A Novel Coronavirus from Patients with Pneumonia in China, 2019. *N. Engl. J. Med.* **2020**, *382*, 727–733. [CrossRef] [PubMed]

4. Gromova, O.A.; Torshin, I.Y.; Semenov, V.A.; Putilina, M.V.; Chuchalin, A.G. Direct and indirect neurological manifestations of COVID-19. *Zhurnal Nevrol. I Psikhiatrii Im. SS Korsakova* **2020**, *120*, 11–21. [CrossRef] [PubMed]

5. Chen, N.; Zhou, M.; Dong, X.; Qu, J.; Gong, F.; Han, Y.; Qiu, Y.; Wang, J.; Liu, Y.; Wei, Y.; et al. Epidemiological and clinical characteristics of 99 cases of 2019 novel coronavirus pneumonia in Wuhan, China: A descriptive study. *Lancet* **2020**, *395*, 507–513. [CrossRef]

6. Guan, W.J.; Ni, Z.Y.; Hu, Y.; Liang, W.H.; Ou, C.Q.; He, J.X.; Liu, L.; Shan, H.; Lei, C.L.; Hui, D.S.; et al. Clinical Characteristics of Coronavirus Disease 2019 in China. *N. Engl. J. Med.* **2020**, *382*, 1708–1720. [CrossRef]

7. Huang, C.; Wang, Y.; Li, X.; Ren, L.; Zhao, J.; Hu, Y.; Zhang, L.; Fan, G.; Xu, J.; Gu, X.; et al. Clinical features of patients infected with 2019 novel coronavirus in Wuhan, China. *Lancet* **2020**, *395*, 497–506. [CrossRef]

8. Liu, W.; Liu, Y.; Xu, Z.; Jiang, T.; Kang, Y.; Zhu, G.; Chen, Z. Clinical characteristics and predictors of the duration of SARS-CoV-2 viral shedding in 140 healthcare workers. *J. Intern. Med.* **2020**, *288*, 725–736. [CrossRef]

9. Serafim, R.B.; Povoa, P.; Souza-Dantas, V.; Kalil, A.C.; Salluh, J.I.F. Clinical course and outcomes of critically ill patients with COVID-19 infection: A systematic review. *Clin. Microbiol. Infect.* **2021**, *27*, 47–54. [CrossRef]

10. Long, Q.X.; Liu, B.Z.; Deng, H.J.; Wu, G.C.; Deng, K.; Chen, Y.K.; Liao, P.; Qiu, J.F.; Lin, Y.; Cai, X.F.; et al. Antibody responses to SARS-CoV-2 in patients with COVID-19. *Nat Med.* **2020**, *26*, 845–848. [CrossRef]

11. Yüce, M.; Filiztekin, E.; Özkaya, K.G. COVID-19 diagnosis—A review of current methods. *Biosens. Bioelectron.* **2021**, *172*, 112752. [CrossRef]

12. Dogan, M.; Kozhaya, L.; Placek, L.; Gunter, C.; Yigit, M.; Hardy, R.; Plassmeyer, M.; Coatney, P.; Lillard, K.; Bukhari, Z.; et al. Novel SARS-CoV-2 specific antibody and neutralization assays reveal wide range of humoral immune response during COVID-19. *medRxiv* **2020**, *4*, 129.

13. Ye, X.; Xiao, X.; Li, B.; Zhu, W.; Li, Y.; Wu, J.; Huang, X.; Jin, J.; Chen, D.; Jin, J.; et al. Low Humoral Immune Response and Ineffective Clearance of SARS-CoV-2 in a COVID-19 Patient with CLL during a 69-Day Follow-Up. *Front Oncol.* **2020**, *10*, 1272. [CrossRef]

14. Jiang, S.; Hillyer, C.; Du, L. Neutralizing Antibodies against SARS-CoV-2 and Other Human Coronaviruses. *Trends Immunol.* **2020**, *41*, 545. [CrossRef]

15. Tomaras, G.D.; Haynes, B.F. HIV-1-specific antibody responses during acute and chronic HIV-1 infection. *Curr. Opin. HIV AIDS* **2009**, *4*, 373–379. [CrossRef]

16. Cobey, S.; Hensley, S.E. Immune history and influenza virus susceptibility. *Curr Opin Virol.* **2017**, *22*, 105–111. [CrossRef]

17. Saphire, E.O.; Schendel, S.L.; Gunn, B.M.; Milligan, J.C.; Alter, G. Antibody-mediated protection against Ebola virus. *Nat. Immunol.* **2018**, *19*, 1169–1178. [CrossRef]

18. Atyeo, C.; Fischinger, S.; Zohar, T.; Slein, M.D.; Burke, J.; Loos, C.; McCulloch, D.J.; Newman, K.L.; Wolf, C.; Yu, J.; et al. Distinct Early Serological Signatures Track with SARS-CoV-2 Survival. *Immunity* **2020**, *53*, 524–532.e524. [CrossRef]

19. Wang, H.; Wu, X.; Zhang, X.; Hou, X.; Liang, T.; Wang, D.; Teng, F.; Dai, J.; Duan, H.; Guo, S.; et al. SARS-CoV-2 Proteome Microarray for Mapping COVID-19 Antibody Interactions at Amino Acid Resolution. *ACS Cent. Sci.* **2020**, *6*, 2238–2249. [CrossRef]

20. Amrun, S.N.; Lee, C.Y.; Lee, B.; Fong, S.W.; Young, B.E.; Chee, R.S.; Yeo, N.K.; Torres-Ruesta, A.; Carissimo, G.; Poh, C.M.; et al. Linear B-cell epitopes in the spike and nucleocapsid proteins as markers of SARS-CoV-2 exposure and disease severity. *EBioMedicine* **2020**, *58*, 102911. [CrossRef]

21. Li, Y.; Lai, D.Y.; Zhang, H.N.; Jiang, H.W.; Tian, X.; Ma, M.L.; Qi, H.; Meng, Q.F.; Guo, S.J.; Wu, Y. Linear epitopes of SARS-CoV-2 spike protein elicit neutralizing antibodies in COVID-19 patients. *Cell Mol. Immunol.* **2020**, *17*, 1095–1097. [CrossRef]

22. Lon, J.R.; Bai, Y.; Zhong, B.; Cai, F.; Du, H. Prediction and evolution of B cell epitopes of surface protein in SARS-CoV-2. *Virol. J.* **2020**, *17*, 165. [CrossRef]

23. Wang, D.; Mai, J.; Zhou, W.; Yu, W.; Zhan, Y.; Wang, N.; Epstein, N.D.; Yang, Y. Immunoinformatic Analysis of T- and B-Cell Epitopes for SARS-CoV-2 Vaccine Design. *Vaccines* **2020**, *8*, 355. [CrossRef] [PubMed]

24. Zheng, H.-Y.; Yang, C.-X.; Zhang, N.; Wang, X.-C.; Yang, X.-P.; Dong, X.-Q.; Zheng, Y.-T. Elevated exhaustion levels and reduced functional diversity of T cells in peripheral blood may predict severe progression in COVID-19 patients. *Cell. Mol. Immunol.* **2020**, *17*, 541–543. [CrossRef] [PubMed]

25. Shu, T.; Ning, W.; Wu, D.; Xu, J.; Han, Q.; Huang, M.; Zou, X.; Yang, Q.; Yuan, Y.; Bie, Y.; et al. Plasma Proteomics Identify Biomarkers and Pathogenesis of COVID-19. *Immunity* **2020**, *53*, 1108–1122.e1105. [CrossRef]

26. Zhang, X.; Tan, Y.; Ling, Y.; Lu, G.; Liu, F.; Yi, Z.; Jia, X.; Wu, M.; Shi, B.; Xu, S.; et al. Viral and host factors related to the clinical outcome of COVID-19. *Nature* **2020**, *583*, 437–440. [CrossRef]

27. Tan, L.; Wang, Q.; Zhang, D.; Ding, J.; Huang, Q.; Tang, Y.Q.; Wang, Q.; Miao, H. Lymphopenia predicts disease severity of COVID-19: A descriptive and predictive study. *Signal Transduct. Target Ther.* **2020**, *5*, 33. [CrossRef]

28. Rapp, J.L.; Lieberman-Cribbin, W.; Tuminello, S.; Taioli, E. Male Sex, Severe Obesity, Older Age, and Chronic Kidney Disease Are Associated With COVID-19 Severity and Mortality in New York City. *Chest* **2020**, *159*, 112–115. [CrossRef]

29. Liang, W.; Liang, H.; Ou, L.; Chen, B.; Chen, A.; Li, C.; Li, Y.; Guan, W.; Sang, L.; Lu, J.; et al. Development and Validation of a Clinical Risk Score to Predict the Occurrence of Critical Illness in Hospitalized Patients With COVID-19. *JAMA Intern. Med.* **2020**, *180*, 1081–1089. [CrossRef]

30. Jiang, H.W.; Li, Y.; Zhang, H.N.; Wang, W.; Yang, X.; Qi, H.; Li, H.; Men, D.; Zhou, J.; Tao, S.C. SARS-CoV-2 proteome microarray for global profiling of COVID-19 specific IgG and IgM responses. *Nat Commun.* **2020**, *11*, 3581. [CrossRef]

31. Jääskeläinen, A.J.; Kuivanen, S.; Kekäläinen, E.; Ahava, M.J.; Loginov, R.; Kallio-Kokko, H.; Vapalahti, O.; Jarva, H.; Kurkela, S.; Lappalainen, M. Performance of six SARS-CoV-2 immunoassays in comparison with microneutralisation. *J. Clin. Virol.* **2020**, *129*, 104512. [CrossRef] [PubMed]

32. Lu, Y.; Li, Z.; Teng, H.; Xu, H.; Qi, S.; He, J.A.; Gu, D.; Chen, Q.; Ma, H. Chimeric peptide constructs comprising linear B-cell epitopes: Application to the serodiagnosis of infectious diseases. *Sci. Rep.* **2015**, *5*, 13364. [CrossRef] [PubMed]

33. Zhang, H.; Song, Z.; Yu, H.; Zhang, X.; Xu, S.; Li, Z.; Li, J.; Xu, H.; Yuan, Z.; Ma, H.; et al. Genome-wide linear B-cell epitopes of enterovirus 71 in a hand, foot and mouth disease (HFMD) population. *J. Clin. Virol.* **2018**, *105*, 41–48. [CrossRef] [PubMed]

34. Sun, B.; Feng, Y.; Mo, X.; Zheng, P.; Wang, Q.; Li, P.; Peng, P.; Liu, X.; Chen, Z.; Huang, H.; et al. Kinetics of SARS-CoV-2 specific IgM and IgG responses in COVID-19 patients. *Emerg. Microbes Infect.* **2020**, *9*, 940–948. [CrossRef] [PubMed]

35. Raghunathan, G.; Smart, J.; Williams, J.; Almagro, J.C. Antigen-binding site anatomy and somatic mutations in antibodies that recognize different types of antigens. *J. Mol. Recognit.* **2012**, *25*, 103–113. [CrossRef] [PubMed]

36. Wang, Y.; Zhang, L.; Sang, L.; Ye, F.; Ruan, S.; Zhong, B.; Song, T.; Alshukairi, A.N.; Chen, R.; Zhang, Z.; et al. Kinetics of viral load and antibody response in relation to COVID-19 severity. *J. Clin. Investig.* **2020**, *130*, 5235–5244. [CrossRef]

37. Solinas, C.; Perra, L.; Aiello, M.; Migliori, E.; Petrosillo, N. A critical evaluation of glucocorticoids in the management of severe COVID-19. *Cytokine Growth Factor Rev.* **2020**, *54*, 8–23. [CrossRef]

38. Miranda, C.; Silva, V.; Capita, R.; Alonso-Calleja, C.; Igrejas, G.; Poeta, P. Implications of antibiotics use during the COVID-19 pandemic: Present and future. *J. Antimicrob Chemother.* **2020**, *75*, 3413–3416. [CrossRef]

39. Prins, H.J.; Duijkers, R.; van der Valk, P.; Schoorl, M.; Daniels, J.M.; van der Werf, T.S.; Boersma, W.G. CRP-guided antibiotic treatment in acute exacerbations of COPD in hospital admissions. *Eur. Respir. J.* **2019**, *53*, 1802014. [CrossRef]

40. Sophie Samue, T.N.; Choi, H.A. Pharmacologic Characteristics of Corticosteroids. *J. Neurocrit. Care* **2017**, *10*, 53–59.

41. Fois, A.G.; Paliogiannis, P.; Scano, V.; Cau, S.; Babudieri, S.; Perra, R.; Ruzzittu, G.; Zinellu, E.; Pirina, P.; Carru, C.; et al. The Systemic Inflammation Index on Admission Predicts In-Hospital Mortality in COVID-19 Patients. *Molecules* **2020**, *25*, 5725. [CrossRef] [PubMed]

42. de la Rica, R.; Borges, M.; Gonzalez-Freire, M. COVID-19: In the Eye of the Cytokine Storm. *Front Immunol.* **2020**, *11*, 558898. [CrossRef] [PubMed]

43. Ragab, D.; Salah-Eldin, H.; Afify, M.; Soliman, W.; Badr, M.H. A case of COVID-19, with cytokine storm, treated by consecutive use of therapeutic plasma exchange followed by convalescent plasma transfusion: A case report. *J. Med. Virol.* **2020**, *93*, 1854–1856. [CrossRef]

44. Fauci, A.S. Mechanisms of the immunosuppressive and anti-inflammatory effects of glucocorticosteroids. *J. Immunopharmacol.* **1978**, *1*, 1–25. [CrossRef]

45. Torres, A.; Sibila, O.; Ferrer, M.; Polverino, E.; Menendez, R.; Mensa, J.; Gabarrús, A.; Sellarés, J.; Restrepo, M.I.; Anzueto, A.; et al. Effect of corticosteroids on treatment failure among hospitalized patients with severe community-acquired pneumonia and high inflammatory response: A randomized clinical trial. *JAMA* **2015**, *313*, 677–686. [CrossRef]

46. Xu, K.; Chen, Y.; Yuan, J.; Yi, P.; Ding, C.; Wu, W.; Li, Y.; Ni, Q.; Zou, R.; Li, X.; et al. Factors Associated with Prolonged Viral RNA Shedding in Patients with Coronavirus Disease 2019 (COVID-19). *Clin. Infect. Dis.* **2020**, *71*, 799–806. [CrossRef]

47. Zmievskaya, E.; Valiullina, A.; Ganeeva, I.; Petukhov, A.; Rizvanov, A.; Bulatov, E. Application of CAR-T Cell Therapy beyond Oncology: Autoimmune Diseases and Viral Infections. *Biomedicines* **2021**, *9*, 59. [CrossRef]

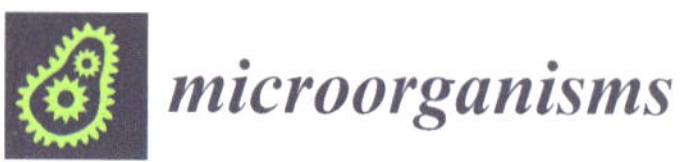 *microorganisms*

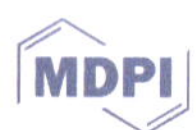

Article

Development and Validation of a Highly Sensitive Multiplex Immunoassay for SARS-CoV-2 Humoral Response Monitorization: A Study of the Antibody Response in COVID-19 Patients with Different Clinical Profiles during the First and Second Waves in Cadiz, Spain

Lucia Olvera-Collantes [1,2,†], Noelia Moares [1,†], Ricardo Fernandez-Cisnal [1,2], Juan P. Muñoz-Miranda [1,2], Pablo Gonzalez-Garcia [2], Antonio Gabucio [1], Carolina Freyre-Carrillo [3], Juan de Dios Jordan-Chaves [3], Teresa Trujillo-Soto [4], Maria P. Rodriguez-Martinez [5], Maria I. Martin-Rubio [6], Eva Escuer [7], Manuel Rodriguez-Iglesias [1,2,4], Cecilia Fernandez-Ponce [1,2,*,‡] and Francisco Garcia-Cozar [1,2,*,‡]

[1] Department of Biomedicine, Biotechnology and Public Health, School of Medicine, University of Cadiz, 11003 Cadiz, Spain; antonio.gabucio@uca.es (A.G.); manuel.rodrigueziglesias@uca.es (M.R.-I.)
[2] Institute of Biomedical Research Cadiz (INIBICA), 11009 Cadiz, Spain
[3] Microbiology Service, Puerto Real University Hospital, 11510 Puerto Real, Spain
[4] Microbiology Service, Puerta del Mar University Hospital, 11009 Cadiz, Spain
[5] La Milagrosa Health Centre, 11406 Jerez de la Frontera, Spain
[6] Jerez Costa Noroeste Health District, 11403 Jerez de la Frontera, Spain
[7] Jerez University Hospital, 11407 Jerez de la Frontera, Spain; eva.escuer.sspa@juntadeandalucia.es
* Correspondence: ceciliamatilde.fernandez@uca.es (C.F.-P.); curro.garcia@uca.es (F.G.-C.); Tel.: +34-620142777 (F.G.-C.)
† These authors contributed equally to this work.
‡ These authors contributed equally to this work.

Citation: Olvera-Collantes, L.; Moares, N.; Fernandez-Cisnal, R.; Muñoz-Miranda, J.P.; Gonzalez-Garcia, P.; Gabucio, A.; Freyre-Carrillo, C.; Jordan-Chaves, J.d.D.; Trujillo-Soto, T.; Rodriguez-Martinez, M.P.; et al. Development and Validation of a Highly Sensitive Multiplex Immunoassay for SARS-CoV-2 Humoral Response Monitorization: A Study of the Antibody Response in COVID-19 Patients with Different Clinical Profiles during the First and Second Waves in Cadiz, Spain. *Microorganisms* 2023, 11, 2997. https://doi.org/10.3390/microorganisms11122997

Academic Editor: Qibin Geng

Received: 31 October 2023
Revised: 4 December 2023
Accepted: 9 December 2023
Published: 16 December 2023

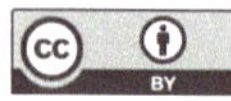

Abstract: There is still a long way ahead regarding the COVID-19 pandemic, since emerging waves remain a daunting challenge to the healthcare system. For this reason, the development of new preventive tools and therapeutic strategies to deal with the disease have been necessary, among which serological assays have played a key role in the control of COVID-19 outbreaks and vaccine development. Here, we have developed and evaluated an immunoassay capable of simultaneously detecting multiple IgG antibodies against different SARS-CoV-2 antigens through the use of Bio-Plex[TM] technology. Additionally, we have analyzed the antibody response in COVID-19 patients with different clinical profiles in Cadiz, Spain. The multiplex immunoassay presented is a high-throughput and robust immune response monitoring tool capable of concurrently detecting anti-S1, anti-NC and anti-RBD IgG antibodies in serum with a very high sensitivity (94.34–97.96%) and specificity (91.84–100%). Therefore, the immunoassay proposed herein may be a useful monitoring tool for individual humoral immunity against SARS-CoV-2, as well as for epidemiological surveillance. In addition, we show the values of antibodies against multiple SARS-CoV-2 antigens and their correlation with the different clinical profiles of unvaccinated COVID-19 patients in Cadiz, Spain, during the first and second waves of the pandemic.

Keywords: SARS-CoV-2; COVID-19; antibody response; IgG antibodies; multiplex immunoassay; monitoring tool

1. Introduction

During the coronavirus disease 2019 (COVID-19) pandemic, caused by severe acute respiratory syndrome coronavirus 2 (SARS-CoV-2), the need for the development of rapid, specific and sensitive detection methods was apparent, being essential for the establishment of an effective prevention and treatment protocol, as well as for the epidemiological monitoring of the disease [1–7].

SARS-CoV-2 is a virus with a single-stranded, positive-sense RNA genome (+ss-RNA) [8]. It consists primarily of four structural proteins: the spike (S) glycoprotein, envelope (E) protein, membrane (M) glycoprotein and nucleocapsid (NC) phosphoprotein [9]. The SARS-CoV-2 spike glycoprotein presents key mutations not found in other coronaviruses, which plays a crucial role in its high infectivity. This protein contains a receptor-binding domain (RBD) in the S1 subunit, responsible for binding to the ACE2 receptor on the surface of host cells, and subsequently allowing the fusion of the virus and cell membranes, which leads to cell infection [10–12].

Most serological tests used for monitoring immune responses against SARS-CoV-2 use one single antigen, such as the NC protein, RBD or S glycoprotein, to be recognized by antibodies present in patient sera [13–15]. As any test can lead to false positives due to sequence similarity between SARS-CoV-2 and other coronaviruses, like SARS-CoV or seasonal human coronavirus [16–18], relying on a multiantigen test may constitute a better option.

This study aims to develop and evaluate a serological multiplex assay capable of simultaneously detecting anti-S1, anti-RBD and anti-NC immunoglobulin G (IgG) antibodies in serum based on the Bio-Plex^{TM} multiplex assay platform, which is a high-throughput tool able to detect several analytes at the same time [19,20]. The immunoassay designed herein makes use of fluorescence-coded magnetic beads, functionalized with either S1, NC or RBD, placed in contact with patient sera to capture the anti-SARS-CoV-2 IgG antibodies that will be detected by means of a labeled anti-IgG antibody.

With the aim of evaluating the sensitivity, specificity and overall quality of the proposed antibody-based immune response monitoring tool for COVID-19, a receiver operating characteristic (ROC) curve analysis was carried out. Moreover, we have studied the relationship between antibody levels against multiple SARS-CoV-2 antigens and the different clinical profiles of unvaccinated COVID-19 patients in Cadiz, Spain, during the first and second waves of the pandemic.

2. Materials and Methods

2.1. Clinical Samples

Peripheral blood samples (n = 165) were obtained from unvaccinated COVID-19 patients at the Puerta del Mar University Hospital (n = 65), Puerto Real University Hospital (n = 10) and a nursing home associated with La Milagrosa Health Center in Jerez de la Frontera (n = 90) during the first and second waves of the pandemic (March to June and November to December of 2020, respectively) in Cadiz, Spain. Moreover, 40 samples obtained before 2020 (prepandemic samples) were retrieved from the Puerta del Mar University Hospital as negative controls. None of the research participants were vaccinated and no exclusion criteria were considered.

Peripheral blood samples were drawn by trained nursing staff from an intravenous cannula using an adaptor device (the BD Vacutainer Luer-Lok^{TM} access device), to which vacuum tubes with a clot-activator collection tube and separating gel were attached. Samples were then promptly centrifuged at 2500× g for 10 min (at 23 °C) in a swinging-bucket centrifuge.

2.2. Bead Functionalization

Binding between SARS-CoV-2 S1 (ACROBiosystems SARS-CoV-2 (COVID-19) S1 protein, Mouse IgG2a Fc Tag), RBD (ACROBiosystems SARS-CoV-2 (COVID-19) S protein RBD, Mouse IgG2a Fc Tag) and NC (ACROBiosystems SARS-CoV-2 (COVID-19) nucleocapsid protein, His Tag) recombinant proteins to the carboxylated bead surface was based on the methodology described in the Bio-Plex Pro^{TM} magnetic COOH Beads Amine Coupling Kit (Bio-Rad, Hercules, CA, USA) instruction manual. Magnetic COOH beads (Bio-Rad,

Hercules, CA, USA), subset #26, #36 and #34, were used to link the S1, RBD and NC, respectively. Beads were washed twice with PBS, and subsequently with Milli-Q water, then magnetically separated and resuspended in HBS-EP (Cytiva®). EDC (Pierce Biotechnology, Thermo Fisher Scientific, Waltham, MA, USA) and Sulfo-NHS (Pierce Biotechnology, Thermo Fisher Scientific, Waltham, MA, USA) reagents were then added and mixed for the activation and stabilization of the beads. Before carrying out two more washes with PBS (with a pH of 7.4), the activated beads were incubated at room temperature in the dark for 20 min. After incubation, the corresponding recombinant SARS-CoV-2 protein (S1 subunit, RBD or NC) was added at 5μM and incubated with stirring at room temperature for 2 h. After magnetic separation, the supernatant was removed and the beads were incubated with ethanolamine for 7 min to inactivate any unused NHS moiety; then, they were washed with PBS (with a pH of 7.4), followed by resuspension in a blocking buffer (PBS (with a pH of 7.4), 10%FBS, 0.02% azida) and stored at 4 °C until further use.

2.3. Multiplex Immunoassay

To perform the serological assays, we used the reagents included in the Bio-Plex Cytokine Reagent Kit (Bio-Rad Laboratories). Patient sera were placed on a 96-well plate in duplicate, then diluted 1:10 in a sample diluent buffer. Subsequently, a mixture containing the desired amount per well of the S1-functionalized beads (subset #26), RBD-functionalized beads (subset#36) and NC-functionalized beads (subset#34), diluted 1:10 in an assay buffer, was prepared and added to each well. The plate was incubated while stirring at 1100 rpm in the dark for 30 min at room temperature. After incubation, 3 washes with wash buffer were carried out. Biotinylated antihuman IgG antibody (Goat antihuman IgG (heavy chain), Antibodies-online) was added to each well and diluted 1:100 in a detection antibody buffer. Afterwards, the 96-well plate was incubated while stirring at 1100 rpm in the dark for 30 min at room temperature, followed by 3 washes with wash buffer.

Fluorescent streptavidin (streptavidin-PE, Bio-Rad Laboratories), diluted 1:100 in an assay buffer, was added to each well. Subsequently, the 96-well plate was incubated again while stirring at 1100 rpm in the dark for 30 min at room temperature, and 3 washes with wash buffer were subsequently carried out. Lastly, the plate was stirred for 30 s to dislodge the beads before detection by the Bio-Plex™ array reader (Bio-Plex 200 Luminex System, Bio-Rad Laboratories) in the Core Biomedical Research Facility from Cadiz University, thus allowing the simultaneous identification of anti-S1, anti-RBD and anti-NC IgG in the patients' samples (Figure 1).

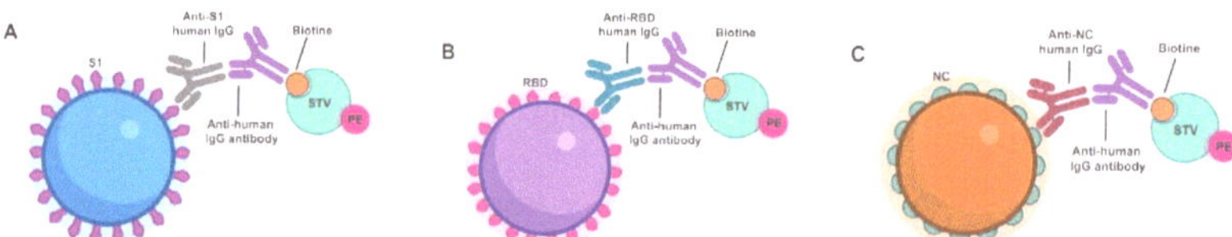

Figure 1. Schematic representation of the multiplex immunoassay developed for anti-S1, anti-RBD and anti-NC IgG antibody detection. Anti-S1 IgG (**A**), anti-RBD IgG (**B**) and/or anti-NC IgG (**C**) antibodies present in patients' sera will bind to the magnetic beads functionalized with each antigen, and were differentially color-coded. Human antibodies captured onto each bead by the corresponding antigen would be recognized by the biotinylated antihuman IgG detection antibody, that will in turn bind fluorescently labeled streptavidin (STV-PE). PE fluorescence corresponding to the amount of antibodies captured by each antigen will be assigned by electronically gating each fluorescently coded bead, thus allowing for the simultaneous detection of IgG antibodies recognizing S1, NC and RBD by the Bio-Plex™ array reader.

2.4. Statistical Analysis

The ROC curve analysis was performed with GraphPad Prism (version 9.0). A total of 98 samples were used for the ROC analysis, of which 40 were prepandemic and 58 were pandemic samples from the Puerta del Mar University Hospital. Abbot Alinity SARS-CoV-2 CLIA immunoassays for anti-NC, anti-S IgG and IgM antibodies were used as reference serological assays [21], with a combined sensitivity and specificity of nearly 100%. As no reference data for anti-RBD antibodies were available at that time, anti-S IgG CLIA data were used as a reference. The availability of CLIA and multiplex results were used as inclusion criteria for the trial.

The Matplotlib package in Python 3 was used to elaborate the scatter plots in order to study the association between anti-S1, anti-NC and anti-RBD IgG values in COVID-19 patients with multiple clinical variables (sex, age, days since a positive PCR, severity of COVID-19 disease, comorbidities and body mass index (BMI)). This package was also used to evaluate the differences in the anti-S1, anti-NC and anti-RBD IgG values between prepandemic ($n = 40$) and COVID-19 patients ($n = 165$). The SciPy package in Python 3 was also used to carry out the Mann–Whitney U test, with a significance level of 5%. Inclusion criteria for the analyses were the availability of data for each patient at the time of data collection; therefore, the number of samples varies according to the variable studied.

3. Results

3.1. Multiplex Immunoassay Detects Anti-SARS-CoV-2 S1, RBD and NC IgG Antibodies with a High Specificity and Sensitivity

In order to determine the specificity and sensitivity of the multiplex immunoassay performed on the Bio-Plex™ platform, as well as to establish the appropriate cut-off values for positivity, an ROC analysis was performed.

The empirical ROC curve analysis for the detection of anti-S1 IgG antibodies (Figure 2A) shows that the multiplex immunoassay performed is capable of detecting anti-S1 IgG antibodies with a high sensitivity (94.34%) and specificity (100%), with a calculated empirical ROC area under the curve (AUC) of 0.9849. The ROC curve analysis for the anti-RBD IgG antibody detection evidences that the immunoassay is able to detect the anti-RBD IgG antibodies with a 94.34% sensitivity and a 100% specificity (Figure 2B), with a calculated empirical ROC AUC of 0.9941. The empirical ROC curve analysis for the detection of the anti-NC IgG antibodies estimates that the multiplex assay is capable of detecting anti-NC IgG antibodies with a 97.96% sensitivity and a 91.84% specificity (Figure 2C), with a calculated empirical ROC AUC of 0.9696. Overall, the multiplex immunoassay performed through the Bio-Plex™ technology displays a very high sensitivity (94.34–97.96%) and specificity (91.84–100%), with a 95% confidence interval.

Nonetheless, in order to determine the cut-off values for the positivity of the different antibodies, the Youden index was calculated. Therefore, it has been finally determined that the cut-off values for the positivity are 25,000 mean fluorescence intensities (MFIs) for the anti-S1 IgG antibodies, 20,000 MFIs for the anti-RBD IgG antibodies and 23,000 MFIs for the anti-NC IgG antibodies (some exceptions will be discussed later).

3.2. Multiplex Immunoassay Can Discriminate between Positive and Negative Samples

To analyze the ability of the multiplex immunoassay to correctly discriminate between positive and negative samples, SARS-CoV-2 anti-S1, anti-NC and anti-RBD IgG antibodies were assayed in the prepandemic samples ($n = 40$) and COVID-19 samples ($n = 165$). As shown in Figure 3, low MFI values below the determined cut-off for positivity were recorded in all prepandemic samples with a p-value < 0.001. Higher MFI values would correlate with high values of anti-S1, anti-NC or anti-RBD IgG antibodies, and low MFI values would indicate the absence, or lower values, of IgG antibodies against SARS-CoV-2. Although the MFI values for anti-S1 and anti-RBD IgG in prepandemic samples are distinctly negative, indicating no prior exposure to the specific antigens or any cross-reactivity, when analyzing the anti-NC IgG antibodies, positive MFI values are detected in some prepandemic samples, stressing the risk of relying on single-antigen detection.

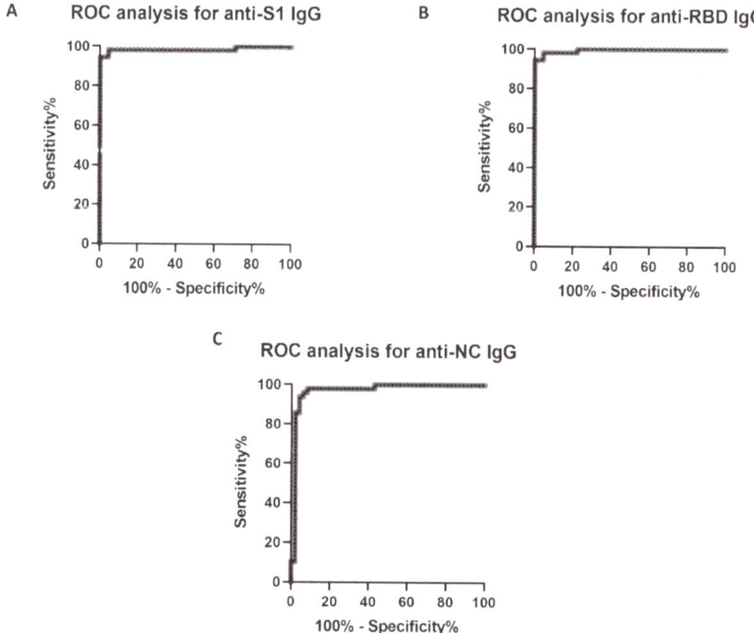

Figure 2. ROC analysis of the performed multiplex immunoassay. ROC curve representation (Black line) for the detection of anti-S1 IgG antibodies (**A**), anti-RBD IgG antibodies (**B**) and anti-NC IgG antibodies (**C**).

3.3. Comparison between Anti-S1, Anti-RBD and Anti-NC IgG Antibody Values by Different Clinical Variables

After successfully establishing our antibody detection assay, we advanced to analyzing patient samples to glean insights into the antibody response. Our goal was to correlate the antibody detection results with a range of clinical parameters, including age groups, sex, days since a positive PCR, disease severity, body mass index (BMI) and comorbidities.

The number of samples in each analysis varied depending on the data available at the time of collection. Prepandemic samples were not used for these analyses.

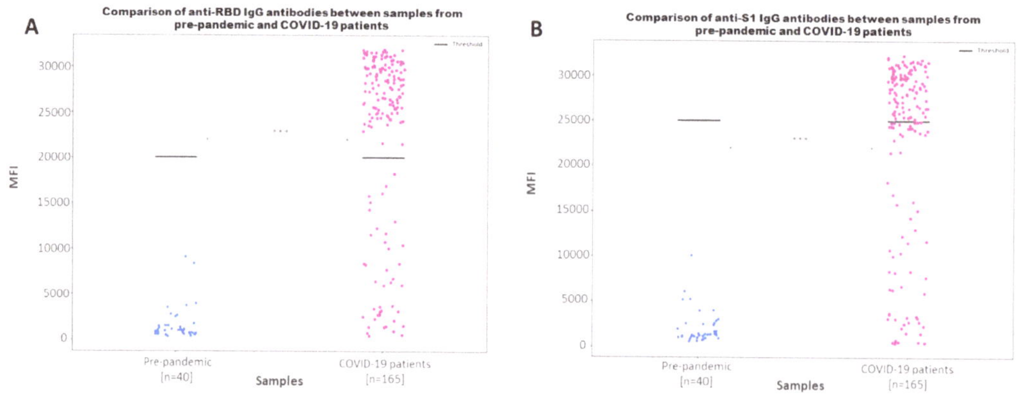

Figure 3. *Cont.*

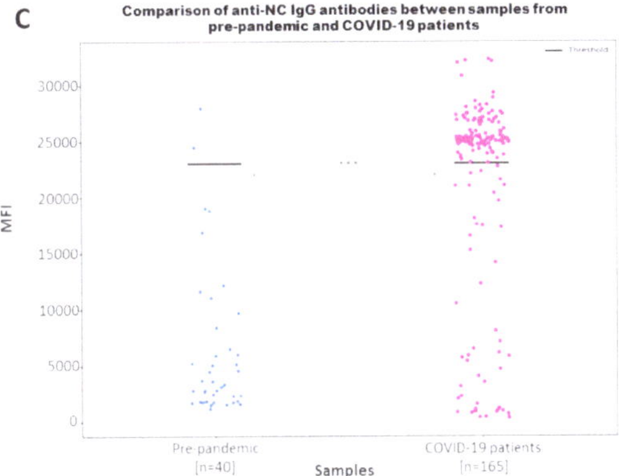

Figure 3. Comparison of antibody values between samples from prepandemic and COVID-19 patients. Scatter plot represents the MFI values for anti-RBD (**A**), anti-S1 (**B**) and anti-NC IgG (**C**). Bold lines represent the assay positivity cut-off value. The *p*-value returned from the Mann–Whitney U test carried out between both groups is shown as asterisks (***), for *p*-values ≤ 0.001.

3.3.1. Antibody Responses by Age and Sex

When comparing the anti-S1, anti-NC and anti-RBD IgG antibody values by age groups (Figure 4) and sex (Figure 5), no statistically significant differences were found (*p*-value > 0.05).

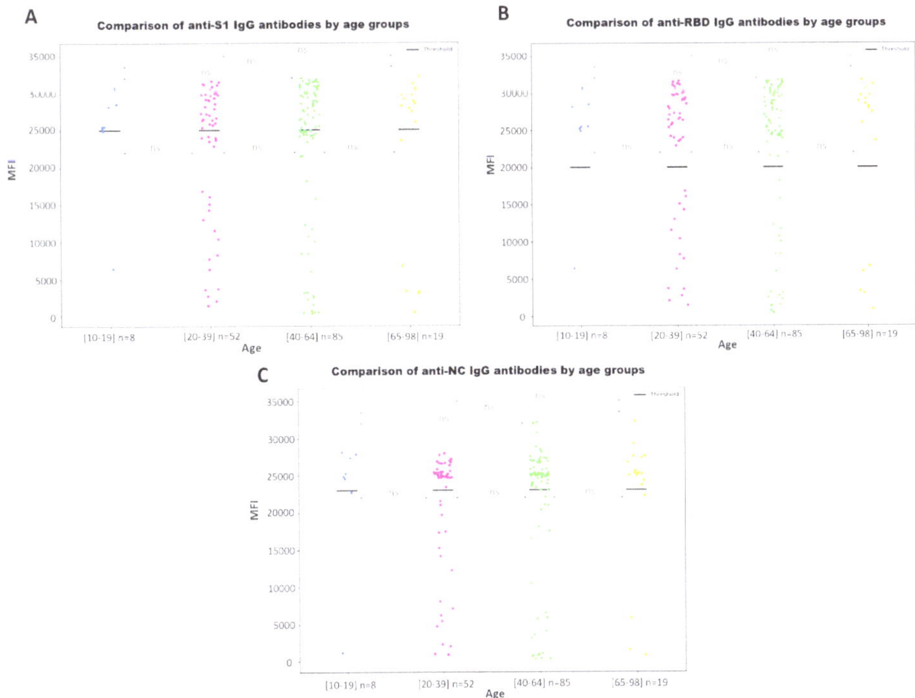

Figure 4. SARS-CoV-2 IgG antibody values by age groups. Scatter plot represents the MFI values for IgG anti-S1 (**A**), anti-RBD (**B**) and anti-NC IgG (**C**) antibodies. Bold lines represent the assay positivity cut-off. No statistically significant differences are represented with 'ns'.

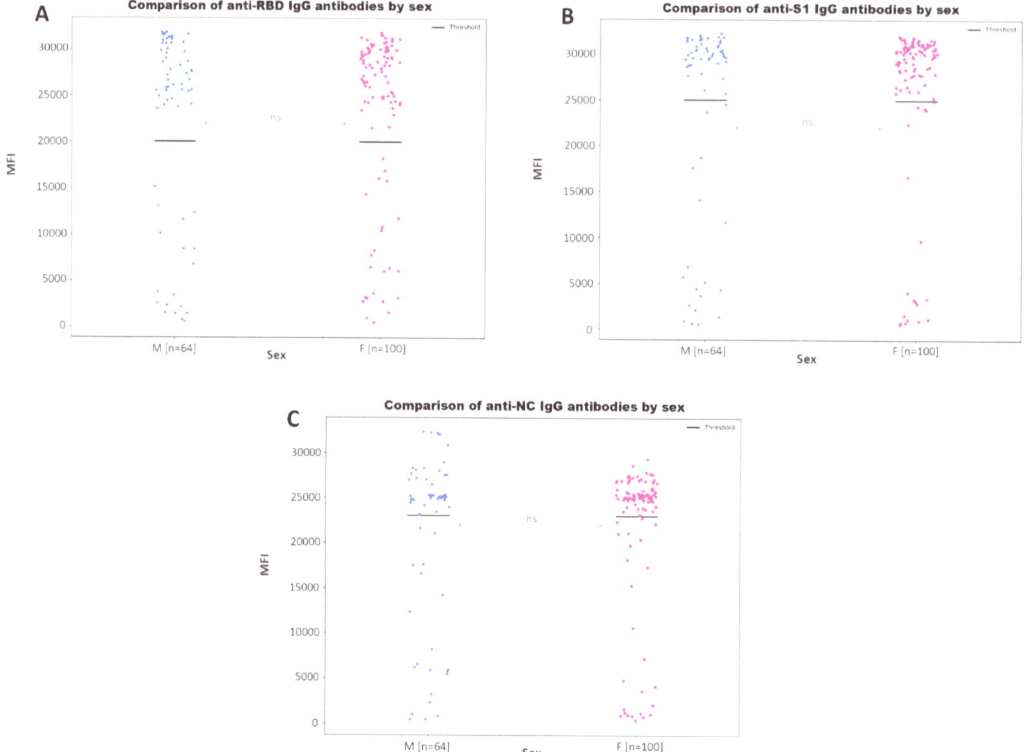

Figure 5. Scatter plot showing the IgG antibody values against SARS-CoV-2 obtained in the multiplex immunoassay according to sex. Scatter plot represents the MFI values for the detection of anti-S1 (**A**), anti-RBD (**B**) and anti-NC IgG (**C**) antibodies. Bold lines represent the assay positivity cut-off. No statistically significant differences are represented with 'ns'.

3.3.2. Antibody Responses by Days since a Positive PCR

When comparing the antibody values among the COVID-19 samples according to the days elapsed after a PCR detection, we found no significant differences for anti-RBD IgG (Figure 6A), while significant differences were found for anti-S1 IgG values (Figure 6B) between the samples drawn on days 0–30 and 91–180 after the PCR detection with those from days 181–343. For the anti-NC antibody (Figure 6C), significant differences were found among all day ranges, with the exception of values from samples obtained on days 0–30 vs. 31–90 since a positive PCR.

3.3.3. Association between Increased SARS-CoV-2 IgG Antibody Response and Disease Severity

Analysis of the relationship between antibody values and COVID-19 severity showed significant differences (p-value < 0.05) for the anti-S1 (Figure 7B) and anti-NC (Figure 7C) antibody values between asymptomatic patients and those who presented with mild, moderate or severe illness. Likewise, we found significant differences among the anti-NC IgG values from asymptomatic patients and patients with critical illness. These results suggested that asymptomatic patients produce a decreased IgG humoral response compared to those experiencing symptoms.

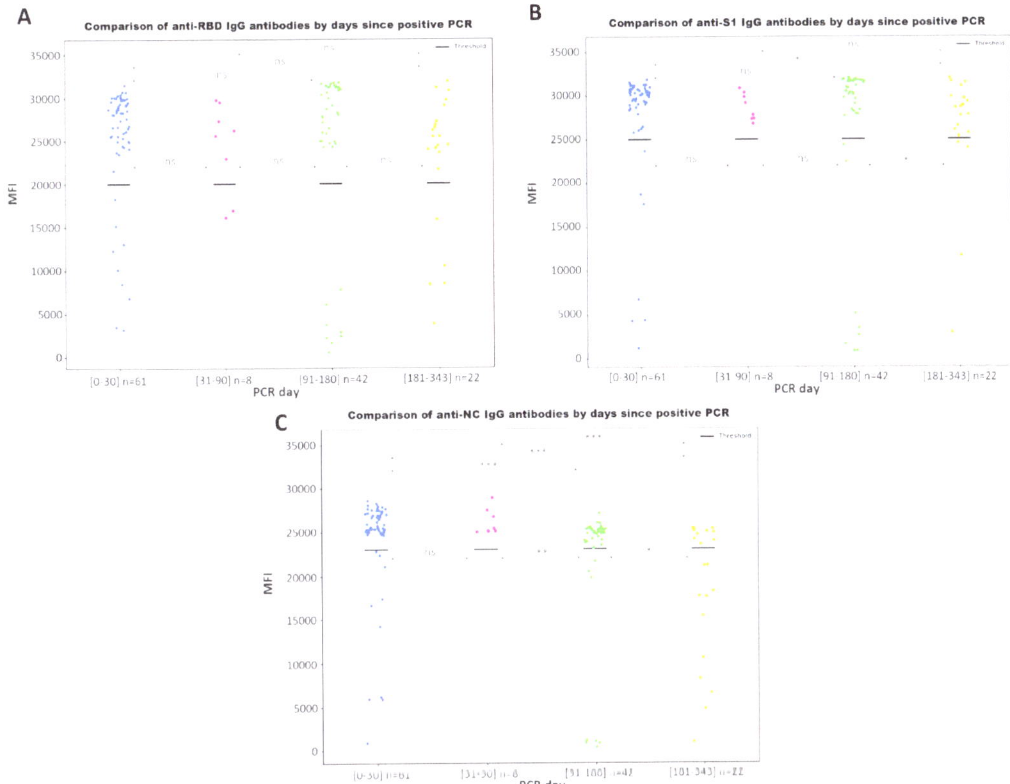

Figure 6. Dynamics of the SARS-CoV-2 antibody values according to the days since a positive PCR. Scatter plot representing the MFI values for the detection of anti-S1 (**A**), anti-RBD (**B**) and anti-NC IgG (**C**) antibodies. Bold lines represent the assay positivity cut-off. Statistical significance returned from the Mann–Whitney U test for each comparison is shown with asterisks (*), (**) or (***), for p-values ≤ 0.05, ≤ 0.01 and ≤ 0.001, respectively. No statistically significant differences are represented with 'ns'.

The classification has been made according to the severity values of respiratory infections and their definitions (SARS-CoV-2) as extracted from the Technical Document "Clinical Management of COVID-19: Hospital Care" (Ministry of Health—Government of Spain).

3.3.4. Negative Association between SARS-CoV-2 Antibody Values and Body Mass Index

Patients with a healthy weight produced a decreased anti-RBD (Figure 8A) and anti-S1 (Figure 8B) IgG humoral profile when compared to overweight and obese patients ($p \leq 0.05$). However, no statistically significant differences were found in the anti-NC antibody values (Figure 8C).

3.3.5. Antibody Responses According to Comorbidities

We additionally searched for a relationship between single comorbidities and the IgG antibody profile. Comorbidities in this study were high blood pressure (HBP), diabetes mellitus (DM), obesity, asthma and allergic rhinitis (AR). Although no statistically significant differences were found when comparing the anti-RBD (Figure 9A) and anti-S1 (Figure 9B) IgG antibody values, those who had AR exhibited a decreased anti-NC IgG humoral response against SARS-CoV-2 (Figure 9C).

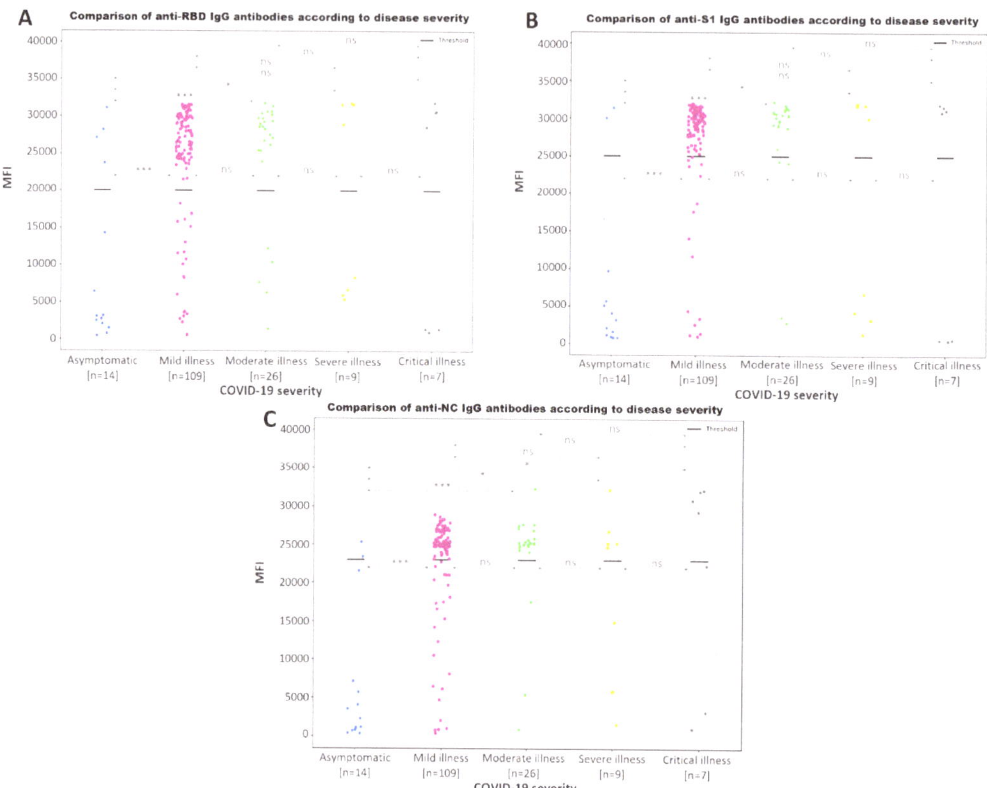

Figure 7. Comparison of the antibody values according to COVID-19 severity. Scatter plot represents the MFI values for anti-S1 (**A**), anti-RBD (**B**) and anti-NC IgG (**C**) antibodies. Bold lines represent the assay positivity cut-off. The *p*-values returned from the Mann–Whitney U test for each comparison is shown as asterisks (*) and (***), for *p*-values ≤ 0.05 and ≤ 0.001, respectively. No statistically significant differences are represented with 'ns'.

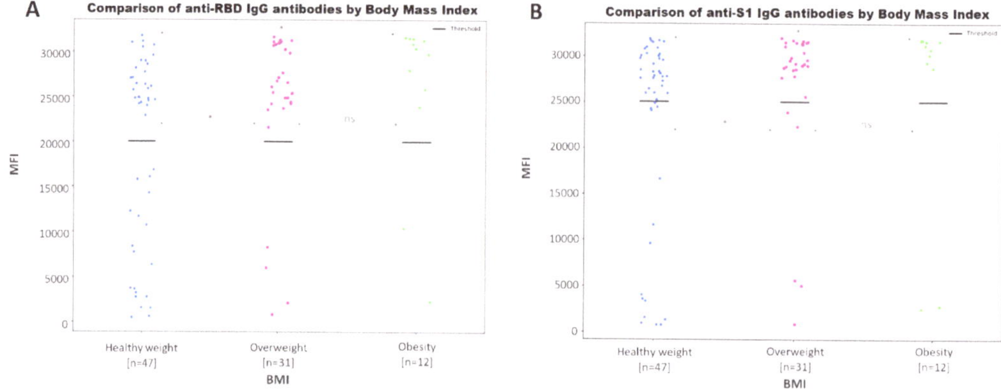

Figure 8. *Cont.*

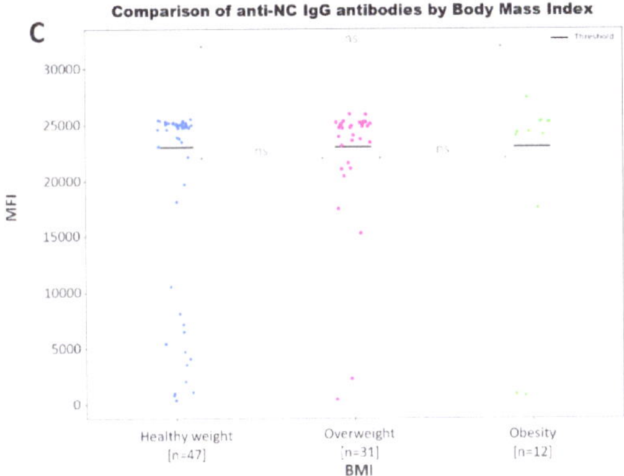

Figure 8. Comparison of different SARS-CoV-2 IgG antibody profiles by body mass index. Scatter plot represents the MFI values for anti-S1 (**A**), anti-RBD (**B**) and anti-NC IgG (**C**) antibodies. Bold lines represent the assay positivity cut-off. The *p*-values returned from the Mann–Whitney U test for each comparison is shown as asterisks (*), for *p*-values ≤ 0.05. No statistically significant differences are represented with 'ns'.

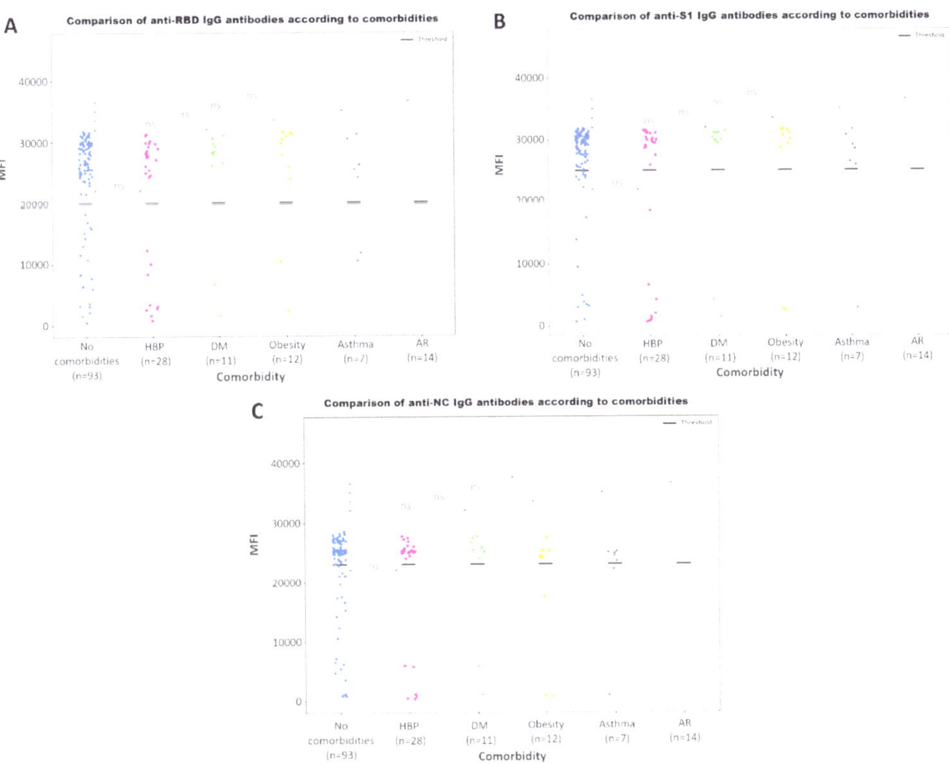

Figure 9. Comparison of antibody values according to comorbidities. Scatter plot represents the MFI values for anti-S1 (**A**), anti-RBD (**B**) and anti-NC IgG (**C**) antibodies. Bold lines represent the assay positivity cut-off. The *p*-values returned from the Mann–Whitney U test for each comparison is shown as asterisks (*), for *p*-values ≤ 0.05. No statistically significant differences are represented with 'ns'.

4. Discussion

Serology tests provide information about the epidemiology of an infection, which make them a fundamental tool for COVID-19 spread control. These tests also provide insights into the protective immunity of individuals against COVID-19 [22–24], and can be used for SARS-CoV-2 vaccine assessment and the development of new therapeutic approaches [25–30].

In order to determine the sensitivity and specificity of the multiplex immunoassay designed in this study, an ROC curve analysis was carried out. All in all, the multiplex assay performed through the Bio-Plex™ technology displayed a very high sensitivity (94.34–97.96%) and specificity (91.84–100%), with a 95% confidence interval.

Interestingly, the MFI values detected in the prepandemic samples were considerably higher for the anti-NC IgG than the anti-S1 and anti-RBD IgG (Figure 3), even exceeding the positivity cut-off values for some samples. It has already been shown that the viral nucleocapsid (N), that serves a general purpose and is not subjected to strong immunological pressure, is more conserved than the spike among coronaviruses, like those causing the common cold, to which there is a very strong exposure in the general population. A broad cross-reactivity against common cold coronaviruses has also been shown for T cell responses for the N protein [31–33]. This hypothesis is strongly supported by the study of Anderson et al. [17], since they found that antibodies against some prepandemic seasonal human coronaviruses cross-reacted with the SARS-CoV-2 spike, RBD and NC proteins (4.2%, 0.93% and 16.2% of the serum samples, respectively). They showed that, while these antibodies were boosted upon SARS-CoV-2 infection, these cross-reactive SARS-CoV-2 antibodies were not associated with immune protection. These findings further stress the rational that, in order to avoid false-positive diagnoses due to anti-NC IgG antibody cross-reactivity, it may be recommended to rely not only on the detection of anti-NC IgG, but also on the detection of IgG antibodies against multiple SARS-CoV-2 epitopes, such as those present on S1 or RBD.

Similar results have been reported from recent studies, in which multiplex immunoassays based on similar approaches were developed and SARS-CoV-2 cross reactive anti-NC IgG antibodies were also found. Interestingly, they reported that multiplex IgG antibody testing increased the specificity and sensitivity compared to single-antigen antibody detection [34–36].

We found no association between the IgG antibody values and age (Figure 4) or sex (Figure 5). Although several studies have analyzed the humoral response to SARS-CoV-2 according to these variables, results are not homogeneous and reach different conclusions [37–40].

Additionally, no substantial differences between anti-S1, anti-NC and anti-RBD IgG antibody values detected through the multiplex immunoassay were found depending on the number of days since the positive PCR test was performed (Figure 6). However, we noted that the anti-S1 IgG antibody values slightly decreased after 6 months following a positive PCR test, while the anti-NC IgG antibody values already decreased after 3 months. Several studies indicate that the concentration of the anti-SARS-CoV-2 IgG antibodies remains readily detectable and elevated for up to 3 months before gradually declining over time. However, in some cases, they can still be reliably detected up to 15 months, and may exhibit long-lasting persistence [41]. Another study reported that antibodies against SARS-CoV-2 sustained for at least 9 months [42].

When comparing the IgG values among patients with different disease severities, we found that symptomatic patients exhibited lower anti-RBD and anti-S1 IgG antibody values than those with mild, moderate or severe symptoms (Figure 7), including critical patients, when the anti-NC antibody values were studied. These results are in line with previous findings, where the correlation between the clinical profiles of individuals and the values of IgG antibodies specific to SARS-CoV-2 was found to be notably stronger in cases of severe illness [37,43–47].

In accordance with past studies [37,38,48], we detected increased anti-S1 and anti-RBD IgG antibody values in overweight or obese individuals when compared with those of normal weight (Figure 8). According to a recent report by the World Obesity Forum [49], there is a clear correlation between the prevalence of obesity in a country and the increased mortality rate associated with COVID-19, even after accounting for age and wealth factors. This suggests that, despite exhibiting strong humoral responses, individuals with higher BMI values are more susceptible to developing severe infectious diseases compared to those who have a healthy weight.

Finally, we studied whether there was an association between COVID-19 patients' comorbidities and IgG antibody values (Figure 9). Although we did not find statistically significant differences for patients with high blood pressure, diabetes mellitus, obesity or asthma, we did find significant variations in anti-NC IgG antibody values for patients affected by allergic rhinitis (AR). The study of Xu et al. [50] reported that none of the included studies reported statistically significant differences between AR and non-AR patients, but their analysis indicated that allergic rhinitis was considered a comorbidity that was associated with reduced severity and lower rates of hospitalization among COVID-19 patients, which may be explained by our findings.

Nevertheless, since this study has a limited cohort size, future studies are needed to support these findings. Moreover, a larger analysis, including information about new SARS-CoV-2 variants of concern (VOC) and vaccinated immune responses, should be performed, as we only studied the IgG response profile of patients exposed to the circulating variants of the first and second waves in Spain, which mainly included the A.2, A.5, B.1 and B.1.177 lineages [51].

All in all, these findings evidence that the Bio-Plex multiplex immunoassay proposed herein is a robust and high-throughput SARS-CoV-2 immune response monitoring tool capable of simultaneously detecting anti-S1, anti-NC and anti-RBD IgG antibodies in serum with a very high sensitivity and specificity. Moreover, the multiplex SARS-CoV-2 immunoassay that we have described offers a versatile and flexible framework that allows for the inclusion of additional antigens specific to emerging SARS-CoV-2 variants, as well as for different applications, such as for tumor, inflammatory or infectious disease immunodiagnostics and surveillance.

Author Contributions: Investigation, L.O.-C. and N.M.; Formal Analysis, L.O.-C. and N.M.; Writing—Original Draft, L.O.-C. and N.M.; Methodology, R.F.-C. and J.P.M.-M.; Validation, R.F.-C., P.G.-G. and A.G.; Data Curation, R.F.-C., P.G.-G. and A.G.; Resources and Clinical Perspective, C.F.-C., J.d.D.J.-C., T.T.-S., M.P.R.-M., M.I.M.-R., E.E. and M.R.-I.; Supervision, C.F.-P. and F.G.-C.; Funding Acquisition, C.F.-P. and F.G.-C.; Writing—Review and Editing, C.F.-P. and F.G.-C.; Project Administration, F.G.-C. All authors have read and agreed to the published version of the manuscript.

Funding: This research was funded by project grant number COV20-00173 of the 2020 Emergency Call for Research Projects about the SARS-CoV-2 virus and the COVID-19 disease of the Institute of Health "Carlos III" from the Spanish Ministry of Science and Innovation, and by project grant number PECART-0096-2020, Consejería de Salud y Familias, Junta de Andalucía, Spain.

Institutional Review Board Statement: The study was conducted in accordance with the Declaration of Helsinki and approved by the Coordinating Committee for the Ethics of Biomedical Research in Andalusia on 06/04/2020 (reference number: S2000408-REV).

Informed Consent Statement: Informed consent was obtained from all subjects involved in the study.

Data Availability Statement: Data are contained within the article.

Acknowledgments: The authors would like to thank the support received by the University of Cadiz through the Plan Propio—UCA, INICIA-INV: Initiation to Research (2022–2023) scholarship granted to Noelia Moares and the FPI UCA (2021) grant given to Lucia Olvera-Collantes. We thank the Spanish Ministry of Universities for the support through the FPU grant (FPU21/03325) to Noelia Moares. We also thank the Core Biomedical Research Facility from the University of Cadiz for the use of relevant instruments.

Conflicts of Interest: The authors declare no conflict of interest.

References

1. Peeling, R.W.; Heymann, D.L.; Teo, Y.-Y.; Garcia, P.J. Diagnostics for COVID-19: Moving from Pandemic Response to Control. *Lancet* **2022**, *399*, 757–768. [CrossRef] [PubMed]
2. Ravi, N.; Cortade, D.L.; Ng, E.; Wang, S.X. Diagnostics for SARS-CoV-2 Detection: A Comprehensive Review of the FDA-EUA COVID-19 Testing Landscape. *Biosens. Bioelectron.* **2020**, *165*, 112454. [CrossRef] [PubMed]
3. Food and Drug Administration. In Vitro Diagnostics EUAs. 2022. Available online: https://www.fda.gov/medical-devices/covid-19-emergency-use-authorizations-medical-devices/in-vitro-diagnostics-euas (accessed on 30 October 2023).
4. Mathur, G.; Mathur, S. Antibody Testing for COVID-19 Can It Be Used as a Screening Tool in Areas With Low Prevalence? *Am. J. Clin. Pathol.* **2020**, *154*, 1–3. [CrossRef] [PubMed]
5. Wiersinga, W.J.; Rhodes, A.; Cheng, A.C.; Peacock, S.J.; Prescott, H.C. Pathophysiology, Transmission, Diagnosis, and Treatment of Coronavirus Disease 2019 (COVID-19): A Review. *JAMA* **2020**, *324*, 782–793. [CrossRef] [PubMed]
6. Drain, P.K. Rapid Diagnostic Testing for SARS-CoV-2. *N. Engl. J. Med.* **2022**, *386*, 264–272. [CrossRef] [PubMed]
7. Bohn, M.K.; Lippi, G.; Horvath, A.; Sethi, S.; Koch, D.; Ferrari, M.; Wang, C.-B.; Mancini, N.; Steele, S.; Adeli, K. Molecular, Serological, and Biochemical Diagnosis and Monitoring of COVID-19: IFCC Taskforce Evaluation of the Latest Evidence. *Clin. Chem. Lab. Med.* **2020**, *58*, 1037–1052. [CrossRef] [PubMed]
8. Wrapp, D.; Wang, N.; Corbett, K.S.; Goldsmith, J.A.; Hsieh, C.-L.; Abiona, O.; Graham, B.S.; McLellan, J.S. Cryo-EM Structure of the 2019-nCoV Spike in the Prefusion Conformation. *Science* **2020**, *367*, 1260–1263. [CrossRef] [PubMed]
9. Khan, M.; Adil, S.F.; Alkhathlan, H.Z.; Tahir, M.N.; Saif, S.; Khan, M.; Khan, S.T. COVID-19: A Global Challenge with Old History, Epidemiology and Progress So Far. *Molecules* **2020**, *26*, 39. [CrossRef]
10. Chambers, J.P.; Yu, J.; Valdes, J.J.; Arulanandam, B.P. SARS-CoV-2, Early Entry Events. *J. Pathog.* **2020**, *2020*, 9238696. [CrossRef]
11. Harrison, A.G.; Lin, T.; Wang, P. Mechanisms of SARS-CoV-2 Transmission and Pathogenesis. *Trends Immunol.* **2020**, *41*, 1100–1115. [CrossRef]
12. Mehta, P.; McAuley, D.F.; Brown, M.; Sanchez, E.; Tattersall, R.S.; Manson, J.J. HLH Across Speciality Collaboration, UK COVID-19: Consider Cytokine Storm Syndromes and Immunosuppression. *Lancet* **2020**, *395*, 1033–1034. [CrossRef] [PubMed]
13. Liu, G.; Rusling, J.F. COVID-19 Antibody Tests and Their Limitations. *ACS Sens.* **2021**, *6*, 593–612. [CrossRef] [PubMed]
14. Qi, H.; Liu, B.; Wang, X.; Zhang, L. The Humoral Response and Antibodies against SARS-CoV-2 Infection. *Nat. Immunol.* **2022**, *23*, 1008–1020. [CrossRef] [PubMed]
15. Vabret, N.; Britton, G.J.; Gruber, C.; Hegde, S.; Kim, J.; Kuksin, M.; Levantovsky, R.; Malle, L.; Moreira, A.; Park, M.D.; et al. Immunology of COVID-19: Current State of the Science. *Immunity* **2020**, *52*, 910–941. [CrossRef] [PubMed]
16. Ward, S.; Lindsley, A.; Courter, J.; Assa'ad, A. Clinical Testing for COVID-19. *J. Allergy Clin. Immunol.* **2020**, *146*, 23–34. [CrossRef] [PubMed]
17. Anderson, E.M.; Goodwin, E.C.; Verma, A.; Arevalo, C.P.; Bolton, M.J.; Weirick, M.E.; Gouma, S.; McAllister, C.M.; Christensen, S.R.; Weaver, J.; et al. Seasonal Human Coronavirus Antibodies Are Boosted upon SARS-CoV-2 Infection but Not Associated with Protection. *Cell* **2021**, *184*, 1858–1864. [CrossRef] [PubMed]
18. Hu, B.; Guo, H.; Zhou, P.; Shi, Z.-L. Characteristics of SARS-CoV-2 and COVID-19. *Nat. Rev. Microbiol.* **2021**, *19*, 141–154. [CrossRef]
19. Surenaud, M.; Manier, C.; Richert, L.; Thiébaut, R.; Levy, Y.; Hue, S.; Lacabaratz, C. Optimization and Evaluation of Luminex Performance with Supernatants of Antigen-Stimulated Peripheral Blood Mononuclear Cells. *BMC Immunol.* **2016**, *17*, 44. [CrossRef]
20. Breen, E.J.; Tan, W.; Khan, A. The Statistical Value of Raw Fluorescence Signal in Luminex xMAP Based Multiplex Immunoassays. *Sci. Rep.* **2016**, *6*, 26996. [CrossRef]
21. Narasimhan, M.; Mahimainathan, L.; Araj, E.; Clark, A.E.; Markantonis, J.; Green, A.; Xu, J.; SoRelle, J.A.; Alexis, C.; Fankhauser, K.; et al. Clinical Evaluation of the Abbott Alinity SARS-CoV-2 Spike-Specific Quantitative IgG and IgM Assays among Infected, Recovered, and Vaccinated Groups. *J. Clin. Microbiol.* **2021**, *59*, e00388-21. [CrossRef]
22. Torretta, S.; Zuccotti, G.; Cristofaro, V.; Ettori, J.; Solimeno, L.; Battilocchi, L.; D'Onghia, A.; Bonsembiante, A.; Pignataro, L.; Marchisio, P.; et al. Diagnosis of SARS-CoV-2 by RT-PCR Using Different Sample Sources: Review of the Literature. *Ear Nose Throat J.* **2021**, *100*, 131S–138S. [CrossRef] [PubMed]
23. Sule, W.F.; Oluwayelu, D.O. Real-Time RT-PCR for COVID-19 Diagnosis: Challenges and Prospects. *Pan Afr. Med. J.* **2020**, *35*, 121. [CrossRef] [PubMed]
24. Stapleton, J.T. Severe Acute Respiratory Syndrome Coronavirus 2 Antibody Testing: Important but Imperfect. *Clin. Infect. Dis.* **2021**, *73*, E3074–E3076. [CrossRef]
25. Smerczak, E. SARS-CoV-2 Antibody Testing: Where Are We Now? *Lab. Med.* **2022**, *53*, E19–E29. [CrossRef] [PubMed]
26. Galipeau, Y.; Greig, M.; Liu, G.; Driedger, M.; Langlois, M.-A. Humoral Responses and Serological Assays in SARS-CoV-2 Infections. *Front. Immunol.* **2020**, *11*, 610688. [CrossRef]
27. Knezevic, I.; Mattiuzzo, G.; Page, M.; Minor, P.; Griffiths, E.; Nuebling, M.; Moorthy, V. WHO International Standard for Evaluation of the Antibody Response to COVID-19 Vaccines: Call for Urgent Action by the Scientific Community. *Lancet Microbe* **2022**, *3*, E235–E240. [CrossRef]

28. Taylor, P.C.; Adams, A.C.; Hufford, M.M.; de la Torre, I.; Winthrop, K.; Gottlieb, R.L. Neutralizing Monoclonal Antibodies for Treatment of COVID-19. *Nat. Rev. Immunol.* **2021**, *21*, 382–393. [CrossRef]
29. Dhawan, M.; Priyanka; Parmar, M.; Angural, S.; Choudhary, O.P. Convalescent Plasma Therapy against the Emerging SARS-CoV-2 Variants: Delineation of the Potentialities and Risks. *Int. J. Surg.* **2022**, *97*, 106204. [CrossRef]
30. Hodgson, S.H.; Mansatta, K.; Mallett, G.; Harris, V.; Emary, K.R.W.; Pollard, A.J. What Defines an Efficacious COVID-19 Vaccine? A Review of the Challenges Assessing the Clinical Efficacy of Vaccines against SARS-CoV-2. *Lancet Infect. Dis.* **2021**, *21*, e26–e35. [CrossRef]
31. Bai, Z.; Cao, Y.; Liu, W.; Li, J. The SARS-CoV-2 Nucleocapsid Protein and Its Role in Viral Structure, Biological Functions, and a Potential Target for Drug or Vaccine Mitigation. *Viruses* **2021**, *13*, 1115. [CrossRef]
32. Rak, A.; Donina, S.; Zabrodskaya, Y.; Rudenko, L.; Isakova-Sivak, I. Cross-Reactivity of SARS-CoV-2 Nucleocapsid-Binding Antibodies and Its Implication for COVID-19 Serology Tests. *Viruses* **2022**, *14*, 2041. [CrossRef] [PubMed]
33. Westphal, T.; Mader, M.; Karsten, H.; Cords, L.; Knapp, M.; Schulte, S.; Hermanussen, L.; Peine, S.; Ditt, V.; Grifoni, A.; et al. Evidence for Broad Cross-Reactivity of the SARS-CoV-2 NSP12-Directed CD4+ T-Cell Response with Pre-Primed Responses Directed against Common Cold Coronaviruses. *Front. Immunol.* **2023**, *14*, 1182504. [CrossRef] [PubMed]
34. Ayouba, A.; Thaurignac, G.; Morquin, D.; Tuaillon, E.; Raulino, R.; Nkuba, A.; Lacroix, A.; Vidal, N.; Foulongne, V.; Le Moing, V.; et al. Multiplex Detection and Dynamics of IgG Antibodies to SARS-CoV2 and the Highly Pathogenic Human Coronaviruses SARS-CoV and MERS-CoV. *J. Clin. Virol.* **2020**, *129*, 104521. [CrossRef] [PubMed]
35. Cook, N.; Xu, L.; Hegazy, S.; Wheeler, B.J.; Anderson, A.R.; Critelli, N.; Yost, M.; McElroy, A.K.; Shurin, M.R.; Wheeler, S.E. Multiplex Assessment of SARS-CoV-2 Antibodies Improves Assay Sensitivity and Correlation with Neutralizing Antibodies. *Clin. Biochem.* **2021**, *97*, 54–61. [CrossRef]
36. den Hartog, G.; Schepp, R.M.; Kuijer, M.; GeurtsvanKessel, C.; van Beek, J.; Rots, N.; Koopmans, M.P.G.; van der Klis, F.R.M.; van Binnendijk, R.S. SARS-CoV-2-Specific Antibody Detection for Seroepidemiology: A Multiplex Analysis Approach Accounting for Accurate Seroprevalence. *J. Infect. Dis.* **2020**, *222*, 1452–1461. [CrossRef]
37. Karachaliou, M.; Moncunill, G.; Espinosa, A.; Castaño-Vinyals, G.; Jiménez, A.; Vidal, M.; Santano, R.; Barrios, D.; Puyol, L.; Carreras, A.; et al. Infection Induced SARS-CoV-2 Seroprevalence and Heterogeneity of Antibody Responses in a General Population Cohort Study in Catalonia Spain. *Sci. Rep.* **2021**, *11*, 21571. [CrossRef]
38. Gudbjartsson, D.F.; Norddahl, G.L.; Melsted, P.; Gunnarsdottir, K.; Holm, H.; Eythorsson, E.; Arnthorsson, A.O.; Helgason, D.; Bjarnadottir, K.; Ingvarsson, R.F.; et al. Humoral Immune Response to SARS-CoV-2 in Iceland. *N. Engl. J. Med.* **2020**, *383*, 1724–1734. [CrossRef]
39. Conti, P.; Younes, A. Coronavirus COV-19/SARS-CoV-2 Affects Women Less than Men: Clinical Response to Viral Infection. *J. Biol. Regul. Homeost. Agents* **2020**, *34*, 339–343. [CrossRef]
40. Garcia-Basteiro, A.L.; Moncunill, G.; Tortajada, M.; Vidal, M.; Guinovart, C.; Jiménez, A.; Santano, R.; Sanz, S.; Méndez, S.; Llupià, A.; et al. Seroprevalence of Antibodies against SARS-CoV-2 among Health Care Workers in a Large Spanish Reference Hospital. *Nat. Commun.* **2020**, *11*, 3500. [CrossRef]
41. Yousefi, Z.; Taheri, N.; Dargahi, M.; Chaman, R.; Binesh, E.; Emamian, M.H.; Jafari, R. Long-Term Persistence of Anti-SARS-COV-2 IgG Antibodies. *Curr. Microbiol.* **2022**, *79*, 96. [CrossRef]
42. He, Z.; Ren, L.; Yang, J.; Guo, L.; Feng, L.; Ma, C.; Wang, X.; Leng, Z.; Tong, X.; Zhou, W.; et al. Seroprevalence and Humoral Immune Durability of Anti-SARS-CoV-2 Antibodies in Wuhan, China: A Longitudinal, Population-Level, Cross-Sectional Study. *Lancet* **2021**, *397*, 1075–1084. [CrossRef] [PubMed]
43. Soares, S.R.; Da Silva Torres, M.K.; Lima, S.S.; De Sarges, K.M.L.; Santos, E.F.D.; De Brito, M.T.F.M.; Da Silva, A.L.S.; De Meira Leite, M.; Da Costa, F.P.; Cantanhede, M.H.D.; et al. Antibody Response to the SARS-CoV-2 Spike and Nucleocapsid Proteins in Patients with Different COVID-19 Clinical Profiles. *Viruses* **2023**, *15*, 898. [CrossRef] [PubMed]
44. Long, Q.-X.; Liu, B.-Z.; Deng, H.-J.; Wu, G.-C.; Deng, K.; Chen, Y.-K.; Liao, P.; Qiu, J.-F.; Lin, Y.; Cai, X.-F.; et al. Antibody Responses to SARS-CoV-2 in Patients with COVID-19. *Nat. Med.* **2020**, *26*, 845–848. [CrossRef] [PubMed]
45. Liao, B.; Chen, Z.; Zheng, P.; Li, L.; Zhuo, J.; Li, F.; Li, S.; Chen, D.; Wen, C.; Cai, W.; et al. Detection of Anti-SARS-CoV-2-S2 IgG Is More Sensitive Than Anti-RBD IgG in Identifying Asymptomatic COVID-19 Patients. *Front. Immunol.* **2021**, *12*, 724763. [CrossRef] [PubMed]
46. Legros, V.; Denolly, S.; Vogrig, M.; Boson, B.; Siret, E.; Rigaill, J.; Pillet, S.; Grattard, F.; Gonzalo, S.; Verhoeven, P.; et al. A Longitudinal Study of SARS-CoV-2-Infected Patients Reveals a High Correlation between Neutralizing Antibodies and COVID-19 Severity. *Cell Mol. Immunol.* **2021**, *18*, 318–327. [CrossRef] [PubMed]
47. Lau, E.H.Y.; Tsang, O.T.Y.; Hui, D.S.C.; Kwan, M.Y.W.; Chan, W.-H.; Chiu, S.S.; Ko, R.L.W.; Chan, K.H.; Cheng, S.M.S.; Perera, R.A.P.M.; et al. Neutralizing Antibody Titres in SARS-CoV-2 Infections. *Nat. Commun.* **2021**, *12*, 63. [CrossRef]
48. Racine-Brzostek, S.E.; Yang, H.S.; Jack, G.A.; Chen, Z.; Chadburn, A.; Ketas, T.J.; Francomano, E.; Klasse, P.J.; Moore, J.P.; McDonough, K.A.; et al. Postconvalescent SARS-CoV-2 IgG and Neutralizing Antibodies Are Elevated in Individuals with Poor Metabolic Health. *J. Clin. Endocrinol. Metab.* **2021**, *106*, e2025–e2034. [CrossRef]
49. Lobstein, T. *COVID-19 and Obesity: The 2021 Atlas*; World Obesity Federation: London, UK, 2021.

50. Xu, C.; Zhao, H.; Song, Y.; Zhou, J.; Wu, T.; Qiu, J.; Wang, J.; Song, X.; Sun, Y. The Association between Allergic Rhinitis and COVID-19: A Systematic Review and Meta-Analysis. *Int. J. Clin. Pract.* **2022**, *2022*, 6510332. [CrossRef]
51. Troyano-Hernáez, P.; Reinosa, R.; Holguín, Á. Evolution of SARS-CoV-2 in Spain during the First Two Years of the Pandemic: Circulating Variants, Amino Acid Conservation, and Genetic Variability in Structural, Non-Structural, and Accessory Proteins. *Int. J. Mol. Sci.* **2022**, *23*, 6394. [CrossRef]

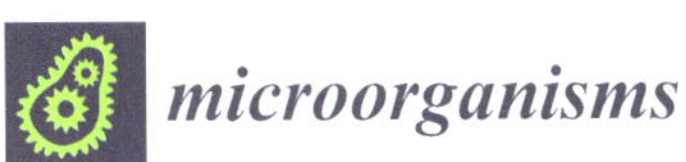 *microorganisms*

MDPI

Article

Humoral Immune Responses in Patients with Severe COVID-19: A Comparative Pilot Study between Individuals Infected by SARS-CoV-2 during the Wild-Type and the Delta Periods

Maria Sukhova [1,2], Maria Byazrova [1,2,3], Artem Mikhailov [1,2], Gaukhar Yusubalieva [4,5], Irina Maslova [6], Tatyana Belovezhets [7], Nikolay Chikaev [7], Ivan Vorobiev [8], Vladimir Baklaushev [4,5] and Alexander Filatov [1,2,*]

[1] Laboratory of Immunochemistry, National Research Center Institute of Immunology, Federal Medical Biological Agency of Russia, 115522 Moscow, Russia; mary.sukhova13@gmail.com (M.S.); mbyazrova@list.ru (M.B.); artem.mihaylov.2001@mail.ru (A.M.)
[2] Department of Immunology, Faculty of Biology, Lomonosov Moscow State University, 119234 Moscow, Russia
[3] Department of Immunology, Peoples' Friendship University of Russia (RUDN University) of Ministry of Science and Higher Education of the Russian Federation, 117198 Moscow, Russia
[4] Laboratory of Cell Technology, Federal Research and Clinical Center for Specialized Types of Medical Care and Medical Technologies of the FMBA of Russia, 115682 Moscow, Russia; gaukhar@gaukhar.org (G.Y.); serpoff@gmail.com (V.B.)
[5] Engelhardt Institute of Molecular Biology, Russian Academy of Sciences, 119991 Moscow, Russia
[6] Clinical Hospital #85, Federal Medical Biological Agency of Russia, 115409 Moscow, Russia; dr.imaslova@gmail.com
[7] Laboratory of Immunogenetics, Institute of Molecular and Cellular Biology, Siberian Branch of the Russian Academy of Sciences, 630090 Novosibirsk, Russia; belovezhec@mcb.nsc.ru (T.B.); na_chik@mcb.nsc.ru (N.C.)
[8] Laboratory of Mammalian Cell Bioengineering, Skryabin Institute of Bioengineering, Research Center of Biotechnology of the Russian Academy of Sciences, 117312 Moscow, Russia; ptichman@gmail.com
* Correspondence: avfilat@yandex.ru

Citation: Sukhova, M.; Byazrova, M.; Mikhailov, A.; Yusubalieva, G.; Maslova, I.; Belovezhets, T.; Chikaev, N.; Vorobiev, I.; Baklaushev, V.; Filatov, A. Humoral Immune Responses in Patients with Severe COVID-19: A Comparative Pilot Study between Individuals Infected by SARS-CoV-2 during the Wild-Type and the Delta Periods. *Microorganisms* **2023**, *11*, 2347. https://doi.org/10.3390/microorganisms11092347

Academic Editor: Qibin Geng

Received: 9 August 2023
Revised: 8 September 2023
Accepted: 9 September 2023
Published: 20 September 2023

Abstract. Since the onset of the COVID-19 pandemic, humanity has experienced the spread and circulation of several SARS-CoV-2 variants that differed in transmissibility, contagiousness, and the ability to escape from vaccine-induced neutralizing antibodies. However, issues related to the differences in the variant-specific immune responses remain insufficiently studied. The aim of this study was to compare the parameters of the humoral immune responses in two groups of patients with acute COVID-19 who were infected during the circulation period of the D614G and the Delta variants of SARS-CoV-2. Sera from 48 patients with acute COVID-19 were tested for SARS-CoV-2 binding and neutralizing antibodies using six assays. We found that serum samples from the D614G period demonstrated 3.9- and 1.6-fold increases in RBD- and spike-specific IgG binding with wild-type antigens compared with Delta variant antigens ($p < 0.01$). Cluster analysis showed the existence of two well-separated clusters. The first cluster mainly consisted of D614G-period patients and the second cluster predominantly included patients from the Delta period. The results thus obtained indicate that humoral immune responses in D614G- and Delta-specific infections can be characterized by variant-specific signatures. This can be taken into account when developing new variant-specific vaccines.

Keywords: SARS-CoV-2; COVID-19; variants of concern; virus neutralization

1. Introduction

During the COVID-19 pandemic, a wide range of aspects of immune response to SARS-CoV-2 was studied and by now, many features for achieving immunity against this virus have been uncovered. Both innate and T-cell immune responses have been shown to play important roles in protection against COVID-19; however, it was firmly established that virus-neutralizing antibodies serve as the most critical factor determining protection from symptomatic SARS-CoV-2 infection [1]. Accordingly, most of the studies during and in the wake of the COVID-19 pandemic have focused on the humoral immune response during the course of the disease and/or vaccination.

The specific humoral response against SARS-CoV-2 has been extensively studied in different scenarios. These include examining the immune response during or shortly after acute infection [2], as well as monitoring the immunity over the following months, upon re-infection or immunization with various vaccines and boosters [3–5]. Both homologous and heterologous vaccination regimens, hybrid vaccination after COVID-19, and breakthrough infection have been tested [6]. In these studies, much attention was paid to the study of the virus-binding and virus-neutralizing activity of sera against a variety of SARS-CoV-2 lineages, ranging from Wuhan-Hu-1 and D614G strains to the latest Omicron variants, such as Omicron BQ.1 and XBB. Numerous data have been collected on the differences between different variants of concern (VOCs) in terms of transmissibility, contagiousness, relative severity of the disease, and their ability to escape from vaccine-induced neutralizing antibodies [7].

Despite a large amount of accumulated data, limited attention has been paid to direct comparison of immunity after COVID-19 caused by the different variants of SARS-CoV-2 [8–10]. In order to fill this knowledge gap, we examined the levels of humoral responses induced by natural infection with SARS-CoV-2 variants causing the COVID-19 in Moscow, Russia. Since the beginning of the COVID-19 pandemic, Moscow has experienced several waves of COVID-19, and the dynamics of circulating SARS-CoV-2 genetic variants in the Moscow region have been closely monitored [11,12]. According to the whole-genome sequencing analyses dating back to May–June 2020, the B.1 variant of SARS-CoV-2 which bears a single D614G substitution in the spike protein was predominant in Moscow [13]. Subsequently, numerous VOCs appeared and began to spread; however, during the COVID-19 wave in October–November 2021, only the Delta (B.1.617.2) variant of SARS-CoV-2 was detected in Moscow [14].

The aim of this study was to compare the effects of acute SARS-CoV-2 infections during the D614G and the Delta waves on the humoral immune response. To address this goal, we investigated the cross-reactivity of the antibodies in these two groups of infected individuals against the antigens from the wild-type and Delta variant. Additionally, the Omicron BA.1 subvariant, which has a high number of mutations in the spike (S) protein was also included as a distant antigen in the study. Notably, as SARS-CoV-2 evolves and new variants emerge, there is a clear need to develop a new, robust and simple method for detecting virus-specific antibodies. In this study, we propose two new cell-based approaches evaluating spike-binding and virus-neutralization activities that can be easily adapted to new antigenic variants.

2. Materials and Methods

2.1. Patients

The study included patients who experienced acute SARS-CoV-2 infection in May–June 2020 ($n = 27$) or October–November 2021 ($n = 21$). All the examined individuals were hospitalized at the Federal Research Clinical Center of the Federal Medical-Biological Agency of Russia (FRCC) and were characterized by moderate or severe course of COVID-19. The inclusion criteria were as follows: a positive rt-qPCR test, presence of antibodies against SARS-CoV-2 nucleocapsid protein, no history of vaccination against SARS-CoV-2, and no history of previous self-reported COVID-19 infection.

2.2. Serum Samples

Serum samples were collected in the acute phase of the disease at a late time point (median 21 days, IQR 18–33) from the onset of the disease. Blood samples were collected into heparinized vacutainer tubes (Sarstedt, Nümbrecht, Germany #04.1927). Blood plasma samples were obtained by centrifugation, aliquoted into collection vials and stored at

$-70\ ^\circ$C. Samples were named according to the patient IDs and tested using six serological assays (Supplementary Figure S1).

2.3. Recombinant Proteins

In-house production of recombinant RBD proteins (residues 319–541) was described earlier [15]. In brief, His-tagged RBD was expressed using the HEK293 cells and purified from cell culture supernatant using affinity chromatography on Ni-NTA agarose resin (Novagen, St. Louis, MO, USA). The RBD from the Wuhan-Hu-1 strain was designated as wild-type (WT) RBD and it matched the RBD from the D614G strain. RBD variants used in the study had the following substitutions: L452R, T478K (Delta); G339D, S371L, S373P, S375F, K417N, N440K, G446S, S477N, T478K, E484A, Q493R, G496S, Q498R, N501Y, Y505H (Omicron BA.1).

Extracellular domain of the human angiotensin-converting enzyme 2 (residues 319–541) was fused to an immunoglobulin G crystallizable fragment (ACE2-Fc) as described earlier [16]. The ACE2-Fc was stably expressed in a DHFR-negative Chinese hamster ovary (CHO) DG-44 cell line (Thermo Fischer Scientific, Waltham, MA, USA) and was purified from the conditioned-culture medium using chromatography on MabSelect SuRe column (Cytiva, Marlborough, MA, USA).

ACE2-Fc was fluorescently labeled using Alexa Fluor 488 NHS Ester Succinimidyl Ester (Thermo Fisher Scientific, A20000) followed by the removal of excess dye by buffer exchange on PD-10 desalting column (Cytiva, #17-0851-01). ACE2-Fc was conjugated to the horseradish peroxidase using HRP Conjugation Kit (Abcam, Cambridge, UK, #Ab102890) according to the manufacturer's instructions.

2.4. ELISA

The levels of RBD-specific IgGs were determined using an in-house ELISA test [17]. In brief, 96-well high-binding ELISA plates (Greiner Bio-One, Kremsmünster, Austria) were coated overnight with 2 µg/mL of recombinant RBD in PBS. Plates were then washed three times and blocked with blocking buffer (Xema Co., Moscow, Russia) for 1 h at room temperature. Serum samples from patients with COVID-19 were 2-fold serially diluted from 1:20 to 1:12,500 in blocking buffer and added into the wells. Plates were then incubated with samples for 1 h at room temperature. After washing in PBS with 0.05% Tween 20, the plates were incubated for 1 h with rabbit anti-human IgG antibody (Jackson Immuno Research, West Grove, PA, USA, Cat# 309-005-008), thoroughly washed and incubated with goat ant-rabbit IgG antibodies conjugated with horseradish peroxidase (Bio-Rad, Hercules, CA, USA, #1721019) for 1 h. ELISA plates were washed 7 times and developed for 10 min with 100 µL of tetramethylbenzidine chromogen solution (Xema Co., Moscow, Russia). The reaction was stopped with 50 µL 1M H2SO4 and absorbance at 450 nm was read with an iMark microplate absorbance reader (Bio-Rad). Each sample was measured in triplicate. To determine the concentration of WT and Delta RBD-specific IgGs, a serial dilution of anti-SARS-CoV-2 RBD-specific human monoclonal antibody iB12 known to recognize both RBD variants equally well was included on each plate, a calibration curve was built and IgG levels were calculated (µg/mL) [15]. When determining the levels of BA.1-specific IgGs, we used high-titer serum as a standard and antibody levels were expressed as relative units (RU). Baseline values for 8 pre-pandemic healthy donor serum samples were derived from the cryopreserved samples collected in 2017–2018.

2.5. Membrane-Based ELISA (mELISA)

HEK293 cells were seeded at a density of 3.6×10^6 cells/100 mm Petri dish (NEST). Next day, cells were transiently transfected with 30 µg of pCAGGS-SΔ19 expression plasmid encoding the spike protein of the D614G strain, Delta or Omicron BA.1 VOC. Spike variants had the following substitutions: T19R, G142D, Δ156–157, R158G, L452R, T478K, D614G, P681R, D950N (Delta); A67V, Δ69–70, T95I, G142D, Δ143–145, Δ211, L212I, ins214EPE, G339D, S371L, S373P, S375F, K417N, N440K, G446S, S477N, T478K, E484A, Q493R, G496S,

Q498R, N501Y, Y505H, T547K, D614G, H655Y, N679K, P681H, N764K, D796Y, N856K, Q954H, N969K, L981F (Omicron BA.1). Transfection was performed by the calcium phosphate method [17].

Seventy-two hours after transfection, cells were harvested and lysed using a standard freeze–thaw protocol [18]. In brief, cells were washed twice with PBS, scraped, and pelleted at 300 g for 10 min. The pellet was resuspended in PBS containing 100 mM PMSF, and lysed in three freeze–thaw cycles. Lysates were clarified at 300 g for 10 min at 4 °C and membrane fraction was pelleted by centrifugation at 30,000 rpm for 90 min at 4 °C. The pellet was resuspended in PBS and protein concentration was determined by measuring the absorbance at 280 nm. ELISA plates (Greiner Bio-One, Kremsmünster, Austria) were coated with 20 µg/well of membrane preparation. The reaction of serum samples with the spike protein in membrane preparations was developed and recorded in the same way as described above when performing RBD-specific ELISA. The antibody binding was measured in OD values. Wells coated with membranes derived from non-transfected HEK293 cells were used as negative controls. All samples were analyzed in duplicate.

2.6. Pseudotyped Virus-Neutralization Assay (pVNA)

Virus-neutralization activity in serum samples was determined using lentiviral particles pseudotyped with the SARS-CoV-2 S protein of the D614G strain or Delta and Omicron BA.1 VOCs. To produce SARS-CoV-2 S-pseudotyped virus-like particles (VLPs), HEK293 cells were co-transfected with three plasmids: lentiviral packaging plasmid pCMVΔ8.2R (Addgene, Teddington, UK), reporter plasmid pUCHR-GFP, and an expression plasmid pCAGGS-SΔ19 encoding the wild-type SARS-CoV-2 spike protein or those of the Delta or Omicron BA.1 VOCs [19].

Transfection was performed by the calcium phosphate method; 72 h after transfection, the supernatants were filtered through a 0.45 µm filter and concentrated 20-fold on Amicon® Ultra-15 ultrafiltration cells with a 100 kDa cutoff (Merck, #UFC910008). Concentrated supernatants were then re-centrifuged at 30,000× g, 8 °C for 150 min. The pellet was resuspended in Opti-MEM medium. Before proceeding to pVNA, VLPs were titrated by limiting dilution with HEK293 cells stably transfected with a plasmid-expressing human ACE2 (HEK293-hACE2). A dose of viral particles which gave 50% green fluorescent protein (GFP)-positive cells was selected for use in the test. For pVNA, all plasma samples were heat-inactivated for 30 min at 56 °C prior to use. Serial dilutions of sera were pre-incubated with VLPs and then added to target cells and co-cultivated for four days. On the fourth day, the cells were re-suspended, and the percentage of GFP-positive cells was measured by flow cytometry. ID_{50} values were calculated using a normalized nonlinear regression with GraphPad Prism software, version 8.4.3. (Sigmoidal, 4PL).

2.7. Flow Cytometry-Based Surrogate Virus-Neutralization Assay (fcVNA)

This method measures the ability of sera to inhibit the binding of Alexa Fluor 488-labeled ACE2-Fc to HEK293 cells transiently expressing the S protein of interest. As described above, HEK293 cells were transiently transfected with pCAGGS-SΔ19 plasmid encoding the S-protein of either the D614G strain, Delta or Omicron BA.1 VOCs.

The HEK293-spike cells (5×10^4 cells/well) were mixed with an equal volume of serial serum dilutions (ranging from 1:2 to 1:64) and incubated for 1 h at room temperature. After washing, the cells were additionally incubated for 1 h with Alexa Fluor 488-labeled ACE2-Fc. Then, the wells were washed twice and the percentage of ACE2-positive cells was measured on a flow cytometer. Before the fcVNA assay, the transfection efficiency was monitored using staining with ACE2-Alexa Fluor 488. Preparations in which the percentage of S^+ cells exceeded 75% were taken for fcVNA assay.

In the absence of serum, ACE2-Alexa Fluor 488 binding was the highest (set to 100%) and when the ACE2-Alexa Fluor 488 binding was completely inhibited, target cells did not produce a fluorescent signal. The results were presented as the serum dilution at which

50% inhibition (ID_{50}) of cell binding was observed, calculated from the Sigmoidal titration plot, 5PL, in the GraphPad Prism program.

2.8. Surrogate Virus-Neutralization Assay (sVNA)

ELISA plates (Greiner Bio-One, Kremsmünster, Austria, #756071) were coated with 2 µg/mL of recombinant RBD diluted in PBS. After incubation overnight, the plates were washed with PBS, containing 0.025% Tween-20 (PBS-T) thrice and blocked with 200 µL/well of 5% BSA-PBS. Serum samples were diluted 1:20 and added to the plates to allow for binding of antibodies to the protein. The plates were incubated for 1 h. After washing, the plates were additionally incubated for 1 h with ACE2-Fc conjugated with horseradish peroxidase (50 ng/mL) [16]. ID_{50} values were calculated as described above.

2.9. Antibody-Dependent NK Cell Activation Assay (ADNKA)

Flat bottom 96-well plates (Greiner Bio-One, Kremsmünster, Austria) were coated with 200 µL 2 µg/mL of recombinant RBD (WT or Delta) in PBS overnight at 4 °C. Plates were blocked with 200 µL/well of 1% of bovine serum albumin with 5% sucrose in PBS for 1 h at RT. After five sequential washes with PBS, serum was added at a dilution of 1:40, incubated for 3 h at 37 °C, and washed 3 times with PBS.

Whole-blood samples from healthy donors were collected into heparinized vacutainer tubes (Sarstedt, #04.1927). PBMCs were isolated by density gradient centrifugation. NK cells were purified from PBMCs by negative selection using the Dynabeads Untouched human NK cells kit (Thermo Fisher Scientific, #11349D).

Immunomagnetically separated NK cells were resuspended in complete DMEM/F12 medium supplemented with 10% FBS (Cytiva, #SV30160.03), and plated at a density of 30,000 cells per well onto the RBD-coated plates in duplicate. After incubation for 6 h at 37 °C, Brefeldin A (5 mg/mL final concentration; Invitrogen, Waltham, MA, USA) was added and cells incubated for another 10 h. Activated NK cells were harvested, fixed, permeabilized using 0.1% saponin, and stained with PE/Cy5-labeled antibody for IFN-γ (Sony, Tokyo, Japan, clone 45.B3).

Each ADNKA was performed with NK cells from a single donor. Cells were analyzed on a CytoFLEX S flow cytometer (Beckman Coulter, Brea, CA, USA). Up to 10×10^5 cells were acquired per sample. Data were analyzed using FlowJo Software (version 10.6.1., Tree Star).

2.10. Statistical Analysis

All assays were carried out in duplicate, with the relevant positive and negative controls. The Kruskal–Wallis H test was used for comparison between multiple groups, and Dunn's multiple comparisons test was performed using GraphPad Prism software, version 8.0.1. or Wilcoxon test for pairwise comparison. $p < 0.05$ was considered statistically significant. All statistical analyses were carried out using GraphPad Prism version 8.4.3 (GraphPad Software, San Diego, CA, USA). Heatmap generation and principal component analysis were performed with ClustVis using normalized data [20]. Data are presented as median values and interquartile ranges (IQR). Levels of statistical significance were denoted as * for $p < 0.05$, ** for $p < 0.01$, *** for $p < 0.001$, **** for $p < 0.0001$, ns for nonsignificant differences.

2.11. Ethics Statement

Written informed consent was obtained from each of the study participants before performing any study procedures. Study protocol was reviewed and approved by the Medical Ethical Committee of FRCC (#4-2020 28 April 2020) and conforms to the ethical guidelines of the 1975 Declaration of Helsinki.

3. Results

3.1. Study Design

Between May 2020 and April 2023, Moscow experienced at least six waves of COVID-19 cases (Figure 1A). Whole-genome sequencing analysis data (available on the GISAID server https://www.gisaid.org, accessed on 10 July 2023) showed a succession of different SARS-CoV-2 genetic variants (Figure 1B). At the early stage of the pandemic, SARS-CoV-2 evolved rather slowly [21] and throughout most of 2020 the B.1 variant was dominant. The B.1 spike protein differed from the Wuhan-Hu-1 isolate only by a single D614G mutation. At the turn of 2020 and 2021, the Alpha appeared briefly and the Beta VOC was also minimally present. At the beginning of 2022, all previous variants were completely replaced by the Delta (B.1.617.2) VOC. Various subvariants of Omicron have been establishing themselves in Russia since early 2022.

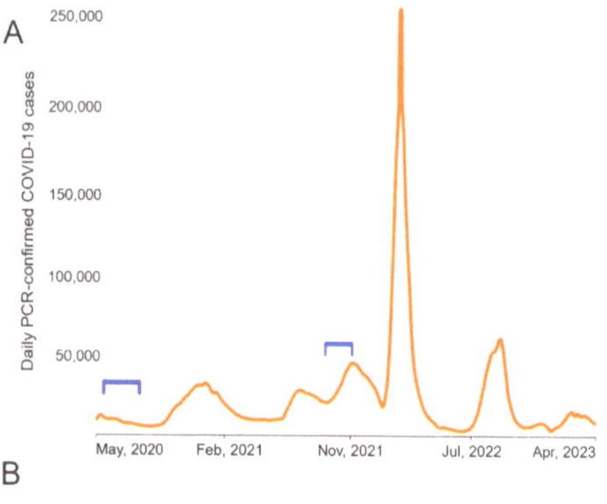

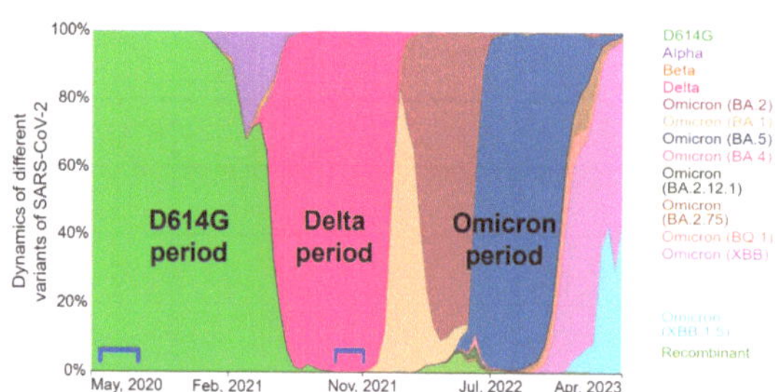

Figure 1. The dynamics of the spread of SARS-CoV-2 variants in Moscow population during the period from May 2020 to April 2023. Numbers of confirmed COVID-19 cases (**A**). Relative prevalence of SARS-CoV2 VOCs. Brackets denote the two periods of infection, D614G and Delta, in the study groups. (**B**) showed a succession of different SARS-CoV-2 genetic variants.

Our study included two groups of patients hospitalized for acute COVID-19. We obtained serum samples from patients who had been infected in May–June 2020 ($n = 27$) or in October–November 2021 ($n = 21$). We did not determine the genotypes of the infecting variants in patients; however, it can be stated with a high degree of certainty that individuals from the May–June 2020 group were infected with D614G strain, and those from the November–December 2021 group were infected with the Delta variant. Accordingly, the groups were classified as "D614G period" and "Delta period".

The demographic characteristics of the patients are summarized in Supplementary Table S1. The two groups of patients were overall similar in terms of age, male/female ratio, and disease severity. The median age was 68 years (IQR 60–72) and 73 years (IQR 63–82) for the D614G-period and Delta-period patients, correspondingly. The study included 18 patients with the moderate form (non-ICU) and 30 patients with the severe (ICU) form of COVID-19. Samples were collected during the acute phase of the disease; the median time between the onset of symptoms and sample collection was 21 days (IQR 18–33).

3.2. RBD- and Spike-Specific IgG Response

Since the RBD region plays a critical role in mediating the interaction between the S protein of the coronavirus and the ACE2 receptor, RBD is the main target for neutralizing antibodies. First of all, we determined the levels of RBD-specific IgGs in serum samples. In a standard ELISA, we used WT and Delta RBDs, which fully corresponded to the antigens in the D614G and Delta periods. For comparative purposes, BA.1 RBD was also included in the analysis. IgGs from the D614G and Delta periods bound well to WT and Delta RBD, but much worse to BA.1 RBD ($p < 0.0001$; Supplementary Figure S2).

Then, we compared anti-RBD IgG levels between the patients from the D614G and Delta periods and studied the cross-reactive activity of antibodies in these two groups. The activity of sera from the D614G period against WT RBD was 3.8 times higher than the cross-reactivity of sera from the Delta period ($p < 0.01$; Figure 2A, left panel). In contrast, the cross-reactivity of sera from the D614G period sera did not differ from the activity of the Delta sera against Delta RBD ($p = 0.1161$; Figure 2A, middle panel). Sera from either period reacted equally poorly with Omicron RBD (D614G vs. Delta period, $p = 0.9909$; Figure 2A, right panel).

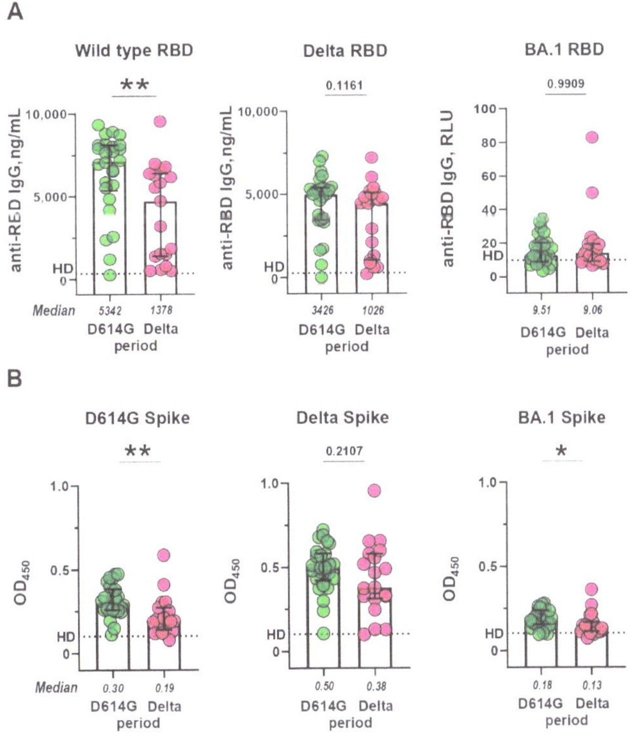

Figure 2. RBD- and S-binding activity of sera from patients with COVID-19 infected during the D614G and Delta periods. (**A**) Levels of serum IgG against WT, Delta, and BA.1 RBD, measured by ELISA. (**B**) Levels of serum IgG against WT, Delta, and BA.1 S protein, measured by mELISA. Dotted lines indicate the cut-off value for differentiating a positive response from a background response in the pre-pandemic samples from healthy donors (HD). ** $p < 0.01$, * $p < 0.05$.

The slight differences in cross-reactivity are probably due to the fact that WT and Delta RBDs differ from each other by only two amino acid substitutions. A more complete antigenic portrait of SARS-CoV-2 is presented on the transmembrane full-length S protein. S-specific antibodies were evaluated using an in-house developed mELISA assay. In this case, we used membrane preparations of HEK293 cells transiently transfected with a construct encoding a variant-specific S protein as an antigen. Similar to RBD-specific IgGs, the serum samples from the D614G and Delta periods showed strong binding to both WT and Delta S proteins, but a much weaker binding to the BA.1 S protein ($p < 0.0001$; Supplementary Figure S3).

Then, we compared the levels of S-specific humoral responses induced by natural infection with SARS-CoV-2 during D614G and Delta periods. The anti-S IgG response in the D614G and Delta groups exhibited a comparable pattern to that observed for anti-RBD IgG (Figure 2B). The sera from the D614G period reacted more preferentially with the homologous WT spike than with heterologous Delta S protein (fold difference 1.96, $p < 0.01$; Figure 2B, left panel), while the Delta period sera were equally reactive towards the heterologous WT and homologous Delta S proteins ($p = 0.2107$; Figure 2B, middle panel). Some statistically significant differences were observed between the D614G- and Delta-period groups in terms of antibodies against the BA.1 S protein ($p < 0.05$; Figure 2B, right panel).

3.3. Virus-Neutralizing Response

To investigate the functionality of antibodies from D614G and Delta periods, we proceeded to evaluate the serum virus-neutralizing activity in pVNA. First, we compared how sera neutralize VLPs pseudotyped with different spike variants. Sera from the D614G period neutralized VLPs bearing the S protein of either WT or Delta variant approximately equally and 3.7 times more potently than the BA.1-pseudotyped VLPs ($p < 0.0001$; Supplementary Figure S4). Sera from the Delta period neutralized VLPs pseudotyped with Delta S protein 3.5 and 3.9 times more effectively than WT- and BA.1-pseudotyped VLPs, respectively ($p < 0.05$, $p < 0.01$; Supplementary Figure S4). No significant differences between serum samples from D614G and Delta period were observed in the level of virus neutralization in pVNA for WT, Delta, and BA.1 variants (Figure 3A).

We further characterized serum samples from the two groups of patients using a flow cytometry-based surrogate virus-neutralization assay (fcVNA) developed in this work. In this method, the S protein transiently expressed on HEK293 cells was used as an antigen and Alexa Fluor 488-conjugated ACE2-Fc fusion protein was used as the detection reagent. Neutralizing antibodies prevent the ACE2-Fc chimera from binding to the cell surface-expressed S protein. Representative flow plots for serum samples with and without neutralizing activity are shown in Supplementary Figure S5A.

The levels of neutralization in fcVNA to each of the S protein (WT, Delta, and BA.1) variants tested were similar across both of the periods of infection (Figure 3B). fcVNA has an advantage over pVNA in terms of ease of setup, but is less sensitive than pVNA. Median values for ID_{50} in the fcVNA ranged from 2.3 to 10.1. Traditional sVNA, which is performed in the ELISA format, has a higher sensitivity. Recombinant RBD from WT, Delta and BA.1 variants was used as the plate-coating antigen and HRP-conjugated ACE2-Fc fusion was used as the detection reagent. Median values for ID_{50} in sVNA ranged from 21.7 to 66.5. Despite the higher sensitivity of sVNA, we were unable to detect differences in virus neutralization between the samples from the D614G and Delta periods (Figure 3C). The sensitivity of the Omicron variant to neutralization by serum samples from infected patients was very low.

3.4. Antibody-Dependent NK Cell Activation Assay (ADNKA)

RBD-specific antibodies, in addition to virus-neutralizing activity, can also have an effect or function associated with NK-cell–mediated antibody-dependent cell-mediated cytotoxicity, thereby contributing to a functional antiviral response [22,23]. To assess the effect of RBD-specific antibodies on NK cell activation, freshly purified NK cells isolated from healthy donor PBMCs were cultured in RBD-coated plates in the presence of serum samples from patients infected during the D614G and Delta periods. We observed RBD-specific Fc-dependent activation of NK cells which was accompanied by the expression of IFN-γ (Supplementary Figure S6). After incubation with serum samples from healthy controls, no more than 1% of NK cells expressed IFN-γ, and this level was established as a baseline.

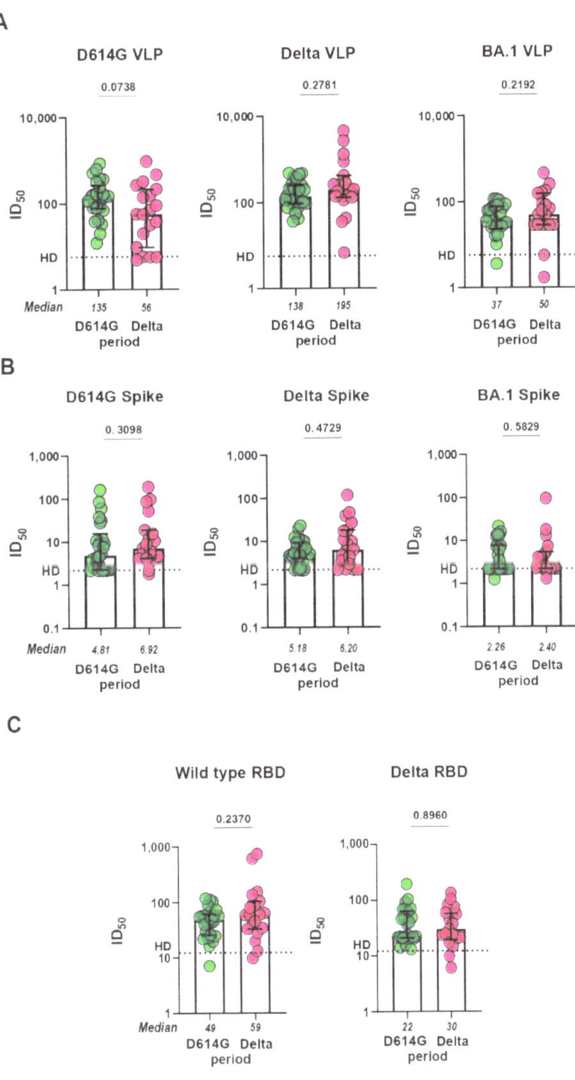

Figure 3. Neutralization antibody titers (ID_{50} values) against SARS-CoV-2 variants for sera from COVID-19 patients infected in the D614G and Delta period. (**A**) Neutralization of VLPs pseudotyped with the S protein from WT, Delta, and BA.1 Omicron variants. (**B**) Antibody-mediated blocking of ACE2-Alexa488 binding to HEK293 cells transiently transfected with S protein from WT, Delta, and BA.1 Omicron variants evaluated in fcVNA. (**C**) Antibody-mediated blocking of ACE2-HRP binding with RBD from WT, Delta, and BA.1 Omicron variants evaluated in sVNA.

Functional RBD-specific antibodies that can induce NK cell activation were found in some serum samples of patients with COVID-19. Of the D614G- and Delta-serum samples, 37% (10/27) and 52% (11/21) had IFN-γ+ NK cells above the baseline when tested against WT RBD, correspondingly, whereas 89% (24/27) and 86% (18/21) of samples exceeded the baseline in ADNKA against the Delta RBD, respectively (Figure 4). The comparison of serum samples from the D614G and Delta periods showed that the levels of ADNKA for these groups did not differ significantly ($p = 0.12$ and $p = 0.96$, respectively).

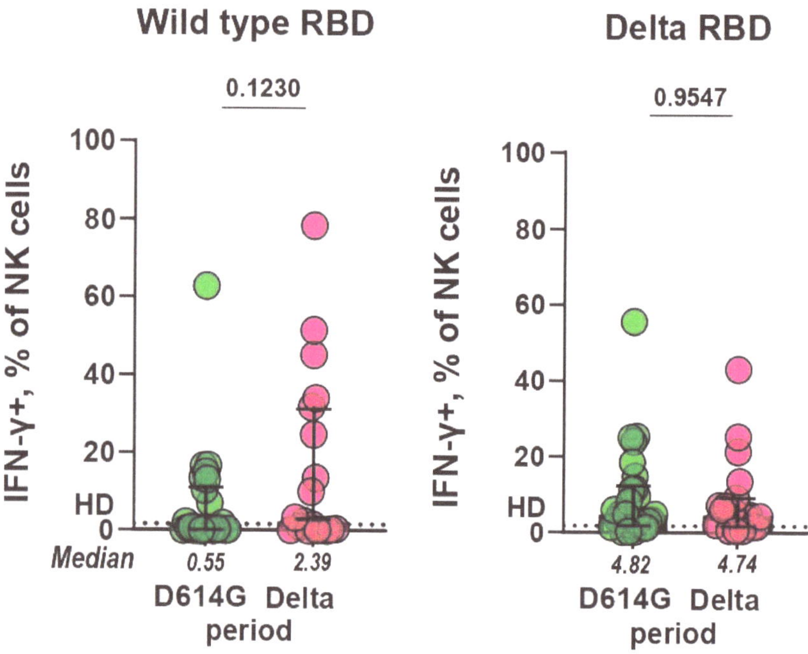

Figure 4. IFN-γ expression by NK cells in ADNKA. Plates were coated with wild-type (**left panel**) or Delta (**right panel**) RBD. NK cells were cultivated on plates in the presence of serum samples (dilution 1:40) from patients infected during D614G and Delta periods.

3.5. Hierarchical Cluster and Principal Component Analyses

Next, we compared the samples from the D614G- and Delta-period groups for individual parameters obtained by various assays, i.e., we set out to examine the full complement of inter-relationships between all the variables. This task was completed by using hierarchical cluster and principal component analyses, which included 45 samples measured by 16 humoral immune response parameters.

The constructed dendrograms indicated the existence of two well-separated clusters (Figure 5A). The first cluster mainly consisted of D614G-period patients (total $n = 24$, D614G and Delta periods $n = 20$ and 4, respectively) and the second cluster predominantly included patients from the Delta period (total $n = 21$, D614G and Delta periods $n = 6$ and 15, respectively). When comparing the samples using principal component analysis, we did not observe well-separated clusters. However, it could be noted that serum samples from the Delta period had significantly greater variability than those from the D614G period. The serum samples from the D614G-period cluster were quite compact and were completely included within the Delta-period cluster.

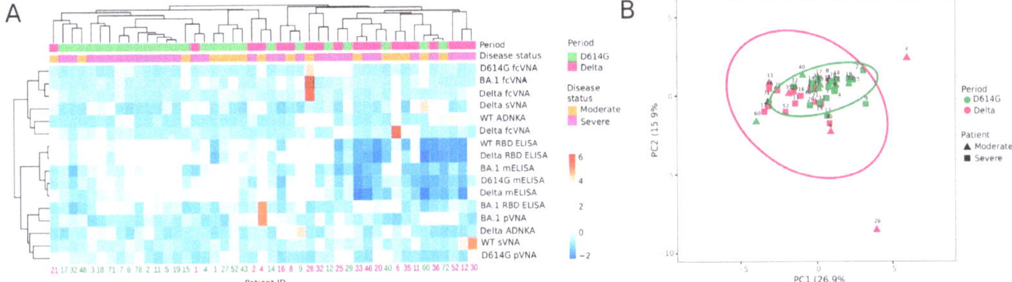

Figure 5. Hierarchical cluster (**A**) and principal component analysis (**B**) of serum samples from patients hospitalized with COVID-19 during D614G and Delta period. (**A**) Columns denote patients with their IDs. Rows correspond to immune response variables. Dendrograms on the top illustrate the clustering of patients. Immune response measurement values are color-coded according to the key shown on the right. (**B**) Principal component analysis of patients with COVID-19. Patient IDs are shown. D614G- and Delta-period clusters are indicated by the ovals. Results are shown for individual samples (symbols) from D614G period (*n* = 26) and Delta period (*n* = 19) patients.

4. Discussion

The vast majority of currently approved COVID-19 vaccines are based on the reference viral strain originally identified in Wuhan. Initially, the developed vaccines successfully protected against COVID-19. However, due to the continuous evolution of SARS-CoV-2 and the emergence of new VOCs, antibodies generated in the vaccinated individuals displayed progressively reduced virus-neutralizing activity against antigenically distinct variants, in particular, Delta and especially against Omicron and its sublineages [24]. Since the protective efficacy of the original vaccines against VOCs has declined, this prompts the development of variant-adapted vaccines. Several variant-adapted vaccines have been developed and approved, for which increased immunogenicity and protection against Omicron-related subvariants have been reported [25]; however, the relative benefits of using variant-adapted vaccines remain controversial [26]. The ambiguity in the use of variant-specific vaccines is compounded by the fact that the development and trials of new vaccines is laborious, complex and expensive. In addition to vaccination, protection against COVID-19 can be achieved by treating with monoclonal antibodies (mAbs) against SARS-CoV-2 antigens. The problem of increased immune escape by the new SARS-CoV-2 variants is common to both variant-specific vaccines and therapeutic mAbs [27], so the study of the cross-reactivity of sera from recovered patients with different SARS-CoV-2 variants can also serve as a valuable resource for the development of novel prophylactic monoclonal antibodies (mAbs).

For variant-specific vaccines, the critical question is whether immunization can induce cross-reactive (cross-neutralizing) antibodies to other variants. This can be easily assessed using animal models [28]. It was shown that variant-specific immunization caused higher activity of neutralizing antibodies against the corresponding variant than against the original strain [10].

An alternative approach to evaluate variant-specific immunization is to compare serum samples from patients who had a prior infection with different SARS-CoV-2 variants in terms of their cross-reactivity. However, only a few detailed reports on this subject have been published [8,9]. In particular, it was demonstrated that Omicron infections lead to increased antibody binding to pre-Omicron S variants [9]; at the same time, sera from the Delta and pre-Delta periods were similar in binding to S protein variants. In order to compare more comprehensively the humoral immunity in patients from the D614G and Delta periods, we used a set of methods, both standard (ELISA, pVNA, and sVNA) and especially designed for this case (fcVNA and mELISA).

Capture antigens used in ELISA should mimic natural antigenic epitopes as much as possible. The S protein is a large transmembrane, heavily glycosylated polypeptide with molecular weight 180–200 kDa. Human HEK293 or Chinese hamster ovary (CHO) cells represent the best option for the production of a soluble extracellular domain of the S protein. However, due to the large size of the S protein, it belongs to a class of difficult-to-express proteins [29,30]. The antigenic portrait of the S protein is most complete when it is present in a prefusion trimerized conformation. However, this conformation is metastable. The prefusion state of the SARS-CoV-2 S trimer protein can be stabilized by the addition of two or six proline residues (S-2P or HexaPro variant) and abolishing the furin cleavage site [31–33]. In addition, depending on the position of the RBD domains, the S trimer can be in several states: closed, partially, or completely open conformation.

When switching to a new variant of the S protein, the production and purification procedure must be adjusted anew. Production of a set of mutant variants of the S protein in its native conformation is a very labor-intensive and expensive process. Thus, the search for alternative ways to obtain S proteins is an urgent task. In this study, we proposed the mELISA method, in which the full-length S protein in the membrane fraction of transfected cells is used as an antigen immobilized on microplates. In this method, the S protein is presented in a native conformation in a tagless form, and its production is very simple and easily adaptable to new mutant variants. The full-length transmembrane S protein from transiently transfected cells possesses the complete antigenic spectrum and in combination with mELISA could represent a rapid production platform for detecting antibodies against mutant variants. The idea to use the transmembrane S protein as ligand instead of isolated recombinant antigen was also used by us in the flow cytometry-based surrogate virus-neutralization assay (fcVNA).

The binding of recombinant ACE2 with the membrane-bound S protein is more consistent with the interaction between the RBD of SARS-CoV-2 with the ACE2, a cell surface receptor of the human host cell, than when a purified recombinant RBD, which is commonly used in sVNA [34], is considered. Since a single, invariant reagent, namely, ACE2-Fc, is used as a labeled probe for various S protein variants, the method can be easily adapted to any S variant. Finally, the protocol of fcVNA allows experiments to be performed on the full-length S protein at a minimal cost. It should be noted that traditional pVNT is more sensitive than sVNT and fcVNA.

For the examined patients, we did not perform genotyping of the SARS-CoV-2 variants they were infected with; however, the time of collection was chosen in such a way as to ensure the variant-specificity of the obtained samples to the greatest extent. Taking into account the published data on SARS-CoV-2 sequencing carried out in Russia, it can be argued that the examined groups represent fairly pure populations that were infected with either D614G or Delta variants. During the first wave of 2020, there were no vaccinated or reinfected patients, and in the wave of 2021, their numbers were still very small and easily separable from the general sample. It would have been of great interest to include patients from the Omicron period in this study; however, subsequent waves were fueled by several Omicron subvariants. In addition, by this time, the percentage of vaccinated people or those infected with previous variants had noticeably increased, and a significant proportion of the population already had some level of immunoreactivity against SARS-CoV-2.

The aim of this study was to determine whether variant-specific infections have a unique molecular signature. Our comparison of patients from the D614G and Delta periods in terms of individual parameters of the humoral response revealed only minimal differences between these groups. This is not surprising, because compared to the D614G strain, the Delta S variant has only nine amino acid substitutions, including two deletions in the S protein and these antigens are more than 98% identical.

However, we found that serum samples from the D614G period reacted with RBD and S from the WT strain 3.9 and 1.6 times more strongly than with the corresponding antigens from the Delta variant. Interestingly, serum samples from the Delta period demonstrated similar levels of IgGs against the WT and Delta variants of RBD and S. This demonstrates that Delta infection is a good inducer of cross-reactive antibodies against a predecessor WT strain. The Omicron infection has recently been found to induce cross-reactive antibodies against heterologous spike variants [9]. We hypothesize that the Delta infection similarly contributed to increased antibody binding to the D614G spike variant.

A more thorough analysis using the antigenic maps showed that the serum samples from D614G and Delta patients were located at a small but distinguishable antigenic distance from each other, and formed distinct clusters [8]. In line with these data, our cluster analysis also showed some differences between the studied groups of patients. Thus, taking into account several humoral parameters, it was possible to identify the signatures of humoral immunity in the D614G- and Delta-period groups. The presented study can be considered as a pilot study. In order to evaluate variant-specific humoral responses more accurately, additional epidemiological studies will be needed.

5. Limitations of the Study

The limitation of this study is the relatively small sample size. In addition, the assignment of the patients to either D614G- or Delta-infected groups was based on the period of disease, but was not directly confirmed by genomic sequencing.

6. Conclusions

The results of our study show that humoral immune responses in D614G- and Delta-specific infections can be characterized by variant-specific signatures. These data can be taken into account when developing new variant-specific vaccines.

Supplementary Materials: The following supporting information can be downloaded at: https://www.mdpi.com/article/10.3390/microorganisms11092347/s1, Table S1: Patients' characteristics; Figure S1: Study design; Figure S2: Reactivity of (A) D614G- and (B) Delta-period serum samples with WT, Delta, and BA.1 RBD in ELISA; Figure S3: Reactivity of (A) D614G- and (B) Delta-period serum samples with WT, Delta, and BA.1 S protein in membrane based ELISA (mELISA); Figure S4: Neutralization antibody titers (ID_{50} values) against VLP pseudotyped with WT-, Delta-, and BA.1-spike variants in pseudotyped virus-neutralization assay (pVNA); Figure S5: Flow cytometry-based surrogate virus-neutralization assay; Figure S6: Representative flow plots of antibody-dependent NK cell activation assay (ADNKA).

Author Contributions: Conceptualization, V.B. and A.F.; methodology, T.B., N.C. and I.V.; validation, G.Y. and M.B.; formal analysis, M.S. and M.B.; investigation, M.S., M.B. and A.M.; resources, G.Y. and I.M.; data curation, G.Y. and I.M.; writing—original draft preparation, M.S.; writing—review and editing, A.F.; visualization, M.S.; supervision, A.F.; project administration, V.B. and A.F.; funding acquisition, V.B. and A.F. All authors have read and agreed to the published version of the manuscript.

Funding: This work was financially supported by the Ministry of Science and Higher Education of the Russian Federation (Agreement No. 075-15-2021-1086, contract No. RF----193021X0015, 15.ИП.21.0015).

Data Availability Statement: The data that support the findings of this study are available from the corresponding author upon reasonable request.

Acknowledgments: We thank Alexander Taranin and Andrey Gorchakov for the helpful discussion and providing reagents.

Conflicts of Interest: The authors declare no conflict of interest.

References

1. Khoury, D.S.; Cromer, D.; Reynaldi, A.; Schlub, T.E.; Wheatley, A.K.; Juno, J.A.; Subbarao, K.; Kent, S.J.; Triccas, J.A.; Davenport, M.P. Neutralizing Antibody Levels Are Highly Predictive of Immune Protection from Symptomatic SARS-CoV-2 Infection. *Nat. Med.* **2021**, *27*, 1205–1211. [CrossRef] [PubMed]
2. Tang, J.; Ravichandran, S.; Lee, Y.; Grubbs, G.; Coyle, E.M.; Klenow, L.; Genser, H.; Golding, H.; Khurana, S. Antibody Affinity Maturation and Plasma IgA Associate with Clinical Outcome in Hospitalized COVID-19 Patients. *Nat. Commun.* **2021**, *12*, 1221. [CrossRef]

3. Ariën, K.K.; Heyndrickx, L.; Michiels, J.; Vereecken, K.; Van Lent, K.; Coppens, S.; Willems, B.; Pannus, P.; Martens, G.A.; Van Esbroeck, M.; et al. Three Doses of BNT162b2 Vaccine Confer Neutralising Antibody Capacity against the SARS-CoV-2 Omicron Variant. *NPJ Vaccines* **2022**, *7*, 35. [CrossRef] [PubMed]

4. Becker, M.; Cossmann, A.; Lürken, K.; Junker, D.; Gruber, J.; Juengling, J.; Ramos, G.M.; Beigel, A.; Wrenger, E.; Lonnemann, G.; et al. Longitudinal Cellular and Humoral Immune Responses after Triple BNT162b2 and Fourth Full-Dose MRNA-1273 Vaccination in Haemodialysis Patients. *Front. Immunol.* **2022**, *13*, 1004045. [CrossRef]

5. Goel, R.R.; Apostolidis, S.A.; Painter, M.M.; Mathew, D.; Pattekar, A.; Kuthuru, O.; Gouma, S.; Hicks, P.; Meng, W.; Rosenfeld, A.M.; et al. Distinct Antibody and Memory B Cell Responses in SARS-CoV-2 Naïve and Recovered Individuals Following MRNA Vaccination. *Sci. Immunol.* **2021**, *6*, eabi6950. [CrossRef] [PubMed]

6. Reynolds, C.J.; Gibbons, J.M.; Pade, C.; Lin, K.-M.; Sandoval, D.M.; Pieper, F.; Butler, D.K.; Liu, S.; Otter, A.D.; Joy, G.; et al. Heterologous Infection and Vaccination Shapes Immunity against SARS-CoV-2 Variants. *Science* **2022**, *375*, 183–192. [CrossRef]

7. Carabelli, A.M.; Peacock, T.P.; Thorne, L.G.; Harvey, W.T.; Hughes, J.; COVID-19 Genomics UK Consortium; De Silva, T.I.; Peacock, S.J.; Barclay, W.S.; De Silva, T.I.; et al. SARS-CoV-2 Variant Biology: Immune Escape, Transmission and Fitness. *Nat. Rev. Microbiol.* **2023**, *21*, 162–177. [CrossRef]

8. Lusvarghi, S.; Pollett, S.D.; Neerukonda, S.N.; Wang, W.; Wang, R.; Vassell, R.; Epsi, N.J.; Fries, A.C.; Agan, B.K.; Lindholm, D.A.; et al. SARS-CoV-2 BA.1 Variant Is Neutralized by Vaccine Booster–Elicited Serum but Evades Most Convalescent Serum and Therapeutic Antibodies. *Sci. Transl. Med.* **2022**, *14*, eabn8543. [CrossRef]

9. Mahalingam, G.; Periyasami, Y.; Arjunan, P.; Subaschandrabose, R.K.; Mathivanan, T.V.; Mathew, R.S.; Devi, R.K.T.; Premkumar, P.S.; Muliyil, J.; Srivastava, A.; et al. Omicron Infection Increases IgG Binding to Spike Protein of Predecessor Variants. *J. Med. Virol.* **2023**, *95*, e28419. [CrossRef]

10. Akache, B.; Renner, T.M.; Stuible, M.; Rohani, N.; Cepero-Donates, Y.; Deschatelets, L.; Dudani, R.; Harrison, B.A.; Gervais, C.; Hill, J.J.; et al. Immunogenicity of SARS-CoV-2 Spike Antigens Derived from Beta & Delta Variants of Concern. *NPJ Vaccines* **2022**, *7*, 118. [CrossRef]

11. Matsvay, A.; Klink, G.V.; Safina, K.R.; Nabieva, E.; Garushyants, S.K.; Biba, D.; Bazykin, G.A.; Mikhaylov, I.M.; Say, A.V.; Zakamornaya, A.I.; et al. Genomic epidemiology of SARS-CoV-2 in Russia reveals recurring cross-border transmission throughout 2020. *PLoS ONE* **2023**, *18*, e0285664. [CrossRef]

12. Komissarov, A.B.; Safina, K.R.; Garushyants, S.K.; Fadeev, A.V.; Sergeeva, M.V.; Ivanova, A.A.; Danilenko, D.M.; Lioznov, D.; Shneider, O.V.; Shvyrev, N.; et al. Genomic Epidemiology of the Early Stages of the SARS-CoV-2 Outbreak in Russia. *Nat. Commun.* **2021**, *12*, 649. [CrossRef] [PubMed]

13. Gushchin, V.A.; Dolzhikova, I.V.; Shchetinin, A.M.; Odintsova, A.S.; Siniavin, A.E.; Nikiforova, M.A.; Pochtovyi, A.A.; Shidlovskaya, E.V.; Kuznetsova, N.A.; Burgasova, O.A.; et al. Neutralizing Activity of Sera from Sputnik V-Vaccinated People against Variants of Concern (VOC: B.1.1.7, B.1.351, P.1, B.1.617.2, B.1.617.3) and Moscow Endemic SARS-CoV-2 Variants. *Vaccines* **2021**, *9*, 779. [CrossRef]

14. Mitrofanova, L.B.; Makarov, I.A.; Gorshkov, A.N.; Runov, A.L.; Vonsky, M.S.; Pisareva, M.M.; Komissarov, A.B.; Makarova, T.A.; Li, Q.; Karonova, T.L.; et al. Comparative Study of the Myocardium of Patients from Four COVID-19 Waves. *Diagnostics* **2023**, *13*, 1645. [CrossRef]

15. Gorchakov, A.A.; Kulemzin, S.V.; Guselnikov, S.V.; Baranov, K.O.; Belovezhets, T.N.; Mechetina, L.V.; Volkova, O.Y.; Najakshin, A.M.; Chikaev, N.A.; Chikaev, A.N.; et al. Isolation of a Panel of Ultra-Potent Human Antibodies Neutralizing SARS-CoV-2 and Viral Variants of Concern. *Cell Discov.* **2021**, *7*, 96. [CrossRef] [PubMed]

16. Kolesov, D.E.; Sinegubova, M.V.; Dayanova, L.K.; Dolzhikova, I.V.; Vorobiev, I.I.; Orlova, N.A. Fast and Accurate Surrogate Virus Neutralization Test Based on Antibody-Mediated Blocking of the Interaction of ACE2 and SARS-CoV-2 Spike Protein RBD. *Diagnostics* **2022**, *12*, 393. [CrossRef] [PubMed]

17. Byazrova, M.G.; Kulemzin, S.V.; Astakhova, E.A.; Belovezhets, T.N.; Efimov, G.A.; Chikaev, A.N.; Kolotygin, I.O.; Gorchakov, A.A.; Taranin, A.V.; Filatov, A.V. Memory B Cells Induced by Sputnik V Vaccination Produce SARS-CoV-2 Neutralizing Antibodies Upon Ex Vivo Restimulation. *Front. Immunol.* **2022**, *13*, 840707. [CrossRef]

18. Tansey, W.P. Freeze-Thaw Lysis for Extraction of Proteins from Mammalian Cells. *Cold Spring Harb. Protoc.* **2006**, *2006*, pdb.prot4614. [CrossRef]

19. Astakhova, E.A.; Byazrova, M.G.; Yusubalieva, G.M.; Kulemzin, S.V.; Kruglova, N.A.; Prilipov, A.G.; Baklaushev, V.P.; Gorchakov, A.A.; Taranin, A.V.; Filatov, A.V. Functional Profiling of In Vitro Reactivated Memory B Cells Following Natural SARS-CoV-2 Infection and Gam-COVID-Vac Vaccination. *Cells* **2022**, *11*, 1991. [CrossRef]

20. Metsalu, T.; Vilo, J. ClustVis: A Web Tool for Visualizing Clustering of Multivariate Data Using Principal Component Analysis and Heatmap. *Nucleic Acids Res.* **2015**, *43*, W566–W570. [CrossRef] [PubMed]

21. Harvey, W.T.; Carabelli, A.M.; Jackson, B.; Gupta, R.K.; Thomson, E.C.; Harrison, E.M.; Ludden, C.; Reeve, R.; Rambaut, A.; COVID-19 Genomics UK (COG-UK) Consortium; et al. SARS-CoV-2 Variants, Spike Mutations and Immune Escape. *Nat. Rev. Microbiol.* **2021**, *19*, 409–424. [CrossRef] [PubMed]

22. Hagemann, K.; Riecken, K.; Jung, J.M.; Hildebrandt, H.; Menzel, S.; Bunders, M.J.; Fehse, B.; Koch-Nolte, F.; Heinrich, F.; Peine, S.; et al. Natural Killer Cell-mediated ADCC in SARS-CoV-2-infected Individuals and Vaccine Recipients. *Eur. J. Immunol.* **2022**, *52*, 1297–1307. [CrossRef] [PubMed]

23. Tong, X.; McNamara, R.P.; Avendaño, M.J.; Serrano, E.F.; García-Salum, T.; Pardo-Roa, C.; Bertera, H.L.; Chicz, T.M.; Levican, J.; Poblete, E.; et al. Waning and Boosting of Antibody Fc-Effector Functions upon SARS-CoV-2 Vaccination. *Nat. Commun.* **2023**, *14*, 4174. [CrossRef]
24. Pérez-Then, E.; Lucas, C.; Monteiro, V.S.; Miric, M.; Brache, V.; Cochon, L.; Vogels, C.B.F.; Malik, A.A.; De La Cruz, E.; Jorge, A.; et al. Neutralizing Antibodies against the SARS-CoV-2 Delta and Omicron Variants Following Heterologous CoronaVac plus BNT162b2 Booster Vaccination. *Nat. Med.* **2022**, *28*, 481–485. [CrossRef]
25. Scheaffer, S.M.; Lee, D.; Whitener, B.; Ying, B.; Wu, K.; Liang, C.-Y.; Jani, H.; Martin, P.; Amato, N.J.; Avena, L.E.; et al. Bivalent SARS-CoV-2 MRNA Vaccines Increase Breadth of Neutralization and Protect against the BA.5 Omicron Variant in Mice. *Nat. Med.* **2023**, *29*, 247–257. [CrossRef]
26. Khoury, D.S.; Docken, S.S.; Subbarao, K.; Kent, S.J.; Davenport, M.P.; Cromer, D. Predicting the Efficacy of Variant-Modified COVID-19 Vaccine Boosters. *Nat. Med.* **2023**, *29*, 574–578. [CrossRef]
27. Cox, M.; Peacock, T.P.; Harvey, W.T.; Hughes, J.; Wright, D.W.; COVID-19 Genomics UK (COG-UK) Consortium; Willett, B.J.; Thomson, E.; Gupta, R.K.; Peacock, S.J.; et al. SARS-CoV-2 variant evasion of monoclonal antibodies based on in vitro studies. *Nat. Rev. Microbiol.* **2023**, *21*, 112–124. [CrossRef]
28. Peng, L.; Renauer, P.A.; Ökten, A.; Fang, Z.; Park, J.J.; Zhou, X.; Lin, Q.; Dong, M.B.; Filler, R.; Xiong, Q.; et al. Variant-Specific Vaccination Induces Systems Immune Responses and Potent in Vivo Protection against SARS-CoV-2. *Cell Rep. Med.* **2022**, *3*, 100634. [CrossRef]
29. Johari, Y.B.; Jaffé, S.R.P.; Scarrott, J.M.; Johnson, A.O.; Mozzanino, T.; Pohle, T.H.; Maisuria, S.; Bhayat-Cammack, A.; Lambiase, G.; Brown, A.J.; et al. Production of Trimeric SARS-CoV-2 Spike Protein by CHO Cells for Serological COVID-19 Testing. *Biotechnol. Bioeng.* **2021**, *118*, 1013–1021. [CrossRef] [PubMed]
30. Riley, T.P.; Chou, H.-T.; Hu, R.; Bzymek, K.P.; Correia, A.R.; Partin, A.C.; Li, D.; Gong, D.; Wang, Z.; Yu, X.; et al. Enhancing the Prefusion Conformational Stability of SARS-CoV-2 Spike Protein Through Structure-Guided Design. *Front. Immunol.* **2021**, *12*, 660198. [CrossRef]
31. Wrapp, D.; Wang, N.; Corbett, K.S.; Goldsmith, J.A.; Hsieh, C.-L.; Abiona, O.; Graham, B.S.; McLellan, J.S. Cryo-EM Structure of the 2019-NCoV Spike in the Prefusion Conformation. *Science* **2020**, *367*, 1260–1263. [CrossRef] [PubMed]
32. Hsieh, C.-L.; Goldsmith, J.A.; Schaub, J.M.; DiVenere, A.M.; Kuo, H.-C.; Javanmardi, K.; Le, K.C.; Wrapp, D.; Lee, A.G.; Liu, Y.; et al. Structure-Based Design of Prefusion-Stabilized SARS-CoV-2 Spikes. *Science* **2020**, *369*, 1501–1505. [CrossRef]
33. Akache, B.; Renner, T.M.; Tran, A.; Deschatelets, L.; Dudani, R.; Harrison, B.A.; Duque, D.; Haukenfrers, J.; Rossotti, M.A.; Gaudreault, F.; et al. Immunogenic and Efficacious SARS-CoV-2 Vaccine Based on Resistin-Trimerized Spike Antigen SmT1 and SLA Archaeosome Adjuvant. *Sci. Rep.* **2021**, *11*, 21849. [CrossRef] [PubMed]
34. Tan, C.W.; Chia, W.N.; Qin, X.; Liu, P.; Chen, M.I.-C.; Tiu, C.; Hu, Z.; Chen, V.C.-W.; Young, B.E.; Sia, W.R.; et al. A SARS-CoV-2 Surrogate Virus Neutralization Test Based on Antibody-Mediated Blockage of ACE2–Spike Protein–Protein Interaction. *Nat. Biotechnol.* **2020**, *38*, 1073–1078. [CrossRef] [PubMed]

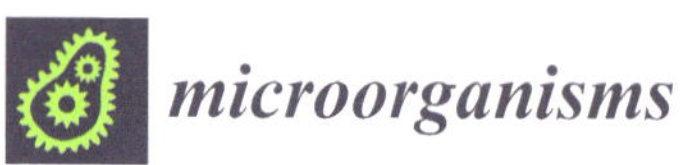

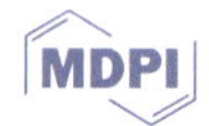

Communication

Diagnosis and Outcomes of Fungal Co-Infections in COVID-19 Infections: A Retrospective Study

Richard Swaney [1], Rutendo Jokomo-Nyakabau [2], Anny A. N. Nguyen [3], Dorothy Kenny [3], Paul G. Millner [2], Mohammad Selim [2], Christopher J. Destache [4,5] and Manasa Velagapudi [5,*]

[1] Internal Medicine/Infectious Diseases, Creighton University School of Medicine, Omaha, NE 68178, USA; richardswaney@creighton.edu

[2] Internal Medicine, Creighton University School of Medicine, Omaha, NE 68178, USA; rutendojokomonyakabau@creighton.edu (R.J.-N.); paulmillner@creighton.edu (P.G.M.); mohammadselim@creighton.edu (M.S.)

[3] School of Medicine, Creighton University, Omaha, NE 68178, USA; annynguyen@creighton.edu (A.A.N.N.)

[4] School of Pharmacy & Health Professions, Creighton University, Omaha, NE 68178, USA; chrisdestache@creighton.edu

[5] Division of Infectious Diseases, Catholic Health Initiative (CHI) Health Creighton University Medical Center, Omaha, NE 68178, USA

* Correspondence: manasavelagapudi@creighton.edu

Abstract: The SARS-CoV-2 pandemic has resulted in a public health emergency with unique complications such as the development of fungal co-infections. The diagnosis of fungal infections can be challenging due to confounding imaging studies and difficulty obtaining histopathology. In this retrospective study, 173 patients with COVID-19 receiving antifungal therapy due to concern for fungal co-infection were evaluated. Patient characteristics, clinical outcomes, and the utility of fungal biomarkers were then evaluated for continuation of antifungal therapy. Data were collected from the electronic health record (EPIC) and analyzed using SPSS (version. 28, IBM, Inc., Armonk, NY, USA) Data are presented as mean ± SD or percentages. A total of 56 COVID-19 patients were diagnosed with fungal co-infection and 117 COVID-19 + patients had no fungal infection. Significantly fewer female patients were in the fungal+ group compared to COVID-19 control patients (29% in fungal+ compared to 51% in controls $p = 0.005$). Fungal diagnostics were all significantly higher in fungal+ patients. These include 1,4-beta-D-glucan (BDG), fungal culture, and bronchoalveolar lavage galactomannan (BAL GM). Intensive care unit hospitalization, mechanical ventilation, and mortality in fungal+ patients with COVID-19 were significantly higher than in control patients. Finally, significantly more fungal+ patients received voriconazole, isavuconazonium, or amphotericin B therapies, whereas control patients received significantly more short-course fluconazole. COVID-19+ patients with fungal co-infection were significantly more likely to be in the ICU and mechanically ventilated, and they result in higher mortality compared to control COVID-19 patients. The use of fungal diagnostics markers were helpful for diagnosis.

Keywords: COVID-19; diagnosis; fungal infection; outcome

Citation: Swaney, R.; Jokomo-Nyakabau, R.; Nguyen, A.A.N.; Kenny, D.; Millner, P.G.; Selim, M.; Destache, C.J.; Velagapudi, M. Diagnosis and Outcomes of Fungal Co-Infections in COVID-19 Infections: A Retrospective Study. *Microorganisms* **2023**, *11*, 2326. https://doi.org/10.3390/microorganisms11092326

Academic Editor: Qibin Geng

Received: 23 August 2023
Revised: 9 September 2023
Accepted: 13 September 2023
Published: 15 September 2023

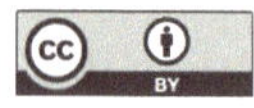

1. Introduction

The SARS-CoV-2 pandemic has resulted in a public health emergency of global concern with a multitude of complications and morbidities. While the effects and consequences of bacterial and viral co-infections have been reported extensively in the literature, there is less understanding of fungal co-infections in patients with COVID-19 [1,2]. The most common fungal infection appears to be COVID-19-associated pulmonary aspergillosis (CAPA), but there have been reports of other fungal co-infections, including, but not limited to, invasive candidiasis, mucormycosis, pneumocystis pneumonia, histoplasmosis, and cryptococcosis [3]. The reported rate of these infections varies greatly between different studies. For CAPA, the prevalence may range anywhere from 3 to 33%; a recent multicenter study reported a prevalence ranging from 1.7 to 26.8% in ICU patients across all centers studied. In comparison, invasive pulmonary aspergillosis was found in up to 15% of clinical and autopsy studies of immunocompetent patients who developed acute respiratory distress syndrome (ARDS) [4]. The incidence of candidemia in COVID-19 patients has been reported as being between 5 and 9% [5,6]. A study in Egypt reported an incidence rate of 7.63% for COVID-19-associated mucormycosis, although incidence is thought to be significantly higher in India [7,8]. Secondary fungal infections are speculated to occur due to the direct impact of SARS-CoV-2 in decreasing the immune response, as well as due to sepsis disrupting the mucosal barriers and sequelae of common COVID-19 treatments such as corticosteroids and prolonged mechanical ventilation [9]. Mortality has been reported to be higher in patients with fungal co-infections such as CAPA, indicating the importance of prompt diagnosis and treatment [10]. One study reported that mortality risk in CAPA patients was almost twice that of non-CAPA patients in the ICU setting [3].

The diagnosis of COVID-19 fungal co-infections can be challenging, as common risk factors seen with invasive fungal disease such as neutropenia, immunosuppression, or malignancy may be absent [11]. Another challenge is the lack of a standardized diagnostic algorithm for co-fungal infections. For example, while CAPA is one of the more well-studied infections, there is still no definitive approach to diagnosing CAPA, and most of the criteria are still speculative [12]. For CAPA, diagnosis is recommended using the presence of clinical features in combination with mycological lab evidence, including aspergillus growth in fungal culture, positive PCR, beta-D-glucan (BDG), and serum or bronchoalveolar lavage (BAL), for detection of *Aspergillus* galactomannan (GM). Bronchoscopy is needed for definitive diagnosis of CAPA; however, concerns of virus aerosolization limited the use of this procedure during the early stages of the pandemic [13]. Although tissue biopsy is considered the gold standard for definitive diagnosis of fungal infection, it is less commonly performed due to the risk of patient complications [10] Sputum, BAL, or tracheal aspirate cultures can be utilized, but carry risks of contamination by upper respiratory flora and possible false positivity [14,15].

Fungal biomarkers such as serum and BAL GM and serum BDG are commonly used but present challenges as well. For instance, serum and BAL GM have shown reduced sensitivities when applied to non-neutropenic COVID-19 patients [13], with one study indicating a sensitivity of 46.9% and 54.5% for serum and BAL GM, respectively [16]. Another problem with BAL GM is its inability to distinguish between *Aspergillus* colonization and actual infection. Serum BDG might exhibit higher sensitivity than GM, but it lacks specificity as it rises in various fungal infections and fails to identify the responsible organisms [17]. These observations underscore the necessity for more comprehensive research and assessment of the diagnostic capabilities of fungal biomarkers in detecting fungal co-infections in COVID-19 patients.

In this study, the effectiveness of fungal biomarkers such as fungal culture, serum BDG, and serum and BAL GM in diagnosing fungal co-infections in COVID-19 patients was assessed along the clinical outcomes of COVID-19 patients with fungal co-infections.

2. Methods

The study was a retrospective, observational study examining patients admitted to hospital with COVID-19 diagnosis who received antifungal therapy. The study population were patients admitted to CHI Health Nebraska hospital centers (inpatient hospital facilities located in Omaha, NE, USA; Council Bluffs, IA, USA; Lincoln, NE, USA; and Grand Island, NE, USA) from June 2020 to December 2021. Inclusion criteria included patients olds than 19 years of age with positive COVID-19 diagnosis through PCR (polymerase chain reaction) testing who received antifungal agents of either fluconazole, voriconazole, isavuconazonium, amphotericin B, micafungin, or itraconazole during their hospitalization. Data were then divided into COVID-19 patients with diagnostic evidence for development of a fungal infection (fungal+) and COVID-19 patients without diagnostic/clinical evidence for fungal infection (controls). Patients were categorized as fungal+ if they had positive fungal biomarker testing, (BDG, *cryptococcus* antigen, urine, and serum *histoplasma* antigen, *histoplasma* antibody, BAL *Aspergillus* GM or positive blood, sputum, or BAL cultures for fungal elements) and received continued treatment for invasive fungal disease after diagnosis. Patients with sputum or BAL cultures positive for *Candida* species were excluded from the positive fungal culture group. Control patients were categorized as those with COVID-19 whose empiric antifungal therapy was discontinued based on negative testing, sputum, BAL cultures positive for candida species only, or lack of clinical parameters for fungal disease.

Patient data were collected from the electronic medical record (EPIC),including demographics (age, gender, and race (Hispanic, African American, White, or Asian)), comorbidities (BMI, history of malignancy, history of solid organ transplant, high dose corticosteroid use 4 weeks prior to admission, use of chronic immunosuppressant therapy, and HIV status), length of hospitalization, need for ICU admission, need for mechanical intubation, need for extracorporeal membrane oxygenation (ECMO), COVID-19 treatment (corticosteroids, remdesivir, tocilizumab, or barcitinib), fungal treatment (voriconazole, posaconazole, isavuconazonium, amphotericin B, fluconazole, micafungin, itraconazole or other antifungal therapy). Patient outcome (treated or expired) was also collected.

Data were collected in Excel and analyzed using SPSS (ver. 28, IBM, Inc., Armonk, NY, USA).

Descriptive data were analyzed using Chi-square or Fisher's exact test. Continuous data were analyzed with unpaired Student t-test. *Apriori* level of significance was $p \leq 0.05$.

3. Results

A total of 177 patients were identified as having a positive COVID-19 diagnosis and use of antifungal therapy during their hospitalization. Four patients were identified as having fungal infections prior to hospitalization for COVID and were thus excluded, resulting in 173 patients in the study. Based on positive fungal testing in which the primary team determined antifungal treatment was necessary, 56 patients were categorized in the fungal+ group. Those categorized as the control group, whose antifungal therapy was discontinued either from negative fungal testing or lack of physician clinical suspicion, included 117 patients.

Table 1 lists relevant demographic data between the two groups. Significantly fewer female patients were in the fungal+ group compared to COVID-19+ control patients (29% in fungal+ compared to 51% in control, $p = 0.005$); however, age, BMI, race, and history of malignancy, neutropenia, or recent immunosuppression use were not significant between the two groups.

Table 1. Study demographics.

Variable Mean ± SD or No (%)	Controls (N = 117)	Fungal+ (N = 56)	*p*-Value
Age (yrs)	58.7 ± 14.9	62.6 ± 11.5	NS
BMI (m²/kg)	33.9 ± 11.2	33.2 ± 7.4	NS
Females	60 (51)	16 (29)	0.005
Race			NS
Hispanic	15 (13)	4 (7)	NS
Black	11 (9)	3 (5)	NS
White	87 (74)	43 (77)	NS
Asian	1 (1)	0 (0)	NS
Other	2 (2)	3 (5)	NS

Table 1. *Cont.*

Variable Mean ± SD or No (%)	Controls (N = 117)	Fungal+ (N = 56)	*p*-Value
Cancer history	12 (10)	4 (7)	NS
Neutropenia	2 (1)	1 (2)	NS
Immunosuppressive therapy	10 (9)	6 (11)	NS

BMI = body mass index; NS = not significant; SD = standard deviation.

Table 2 outlines the comparison between the fungal+ group and the control group in hospital management and outcomes. Significantly more fungal+ COVID-19 patients were hospitalized in the intensive care unit compared to control patients (95% in fungal+ compared to 68% in control, $p < 0.001$). Significantly more fungal+ patients were mechanically ventilated compared to control patients (91% compared to 54%, $p < 0.001$). The duration of mechanical ventilation averaged 4.5 days longer in fungal+ patients but did not reach statistical significance. Significantly more fungal+ patients underwent bronchoscopy compared to control patients (64% compared to 34%, $p < 0.001$). Finally, the mortality rate in fungal+ patients with COVID-19 was significantly higher (63%) compared to the control COVID-19 patients (42%, $p = 0.010$). There were five control patients and three fungal+ patients who received ECMO therapy. Treatment of COVID-19 with remdesivir and immune modulators were not significantly different between the two groups of patients; however, all fungal+ patients with COVID-19 received corticosteroids compared to 89% in the control group, $p = 0.01$. Significantly more fungal+ patients received concurrent antimicrobial therapy compared to control patients (98% in fungal+ compared to 83% in control, $p = 0.002$).

Table 2. Comparison of study results.

Variable Mean ± SD or No (%)	Controls (N = 117)	Fungal+ (N = 56)	*p*-Value
ICU bed	80 (68)	53 (95)	<0.001
Mechanical ventilation	63 (54)	51 (91)	<0.001
Bronchoscopy procedure	42 (34)	36 (64)	<0.001
Mortality rate	51 (42)	35 (63)	0.010
Antimicrobial therapy	97 (83)	55 (98)	0.002
Corticosteroid use	105 (89)	56 (100)	0.01
Remdesivir use	87 (74)	48 (86)	NS
Tocilizumab use	24 (21)	18 (32)	NS
Baricitinib use	28 (24)	10 (18)	NS
Fungal diagnostics			
Beta-D-glucan (BDG)	7 (6)	19 (34)	<0.001
Culture	3 (6)	41 (73)	<0.001
BAL Galactomannan (GM)	1 (2)	28 (50)	<0.001
Fungal treatment			
Voriconazole	35 (30)	45 (80)	<0.001
Isuvoconazole	1 (1)	5 (9)	<0.007
Amphotericin B	1 (1)	5 (9)	<0.007
Fluconazole	59 (50)	8 (14)	<0.001
Micafungin	27 (23)	10 (18)	NS
Others	15 (13)	5 (9)	NS

Table 2. *Cont.*

Variable Mean ± SD or No (%)	Controls (N = 117)	Fungal+ (N = 56)	*p*-Value
CAPA diagnosed	0 (0)	28 (50)	<0.001
Length of hospitalization (d)	25.6 ± 20.1	27 ± 17.9	NS

NS = not significant; CAPA = COVID-19-associated pulmonary aspergillosis; BAL = bronchoalveolar lavage; ICU = intensive care unit.

Fungal diagnostics were all significantly higher in fungal+ patients. These include BDG, fungal culture and BAL GM. Fungus species isolated from positive cultures are available in Table 3.

Table 3. Fungal culture identification.

Fungal Pathogen Cultured	No. (%)
Aspergillus species	27 (65%)
Candida species on blood culture	9 (21%)
Cryptococcus	2 (1%)
Fusarium	1 (<1%)
Histoplasmosis	1 (<1%)
Other (mold not identified)	1 (<1%)

Fungal culture positivity was significantly different between the fungal+ and control groups. Of the patients in the fungal+ group with positive fungal cultures (73%), aspergillus was the most frequently isolated organism (66%), followed by *Candida* blood stream infections (22%). *Cryptococcus neoformans* was isolated in two cases, while *Histoplasma* and *Fusarium* was isolated in one case each. In one instance, a mold was isolated which was not able to be further identified. Other diagnostic tests, including *cryptococcal* antigen, serum and urinary *histoplasma* antigen, and *histoplasma* antibody, were not performed in both groups of COVID-19 patients.

Fungal+ patients received significantly more voriconazole, isavuconazonium, or amphotericin B therapies, whereas control patients received significantly more fluconazole. Significantly more fungal+ patients were diagnosed with CAPA (50%), whereas none of the control patients received this diagnosis, $p < 0.001$. Finally, length of hospitalization averaged 27 days in fungal+ patients and was not different from COVID-19 patients without fungal infections averaging 25 days.

4. Discussion

According to the existing literature, the simultaneous presence of fungal co-infection in individuals with COVID-19 poses a significant danger, particularly for those with preexisting conditions. This can result in the worsening of complications and ultimately lead to a higher mortality rate [18]. The virus is known to cause immune dysregulation, an overproduction of pro-inflammatory cytokines, a weakened cell-mediated immunity, and a decrease in CD4 and CD8+ T-cells, all of which can increase the likelihood of invasive fungal infections [19–21]. Fungal co-infections in patients with COVID-19 have non-specific imaging findings. These patients are at high risk of progression to ARDS and bacterial infections that can mimic fungal infections [22], making the diagnosis challenging.

Here, 56 patients who were treated with COVID-19 and fungal co-infections were compared with patients who did not have a fungal co-infection. This study used a variety of fungal biomarkers, including serum BDG and BAL GM, and respiratory cultures to help confirm fungal infections in suspected populations with COVID-19 infections. While serum BDG is a non-specific test with high negative predictive value, the risk of false positivity can deter physicians from using it to accurately diagnose and treat patients for fungal co-infections [23]. Our study demonstrated a statistically significant correlation in elevated BDG assays and the decision to treat patients for invasive fungal infections. In the fungal+ group, however, BDG was not the only positive fungal biomarker when deciding to treat fungal infections. All patients in the fungal+ group with positive BDG also had either a BAL GM or were fungal culture-positive before deciding to continue treatment. On the other hand, the control group had seven patients with positive BDG assay without any other positive biomarkers. In these patients, the decision was made to stop antifungal therapy. This study supports the role of BDG as an adjunctive test for determining fungal co-infection in COVID-19 patients.

While diagnosis of confirmed fungal infections requires histopathological diagnosis, this was not performed in this study and is not frequently used in real-world settings. Fungal cultures are a strong alternative to histopathological testing and allow for less invasive bronchoscopic procedures with less risk of complications. Our study demonstrated that positive fungal cultures allowed physicians to confidently diagnosis and treat patients of COVID-19 with fungal co-infections. Furthermore, the fungal+ group had positive fungal cultures in addition to the fungal biomarkers. Using these tests together allowed for a higher degree of suspicion of true infection, i.e., rather than fungal culture alone, in determining true infection versus colonization/false positivity when treating the patient group. This study highlights the importance of obtaining fungal culture to guiding the decision to treat patients with fungal co-infections.

Of the patients in the fungal+ group with positive fungal cultures, *Aspergillus* was the most frequently isolated organism (n = 27), followed by *Candida* fungemia (n = 9). This study is consistent with other studies which outline aspergillosis as the most common fungal co-infection in COVID-19 infections, followed by candidemia. Of note, two cases of identified *Cryptococcal* fungemia were found. The association between COVID-19 infections and *Cryptococcal* fungemia has not been widely reported and warrants future studies. Although COVID-19-associated mucormycosis have been identified in the literature, none were identified on our retrospective study.

First line treatment for invasive aspergillosis infections includes voriconazole or isavuconazonium. Primary treatment for invasive candidemia includes fluconazole and echinocandins. Amphotericin B is usually reserved for severe infections refractory to primary treatments due to the severe side-effect profile. Comparison of antifungal agents used in the fungal+ group versus the control group demonstrated a significantly increased use of voriconazole, isavuconazonium, and amphotericin B in the fungal+ group and a significantly increased use of fluconazole for the control group. This discrepancy in antifungal agents used between groups could be due to concern for the adverse effects of voriconazole and amphotericin B, in which case their use would be limited in patients with confirmed diagnosis only through positive cultures, or in patients with higher degrees of suspicion. Conversely, the increased use of fluconazole may be due to lower concern for infection, less severe adverse effects, and their potential use for non-invasive fungal infections such as vulvovaginal candidiasis or oral thrush.

Immune modulating therapy is an important risk factor in the development of fungal infections. Corticosteroids, which are recommended in COVID-19 treatment, pose a risk of immunosuppression and the development of fungal infections. Previous studies have identified corticosteroid use in patients with severe influenza infections as a risk for the development of invasive pulmonary aspergillosis [24]. Furthermore, immunomodulators are recommended in COVID-19 treatment to help reduce the hyperactive inflammatory response [25]. The risk of these immunomodulators for invasive fungal infections is of interest. Our study looked at the use of corticosteroids, baricitinib, and tocilizumab in patients treated with COVID-19 and found no statistically significant increase in risk with respect to positive fungal testing and treatment for COVID-19 fungal co-infection.

A limitation of our study was its lack of insight into the doses and duration of these immunosuppressive medications. Further research into the dosing of corticosteroids and the risk of developing COVID-19 fungal co-infections could be a useful area of research in the future.

Another limitation was the retrospective nature of the study. Further prospective studies should be performed to help remove sampling bias.

5. Conclusions

Prompt recognition with the use of fungal biomarkers and treatments for fungal co-infection with COVID19 is key to reducing delays in diagnosis and treatment to prevent complications and death from these infections. In cases of COVID-19 and fungal co-infection, the likelihood of positive fungal biomarkers such as BDG and GM was higher. Although the use of these biomarkers for diagnosis was not common among COVID-positive patients, those who did undergo testing were found to have a greater chance of testing positive for fungal infection. In such cases, fungal culture was often used to prompt antifungal therapy, with voriconazole treatment being the most common course of action.

Author Contributions: M.V., C.J.D., R.S., P.G.M., M.S. and R.J.-N.: Conceptualization, Methodology, Writing—Original Draft; A.A.N.N., D.K., R.S., C.J.D., M.V. and R.J.-N.: Data Curation, Writing; M.V., C.J.D. and R.S.: Supervision, Project Administration. All authors have read and agreed to the published version of the manuscript.

Funding: This research received no external funding.

Institutional Review Board Statement: The study was conducted in accordance with the Declaration of Helsinki and approved by the In-stitutional Review Board of Creighton University on 18 October 2021 (IRB #2002584).

Informed Consent Statement: Not applicable.

Data Availability Statement: To interested parties upon request.

Conflicts of Interest: The authors declare no conflict of interest.

References

1. Chiurlo, M.; Mastrangelo, A.; Ripa, M.; Scarpellini, P. Invasive Fungal Infections in Patients with COVID-19: A Review on Pathogenesis, Epidemiology, Clinical Features, Treatment, and Outcomes. *New Microbiol.* **2021**, *44*, 71–83. [PubMed]
2. Lai, C.C.; Yu, W.L. COVID-19 Associated with Pulmonary Aspergillosis: A Literature Review. *J. Microbiol. Immunol. Infect.* **2021**, *54*, 46–53. [CrossRef]
3. Prattes, J.; Wauters, J.; Giacobbe, D.R.; Salmanton-García, J.; Maertens, J.; Bourgeois, M.; Reynders, M.; Rutsaert, L.; Van Regenmortel, N.; Lormans, P.; et al. Risk Factors and Outcome of Pulmonary Aspergillosis in Critically Ill Coronavirus Disease 2019 Patients—A Multinational Observational Study by the European Confederation of Medical Mycology. *Clin. Microbiol. Infect.* **2022**, *28*, 580–587. [CrossRef] [PubMed]
4. Tudesq, J.J.; Peyrony, O.; Lemiale, V.; Azoulay, E. Invasive Pulmonary Aspergillosis in Nonimmunocompromised Hosts. *Semin. Respir. Crit. Care Med.* **2019**, *40*, 540–547. [CrossRef]
5. Bishburg, E.; Okoh, A.; Nagarakanti, S.R.; Lindner, M.; Migliore, C.; Patel, P. Fungemia in COVID-19 ICU Patients, a Single Medical Center Experience. *J. Med. Virol.* **2021**, *93*, 2810–2814. [CrossRef]
6. Blaize, M.; Raoelina, A.; Kornblum, D.; Kamus, L.; Lampros, A.; Berger, M.; Demeret, S.; Constantin, J.M.; Monsel, A.; Mayaux, J.; et al. Occurrence of Candidemia in Patients with COVID-19 Admitted to Five ICUs in France. *J. Fungi* **2022**, *8*, 678. [CrossRef] [PubMed]
7. Farghly Youssif, S.; Abdelrady, M.M.; Thabet, A.A.; Abdelhamed, M.A.; Gad, M.O.A.; Abu-Elfatth, A.M.; Saied, G.M.; Goda, I.; Algammal, A.M.; Batiha, G.E.S.; et al. COVID-19 Associated Mucormycosis in Assiut University Hospitals: A Multidisciplinary Dilemma. *Sci. Rep.* **2022**, *12*, 10494. [CrossRef]
8. Singh, A.K.; Singh, R.; Joshi, S.R.; Misra, A. Mucormycosis in COVID-19: A Systematic Review of Cases Reported Worldwide and in India. Diabetes Metab. *Syndr. Clin. Res. Rev.* **2021**, *15*, 102146. [CrossRef]
9. Oh, K.H.; Lee, S.H. COVID-19 and Fungal Diseases. *Antibiotics* **2022**, *11*, 803. [CrossRef]
10. Koehler, P.; Bassetti, M.; Chakrabarti, A.; Chen, S.C.; Colombo, A.L.; Hoenigl, M.; Klimko, N.; Lass-Flörl, C.; Oladele, R.O.; Vinh, D.C.; et al. Defining and Managing COVID-19-Associated Pulmonary Aspergillosis: The 2020 ECMM/ISHAM Consensus Criteria for Research and Clinical Guidance. *Lancet Infect. Dis.* **2021**, *21*, e149–e162. [CrossRef]
11. Paramythiotou, E.; Dimopoulos, G.; Koliakos, N.; Siopi, M.; Vourli, S.; Pournaras, S.; Meletiadis, J. Epidemiology and Incidence of COVID-19-Associated Pulmonary Aspergillosis (CAPA) in a Greek Tertiary Care Academic Reference Hospital. *Infect. Dis. Ther.* **2021**, *10*, 1779–1792. [CrossRef] [PubMed]

12. Lamoth, F. Invasive Aspergillosis in Coronavirus Disease 2019: A Practical Approach for Clinicians. *Curr. Opin. Infect. Dis.* **2022**, *35*, 163–169. [CrossRef] [PubMed]
13. Shishido, A.A.; Mathew, M.; Baddley, J.W. Overview of COVID-19-Associated Invasive Fungal Infection. *Curr. Fungal Infect. Rep.* **2022**, *16*, 87–97. [CrossRef] [PubMed]
14. Dimopoulos, G.; Almyroudi, M.P.; Myrianthefs, P.; Rello, J. COVID-19-Associated Pulmonary Aspergillosis (CAPA). *J. Intensive Med.* **2021**, *1*, 71–80. [CrossRef] [PubMed]
15. Baddley, J.W.; Thompson, G.R.; Chen, S.C.A.; White, P.L.; Johnson, M.D.; Nguyen, M.H.; Schwartz, I.S.; Spec, A.; Ostrosky-Zeichner, L.; Jackson, B.R.; et al. Coronavirus Disease 2019-Associated Invasive Fungal Infection. *Open Forum Infect. Dis.* **2021**, *8*, ofab510. [CrossRef]
16. Ghazanfari, M.; Yazdani Charati, J.; Davoodi, L.; Arastehfar, A.; Moazeni, M.; Abastabar, M.; Haghani, I.; Mayahi, S.; Hoenigl, M.; Pan, W.; et al. Comparative Analysis of Galactomannan Lateral Flow Assay, Galactomannan Enzyme Immunoassay and BAL Culture for Diagnosis of COVID-19-Associated Pulmonary Aspergillosis. *Mycoses* **2022**, *65*, 960–968. [CrossRef]
17. Fekkar, A.; Lampros, A.; Mayaux, J.; Poignon, C.; Demeret, S.; Constantin, J.M.; Marcelin, A.G.; Monsel, A.; Luyt, C.E.; Blaize, M.; et al. Occurrence of Invasive Pulmonary Fungal Infections in Patients with Severe COVID-19 Admitted to the ICU. *Am. J. Respir. Crit. Care Med.* **2021**, *203*, 307–317. [CrossRef]
18. Seyedjavadi, S.S.; Bagheri, P.; Nasiri, M.J.; Razzaghi-Abyaneh, M.; Goudarzi, M. Fungal Infection in Co-infected Patients With COVID-19: An Overview of Case Reports/Case Series and Systematic Review. *Front. Microbiol.* **2022**, *13*, 888452. [CrossRef]
19. Hughes, S.; Troise, O.; Donaldson, H.; Mughal, N.; Moore, L.S. Bacterial and Fungal Coinfection Among Hospitalized Patients with COVID-19: A Retrospective Cohort Study in a UK Secondary-Care Setting. *Clin. Microbiol. Infect.* **2020**, *26*, 1395–1399. [CrossRef]
20. Farhan, C.; Sohail, M.U.; Abdelhafez, I.; Salman, S.; Attique, Z.; Kamareddine, L.; Al-Asmakh, M. SARS-CoV-2 and Immune-Microbiome Interactions: Lessons from Respiratory Viral Infections. *Int. J. Infect. Dis.* **2021**, *105*, 540–550. [CrossRef]
21. Rawson, T.M.; Moore, L.S.; Zhu, N.; Ranganathan, N.; Skolimowska, K.; Gilchrist, M.; Satta, G.; Cooke, G.; Holmes, A. Bacterial and Fungal Coinfection in Individuals with Coronavirus: A Rapid Review to Support COVID-19 Antimicrobial Prescribing. *Clin. Infect. Dis.* **2020**, *71*, 2459–2468. [CrossRef] [PubMed]
22. Kato, S.; Ishiwata, Y.; Aoki, R.; Iwasawa, T.; Hagiwara, E.; Ogura, T.; Utsunomiya, D. Imaging of COVID-19: An Update of Current Evidence. *Diagn. Interv. Imaging* **2021**, *102*, 493–500. [CrossRef] [PubMed]
23. Finkelman, M.A. Specificity Influences in $(1{\rightarrow}3)$-β-d-Glucan-Supported Diagnosis of Invasive Fungal Disease. *J. Fungi* **2020**, *7*, 14. [CrossRef] [PubMed]
24. Huang, L.; Zhang, N.; Huang, X.; Xiong, S.; Feng, Y.; Zhang, Y. Invasive Pulmonary Aspergillosis in Patients with Influenza Infection: A Retrospective Study and Review of the Literature. *Clin. Resp. J.* **2019**, *13*, 202–211. [CrossRef] [PubMed]
25. Montazersaheb, S.; Hosseiniyan Khatibi, S.M.; Hejazi, M.S.; Tarhriz, V.; Farjami, A.; Ghasemian Sorbeni, F.; Farahzadi, R.; Ghasemnejad, T. COVID-19 Infection: An Overview on Cytokine Storm and Related Interventions. *Virol. J.* **2022**, *19*, 92. [CrossRef]

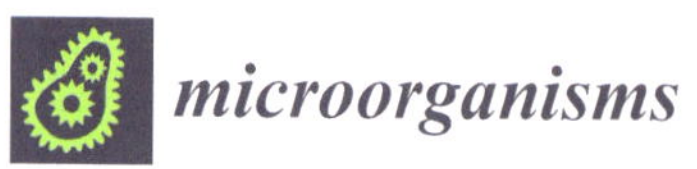

microorganisms

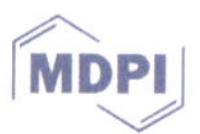

Article

Exploring the Synergistic Potential of Radiomics and Laboratory Biomarkers for Enhanced Identification of Vulnerable COVID-19 Patients

Catharina Gerhards [1,*], Verena Haselmann [1], Samuel F. Schaible [2], Volker Ast [1], Maximilian Kittel [1], Manfred Thiel [3], Alexander Hertel [2], Stefan O. Schoenberg [2], Michael Neumaier [1,†] and Matthias F. Froelich [2,†]

[1] Institute for Clinical Chemistry, Medical Faculty Mannheim of the University of Heidelberg, Theodor Kutzer Ufer 1-3, 68167 Mannheim, Germany

[2] Department of Radiology and Nuclear Medicine, University Medical Center Mannheim, Medical Faculty Mannheim of the University of Heidelberg, Theodor-Kutzer-Ufer 1-3, 68167 Mannheim, Germany

[3] Department of Anaesthesiology and Surgical Intensive Care Medicine, Medical Faculty Mannheim of the University of Heidelberg, Theodor-Kutzer-Ufer 1-3, 68167 Mannheim, Germany

[*] Correspondence: catharina.gerhards@umm.de; Tel.: +49-621-383-8414; Fax: +49-621-383-1946

[†] These authors contributed equally to this work.

Abstract: Background: Severe courses and high hospitalization rates were ubiquitous during the first pandemic SARS-CoV-2 waves. Thus, we aimed to examine whether integrative diagnostics may aid in identifying vulnerable patients using crucial data and materials obtained from COVID-19 patients hospitalized between 2020 and 2021 ($n = 52$). Accordingly, we investigated the potential of laboratory biomarkers, specifically the dynamic cell decay marker cell-free DNA and radiomics features extracted from chest CT. Methods: Separate forward and backward feature selection was conducted for linear regression with the Intensive-Care-Unit (ICU) period as the initial target. Three-fold cross-validation was performed, and collinear parameters were reduced. The model was adapted to a logistic regression approach and verified in a validation naïve subset to avoid overfitting. Results: The adapted integrated model classifying patients into "ICU/no ICU demand" comprises six radiomics and seven laboratory biomarkers. The models' accuracy was 0.54 for radiomics, 0.47 for cfDNA, 0.74 for routine laboratory, and 0.87 for the combined model with an AUC of 0.91. Conclusion: The combined model performed superior to the individual models. Thus, integrating radiomics and laboratory data shows synergistic potential to aid clinic decision-making in COVID-19 patients. Under the need for evaluation in larger cohorts, including patients with other SARS-CoV-2 variants, the identified parameters might contribute to the triage of COVID-19 patients.

Keywords: COVID-19; SARS-CoV-2; coronavirus infection; integrative medicine; intensive care units; thoracic radiography; cell-free nucleic acid; algorithms

Citation: Gerhards, C.; Haselmann, V.; Schaible, S.F.; Ast, V.; Kittel, M.; Thiel, M.; Hertel, A.; Schoenberg, S.O.; Neumaier, M.; Froelich, M.F. Exploring the Synergistic Potential of Radiomics and Laboratory Biomarkers for Enhanced Identification of Vulnerable COVID-19 Patients. *Microorganisms* **2023**, *11*, 1740. https://doi.org/10.3390/microorganisms11071740

Academic Editors: Qibin Geng and José Ramón Blanco

Received: 17 June 2023
Revised: 23 June 2023
Accepted: 29 June 2023
Published: 3 July 2023

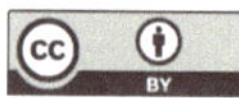

1. Introduction

The pandemic spread of severe acute respiratory syndrome coronavirus type 2 (SARS-CoV-2) and the emergence of coronavirus disease 2019 (COVID-19) has had enormous global health and socio-economic consequences and high infectivity as well as hospitalization rates have put hospital bed and Intensive-Care-Unit (ICU) capacities under enormous stress during the first pandemic waves [1]. Accordingly, the rapid identification of disease severity enabling triaging of patients is an essential clinical aspect and requires a multidisciplinary approach to optimize the diagnostic potential. Various routine laboratory parameters associated with disease severity have already been described, but an integrative approach including Radiomics and cfDNA is missing so far. Among those, C-reactive protein (CRP), activated partial thromboplastin time (PTT), D-dimer, and lactate dehydrogenase (LDH) have been reported [2–4]. Moreover, previous studies have shown an association between increased cell-free DNA (cfDNA) and a severe course of

COVID-19 [5,6]. In this study, we intended to identify suitable markers associated with intensive care requirements. The routine laboratory parameters examined in other studies were further augmented by quantified cfDNA in our work as a dynamic marker of cell decay. Since we anticipated increased cell death of lung tissue, especially in the presence of lung consolidations, this study was called "Laboratory Assessment of Ground Glass Opacities" (LAGGO), emphasizing the interdisciplinary aspect of the work.

While blood-bourne laboratory parameters serve as surrogate markers for monitoring various organ functions, the chest's computed tomography (CT) adds important diagnostic topological information on lung involvement in COVID-19 patients [7]. Tsang et al. have developed the SARS severity score to estimate the severity of lung involvement semi-quantitatively [8]. Additionally, the Radiological Society of North America has developed a structured reporting system that classifies findings related to COVID-19 [9]. Radomics analysis of COVID-19 CTs aims to quantify lung involvement in a fully automatic and reader-independent fashion. Thanks to recent advances in deep-learning-based machine vision, the software can aid the image segmentation necessary for radiomics analyses [10]. Radiomics is an innovative and rapidly evolving field, including the extraction and analysis of quantitative features from medical imaging. By converting an image into mineable data, radiomics complements the traditional visual interpretation and enables a quantitative evaluation of radiological images. In this manner, radiological data can be leveraged not only for qualitative evaluation but also in the form of diverse quantitative datasets to enable personalized patient predictions. This presents many opportunities for analysing radiological data, particularly in assessing tumor diseases, where it is commonly applied. However, ongoing research is necessary to prove the promising potential of radiomics with regard to acquisition protocols, segmentations, and feature extractions [11].

Therefore, so far, the use of radiomics is not widely adopted in the clinical setting, yet [12]. Both laboratory medicine and radiology provide complementary diagnostic value in various stages of COVID-19. Thus, we investigated the potential value of integrated diagnostics in estimating the likelihood of ICU admission to aid in planning ICU capacities in managing Corona cases.

For this purpose, we utilized conserved residual specimens obtained during the initial SARS-CoV-2 pandemic outbreaks to quantify cfDNA and reanalyzed previously acquired data to retrospectively evaluate the significance of specific biomarkers in predicting a severe hospitalized COVID-19 course. Thus, in this study, we present biomarkers that potentially allow discrimination between ICU requirements and normal inpatient treatment in cases of infection with the first SARS-CoV-2 variants in Germany.

The primary objective of this investigation is to establish a suitable algorithm for identifying distinct laboratory and radiology parameters correlated with the need for intensive care unit (ICU) admission (aim I). Subsequently, a verification of the selected parameters via an alternative method is required (aim II). Furthermore, in case of a substantial number of parameters, selecting the most significant ones has to be performed via an algorithm (aim III). Finally, the individual radiomics, RSNA Score, routine laboratory, cfDNA and combined variables have to be compared in their predictive power (aim IV).

2. Materials and Methods

2.1. Participant Recruitment

From May 2020 to September 2021, SARS-CoV-2 patients aged 18 or older previously confirmed by qPCR were enrolled in the LAGGO (Laboratory Assessment of Ground Glass Opacities) study at the University Medical Center Mannheim, Germany (see Figure 1). Informed written consent was obtained from each subject ($n = 52$). The Institutional Review Board (2020-541N) approved the study protocol, and the study was conducted in accordance with the Declaration of Helsinki. During the initial wave of the SARS-CoV-2 pandemic, we deemed it inappropriate to obtain informed consent when requiring intensive care treatment based on ethical considerations. Therefore, the study inclusion was conducted retrospectively after the completion of treatment. Considering this aspect and the high mortality rate, this accounts for the limited number of participants. We have to address this point in the study's limitations.

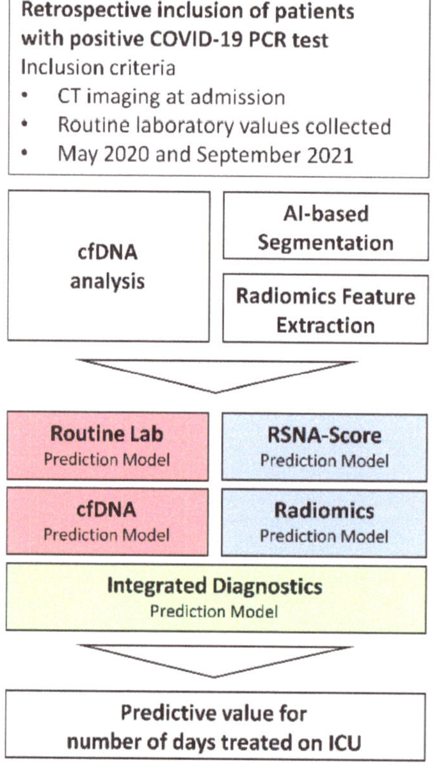

Figure 1. Study concept.

Figure 1: Presentation of the study concept and the research objectives. The inclusion criterion in the study was the diagnosis of COVID-19 based on a positive qRT-PCR result of a nasopharyngeal swab. Radiological chest CT data were segmented and radiomically analyzed. In addition, the patient's routine laboratory was evaluated, and cfDNA was prospectively isolated and quantified. Radiological and laboratory features were selected separately for predicting the duration of intensive care. Before inclusion in an integrated prediction model, the existence of collinearities was reduced using a minimal redundancy algorithm. The final model intends to indicate the patient outcome by predicting an intensive care requirement and facilitating clinical decisions.

2.2. Routine Laboratory Analysis

Blood count was measured on Sysmex XN-9000 (Sysmex, Hamburg, Germany) platform. Hemostaseological parameters were determined on the CS-5100 analyzer (Sysmex, Hamburg, Germany). Clinical chemistry biomarkers were measured on an Atellica-CH Analyzer (Siemens Healthcare GmbH, Eschborn, Germany). For all measurements, the dedicated reagent systems were used according to the manufacturers' recommendations and after internal verification in compliance with DIN EN ISO 15189 in an accredited laboratory. Pre-analytical quality was subsequently judged by centrifugation using the hemolysis assessment system of the analyzer platform on an ordinal scale ranging from no (0) to significant hemolysis (5)). For samples exceeding the value "1", the results for LDH and ASAT were not used in the respective samples since an influence with regard to increased values is described [13,14]. Although the manufacturer does not specify any restrictions in the corresponding instructions, we decided to enhance the quality of the preanalytic by the mentioned procedure. Blood gas analyses (BGA) from arterial and venous blood were conducted under point-of-care-testing conditions.

2.3. Sample Collection and cfDNA Analysis

For the isolation of cfDNA, ethylene diamine tetraacetic acid (EDTA) plasma obtained when clinically indicated was processed within 4 h of blood collection. Specimens were centrifuged at $1600 \times g$ for 10 min at 20 °C. The supernatant was transferred to a new 15 mL tube and centrifuged at $3000 \times g$ for 10 min. Optical control for hemolysis was performed, and insofar as it was visually detectable, the sample was excluded. The final supernatant was stored at −80 °C until the isolation of the cfDNA. CfDNA was isolated using the Qiagen QIAmp Circulating Nucleic Acid Kit (Qiagen, Hilden, Germany) according to the manufacturer's instructions without modifications. For cfDNA isolation, the maximal plasma volume processed from the subject's specimen was utilized (range 0.4 and 1.5 mL). The quantification of the cfDNA was performed by means of a Qubit Fluorometer and Qubit cfDNA HS Assay Kit (Invitrogen, Los Angeles, CA, USA) and the results was normalized via a control with known concentration included in each measurement. In addition, the determined concentration was recalculated in relation to the input volume and reported as ng per mL plasma.

2.4. Chest CT Imaging

All patients in this study underwent native or contrast-enhanced CT imaging of the chest. The scans were performed on either a SOMATOM Definition AS, SOMATOM Definition Flash or a SOMATOM Definition 64 (Siemens Healthcare GmbH, Erlangen, Germany). Depending on the history, clinical presentation and possible comorbidities, patients were scanned using one of the following protocols: Low-dose CT, routine non-contrast-enhanced CT, contrast-enhanced CT or CT pulmonary angiography. In total, 74.54% of scans were performed with contrast agents, of which 58.54% were performed as arterial phase CT. Imeron 300 (Bracco Imaging S.p.A., Milan, Italy) was used as a contrast agent in a dose adjusted for CT protocol and weight.

2.5. Chest CT Imaging Analysis

CTs were analyzed by a resident radiologist, using a semi-quantitative score to quantify pathological changes in the lung parenchyma. To calculate the score, each lung is divided into three sections and scored from 0–4 with regard to severity. For 25% involvement, one point is given per section. Then the sum of all six sections is added, resulting in a score from 0 to 24 [9]. Furthermore, CTs were analyzed quantitatively with radiomics methods using the research application MM Radiomics Frontier Prototype 1.2.6. (August 2016, Siemens Healthcare GmbH, Erlangen, Germany) within syngo.via VB60A (May 2021, Siemens Healthcare GmbH, Erlangen, Germany). To extract radiomics features, segmentation of CT scans is necessary [13]. Segmentation was collected in an automated fashion using the deep-learning-based research segmentation application CT Pneumonia Analysis prototype 2.5.2 (April 2021, Siemens Healthcare GmbH, Erlangen, Germany). This software is currently classified as "for research use only". A binWidth of 25, a 512 × 512 matrix, voxelArrayShift of 0 was applied. For the analysis, pyradiomics version 2.1.0 was applied. Only original radiomics features were included in the analysis.

2.6. Performance of Feature Selection and Statistical Analysis

For identifying adequate parameters associated with a severe course, we opted for an algorithm-based training of a model. A multivariate linear regression with internal 3-fold cross-validation was performed to construct a linear model initially predicting the duration of intensive care in days. It was adapted into a categorizing model dividing subjects into "ICU" versus "no-ICU-demand". This was realized separately for laboratory and radiological data based on a stepwise forward and backward feature selection to create a linear regression model with "ICU period in days" as the initial training target. With regard to the routine laboratory, all mentioned parameters exclusive to cfDNA were used for internal cross-validation comprising three sub-datasets randomly split (each consisting of $n = 22$ for the training and $n = 10$ for the validation). The training was always performed on 22 subjects and validated in the unaffected cohort. This was repeated successively with different cohort formations to obtain a more representative selection despite the limited number of participants. In addition, we used two selection methods-forward and backward selection. The forward selection is a method using subsets of features to train the model, starting with one variable, and adding further variables in each iteration until no model improvement can be achieved. Regarding backward selection all parameters are used initially and then reduced until the model deteriorates due to the omission of variables.

Due to the high number of variables identified, especially for Radiomics, a further reduction before integration into a model was essential. Therefore, a ranking was implemented via the frequencies of feature selection in the sub-datasets resulting in values between 0–3 (0: not selected in a sub-dataset; 3: selected in all three datasets). We excluded parameters selected only once or less.

Moreover, we used a random forest algorithm to verify the selected laboratory parameters and to examine the relevance of cfDNA predicting the regression target "ICU period". The algorithm creates shadow variables for each real variable by permutation and compares the importance of the real variable with the maximum importance of all shadow variables. If the real variable shows higher importance than the corresponding shadow variable, the algorithm assigns high importance to the feature [14,15]. The feature selection was performed identically for the radiological parameters.

Furthermore, we first created separate correlation plots for radiomics and laboratory data in R Studio to identify collinearities using the "library(corrplot)". Subsequently, we applied a minimal redundancy algorithm utilizing the following commands, among others "findCorrelation", "library(heatmap)") to reduce redundant parameters as a combination of collinear variables would not enhance the predictive potential. The selection of initial parameters, including clustering of strongly correlated variables (shown in dark brown), is presented as the first correlation plot in the results. Following the reduction of parameters using the algorithm, a second visualization in the form of a correlation plot is provided. These parameters were then used for singular radiomics or laboratory models and the integrative model.

After the variable reduction, the maintaining potential to classify subjects was illustrated by a heatmap performing unsupervised clustering based on the final parameters (R package "pheatmap"). The application of the validation dataset served to prove the maintenance of classification potential and not to determine the model's power, as this would lead to overfitting (Supplemental Material). Due to the Root Mean Square Error (RMSE) of predicted and actual days in ICU, even in our validation cohort, the model was adapted to a logistic regression approach with the clinical decision endpoint "ICU stay yes/no" and a cut-off for this categorization has been selected based on this RMSE.

The final verification and the determination of the accuracies of the integrative model were realized with a training and validation independent test cohort. In addition to establishing an integrative model, we compared individual cfDNA, RSNA score, radiomics or routine laboratory models with the combined model. The prediction of ICU needs was performed using the test cohort in R-Studio. To accomplish this, we applied the previously trained and validated models on the test cohort as a logistic model. The algorithm employed classified values above six as indicating "ICU need" and values below six as indicating "regular inpatient treatment".

Additionally, we conducted a ROC analysis to compare true positives with false positives based on the test cohort ("library(ROCR)"). This analysis was performed for different models, and the Area under the Curve (AUC) was calculated. Patient's symptoms were not included in the model but compared between ICU and non-ICU cohorts. All statistical analyses, including comparing demographics, COVID-19 symptoms, treatment and laboratory parameters of ICU and non-ICU cohorts, were performed using R statistics software (Version 4.1.2) [16]. Cohort comparisons of non-normally distributed continuous variables were performed by the Kruskal-Wallis rank sum test, and normally distributed continuous variables were compared via regular ANOVA test. Categorical variables are presented as frequency and percentage. For the comparison of categorical variables, a Fisher exact test was performed. p-values < 0.05 were considered significant.

3. Results

3.1. Demographics and Clinical Aspects

For the assessment of the diversity of the disease in COVID-19 severity and treatment, a comparison between the ICU- and non-ICU cohorts was performed. Moreover, this comparison revealed significantly elevated laboratory parameters in cases requiring ICU admission (Table 1/Figure 2). Participants in whom CT could be assessed for pulmonary embolism were not observed to have a central or distal embolism.

Table 1. Patient collective overview.

	All Patients	**Non-ICU Cohort**	**ICU Cohort**	p **Value**
	$n = 52$	$n = 16$	$n = 36$	
Age (mean (SD))	68.46 (13.56)	73.38 (14.94)	66.28 (12.50)	0.081
Gender F/M (%)	22/31 (42.3/57.7)	10/6 (62.5/37.5)	12/25 (33.3/66.7)	0.070
Symptoms				
Fever (%)	14 (30.4)	3 (20.0)	11 (35.5)	0.331
Subfebrile (%)	1 (2.2)	1 (6.7)	0 (0.0)	0.326
Night sweat (%)	1 (2.2)	0 (0.0)	1 (3.2)	1.000
Reduced condition (%)	4 (8.7)	2 (13.3)	2 (6.5)	0.587
Diarrhoea (%)	5 (10.9)	2 (13.3)	3 (9.7)	1.000
Cough (%)	16 (34.8)	5 (33.3)	11 (35.5)	1.000
Sore throat (%)	2 (4.3)	0 (0.0)	2 (6.5)	1.000
Dyspnea (%)	16 (34.8)	6 (40.0)	10 (32.3)	0.744
Fatigue (%)	7 (15.2)	2 (13.3)	5 (16.1)	1.000
Nausea (%)	2 (4.3)	0 (0.0)	2 (6.5)	1.000
Anosmia (%)	3 (6.5)	1 (6.7)	2 (6.5)	1.000
Ageusia (%)	4 (8.7)	1 (6.7)	3 (9.7)	1.000
Severity-Score (mean (SD))	1.65 (1.17)	1.60 (1.02)	1.68 (1.26)	0.837
Treatment				
ICU days (mean (SD))	9.52 [0.00, 22.66]	0.00 [0.00, 0.00]	16.17 [7.92, 27.06]	**<0.001**
Deceased (%)	3 (5.9)	0 (0.0)	3 (8.6)	0.543
Ventilation (%)	24 (46.2)	0 (0.0)	24 (66.7)	**<0.001**
CVC (%)	28 (53.8)	0 (0.0)	28 (77.8)	**<0.001**
Reanimation (%)	5 (9.6)	0 (0.0)	5 (13.9)	0.308
ICU complex (%)	28 (53.8)	0 (0.0)	28 (77.8)	**<0.001**
Transfusion				
erythrocytes/platelets (%)	12 (23.1)	0 (0.0)	12 (33.3)	**0.010**
plasma (%)	1 (1.9)	0 (0.0)	1 (2.8)	1.000
ECMO (%)	6 (11.5)	0 (0.0)	6 (16.7)	0.160
Hemodiafiltration (%)	9 (17.3)	1 (6.2)	8 (22.2)	0.245
Tracheostomy (%)	11 (21.2)	0 (0.0)	11 (30.6)	**0.012**
Operation (%)	9 (17.3)	1 (6.2)	8 (22.2)	0.245

Table 1. *Cont.*

	All Patients	Non-ICU Cohort	ICU Cohort	*p* Value
Laboratory parameters				
cfDNA (median [IQR]), ng/mL	118.85 [70.58, 292.87]	68.54 [25.73, 93.33]	220.18 [102.19, 25.54]	**<0.001**
Quick (mean (SD)), %	87.75 (17.47)	90.69 (12.32)	86.44 (19.34)	0.424
PTT (median [IQR]), sec.	25.70 [22.03, 34.92]	23.60 [22.17, 26.30]	27.15 [21.65, 38.85]	0.115
D-dimer (median [IQR]), mg/L	1.63 [0.76, 3.90]	1.49 [0.96, 1.73]	1.93 [0.72, 4.06]	0.619
Fibrinogen (mean (SD)), g/L	6.33 (1.91)	5.08 (NA)	6.37 (1.94)	NA
Platelets (mean (SD)), 10^9/L	270.06 (121.64)	254.25 (130.85)	277.08 (118.57)	0.537
RBC (mean (SD)), 10^{12}/L	3.49 (0.71)	3.75 (0.61)	3.38 (0.73)	0.084
Hemoglobin (mean (SD)), g/dL	10.31 (2.18)	10.71 (2.13)	10.14 (2.21)	0.389
MCV (mean (SD)), fl	88.44 (7.36)	84.06 (7.14)	90.38 (6.66)	**0.003**
MCH (median [IQR]), pg	30.10 [28.62, 31.02]	29.05 [27.88, 30.22]	30.65 [29.23, 31.27]	**0.026**
MCHC (mean (SD)), g/dL	33.49 (1.34)	33.92 (1.36)	33.29 (1.31)	0.118
WBC (median [IQR]), 10^9/L	8.71 [6.26, 11.65]	5.86 [3.92, 8.32]	9.66 [7.94, 15.05]	**<0.001**
CRP (median [IQR]), mg/L	83.50 [41.75, 149.75]	38.50 [27.00, 76.75]	95.55 [64.00, 173.00]	**0.001**
GFR (mean (SD)), mL/min/1.73 m^2	62.69 (32.35)	62.94 (34.60)	62.58 (31.81)	0.971
Creatinine (median [IQR]), mg/dL	1.03 [0.73, 1.62]	0.92 [0.68, 1.25]	1.03 [0.75, 1.85]	0.258
Urea (median [IQR]), mg/dL	49.10 [37.55, 90.22]	35.60 [30.92, 58.75]	52.45 [41.45, 96.95]	**0.012**
AST (median [IQR]), U/L	38.00 [27.00, 61.00]	29.00 [26.00, 38.00]	48.00 [32.50, 77.75]	**0.016**
ALT (median [IQR]), U/L	32.00 [23.00, 60.00]	26.00 [17.00, 40.00]	39.50 [24.75, 61.50]	0.094
GGT (median [IQR]), U/L	96.00 [37.00, 161.00]	45.00 [28.00, 107.00]	131.00 [38.75, 181.75]	**0.014**
Cholinesterase (mean (SD)), U/L	5722.41 (2140.03)	6459.33 (1974.75)	5588.42 (2169.98)	0.366
Albumin (mean (SD)), g/L	24.13 (5.48)	29.62 (4.02)	21.84 (4.27)	**<0.001**
Bilirubin (median [IQR]), mg/dL	0.41 [0.30, 0.67]	0.44 [0.28, 0.53]	0.40 [0.30, 0.82]	0.464
LDH (median [IQR]), U/L	382.00 [293.50, 447.00]	331.00 [228.00, 389.50]	399.50 [323.50, 469.25]	**0.016**

Presentation of demographic data, initial symptoms, treatment characteristics and laboratory parameters. Non-normally distributed continuous variables were compared by a Kruskal-Wallis rank sum test. For categorical variables, a Fisher exact test was performed. *p*-values < 0.05 were considered significant and are highlighted in bold and underlined.

Patient 1: 62y, male

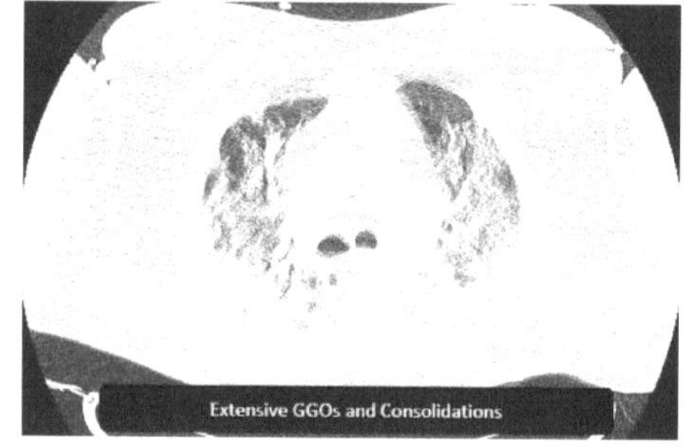

cfDNA	3226.36 ng/ml
aPTT	40.6 s
Albumin	19.7 g/l
CRP	203 mg/l
CT-COVID-Score	30

Patient 2: 77y, male

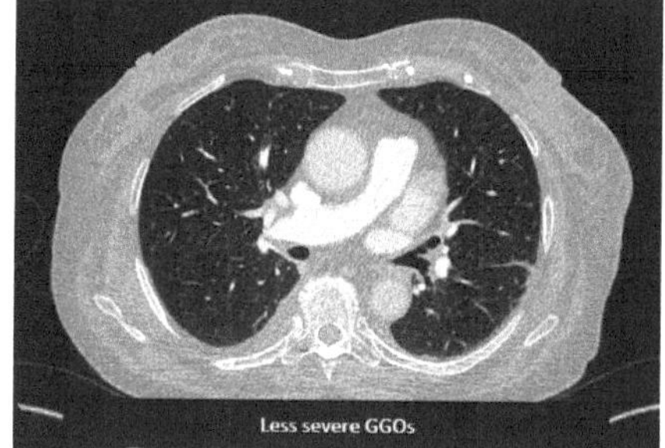

cfDNA	18.9 ng/ml
aPTT	22.1 s
Albumin	31.0 g/l
CRP	24 mg/l
CT-COVID-Score	3

Figure 2. Two example patients enrolled in the LAGGO study.

Exemplary presentation of two test persons with severe and mild progression.

3.2. Prognostic Value of Laboratory Parameters

Creation of the Laboratory Prediction Model

Differences in laboratory parameters between the ICU and non-ICU cohorts are summarised in Table 1. Moreover, the training and cross-validation described in more detail in the methods were performed with a dataset comprising three sub-datasets (Table 2). The most frequent parameters, PTT, albumin, GGT and CRP, and ALT, platelets, and WBC, were selected in two training sets and were included in further analysis.

Table 2. Cross-validation of prediction models for routine laboratory parameters and Radiomics.

Internal Cross-Validation I				
Laboratory Values	**Dataset 1** *Training n = 23* *Validation n = 9*	**Dataset 2** *Training n = 22* *Validation n = 10*	**Dataset 3** *Training n = 22* *Validation n = 10*	**Ranking** *frequencies*
partial thromboplastin time	0.364	0.156	0.003	3
Albumin	0.198	0.656	0.679	3
C-reactive protein	0.903	0.712	0.462	3
gamma-glutamyltransferase	0.224	0.517	0.158	3
alanine aminotransferase	0.286		0.163	2
Platelets		0.850	0.806	2
white blood cells	0.375	0.467		2
Urea			0.344	1
glomerular filtration rate			0.065	1
creatinine			0.512	1
red blood cells			0.736	1
mean corpuscular hemoglobin concentration			0.482	1
lactate dehydrogenase	0.495			1
Internal cross-validation II				
Radiomics	**dataset 1** *training n = 20* *validation n = 10*	**dataset 2** *training n = 20* *validation n = 10*	**dataset 3** *training n = 20* *validation n = 10*	**Ranking** *frequencies*
original_firstorder_10Percentile	0.921	0.643	0.508	3
original_gldm_LargeDependenceLowGrayLevelEmphasis	0.236	0.565	0.484	3
original_shape_Maximum2DdiameterSlice	0.355		0.871	2
original_firstorder_Energy	0.707		0.724	2
original_firstorder_TotalEnergy		0.050	0.673	2
original_glcm_ClusterShade	0.299		0.923	2
original_glcm_DifferenceVariance		0.325	0.972	2
original_glrlm_RunEntropy	0.590		0.967	2
original_glrlm_RunLengthNonUniformity	0.891	0.925		2
original_ngtdm_Busyness		0.117	0.493	2
original_ngtdm_Contrast	0.454	0.050		2
original_shape_Elongation		0.277	0.654	2
original_shape_Flatness	0.214	0.387		2
original_shape_LeastAxisLength		0.094	0.462	2
original_shape_MajorAxisLength		0.461	0.961	2
original_shape_Maximum3Ddiameter	0.519		0.823	2
original_firstorder_90Percentile	0.576			1
original_glcm_DifferenceEntropy	0.942			1
original_glcm_MaximumProbability	0.849			1
original_gldm_DependenceNonUniformity	0.905			1
original_gldm_SmallDependenceHighGrayLevelEmphasis	0.235			1
original_glszm_GrayLevelNonUniformity	0.731			1
original_glszm_ZoneEntropy	0.524			1
original_shape_SphericalDisproportion	0.328			1
original_shape_VoxelVolume	0.251			1
original_glcm_ClusterTendency		0.941		1
original_glcm_Imc1		0.254		1
original_glcm_MCC		0.022		1
original_gldm_GrayLevelNonUniformity		0.946		1
original_gldm_SmallDependenceEmphasis		0.577		1
original_glszm_GrayLevelVariance		0.382		1
original_ngtdm_Complexity		0.229		1
original_shape_MinorAxisLength		0.318		1
original_shape_SurfaceVolumeRatio		0.037		1
original_firstorder_Skewness			0.564	1
original_glrlm_GrayLevelNonUniformity			0.726	1
original_glszm_GrayLevelNonUniformityNormalized			0.922	1
original_glszm_LowGrayLevelZoneEmphasis			0.666	1
original_glszm_SizeZoneNonUniformity			0.492	1
original_shape_Compactness1			0.347	1
original_shape_Maximum2DdiameterRow			0.270	1

The difference in the number of subjects in the laboratory ($n = 32$) and radiological ($n = 30$) cross-validation was because two subjects did not receive a chest CT during routine care. p-values for the "Laboratory values" and "Radiomics" are presented and variables were excluded from further analysis at a frequency of 1.

In addition, the feature selection was methodically verified using a random forest analysis with the same target as our regression model (ICU stay). This was done to verify the importance of the variables selected by forward and backward feature selection. In the following, the previously selected parameters were used, but due to the high importance of cfDNA, cfDNA was included in the further establishment of the prediction model (Figure 3).

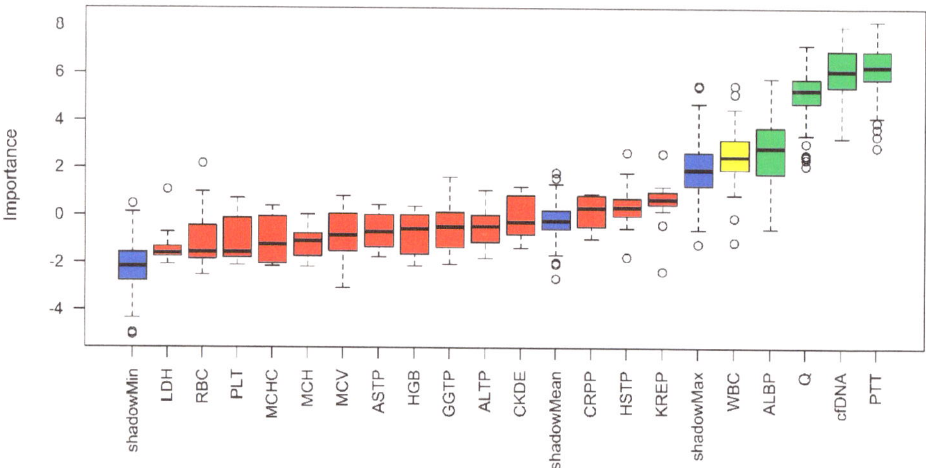

Figure 3. Random–Forest Approach estimating the variable importance for predicting ICU days.

High importance is illustrated by green, medium by yellow and low by red. In addition, the minimum, mean, and maximum importance of the shadow variables are shown in blue. Parameters with a lower relevance for predicting the duration of intensive care requirements than the maximum shadow variable have been assigned low importance.

Furthermore, we considered the first BGA results of the subjects and examined the results. The parameters were investigated for their suitability as predictors of ICU admission via unsupervised clustering in Supplemental S1. Here, no clear differentiation between normal inpatients to long–term intensive care patients could be observed as the values were either similar among the groups (see pH variation) or showed heterogeneities within all subcohorts.

3.3. Prognostic Value of Radiological Parameters
Creation of the Radiological Prediction Model

The radiomics data were equally cross − validated ($n = 30$), and the ranking was performed equivalently as previously described. Due to the high diversity of radiomics, the algorithm selected more parameters per dataset than for the laboratory data. Details of all identified parameters of each sub-dataset are presented in Table 2. 16 parameters were selected for establishing a model predicting ICU stay (original_firstorder_10Percentile, original_gldm_LargeDependenceLowGrayLevelEmphasis, original_shape_Maximum2D DiameterSlice, original_firstorder_Energy, original_firstorder_TotalEnergy, original_glcm_ ClusterShade, original_glcm_DifferenceVariance, original_glrlm_RunEntropy, original_glrlm_ RunLengthNonUniformity, original_ngtdm_Busyness, original_ngtdm_Contrast, original_shape_Elongation, original_shape_Flatness, original_shape_LeastAxisLength, original_shape_MajorAxisLength, original_shape_Maximum3DDiameter). Therefore, a reduction of the selected parameters was essential, as described in the following.

In addition, the CT COVID Severity (RSNA) score was used as a variable to predict ICU stay.

3.4. Prognostic Value of Integrated Diagnostics

The radiological and laboratory parameters were examined for collinearities before integration into the final models, as a reduction of features was essential. Since various correlations were identified, we applied a redundancy reduction algorithm (Figure 4). For this purpose, separate correlation matrices were initially created for radiomic parameters (Figure 4A) and laboratory parameters (Figure 4C). A high correlation between parameters is illustrated by a dark color. After applying the "findCorrelation" command, which identifies collinear parameters and removes one of the two variables, updated correlation plots were generated for the remaining radiomic parameters (Figure 4B) and laboratory parameters (Figure 4D). Finally, seven laboratory (albumin, ALT, GGT, platelets, PTT, CRP and cfDNA) and six radiomics parameters (original_glcm_CLusterShade, original_gldm_LargeDependenceLowGrayLevelEmphasis, original_glrlm_RunEntropy, original_shape_Elongation, original_shape_MajorAxisLength and original_ngtdm_Busyness) were integrated in the combined model.

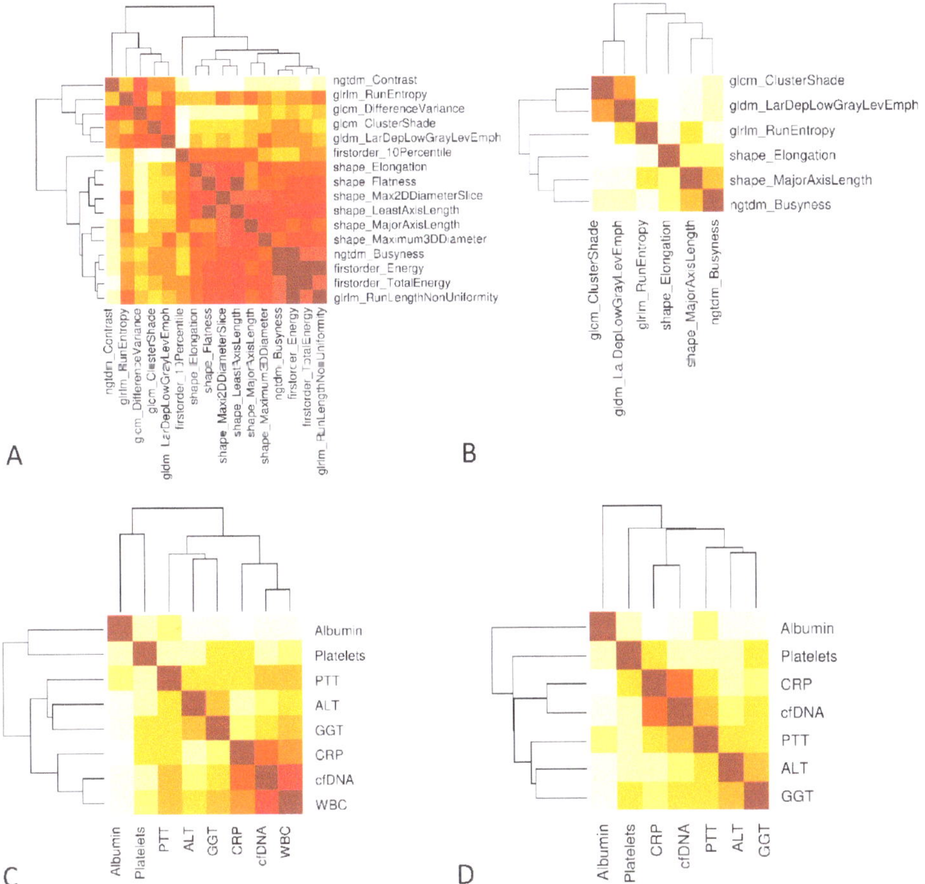

Figure 4. Reduction of collinearity. (**A**) Correlation plot to identify potential clusters of radiomics. The degree of correlation is classified by the brightness of the colors (dark brown corresponds to a high correlation). (**B**) Clustering was reduced by the use of a minimal redundancy algorithm. (**C**) Correlation plot of laboratory parameters. (**D**) Exclusion of "white blood cells" because of the highest correlation with CRP. (**B,D**) Variables were included in the final integrative model.

After successfully identifying suitable parameters, we created a heatmap illustrating the unsupervised clustering of the combined dataset. We applied the model to our cross-validation dataset (Supplemental S1) to verify the selected variables even after the previously described variable reduction.

Moreover, the period in ICU predicted by the integrative model was compared to the actual days in an independent test cohort ($n = 15$, Figure 5). The Root Mean Square (RMSE) of the deviations between the actual and predicted days was 5.3 days in the cross-validation set and 12.3 days in the test-cohort set (outliner V5 is excluded as the training set is not representative of values above 40 days). The application on the validation cohort only served to verify the variable selection even after reducing the initial parameters and not to assess the model's power, as this would cause overfitting. Based on these results, revealing limitations in the linear prediction of shorter ICU stay even in the validation cohort, the linear approach had to be adapted via a categorization into likely ICU and unlikely ICU with six days as a decision cut-off between intensive care and normal care treatment.

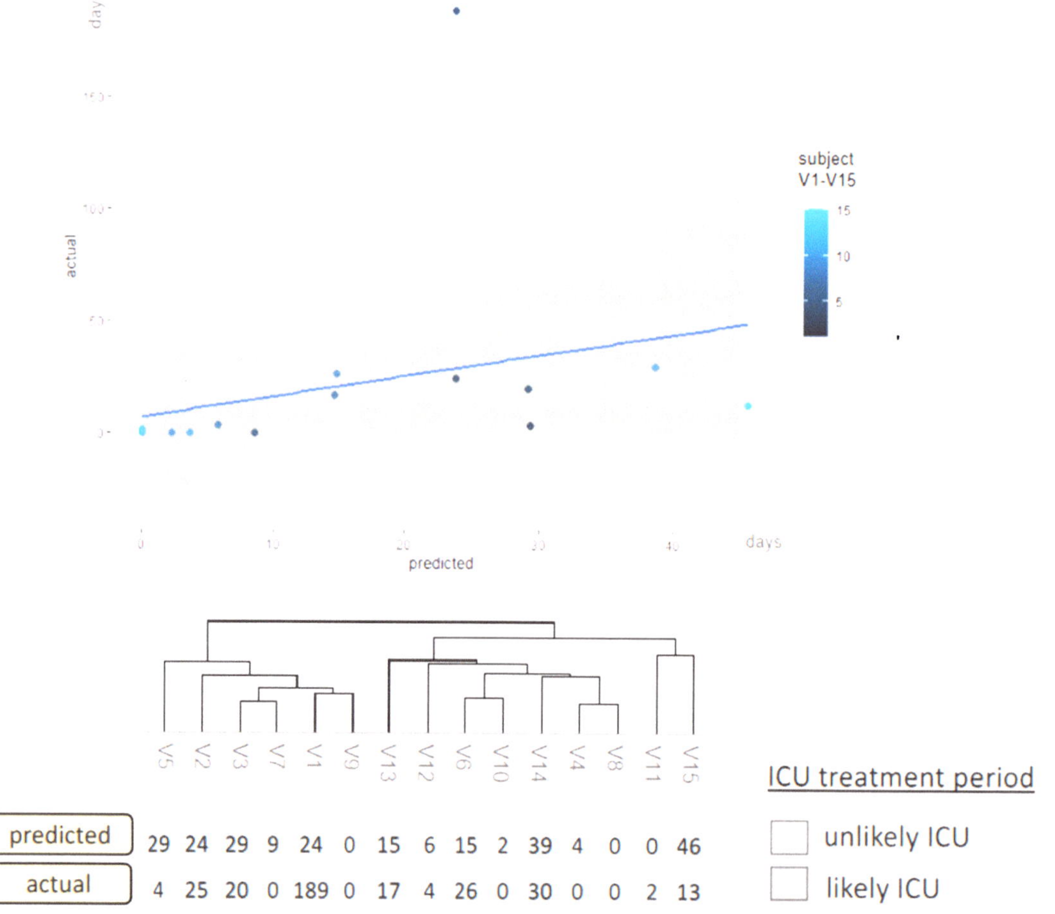

Figure 5. The integrative model applied to the validation-independent test set.

Correlation between actual and predicted ICU treatment applied to a second dataset not affected by cross-validation. The predicted days are compared to the actual days, and the model is categorized as described previously. X-axis: predicted ICU days, y-axis:

actual ICU days for the validation-naïve patients V1–V15. Only the categorizing version represents the final model. Thus, the light-colored patients would have a recommendation for normal inpatient treatment, and the dark-colored patients would have a referral for ICU treatment.

The cut-off was based on the RMSE in the validation set and was finally tested in a validation-independent cohort. Two false positives were identified in the test cohort resulting in an AUC of 0.91 in ROC analysis (Figure 6). Compared to singular models (RSNA, cfDNA, Radiomics, Routine lab), the integrated model demonstrates the highest predictive potency for intensive care requirements (accuracy = 0.87, Table 3). The accuracies were determined using the independent test set not used for prior cross-validation.

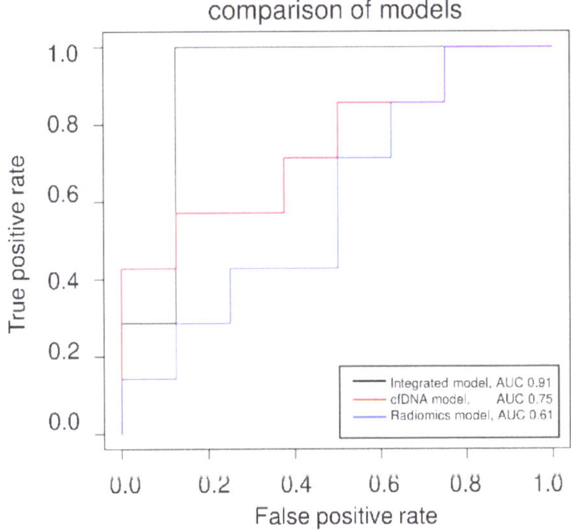

Figure 6. ROC analysis of the categorized approach.

Table 3. Accuracies of regression models.

Prediction of ICU Demand	
Model	**Accuracy**
cfDNA	0.47
Radiomics	0.54
Routine lab	0.74
Integrated diagnostics	0.87

ROC analysis of the cfDNA model, the Radiomics model, and the integrated model applying the categorized approach predicting ICU demand (yes/no).

4. Discussion

This study assessed several diagnostic models for predicting the requirement of intensive care treatment in COVID-19 patients. The special aspect of our model is the integration of routine laboratory, cfDNA, and radiomics, which was intended to increase the diagnostic potential and has thus been trained, validated, and verified in independent datasets. Our results show a synergistic potential of laboratory and radiological parameters to support clinical decision-making in COVID-19 patients.

These results align with published literature but gain additional insights using a truly interdisciplinary diagnostic assessment. Some studies have focused on differentiating

COVID-19 pneumonia from other lung conditions [17]. Subsequently, the prognostic value of radiomics based on initial CT scans was investigated by Zhang et al., who proposed an AI-based radiomics nomogram to predict disease progression in COVID-19 patients [18]. Similarly, Lassau et al. have shown via AI-deep-learning mechanisms that the severity of COVID-19 can be predicted by integrating CT scan data and biological and clinical parameters [19]. Some other studies have also dealt with outcome parameters such as hospitalization, patient management, or organ involvement, such as acute renal failure in COVID-19.

In some cases, as in our work, cell decay markers (LDH instead of cfDNA), acute phase parameters (CRP, WBC), and quantitative lung parenchyma data were identified as possible predictors. Thus, the selection of our potential predictors is partially supported by results published in other studies [20–22]. Nevertheless, combining radiomics, routine laboratory, and cfDNA represents a new aspect.

Concerning the prognostic value of initial routine laboratory values, the prognostic value of D-dimers has been described extensively [23,24]. Initial hypercoagulability with the transition to the consumptive stage of disseminated intravascular coagulopathy (DIC) has been reported [25–27]. Moreover, Gatto et al. showed a frequent occurrence of pulmonary embolism between days 1 and 47 of hospitalization, occurring in the majority on day 10 [27]. We evaluated the CT images in temporal proximity to the first available blood sampling for the presence of central or distal pulmonal embolism. In those that could be assessed for pulmonary embolism, none were demonstrated. As we used the closest available initial laboratory to identify appropriate treatment predictors, this could explain why pulmonary embolism was not present then. Even Gatto et al. described a high variability of the incidence of pulmonal embolism in COVID-19, thus supporting our result [27]. This may explain why D-dimers were not identified as a marker for predicting the need for intensive care treatment in our study. Still, platelets and PTT were included in the final integrative model emphasizing the importance of hemostaseological diagnostic findings in COVID-19. In addition, models for predicting mortality that combines laboratory or radiological parameters with clinical aspects have already been established via comparable machine-learning approaches [28,29]. Thus, the potential of AI-based algorithms has been demonstrated and can be expanded for interdisciplinary approaches combining laboratory and radiomics values [28]. Predictive endpoints in the previous study by Yu et al. were the need for ventilation and, ultimately, patient mortality. However, our study presents a tool that might help clinicians triage COVID-19 patients upon initial presentation.

For this reason, we have adapted the initial target to predict ICU duration into a categorizing approach and propose a model that might help physicians in emergency departments to distinguish between ICU and normal care demand. Chieregato et al. emphasize that classification into ICU/non-ICU depicts an endpoint representing clinical decision support, a conclusion we would like to emphasize with our results. In addition, the high variation of clinical symptoms was addressed by Chieregato et al. Thus we adopt a purely apparative diagnostic approach [30]. Moreover, we can support this with our results, as there was no significant difference in initial symptom-based severity score between the ICU- and non-ICU cohorts.

Furthermore, in this study, we augmented routine laboratory parameters used in the mentioned previous studies by cfDNA, a dynamic marker of cell decay. Regarding cfDNA, Cavalier et al. have already described nucleosomal cfDNA to predict requirements for ICU care, underlining the relevance of cfDNA for ICU prediction [5]. We demonstrated significant differences between the cfDNA concentrations in normal and intensive care units ($p < 0.001$), and the importance of predicting ICU demand was verified via the random forest approach.

Moreover, a study by Giraudo et al. presents a radiomics model for predicting ICU transfer [30]. Our results may indicate the elevated diagnostic accuracy of an integrated, multimodal approach for COVID-19 diagnostic evaluation. This can be explained by the additional information offered by routine labs on extrapulmonary organ damage as a compound increased risk of ICU treatment. The results highlight the need for an integrated assessment of interdisciplinary diagnostic data to stratify the planning of treatment capacities better and potentially achieve better clinical outcomes.

Yet, this study must be interpreted with some limitations. First, the results presented are from a small collective due to many deceased patients during the first global spread of COVID-19, and explicit patient consent was required for cfDNA testing from residual routine care material. Due to the prospective part of the laboratory analysis, not all in-house data could be used for our model, which would have increased the generalizability of our results. In particular, the assessment in a naïve cohort has to be expanded in follow-up studies, as we had to minimize this in favor of the training and validation cohort. Still, we extracted important material and data from the first pandemic waves. We were able to present the applicability of cfDNA and machine-learning algorithms for the stratification of ICU capacities. Thus, this can now be used to extrapolate information from past scenarios that may apply to future variants potentially associated with elevated hospitalization rates again. In a subsequent approach with significantly larger datasets, we aim to evaluate the model's potential for other SARS-CoV-2 variants. To ensure a higher number of participants, we will assess the necessity of cfDNA in this model. A potential focus on radiomics and routine laboratory parameters could enable its applicability in smaller centers that may not practice these isolation methods and quantification. A purely retrospective analysis would enable the utilization of a larger dataset for testing the model, enhancing the significance, robustness, and generalizability of the potential predictors presented in this study. Additionally, we are considering testing the model on other respiratory diseases to determine whether it is a general model for infectious respiratory diseases or specific to COVID-19.

Considering the selected parameters for the model, further limitations can be discussed. One aspect is the influence of anticoagulatory medication, such as heparin, used in intensive care cohorts. However, when considering the aPTT of both cohorts, no significant difference could be observed, suggesting no influence of heparin on the variable selection. In addition to indicating organ damage, a simultaneous elevation of AST, LDH, and cfDNA may also point to in-vitro hemolysis as a potential confounding factor. To minimize this pre-analytical factor, visual control and photometric evaluation of the sample quality were performed before the analyses ensuring the validity of the results.

Furthermore, there was a certain degree of heterogeneity with regard to the imaging data. Yet, most cases were scanned at one scanner with one standardized protocol. However, a remaining bias cannot be fully ruled out.

With regard to the cfDNA isolation method, it has been shown that the final elution volume and elution steps can be adjusted when the initial plasma volume is low [31]. Since we did not apply these adjustments, this influence on concentration values should be considered when comparing the results with other studies. In addition, a fluorometric approach was used for the concentration measurements, as this is a more cost-effective method and easier to implement in routine diagnostic procedures. In this context, the influence of the carrier RNA contained in the isolation kit may be considered. However, as all samples were treated identically, this does not affect the comparison of our ICU and non-ICU cohorts, ensuring significant differences remain valid. In addition, it is well known that patients with significantly elevated BMI suffer from more severe diseases requiring intensive care treatment [32]. As cfDNA levels are known to correlate with body weight, this might also elevate cfDNA levels in addition to infection-associated cell damage [33].

Moreover, pathognomonic symptoms have been included in various other scoring systems [34,35]. Our cohort's clinical data points of initial symptoms revealed no significant difference among the sub-cohorts. Due to this low discrimination potential, the clinical variables were not included. Furthermore, it could be argued that the pulmonary oxygenation capacity influences clinical disease progression. However, reliable BGA requires arterial blood sampling, which is often difficult to achieve outside intensive care environments, suggesting limited applicability. Equally, including BGA data from non-arterial samples, regularly done during hospital admission, did not provide relevant predictive information for predicting ICU stay. For these reasons, we did not include BGA while still focusing on our model's radiomics evaluation of lung imaging and the laboratory parameters.

Finally, we established an integrative linear prediction model for the requirement of ICU admission. Based on our cross-validation set, the model was not capable of correctly predicting impending shorter ICU stays of up to 6 days. For this reason, we have resorted to a categorization model of "ICU stay likely/unlikely" with a cut-off at six days of predicted ICU stay. The cut-off is based on the mean deviations of predicted and actual days in ICU in our cross-validation set and was further applied to a validation-naive set with high accuracy. This approach is intended to assist medical staff in assessing the probable demand for intensive treatment during their patients' initial presentation. The ROC analysis shows a clear superiority of the integrated model compared to the isolated assessment of the biomarkers. We also conclude that cfDNA is a complementary but not essential parameter in this categorized approach. Nevertheless, cfDNA was identified to be significantly elevated in patients requiring intensive care, confirming its potential as a dynamic marker of severe disease.

5. Conclusions

In conclusion, we have identified radiomics and laboratory biomarkers associated with a severe COVID-19 course via feature selection algorithms (aim I). The selected parameters have been verified by a random forest approach (aim II), and collinear parameters were reduced via a minimal redundancy algorithm (aim III). Moreover, our results might suggest a solution for a difficult clinical decision-making problem in patients experiencing severe COVID-19, namely, predicting whether a patient on time of admission to the hospital might need ICU treatment shortly. An interdisciplinary approach of integrated diagnostics using laboratory medicine and radiology biomarkers was used to establish this clinical prediction model and was superior to single models (aim IV). Therefore, we propose to study the potentially improved efficiency of ICU capacities using prediction algorithms. Particularly, in scenarios of rapidly rising global infection rates and concomitant hospitalizations, this approach of facilitating triaging vulnerable patients might be relevant.

Supplementary Materials: The following supporting information can be downloaded at: https://www.mdpi.com/article/10.3390/microorganisms11071740/s1, Supplemental S1: Blood gas analysis to predict ICU days; Supplemental S2: Verification of reduced features via unsupervised clustering in our validation set.

Author Contributions: C.G.: Conceptualization, Methodology, Data curation, Resources, Writing—Original Draft, Writing—Review & Editing, Visualization, Project administration; V.H.: Writing—Original Draft, Writing—Review & Editing; S.F.S.: Conceptualization, Methodology, Data curation, Resources, Writing—Original Draft, Writing—Review & Editing, Visualization, Project administration; V.A.: Data curation, Writing—Original Draft, Writing—Review & Editing; M.K.: Writing—Original Draft, Writing—Review & Editing; M.T.: Patient recruitment, Writing—Original Draft, Writing—Review & Editing; A.H.: Data curation, Writing—Original Draft, Writing—Review & Editing; S.O.S.: Conceptualization, Methodology, Data curation, Resources, Writing—Original Draft, Writing—Review & Editing, Supervision; M.N.: Conceptualization, Methodology, Data curation, Resources, Writing—Original Draft Review & Editing, Supervision; M.F.F.: Conceptualization, Methodology, Data curation, Resources, Writing—Original Draft, Writing—Review & Editing, Visualization, Project administration. All authors have read and agreed to the published version of the manuscript.

Funding: Ministry of Science, Research and Arts, Baden-Württemberg, Germany: "Measures to combat the coronavirus SARS-CoV-2 pandemic in the field of medical research", special funding program COVID-19 (Chap. 1499 TG 93), (MA10).

Institutional Review Board Statement: Institutional Review Board (2020-541N) approved the study protocol, and the study was conducted in accordance with the Declaration of Helsinki.

Informed Consent Statement: Informed written consent was obtained from each subject.

Data Availability Statement: The data presented in this study are available on request from the corresponding author.

Acknowledgments: We thank Andreas Teufel for organizing the ethical requirements at the Institutional Review Board. We thank Ameli Götz for aliquoting the samples and performance of further cfDNA analysis, Sonika Rao for conducting the routine laboratory data query, and Caterina Hassler for recording clinical symptoms. Further, we thank Sebastian Faby and Andreas Wimmer from Siemens Healthineers for supporting the research applications. Finally, we thank all of the study participants.

Conflicts of Interest: The authors have declared no conflict of interest.

Abbreviations

ALAT	Alanine aminotransferase
aPTT	activated partial thromboplastin time
ARDS	Acute respiratory distress syndrome
ASAT	Aspartate aminotransferase
BGA	Blood gas analysis
cfDNA	Circulation free Deoxyribonucleic acid
CAHA	COVID-19-associated hemostatic abnormalities
COVID-19	Coronavirus disease 2019
CRP	C-reactive protein
CT	Computed tomography
DIC	Disseminated intravascular coagulopathy
EDTA	Ethylene diamine tetraacetic acid
GFR	Glomerular filtration rate
GGT	Gamma-glutamyltransferase
ICU	Intensive Care Unit
IL	Interleukin
ISTH	International Society of Thrombosis and Hemostatic
LC	Lymphocyte count
LDH	Lactate dehydrogenase
MCH	Mean corpuscular hemoglobin
MCHC	Mean corpuscular hemoglobin concentration,
MCV	Mean corpuscular volume
MOF	Multiple organ failure
NC	Neutrophil count
NLR	Neutrophil: lymphocyte ratio
PCT	Procalcitonin
PE	Pulmonary embolism
qPCR	quantitative polymerase chain reaction
RSNA	Radiological Society of North America
SARS-CoV-2	Severe acute respiratory syndrome coronavirus type 2
WBC	White blood cells

References

1. Mouffak, S.; Shubbar, Q.; Saleh, E.; El-Awady, R. Recent advances in management of COVID-19: A review. *Biomed. Pharmacother.* **2021**, *143*, 112107. [CrossRef]
2. Wang, Q.; Cheng, J.; Shang, J.; Wang, Y.; Wan, J.; Yan, Y.Q.; Liu, W.B.; Zhang, H.P.; Wang, J.P.; Wang, X.Y.; et al. Clinical value of laboratory indicators for predicting disease progression and death in patients with COVID-19: A retrospective cohort study. *BMJ Open* **2021**, *11*, e043790. [CrossRef]
3. Bivona, G.; Agnello, L.; Ciaccio, M. Biomarkers for Prognosis and Treatment Response in COVID-19 Patients. *Ann. Lab. Med.* **2021**, *41*, 540–548. [CrossRef]
4. Guan, X.; Zhang, B.; Fu, M.; Li, M.; Yuan, X.; Zhu, Y.; Peng, J.; Guo, H.; Lu, Y. Clinical and inflammatory features based machine learning model for fatal risk prediction of hospitalized COVID-19 patients: Results from a retrospective cohort study. *Ann. Med.* **2021**, *53*, 257–266. [CrossRef]

5. Cavalier, E.; Guiot, J.; Lechner, K.; Dutsch, A.; Eccleston, M.; Herzog, M.; Bygott, T.; Schomburg, A.; Kelly, T.; Holdenrieder, S. Circulating Nucleosomes as Potential Markers to Monitor COVID-19 Disease Progression. *Front. Mol. Biosci.* **2021**, *8*, 600881. [CrossRef]

6. Hammad, R.; Eldosoky, M.A.E.R.; Fouad, S.H.; Elgendy, A.; Tawfeik, A.M.; Alboraie, M.; Abdelmaksoud, M.F. Circulating cell-free DNA, peripheral lymphocyte subsets alterations and neutrophil lymphocyte ratio in assessment of COVID-19 severity. *Innate Immun.* **2021**, *27*, 240–250. [CrossRef] [PubMed]

7. Rubin, G.D.; Ryerson, C.J.; Haramati, L.B.; Sverzellati, N.; Kanne, J.P.; Raoof, S.; Schluger, N.W.; Volpi, A.; Yim, J.J.; Martin, I.B.K.; et al. The Role of Chest Imaging in Patient Management during the COVID-19 Pandemic: A Multinational Consensus Statement from the Fleischner Society. *Radiology* **2020**, *296*, 172–180. [CrossRef]

8. Ooi, G.C.; Khong, P.L.; Müller, N.L.; Yiu, W.C.; Zhou, L.J.; Ho, J.C.; Lam, B.; Nicolaou, S.; Tsang, K.W. Severe Acute Respiratory Syndrome: Temporal Lung Changes at Thin-Section CT in 30 Patients. *Radiology* **2004**, *230*, 836–844. [CrossRef] [PubMed]

9. Simpson, S.; Kay, F.U.; Abbara, S.; Bhalla, S.; Chung, J.H.; Chung, M.; Henry, T.S.; Kanne, J.P.; Kligerman, S.; Ko, J.P.; et al. Radiological Society of North America Expert Consensus Document on Reporting Chest CT Findings Related to COVID-19: Endorsed by the Society of Thoracic Radiology, the American College of Radiology, and RSNA. *Radiol. Cardiothorac. Imaging* **2020**, *2*, e200152. [CrossRef]

10. Gouda, W.; Yasin, R. COVID-19 disease: CT Pneumonia Analysis prototype by using artificial intelligence, predicting the disease severity. *Egypt. J. Radiol. Nucl. Med.* **2020**, *51*, 196. [CrossRef]

11. van Timmeren, J.E.; Cester, D.; Tanadini-Lang, S.; Alkadhi, H.; Baessler, B. Radiomics in medical imaging—"how-to" guide and critical reflection. *Insights Imaging* **2020**, *11*, 91. [CrossRef]

12. Lippi, G.; Luca Salvagno, G.; Montagnana, M.; Brocco, G.; Guidi, G.C. Influence of hemolysis on routine clinical chemistry testing. *Clin. Chem. Lab. Med. CCLM* **2006**, *44*, 311–316. [CrossRef] [PubMed]

13. Simundic, A.-M.; Baird, G.; Cadamuro, J.; Costelloe, S.J.; Lippi, G. Managing hemolyzed samples in clinical laboratories. *Crit. Rev. Clin. Lab. Sci.* **2020**, *57*, 1–21. [CrossRef] [PubMed]

14. Degenhardt, F.; Seifert, S.; Szymczak, S. Evaluation of variable selection methods for random forests and omics data sets. *Brief. Bioinform.* **2019**, *20*, 492–503. [CrossRef] [PubMed]

15. Acharjee, A.; Larkman, J.; Xu, Y.; Cardoso, V.R.; Gkoutos, G.V. A random forest based biomarker discovery and power analysis framework for diagnostics research. *BMC Med. Genom.* **2020**, *13*, 178. [CrossRef]

16. R: A Language and Environment for Statistical Computing. Statistical Software. Available online: https://posit.co/downloads/ (accessed on 25 June 2023).

17. Liu, H.; Ren, H.; Wu, Z.; Xu, H.; Zhang, S.; Li, J.; Hou, L.; Chi, R.; Zheng, H.; Chen, Y.; et al. CT radiomics facilitates more accurate diagnosis of COVID-19 pneumonia: Compared with CO-RADS. *J. Transl. Med.* **2021**, *19*, 29. [CrossRef]

18. Zhang, M.; Zeng, X.; Huang, C.; Liu, J.; Liu, X.; Xie, X.; Wang, R. An AI-based radiomics nomogram for disease prognosis in patients with COVID-19 pneumonia using initial CT images and clinical indicators. *Int. J. Med. Inf.* **2021**, *154*, 104545. [CrossRef]

19. Lassau, N.; Ammari, S.; Chouzenoux, E.; Gortais, H.; Herent, P.; Devilder, M.; Soliman, S.; Meyrignac, O.; Talabard, M.P.; Lamarque, J.P.; et al. Integrating deep learning CT-scan model, biological and clinical variables to predict severity of COVID-19 patients. *Nat. Commun.* **2021**, *12*, 634. [CrossRef]

20. Hectors, S.J.; Riyahi, S.; Dev, H.; Krishnan, K.; Margolis, D.J.A.; Prince, M.R. Multivariate analysis of CT imaging, laboratory, and demographical features for prediction of acute kidney injury in COVID-19 patients: A Bi-centric analysis. *Abdom. Radiol.* **2021**, *46*, 1651–1658. [CrossRef]

21. Weikert, T.; Rapaka, S.; Grbic, S.; Re, T.; Chaganti, S.; Winkel, D.J.; Anastasopoulos, C.; Niemann, T.; Wiggli, B.J.; Bremerich, J.; et al. Prediction of Patient Management in COVID-19 Using Deep Learning-Based Fully Automated Extraction of Cardiothoracic CT Metrics and Laboratory Findings. *Korean J. Radiol.* **2021**, *22*, 994. [CrossRef]

22. Do, T.D.; Skornitzke, S.; Merle, U.; Kittel, M.; Hofbaur, S.; Melzig, C.; Kauczor, H.U.; Wielpütz, M.O.; Weinheimer, O. COVID-19 pneumonia: Prediction of patient outcome by CT-based quantitative lung parenchyma analysis combined with laboratory parameters. *PLoS ONE* **2022**, *17*, e0271787. [CrossRef]

23. Naymagon, L.; Zubizarreta, N.; Feld, J.; van Gerwen, M.; Alsen, M.; Thibaud, S.; Kessler, A.; Venugopal, S.; Makki, I.; Qin, Q.; et al. Admission D-dimer levels, D-dimer trends, and outcomes in COVID-19. *Thromb. Res.* **2020**, *196*, 99–105. [CrossRef]

24. Zhang, L.; Yan, X.; Fan, Q.; Liu, H.; Liu, X.; Liu, Z.; Zhang, Z. D-dimer levels on admission to predict in-hospital mortality in patients with COVID-19. *J. Thromb. Haemost.* **2020**, *18*, 1324–1329. [CrossRef] [PubMed]

25. Fernandez-Botran, R.; Furmanek, S.; Ambadapoodi, R.S.; Expósito González, E.; Cahill, M.; Carrico, R.; Akca, O.; Ramírez, J.A. Association and predictive value of biomarkers with severe outcomes in hospitalized patients with SARS-CoV-2 infection. *Cytokine* **2022**, *149*, 155755. [CrossRef]

26. Hoteit, L.; Deeb, A.-P.; Andraska, E.A.; Kaltenmeier, C.; Yazdani, H.O.; Tohme, S.; Neal, M.D.; Mota, R.I. The Pathobiological Basis for Thrombotic Complications in COVID-19: A Review of the Literature. *Curr. Pathobiol. Rep.* **2021**, *9*, 107–117. [CrossRef] [PubMed]

27. Gatto, M.C.; Oliva, A.; Palazzolo, C.; Picariello, C.; Garascia, A.; Nicastri, E.; Girardi, E.; Antinori, A. Efficacy and Safety of Anticoagulant Therapy in COVID-19-Related Pulmonary Embolism with Different Extension. *Biomedicines* **2023**, *11*, 1282. [CrossRef] [PubMed]

28. Yu, L.; Halalau, A.; Dalal, B.; Abbas, A.E.; Ivascu, F.; Amin, M.; Nair, G.B. Machine learning methods to predict mechanical ventilation and mortality in patients with COVID-19. *PLoS ONE* **2021**, *16*, e0249285. [CrossRef]

29. Chieregato, M.; Frangiamore, F.; Morassi, M.; Baresi, C.; Nici, S.; Bassetti, C.; Bnà, C.; Galelli, M. A hybrid machine learning/deep learning COVID-19 severity predictive model from CT images and clinical data. *Sci. Rep.* **2022**, *12*, 4329. [CrossRef]

30. Giraudo, C.; Frattin, G.; Fichera, G.; Motta, R.; Stramare, R. A practical integrated radiomics model predicting intensive care hospitalization in COVID-19. *Crit. Care* **2021**, *25*, 145. [CrossRef]

31. Bronkhorst, A.J.; Ungerer, V.; Holdenrieder, S. Comparison of methods for the quantification of cell-free DNA isolated from cell culture supernatant. *Tumor Biol.* **2019**, *41*, 101042831986636. [CrossRef]

32. Simonnet, A.; Chetboun, M.; Poissy, J.; Raverdy, V.; Noulette, J.; Duhamel, A.; Labreuche, J.; Mathieu, D.; Pattou, F.; Jourdain, M. High Prevalence of Obesity in Severe Acute Respiratory Syndrome Coronavirus-2 (SARS-CoV-2) Requiring Invasive Mechanical Ventilation. *Obesity* **2020**, *28*, 1195–1199. [CrossRef]

33. Nishimoto, S.; Fukuda, D.; Higashikuni, Y.; Tanaka, K.; Hirata, Y.; Murata, C.; Kim-Kaneyama, J.R.; Sato, F.; Bando, M.; Yagi, S.; et al. Obesity-induced DNA released from adipocytes stimulates chronic adipose tissue inflammation and insulin resistance. *Sci. Adv.* **2016**, *2*, e1501332. [CrossRef] [PubMed]

34. Menni, C.; Valdes, A.M.; Freidin, M.B.; Sudre, C.H.; Nguyen, L.H.; Drew, D.A.; Ganesh, S.; Varsavsky, T.; Cardoso, M.J.; El-Sayed Moustafa, J.S.; et al. Real-time tracking of self-reported symptoms to predict potential COVID-19. *Nat. Med.* **2020**, *26*, 1037–1040. [CrossRef] [PubMed]

35. Gerhards, C.; Thiaucourt, M.; Kittel, M.; Becker, C.; Ast, V.; Hetjens, M.; Neumaier, M.; Haselmann, V. Longitudinal assessment of anti-SARS-CoV-2 antibody dynamics and clinical features following convalescence from a COVID-19 infection. *Int. J. Infect. Dis.* **2021**, *107*, 221–227. [CrossRef] [PubMed]

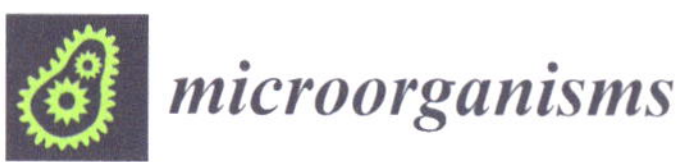 *microorganisms*

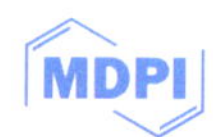

Review

A Dual Pharmacological Strategy against COVID-19: The Therapeutic Potential of Metformin and Atorvastatin

Luis Adrián De Jesús-González [1,2,*], Rosa María del Ángel [2,*], Selvin Noé Palacios-Rápalo [2], Carlos Daniel Cordero-Rivera [2], Adrián Rodríguez-Carlos [1], Juan Valentin Trujillo-Paez [1], Carlos Noe Farfan-Morales [3], Juan Fidel Osuna-Ramos [4], José Manuel Reyes-Ruiz [5,6], Bruno Rivas-Santiago [1], Moisés León-Juárez [7], Ana Cristina García-Herrera [1], Adriana Clara Ramos-Cortes [1], Erika Alejandra López-Gándara [1] and Estefanía Martínez-Rodríguez [1]

[1] Unidad de Investigación Biomédica de Zacatecas, Instituto Mexicano del Seguro Social, Zacatecas 98000, Mexico; rdz.carlos09@hotmail.com (A.R.-C.); taneiro87@hotmail.com (J.V.T.-P.); rondo_vm@yahoo.com (B.R.-S.); ana.garciaher@imss.gob.mx (A.C.G.-H.); ramcor16@hotmail.com (A.C.R.-C.); erykagandara@gmail.com (E.A.L.-G.); estefania_940@yahoo.com.mx (E.M.-R.)

[2] Department of Infectomics and Molecular Pathogenesis, Center for Research and Advanced Studies (CINVESTAV-IPN), Mexico City 07360, Mexico; selvin.palacios@cinvestav.mx (S.N.P.-R.); carlos.cordero@cinvestav.mx (C.D.C.-R.)

[3] Departamento de Ciencias Naturales, Universidad Autónoma Metropolitana (UAM), Unidad Cuajimalpa, Ciudad de México 05348, Mexico; carlos.farfan@cinvestav.mx

[4] Facultad de Medicina, Universidad Autónoma de Sinaloa, Culiacán 80019, Mexico; osunajuanfidel.fm@uas.edu.mx

[5] División de Investigación en Salud, Unidad Médica de Alta Especialidad, Hospital de Especialidades No. 14, Centro Médico Nacional "Adolfo Ruiz Cortines", Instituto Mexicano del Seguro Social (IMSS), Veracruz 91897, Mexico; jose.reyesr@imss.gob.mx

[6] Facultad de Medicina, Región Veracruz, Universidad Veracruzana (UV), Veracruz 91700, Mexico

[7] Laboratorio de Virología Perinatal y Diseño Molecular de Antígenos y Biomarcadores, Departamento de Inmunobioquímica, Instituto Nacional de Perinatología, Ciudad de México 11000, Mexico; moisesleoninper@gmail.com

* Correspondence: luis.dejesus@cinvestav.mx (L.A.D.J.-G.); rmangel@cinvestav.mx (R.M.d.Á.); Tel.: +52-492-9226-019 (L.A.D.J.-G.)

Citation: De Jesús-González, L.A.; del Ángel, R.M.; Palacios-Rápalo, S.N.; Cordero-Rivera, C.D.; Rodríguez-Carlos, A.; Trujillo-Paez, J.V.; Farfan-Morales, C.N.; Osuna-Ramos, J.F.; Reyes-Ruiz, J.M.; Rivas-Santiago, B.; et al. A Dual Pharmacological Strategy against COVID-19: The Therapeutic Potential of Metformin and Atorvastatin. *Microorganisms* **2024**, *12*, 383. https://doi.org/10.3390/microorganisms12020383

Academic Editor: Qibin Geng

Received: 29 December 2023
Revised: 31 January 2024
Accepted: 11 February 2024
Published: 13 February 2024

Abstract: Metformin (MET) and atorvastatin (ATO) are promising treatments for COVID-19. This review explores the potential of MET and ATO, commonly prescribed for diabetes and dyslipidemia, respectively, as versatile medicines against SARS-CoV-2. Due to their immunomodulatory and antiviral capabilities, as well as their cost-effectiveness and ubiquitous availability, they are highly suitable options for treating the virus. MET's effect extends beyond managing blood sugar, impacting pathways that can potentially decrease the severity and fatality rates linked with COVID-19. It can partially block mitochondrial complex I and stimulate AMPK, which indicates that it can be used more widely in managing viral infections. ATO, however, impacts cholesterol metabolism, a crucial element of the viral replicative cycle, and demonstrates anti-inflammatory characteristics that could modulate intense immune reactions in individuals with COVID-19. Retrospective investigations and clinical trials show decreased hospitalizations, severity, and mortality rates in patients receiving these medications. Nevertheless, the journey from observing something to applying it in a therapeutic setting is intricate, and the inherent diversity of the data necessitates carefully executed, forward-looking clinical trials. This review highlights the requirement for efficacious, easily obtainable, and secure COVID-19 therapeutics and identifies MET and ATO as promising treatments in this worldwide health emergency.

Keywords: COVID-19; metformin; atorvastatin; antiviral drugs; pharmacological repositioning

1. Introduction

SARS-CoV-2, the etiological agent of COVID-19 disease, has generated an unprecedented epidemic, putting enormous strain on healthcare systems around the world. Despite the widespread use of multiple vaccines, the recurrence of symptomatic cases underscores the necessity of practical treatment approaches against this virus [1,2]. Although vaccines are the primary prevention method, the appearance of viral variants and the risk of inadequate immune responses in some people underline the need for effective therapy [3]. The Food and Drug Administration (FDA) of the United States has approved and permitted the emergency use of medications to treat COVID-19. These cover many therapeutic techniques, from direct antiviral medicines to immunomodulatory [1,4].

On the other hand, the genetic diversity of SARS-CoV-2 is a decisive factor in its infective capacity and transmission dynamics in the human population. Because its RNA polymerase lacks proofreading mechanisms during replication, it has an inherent propensity to accumulate mutations as a single-stranded RNA virus. When these mutations occur in essential areas, such as the S protein, they are critical because they play a role in the virion entry into host cells, affecting the primary target of immune responses and antiviral medicines [5].

Reevaluating current medications for new therapeutic applications has emerged as a critical tactic in this setting. This review focuses on repositioning metformin (MET) and atorvastatin (ATO) as prospective COVID-19 therapy candidates. Traditionally used to treat diabetes [6,7] and dyslipidemia [8,9], these medicines have been demonstrated to have immunomodulatory and antiviral effects that may be useful in treating SARS-CoV-2 infection [10–16].

It is necessary to find treatments that are safe, effective, and easy to obtain. With their well-known security features and wide availability, MET and ATO offer a unique chance. This review carefully examines the pharmacological basis of both drugs and the latest information on COVID-19 and its antiviral properties.

2. Fundamentals and Mechanisms: An In-Depth Analysis of the Pharmacology of Metformin and Atorvastatin

MET (N, N-dimethylbiguanide) is one of the most prescribed drugs worldwide. It is used for treating diabetes, prediabetes, gestational diabetes, polycystic ovarian syndrome, cancer, HIV-associated diabetes, and cardiac ischemia [17]. During the 1920s, guanidine, the active component of Galega officinalis, was used to synthesize multiple antidiabetic compounds, including the main biguanides, MET, and phenformin [18]. Still, MET distinguishes itself due to its favorable profile in treating type 2 diabetes. The structure of biguanides consists of two guanidine groups linked by a methylene bridge (-CH2-). MET has demonstrated a higher safety margin concerning severe complications such as lactic acidosis. Its therapeutic range in hepatic concentrations varies between 10 and 40 μM in type 2 diabetic patients [19]. MET lowers the basal and postprandial plasma glucose (PPG) as a biguanide agent [20]. MET actions ameliorate insulin resistance by inhibiting principally hepatic gluconeogenesis, reducing intestinal glucose adsorption, and improving glucose uptake and utilization. Within the liver, the principal effect of MET is a reduction in the hepatic glucose output. Besides lowering blood glucose levels, MET has additional health benefits, including weight reduction, reducing plasma lipid levels, and preventing some microvascular complications [21]. The drug is not metabolized and is widely distributed into the body tissues, including the intestine, liver, and kidney, by organic cation transporters [22].

MET's antidiabetic effect is due to the partial reduction of the activity of the respiratory chain on mitochondrial complex I through interfering with electron transfer and ATP production [6,7]. Interestingly, MET inhibits the mitochondrial glycerophosphate (mGPD) activity and mitochondrial respiration from glycerol-3-phosphate at lower concentrations than those affecting complex I [23]. This mechanism leads to other downstream events, including the activation of adenosine monophosphate kinase (AMPK), inhibition of 1,6-bisphosphatase, and glucagon signaling [24].

The defined mechanism of MET action is AMPK activation, inhibiting the liver's critical enzymes involved in gluconeogenesis and glycogen synthesis while stimulating insulin signaling and glucose transport in muscles [24]. AMPK regulates the cellular and organ metabolism, where any decrease in hepatic energy leads to the activation of AMPK by increasing the adenosine monophosphate (AMP) to adenosine triphosphate (ATP) AMP:ATP and adenine diphosphate (ADP) ADP·ATP ratios, as regulated by adenylate cyclase. AMP binds to the sensing domain, where it allosterically activates AMPK. Also, AMP causes the inhibition of the dephosphorylation of Thr172 on the γ subunits [25].

AMPK activation requires the phosphorylation of Thr172 of the catalytic α-subunit, which is regulated upstream by the tumor suppressor serine/threonine kinase 11 (STK11/LKB1) [26] and by the Ca2+ calmodulin-dependent kinase kinases CaMKK-α and -β [27]. The LKB1 pathway regulates downstream the phosphorylation of the transducer of regulated CREB activity 2 (TORC2) [28]. The activated AMPK cascade is a metabolic switch sensor in cells that switches from an anabolic to a catabolic state, switching off the ATP-consuming synthetic pathways and restoring the energy balance by switching on the uptake of glucose and fatty acids [29].

Similar to all medicines, MET can cause side effects, including nausea, vomiting, diarrhea, indigestion, heartburn, flatulence, weakness, myalgia, chest discomfort, palpitations, flushing, headache, lightheadedness, dyspnea, a flu-like condition, reduced vitamin B12 levels, increased diaphoresis and cutaneous side effects [30]. MET is contraindicated in patients with severe renal failure as there is an increased risk of lactic acidosis [31].

On the other hand, ATO is a statin that inhibits 3-hydroxy-3-methyl-glutaryl-CoA (HMG-CoA) reductase (HMGCR). In 1980, it was shown that mevastatin, formerly called ML-236B or compactin, markedly lowers the levels of low-density lipoprotein (LDL) cholesterol [32] and apolipoprotein B (apo-B). ATO is a synthetic variant of this statin, approved in 1996 [8].

ATO exhibits a potent competitive inhibitory effect on the activity of the enzyme HMGCR, which plays a pivotal role in the biosynthesis of cholesterol in the liver. By inhibiting this enzyme, ATO decreases the production of cholesterol. HMGCR inhibition has a rate-limiting effect in the cholesterol synthesis pathway through converting 3-hydroxy-3-methyl glutaryl-CoA (HMG-CoA) into mevalonate, the precursor of cholesterol and other sterols [33]. Consequently, hepatocytes lead to increased production (upregulation) of LDL receptors on their surface, enhancing the uptake and clearance of LDL cholesterol from the bloodstream [8,9].

This reduction in the LDL cholesterol levels helps mitigate the risk of cardiovascular diseases associated with high cholesterol. ATV can also raise the HDL cholesterol levels and decrease triglycerides [18]. The common side effects of ATV happen in more than 1 in 100 people, including gastrointestinal, nausea, bloating, diarrhea or constipation, hepatitis, myalgia, and myopathy [19].

This reduction in the LDL cholesterol levels helps mitigate the risk of cardiovascular diseases associated with high cholesterol. ATO can also raise the HDL cholesterol levels and decrease triglycerides [34]. The common side effects of ATO happen in more than 1 in 100 people, including gastrointestinal, nausea, bloating, diarrhea or constipation, hepatitis, myalgia, and myopathy [35].

3. Antiviral Properties of Metformin and Atorvastatin

MET and ATO are hypoglycemic and hypolipidemic drugs [8,23], respectively. MET interferes with various stages of the viral life cycle (Table 1). Furthermore, MET impacts host cell metabolism, and the immune response might contribute to its antiviral effects. In addition, the drugs' hypolipidemic effects may contribute to many viruses requiring cholesterol or other lipids for an efficient replicative cycle (Table 2) [36]. In vitro and in vivo studies show that both drugs efficiently inhibit the infection of a diverse group of viruses such as IAV, HCV, HBV, HPV, HSV, HIV, Rotavirus, and KSHV [37–40], as well as some RNA viruses such as DENV, ZIKV, YFV [41], including SARS-CoV-2 [42].

Table 1. MET is a broad-spectrum antiviral because it inhibits the replicative cycle of different viruses.

Group Baltimore (Class)	Virus (Family)	Model	Antiviral Effect
I (dsDNA)	HPV	In vitro, in vivo, and patients	MET promotes HPV-HNSCC and cervical cancer cell apoptosis. It can also increase CD8+ Teff and FoxP3+ Tregs in the TME, suggesting an immunomodulatory effect [38,43].
	HSV	In vitro	Co-administration of C-REV (attenuated oncolytic HSV-1) and MET produces an antitumor effect and prolonged survival in mice. Additionally, it improves systemic antitumor immunity [44].
	KSHV	In vitro	MET induces apoptosis in primary effusion lymphoma (KSHV-associated aggressive B-cell lymphoma) cells [45].
III (dsRNA)	Rotavirus (Reoviridae)	In vitro and in vivo	MET inhibits the Rotavirus gene and protein expression in Caco-2 cells. Furthermore, MET mitigates intestinal lesions caused by Rotavirus [39].
	SARS-CoV-2	In vitro and patients	MET effectively inhibits viral replication of SARS-CoV-2 after 48 h of drug exposure without cytotoxic effect in Vero [11], Calu3, and Caco2 cells by up to 99% [42].
IV (ssRNA+)	DENV	In vitro and in vivo	MET inhibited ZIKV infection in Huh-7, C20, and U-87 cells but inhibited DENV and YFV infection in Huh-7 cells more effectively.
	ZIKV YFV		During DENV infection alone, MET increased the survival of male AG129 mice, reducing severe signs of the disease [41,46].
	HCV	In vitro	Simvastatin and MET inhibited cell growth and HCV infection in Huh7.5 cells. Furthermore, MET increased cell death markers, activated type I interferon signaling, and inhibited HCV replication through AMPK activation [47,48].
V (ssRNA-)	IAV	In vitro, in vivo, and patients	Studies showed that MET inhibits viral replication and cytokine expression induced by IAV. MET treatment was associated with decreased influenza-related mortality in diabetic patients [49].
VI (ssRNA-RT)	HIV	Patients	Co-administration of antiretrovirals and MET in patients with HIV decreased the infiltration of CD4 + T cells in the colon and the activation/phosphorylation of mTOR. Additionally, decreased HIV-RNA/HIV-DNA ratios, a surrogate marker of viral transcription [50]. Co-administration of dolutegravir and MET in patients with HIV and diabetes improves the control of both conditions, with a reduction in viral load and control of HgbA1C [51].
VII (dsDNA-RT)	HBV	In vitro	MET shows an HBV-associated inhibitory effect by negatively regulating the HULC/p18/miR-200a/ZEB1 signaling pathway [40].

The reason why MET and ATO are antiviral drugs is related to lipid metabolism [8,24]. Like SARS-CoV-2 and other RNA and DNA viruses, the viral cycle depends on lipid metabolism, especially on molecules like cholesterol and the formation of lipid droplets, which are essential for the replication cycles of many viruses [52].

For example, during the infection of different RNA viruses, such as SARS-CoV-2, lipids are necessary during the replicative cycle. Upon viral entry, lipid bilayers of the virus envelope obtained from the endoplasmic reticulum (ER) membrane participate in viral attachment and fusion. Second, an increase in cholesterol and fatty acid synthesis leads to the formation of invaginations of the ER membrane called replicative complexes (RCs), where viral translation and replication occur. In the next step, a combination of cholesterol-rich RCs used as a scaffold and the accumulation of lipid droplets (LDs) serve as the packaging for the viral genome and the formation of the nucleocapsid and contribute to the assembly of the progeny. Finally, the nucleocapsid buds through the ER membrane, completing the assembly of the virions. Virions are transported through the exocytic pathway to the Golgi complex for maturation and release from the infected cell [41,52–54].

The molecular mechanism of action of MET remains partly unknown. However, it has been suggested that, being a cation, it accumulates in the mitochondria due to the electrical gradient of the internal membrane, inhibiting complex I of the mitochondrial respiratory chain [55,56]. Therefore, MET inhibits mitochondrial ATP synthesis and consequently causes the indirect activation of AMPK, which is sensitive to ATP depletion, affecting fatty acid synthesis. Furthermore, MET directly reduces the synthesis of cholesterol and fatty acids (enzymatic inactivation) through the SREBP pathway, involving the lipid requirements of the virus. On the other hand, MET also induces the interferon-mediated response through AMPK [41,52,53].

Mainly, the antiviral mechanism of MET has been associated with the activation of the AMPK protein [24], which is attenuated in the early stages of infection by some viruses, such as DENV [57], promoting a decrease in intracellular lipids [23]. On the other hand, MET also inhibits the replication of DNA viruses, such as hepatitis B virus (HBV) [37], through the repression of genes related to viral transcription [58]. Likewise, MET with Entecavir (a guanosine nucleoside analog) inhibited HBV replication more significantly than the treatments alone [40,58]. Thus, MET promises to be a potential antiviral therapy, especially with other drugs [52].

Table 2. ATO is a broad-spectrum antiviral because it inhibits the cycle replicative of different viruses.

Group Baltimore (Class)	Virus (Family)	Model	Antiviral Effect
IV (ssRNA+)	SARS-CoV-2	In silico, in vitro, and patients	Molecular docking analyses reveal that ATO could bind to the virus's Mpro protease, Spike protein, and RNA-dependent RNA polymerase [59–61]. ATO showed antiviral activity against the D614G, Delta, and Mu variants of SARS-CoV-2 in Vero E6 cells through pre-post, pre-infection, and post-infection treatments [61–63].
	DENV	In vivo and in vitro	ATO reduced flaviviruses' viral titer and cytopathic effect in Huh-7, Vero, MDCK, and neural stem/progenitor cells. ATO reduced clinical signs and increased survival of AG129 mice [53,64–68].
	ZIKV YFV		ATO inhibits nuclear-cytoplasmic transport of viral proteins, inhibiting DENV viral replication [65].
	HCV	In vitro, and Patients	ATO suppresses HCV replication and has synergistic action with interferon. Additionally, it is associated with a 49% reduction in the incidence of hepatocellular carcinoma [69–72].
V (ssRNA-)	CV	In vivo	ATO reduced pathological features in the myocardium of mice infected with CVB3m and inhibited viral replication [73].
	IAV	In vitro	ATO inhibits the formation of lipid droplets by IAV, suppressing virus replication [74,75].
	RABV	In vitro	ATO inhibits the formation of lipid droplets by RABV, suppressing virus replication [76].
VI (ssRNA-RT)	HIV	Patients	ATO is safe in patients with HIV, reduces virus-associated inflammation, reduces the activation of CD8$^+$ and CD4$^+$ T cells, and prevents viral rebound [75–81] [77–83].

Recently, it has been shown that AMPK stabilizes ACE2 receptor expression upon phosphorylation of Ser360 [84]. It has been reported that phosphorylation of the ACE2 receptor promotes conformational and functional changes that would prevent SARS-CoV-2 from binding to host cells [84]. Furthermore, it is well known that ACE2 has an essential role in the anti-inflammatory immune response [85]. However, the entry of SARS-CoV-2 through interaction with ACE2 downregulates its expression, causing a pro-inflammatory effect [86,87]. Therefore, these data suggest that MET is an excellent therapeutic strategy against COVID-19, not only because it inhibits virus replication and entry but also because it could decrease the severe effects of the disease (Figure 1).

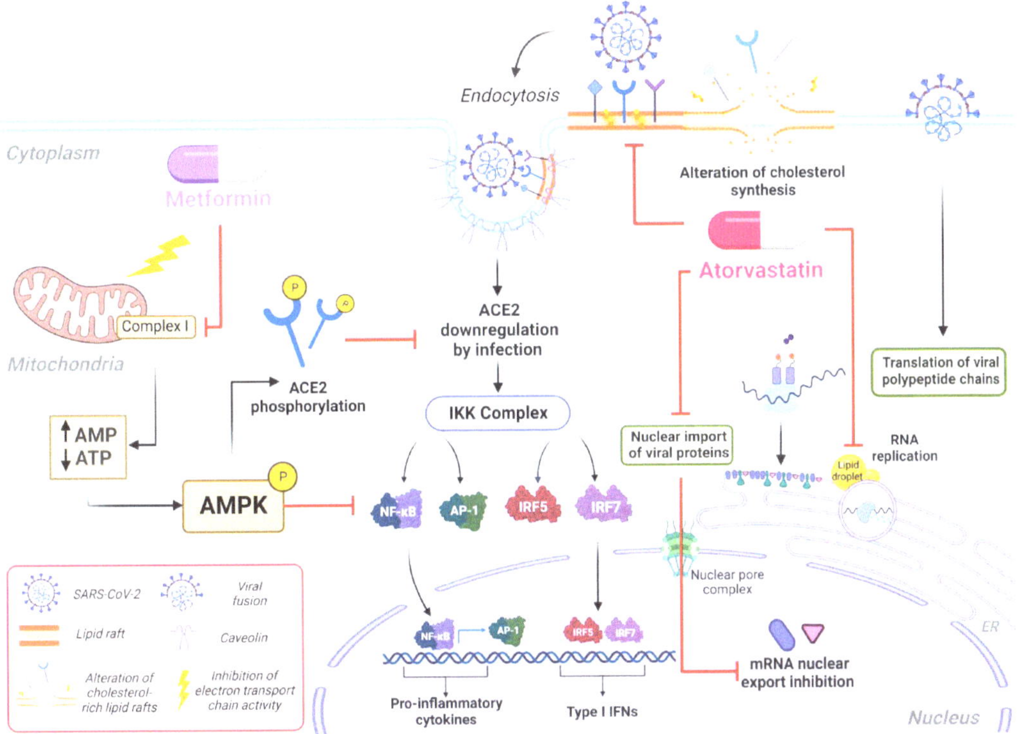

Figure 1. Antiviral capabilities of the MET and ATO drugs. The antiviral mechanism of MET is associated with inhibiting the electron transport chain, which helps the phosphorylation of AMPK and, subsequently, of the ACE2 receptor, preventing the entry of SARS-CoV2. On the other hand, it has been observed that viral entry causes a decrease in ACE2, triggering an exacerbating pro-inflammatory immune response. This allows us to suppose that MET can prevent viral entry and replication and the pro-inflammatory events caused by the disease. Like other statins, ATO has been associated mainly with intracellular lipid depletion, which can affect different viral stages, such as viral entry and replication. One of its effects may be the destabilization of lipid rafts, where viral receptors are anchored, and the decrease in lipids in the endoplasmic reticulum that allows the formation of new viral particles. Also, ATO can prevent the transport of viral proteins to the nucleus by preventing the sequestration of cellular messenger RNA, decreasing viral replication.

Interestingly, ATO is another drug with antiviral properties that inhibits lipid synthesis, affecting viral replication, as does MET [8,62,74]. However, studies in cancer cells have revealed that inhibition of lipid synthesis affects the prenylation of small GTPase proteins involved in actin cytoskeleton remodeling, affecting metastasis and intracellular transport [88]. Additionally, statins, including atorvastatin, have affected various cellular pathways during cellular transformation, such as in lung cancer. They observed its effect on survival pathways, pro-apoptotic signaling, chemotactic control, and angiogenesis. Therefore, atorvastatin could play a role in treating this type of cancer [89]. Due to this, Segatori et al., 2021 studied the effect of ATO treatment on nuclear import, demonstrating that ATO can reduce the nuclear localization of nuclear transport receptor proteins such as karyopherin alpha 2 (KPNA2) [63]. On the other hand, they found that the combination of ATO with ivermectin (an antiparasitic drug that blocks importin α/β pathway-dependent nuclear import [90]) more significantly inhibits the nuclear import of KPNA2 [63], suggesting that ATO in combination with ivermectin could be used as an antiviral treatment against viruses that import proteins into the nucleus, such as flaviviruses, influenza viruses and SARS-CoV-2.

Particularly, ATO can block the nuclear import of Huh7 cells, promoting the cytoplasmic accumulation of KPNA1 and KPNA2, as well as a nuclear import dependent on these pathways [65]. Moreover, ATO treatment can block the nuclear import of NS5 polymerase and NS3 viral protease of DENV-2. Importantly, in this work, we report that combining ATO with ivermectin significantly protects male AG129 mice from Dengue disease compared to a single ATO treatment, in addition to reducing the nuclear localization of NS3 in mouse brain tissue cells [65]. We suggest that the pleiotropic effects of ATO may affect the establishment of infection and viral replication.

On the other hand, we have tested combinations of ATO/ezetimibe and MET/ATO (unpublished data) in in vitro and in vivo models. These combinations show better antiviral capacity against viruses, for example, DENV, ZIKV, and YFV infections, than using a single drug alone [53]. Therefore, these drug combinations would be interesting to test in patients. Together, these results strongly suggest that MET and ATO should be considered possible treatments for COVID-19. On the other hand, we have tried combinations of ATO/ezetimibe [10], ivermectin/ATO [17], and MET/ATO (unpublished data) in in vitro and in vivo models. These combinations show better antiviral capacity against viruses, for example, DENV, ZIKV, and YFV infections, than using a single drug alone. Therefore, this drug is a combination that would be interesting to test in patients. Together, these results strongly suggest that MET and ATO should be considered possible treatments for COVID-19.

4. The Impact of Metformin and Atorvastatin on the Immune Response

The term "Immunomodulators" pertains to drugs that modify the immune system's response. These essential medications combat various conditions, such as infectious diseases, tumors, and primary or secondary immunodeficiency. However, these molecules may have differential impacts involved in the given pathology. Some reports have shown that immune modulators can decrease the morbidity and mortality in severely affected patients during viral infections [91]. The antiviral activity of MET is due, in part, to its immunostimulatory effects [92]. These effects mainly depend on AMP-activated protein kinase (AMPK) activation, as described above. Briefly, the activation of MAPK increases mTOR signaling by phosphorylating TSC2 and RAPTOR, a crucial connection between immune function and metabolism [93].

Additionally, this response can inhibit the NF-κB pathway, a master regulator of the inflammatory response [94]. For instance, several studies have demonstrated in animal models that MET decreases inflammatory cytokines, such as IL-1β, IL-6, and TNFα, and increases anti-inflammatory via IL-10 expression [92,93,95]. Thus, it protects against acute lung injuries or can suppress the cytokine storm produced by severe COVID-19 [96].

On the other hand, MET modulates the differentiation and activation effects of various immune cells. Macrophages exhibit two primary phenotypes: pro-inflammatory (M1) and "alternatively" activated (M2) macrophages. These distinct macrophage phenotypes are primarily pro-inflammatory responses or the resolution of inflammation [97]. In vitro, MET can have anti-inflammatory preferences. Thus, the response in macrophages stimulated with LPS decreases the TNF-α, IL-6, MCP-1, ROS, and pro-IL-1β while boosting IL-10 expression [98]. However, MET in a cancer environment induces a shift from M2 to M1 polarization of macrophages [99]. This provides evidence of MET's ability to enhance the balance between M1 and M2 macrophages. In addition, MET has demonstrated a reduction in the neutrophil count in patients with diabetes and polycystic ovarian disease. Furthermore, MET modulates the function of neutrophils by decreasing the formation of neutrophil extracellular traps (NETs) [100]. This effect is particularly relevant considering the involvement of neutrophils in various complications of SARS-CoV-2 infection [101].

The adaptive immune response begins with the recognition of specific antigens, marking the commencement of a cascade that transforms naive T cells into effector T cells. These effector cells can differentiate into T-helper cells (CD4) or cytotoxic T cells (CD8). In the MET-treated mouse model, the T-helper response showed a decrease in the levels of Th1 and Th17 cytokines profile through the downregulation of T-box and RORγt transcription factors [102]. Also, upregulation of the anti-inflammatory or immunosuppressive response has been reported, characterized by increased Th2 and T-regulatory cell subpopulations, respectively. Moreover, some reports have demonstrated that MET reduced the levels of autoantibodies in relevant autoimmune disease models. Similarly, MET has shown favorable outcomes in the context of cancer, such as reduced tumor progression and, in some cases, complete tumor eradication. This beneficial effect is attributed to enhancing the downregulation of the immunosuppressive T-regulatory cells and the upregulation of T memory cells [103,104].

Although the immunomodulatory effect of ATO has been less studied than that of MET, statins appear to play a crucial role in modulating the immune response at various levels. The growing body of evidence has identified statins as potential anti-inflammatory agents. As described above, several cholesterol metabolites and their associated nuclear receptors can regulate the immune system.

The in vitro studies investigating the impact of ATO on inflammatory cytokines, such as IL-6 and IL-1β, suggest a potential role in reducing their concentrations [105]. If applicable in vivo, this could imply that statins, like ATO, may possess the ability to mitigate the pro-inflammatory effects of these cytokines within tissues. For instance, the use of ATO in Multiple Sclerosis increased the levels of IL-4, IL-10, and TGF-β, while IL-17 and TNF-α decreased compared to the control group [106]. Similarly, in Kawasaki disease, ATO exhibited inhibitory effects in producing soluble mediators of inflammation, including IL-2 and TNF-α, impacting T cell proliferation [107].

Additional studies have highlighted the substantial immune-suppressive effects of statins on adaptive immune cells, leading to a decrease in the T cell quantity, impairment of antigen-presenting cell activation of T cells, and a shift toward Th2 cytokines, potentially resolving autoimmunity. Moreover, some reports have demonstrated an influence on humoral immunity in healthy individuals through the short-term statin administration, potentially leading to improved vaccine efficacy and immunomodulatory actions. This warrants further investigation to fully understand their implications in various health conditions [108–110].

5. Retrospective Studies and Clinical Trials That Have Evaluated the Potential for Use of Metformin and Atorvastatin during COVID-19

Several retrospective studies have examined the efficacy of specific drugs, such as MET and ATO, in combating COVID-19. These findings indicate that MET, a medication routinely recommended for diabetes, may have additional beneficial effects outside its typical application. Notably, diabetic individuals who were already undergoing MET therapy when diagnosed with COVID-19 showed a propensity for improved clinical results. Based on these investigations, it was found that these people had a diminished likelihood of developing severe manifestations of COVID-19. Additionally, they saw a decrease in the necessity for admission to intensive care units due to progression and severity and a lower mortality rate in comparison to individuals who were not using the medication. These findings are noteworthy as they indicate that MET can be used not only as a treatment for diabetes but also as a potential aid in mitigating the severity of COVID-19 [12,111–113].

On the other hand, dysbiosis in the intestinal microbiota has been described as contributing to the appearance and progression of many viral diseases, including COVID-19 and its subsequent manifestations (long COVID) [114]. MET has been shown to modulate the intestinal microbiota in patients with COVID-19, increasing the alpha diversity of bacteria, which contributes to the modulation of the immune response and reduces the appearance of long COVID cases [14,115,116].

However, research has also been conducted on ATO, a statin recognized for its role in cholesterol regulation, concerning COVID-19. Several retrospective cohort studies have indicated that this medication may be linked to a reduction in both COVID-19 mortality and progression. Despite the encouraging nature of these findings, they must be interpreted critically on account of the inherent limitations of these research studies [117–119]. In addition, it has been described that it can modulate the immune response of patients with COVID-19, preventing the appearance of long COVID, and as a treatment for this [120,121].

However, it is essential to consider these findings within the context of the methodological limitations of the studies and the need for further research, preferably through prospective clinical trials, to confirm these effects and better understand how these drugs can be used effectively against COVID-19.

5.1. Clinical Trials with Metformin

Several clinical trials have been conducted to investigate MET usage during COVID-19. A summary of them and their main findings are presented in Table 3.

Table 3. Clinical trials with MET.

Authors	Sample size (Patients)	Dosage	Primary Outcomes
Reis et al., 2022 [10].	421	750 mg (extended-release) twice daily for ten days	Presence of side effects and interruptions. Hospitalization in 8 of 168 patients (4.8%) (MET group) vs. 14 of 179 patients (7.8%) (control group).
Ventura-López et al., 2022 [11].	20	620 mg twice daily for 14 days vs. placebo *	MET significantly reduced viral load (93.2%) in 3.3 days and decreased hospitalization time to 8.8 days and supplemental oxygen requirement. Changes were observed in AST, lymphocytes, neutrophils, D-dimer, CRP, DHL, and IgG biomarkers. The average hospitalization time was 8.8 days for the MET group and 9.8 days for the placebo group. Safety was comparable between groups, with no serious adverse events or hypoglycemia. No adverse events occurred.
Bramante et al., 2022 [13].	1431	They tested three drugs. Immediate-release MET was administered for 1–6 days (750 mg) and 7–14 days (1500 mg per day), ivermectin 390 to 470 µg per kilogram per day for three days, and fluvoxamine at 50 mg twice a day for 14 days.	None of the medications were effective in preventing hypoxia, ICU visits, hospitalization, or death. However, the authors mention that in the case of MET, there was a trend of benefits for preventing the severe form.
Bramante et al., 2023 [14].	1126		MET reduced the incidence of post-COVID-19 (4.1% absolute reduction)
Boulware et al., 2023 [122].	1323	MET 1000 mg/day on days 2 to 5; 1500 mg/day on days 6 to 14 *	42% reduction in ER visits, hospitalizations and deaths by day 14, and 58% reduction in hospitalizations and deaths by day 28 42% reduction in long COVID in 10 months Decrease in viral load compared to placebo

* These doses of MET showed better results in the treatment of COVID-19.

Evidence suggests that MET may be clinically beneficial for patients with COVID-19. For instance, Reis et al., 2022 conducted a randomized, placebo-controlled clinical trial in Brazil to determine the possible use of MET during COVID-19. The researchers enrolled 421 adults during different waves of SARS-CoV-2 variants to evaluate whether extended-release MET at a dose of 750 mg twice daily would provide benefits over placebo, even in patients already taking 1000 mg of immediate-release MET for conditions such as diabetes, prediabetes, weight loss, polycystic ovary syndrome, or nonalcoholic fatty liver disease. The relative risk of hospitalization or prolonged emergency service visit with MET was 1.03 (95% Bayesian credible interval, 0.64 to 1.66). In this trial, patients were started on MET at 1500 mg daily without dose adjustment, which may have caused side effects and discontinuations. However, hospitalization occurred in 8 of 168 patients (4.8%) in the MET group and 14 of 179 patients (7.8%) in the control group [10]. The authors suggest that MET was crucial in early treatment during the health crisis caused by COVID-19.

Another study was carried out by Ventura-López et al., 2022. The authors claim that MET is a therapeutic option for COVID-19 patients. They first evaluated the impact of MET in an in vitro model using lung cells infected with SARS-CoV-2 clinically isolated (alpha, delta, and epsilon variants of SARS-CoV-2). In the in vitro aspect, MET effectively inhibited viral replication after 48 h of exposure (IC50 189.8 µM) without showing toxicity up to doses of 100 µM and was effective against the variants studied [11].

The clinical trial in patients with SARS-CoV-2 infection and diagnosis of type 2 diabetes mellitus, performed as an adaptive, randomized, prospective, longitudinal, double-blind, multicenter, phase IIb study, compared MET administered at 620 mg twice daily for 14 days vs. placebo. In patients treated with MET, changes were observed in the levels of AST (33.8 to 31.5 U/L), lymphocytes (8.1 to 17%), neutrophils (85.2 to 76.2%), D-dimer (480 to 634 ng/mL), CPR (4.16 to 0.10 mg/L), DHL (257.5 to 256.5 µL/L) and IgG (969 to 781 mg/dL) from the beginning to the end of the study. Additionally, the MET group showed a notable reduction in the viral load, decreasing by 93.2% in just 3.3 days, compared to a 78.3% reduction in 5.6 days in the placebo group. The average hospitalization time was shorter in the MET group (8.8 days) compared to the placebo group (9.8 days), and the patients treated with MET required less supplemental oxygen (5.9 vs. 10.6 points) [11]. The average hospitalization time was shorter in the MET group (8.8 days) compared to the placebo group (9.8 days), and the patients treated with MET required less supplemental oxygen (5.9 vs. 10.6 points) [11]. Regarding safety, mild adverse events were recorded in both groups, with no incidences of hypoglycemia. This study highlights the potential efficacy of MET in decreasing the SARS-CoV-2 viral load and improving the clinical outcomes in patients with COVID-19 and type 2 diabetes mellitus [11].

Clinical studies were conducted by Bramante et al. in 2022, with a phase 3, double-blind, randomized, and placebo-controlled design. They tested the effectiveness of three repurposed drugs (MET, ivermectin, and fluvoxamine) in 1431 US patients with COVID-19 to prevent severe disease cases in non-hospitalized adults. The patients were between 30 and 85 years old, and all were overweight or obese. The outcome variables evaluated were hypoxia (≤93% oxygen saturation on home oximetry), emergency department visits, hospitalization, or death. The groups received the trial drugs according to the following doses: immediate-release MET administered with a dose escalation over six days to 1500 mg per day for 14 days, ivermectin at an amount of 390 to 470 µg per kilogram per day for three days, and fluvoxamine at a dose of 50 mg twice a day for 14 days [13].

Additionally, patients were asked to record the severity of their daily symptoms in paper diaries over 14 days. Neither overall signs nor specific symptoms of COVID-19 were reduced more rapidly with placebo than with any of the trial drugs. This study highlights no serious adverse events related to the medication [13].

Ultimately, the clinical trial concluded that none of the medications were effective in preventing hypoxia, ICU visits, hospitalization, or death. However, the authors mention that in the case of MET, there was a trend of benefit for the prevention of the severe form, according to their criteria (visit to the emergency department, hospitalization, or death), so they argue that more studies are needed with different doses or other populations to determine if any of the antiviral mechanisms (reduction of hepatitis C viral load [123]) or anti-inflammatory have clinical activity in the treatment of COVID-19 [13].

Derived from the previous study, two more studies were generated. In one of them, the authors followed up for up to 300 days with 1126 participants from the original study, who received MET plus ivermectin (group 1), MET plus fluvoxamine (group 2), MET plus placebo (group 3), ivermectin plus placebo (group 4), fluvoxamine plus placebo (group 5) or placebo plus placebo (group 6)), and they found that MET reduced the incidence of post-COVID-19 (4.1% absolute reduction) compared to the placebo. The main post-COVID-

19 symptoms were fatigue, difficulty focusing, difficulty sleeping, difficulty breathing, headache, loss of taste, and depression [14].

The latest work was presented during a conference on retroviruses and opportunistic diseases in the USA by Boulware et al., 2023. In this work, they mention that MET has in vitro activity against SARS-CoV-2. Furthermore, they mention that in a randomized phase 3, quadruple-blind, placebo-controlled trial in 1323 participants, MET (1000 mg/day on days 2 to 5; 1500 mg/day on days 6 to 14) resulted in a 42% reduction in ER visits, hospitalizations, and deaths on day 14, a 58% reduction in hospitalizations and deaths on day 28, and a 42% reduction in long COVID in 10 months [122].

Additionally, they mention that MET reduced the viral load by 4.4 times compared to the placebo from baseline to follow-up (5, 10, and 14 days). The antiviral effect increased with an increasing MET dose on days 6 to 14. Conversely, they mention that the antiviral effect was more significant in the unvaccinated group (mean -0.95 log copies/mL) than in the vaccinated group (mean -0.39 log copies/mL). There were no changes in the viral load versus the placebo for ivermectin or fluvoxamine [122].

Finally, the authors conclude that MET reduced the viral load of SARS-CoV-2 in this clinical trial. The temporal relationship with dose titration suggests a dose-dependent effect. The magnitude of the antiviral effect was similar to that of nirmatrelvir on day five and more significant than that of nirmatrelvir on day ten. And they emphasize that MET is safe, widely available, and has few contraindications [122].

5.2. Clinical Trials with Atorvastatin

Several clinical trials investigated ATO usage during COVID-19. The following is a summary of them and their principal findings (Table 4).

Table 4. Clinical trials with ATO.

Authors	Sample Size	Dosage	Primary Outcomes
Davoodi et al., 2021 [15].	40	40 mg ATO + 400/100 mg lopinavir/ritonavir (group 1) or 400/100 mg lopinavir/ritonavir for 5 days *	The duration of hospitalization was significantly reduced in the lopinavir/ritonavir + ATO group.
BMJ 2022 [16].	605	20 mg oral ATO once daily and placebo each for 30 days	90 (31%) patients died in the ATO group and 103 (35%) in the placebo group. Venous thromboembolism rates were 2% ($n = 6$) in the ATO group and 3% ($n = 9$) in the placebo group. ATO is safe with few adverse effects. Reduction in levels of white blood cells, platelets, and D-dimer in patients treated with ATO

* These doses of MET showed better results in the treatment of COVID-19.

On the other hand, ATO, a statin used to reduce cholesterol levels, has been researched due to its anti-inflammatory and anticoagulant properties. Davoodi et al., 2021 conducted a randomized controlled clinical trial on 40 Iranian adults hospitalized with COVID-19. Patients were randomly assigned (1:1) to a treatment group receiving ATO 40 mg + lopinavir/ritonavir 400/100 mg or a control group receiving lopinavir/ritonavir alone. ATO was administered as one tablet daily. In the case of lopinavir/ritonavir, it was administered twice daily. Both treatments were administered for five days [15].

The primary outcome of the trial was the length of hospitalization; the secondary outcomes were the need for interferon or immunoglobulin, receipt of invasive mechanical ventilation, O2 saturation (O2 sat), and C-reactive protein (CRP) level, assessed at baseline and on the sixth day of treatment [15].

The CRP level decreased significantly in the lopinavir/ritonavir + ATO group ($p < 0.0001$, Cohen's d = 0.865) so that there was a significant difference in the CRP level on the sixth day between the two groups ($p = 0.01$). However, there was no significant difference in O2 sat on day 6. Although the duration of hospitalization in the lopinavir/ritonavir + ATO group was significantly reduced compared with the control group (p = 0.012), there was no significant difference in the invasive mechanical ventilation, receipt, and need for interferon and immunoglobulin. The authors conclude that combining ATO + lopinavir/ritonavir may be more effective than lopinavir/ritonavir in treating adult patients hospitalized with COVID-19 [15].

In another randomized controlled trial published in *The BMJ*, in 11 hospitals in Iran, 605 patients >18 years of age with COVID-19 admitted to the ICU participated. ATO 20 mg was administered orally once daily versus placebo; follow-up was performed for 30 days from randomization, regardless of the hospital discharge status [16].

Death occurred in 90 (31%) patients in the ATO group and 103 (35%) in the placebo group (odds ratio 0.84, 95% confidence interval 0.58 to 1.22). The venous thromboembolism rates were 2% (n = 6) in the ATO group and 3% (n = 9) in the placebo group (odds ratio 0.71, 95% confidence interval: 0.24 to 2.06). Myopathy was not diagnosed clinically in either group. The liver enzyme levels increased (2%) in five patients assigned to ATO and six assigned to placebo (odds ratio 0.85, 95% confidence interval 0.25 to 2.81). The main drugs in the co-treatment were aspirin and antivirals such as remdesivir and favipiravir [16].

The authors conclude that ATO was not associated with a significant reduction in composite venous or arterial thrombosis, extracorporeal membrane oxygenation treatment, or all-cause mortality compared with placebo. However, the treatment was found to be safe. The overall event rates were lower than expected, so a clinically significant treatment effect cannot be excluded. Furthermore, they found a slight reduction in white blood cells, platelets, and D-dimer levels in the patients treated with ATO [16].

Visos-Varela et al., 2023 analyzed the chronic use of statins (simvastatin, lovastatin, pravastatin, fluvastatin, ATO, rosuvastatin, and pitavastatin) and severe outcomes of COVID-19 (risk of hospitalization and mortality), progression to severe consequences and susceptibility to the virus. The study evaluated the risk of hospitalization, mortality, progression, and susceptibility to COVID-19. They collected data on 2821 hospitalized cases, 26,996 non-hospitalized cases, and 52,318 controls [121].

Chronic use of ATO was associated with a decreased risk of hospitalization (adjusted odds ratios [aOR] = 0.83; 95% confidence interval [CI]: 0.74–0.92) and mortality (aOR = 0.70; 95% CI: 0.53–0.93), partly attributable to a lower risk of susceptibility to the virus (aOR = 0.91; 95% CI: 0.86–0.96) [121].

On the other hand, simvastatin was associated with a reduced mortality risk (aOR = 0.59, 95% CI: 0.40–0.87). The large degree of heterogeneity observed in the estimated OR of the different statins suggests that there was no class effect. In conclusion, the authors suggest that chronic use of ATO (and, to a lesser extent, simvastatin) is associated with a decreased risk of severe COVID-19 outcomes [121].6. Conclusions and Future Perspectives

The possibility of MET and ATO as therapeutic therapies for COVID-19 is highly promising. These medications, commonly used for treating diabetes and dyslipidemia, have shown notable immunomodulatory and antiviral effects that could be crucial against SARS-CoV-2. Ensuring effective, widely available, and safe treatments is especially critical during the current worldwide health emergency.

Notably, the cost-effectiveness of these treatments must not be disregarded. MET and ATO, being generic pharmaceuticals, represent a cost-efficient [124,125] substitute for more recent, trademarked anti-SARS-CoV-2 medications like Paxlovid® [126]. Their FDA and Cofepris (Mexico) approvals for diabetes management demonstrate their thorough examinations for safety and effectiveness [127,128], which increases confidence in their use for COVID-19 based on positive results from earlier clinical trials.

The role of MET extends beyond managing diabetes, as its antidiabetic actions can potentially reduce the severity and mortality of COVID-19. Through the partial inhibition of mitochondrial complex I and the activation of AMPK, MET enhances insulin sensitivity and has possible antiviral properties. Moreover, the capacity of ATO to reduce cholesterol levels and regulate immunological responses could be quite beneficial, particularly in severe instances of COVID-19 that are distinguished by an excessively aggressive immune response.

The available evidence, however varied, tends to favor optimism. Several research studies suggest that using MET and ATO can effectively reduce the severity and mortality of COVID-19, while some studies advise interpreting the results with caution. The documented advantages in specific patient cohorts, such as decreased hospitalizations and mortality rates, underscore their potential to impact patient outcomes effectively.

However, the journey from observation to clinical implementation is fraught with obstacles. The presence of diverse study approaches and patient demographics necessitates meticulous data analysis. Conducting prospective randomized controlled trials is crucial for confirming these results and finding the most efficient use of MET and ATO in treating COVID-19. Furthermore, considering the wide range of possible adverse effects, it is necessary to reevaluate these treatments' widely recognized safety profiles in COVID-19.

Amidst the ongoing challenges posed by the COVID-19 pandemic, repurposing MET and ATO is a promising and innovative gesture. Due to their cost-effectiveness, wide availability, and extensive safety records, they are highly suitable for reapplication. Nevertheless, this endeavor necessitates thorough investigation, precise examination, and a steadfast commitment to comprehending their significance in the COVID-19 storyline. By following this road, we will be able to fully utilize the therapeutic capabilities of MET and ATO, providing a more promising future in this ongoing global health crisis.

Author Contributions: Conceptualization: L.A.D.J.-G., R.M.d.Á., S.N.P.-R., C.D.C.-R. and C.N.F.-M.; funding acquisition: L.A.D.J.-G. and R.M.d.Á.; investigation: A.R.-C., J.V.T.-P., C.N.F.-M., J.F.O.-R., J.M.R.-R., B.R.-S., M.L.-J. and A.C.G.-H.; supervision: L.A.D.J.-G., R.M.d.Á., S.N.P.-R., C.D.C.-R. and C.N.F.-M.; visualization: B.R.-S., M.L.-J., A.C.G.-H., A.C.R.-C., E.A.L.-G. and E.M.-R.; writing—review and editing: A.R.-C., J.V.T.-P., C.N.F.-M., J.F.O.-R., J.M.R.-R., B.R.-S., M.L.-J. and A.C.G.-H. All authors have read and agreed to the published version of the manuscript.

Funding: This research was funded by grants Pronaii 302979 and A1-S-9005 CONAHCyT (México) from R.M.D.Á. Additionally, it was funded by FUNDACIÓN IMSS, AC (LADJG). However, the funders had no role in study design, data collection, analysis, publication decision, or article preparation.

Acknowledgments: L.A.D.J.-G., R.M.d.Á., A.R.-C., C.N.F.-M., J.F.O.-R., J.M.R.-R., B.R.-S. and M.L.-J. acknowledge their membership of the National System of Research (SNI CONAHCyT). SPR, CDCR, and JVTP appreciate the scholarship provided by CONAHCyT for doctoral or postdoctoral studies. We also thank the MDPI editorial board for their advice. The vatillos team.

Conflicts of Interest: The authors declare no conflicts of interest.

References

1. Cascella, M.; Rajnik, M.; Aleem, A.; Dulebohn, S.C.; Di Napoli, R. Features, Evaluation, and Treatment of Coronavirus (COVID-19). In *StatPearls*; StatPearls Publishing: Treasure Island, FL, USA, 2023.

2. Reyes-Ruiz, J.M.; García-Hernández, O.; Martínez-Mier, G.; Osuna-Ramos, J.F.; De Jesús-González, L.A.; Farfan-Morales, C.N.; Palacios-Rápalo, S.N.; Cordero-Rivera, C.D.; Ordoñez-Rodríguez, T.; Ángel, R.M.d. The Role of Aspartate Aminotransferase-to-Lymphocyte Ratio Index (ALRI) in Predicting Mortality in SARS-CoV-2 Infection. *Microorganisms* **2023**, *11*, 2894. [CrossRef]

3. Li, G.; Hilgenfeld, R.; Whitley, R.; De Clercq, E. Therapeutic Strategies for COVID-19: Progress and Lessons Learned. *Nat. Rev. Drug Discov.* **2023**, *22*, 449–475. [CrossRef] [PubMed]

4. Kumari, M.; Lu, R.-M.; Li, M.-C.; Huang, J.-L.; Hsu, F.-F.; Ko, S.-H.; Ke, F.-Y.; Su, S.-C.; Liang, K.-H.; Yuan, J.P.-Y.; et al. A Critical Overview of Current Progress for COVID-19: Development of Vaccines, Antiviral Drugs, and Therapeutic Antibodies. *J. Biomed. Sci.* **2022**, *29*, 68. [CrossRef] [PubMed]

5. Akkiz, H. Implications of the Novel Mutations in the SARS-CoV-2 Genome for Transmission, Disease Severity, and the Vaccine Development. *Front. Med.* **2021**, *8*, 636532. [CrossRef] [PubMed]

6. El-Mir, M.Y.; Nogueira, V.; Fontaine, E.; Avéret, N.; Rigoulet, M.; Leverve, X. Dimethylbiguanide Inhibits Cell Respiration via an Indirect Effect Targeted on the Respiratory Chain Complex I. *J. Biol. Chem.* **2000**, *275*, 223–228. [CrossRef] [PubMed]

7. Hawley, S.A.; Ross, F.A.; Chevtzoff, C.; Green, K.A.; Evans, A.; Fogarty, S.; Towler, M.C.; Brown, L.J.; Ogunbayo, O.A.; Evans, A.M.; et al. Use of Cells Expressing Gamma Subunit Variants to Identify Diverse Mechanisms of AMPK Activation. *Cell Metab.* **2010**, *11*, 554–565. [CrossRef] [PubMed]

8.   Conde, K.; Pineda, G.; Newton, R.S.; Fernandez, M.L. Hypocholesterolemic Effects of 3-Hydroxy-3-Methylglutaryl Coenzyme A (HMG-CoA) Reductase Inhibitors in the Guinea Pig: Atorvastatin versus Simvastatin. *Biochem. Pharmacol.* **1999**, *58*, 1209–1219. [CrossRef] [PubMed]
9.   Chong, P.H.; Seeger, J.D. Atorvastatin Calcium: An Addition to HMG-CoA Reductase Inhibitors. *Pharmacotherapy* **1997**, *17*, 1157–1177. [CrossRef] [PubMed]
10. Reis, G.; Silva, E.A.d.S.M.; Silva, D.C.M.; Thabane, L.; Milagres, A.C.; Ferreira, T.S.; dos Santos, C.V.Q.; Neto, A.D.d.F.; Callegari, E.D.; Savassi, L.C.M.; et al. Effect of Early Treatment with Metformin on Risk of Emergency Care and Hospitalization among Patients with COVID-19: The TOGETHER Randomized Platform Clinical Trial. *Lancet Reg. Health Am.* **2022**, *6*, 100142. [CrossRef]
11. Ventura-López, C.; Cervantes-Luevano, K.; Aguirre-Sánchez, J.S.; Flores-Caballero, J.C.; Alvarez-Delgado, C.; Bernaldez-Sarabia, J.; Sánchez-Campos, N.; Lugo-Sánchez, L.A.; Rodríguez-Vázquez, I.C.; Sander-Padilla, J.G.; et al. Treatment with Metformin Glycinate Reduces SARS-CoV-2 Viral Load: An in Vitro Model and Randomized, Double-Blind, Phase IIb Clinical Trial. *Biomed. Pharmacother.* **2022**, *152*, 113223. [CrossRef]
12. Bramante, C.T.; Ingraham, N.E.; Murray, T.A.; Marmor, S.; Hovertsen, S.; Gronski, J.; McNeil, C.; Feng, R.; Guzman, G.; Abdelwahab, N.; et al. Metformin and Risk of Mortality in Patients Hospitalised with COVID-19: A Retrospective Cohort Analysis. *Lancet Healthy Longev.* **2021**, *2*, e34–e41. [CrossRef] [PubMed]
13. Bramante, C.T.; Huling, J.D.; Tignanelli, C.J.; Buse, J.B.; Liebovitz, D.M.; Nicklas, J.M.; Cohen, K.; Puskarich, M.A.; Belani, H.K.; Proper, J.L.; et al. Randomized Trial of Metformin, Ivermectin, and Fluvoxamine for COVID-19. *N. Engl. J. Med.* **2022**, *387*, 599–610. [CrossRef] [PubMed]
14. Bramante, C.T.; Buse, J.B.; Liebovitz, D.M.; Nicklas, J.M.; Puskarich, M.A.; Cohen, K.; Belani, H.K.; Anderson, B.J.; Huling, J.D.; Tignanelli, C.J.; et al. Outpatient Treatment of COVID-19 and Incidence of Post-COVID-19 Condition over 10 Months (COVID-OUT): A Multicentre, Randomised, Quadruple-Blind, Parallel-Group, Phase 3 Trial. *Lancet Infect. Dis.* **2023**, *23*, 1119–1129. [CrossRef] [PubMed]
15. Davoodi, L.; Jafarpour, H.; Oladi, Z.; Zakariaei, Z.; Tabarestani, M.; Ahmadi, B.M.; Razavi, A.; Hessami, A. Atorvastatin Therapy in COVID-19 Adult Inpatients: A Double-Blind, Randomized Controlled Trial. *Int. J. Cardiol. Heart Vasc.* **2021**, *36*, 100875. [CrossRef] [PubMed]
16. Investigators, I.-S. Atorvastatin versus Placebo in Patients with COVID-19 in Intensive Care: Randomized Controlled Trial. *BMJ* **2022**, *376*, e068407. [CrossRef]
17. Nasri, H.; Rafieian-Kopaei, M. Metformin: Current Knowledge. *J. Res. Med. Sci.* **2014**, *19*, 658–664. [PubMed]
18. Bailey, C.J.; Turner, R.C. Metformin. *N. Engl. J. Med.* **1996**, *334*, 574–579. [CrossRef] [PubMed]
19. Sum, C.F.; Webster, J.M.; Johnson, A.B.; Catalano, C.; Cooper, B.G.; Taylor, R. The Effect of Intravenous Metformin on Glucose Metabolism during Hyperglycaemia in Type 2 Diabetes. *Diabet. Med.* **1992**, *9*, 61–65. [CrossRef]
20. Scarpello, J.H.B.; Howlett, H.C.S. Metformin Therapy and Clinical Uses. *Diab. Vasc. Dis. Res.* **2008**, *5*, 157–167. [CrossRef]
21. DeFronzo, R.A.; Goodman, A.M. Efficacy of Metformin in Patients with Non-Insulin-Dependent Diabetes Mellitus. *N. Engl. J. Med.* **1995**, *333*, 541–549. [CrossRef]
22. Giannarelli, R.; Aragona, M.; Coppelli, A.; Del Prato, S. Reducing Insulin Resistance with Metformin: The Evidence Today. *Diabetes Metab.* **2003**, *29*, 6S28–6S35. [CrossRef]
23. Madiraju, A.K.; Erion, D.M.; Rahimi, Y.; Zhang, X.-M.; Braddock, D.T.; Albright, R.A.; Prigaro, B.J.; Wood, J.L.; Bhanot, S.; MacDonald, M.J.; et al. Metformin Suppresses Gluconeogenesis by Inhibiting Mitochondrial Glycerophosphate Dehydrogenase. *Nature* **2014**, *510*, 542–546. [CrossRef]
24. LaMoia, T.E.; Shulman, G.I. Cellular and Molecular Mechanisms of Metformin Action. *Endocr. Rev.* **2021**, *42*, 77–96. [CrossRef]
25. Xiao, B.; Heath, R.; Saiu, P.; Leiper, F.C.; Leone, P.; Jing, C.; Walker, P.A.; Haire, L.; Eccleston, J.F.; Davis, C.T.; et al. Structural Basis for AMP Binding to Mammalian AMP-Activated Protein Kinase. *Nature* **2007**, *449*, 496–500. [CrossRef]
26. Hawley, S.A.; Boudeau, J.; Reid, J.L.; Mustard, K.J.; Udd, L.; Mäkelä, T.P.; Alessi, D.R.; Hardie, D.G. Complexes between the LKB1 Tumor Suppressor, STRAD Alpha/Beta and MO25 Alpha/Beta Are Upstream Kinases in the AMP-Activated Protein Kinase Cascade. *J. Biol.* **2003**, *2*, 28. [CrossRef] [PubMed]
27. Hawley, S.A.; Pan, D.A.; Mustard, K.J.; Ross, L.; Bain, J.; Edelman, A.M.; Frenguelli, B.G.; Hardie, D.G. Calmodulin-Dependent Protein Kinase Kinase-Beta Is an Alternative Upstream Kinase for AMP-Activated Protein Kinase. *Cell Metab.* **2005**, *2*, 9–19. [CrossRef] [PubMed]
28. Shaw, R.J.; Lamia, K.A.; Vasquez, D.; Koo, S.-H.; Bardeesy, N.; Depinho, R.A.; Montminy, M.; Cantley, L.C. The Kinase LKB1 Mediates Glucose Homeostasis in Liver and Therapeutic Effects of Metformin. *Science* **2005**, *310*, 1642–1646. [CrossRef] [PubMed]
29. Fullerton, M.D.; Galic, S.; Marcinko, K.; Sikkema, S.; Pulinilkunnil, T.; Chen, Z.-P.; O'Neill, H.M.; Ford, R.J.; Palanivel, R.; O'Brien, M.; et al. Single Phosphorylation Sites in Acc1 and Acc2 Regulate Lipid Homeostasis and the Insulin-Sensitizing Effects of Metformin. *Nat. Med.* **2013**, *19*, 1649–1654. [CrossRef]
30. Badr, D.; Kurban, M.; Abbas, O. Metformin in Dermatology: An Overview. *J. Eur. Acad. Dermatol. Venereol.* **2013**, *27*, 1329–1335. [CrossRef]
31. Frid, A.; Sterner, G.N.; Löndahl, M.; Wiklander, C.; Cato, A.; Vinge, E.; Andersson, A. Novel Assay of Metformin Levels in Patients with Type 2 Diabetes and Varying Levels of Renal Function: Clinical Recommendations. *Diabetes Care* **2010**, *33*, 1291–1293. [CrossRef]

32. Endo, A. The Discovery and Development of HMG-CoA Reductase Inhibitors. *J. Lipid Res.* **1992**, *33*, 1569–1582. [CrossRef] [PubMed]
33. Goldstein, J.L.; Brown, M.S. Regulation of the Mevalonate Pathway. *Nature* **1990**, *343*, 425–430. [CrossRef] [PubMed]
34. Roglans, N.; Verd, J.C.; Peris, C.; Alegret, M.; Vázquez, M.; Adzet, T.; Díaz, C.; Hernández, G.; Laguna, J.C.; Sánchez, R.M. High Doses of Atorvastatin and Simvastatin Induce Key Enzymes Involved in VLDL Production. *Lipids* **2002**, *37*, 445–454. [CrossRef] [PubMed]
35. Wierzbicki, A.S. Atorvastatin. *Expert Opin. Pharmacother.* **2001**, *2*, 819–830. [CrossRef] [PubMed]
36. Carro, A.C.; Damonte, E.B. Requirement of Cholesterol in the Viral Envelope for Dengue Virus Infection. *Virus Res.* **2013**, *174*, 78–87. [CrossRef] [PubMed]
37. Xun, Y.-H.; Zhang, Y.-J.; Pan, Q.-C.; Mao, R.-C.; Qin, Y.-L.; Liu, H.-Y.; Zhang, Y.-M.; Yu, Y.-S.; Tang, Z.-H.; Lu, M.-J.; et al. Metformin Inhibits Hepatitis B Virus Protein Production and Replication in Human Hepatoma Cells. *J. Viral. Hepat.* **2014**, *21*, 597–603. [CrossRef] [PubMed]
38. Hoppe-Seyler, K.; Herrmann, A.L.; Däschle, A.; Kuhn, B.J.; Strobel, T.D.; Lohrey, C.; Bulkescher, J.; Krijgsveld, J.; Hoppe-Seyler, F. Effects of Metformin on the Virus/Host Cell Crosstalk in Human Papillomavirus-Positive Cancer Cells. *Int. J. Cancer* **2021**, *149*, 1137–1149. [CrossRef] [PubMed]
39. Zhang, R.; Feng, C.; Luo, D.; Zhao, R.; Kannan, P.R.; Yin, Y.; Iqbal, M.Z.; Hu, Y.; Kong, X. Metformin Hydrochloride Significantly Inhibits Rotavirus Infection in Caco2 Cell Line, Intestinal Organoids, and Mice. *Pharmaceuticals* **2023**, *16*, 1279. [CrossRef]
40. Jiang, Z.; Liu, H. Metformin Inhibits Tumorigenesis in HBV-Induced Hepatocellular Carcinoma by Suppressing HULC Overexpression Caused by HBX. *J. Cell Biochem.* **2018**, *119*, 4482–4495. [CrossRef]
41. Farfan-Morales, C.N.; Cordero-Rivera, C.D.; Osuna-Ramos, J.F.; Monroy-Muñoz, I.E.; De Jesús-González, L.A.; Muñoz-Medina, J.E.; Hurtado-Monzón, A.M.; Reyes-Ruiz, J.M.; del Ángel, R.M. The Antiviral Effect of Metformin on Zika and Dengue Virus Infection. *Sci. Rep.* **2021**, *11*, 8743. [CrossRef]
42. Parthasarathy, H.; Tandel, D.; Siddiqui, A.H.; Harshan, K.H. Metformin Suppresses SARS-CoV-2 in Cell Culture. *Virus Res.* **2022**, *323*, 199010. [CrossRef]
43. Curry, J.M.; Johnson, J.; Mollaee, M.; Tassone, P.; Amin, D.; Knops, A.; Whitaker-Menezes, D.; Mahoney, M.G.; South, A.; Rodeck, U.; et al. Metformin Clinical Trial in HPV+ and HPV- Head and Neck Squamous Cell Carcinoma: Impact on Cancer Cell Apoptosis and Immune Infiltrate. *Front. Oncol.* **2018**, *8*, 436. [CrossRef] [PubMed]
44. Abdelmoneim, M.; Eissa, I.R.; Aboalela, M.A.; Naoe, Y.; Matsumura, S.; Sibal, P.A.; Bustos-Villalobos, I.; Tanaka, M.; Kodera, Y.; Kasuya, H. Metformin Enhances the Antitumor Activity of Oncolytic Herpes Simplex Virus HF10 (Canerpaturev) in a Pancreatic Cell Cancer Subcutaneous Model. *Sci. Rep.* **2022**, *12*, 21570. [CrossRef] [PubMed]
45. Granato, M.; Gilardini Montani, M.S.; Romeo, M.A.; Santarelli, R.; Gonnella, R.; D'Orazi, G.; Faggioni, A.; Cirone, M. Metformin Triggers Apoptosis in PEL Cells and Alters Bortezomib-Induced Unfolded Protein Response Increasing Its Cytotoxicity and Inhibiting KSHV Lytic Cycle Activation. *Cell. Signal.* **2017**, *40*, 239–247. [CrossRef] [PubMed]
46. Wang, X.; Wang, H.; Yi, P.; Baker, C.; Casey, G.; Xie, X.; Luo, H.; Cai, J.; Fan, X.; Soong, L.; et al. Metformin Restrains ZIKV Replication and Alleviates Virus-Induced Inflammatory Responses in Microglia. *Int. Immunopharmacol.* **2023**, *121*, 110512. [CrossRef]
47. del Campo, J.A.; García Valdecasas, M.; Gil Gómez, A.; Rojas Alvarez-Ossorio, M.A.; Gallego, P.; Ampuero Herrojo, J.; Gallego Durán, R.; Pastor, H.; Grande, L.; Padillo Ruiz, F.J.; et al. Simvastatin and Metformin Inhibit Cell Growth in Hepatitis C Virus Infected Cells via mTOR Increasing PTEN and Autophagy. *PLoS ONE* **2018**, *13*, e0191805. [CrossRef]
48. Tsai, W.-L.; Chang, T.-H.; Sun, W.-C.; Chan, H.-H.; Wu, C.-C.; Hsu, P.-I.; Cheng, J.-S.; Yu, M.-L. Metformin Activates Type I Interferon Signaling against HCV via Activation of Adenosine Monophosphate-Activated Protein Kinase. *Oncotarget* **2017**, *8*, 91928–91937. [CrossRef]
49. Lee, H.S.; Noh, J.Y.; Song, J.Y.; Cheong, H.J.; Kim, W.J. Metformin Reduces the Risk of Developing Influenza A Virus Related Cardiovascular Disease. *Heliyon* **2023**, *9*, e20284. [CrossRef]
50. Planas, D.; Pagliuzza, A.; Ponte, R.; Fert, A.; Marchand, L.R.; Massanella, M.; Gosselin, A.; Mehraj, V.; Dupuy, F.P.; Isnard, S.; et al. LILAC Pilot Study: Effects of Metformin on mTOR Activation and HIV Reservoir Persistence during Antiretroviral Therapy. *EBioMedicine* **2021**, *65*, 103270. [CrossRef]
51. Masich, A.M.; Thompson, L.; Fulco, P.P. Bictegravir and Metformin Drug-Drug Interaction in People with Human Immunodeficiency Virus (HIV). *Infect. Dis. Rep.* **2023**, *15*, 231–237. [CrossRef]
52. Farfan-Morales, C.N.; Cordero-Rivera, C.D.; Reyes-Ruiz, J.M.; Hurtado-Monzón, A.M.; Osuna-Ramos, J.F.; González-González, A.M.; De Jesús-González, L.A.; Palacios-Rápalo, S.N.; del Ángel, R.M. Anti-Flavivirus Properties of Lipid-Lowering Drugs. *Front. Physiol.* **2021**, *12*, 749770. [CrossRef]
53. Osuna-Ramos, J.F.; Farfan-Morales, C.N.; Cordero-Rivera, C.D.; De Jesús-González, L.A.; Reyes-Ruiz, J.M.; Hurtado-Monzón, A.M.; Palacios-Rápalo, S.N.; Jiménez-Camacho, R.; Meraz-Ríos, M.A.; Del Ángel, R.M. Cholesterol-Lowering Drugs as Potential Antivirals: A Repurposing Approach against Flavivirus Infections. *Viruses* **2023**, *15*, 1465. [CrossRef]
54. Herrera-Moro Huitron, L.; De Jesús-González, L.A.; Martínez-Castillo, M.; Ulloa-Aguilar, J.M.; Cabello-Gutierrez, C.; Helguera-Repetto, C.; Garcia-Cordero, J.; León Juárez, M. Multifaceted Nature of Lipid Droplets in Viral Interactions and Pathogenesis. *Microorganisms* **2023**, *11*, 1851. [CrossRef] [PubMed]

55. Owen, M.R.; Doran, E.; Halestrap, A.P. Evidence That Metformin Exerts Its Anti-Diabetic Effects through Inhibition of Complex 1 of the Mitochondrial Respiratory Chain. *Biochem. J.* **2000**, *348 Pt 3*, 607–614. [CrossRef] [PubMed]

56. Fontaine, E. Metformin-Induced Mitochondrial Complex I Inhibition: Facts, Uncertainties, and Consequences. *Front. Endocrinol.* **2018**, *9*, 753. [CrossRef] [PubMed]

57. Soto-Acosta, R.; Bautista-Carbajal, P.; Cervantes-Salazar, M.; Angel-Ambrocio, A.H.; Del Angel, R.M. DENV Up-Regulates the HMG-CoA Reductase Activity through the Impairment of AMPK Phosphorylation: A Potential Antiviral Target. *PLoS Pathog.* **2017**, *13*, e1006257. [CrossRef] [PubMed]

58. Honda, M.; Shirasaki, T.; Terashima, T.; Kawaguchi, K.; Nakamura, M.; Oishi, N.; Wang, X.; Shimakami, T.; Okada, H.; Arai, K.; et al. Hepatitis B Virus (HBV) Core-Related Antigen During Nucleos(t)ide Analog Therapy Is Related to Intra-Hepatic HBV Replication and Development of Hepatocellular Carcinoma. *J. Infect. Dis.* **2016**, *213*, 1096–1106. [CrossRef] [PubMed]

59. Sharma, T.; Abohashrh, M.; Baig, M.H.; Dong, J.-J.; Alam, M.M.; Ahmad, I.; Irfan, S. Screening of Drug Databank against WT and Mutant Main Protease of SARS-CoV-2: Towards Finding Potential Compound for Repurposing against COVID-19. *Saudi J. Biol. Sci.* **2021**, *28*, 3152–3159. [CrossRef] [PubMed]

60. Kumar, V.; Liu, H.; Wu, C. Drug Repurposing against SARS-CoV-2 Receptor Binding Domain Using Ensemble-Based Virtual Screening and Molecular Dynamics Simulations. *Comput. Biol. Med.* **2021**, *135*, 104634. [CrossRef]

61. Duarte, R.R.R.; Copertino, D.C.; Iñiguez, L.P.; Marston, J.L.; Bram, Y.; Han, Y.; Schwartz, R.E.; Chen, S.; Nixon, D.F.; Powell, T.R. Identifying FDA-Approved Drugs with Multimodal Properties against COVID-19 Using a Data-Driven Approach and a Lung Organoid Model of SARS-CoV-2 Entry. *Mol. Med.* **2021**, *27*, 105. [CrossRef]

62. Zapata-Cardona, M.I.; Flórez-Álvarez, L.; Zapata-Builes, W.; Guerra-Sandoval, A.L.; Guerra-Almonacid, C.M.; Hincapié-García, J.; Rugeles, M.T.; Hernandez, J.C. Atorvastatin Effectively Inhibits Ancestral and Two Emerging Variants of SARS-CoV-2 in Vitro. *Front. Microbiol.* **2022**, *13*, 721103. [CrossRef]

63. Segatori, V.I.; Garona, J.; Caligiuri, L.G.; Bizzotto, J.; Lavignolle, R.; Toro, A.; Sanchis, P.; Spitzer, E.; Krolewiecki, A.; Gueron, G.; et al. Effect of Ivermectin and Atorvastatin on Nuclear Localization of Importin Alpha and Drug Target Expression Profiling in Host Cells from Nasopharyngeal Swabs of SARS-CoV-2-Positive Patients. *Viruses* **2021**, *13*, 2084. [CrossRef]

64. Bryan-Marrugo, O.L.; Arellanos-Soto, D.; Rojas-Martinez, A.; Barrera-Saldaña, H.; Ramos-Jimenez, J.; Vidaltamayo, R.; Rivas-Estilla, A.M. The Anti-dengue Virus Properties of Statins May Be Associated with Alterations in the Cellular Antiviral Profile Expression. *Mol. Med. Rep.* **2016**, *14*, 2155–2163. [CrossRef] [PubMed]

65. Palacios-Rápalo, S.N.; Farfan-Morales, C.N.; Cordero-Rivera, C.D.; De Jesús-González, L.A.; Reyes-Ruiz, J.M.; Meraz-Ríos, M.A.; Del Ángel, R.M. An Ivermectin—Atorvastatin Combination Impairs Nuclear Transport Inhibiting Dengue Infection in Vitro and in Vivo. *iScience* **2023**, *26*, 108294. [CrossRef] [PubMed]

66. Españo, E.; Kim, J.-K. Effects of Statin Combinations on Zika Virus Infection in Vero Cells. *Pharmaceutics* **2022**, *15*, 50. [CrossRef] [PubMed]

67. Stoyanova, G.; Jabeen, S.; Landazuri Vinueza, J.; Ghosh Roy, S.; Lockshin, R.A.; Zakeri, Z. Zika Virus Triggers Autophagy to Exploit Host Lipid Metabolism and Drive Viral Replication. *Cell Commun. Signal.* **2023**, *21*, 114. [CrossRef]

68. Wani, M.A.; Mukherjee, S.; Mallick, S.; Akbar, I.; Basu, A. Atorvastatin Ameliorates Viral Burden and Neural Stem/Progenitor Cell (NSPC) Death in an Experimental Model of Japanese Encephalitis. *J. Biosci.* **2020**, *45*, 77. [CrossRef]

69. Ikeda, M.; Kato, N. Life Style-Related Diseases of the Digestive System: Cell Culture System for the Screening of Anti-Hepatitis C Virus (HCV) Reagents: Suppression of HCV Replication by Statins and Synergistic Action with Interferon. *J. Pharmacol. Sci.* **2007**, *105*, 145–150. [CrossRef] [PubMed]

70. Ikeda, M.; Abe, K.; Yamada, M.; Dansako, H.; Naka, K.; Kato, N. Different Anti-HCV Profiles of Statins and Their Potential for Combination Therapy with Interferon. *Hepatology* **2006**, *44*, 117–125. [CrossRef] [PubMed]

71. Todorovska, B.; Caloska-Ivanova, V.; Dimitrova-Genadieva, M.; Trajkovska, M.; Popova-Jovanovska, R.; Grivceva-Stardelova, K.; Licoska-Josifovic, F.; Andreevski, V.; Curakova-Ristovska, E.; Joksimovic, N. Atorvastatin in Combination with Pegylated Interferon and Ribavirin Provided High Rate of Sustained Virological Response in Patients with Genotype 3 Hepatitis C Virus. *Open Access Maced. J. Med. Sci.* **2019**, *7*, 1641–1648. [CrossRef]

72. Simon, T.G.; Bonilla, H.; Yan, P.; Chung, R.T.; Butt, A.A. Atorvastatin and Fluvastatin Are Associated with Dose-Dependent Reductions in Cirrhosis and Hepatocellular Carcinoma, among Patients with Hepatitis C Virus: Results from ERCHIVES. *Hepatology* **2016**, *64*, 47–57. [CrossRef]

73. Guan, J.; Sun, X.; Liang, Y.; Dong, W.; Zhang, L.; Zhu, J.; Wang, G. Atorvastatin Attenuates Coxsackie Virus B3m-Induced Viral Myocarditis in Mice. *J. Cardiovasc. Pharmacol.* **2010**, *56*, 540–547. [CrossRef]

74. Episcopio, D.; Aminov, S.; Benjamin, S.; Germain, G.; Datan, E.; Landazuri, J.; Lockshin, R.A.; Zakeri, Z. Atorvastatin Restricts the Ability of Influenza Virus to Generate Lipid Droplets and Severely Suppresses the Replication of the Virus. *FASEB J.* **2019**, *33*, 9516–9525. [CrossRef]

75. Ianevski, A.; Yao, R.; Zusinaite, E.; Lysvand, H.; Oksenych, V.; Tenson, T.; Bjørås, M.; Kainov, D. Active Components of Commonly Prescribed Medicines Affect Influenza A Virus-Host Cell Interaction: A Pilot Study. *Viruses* **2021**, *13*, 1537. [CrossRef]

76. Zhao, J.; Zeng, Z.; Chen, Y.; Liu, W.; Chen, H.; Fu, Z.F.; Zhao, L.; Zhou, M. Lipid Droplets Are Beneficial for Rabies Virus Replication by Facilitating Viral Budding. *J. Virol.* **2022**, *96*, e0147321. [CrossRef] [PubMed]

77. Mystakelis, H.A.; Wilson, E.; Laidlaw, E.; Poole, A.; Krishnan, S.; Rupert, A.; Welker, J.L.; Gorelick, R.J.; Lisco, A.; Manion, M.; et al. An Open Label Randomized Controlled Trial of Atorvastatin versus Aspirin in Elite Controllers and Antiretroviral-Treated People with HIV. *AIDS* **2023**, *37*, 1827–1835. [CrossRef] [PubMed]

78. Overton, E.T.; Sterrett, S.; Westfall, A.O.; Kahan, S.M.; Burkholder, G.; Zajac, A.J.; Goepfert, P.A.; Bansal, A. Effects of Atorvastatin and Pravastatin on Immune Activation and T-Cell Function in Antiretroviral Therapy-Suppressed HIV-1-Infected Patients. *AIDS* **2014**, *28*, 2627–2631. [CrossRef] [PubMed]

79. Ganesan, A.; Crum-Cianflone, N.; Higgins, J.; Qin, J.; Rehm, C.; Metcalf, J.; Brandt, C.; Vita, J.; Decker, C.F.; Sklar, P.; et al. High Dose Atorvastatin Decreases Cellular Markers of Immune Activation without Affecting HIV-1 RNA Levels: Results of a Double-Blind Randomized Placebo Controlled Clinical Trial. *J. Infect. Dis.* **2011**, *203*, 756–764. [CrossRef] [PubMed]

80. Negredo, E.; Clotet, B.; Puig, J.; Pérez-Alvarez, N.; Ruiz, L.; Romeu, J.; Moltó, J.; Rey-Joly, C.; Blanco, J. The Effect of Atorvastatin Treatment on HIV-1-Infected Patients Interrupting Antiretroviral Therapy. *AIDS* **2006**, *20*, 619–621. [CrossRef] [PubMed]

81. Riestenberg, R.A.; Furman, A.; Cowen, A.; Pawlowksi, A.; Schneider, D.; Lewis, A.A.; Kelly, S.; Taiwo, B.; Achenbach, C.; Palella, F.; et al. Differences in Statin Utilization and Lipid Lowering by Race, Ethnicity, and HIV Status in a Real-World Cohort of Persons with Human Immunodeficiency Virus and Uninfected Persons. *Am. Heart J.* **2019**, *209*, 79–87. [CrossRef] [PubMed]

82. Negredo, E.; Puigdomènech, I.; Marfil, S.; Puig, J.; Pérez-Alvarez, N.; Ruiz, L.; Rey-Joly, C.; Clotet, B.; Blanco, J. Association between HIV Replication and Cholesterol in Peripheral Blood Mononuclear Cells in HIV-Infected Patients Interrupting HAART. *J. Antimicrob. Chemother.* **2008**, *61*, 400–404. [CrossRef]

83. Calza, L.; Trapani, F.; Bartoletti, M.; Manfredi, R.; Colangeli, V.; Borderi, M.; Grossi, G.; Motta, R.; Viale, P. Statin Therapy Decreases Serum Levels of High-Sensitivity C-Reactive Protein and Tumor Necrosis Factor-α in HIV-Infected Patients Treated with Ritonavir-Boosted Protease Inhibitors. *HIV Clin. Trials* **2012**, *13*, 153–161. [CrossRef]

84. Zhang, J.; Dong, J.; Martin, M.; He, M.; Gongol, B.; Marin, T.L.; Chen, L.; Shi, X.; Yin, Y.; Shang, F.; et al. AMP-Activated Protein Kinase Phosphorylation of Angiotensin-Converting Enzyme 2 in Endothelium Mitigates Pulmonary Hypertension. *Am. J. Respir. Crit. Care Med.* **2018**, *198*, 509–520. [CrossRef]

85. Simões e Silva, A.; Silveira, K.; Ferreira, A.; Teixeira, M. ACE2, Angiotensin-(1-7) and Mas Receptor Axis in Inflammation and Fibrosis. *Br. J. Pharmacol.* **2013**, *169*, 477–492. [CrossRef]

86. Gheblawi, M.; Wang, K.; Viveiros, A.; Nguyen, Q.; Zhong, J.-C.; Turner, A.J.; Raizada, M.K.; Grant, M.B.; Oudit, G.Y. Angiotensin-Converting Enzyme 2: SARS-CoV-2 Receptor and Regulator of the Renin-Angiotensin System. *Circ. Res.* **2020**, *126*, 1456–1474. [CrossRef]

87. Bian, J.; Li, Z. Angiotensin-Converting Enzyme 2 (ACE2): SARS-CoV-2 Receptor and RAS Modulator. *Acta Pharm. Sin. B* **2021**, *11*, 1–12. [CrossRef]

88. Chi, X.; Wang, S.; Huang, Y.; Stamnes, M.; Chen, J.-L. Roles of Rho GTPases in Intracellular Transport and Cellular Transformation. *Int. J. Mol. Sci.* **2013**, *14*, 7089–7108. [CrossRef]

89. Marcianò, G.; Palleria, C.; Casarella, A.; Rania, V.; Basile, E.; Catarisano, L.; Vocca, C.; Bianco, L.; Pelaia, C.; Cione, E.; et al. Effect of Statins on Lung Cancer Molecular Pathways: A Possible Therapeutic Role. *Pharmaceuticals* **2022**, *15*, 589. [CrossRef]

90. Wagstaff, K.M.; Sivakumaran, H.; Heaton, S.M.; Harrich, D.; Jans, D.A. Ivermectin Is a Specific Inhibitor of Importin α/β-Mediated Nuclear Import Able to Inhibit Replication of HIV-1 and Dengue Virus. *Biochem. J.* **2012**, *443*, 851–856. [CrossRef]

91. Chen, L.Y.C.; Quach, T.T.T. Combining Immunomodulators and Antivirals for COVID-19. *Lancet Microbe* **2021**, *2*, e233. [CrossRef]

92. Chen, X.; Guo, H.; Qiu, L.; Zhang, C.; Deng, Q.; Leng, Q. Immunomodulatory and Antiviral Activity of Metformin and Its Potential Implications in Treating Coronavirus Disease 2019 and Lung Injury. *Front. Immunol.* **2020**, *11*, 2056. [CrossRef]

93. Foretz, M.; Guigas, B.; Bertrand, L.; Pollak, M.; Viollet, B. Metformin: From Mechanisms of Action to Therapies. *Cell Metab.* **2014**, *20*, 953–966. [CrossRef]

94. Chaudhary, S.C.; Kurundkar, D.; Elmets, C.A.; Kopelovich, L.; Athar, M. Metformin, an Antidiabetic Agent Reduces Growth of Cutaneous Squamous Cell Carcinoma by Targeting mTOR Signaling Pathway†. *Photochem. Photobiol.* **2012**, *88*, 1149–1156. [CrossRef]

95. Marcucci, F.; Romeo, E.; Caserta, C.A.; Rumio, C.; Lefoulon, F. Context-Dependent Pharmacological Effects of Metformin on the Immune System. *Trends Pharmacol. Sci.* **2020**, *41*, 162–171. [CrossRef]

96. Huang, C.; Wang, Y.; Li, X.; Ren, L.; Zhao, J.; Hu, Y.; Zhang, L.; Fan, G.; Xu, J.; Gu, X.; et al. Clinical Features of Patients Infected with 2019 Novel Coronavirus in Wuhan, China. *Lancet* **2020**, *395*, 497–506. [CrossRef]

97. Mills, C. M1 and M2 Macrophages: Oracles of Health and Disease. *CRI* **2012**, *32*, 463–488. [CrossRef]

98. Kelly, B.; Tannahill, G.M.; Murphy, M.P.; O'Neill, L.A.J. Metformin Inhibits the Production of Reactive Oxygen Species from NADH:Ubiquinone Oxidoreductase to Limit Induction of Interleukin-1β (IL-1β) and Boosts Interleukin-10 (IL-10) in Lipopolysaccharide (LPS)-Activated Macrophages *. *J. Biol. Chem.* **2015**, *290*, 20348–20359. [CrossRef]

99. Ding, L.; Liang, G.; Yao, Z.; Zhang, J.; Liu, R.; Chen, H.; Zhou, Y.; Wu, H.; Yang, B.; He, Q. Metformin Prevents Cancer Metastasis by Inhibiting M2-like Polarization of Tumor Associated Macrophages. *Oncotarget* **2015**, *6*, 36441–36455. [CrossRef]

100. Saito, A.; Koinuma, K.; Kawashima, R.; Miyato, H.; Ohzawa, H.; Horie, H.; Yamaguchi, H.; Kawahira, H.; Mimura, T.; Kitayama, J.; et al. Metformin May Improve the Outcome of Patients with Colorectal Cancer and Type 2 Diabetes Mellitus Partly through Effects on Neutrophil Extracellular Traps. *BJC Rep.* **2023**, *1*, 20. [CrossRef]

101. Li, J.; Zhang, K.; Zhang, K.; Zhang, Y.; Gu, Z.; Huang, C. Neutrophils in COVID-19: Recent Insights and Advances. *Virol. J.* **2023**, *20*, 169. [CrossRef]

102. Sun, Y.; Tian, T.; Gao, J.; Liu, X.; Hou, H.; Cao, R.; Li, B.; Quan, M.; Guo, L. Metformin Ameliorates the Development of Experimental Autoimmune Encephalomyelitis by Regulating T Helper 17 and Regulatory T Cells in Mice. *J. Neuroimmunol.* **2016**, *292*, 58–67. [CrossRef]

103. Liu, X.; Yu, P.; Xu, Y.; Wang, Y.; Chen, J.; Tang, F.; Hu, Z.; Zhou, J.; Liu, L.; Qiu, W.; et al. Metformin Induces Tolerogenicity of Dendritic Cells by Promoting Metabolic Reprogramming. *Cell Mol. Life Sci.* **2023**, *80*, 283. [CrossRef]

104. Cortés, M.; Brischetto, A.; Martinez-Campanario, M.C.; Ninfali, C.; Domínguez, V.; Fernández, S.; Celis, R.; Esteve-Codina, A.; Lozano, J.J.; Sidorova, J.; et al. Inflammatory Macrophages Reprogram to Immunosuppression by Reducing Mitochondrial Translation. *Nat. Commun.* **2023**, *14*, 7471. [CrossRef]

105. Wiklund, O.; Mattsson-Hultén, L.; Hurt-Camejo, E.; Oscarsson, J. Effects of Simvastatin and Atorvastatin on Inflammation Markers in Plasma. *J. Intern. Med.* **2002**, *251*, 338–347. [CrossRef] [PubMed]

106. Al-Kuraishy, H.M.; Al-Gareeb, A.I.; Saad, H.M.; Batiha, G.E.-S. The Potential Therapeutic Effect of Statins in Multiple Sclerosis: Beneficial or Detrimental Effects. *Inflammopharmacology* **2023**, *31*, 1671–1682. [CrossRef] [PubMed]

107. Blankier, S.; McCrindle, B.W.; Ito, S.; Yeung, R.S.M. The Role of Atorvastatin in Regulating the Immune Response Leading to Vascular Damage in a Model of Kawasaki Disease. *Clin. Exp. Immunol.* **2011**, *164*, 193–201. [CrossRef] [PubMed]

108. Sorathia, N.; Al-Rubaye, H.; Zal, B. The Effect of Statins on the Functionality of CD4+CD25+FOXP3+ Regulatory T-Cells in Acute Coronary Syndrome: A Systematic Review and Meta-Analysis of Randomised Controlled Trials in Asian Populations. *Eur. Cardiol.* **2019**, *14*, 123–129. [CrossRef] [PubMed]

109. Fessler, M.B. Regulation of Adaptive Immunity in Health and Disease by Cholesterol Metabolism. *Curr. Allergy Asthma Rep.* **2015**, *15*, 48. [CrossRef]

110. Sheridan, A.; Wheeler-Jones, C.P.D.; Gage, M.C. The Immunomodulatory Effects of Statins on Macrophages. *Immuno* **2022**, *2*, 317–343. [CrossRef]

111. Pedrosa, A.R.; Martins, D.C.; Rizzo, M.; Silva-Nunes, J. Metformin in SARS-CoV-2 Infection: A Hidden Path—From Altered Inflammation to Reduced Mortality. A Review from the Literature. *J. Diabetes Complicat.* **2023**, *37*, 108391. [CrossRef] [PubMed]

112. Scheen, A.J. Metformin and COVID-19: From Cellular Mechanisms to Reduced Mortality. *Diabetes Metab.* **2020**, *46*, 423–426. [CrossRef]

113. Petakh, P.; Griga, V.; Mohammed, I.B.; Loshak, K.; Poliak, I.; Kamyshnyiy, A. Effects of Metformin, Insulin on Hematological Parameters of COVID-19 Patients with Type 2 Diabetes. *Med. Arch.* **2022**, *76*, 329–332. [CrossRef]

114. Moreno-Corona, N.C.; López-Ortega, O.; Pérez-Martínez, C.A.; Martínez-Castillo, M.; De Jesús-González, L.A.; León-Reyes, G.; León-Juárez, M. Dynamics of the Microbiota and Its Relationship with Post-COVID-19 Syndrome. *Int. J. Mol. Sci.* **2023**, *24*, 14822. [CrossRef]

115. Petakh, P.; Kamyshna, I.; Nykyforuk, A.; Yao, R.; Imbery, J.F.; Oksenych, V.; Korda, M.; Kamyshnyi, A. Immunoregulatory Intestinal Microbiota and COVID-19 in Patients with Type Two Diabetes: A Double-Edged Sword. *Viruses* **2022**, *14*, 477. [CrossRef]

116. Petakh, P.; Kamyshna, I.; Oksenych, V.; Kainov, D.; Kamyshnyi, A. Metformin Therapy Changes Gut Microbiota Alpha-Diversity in COVID-19 Patients with Type 2 Diabetes: The Role of SARS CoV 2 Variants and Antibiotic Treatment. *Pharmaceuticals* **2023**, *16*, 904. [CrossRef]

117. Rodriguez-Nava, G.; Trelles-Garcia, D.P.; Yanez-Bello, M.A.; Chung, C.W.; Trelles-Garcia, V.P.; Friedman, H.J. Atorvastatin Associated with Decreased Hazard for Death in COVID-19 Patients Admitted to an ICU: A Retrospective Cohort Study. *Crit. Care* **2020**, *24*, 429. [CrossRef]

118. Kouhpeikar, H.; Khosaravizade Tabasi, H.; Khazir, Z.; Naghipour, A.; Mohammadi Moghadam, H.; Forouzanfar, H.; Abbasifard, M.; Kirichenko, T.V.; Reiner, Ž.; Banach, M.; et al. Statin Use in COVID-19 Hospitalized Patients and Outcomes: A Retrospective Study. *Front. Cardiovasc. Med.* **2022**, *9*, 820260. [CrossRef] [PubMed]

119. Haji Aghajani, M.; Moradi, O.; Azhdari Tehrani, H.; Amini, H.; Pourheidar, E.; Hatami, F.; Rabiei, M.M.; Sistanizad, M. Promising Effects of Atorvastatin on Mortality and Need for Mechanical Ventilation in Patients with Severe COVID-19; a Retrospective Cohort Study. *Int. J. Clin. Pract.* **2021**, *75*, e14434. [CrossRef] [PubMed]

120. Schieffer, E.; Schieffer, B. The Rationale for the Treatment of Long-Covid Symptoms—A Cardiologist's View. *Front. Cardiovasc. Med.* **2022**, *9*, 992686. [CrossRef]

121. Visos-Varela, I.; Zapata-Cachafeiro, M.; Pintos-Rodríguez, S.; Bugarín-González, R.; González-Barcala, F.J.; Herdeiro, M.T.; Piñeiro-Lamas, M.; Figueiras, A.; Salgado-Barreira, Á. Outpatient Atorvastatin Use and Severe COVID-19 Outcomes: A Population-Based Study. *J. Med. Virol.* **2023**, *95*, e28971. [CrossRef] [PubMed]

122. Boulware, D.R.; Bramante, C.; Pullen, M.; Buse, J.; Odde, D.; Mehta, T.; Murray, T.A. Metformin Reduced SARS-CoV-2 Viral Load in a Phase 3 Randomized Clinical Trial. *Top. Antivir. Med.* **2023**, *31*, 70.

123. Yu, J.-W.; Sun, L.-J.; Zhao, Y.-H.; Kang, P.; Yan, B.-Z. The Effect of Metformin on the Efficacy of Antiviral Therapy in Patients with Genotype 1 Chronic Hepatitis C and Insulin Resistance. *Int. J. Infect. Dis.* **2012**, *16*, e436–e441. [CrossRef]

124. Lv, Z.; Guo, Y. Metformin and Its Benefits for Various Diseases. *Front. Endocrinol.* **2020**, *11*, 191. [CrossRef] [PubMed]

125. Tárraga López, P.J.; Celada Rodríguez, A.; Cerdán Oliver, M.; Solera Albero, J.; Ocaña López, J.M.; de Miguel Clavé, J. Análisis coste-efectividad de atorvastatina frente a simvastatina como tratamiento hipolipemiante en pacientes hipercolesterolémicos en atención primaria. *Aten Primaria* **2001**, *27*, 18–24. [CrossRef] [PubMed]

126. Pepperrell, T.; Ellis, L.; Wang, J.; Hill, A. Barriers to Worldwide Access for Paxlovid, a New Treatment for COVID-19. *Open Forum Infect. Dis.* **2022**, *9*, ofac174. [CrossRef] [PubMed]

127. Corcoran, C.; Jacobs, T.F. Metformin. In *StatPearls*; StatPearls Publishing: Treasure Island, FL, USA, 2023.
128. DOF—Diario Oficial de La Federación. Available online: https://www.dof.gob.mx/nota_detalle.php?codigo=5588819&fecha=10/03/2020#gsc.tab=0 (accessed on 13 June 2023).

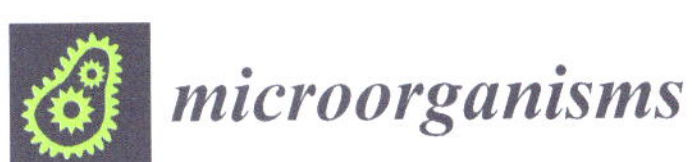

microorganisms

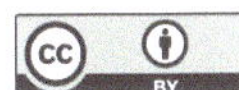

Article

Early Fluvoxamine Reduces the Risk for Clinical Deterioration in Symptomatic Outpatients with COVID-19: A Real-World, Retrospective, before–after Analysis

Aristotelis Tsiakalos [1,*], Panayiotis D. Ziakas [2], Eleni Polyzou [3], Georgios Schinas [3] and Karolina Akinosoglou [3]

[1] Leto General, Maternity & Gynecology Clinic, 11524 Athens, Greece
[2] Department of Medicine, Brown University, Providence, RI 02912, USA; pd.ziakas@gmail.com
[3] Dept of Internal Medicine and Infectious Diseases, Medical School, University General Hospital of Patras, University of Patras, 26504 Rio, Greece; polyzou.el@gmail.com (E.P.); georg.schinas@gmail.com (G.S.); akin@upatras.gr (K.A.)
* Correspondence: atsiakalos@gmail.com

Abstract: Fluvoxamine, a selective serotonin reuptake inhibitor with anti-inflammatory properties, has gained attention as a repurposed drug to treat COVID-19. We aimed to explore the potential benefit of fluvoxamine on outpatients with early SARS-CoV-2 infection. We performed a retrospective study of fluvoxamine adult outpatients with symptomatic COVID-19 disease of early onset (<5 days), in the context of an infectious diseases private practice, between September–December 2021, in Greece. Patients with disease duration $\geq$5 days, dyspnea and/or hypoxemia with oxygen saturation <94% in room air and pregnancy were excluded from the analysis. In total, 103 patients, 54 males/49 females with a median age of 47 years (39–56), were included in this study. Patient characteristics were balanced before and after the introduction of fluvoxamine. Two patients in the fluvoxamine arm (3.8%; 95% CI 0.4–13) had clinical deterioration compared to 8 patients in the standard of care group (16%; 95% CI 7.2–29.1, $p < 0.04$). After controlling for age, sex, body mass index > 30 and vaccination status, fluvoxamine was independently associated with a lower risk of clinical deterioration (adj. OR 0.12; 95% CI 0.02–0.70, $p < 0.02$). Adding on fluvoxamine to treatment for early symptomatic COVID-19 patients may protect them from clinical deterioration and hospitalization, and it is an appealing low-cost, low-toxicity option in the community setting and warrants further investigation.

Keywords: coronavirus; COVID-19; SARS-CoV-2; fluvoxamine; vaccine

Citation: Tsiakalos, A.; Ziakas, P.D.; Polyzou, E.; Schinas, G.; Akinosoglou, K. Early Fluvoxamine Reduces the Risk for Clinical Deterioration in Symptomatic Outpatients with COVID-19: A Real-World, Retrospective, before–after Analysis. *Microorganisms* **2023**, *11*, 2073. https://doi.org/10.3390/microorganisms11082073

Academic Editor: Qibin Geng

Received: 29 June 2023
Revised: 6 August 2023
Accepted: 9 August 2023
Published: 12 August 2023

1. Introduction

In March 2020, the World Health Organization declared the COVID-19 pandemic, caused by the SARS-CoV-2 virus, a global emergency. Since then, the number of persons affected worldwide has markedly increased, putting pressure on health systems and health-care budgets worldwide. The clinical manifestations show a biphasic course of initial viral replication and toxicity, later followed by a phase of hyperinflammatory response, reflected in severe respiratory distress and commonly multiorgan failure [1]. In this context, early antiviral and later concomitant anti-inflammatory intervention represent the mainstay of therapeutic management in these patients. Much attention has been drawn to populations at risk for poor outcomes, including patients with multiple comorbidities, immunocompromised, over-aged, obese patients, and pregnant women who are at risk of progression to severe disease [2]. The presence of underlying systemic disease, on top of increased age, seems to have an additive effect on worsening outcomes [2]. Thus, early identification and prompt intervention in this context are pivotal to avoid rapid clinical deterioration and ensure optimal outcomes.

Currently, clinical research and experience have provided outpatients at risk for worse outcomes with successful therapeutic options embedded in living guidelines [3]. Current options include nirmatrevir/ritonavir, molnupiravir, or a 3-day course of remdesivir in the form of outpatient parenteral antimicrobial therapy [3]. However, national policies as to eligibility criteria pertaining to drug disposal and administration remain diverse, vastly due to associated cost, while global socio-economic inequalities do now ensure for worldwide distribution [4]. Divergence in medical technology in the absence of time for generic development calls for a parallel road of action in low and middle-income countries where stringent budgets drive health policies [5,6]. The idea of repurposing existing drugs is quite appealing in the setting of the COVID-19 pandemic, especially in limited-resource settings. Success has been variable, despite the effort and time spent by researchers in numerous clinical trials across more than 100 countries [7].

A number of prior observational cohort studies of patients with COVID-19 have reported a reduced number of deaths or need for mechanical ventilation in the acute care setting, with subsequent reduced risk of emergency department or hospital visits among those taking antidepressants [8]. Preclinical evidence has also demonstrated the in vitro efficacy of several SSRIs against various variants of SARS-CoV-2, both in human and nonhuman host cells [9]. Fluvoxamine, a selective serotonin reuptake inhibitor approved for the treatment of obsessive-compulsive disorder, is shown to have significant anti-inflammatory properties in animal models and in vitro studies [10–12]. Recent work supported the antiviral and anti-inflammatory properties of fluoxetine in a mouse model of SARS-CoV-2 infection and its in vitro antiviral activity against different variants of concern, including Omicron BA.5 [13]. The lung presents a high serotonin transporter expression in humans, suggesting that potent vasoconstrictor serotonin bioavailability is possibly primarily regulated by the serotonin transporter in the lung endothelium [14]. Thus, one can assume that antidepressants such as fluvoxamine may affect COVID-19 lung function via various mechanisms. Specifically, even before the COVID-19 pandemic, fluvoxamine has been shown to possess anti-inflammatory properties in murine models of septic shock [15]. This process is possibly mediated by the sigma-1 receptor pathway of cytokine release [12]. Another mechanism via which fluvoxamine exerts beneficial effects includes the acid sphingomyelinase/ceramide (ASM) pathway [12]. Inhibition of the ASM/ceramide system by specific antidepressants such as fluvoxamine or fluoxetine prevents infection of Vero E6 cells with SARS-CoV-2 [16]. When reconstitution of ceramides in cells is treated with these specific antidepressants, infection restoration occurs [16]. Other pathways include increased melatonin, modulation of lysosomal viral trafficking, platelet regulation, and activity against the endothelium [12].

Several randomized trials on outpatient COVID-19 cases implied a benefit in averting clinical deterioration and/or hospitalizations [17,18]. To date, however, the COVID-19 Treatment Guidelines Panel does not recommend either for or against its use, given the lack of sufficient evidence [3]. Nonetheless, the drug remains a compelling option for early COVID-19 due to its low cost, the oral route of administration, and the known safety profile, which may render fluvoxamine a cost-effective alternative to oral antivirals for COVID-19 [19,20]. Our study aims to investigate the effect of early fluvoxamine treatment in symptomatic outpatients with COVID-19, with a hypothesis that prompt fluvoxamine administration, as a supplementary treatment to the standard care, reduces the risk for clinical deterioration in these patients.

2. Materials and Methods

We performed a retrospective, before–after analysis of COVID-19 patient data, treated in an outpatient setting between September 2021 and December 2021, at a private infectious disease clinic in Athens, Greece. The analysis included adult patients living in the community with a confirmed SARS-CoV-2 polymerase chain reaction (PCR) or rapid antigen test who had a symptomatic infection with recent onset (<5 days). Inclusion criteria were the presence of fever >38 °C on at least one occasion and/or respiratory symptoms (cough and/or shortness of breath). Patients with long-lasting symptoms (≥5 days), existing comorbidities with impaired performance status before testing positive for SARS-CoV-2 or oxygen saturation of less than 94% at baseline assessment, as well as pregnant individuals, were excluded from this study since they were referred to allocated COVID-19 hospital services in the Athens metropolitan area. Patients were instructed to self-isolate, equip with a thermometer, a pulse oximeter, and a blood pressure monitor via a healthy relative or a proxy pharmacist, per the guidelines advice for mild and moderate disease [21]. During the first contact, eligible patients were instructed to start their treatment the same day. Before the introduction of fluvoxamine, patients were assigned to oral inhalation of budesonide 800 milligrams(mg) twice daily for 14 days and over-the-counter acetaminophen up to 4 times daily—maximum 4 grams (g) per day. Inhaled budesonide was shown to shorten the time to recovery, reduce emergency visits, have a potential benefit on hospitalizations and minimal side-effects [22–24], and it is a therapeutic option for early outpatient treatment of adult patients with COVID-19 per the National Public Health Organization algorithm [21]. Anticoagulation prophylaxis with low-molecular-weight heparin (enoxaparin 4000 IU SC once daily) was added for symptomatic high-risk patients with a history of thrombosis, known thrombophilia or cancer, obesity or advanced age (>65 years) in accordance with the local hematology association guidelines. Fluvoxamine was added as an off-label option after November 2021 at a dose of 100 mg twice daily for a 10-day course based on recently published evidence from two randomized-controlled trials [17,18]. Patients were instructed to provide daily updates of their status on a 24/7 basis. On day 5 after initiation of symptoms, treated patients were instructed to have a laboratory assessment including laboratory inflammation markers, cardiac enzymes and thrombosis biomarkers: a complete blood count, C-reactive protein (CRP) and ferritin levels, troponin, creatine phosphokinase (CPK) and lactate dehydrogenase levels and a quantitative D-dimer assay [25–28]. All patients were screened by phone and/or e-mail and provided informed consent, typically through electronic means.

The primary outcome was clinical deterioration defined by worsening dyspnea with oxygen saturation <94% on room air and the development of pneumonia with or without the need for hospitalization. Data on patients referred to hospital care were updated after discharge.

We analyzed data using Stata 17 (College Station, TX, USA) software. Continuous variables were compared using the non-parametric Mann–Whitney test. For categorical outcomes, Fisher's exact test was used. To measure the association of fluvoxamine with outcome, we reported Odds Ratios (OR) with 95% confidence intervals (95% CIs) using a modified logistic regression framework to compensate for small samples and rare events [29]. Significance was set to $\alpha < 0.05$.

3. Results

Between 1 September 2021 and 31 December 2021, a total of 129 adults with a positive PCR or rapid antigen test for COVID-19 were evaluated. A total of 20 were excluded upon initial screening (9 asymptomatic and 11 pregnancies); six denied receiving the proposed treatment (2 in the standard of care and 4 in the fluvoxamine arm). Of 129 screened, 103 adults (54 male, 52%) were finally analyzed. Their median age was 47 years (range 39–56), with 15% over 65. Fifty (49%) had an underlying chronic condition, including obesity (22% with BMI > 30), hypertension (17%), diabetes mellitus (11%), autoimmunity (8%), dyslipidemia (9%), neurologic disorder (5%) or cancer (4%). Seventy-eight (76%) were fully vaccinated, and 26 (25%) had received a booster shot.

A total of 53 patients initiated fluvoxamine treatment at a dose of 100 mg bid. There were no statistically significant differences in patient demographics, presentation, standard of care and comorbidities after the introduction of fluvoxamine, as shown in Table 1, except for obesity, which was more prevalent in the fluvoxamine group (28% vs. 14%, with marginal significance $p = 0.10$).

Table 1. Patient characteristics and outcome before and after initiating fluvoxamine as an add-on to the standard-of-care (SOC), early outpatient care for symptomatic COVID-19.

	Fluvoxamine + SOC (N = 53)	SOC (N = 50)	p
Median Age (years)	45 (IQR 41–55)	49 (IQR 39–60)	0.65
Male Gender n (%)	25 (47)	29 (58)	0.33
BMI (kg/m^2)			
Median	26.4 (24.0–31.3)	25.8 (23.6–28.3)	0.25
Comorbidities n (%)			
Obesity (BMI > 30)	15 (28)	7 (14)	0.10
Hypertension	10(19)	7 (14)	0.60
Diabetes	5(9)	6(12)	0.76
Dyslipidemia	6(11)	3(6)	0.49
Autoimmunity	5(9)	3(6)	0.72
Neurologic	3(9)	2(4)	1
Thrombophilia	3(6)	0	0.24
Cancer	3(6)	0	0.24
COPD	1(2)	1(2)	1
Other	28(53)	22(44)	0.43
Vaccination n (%)			
Fully vaccinated	38 (72)	40 (80)	0.37
Booster shot	16 (30)	10 (20)	0.26
Treatment n (%)			
Enoxaparin prophylaxis	15 (28)	11 (22)	0.50
Budesonide	53 (100)	50 (100)	1
Outcome n (%)			
Clinical deterioration	2 (4%)	8 (16%)	0.048
Hospitalization/ICU	1/0	6/1	0.05
Deaths	0 (0)	0 (0)	-

BMI: Body Mass Index; ICU: Intensive Care Unit; IQR: Interquartile Range.

All patients were followed from COVID-19 documentation to the resolution of symptoms or deterioration requiring hospital care. Eight patients (7%) were hospitalized, six due to progressive hypoxemia and one due to hypoxemia and acute deep vein thrombosis. One required mechanical ventilation and ICU support. All 8 patients were discharged from the hospital and were alive on the last follow-up. Two additional patients developed hypoxemia and pneumonia and were treated successfully as outpatients with empirical antimicrobial coverage. Of the 10 patients with the primary outcome, two patients (3.8 percent; 95% CI 0.4 to 13.0) had a clinical deterioration in the fluvoxamine group vs. eight (16 percent; 95% CI 7.2 to 29.1) in the standard of care, corresponding to a lower risk for clinical deterioration (crude Odds Ratio 0.24; 95% confidence interval 0.06–1.05, p 0.06). For a baseline risk of 16% for clinical deterioration in the standard care group, the calculated number needed to treat to benefit (NNTB) was 9, with a wide 95% confidence interval (4.2 to 118.6). After age–sex adjustment, BMI and vaccination status controlling (Table 2), the use of fluvoxamine showed significant protection against clinical deterioration (adjusted Odds Ratio 0.12; 95% confidence interval 0.02–0.70, p 0.02). Vaccination was protective, and obesity adversely correlated with outcome.

Laboratory assessment on day 5 showed no significant differences between treatment arms in complete blood counts and biochemistry parameters, except for lymphocyte count (Table 3).

In the fluvoxamine group, 50/53 (94%) completed 10 days of therapy. Seven patients (13%) reported dizziness and nausea during fluvoxamine treatment, which led to early discontinuation (<5 days) in four patients (8%).

Table 2. Association of fluvoxamine use with clinical deterioration, crude (unadjusted) and adjusted estimates.

All Patients (n = 103)	Odds Ratio	95% Confidence Interval	p
Unadjusted effect			
Fluvoxamine	0.24	0.06–1.05	0.06
Adjusted effects			
Fluvoxamine	0.12	0.02–0.70	0.02
Age	1.05	0.99–1.11	0.08
female gender	0.82	0.20–3.34	0.77
BMI > 30	8.2	1.55–43.11	0.01
Full vaccination	0.17	0.03–0.84	0.03

Odds Ratio < 1 denotes a favorable effect.

Table 3. Comparison of laboratory profile on day 5.

	Fluvoxamine + SOC (N = 53)	SOC (N = 50)	p
Complete blood count (CBC)			
White Blood Cell count (/μL)	5520 (IQR 4680–6300)	5383 (IQR 4500–6600)	0.75
Lymphocyte count (/μL)	1862 (IQR 1451–2211)	1638 (IQR 1210–2005)	0.03
Lymphocyte count < 1000 (/μL) [†]	1(2%)	4(8%)	0.20
Hemoglobin (g/dL)	14 (IQR 13.1–15.0)	14 (IQR 12.6–15.2)	0.49
Platelet count ($\times 10^3$/μL)	214 (IQR 180–267)	199 (171–276)	0.63
Biochemistry/Biomarkers			
C-reactive protein (mg/L)	4 (IQR 2.4–8.9)	4.6 (IQR 3.1–16)	0.15
C-reactive protein > 5 mg/L	22 (42%)	23 (46%)	0.69
C-reactive protein > 100 mg/L [†]	0	3 (20%)	0.11
Serum ferritin (ng/mL)	132(IQR 72–199)	122(IQR 70–188)	0.9
Serum ferritin > 1000 (ng/mL) [†]	0	1(2%)	0.49
Lactate dehydrogenase (LDH) U/L	165(IQR 140–201)	166 (IQR 118–193)	0.43
Creatine phosphokinase (CPK) U/L	87(66–115)	77(44–118)	0.20
Troponin assay > 0.40 ng/mL	0	0	
D-dimer assay > 500 μg/mL	9 (17%)	16 (32%)	0.11

[†] Cut-off designated as laboratory evidence of severe COVID-19 disease by local guidelines [21].

4. Discussion

In this retrospective before–after analysis, we found that add-on fluvoxamine to the standard of care was associated with a reduction in clinical deterioration for symptomatic outpatients with confirmed COVID-19. Four percent of patients taking fluvoxamine had a clinical deterioration as opposed to 16 percent of patients who did not. This study, albeit small and retrospective, adds to the recent literature that implies a benefit of using fluvoxamine to treat COVID-19 in the outpatient setting. While our findings align with previous research, our study contributes to the existing literature by providing real-world evidence, which is crucial for validating findings from controlled settings.

A number of previous studies have provided supportive evidence that oral fluvoxamine cuts the risk for clinical deterioration when used early after COVID-19 diagnosis in the outpatient setting with an excellent safety profile and limited side effects, including mild nausea, abdominal discomfort and sleep disturbances [17,18]. In a placebo-controlled study (STOP COVID trial) in the St Louis metropolitan area, none out of 80 patients randomized to fluvoxamine (100 mg up to 3 times daily for 15 days) showed clinical deterioration compared to 6 of 72 (8.3%) patients in the placebo group [17]. Even though statistical differences were detected, the sample size was small; hence, conclusions were rather fragile. A second larger randomized-controlled study of oral fluvoxamine (100 mg twice daily for ten days) across 11 clinical sites in Brazil (TOGETHER trial) found that the composite outcome of either requiring observation in an emergency setting or admission to a tertiary hospital was lower in the fluvoxamine arm (79/741, 11%) compared to the placebo arm (119/756,

16%) [18]. In this setting, prolonged observation was used as a proxy for hospitalization because hospital beds were fully occupied during this phase of the pandemic in Brazil. However, when viral clearance, all-cause hospitalization, time to hospitalization, number of days in the hospital, time to recovery, days of mechanical ventilation or mortality were examined, no significant differences between fluvoxamine and placebo were observed [18,30]. In comparison to these findings, a follow-up study from the same group investigating the combination of fluvoxamine and inhaled budesonide observed a significant reduction in the composite outcome of emergency setting retention for COVID-19 or hospitalization due to disease progression compared to placebo (1.8% vs. 3.7%; relative risk 0.50, 95% credible interval 0.25 to 0.92) [31]. A third, retrospective cohort US study of deidentified electronic health record data across 87 health centers used propensity score matching and found that fluoxetine or fluvoxamine may reduce mortality from COVID-19 from 13.3% in matched controls to 10% in the fluoxetine or fluvoxamine treated (a significant relative risk reduction by 26%) [8]. This finding came in agreement with other authors from smaller studies finding reduced mortality in patients receiving fluvoxamine, especially the earlier given in the course of the disease [32–35]. Recent systematic reviews and meta-analyses confirmed that fluvoxamine significantly and substantially reduces hospitalization risk among outpatients with COVID-19 [35–38]. Benefits also extended to patients admitted to intensive care units. A prospective cohort study of critically ill COVID-19 patients reported a significant association between the 15-day use of fluvoxamine prescribed at a daily dose of 300 mg and reduced mortality [39]. Real-world data from Africa, including 316 patients, of whom 94 received fluvoxamine in addition to standard care, showed that fluvoxamine use was significantly associated with reduced mortality (AHR = 0.32; $p < 0.001$, NNT = 4.4) and with increased complete symptom resolution (AOR = 2.56; $p < 0.001$, NNT = 4.44) [15]. These effects were irrespective of clinical characteristics, including vaccination status. There was a trend toward greater side effects with fluvoxamine (7.45% vs. 3.15%; $p = 0.06$); however, the majority were mild in severity, and none required regimen discontinuation. A ten-day course of 100 mg per day was well tolerated and related to reduced mortality and increased symptom resolution without an increase in time to hospital discharge [15]. Nonetheless, psychotropic drugs, including other selective serotonin reuptake inhibitors, often lack a significant or similar association with outcomes [8,33,40]. The reason for this discrepancy may lie in underlying mechanisms of action [12].

In turn, the COVID-OUT trial failed to show a significant effect of fluvoxamine in preventing disease progression with an adjusted odds ratio of 0.94 (95% CI, 0.66 to 1.36) for the composite outcome of SpO2 of 93% or less on room air, emergency department visit, hospitalization or death [41]. In their subsequent long-term follow-up report, the authors found that there was no significant effect on long COVID incidence with fluvoxamine compared to placebo after 10 months [42]. Likewise, a recent study by McCarthy et al. failed to show any benefits, reporting results from the Accelerating COVID-19 Therapeutic Interventions and Vaccines (ACTIV-6) platform randomized clinical trial [43]. Similar to our study, high-risk comorbidities, including obesity, hypertension, asthma and diabetes, were common, and 67% of patients had received at least two vaccine doses. Results showed no significant benefit as to the median time to sustained recovery, similar to comparable rates of hospitalization, urgent care visit, emergency department visit or death through day 28 [43].

Interpretation of these conflicting results should be made with caution. The reason for this variability in many studies lies in their diverse geographic locations, different circulating variants, time periods, variable baseline risks of progression to severe disease and vaccination rates. Some also used differing dosing regimens and assessed different clinical outcomes, and their utility strongly differs between doctors and patients. Using composite outcomes can enhance statistical methods but also prove problematic. Using patient-centered and reported outcomes such as disability, discomfort and death is more meaningful than outcomes of health resource utilization or their proxies, which can be influenced by institutional bed availability and individual caregiver practices. Another explanation could be owing to the change in the severity of COVID-19 over different dominating variants. Hence, currently, the less severe disease does not easily allow for clinical difference detection, even though we managed to do so.

Despite potential benefits, a note of caution should be added concerning potential drug–drug interactions when prescribing for fluvoxamine [44]. The latter is a potent modulator of cytochrome P450 family enzymes. Hence, its administration can variably increase exposure to co-medications metabolized by this enzyme [45]. Candidate population usually bears multiple comorbidities, and polypharmacy remains an issue. Although the duration of administration is short, CYP inhibition is expected to occur immediately. Hence, the potential need for titration of co-medication (e.g., antiepileptics, neuroleptics, etc.) based on expected clinical response should not be ignored, since dose adjustment may potentially destabilize the patient. Serotonin toxicity, as well as QTc prolongation, must also be screened for in these patients. Other adverse events, including gastrointestinal disturbances, are minor and rarely lead to regime discontinuation.

Considering our analysis in combination with safety data, worldwide accessibility and the current price of approximately USD 1 per day [46], fluvoxamine may be a reasonable option for high-risk outpatients who do not have access to SARS-CoV-2 direct antivirals, monoclonal antibodies or compassionate use in the context of clinical trials. It is estimated that even at a number to treat of 200 patients (i.e., ARR of 0.5%), the corresponding cost to prevent admission would only be USD 2800 [35]. In a recent cost–consequence model, administering a 10-day course of fluvoxamine to COVID-19 outpatients at high risk for poor outcomes is substantially cost-saving, saving USD 232 and 0.15 hospitalization days per patient compared with standard of care in the US [47]. However, as previously stated, need for hospitalization, ICU care and post-acute covid syndrome-related expenditure, which mainly drives costs in such models, can be misleading [47].

That said, our study also highlighted the importance of obesity and vaccination on COVID-19 outcomes. Obesity is a well-recognized risk factor for poor outcomes in patients with COVID-19 [48,49]. In a recent meta-analysis including a total of 208 studies with 3,550,997 participants from over 32 countries, patients with obesity were at increased risk of both COVID-19-related hospitalizations (OR 1.72) and death (OR 1.25). Extreme obesity increases the risk of COVID-19-related hospitalizations and death (OR 2.53 and 2.06, respectively) [49]. This can be attributed to several reasons. First, adipose tissue is rich in ACE2 receptors, which represent a port of entry for SARS-CoV-2 to human cells and a consequent reservoir for viral replication [50]. Second, obesity per se has been shown to cause immune dysregulation and increase the susceptibility to infection while increasing inflammation of the parenchyma and bronchi [51]. Last, obesity decreases lung capacity and reserve, making mechanical ventilation even more difficult.

Vaccination has been found to have a protective effect in our cohort of patients with regard to progression to severe disease. This comes as no surprise as vaccination roll-out programs, including primary series and booster doses, have halted the course of the pandemic worldwide. Vaccine effectiveness for the primary series at baseline was 92% for hospitalizations and 91% for mortality, while for booster doses, vaccine effectiveness at baseline was 70% against infections and 89% against hospitalizations [52]. At the time this study was carried out, booster shots had just begun to be recommended and performed in Greece, and the expected vaccine efficacy from primary doses was 79% and 86% for hospitalizations and mortality, respectively. Even so, completion of the primary series seems to provide adequate protection against progression to severe disease and adverse outcomes.

Last, we also showed that patients receiving fluvoxamine presented a faster restoration of lymphocyte count levels. Severe lymphopenia is a well-recognized marker for the severity of COVID-19 disease [53,54]. It has been associated with a high prevalence of known risk factors for worse outcomes, as highlighted in many studies [55]. It has also been associated with a hyper-inflammatory response characterized by increased serum levels of acute phase proteins and pro-inflammatory mediators [56]. The exact reasons for such an event remain elusive. However, possible explanations could be that SARS-CoV-2 directly infects replication of inflammatory monocytes and lymphocytes, leading to apoptosis of T lymphocytes in vitro.

Additionally, SARS-CoV-2 has been detected in the peripheral blood mononuclear cells and postmortem lung tissues of COVID-19 patients [57]. There is increasing evidence of bone marrow suppression due to SARS-CoV-2 infection of hematopoietic stem cells [58], while thymus suppression has also been proposed [59]. Lymphopenia recovery is variable in COVID-19 patients. Previous studies have shown that lymphopenia may persist for weeks after acute disease [60]. Recently, published data have provided evidence of increased mortality in COVID-19 patients with persistently decreased levels of absolute lymphocyte count, while survivors experience lymphocyte recovery with sepsis [61]. Residual immunosuppression may be a cause of secondary infections and worse outcomes.

There are several limitations to be reported in this study. It is a retrospective cohort study with a pre-post analysis that cannot compete with a randomized trial recruiting patients prospectively. Additionally, the size of the study and the rarity of the primary outcome, especially in the fluvoxamine arm, render a multivariable analysis a challenge. To correct for bias related to small size and rare events, we used a penalized maximum likelihood estimation method to adjust for confounders [62,63], yet the effects are fragile, as seen with previous fluvoxamine studies [17]. Finally, a significant association between fluvoxamine and clinical deterioration may imply but does not prove a causal link, as complex clinical interactions may be present and spurious associations can arise. Despite its limitations, our study adds to the plausible evidence that fluvoxamine at least warrants further investigation in the treatment of COVID-19. Our analysis spans 4 months of observation in a private practice setting in the Athens metropolitan area, with a uniform handling of outpatients compliant with the local guidelines [21], resulting in well-balanced characteristics before and after fluvoxamine was added. Furthermore, the study is an example of the shift towards a more pragmatic approach of minimal in-person contact and self-reported outcomes, a growing and efficient practice during the pandemic [17,64,65].

5. Conclusions

The combination of the low-cost, oral route of administration with limited adverse events renders fluvoxamine a promising candidate for early outpatient use, particularly in limited resource settings. Furthermore, the anti-inflammatory properties of fluvoxamine are not expected to be related to circulating COVID-19 variants and may be useful regardless of the dominant strain. The track record of repurposing drugs to combat COVID-19 was of limited success, but fluvoxamine will remain in the spotlight insofar as supporting evidence accumulates. Our study contributes to the existing body of literature by offering robust real-world evidence that underscores the efficacy of early administration of fluvoxamine as an adjuvant treatment for COVID-19 and suggests a potential immunomodulatory role for its use in this context.

Author Contributions: A.T. and P.D.Z. conceived the idea, A.T. and P.D.Z. collected and analyzed data, A.T., P.D.Z., K.A., E.P. and G.S. wrote the manuscript, K.A. and P.D.Z. critically corrected the manuscript, A.T. oversaw the study. All authors have read and agreed to the published version of the manuscript.

Funding: This research received no external funding.

Data Availability Statement: The data presented in this study are available on request from the corresponding author. The data are not publicly available due to privacy and ethical constraints.

Conflicts of Interest: The authors declare no conflict of interest.

References

1. Chalmers, J.D.; Chotirmall, S.H. Rewiring the Immune Response in COVID-19. *Am. J. Respir. Crit. Care Med.* **2020**, *202*, 784–786. [CrossRef]
2. Russell, C.D.; Lone, N.I.; Baillie, J.K. Comorbidities, multimorbidity and COVID-19. *Nat. Med.* **2023**, *29*, 334–343. [CrossRef] [PubMed]
3. National Institutes of Health. COVID-19 TREATMENT GUIDELINES. Available online: https://www.covid19treatmentguidelines.nih.gov/ (accessed on 15 April 2023).

4.   Usher, A.D. The global COVID-19 treatment divide. *Lancet* **2022**, *399*, 779–782. [CrossRef]

5.   Maxwell, D.; Sanders, K.C.; Sabot, O.; Hachem, A.; Llanos-Cuentas, A.; Olotu, A.; Gosling, R.; Cutrell, J.B.; Hsiang, M.S. COVID-19 Therapeutics for Low- and Middle-Income Countries: A Review of Candidate Agents with Potential for Near-Term Use and Impact. *Am. J. Trop. Med. Hyg.* **2021**, *105*, 584–595. [CrossRef] [PubMed]

6.   Lancet Commission on COVID-19 Vaccines and Therapeutics Task Force Members. Urgent needs of low-income and middle-income countries for COVID-19 vaccines and therapeutics. *Lancet* **2021**, *397*, 562–564. [CrossRef] [PubMed]

7.   Chakraborty, C.; Sharma, A.R.; Bhattacharya, M.; Agoramoorthy, G.; Lee, S.S. The Drug Repurposing for COVID-19 Clinical Trials Provide Very Effective Therapeutic Combinations: Lessons Learned From Major Clinical Studies. *Front. Pharmacol.* **2021**, *12*, 704205. [CrossRef]

8.   Oskotsky, T.; Maric, I.; Tang, A.; Oskotsky, B.; Wong, R.J.; Aghaeepour, N.; Sirota, M.; Stevenson, D.K. Mortality Risk among Patients with COVID-19 Prescribed Selective Serotonin Reuptake Inhibitor Antidepressants. *JAMA Netw. Open* **2021**, *4*, e2133090. [CrossRef] [PubMed]

9.   Zimniak, M.; Kirschner, L.; Hilpert, H.; Geiger, N.; Danov, O.; Oberwinkler, H.; Steinke, M.; Sewald, K.; Seibel, J.; Bodem, J. The serotonin reuptake inhibitor Fluoxetine inhibits SARS-CoV-2 in human lung tissue. *Sci. Rep.* **2021**, *11*, 5890. [CrossRef]

10.   Rosen, D.A.; Seki, S.M.; Fernández-Castañeda, A.; Beiter, R.M.; Eccles, J.D.; Woodfolk, J.A.; Gaultier, A. Modulation of the sigma-1 receptor-IRE1 pathway is beneficial in preclinical models of inflammation and sepsis. *Sci. Transl. Med.* **2019**, *11*, eaau5266. [CrossRef]

11.   Rafiee, L.; Hajhashemi, V.; Javanmard, S.H. Fluvoxamine inhibits some inflammatory genes expression in LPS/stimulated human endothelial cells, U937 macrophages, and carrageenan-induced paw edema in rat. *Iran. J. Basic. Med. Sci.* **2016**, *19*, 977–984.

12.   Hashimoto, Y.; Suzuki, T.; Hashimoto, K. Mechanisms of action of fluvoxamine for COVID-19: A historical review. *Mol. Psychiatry* **2022**, *27*, 1898–1907. [CrossRef]

13.   Pericat, D.; Leon-Icaza, S.A.; Sanchez Rico, M.; Muhle, C.; Zoicas, I.; Schumacher, F.; Planes, R.; Mazars, R.; Gros, G.; Carpinteiro, A.; et al. Antiviral and Anti-Inflammatory Activities of Fluoxetine in a SARS-CoV-2 Infection Mouse Model. *Int. J. Mol. Sci.* **2022**, *23*, 13623. [CrossRef]

14.   Adnot, S.; Houssaini, A.; Abid, S.; Marcos, E.; Amsellem, V. Serotonin transporter and serotonin receptors. *Handb. Exp. Pharmacol.* **2013**, *218*, 365–380. [CrossRef]

15.   Kirenga, B.J.; Mugenyi, L.; Sanchez-Rico, M.; Kyobe, H.; Muttamba, W.; Mugume, R.; Mwesigwa, E.; Kalimo, E.; Nyombi, V.; Segawa, I.; et al. Association of fluvoxamine with mortality and symptom resolution among inpatients with COVID-19 in Uganda: A prospective interventional open-label cohort study. *Mol. Psychiatry* **2023**, *epub ahead of print*. [CrossRef]

16.   Carpinteiro, A.; Edwards, M.J.; Hoffmann, M.; Kochs, G.; Gripp, B.; Weigang, S.; Adams, C.; Carpinteiro, E.; Gulbins, A.; Keitsch, S.; et al. Pharmacological Inhibition of Acid Sphingomyelinase Prevents Uptake of SARS-CoV-2 by Epithelial Cells. *Cell Rep. Med.* **2020**, *1*, 100142. [CrossRef] [PubMed]

17.   Lenze, E.J.; Mattar, C.; Zorumski, C.F.; Stevens, A.; Schweiger, J.; Nicol, G.E.; Miller, J.P.; Yang, L.; Yingling, M.; Avidan, M.S.; et al. Fluvoxamine vs Placebo and Clinical Deterioration in Outpatients with Symptomatic COVID-19: A Randomized Clinical Trial. *JAMA* **2020**, *324*, 2292–2300. [CrossRef]

18.   Reis, G.; Dos Santos Moreira-Silva, E.A.; Silva, D.C.M.; Thabane, L.; Milagres, A.C.; Ferreira, T.S.; Dos Santos, C.V.Q.; de Souza Campos, V.H.; Nogueira, A.M.R.; de Almeida, A.; et al. Effect of early treatment with fluvoxamine on risk of emergency care and hospitalisation among patients with COVID-19: The TOGETHER randomised, platform clinical trial. *Lancet Glob. Health* **2022**, *10*, e42–e51. [CrossRef]

19.   Finley, A. Is Fluvoxamine the Covid Drug We've Been Waiting for? Available online: https://www.wsj.com/articles/is-fluvoxamine-the-covid-miracle-drug-we-have-been-waiting-for-oral-pill-cheap-hospitalization-11640726605 (accessed on 14 January 2022).

20.   Fergal, P.M.; Gilmar, R.; Kristian, T.; Jamie, I.F.; Christina, M.G.; David, R.B.; Edward, J.M.; TOGETHER Investigators. Early Treatment with Fluvoxamine among Patients with COVID-19: A Cost-Consequence Model. *medRxiv* **2021**. [CrossRef]

21.   National Public Health Organization. Guidelines for Healthcare Professionals and Areas of Healthcare Services. Therapeutic Algorithm for Adult Non-Hospitalized Patients with COVID-19. Available online: https://eody.gov.gr/neos-koronaios-covid-19/ (accessed on 1 August 2022).

22.   Yu, L.M.; Bafadhel, M.; Dorward, J.; Hayward, G.; Saville, B.R.; Gbinigie, O.; Van Hecke, O.; Ogburn, E.; Evans, P.H.; Thomas, N.P.B.; et al. Inhaled budesonide for COVID-19 in people at high risk of complications in the community in the UK (PRINCIPLE): A randomised, controlled, open-label, adaptive platform trial. *Lancet* **2021**, *398*, 843–855. [CrossRef]

23.   Ramakrishnan, S.; Nicolau, D.V., Jr.; Langford, B.; Mahdi, M.; Jeffers, H.; Mwasuku, C.; Krassowska, K.; Fox, R.; Binnian, I.; Glover, V.; et al. Inhaled budesonide in the treatment of early COVID-19 (STOIC): A phase 2, open-label, randomised controlled trial. *Lancet Respir. Med.* **2021**, *9*, 763–772. [CrossRef] [PubMed]

24.   Ebell, M.H. Inhaled Budesonide Reduces the Risk of Emergency Department Evaluation or Hospitalization in Early COVID-19. *Am. Fam. Physician* **2021**, *104*, 207–208.

25.   Zhou, F.; Yu, T.; Du, R.; Fan, G.; Liu, Y.; Liu, Z.; Xiang, J.; Wang, Y.; Song, B.; Gu, X.; et al. Clinical course and risk factors for mortality of adult inpatients with COVID-19 in Wuhan, China: A retrospective cohort study. *Lancet* **2020**, *395*, 1054–1062. [CrossRef]

26. Guan, W.-j.; Ni, Z.-y.; Hu, Y.; Liang, W.-h.; Ou, C.-q.; He, J.-x.; Liu, L.; Shan, H.; Lei, C.-l.; Hui, D.S.C.; et al. Clinical Characteristics of Coronavirus Disease 2019 in China. *N. Engl. J. Med.* **2020**, *382*, 1708–1720. [CrossRef]

27. Huang, C.; Wang, Y.; Li, X.; Ren, L.; Zhao, J.; Hu, Y.; Zhang, L.; Fan, G.; Xu, J.; Gu, X.; et al. Clinical features of patients infected with 2019 novel coronavirus in Wuhan, China. *Lancet* **2020**, *395*, 497–506. [CrossRef]

28. Wang, D.; Hu, B.; Hu, C.; Zhu, F.; Liu, X.; Zhang, J.; Wang, B.; Xiang, H.; Cheng, Z.; Xiong, Y.; et al. Clinical Characteristics of 138 Hospitalized Patients with 2019 Novel Coronavirus-Infected Pneumonia in Wuhan, China. *JAMA* **2020**, *323*, 1061–1069. [CrossRef]

29. Coveney, J. FIRTHLOGIT: Stata Module to Calculate Bias Reduction in Logistic Regression. Available online: https://EconPapers.repec.org/RePEc:boc:bocode:s456948 (accessed on 15 April 2023).

30. Reis, G.; Mills, E. Fluvoxamine for the treatment of COVID-19—Author's reply. *Lancet Glob. Health* **2022**, *10*, e333. [CrossRef] [PubMed]

31. Reis, G.; Dos Santos Moreira Silva, E.A.; Medeiros Silva, D.C.; Thabane, L.; de Souza Campos, V.H.; Ferreira, T.S.; Quirino Dos Santos, C.V.; Ribeiro Nogueira, A.M.; Figueiredo Guimaraes Almeida, A.P.; Cançado Monteiro Savassi, L.; et al. Oral Fluvoxamine with Inhaled Budesonide for Treatment of Early-Onset COVID-19: A Randomized Platform Trial. *Ann. Intern. Med.* **2023**, *176*, 667–675. [CrossRef]

32. Hoertel, N. Do the Selective Serotonin Reuptake Inhibitor Antidepressants Fluoxetine and Fluvoxamine Reduce Mortality among Patients with COVID-19? *JAMA Netw. Open* **2021**, *4*, e2136510. [CrossRef]

33. Fico, G.; Isayeva, U.; De Prisco, M.; Oliva, V.; Sole, B.; Montejo, L.; Grande, I.; Arbelo, N.; Gomez-Ramiro, M.; Pintor, L.; et al. Psychotropic drug repurposing for COVID-19: A Systematic Review and Meta-Analysis. *Eur. Neuropsychopharmacol.* **2023**, *66*, 30–44. [CrossRef]

34. Boretti, A. Effectiveness of fluvoxamine at preventing COVID-19 infection from turning severe. *Eur. Neuropsychopharmacol.* **2023**, *67*, 83–85. [CrossRef] [PubMed]

35. Lee, T.C.; Vigod, S.; Bortolussi-Courval, E.; Hanula, R.; Boulware, D.R.; Lenze, E.J.; Reiersen, A.M.; McDonald, E.G. Fluvoxamine for Outpatient Management of COVID-19 to Prevent Hospitalization: A Systematic Review and Meta-analysis. *JAMA Netw. Open* **2022**, *5*, e226269. [CrossRef] [PubMed]

36. Marcec, R.; Dodig, V.M.; Likic, R. A meta-analysis regarding fluvoxamine and hospitalization risk of COVID-19 patients: TOGETHER making a difference. *J. Infect.* **2023**, *86*, 154–225. [CrossRef] [PubMed]

37. Wen, W.; Chen, C.; Tang, J.; Wang, C.; Zhou, M.; Cheng, Y.; Zhou, X.; Wu, Q.; Zhang, X.; Feng, Z.; et al. Efficacy and safety of three new oral antiviral treatment (molnupiravir, fluvoxamine and Paxlovid) for COVID-19: A meta-analysis. *Ann. Med.* **2022**, *54*, 516–523. [CrossRef]

38. Deng, J.; Rayner, D.; Ramaraju, H.B.; Abbas, U.; Garcia, C.; Heybati, K.; Zhou, F.; Huang, E.; Park, Y.J.; Moskalyk, M. Efficacy and safety of selective serotonin reuptake inhibitors in COVID-19 management: A systematic review and meta-analysis. *Clin. Microbiol. Infect.* **2023**, *29*, 578–586. [CrossRef]

39. Calusic, M.; Marcec, R.; Luksa, L.; Jurkovic, I.; Kovac, N.; Mihaljevic, S.; Likic, R. Safety and efficacy of fluvoxamine in COVID-19 ICU patients: An open label, prospective cohort trial with matched controls. *Br. J. Clin. Pharmacol.* **2022**, *88*, 2065–2073. [CrossRef]

40. Rahman, M.M.; Mahi, A.M.; Melamed, R.; Alam, M.A.U. Effects of Antidepressants on COVID-19 Outcomes: Retrospective Study on Large-Scale Electronic Health Record Data. *Interact. J. Med. Res.* **2023**, *12*, e39455. [CrossRef] [PubMed]

41. Bramante, C.T.; Huling, J.D.; Tignanelli, C.J.; Buse, J.B.; Liebovitz, D.M.; Nicklas, J.M.; Cohen, K.; Puskarich, M.A.; Belani, H.K.; Proper, J.L.; et al. Randomized Trial of Metformin, Ivermectin, and Fluvoxamine for COVID-19. *N. Engl. J. Med.* **2022**, *387*, 599–610. [CrossRef]

42. Bramante, C.T.; Buse, J.B.; Liebovitz, D.M.; Nicklas, J.M.; Puskarich, M.A.; Cohen, K.; Belani, H.K.; Anderson, B.J.; Huling, J.D.; Tignanelli, C.J.; et al. Outpatient treatment of COVID-19 and incidence of post-COVID-19 condition over 10 months (COVID-OUT): A multicentre, randomised, quadruple-blind, parallel-group, phase 3 trial. *Lancet Infect. Dis.* **2023**, *epub ahead of print*. [CrossRef]

43. McCarthy, M.W.; Naggie, S.; Boulware, D.R.; Lindsell, C.J.; Stewart, T.G.; Felker, G.M.; Jayaweera, D.; Sulkowski, M.; Gentile, N.; Bramante, C.; et al. Effect of Fluvoxamine vs Placebo on Time to Sustained Recovery in Outpatients with Mild to Moderate COVID-19: A Randomized Clinical Trial. *JAMA* **2023**, *329*, 296–305. [CrossRef]

44. Marzolini, C.; Marra, F.; Boyle, A.; Khoo, S.; Back, D.J. Fluvoxamine for the treatment of COVID-19. *Lancet Glob Health* **2022**, *10*, e331. [CrossRef]

45. van Harten, J. Overview of the pharmacokinetics of fluvoxamine. *Clin. Pharmacokinet.* **1995**, *29* (Suppl. 1), 1–9. [CrossRef]

46. Fluvoxamine Prices GoodRx. Available online: https://www.ramq.gouv.qc.ca/en/media/12091 (accessed on 15 April 2023).

47. Mills, F.P.; Reis, G.; Wilson, L.A.; Thorlund, K.; Forrest, J.I.; Guo, C.M.; Boulware, D.R.; Mills, E.J. Early Treatment with Fluvoxamine among Patients with COVID-19: A Cost-Consequence Model. *Am. J. Trop. Med. Hyg.* **2023**, *108*, 101–106. [CrossRef] [PubMed]

48. Arulanandam, B.; Beladi, H.; Chakrabarti, A. Obesity and COVID-19 mortality are correlated. *Sci. Rep.* **2023**, *13*, 5895. [CrossRef] [PubMed]

49. Sawadogo, W.; Tsegaye, M.; Gizaw, A.; Adera, T. Overweight and obesity as risk factors for COVID-19-associated hospitalisations and death: Systematic review and meta-analysis. *BMJ Nutr. Prev. Health* **2022**, *5*, 10–18. [CrossRef] [PubMed]

50. Sattar, N.; McInnes, I.B.; McMurray, J.J.V. Obesity Is a Risk Factor for Severe COVID-19 Infection: Multiple Potential Mechanisms. *Circulation* **2020**, *142*, 4–6. [CrossRef] [PubMed]
51. Dicker, D.; Bettini, S.; Farpour-Lambert, N.; Fruhbeck, G.; Golan, R.; Goossens, G.; Halford, J.; O'Malley, G.; Mullerova, D.; Ramos Salas, X.; et al. Obesity and COVID-19: The Two Sides of the Coin. *Obes. Facts* **2020**, *13*, 430–438. [CrossRef]
52. Wu, N.; Joyal-Desmarais, K.; Ribeiro, P.A.B.; Vieira, A.M.; Stojanovic, J.; Sanuade, C.; Yip, D.; Bacon, S.L. Long-term effectiveness of COVID-19 vaccines against infections, hospitalisations, and mortality in adults: Findings from a rapid living systematic evidence synthesis and meta-analysis up to December, 2022. *Lancet Respir. Med.* **2023**, *11*, 439–452. [CrossRef]
53. Huang, I.; Pranata, R. Lymphopenia in severe coronavirus disease-2019 (COVID-19): Systematic review and meta-analysis. *J. Intensive Care* **2020**, *8*, 36. [CrossRef]
54. Zhao, Q.; Meng, M.; Kumar, R.; Wu, Y.; Huang, J.; Deng, Y.; Weng, Z.; Yang, L. Lymphopenia is associated with severe coronavirus disease 2019 (COVID-19) infections: A systemic review and meta-analysis. *Int. J. Infect. Dis.* **2020**, *96*, 131–135. [CrossRef]
55. Niu, J.; Sareli, C.; Mayer, D.; Visbal, A.; Sareli, A. Lymphopenia as a Predictor for Adverse Clinical Outcomes in Hospitalized Patients with COVID-19: A Single Center Retrospective Study of 4485 Cases. *J. Clin. Med.* **2022**, *11*, 700. [CrossRef]
56. Diao, B.; Wang, C.; Tan, Y.; Chen, X.; Liu, Y.; Ning, L.; Chen, L.; Li, M.; Liu, Y.; Wang, G.; et al. Reduction and Functional Exhaustion of T Cells in Patients with Coronavirus Disease 2019 (COVID-19). *Front. Immunol.* **2020**, *11*, 827. [CrossRef]
57. Pontelli, M.C.; Castro, I.A.; Martins, R.B.; La Serra, L.; Veras, F.P.; Nascimento, D.C.; Silva, C.M.; Cardoso, R.S.; Rosales, R.; Gomes, R.; et al. SARS-CoV-2 productively infects primary human immune system cells in vitro and in COVID-19 patients. *J. Mol. Cell Biol.* **2022**, *14*, mjac021. [CrossRef]
58. Ratajczak, M.Z.; Kucia, M. SARS-CoV-2 infection and overactivation of Nlrp3 inflammasome as a trigger of cytokine "storm" and risk factor for damage of hematopoietic stem cells. *Leukemia* **2020**, *34*, 1726–1729. [CrossRef]
59. He, Z.; Zhao, C.; Dong, Q.; Zhuang, H.; Song, S.; Peng, G.; Dwyer, D.E. Effects of severe acute respiratory syndrome (SARS) coronavirus infection on peripheral blood lymphocytes and their subsets. *Int. J. Infect. Dis.* **2005**, *9*, 323–330. [CrossRef] [PubMed]
60. Varghese, J.; Sandmann, S.; Ochs, K.; Schrempf, I.M.; Frommel, C.; Dugas, M.; Schmidt, H.H.; Vollenberg, R.; Tepasse, P.R. Persistent symptoms and lab abnormalities in patients who recovered from COVID-19. *Sci. Rep.* **2021**, *11*, 12775. [CrossRef]
61. Drewry, A.M.; Samra, N.; Skrupky, L.P.; Fuller, B.M.; Compton, S.M.; Hotchkiss, R.S. Persistent lymphopenia after diagnosis of sepsis predicts mortality. *Shock* **2014**, *42*, 383–391. [CrossRef]
62. Firth, D. Bias reduction of maximum likelihood estimates. *Biometrika* **1993**, *80*, 27–38. [CrossRef]
63. Heinze, G.; Schemper, M. A solution to the problem of separation in logistic regression. *Stat. Med.* **2002**, *21*, 2409–2419. [CrossRef] [PubMed]
64. Berwanger, O. Antithrombotic Therapy for Outpatients with COVID-19: Implications for Clinical Practice and Future Research. *JAMA* **2021**, *326*, 1685–1686. [CrossRef]
65. Talasaz, A.H.; Sadeghipour, P.; Kakavand, H.; Aghakouchakzadeh, M.; Kordzadeh-Kermani, E.; Van Tassell, B.W.; Gheymati, A.; Ariannejad, H.; Hosseini, S.H.; Jamalkhani, S.; et al. Recent Randomized Trials of Antithrombotic Therapy for Patients with COVID-19: JACC State-of-the-Art Review. *J. Am. Coll. Cardiol.* **2021**, *77*, 1903–1921. [CrossRef]

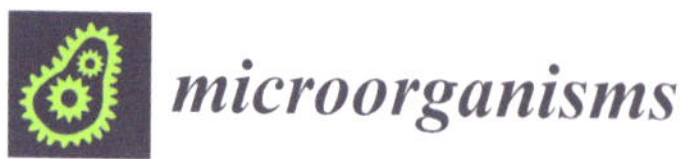 *microorganisms*

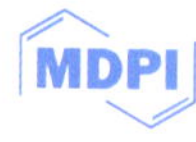

Article

Cold Atmospheric Helium Plasma in the Post-COVID-19 Era: A Promising Tool for the Disinfection of Silicone Endotracheal Prostheses

Diego Morais da Silva [1], Fellype Do Nascimento [2], Noala Vicensoto Moreira Milhan [1], Maria Alcionéia Carvalho de Oliveira [1], Paulo Francisco Guerreiro Cardoso [3], Daniel Legendre [4], Fabio Gava Aoki [5], Konstantin Georgiev Kostov [2] and Cristiane Yumi Koga-Ito [1,*]

[1] Institute of Science and Technology, São Paulo State University (UNESP),
    São José dos Campos 12227-010, SP, Brazil; diego.m.silva@unesp.br (D.M.d.S.);
    milhan.noala@gmail.com (N.V.M.M.); macoliveira12@gmail.com (M.A.C.d.O.)
[2] Faculty of Engineering, São Paulo State University (UNESP), Guaratinguetá 12516-410, SP, Brazil;
    fellype@gmail.com (F.D.N.); konstantin.kostov@unesp.br (K.G.K.)
[3] Division of Thoracic Surgery, Instituto do Coração, Hospital das Clínicas HCFMUSP, Faculdade de Medicina,
    Universidade de São Paulo, São Paulo 01246-903, SP, Brazil; cardosop@gmail.com
[4] Adib Jatene Foundation, Dante Pazzanese Institute of Cardiology, São Paulo 04012-909, SP, Brazil;
    daniel@fajbio.com.br
[5] Institute of Science and Technology, Federal University of São Paulo (UNIFESP),
    São José dos Campos 12231-280, SP, Brazil; fgaoki@unifesp.br
*   Correspondence: cristiane.koga-ito@unesp.br

Citation: Silva, D.M.d.;
Do Nascimento, F.; Milhan, N.V.M.;
Oliveira, M.A.C.d.; Cardoso, P.F.G.;
Legendre, D.; Aoki, F.G.; Kostov,
K.G.; Koga-Ito, C.Y. Cold
Atmospheric Helium Plasma in the
Post-COVID-19 Era: A Promising
Tool for the Disinfection of Silicone
Endotracheal Prostheses.
Microorganisms **2024**, *12*, 130.
https://doi.org/10.3390/
microorganisms12010130

Academic Editor: Qibin Geng

Received: 15 December 2023
Revised: 4 January 2024
Accepted: 6 January 2024
Published: 9 January 2024

Abstract: Despite the excellent properties of silicone endotracheal prostheses, their main limitation is the formation of a polymicrobial biofilm on their surfaces. It can cause local inflammation, interfering with the local healing process and leading to further complications in the clinical scenario. The present study evaluated the inhibitory effect of cold atmospheric plasma (CAP) on multispecies biofilms grown on the silicone protheses' surfaces. In addition to silicone characterization before and after CAP exposure, CAP cytotoxicity on immortalized human bronchial epithelium cell line (BEAS-2B) was evaluated. The aging time test reported that CAP could temporarily change the silicone surface wetting characteristics from hydrophilic (80.5°) to highly hydrophilic (<5°). ATR-FTIR showed no significant alterations in the silicone surficial chemical composition after CAP exposure for 5 min. A significant log reduction in viable cells in monospecies biofilms (log CFU/mL) of *C. albicans*, *S. aureus*, and *P. aeruginosa* (0.636, 0.738, and 1.445, respectively) was detected after CAP exposure. Multispecies biofilms exposed to CAP showed significant viability reduction for *C. albicans* and *S. aureus* (1.385 and 0.831, respectively). The protocol was not cytotoxic to BEAS-2B. CAP can be a simple and effective method to delay multispecies biofilm formation inside the endotracheal prosthesis.

Keywords: multispecies biofilm; non-thermal plasma; endotracheal tubes; silicone prosthesis; COVID-19

1. Introduction

Tracheal stenosis is a clinical condition characterized by a reduction in the central airway diameter through a congenital or acquired pathological process. The COVID-19 pandemic produced a high number of patients submitted to intubation and prolonged mechanical ventilation worldwide, resulting in higher percentages of laryngotracheal stenosis [1–4]. Commonly, patients with tracheal stenosis after COVID-19 cannot undergo tracheal resection since maturation of the stenosis, as well as a reduction in inflammation, needs to be achieved before the procedure [5]. Additionally, the recurrence of tracheal stenosis is a risk during the first three months after surgery [6]. The prevalence of post-intubation tracheal stenosis in retrospective studies ranges from 6% to 20% and that of post-tracheostomy from 0.6% to 21% [7].

Patients with benign tracheal stenosis or tracheal tumors who are not eligible, either temporarily or permanently, for definitive treatment via tracheal surgical resection are considered for airway stenting to maintain airway patency. Silicone airway stents are widely used for their safety, patient tolerance, easy handling, and lower cost than that of self-expanding stents. The silicone T-tube was introduced in 1965 [8]. It requires a tracheostomy for anchoring the horizontal limb of the prosthesis that is occluded by a removable silicone cap. The straight-studded silicone stent was introduced in 1990 [9] and does not require a tracheostomy. Both are used as endoluminal support for the trachea, enabling breathing and phonation through the natural airway, thus improving quality of life [10].

Medical-grade silicone (MGS) is the primary material in endotracheal prostheses. MGS has attractive properties such as chemical inertness, water and temperature resistance, biocompatibility, and flexibility [11]. The constant contact between the inhaled air passing through the airway prosthesis and the tracheal underlying mucosa promotes the accumulation of biofilms composed of bacteria and fungi. The interaction between the polymicrobial biofilm and the surrounding mucosa can potentially aggravate the severity of the stenosis [10,12,13]. *Staphylococcus aureus*, *Pseudomonas aeruginosa*, and *Candida albicans* are the main microorganisms in the polymicrobial biofilm formed inside the patient's silicone prosthesis implant [14]. Biofilm formation usually takes approximately seven days, and severe complications such as pneumonia or sepsis can occur [15]. On the other hand, the MGS degradation promoted by the polymicrobial biofilm is progressive, requiring the prosthesis to be changed every 6 to 12 months after implantation. This can negatively impact the patient's quality of life and induce higher costs [16,17].

Previous studies focused on modifying the MGS surface to promote antimicrobial activity. Silver ions and nanoparticles were used as an alternative approach and were effective against *Escherichia coli*, *P. aeruginosa*, and *Staphylococcus aureus*. The limitations of these methods are the potential cytotoxicity and mucus accumulation on the silver-coated surface, which can reduce its antimicrobial properties [18].

Cold atmospheric plasma (CAP) stands for a low-temperature ($<40\ °C$) gas discharge plasma with extensive applications in the medical and biomedical fields [19–22]. The literature has already reported microbial inactivation due to the reactive oxygen and nitrogen reactive species (RONS) and UV radiation produced by CAP. The antimicrobial effect was observed on several species of bacteria and fungi, including *S. aureus*, *P. aeruginosa*, and *C. albicans* [23–25]. CAP can be delivered through long, flexible plastic tubes [26,27], enabling clinical use. Moreover, previous studies reported that CAP has low toxicity to mammalian cells [28,29].

This pre-clinical in vitro study focused on the effect of the Helium-CAP over mono-species and multispecies biofilms grown on the MGS surface in a laboratory setting, which mimics what is clinically observed inside the T-tube. The CAP treatment's effects on biofilms' viability were assessed, along with the possible surface changes on the MGS caused by CAP. Lastly, the cytotoxicity of the protocol was tested using a BEAS-2B immortalized human bronchial epithelium cell line. The motivation of this study is to develop a protocol for CAP treatment that can be applied directly to the external limb of the T-tube during outpatient visits, aiming to control the biofilm proliferation in the lumen of the silicone prosthesis. Such features can prolong the prosthesis' durability, reduce the interaction between the biofilm and the adjacent mucosa, and enhance the local healing process.

2. Materials and Methods

The MGS samples were prepared in disks measuring 8 mm in diameter and 2 mm in height. The specimens had the same chemical composition as T-tube implants. They were used to perform the surface characterization of silicone before and after the plasma treatment and the microbiological assays. Before treatment, all samples were washed in an ultrasonic bath by immersion for 10 min in water and 10 min in isopropyl alcohol. After that, another step of water washing was performed for 10 min. Finally, the samples were sterilized in an autoclave for 20 min packed in a medical-grade sheet. The MGS samples were stored in a dry place until the experiments.

2.1. Characterization of CAP Interactions with the MGS Surface

Figure 1 illustrates the configuration of the CAP system used to treat MGS samples. The device was described in [24]. It mainly consists of a dielectric barrier discharge (DBD) type reactor, composed of a metallic pin electrode placed inside a closed-end quartz tube, which, in turn, is placed inside a dielectric enclosure. The working gas (helium, 99.2% purity) is fed into the chamber and flushed to the ambient air through a 1 m long and flexible plastic tube connected to the reactor output (inner and outer diameter equal to 2.0 mm and 4.0 mm, respectively). A copper wire with a diameter of 0.5 mm was installed inside the plastic tube and placed a few millimeters inside the reactor to avoid contact with the quartz tube. The other tip of the copper wire terminates 2 mm before the output tip of the plastic tube. The high voltage is turned on when the working gas flows, and a primary discharge is ignited inside the DBD reactor. The latter polarizes the copper wire, and a small plasma jet is ignited at the end of the plastic tube.

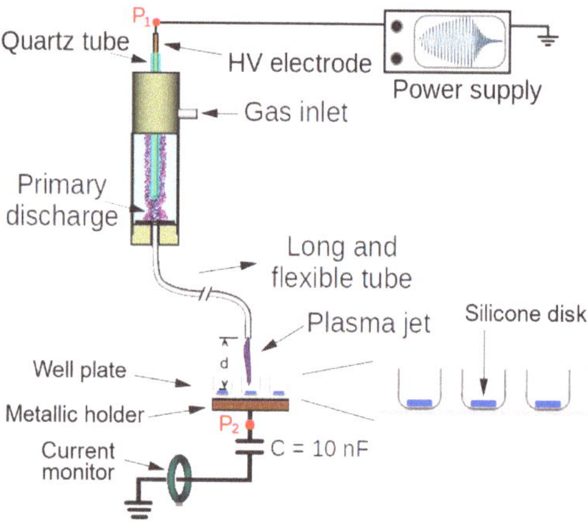

Figure 1. Scheme for CAP generation and MSG treatment.

A commercial AC generator from GBS Elektronik GmbH (model Minipuls4) was used as the power source to generate the CAP. It was used to produce an amplitude-modulated high-voltage (HV) waveform that consists of a sinusoidal "burst" with an oscillation frequency of 31.7 kHz, followed by a voltage-off interval, which repeats at a repetition period (T) equal to 1.2 ms. Such an AC generator was chosen due to its versatility in setting up the main operating parameters (voltage waveform, amplitude, and frequency), allowing us to test different combinations. In previous studies, we have found the operating parameters that do not heat up the target and provide good antimicrobial efficacy [25]. The discharge power for the configuration shown in Figure 1 was calculated by measuring the HV input at point P1 and the voltage on the capacitor at point P_2 [24]. Thus, the discharge power obtained in the current configuration was 436 ± 2 mW.

MGS samples were placed inside a 24-well plate at a distance d = 5.0 mm from the plasma outlet. The employed gas flow rate was 2.0 SLM. Aiming to study the interaction between the CAP and the MGS, as well as the behavior of the MGS surface after 2 min of plasma exposure, the CAP was generated by applying HV with a peak-to-peak amplitude of 17.2 kV to the pin-electrode, which is nearly 40% higher than the value employed for the treatment of biofilms. This value was chosen to simulate an extreme case and evaluate the possibility of material damage due to plasma exposure. The samples were characterized by wettability measurements and attenuated the total reflectance mode of Fourier transform infrared spectroscopy (ATR-FTIR) before and after CAP treatment. To assess the water contact angle (WCA), the samples were analyzed using an F300 Rame-Hart goniometer (Rame-hart, Washington, DC, USA). Six WCA measurements were performed, one before plasma exposure and five after the treatment (at time instants of 0 min, 15 min, 30 min, 1 h, and 2 h). Due to the small sample size, different samples were used for each WCA measurement. To analyze possible changes in the surface chemistry of the MGS samples exposed to CAP treatment, ATR-FTIR spectra were recorded before and right after the CAP exposure. Such measurements were carried out using the ATR mode of a Lambda-100 spectrometer (Perkin-Elmer, Shelton, CT, USA) in the region between 4000 and 400 cm^{-1}, with a 4 cm^{-1} resolution averaged over 16 scans.

2.2. Formation of Monospecies Biofilms on MGS Surfaces

Reference strains (Table 1) were plated in Brain Heart Infusion (BHI) agar for bacteria or Sabouraud agar for fungi. The plates were incubated for 24 h at 37 °C under aerobiosis. After, standardized suspensions (1×10^7 CFU/mL) were prepared in sterile saline (NaCl 0.9%) with the aid of a spectrophotometer (AJX-1600, Micronal, São Paulo, SP, Brazil). The optical density and the wavelength adopted for each microorganism are shown in Table 1. Sterile MGS specimens were transferred to a 24-well plate, and 2.0 mL of brain heart infusion (BHI) broth and 200 μL of the microbial inoculum were added to each well. The plates were incubated for 48 h at 37 °C under aerobiosis and agitation (120 rpm). The culture medium was refreshed after 24 h.

Table 1. Data on the reference strains used for biofilm formation and parameters of optical density (O.D) and wavelength (λ) adopted for standardized suspension preparation (1×10^7 CFU/mL).

Microorganism	Reference Number	Optical Density	Wavelength (nm)
Candida albicans	ATCC 18804	0.760	530
Pseudomonas aeruginosa	ATCC 27853	0.130	600
Staphylococcus aureus	ATCC 6538	0.249	490

2.3. Formation of Multispecies Biofilms on MGS Surfaces

The microbial suspensions were obtained as described in Section 2.2. The multispecies biofilms were grown on the surface of MGS inside a 24-well plate. In total, 2.0 mL of BHI broth + 2.5% Bovine Serum Albumin (BSA) were added to each well. Then, 200 μL of the *C. albicans* and *S. aureus* inoculum were added, followed by 20 μL of *P. aeruginosa* inoculum. The plates were incubated for 48 h at 37 °C under aerobiosis and agitation (120 rpm). The culture medium was refreshed after 24 h.

2.4. CAP Treatment of the Biofilms Formed on MGS

Each well containing the biofilms was separately exposed to He-CAP treatment for 5 min. CAP was produced by the device described in Figure 1 under the same conditions employed to study the interaction between the plasma and the MGS, with a voltage amplitude of 12.3 kV p-p. For the CAP treatment, each sample was placed exactly in the geometrical center of the well (from a 24-well plate), as seen in Figure 2. The distance between the sample surface and the CAP output was 0.5 cm.

Biofilms were also flushed via He gas flow without plasma ignition for comparative purposes.

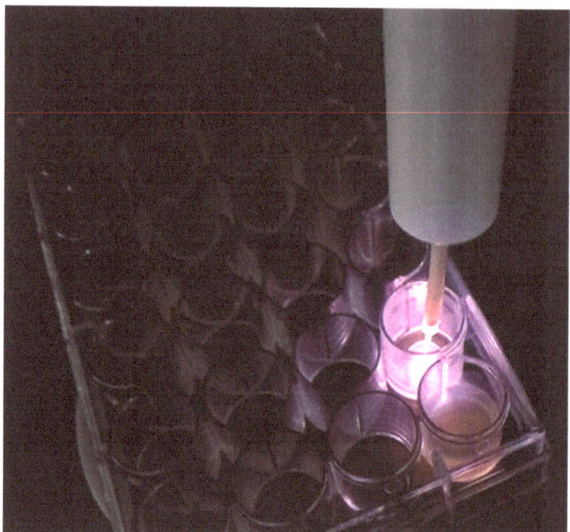

Figure 2. Application of the cold atmospheric plasma jet on the sample surface inside a well (24-well plate), with a distance of 0.5 cm between the plasma outlet and the sample.

2.5. Determination of Viable Cell Counts

After the CAP exposure, the biofilms were recovered from the MGS specimens via sonication (amplitude of 50%) in 3 cycles of 10 s pulse on, intercalated with 20 s pulse off. Finally, the suspensions were serially diluted and plated in specific agar to determine viable cell counts (CFU/mL), according to Table 2. The experiments were performed in triplicate on three independent occasions ($n = 9$). The data obtained were analyzed statistically using the Shapiro–Wilk normality test and compared using the Mann–Whitney test. The level of significance was set at 5%.

Table 2. Description of each culture media used for viable cell recovery from mono- and multispecies biofilms.

	Microorganism	**Culture Medium**
	C. albicans	Sabouraud agar
Monospecies biofilm	*P. aeruginosa*	Brain Heart Infusion (BHI) agar
	S. aureus	Brain Heart Infusion (BHI) agar
	C. albicans	CHROMagar
Multispecies biofilm	*P. aeruginosa*	Cetrimide agar
	S. aureus	Mannitol agar

2.6. Cytotoxicity Analysis

The cell line BEAS-2B was selected to be used in this study to evaluate the toxicity of the CAP exposure protocol on the human bronchial epithelium. The cytotoxicity analysis was based on ISO 10993-5/2009 [30]. The cells were incubated in Gibco™ LHC-9 medium (Thermo Fisher, Waltham, MA, USA) and kept incubated at 37 °C and 5% CO_2 until they reached the desired confluence. To evaluate the cytotoxicity, 4×10^4 cells per well were plated in 24-well plates. The experiments were performed in duplicate ($n = 12$). For the treatment, 200 μL of the new medium was added to the wells to prevent them from drying out, and the cells were exposed to the products of CAP generated inside the T-tube.

Figure 3 shows the schematic for producing and applying the He CAP inside the tracheal T-tube. For this assay, the flexible tube from the CAP device was inserted horizontally inside the extratracheal portion. The 24-well plate was positioned under the T-tube vertical portion so that the distance between the CAP generated inside the T-tube and the cells was 2.0 cm. This configuration was used to study the effects of the CAP products on BEAS-2B cells. The treatment parameters were 31.7 kHz of frequency, 12.3 kV of voltage amplitude, and 2.0 SLM of helium gas flow, and the treatment group was exposed to CAP for 5 min. In the control group, the cells were not exposed to plasma.

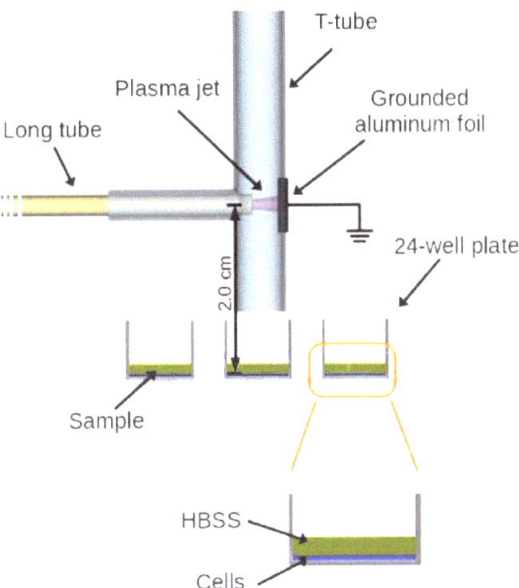

Figure 3. Schematic of the experimental setup to generate CAP inside the T-tube during the cytotoxicity test.

After CAP exposure of each well, 1 mL of the new medium was added to the wells. After 24 h, the medium was removed, the MTT reagent ((3-4,5-dimethylthiazol-2yl)-2,5-diphenyl-tetrazolium, Sigma, St. Louis, MI, USA) was added, and the plates were kept in agitation for 10 min. The optical density of the resulting solution was measured using a spectrophotometer at 570 nm. The control group normalized the obtained absorbance (=100%). The obtained data were evaluated in the GraphPad Prism software, version 8 (GraphPad Software, Inc., La Jolla, CA, USA). Cytotoxicity classification was based on the cell viability percentage, where values above 70% were considered non-cytotoxic [31].

2.7. Statistical Analysis

The collected data were statistically evaluated using GraphPad Prism version 8 (GraphPad Software, Inc., La Jolla, CA, USA). The normal data distribution was evaluated, and the most appropriate statistical tests were selected and applied. The significance level of 5% was adopted for all the tests.

3. Results
3.1. MGS Surface Characterization after CAP Exposure

The WCA behavior measured on the surface of the MGS samples after exposure to CAP treatment is presented in Figure 4. Images of the water droplets on the MGS samples are shown in Figure 5. Non-treated specimens have a WCA of 80.5°, i.e., exhibiting a less hydrophilic surface when compared to the control. The sample analyzed immediately after the CAP exposure showed a WCA < 5°, indicating that CAP changed the MGS surface properties to a highly hydrophilic surface. The MGS surface characteristics after CAP exposure, that is, WCA < 5°, were maintained for approximately 15 min. After 30 min, the WCA increased to 15.2°, and this increasing trend was also observed for the sample analyzed after one hour, two hours, and four hours, showing a WCA of 17.6°, 44.6° and 53.2°, respectively.

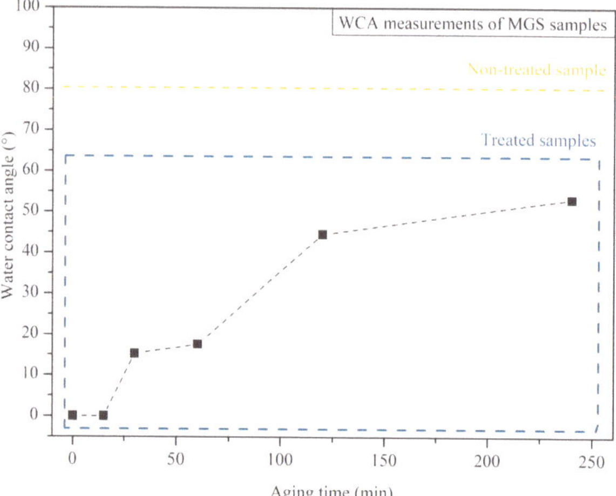

Figure 4. Aging time test of MGS samples after the treatment of CAP. The period of analysis varies between 0 min and 4 h. The WCA of the non-treated sample is displayed in a box inside the graphic for comparison purposes.

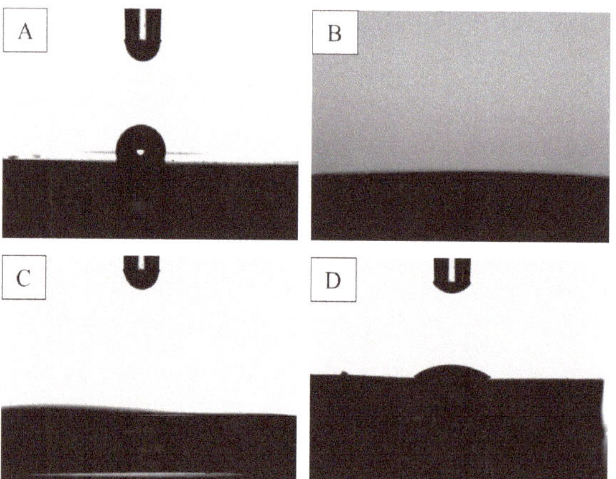

Figure 5. WCA measurement images showing the behavior of MGS surfaces in contact with water droplets at different times: (**A**) before CAP exposure; (**B**) right after CAP exposure; (**C**) 15 min after CAP exposure; (**D**) 4 h after CAP exposure.

Figure 6 shows the spectra obtained from the ATR-FTIR analysis of non-treated and CAP-treated samples. This analysis aimed to look for possible changes in the MGS compositional properties before and after plasma irradiation. Table 3 contributes to the spectra analysis, presenting the correlation between the detected bands and the main functional groups on the MGS surface. The spectra of both samples demonstrate the C-H stretching band at 2962.3 cm^{-1}, the asymmetric stretching of methyl groups at 1412 cm^{-1} characteristic for Si-CH$_3$, and the symmetric stretching of the same group at 1258 cm^{-1}. Finally, the typical bands at 800–1000 cm^{-1} are attributed to the Si-O-Si bond stretching [32].

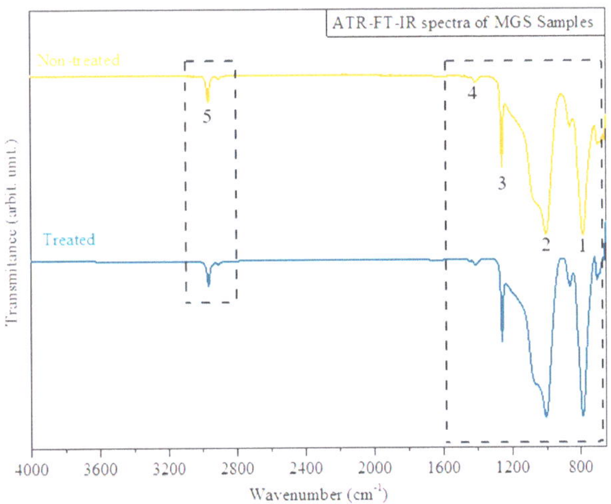

Figure 6. ATR-FTIR spectra of treated (blue) and non-treated (yellow) MGS samples. Numbers 1 and 2 represent $-CH_3$ of $SiCH_3$ bands; 3 and 4 represent Si–O–Si bands; and 5 is related to C–H bands.

Table 3. Attribution to the bands identified in the ATR-FTIR analysis.

Functional Group	Wavenumber (cm^{-1})	Peak #	Reference
$-CH_3$ of $SiCH_3$	1258 and 1412	1, 2	
Si–O–Si	800–1000	3, 4	[33]
C–H	2962.3	5	

3.2. Antimicrobial Activity of CAP

The effect of CAP on the monospecies biofilms of *C. albicans*, *P. aeruginosa*, and *S. aureus* formed on the MGS surface can be observed in Figure 7. The *C. albicans* CAP-treated group demonstrated an average count of viable cells of 1.362×10^6 (CFU/mL), while the control group was 3.151×10^5 (CFU/mL). The treatment resulted in a statistically significant log reduction of 0.636 (*T*-test, $p < 0.0001$). The plasma-treated *P. aeruginosa* group presented an average count of viable cells of 1.42×10^6 (CFU/mL), while the average value of the control group was 3.955×10^7 (CFU/mL). In this way, there was a statistically significant log reduction of 1.445 (Mann–Whitney test, $p < 0.0001$). *S. aureus* monospecies biofilm counts of viable cells of 5.194×10^6 (CFU/mL) and 2.844×10^7 (CFU/mL) were observed for treated and control groups, respectively, with a statistically significant log reduction of 0.738 (*T*-test, $p < 0.05$).

Multispecies biofilms composed of *C. albicans*, *P. aeruginosa*, and *S. aureus* were also treated with CAP. Figure 8 shows the obtained results. The average count of *C. albicans* viable cells recovered from plasma-treated biofilm was 6.333×10^3 (CFU/mL), while that from multispecies biofilm control was 1.571×10^5 (CFU/mL), indicating a statistically significant log reduction of 1.358 (Mann–Whitney test, $p < 0.0001$). Plasma-treated *P. aeruginosa* biofilms had 1.551×10^5 (CFU/mL) viable cells, while 1.655×10^5 (CFU/mL) viable cells were recovered from the control biofilm. Thus, *P. aeruginosa* showed a slight log reduction of 0.028 ($p > 0.05$). The average value of *S. aureus* viable cells recovered from the plasma-treated and the control groups was 1.0×10^3 (CFU/mL) and 6.77×10^3 (CFU/mL), respectively. There was a statistically significant log reduction of 0.83 (Mann–Whitney test, $p < 0.0001$).

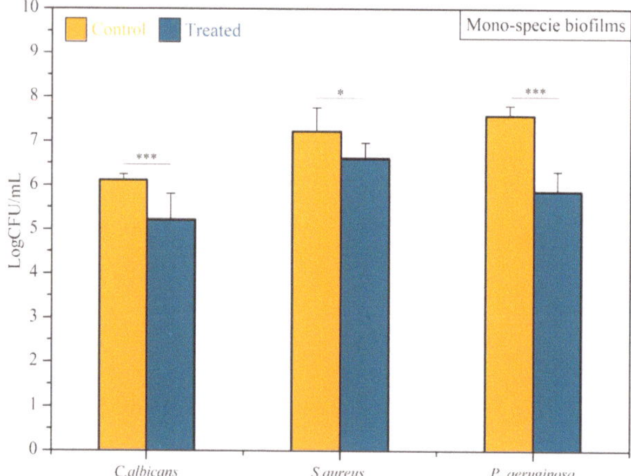

Figure 7. Antibiofilm efficacy of CAP on *Candida albicans, Staphylococcus aureus, and Pseudomonas aeruginosa* monospecies biofilms. Results expressed in the logarithm of colony-forming units per milliliter (log CFU/mL). *T*-test *** $p < 0.0001$ and * $p < 0.05$.

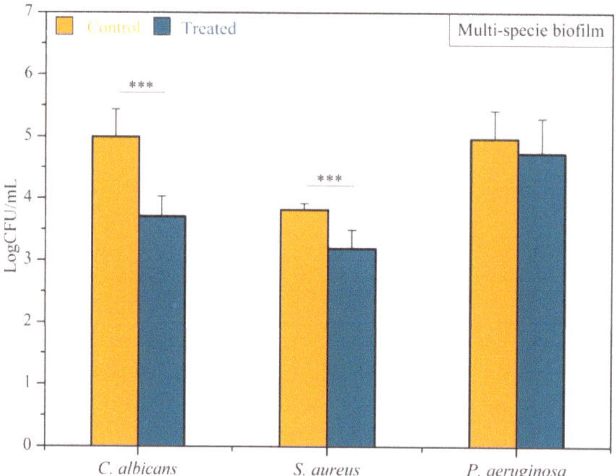

Figure 8. Antibiofilm efficacy of CAP on *C. albicans, P. aeruginosa, and S. aureus* multispecies biofilms. Results are expressed in the logarithm of colony-forming units per milliliter (CFU/mL). Mann–Whitney test, *** indicates $p < 0.0001$.

3.3. Cytotoxicity Test

The results of the cytotoxicity test using the BEAS-2B cells are presented in Figure 9. The viability of the cells exposed to CAP generated inside the T-tube was 95.76%. Thus, the protocol with antimicrobial activity can be considered non-cytotoxic (viability > 70%).

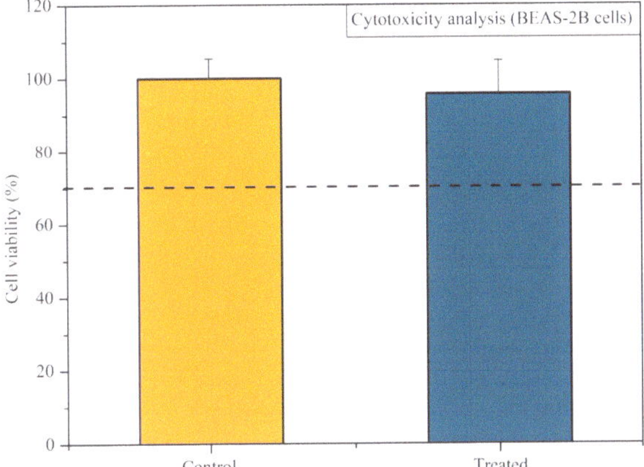

Figure 9. Cytotoxicity analysis of CAP expressed in cell viability (control 100%). The BEAS-2B cells were exposed to CAP generated inside the T-tube for 5 min. The cell viability was determined 24 h after CAP exposure. The dashed line represents 70% of cell viability.

4. Discussion

The increase in tracheal stenosis cases related to previous episodes of COVID-19 emerged as an alarming reality after the pandemic. Beyouglu et al. (2022) reported that the intubation time of patients with COVID-19 is significantly longer when compared to that of patients with other conditions, which further increases the occurrence of tracheal stenosis and the subsequent use of silicone endotracheal prostheses [34]. To avoid the prostheses changing every 6 to 12 months after implantation, alternative treatments that do not negatively interfere with the properties of MGS and present disinfection properties are needed. This study investigated CAP as an antimicrobial tool for removing biofilm commonly found in silicone endotracheal prostheses.

In the first stage, MGS surface characterization was performed after CAP exposure. The WCA increased steadily with time after the CAP treatment. In contrast, in the period studied, it did not recover to the same WCA before CAP exposure (80.5°). Thus, the plasma treatment temporarily changes the MGS surfaces, making them highly hydrophilic; halfway through the treatment, the WCA increases but does not reach the same contact angle as the non-treated sample. After the treatment, the MGS surface at 4 h is still more hydrophilic than the untreated MGS.

Regarding the ATR-FTIR measurements, comparing both spectra, no significant differences were observed in the treated MGS sample compared to the untreated one. This is a positive result, as it shows that the plasma interacts with the MGS material, changing its surface energy without causing any change in its chemical composition or structure.

The hydrophobicity changes highlighted in the WCA analysis can be attributed to the interaction between the MGS surfaces and the RONS produced by CAP [35], leading to the formation of polar groups. Conversely, the ATR-FTIR analysis did not detect these plasma-induced polar groups. However, we should consider that when an internal reflection element is used in ATR-FTIR analysis, the IR beam detects chemical groups to the depth of 0.5–5 µm [36]. So, suppose the plasma modification is limited only to the sample surface. In that case, the ATR-FTIR will probably not be able to detect any changes because it integrates the material response over a much broader depth. On the other hand, the behavior highlighted in the WCA aging test on the MGS surface occurs in the outermost surface layers (few nm) that were affected by the plasma. In this sense, further analyses more sensitive in detecting chemical changes on the MGS surfaces may clarify some of our findings.

To the best of our knowledge, the usage of CAP to treat biofilms on MGS surfaces at our set-up conditions has not been previously reported. However, biofilms treated with CAP on different substrates have already been investigated, and this will be a parameter to discuss our results.

In a previous study, *S. aureus* (ATCC 33591) and *P. aeruginosa* (ATCC 27853) biofilms formed on collagen membranes and were treated with CAP for 5 min with 15 mm of working distance. The treatment against these biofilms was as effective as the treatment performed in our study. The authors observed higher *S. aureus* log reduction than our experiments for the same microorganism [37]. However, it is worth mentioning that we used a different *S. aureus* strain, which could justify some differences in the data. In this previous work, the reported log reduction for *P. aeruginosa* biofilm was lower than the decrease observed in our experiments for the same strain (ATCC 27853). These results indicate that reducing the working distance to 5 mm improves the antimicrobial effectiveness of *P. aeruginosa* biofilm.

The findings in the literature regarding CAP treatment against *C. albicans*, using similar parameters, are available to ATCC 18804. Inhibition zones of 2.0 and 2.5 cm were reached after 150 s treatment [23]. Another study with *C. albicans* strain SC 5314 reported a 2-log reduction when CAP was applied using the same parameters used in the present study and 15 mm of working distance [38]. It is well known that this strain is very virulent, reinforcing the antifungal potential of CAP treatment, as well as its antibacterial effect.

Our study also demonstrated the potential of CAP for treating multispecies biofilms, which more closely reflects the clinical situation of endotracheal prostheses. *P. aeruginosa* was the only microorganism that did not show a statistically significant reduction after the treatment of multispecies biofilms. This finding probably occurred due to *P. aeruginosa*'s dispersal in the polymeric extracellular matrices within *C. albicans* and *S. aureus*, with no or little interaction between *P. aeruginosa* and CAP reactive species. Similarly, the literature reports a high resistance of *P. aeruginosa* to different antibiotics, such as tobramycin and ciprofloxacin. This behavior can be attributed to the disposal of *P. aeruginosa* throughout the biofilm architecture due to the hypoxic and low metabolic conditions known as contributors to antimicrobial resistance [39]. The low reduction in viable *P. aeruginosa* cells recovered from the multispecies biofilm treatment with CAP may be due to the same reason. Once the three microorganisms are part of the same biofilm structure, the disposal of each throughout the biofilm architecture and the competition between them can create the same hypoxic environment, leading to low metabolic conditions, and possibly increasing the *P. aeruginosa* resistance to the CAP treatment. Sequential applications of CAP can be an alternative to enhance the antibacterial activity against *P. aeruginosa* in multispecies biofilms. As this study did not explore the sequential application of CAP, further studies are necessary to better understand its effects on *P. aeruginosa* in multispecies biofilms.

In addition to being antimicrobial, the proposed protocol was not cytotoxic to tracheal cells (BEAS-2B) in the conditions of this study. We emphasize that we focused on exposing the MGS used in T-tubes to CAP and not directly to the cells, simulating a clinical situation where the CAP jet will be directed to the contaminated prosthesis. We observed that a controlled application of CAP in the prosthesis is unlikely to cause harm to the epithelial cells adjacent to and outside the wall of the T-tube. Future studies are necessary to clarify the distribution of RONs inside the tube and to check the improvement in antimicrobial activity after sequential exposures since promising findings have already been obtained after only one application.

5. Conclusions

In conclusion, CAP exposure of MGS samples enhances the surface hydrophilic properties from hydrophilic (WCA = 80.5°) to highly hydrophilic (WCA < 5°). The plasma-jet-induced changes on the surface of the sample were not permanent. ATR-FTIR analysis did not show any significant differences between CAP-treated and non-treated samples, essentially indicating only a modification on the surface of the sample. CAP showed an effective inhibitory effect on all monospecies biofilms formed on MGS surfaces. It also demonstrated antimicrobial efficacy against *C. albicans* and *S. aureus* cells in the multispecies biofilm. The cytotoxicity test showed that the protocol is not cytotoxic for BEAS-2B cells when CAP is generated inside the T-tube. Future studies are required to better understand CAP's potential and limitations in controlling the polymicrobial biofilms inside an endotracheal prosthesis and to make further improvements to the protocol. However, with the findings of this in vitro study, it is already possible to state that CAP is a suitable tool for the disinfection of MGS surfaces and, therefore, promising for the disinfection of silicone endotracheal prostheses.

Author Contributions: Conceptualization, C.Y.K.-I., K.G.K., P.F.G.C., D.L., F.G.A. and D.M.d.S.; methodology, C.Y.K.-I., K.G.K., D.M.d.S., N.V.M.M., F.D.N. and M.A.C.d.O.; software, D.M.d.S., F.D.N., N.V.M.M.; formal analysis, C.Y.K.-I., D.M.d.S., F.D.N. and N.V.M.M.; investigation, D.M.d.S., F.D.N., N.V.M.M. and M.A.C.d.O.; resources, C.Y.K.-I., K.G.K., D.M.d.S., F.D.N. and N.V.M.M.; data curation, C.Y.K.-I., K.G.K., D.M.d.S., N.V.M.M. and F.D.N.; writing—original draft preparation, C.Y.K.-I., K.G.K., D.M.d.S., N.V.M.M. and F.D.N.; writing—review and editing, C.Y.K.-I., K.G.K., F.G.A., D.M.d.S., N.V.M.M., F.D.N., M.A.C.d.O., P.F.G.C. and D.L.; supervision, C.Y.K.-I., K.G.K. and F.G.A.; project administration, C.Y.K.-I.; funding acquisition, C.Y.K.-I., K.G.K., D.M.d.S., N.V.M.M. and F.D.N. All authors have read and agreed to the published version of the manuscript.

Funding: This work was supported by the São Paulo State Research Foundation (FAPESP), grant numbers 2019/05856-7, 2021/02680-5, 2020/09481-5, 2021/00046-7; the Coordination for the Improvement of Higher Education (CAPES) under Print and DS programs; and the Brazilian National Council for Scientific and Technological Development, grant numbers 309762/2021-9, 308127/2018-8, and 310608/2021-0.

Data Availability Statement: The data that support the findings of this study are available from the corresponding author upon reasonable request.

Conflicts of Interest: The authors declare no conflict of interest.

References

1. Piazza, C.; Filauro, M.; Dikkers, F.G.; Nouraei, S.A.R.; Sandu, K.; Sittel, C.; Amin, M.R.; Campos, G.; Eckel, H.E.; Peretti, G. Long-Term Intubation and High Rate of Tracheostomy in COVID-19 Patients Might Determine an Unprecedented Increase of Airway Stenoses: A Call to Action from the European Laryngological Society. *Eur. Arch. Oto-Rhino-Laryngol.* **2021**, *278*, 1–7. [CrossRef]
2. Esteller-Moré, E.; Ibañez, J.; Matiñó, E.; Ademà, J.M.; Nolla, M.; Quer, I.M. Prognostic Factors in Laryngotracheal Injury Following Intubation and/or Tracheotomy in ICU Patients. *Eur. Arch. Oto-Rhino-Laryngol. Head Neck* **2005**, *262*, 880–883. [CrossRef] [PubMed]
3. Mattioli, F.; Marchioni, A.; Andreani, A.; Cappiello, G.; Fermi, M.; Presutti, L. Post-Intubation Tracheal Stenosis in COVID-19 Patients. *Eur. Arch. Oto-Rhino-Laryngol.* **2021**, *278*, 847–848. [CrossRef] [PubMed]
4. Alturk, A.; Bara, A.; Darwish, B. Post-Intubation Tracheal Stenosis after Severe COVID-19 Infection: A Report of Two Cases. *Ann. Med. Surg.* **2021**, *67*, 102468. [CrossRef]
5. Auchincloss, H.G.; Wright, C.D. Complications after Tracheal Resection and Reconstruction: Prevention and Treatment. *J. Thorac. Dis.* **2016**, *8*, S160–S167. [PubMed]
6. Rorris, F.P.; Chatzimichali, E.; Liverakou, E.; Antonopoulos, C.N.; Balis, E.; Kotsifas, C.; Stratakos, G.; Koutsoukou, A.; Zisis, C. Tracheal Resection in Patients Post–COVID-19 Is Associated with High Reintervention Rate and Early Restenosis. *JTCVS Tech.* **2023**, *18*, 157–163. [CrossRef] [PubMed]
7. Ershadi, R.; Rafieian, S.; Sarbazzadeh, J.; Vahedi, M. Tracheal Stenosis Following Mild-to-Moderate COVID-19 Infection without History of Tracheal Intubation: A Case Report. *Gen. Thorac. Cardiovasc. Surg.* **2022**, *70*, 303–307. [CrossRef]
8. Montgomery, W.W. T-Tube Tracheal Stent. *Arch. Otolaryngol.* **1965**, *82*, 320–321. [CrossRef]
9. Dumon, J.-F. A Dedicated Tracheobronchial Stent. *Chest* **1990**, *97*, 328–332. [CrossRef]
10. Bibas, B.J.; Terra, R.M.; Oliveira Junior, A.L.; Tamagno, M.F.L.; Minamoto, H.; Cardoso, P.F.G.; Pêgo-Fernandes, P.M. Predictors for Postoperative Complications After Tracheal Resection. *Ann. Thorac. Surg.* **2014**, *98*, 277–282. [CrossRef]
11. Ding, K.; Wang, Y.; Liu, S.; Wang, S.; Mi, J. Preparation of Medical Hydrophilic and Antibacterial Silicone Rubberviasurface Modification. *RSC Adv.* **2021**, *11*, 39950–39957. [CrossRef] [PubMed]
12. Lee, J.M.; Hashmi, N.; Bloom, J.D.; Tamashiro, E.; Doghramji, L.; Sarani, B.; Palmer, J.N.; Cohen, N.A.; Mirza, N. Biofilm Accumulation on Endotracheal Tubes Following Prolonged Intubation. *J. Laryngol. Otol.* **2012**, *126*, 267–270. [CrossRef] [PubMed]

13. Fusconi, M.; lo Vasco, V.R.; Delfini, A.; de Virgilio, A.; Taddei, A.R.; Vassalli, C.; Conte, M.; del Sette, F.; Benincasa, A.T.; de Vincentiis, M. Is Montgomery Tracheal Safe-T-Tube Clinical Failure Induced by Biofilm? *Otolaryngol.-Head Neck Surg.* **2013**, *149*, 269–276. [CrossRef] [PubMed]

14. Nouraei, S.A.R.; Petrou, M.A.; Randhawa, P.S.; Singh, A.; Howard, D.J.; Sandhu, G.S. Bacterial Colonization of Airway Stents. *Arch. Otolaryngol. Head Neck Surg.* **2006**, *132*, 1086. [CrossRef] [PubMed]

15. Raveendra, N.; Rathnakara, S.H.; Haswani, N.; Subramaniam, V. Bacterial Biofilms on Tracheostomy Tubes. *Indian J. Otolaryngol. Head Neck Surg.* **2021**, *74*, 4995–4999. [CrossRef] [PubMed]

16. Bibas, B.J.; Cardoso, P.F.G.; Salati, M.; Minamoto, H.; Luiz Tamagno, M.F.; Terra, R.M.; Pêgo-Fernandes, P.M. Health-Related Quality of Life Evaluation in Patients with Non-Surgical Benign Tracheal Stenosis. *J. Thorac. Dis.* **2018**, *10*, 4782–4788. [CrossRef] [PubMed]

17. Mazhar, K.; Gunawardana, M.; Webster, P.; Hochstim, C.; Koempel, J.; Kokot, N.; Sinha, U.; Rice, D.; Baum, M. Bacterial Biofilms and Increased Bacterial Counts Are Associated with Airway Stenosis. *Otolaryngol.-Head Neck Surg.* **2014**, *150*, 834–840. [CrossRef]

18. Chen, X.; Ling, X.; Liu, G.; Xiao, J. Antimicrobial Coating: Tracheal Tube Application. *Int. J. Nanomed.* **2022**, *17*, 1483–1494. [CrossRef]

19. Martusevich, A.K.; Surovegina, A.V.; Bocharin, I.V.; Nazarov, V.V.; Minenko, I.A.; Artamonov, M.Y. Cold Argon Athmospheric Plasma for Biomedicine: Biological Effects, Applications and Possibilities. *Antioxidants* **2022**, *11*, 1262. [CrossRef]

20. Miebach, L.; Poschkamp, B.; van der Linde, J.; Bekeschus, S. Medical Gas Plasma—A Potent ROS-Generating Technology for Managing Intraoperative Bleeding Complications. *Appl. Sci.* **2022**, *12*, 3800. [CrossRef]

21. Bekeschus, S.; Saadati, F.; Emmert, S. The Potential of Gas Plasma Technology for Targeting Breast Cancer. *Clin. Transl. Med.* **2022**, *12*, e1022. [CrossRef] [PubMed]

22. Duarte, S.; Panariello, B.H.D. Comprehensive Biomedical Applications of Low Temperature Plasmas. *Arch. Biochem. Biophys.* **2020**, *693*, 108560. [CrossRef] [PubMed]

23. Kostov; Borges, A.C.; Koga-Ito, C.Y.; Nishime, T.M.C.; Prysiazhnyi, V.; Honda, R.Y. Inactivation of Candida Albicans by Cold Atmospheric Pressure Plasma Jet. *IEEE Trans. Plasma Sci.* **2015**, *43*, 770–775. [CrossRef]

24. Kostov; Nishime, T.M.C.; Machida, M.; Borges, A.C.; Prysiazhnyi, V.; Koga-Ito, C.Y. Study of Cold Atmospheric Plasma Jet at the End of Flexible Plastic Tube for Microbial Decontamination. *Plasma Process. Polym.* **2015**, *12*, 1383–1391. [CrossRef]

25. Borges, A.C.; Lima, G.D.M.G.; Nishime, T.M.C.; Gontijo, A.V.L.; Kostov, K.G.; Koga-Ito, C.Y. Amplitude-Modulated Cold Atmospheric Pressure Plasma Jet for Treatment of Oral Candidiasis: In Vivo Study. *PLoS ONE* **2018**, *13*, e0199832. [CrossRef] [PubMed]

26. Bastin, O.; Thulliez, M.; Servais, J.; Nonclercq, A.; Delchambre, A.; Hadefi, A.; Devière, J.; Reniers, F. Optical and Electrical Characteristics of an Endoscopic DBD Plasma Jet. *Plasma Med.* **2020**, *10*, 71–90. [CrossRef]

27. Decauchy, H.; Pavy, A.; Camus, M.; Fouassier, L.; Dufour, T. Cold Plasma Endoscopy Applied to Biliary Ducts: Feasibility Risk Assessment on Human-like and Porcine Models for the Treatment of Cholangiocarcinoma. *J. Phys. D Appl. Phys.* **2022**, *55*, 455401. [CrossRef]

28. Kondeti, V.S.S.K.; Phan, C.Q.; Wende, K.; Jablonowski, H.; Gangal, U.; Granick, J.L.; Hunter, R.C.; Bruggeman, P.J. Long-Lived and Short-Lived Reactive Species Produced by a Cold Atmospheric Pressure Plasma Jet for the Inactivation of Pseudomonas Aeruginosa and Staphylococcus Aureus. *Free Radic. Biol. Med.* **2018**, *124*, 275–287. [CrossRef]

29. Mrochen, D.M.; Miebach, L.; Skowski, H.; Bansemer, R.; Drechsler, C.A.; Hoffmann, U.; Hein, M.; Mamat, U.; Gerling, T.; Schaible, U.; et al. Toxicity and Virucidal Activity of a Neon-Driven Micro Plasma Jet on Eukaryotic Cells and a Coronavirus. *Free Radic. Biol. Med.* **2022**, *191*, 105–118. [CrossRef]

30. *ISO 10993-5 2009*; Biological Evaluation of Medical Devices—Part 5: Tests for in Vitro Cytotoxicity. International Organization for Standardization: Geneva, Switzerland, 2009.

31. Jablonská, E.; Kubásek, J.; Vojtěch, D.; Ruml, T.; Lipov, J. Test Conditions Can Significantly Affect the Results of in Vitro Cytotoxicity Testing of Degradable Metallic Biomaterials. *Sci. Rep.* **2021**, *11*, 6628. [CrossRef]

32. Ceresa, C.; Tessarolo, F.; Maniglio, D.; Tambone, E.; Carmagnola, I.; Fedeli, E.; Caola, I.; Nollo, G.; Chiono, V.; Allegrone, G.; et al. Medical-Grade Silicone Coated with Rhamnolipid R89 Is Effective against *Staphylococcus* spp. Biofilms. *Molecules* **2019**, *24*, 3843. [CrossRef] [PubMed]

33. Salih, S.I.; Oleiwi, J.K.; Ali, H.M. Study the Mechanical Properties of Polymeric Blends (SR/PMMA) Using for Maxillofacial Prosthesis Application. In *Proceedings of the IOP Conference Series: Materials Science and Engineering*; Institute of Physics Publishing: Bristol, UK, 2018; Volume 454.

34. Beyoglu, M.A.; Sahin, M.F.; Turkkan, S.; Yazicioglu, A.; Yekeler, E. Complex Post-Intubation Tracheal Stenosis in Covid-19 Patients. *Indian J. Surg.* **2022**, *84*, 805–813. [CrossRef] [PubMed]

35. Liu, G.; Shi, F.; Wang, Q.; Zhang, Z.; Guo, J.; Zhuang, J. Penetration Effect of the KINPen Plasma Jet Investigated with a 3D Agar-Entrapped Bacteria Model. *Microchem. J.* **2022**, *183*, 107973. [CrossRef]

36. Tiernan, H.; Byrne, B.; Kazarian, S.G. ATR-FTIR Spectroscopy and Spectroscopic Imaging for the Analysis of Biopharmaceuticals. *Spectrochim. Acta Part A Mol. Biomol. Spectrosc.* **2020**, *241*, 118636. [CrossRef] [PubMed]

37. Oliveira, M.A.C.D.; Lima, G.D.M.G.; Nishime, T.M.C.; Gontijo, A.V.L.; Menezes, B.R.C.D.; Caliari, M.V.; Kostov, K.G.; Koga-Ito, C.Y. Inhibitory Effect of Cold Atmospheric Plasma on Chronic Wound-Related Multispecies Biofilms. *Appl. Sci.* **2021**, *11*, 5441. [CrossRef]

38. Borges, A.C.; Castaldelli Nishime, T.M.; Kostov, K.G.; de Morais Gouvêa Lima, G.; Lacerda Gontijo, A.V.; de Carvalho, J.N.M.M.; Yzumi Honda, R.; Yumi Koga-Ito, C. Cold Atmospheric Pressure Plasma Jet Modulates Candida Albicans Virulence Traits. *Clin. Plasma Med.* **2017**, *7–8*, 9–15. [CrossRef]
39. Maurice, N.M.; Bedi, B.; Sadikot, R.T. Pseudomonas Aeruginosa Biofilms: Host Response and Clinical Implications in Lung Infections. *Am. J. Respir. Cell Mol. Biol.* **2018**, *58*, 428–439. [CrossRef]

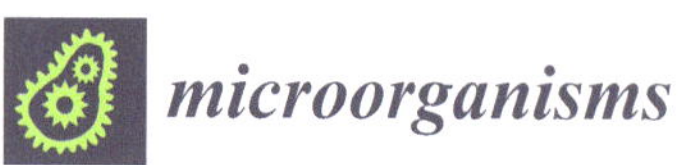 *microorganisms*

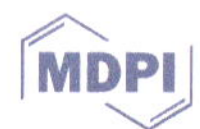

Article

Natural Product Cordycepin (CD) Inhibition for NRP1/CD304 Expression and Possibly SARS-CoV-2 Susceptibility Prevention on Cancers

Ting Li [1,2,†], Na Luo [1,2,†], Jiewen Fu [1,2], Jiaman Du [1], Zhiying Liu [1], Qi Tan [1], Meiling Zheng [1], Jiayue He [1], Jingliang Cheng [1], Dabing Li [1,2,*] and Junjiang Fu [1,*]

1   Key Laboratory of Epigenetics and Oncology, The Research Center for Preclinical Medicine, Southwest Medical University, Luzhou 646000, China; 20220199120034@stu.swmu.edu.cn (T.L.); 20220199120033@stu.swmu.edu.cn (N.L.); fujiewen@swmu.edu.cn (J.F.); 20190199120004@stu.swmu.edu.cn (J.D.); 20210199120022@stu.swmu.edu.cn (Z.L.); 20210199120024@stu.swmu.edu.cn (Q.T.); zhengmeiling@swmu.edu.cn (M.Z.); hejieyue@swmu.edu.cn (J.H.); jingliangc@swmu.edu.cn (J.C.)

2   School of Basic Medical Sciences, Southwest Medical University, Luzhou 646000, China

*   Correspondence: lidabing@swmu.edu.cn (D.L.); fujunjiang@swmu.edu.cn (J.F.); Tel./Fax: +86-830-3160283 (J.F.)

†   These authors contributed equally to this work.

Abstract: NRP1/CD304 is a typical membrane-bound co-receptor for the vascular endothelial cell growth factor (VEGF), semaphorin family members, and viral SARS-CoV-2. Cordycepin (CD) is a natural product or active gradient from traditional Chinese medicine (TCM) from *Cordyceps militaris* Link and *Ophiocordyceps* sinensis (Berk.). However, NRP1 expression regulation via CD in cancers and the potential roles and mechanisms of SARS-CoV-2 infection are not clear. In this study, online databases were analyzed, Western blotting and quantitative RT-PCR were used for NRP1 expression change via CD, molecular docking was used for NRP/CD interaction, and a syncytial formation assay was used for CD inhibition using a pseudovirus SARS-CoV-2 entry. As a result, we revealed that CD inhibits NRP1 expressed in cancer cells and prevents viral syncytial formation in 293T-hACE2 cells, implying the therapeutic potential for both anti-cancer and anti-viruses, including anti-SARS-CoV-2. We further found significant associations between NRP1 expressions and the tumor–immune response in immune lymphocytes, chemokines, receptors, immunostimulators, immune inhibitors, and major histocompatibility complexes in most cancer types, implying NRP1's roles in both anti-cancer and anti-SARS-CoV-2 entry likely via immunotherapy. Importantly, CD also downregulated the expression of NRP1 from lymphocytes in mice and downregulated the expression of A2AR from the lung cancer cell line H1975 when treated with CD, implying the NRP1 mechanism probably through immuno-response pathways. Thus, CD may be a therapeutic component for anti-cancer and anti-viral diseases, including COVID-19, by targeting NRP1 at least.

Keywords: the *NRP1/CD304* gene; SARS-CoV-2; cancers; cordycepin (CD); therapeutics

1. Introduction

The NRP1 (Neuropilin 1, OMIM: 602069), CD304/VEGF165R/NRP/vascular endothelial cell growth factor 165 receptor, is a typical membrane-bound co-receptor for both members of the semaphorin family and vascular endothelial growth factor (VEGF) [1–4]. NRP1 is a cytogenetic located on the human chromosome 10p11.22. NRP1 encodes the deduced 923-amino acid protein with a molecular mass of 103,134 Da (NM_003873.7, NP_003864.5) containing an N-terminal signal sequence, a transmembrane region, an ectodomain, and a cytoplasmic domain, which is consistent to the structure of cell surface receptors [5]. These specific domains participated in different signaling pathways and versatile roles controlling survival, migration, and invasion, as well as angiogenesis and axon guidance, through binding

Citation: Li, T.; Luo, N.; Fu, J.; Du, J.; Liu, Z.; Tan, Q.; Zheng, M.; He, J.; Cheng, J.; Li, D.; et al. Natural Product Cordycepin (CD) Inhibition for NRP1/CD304 Expression and Possibly SARS-CoV-2 Susceptibility Prevention on Cancers. *Microorganisms* **2023**, *11*, 2953. https://doi.org/10.3390/microorganisms11122953

Academic Editor: Qibin Geng

Received: 13 November 2023
Revised: 1 December 2023
Accepted: 2 December 2023
Published: 10 December 2023

ligands to co-receptors, including VEGF and semaphorin family members [3,4]. For example, in breast cancer cells MDA-MB-231, CRISPR-Cas9 knocking out the *NRP1* gene was reported to have a pronounced reduction in lung metastasis [6].

Cantuti-Castelvetri et al. [7] and Daly et al. [8] found that NRP1 can act as a receptor to mediate severe acute respiratory syndrome coronavirus 2 (SARS-CoV-2) invading host cells [9]. As we well know, SARS-CoV-2 caused the severe coronavirus disease 2019 (COVID-19), leading to a global pandemic since the outbreak at the end of 2019 [10–12]. Unlike the S-protein of SARS-CoV, the SARS-CoV-2 S-protein has a polybasic sequence domain (Arg-Arg-Ala-Arg) (the C-end rule, CendR) at the S1-S2 boundary that facilitates the cleavage via furin [13], an enzyme convertase that catalyzes the conversion of a substance to its active state. Thus, SARS-CoV-2 can easily enter the host cells with the aid of NRP1, nourishing its infectivity and promoting its tropism [14]. In addition, cells from the bronchioalveolar lavage of COVID-19 patients showed an increase in NRP1 RNA expressions in SARS-CoV-2 positive cells but not in uninfected cells [7], further enhancing SARS-CoV-2 entry. Tumor necrosis factor α (TNFα) and interleukin-1β (IL-1β) increased the expression of NRP2, an isoform of NRP1, and promoted SARS-CoV-2 proliferation and S-protein binding, thus revealing proinflammatory cytokines such as TNFα for the contribution of SARS-CoV-2 proliferation in host human cells [15]. Meanwhile, Wang et al. [16] reported that NRP1 is highly expressed in macrophages and dendritic cells (DCs) from inside myeloid lineage cells but not in CD4+ T cells, acting as an inhibitor of HIV-1 infectivity.

Gene polymorphisms within the receptors/co-receptors of SARS-CoV-2, including NRP1 (rs10080), were reported to associate with variable COVID-19 outcomes across ethnicities [17,18]. Mutating NRP1 novel interaction sites, located in the vestigial plasminogen–apple–nematode (PAN) domain, were recently reported to reduce the S-protein of SARS-CoV-2 internalization [19], although another reported that the binding affinity is almost the same after mutation at some NRP1 sites (rs141633354, rs142121081, rs145954532, rs200660300, rs200028992, rs369312020, rs370551432, rs370641686, and rs370117610) via molecular docking [20].

Nevertheless, targeting NRP1 could be a potential approach to preventing SARS-CoV-2 entry [21,22] and for developing potential anti-tumor drugs [23,24], with a peptide-based inhibition in anti-angiogenesis, anti-proliferation, and anti-migration of tumor cells [25]. In addition, NRP1 also facilitated other various viruses' invasion and replication, such as the Epstein–Barr virus (EBV) [26], the pseudorabies virus (PRV) [27], the mouse cytomegalovirus (mCMV) [28], and the retroviruses for the human T cell lymphotropic virus-1 (HTLV-1) and HTLV-2 [29].

Small-molecule inhibitors for the S-protein in SARS-CoV-2 may bind to NRP1 [30]. In silico analysis found that interfering with SARS-CoV-2 binds to NRP1 via small molecules of natural products seem to be potential candidates as novel anti-viral agents [31–34]. Folic acid, leucovorin, and alimemazine may have the potential to prevent SARS-CoV-2 internalization by interacting with the S-protein/NRP1 complex [35,36]. Targeting NRP1 with small molecules would thus have the potential to interfere with SARS-CoV-2 invasion [37]. However, NRP1 expression in pan-cancers, its regulation, and the potential role of SARS-CoV-2-infected cancer patients are not clear. It is essential to identify novel small molecules from natural products or traditional Chinese medicine (TCM) with anti-tumor functions that can modulate the expression of host cell entry regulators for interfering with SARS-CoV-2 entry [14,30,38]. Cordycepin (CD) is an active gradient or natural product from traditional Chinese medicine (TCM) from *Cordyceps militaris* Link and *Ophiocordyceps sinensis* (Berk.). Cordycepin (CD), an adenosine derivative, processes a diverse, broad spectrum of biological/pharmacological activities, such as anti-cancer, antimetastatic, anti-viral, antiprotozoal, antimalarial, antimicrobial, insecticidal, anti-inflammatory, antioxidant, and immunomodulatory/immunoregulatory [39–41].

However, NRP1 expression regulation by CD in cancers, and the potential role and mechanism of SARS-CoV-2 infection are not clear [42,43]. In this study, we analyzed the NRP1 expressions and viral syncytial formation in cancer cell lines. Molecular docking was used to investigate NRP/CD interaction. The changes in the immune molecules from lymphocytes in mice when treated with CD were also conducted. Thus, CD may be a therapeutic component for SARS-CoV-2 and cancers by at least targeting NRP1.

2. Materials and Methods

2.1. Online Databases

An integrated repository portal for tumor–immune system interactions (TISIDB) was applied to perform the correlations between abundance in tumor-infiltrating lymphocytes (TILs) and NRP1 expression (http://cis.hku.hk/TISIDB/browse.php?gene=NRP1) (accessed on 1 January 2023) [44]. The sequences for the *NRP1* gene from GenBank NM_003873.7 in the National Center for Biotechnology Information (NCBI) were used to design quantitative RT-PCR primers [11]. Primer 3 (v. 0.4.0) was used to design NRP1 PCR primers and other gene primers (https://bioinfo.ut.ee/primer3-0.4.0/) (accessed on 1 January 2023) [45].

2.2. Antibodies and Reagents

The NRP1 antibody was purchased from the company of Santa Cruz Biotechnology (sc-5307, Dallas, TX, USA). β-actin and HSP70 antibodies served as an internal control. The CD was previously described [38] and purchased from Must Bio-Technology Co., Ltd., Chengdu, China. Fetal bovine serum (FBS) (cat.no.: A6907) was purchased from Invigentech (Irvine, CA, USA). The Roswell Park Memorial Institute (RPMI) 1640 medium (cat. no.: C3010-0500) or Dulbecco's modified Eagle's medium (DMEM) (cat. no.: C3113-0500) plus a 10% FBS was used for cell culture [40,46,47].

2.3. Cell Culture

The indicated cancer cells (H1975, BT549, PC3, and 22RV1) were used, and cultured conditions for cells have been previously described using an RPMI 1640 medium or a DMEM medium with a 10% FBS with antibiotics at 37 °C in a 5% CO_2 [38,48]. In addition, the 293T-hACE2 cell lines were gifted from Professor Xianghui Fu [49] and cultured using the DMEM medium with a 10% FBS with antibiotics at 37 °C in a 5% CO_2.

2.4. CD Treatments and Isolation of Mouse Lymphocytes

BALB/c female mice, which were purchased at Tengxin Biotechnology Co., Ltd. (Chongqing, China), were fed under a constant temperature at 22 °C, 50–60% humidity, and a light/dark cycle for 12 h according to the feeding standard. Six BALB/c female mice were selected and divided into two groups: the experimental and control groups. The mice (10 weeks old, about 24 g) were injected CD with 25 mg/kg/mouse (three mice per group) through the caudal vein and showed no abnormalities, which were observed once every 12 h. After 24 h, sodium pentobarbital (200 mg/kg body weight) was injected intraperitoneally in the experimental group and euthanized. Death presenting no heartbeat after anesthesia, dilated pupils, or cervical dislocation were confirmed as non-vital signs.

A CD (0.006 mg/μL) solution (containing 20% DMSO, 30% polyethylene glycol 400, 5% Tween 80, and 63% NaCl) with 25 mg/kg (CD/mouse) was injected into mice. After 24 h, T cells were isolated from the spleens of mice using our mouse T cell isolationprotocol (>95% purity) with the red blood cell lysate. For details, the spleens of the sacrificed mice were isolated, ground, and filtered using cell strainers (size: 100 μM, cat. no.: 15-1100; Biologix Group Ltd., Camarillo, CA, USA) under an ice bath, then collected into a 15 mL tube and centrifuged. The supernatant was lysed with an iced 1×red blood cell lysis solution (150 mM NH4Cl, 10 mM $KHCO_3$, and 0.1 mM EDTA) and mixed well. After lysis for 5–8 min on ice, the reaction was terminated by a cold 1 × PBS. After centrifugation, the supernatant was mixed with ice 1 × PBS, and the debris was discarded. Then, each sample containing mouse lymphocytes was used for protein and RNA extraction, respectively.

2.5. Western Blotting

After treatments with indicated drugs (0, 10, 20, and 40 μM), the cells were washed and lysed with an ice-cold 1 × EBC buffer (20 mM Tris-HCl pH8.0, 125 mM NaCl, 2 mM EDTA, 0.5% NP-40, and protease inhibitors). Then, the 2× SDS (sodium dodecyl sulfate) buffer was added, and the extracted samples were boiled at 100 °C for 5 min. About 50 μg samples in each well were taken for SDS–PAGE electrophoresis, and proteins were separated into 8% or 10% gels according to the molecular weight sizes of proteins with a voltage of 100 V for 2 h. After electrophoresis, the proteins were transferred into the PVDF membranes (polyvinylidene fluoride) with a voltage of 100 V for 2 h. The 1 × TBST (Tris-buffered saline with Tween 20, 137 mM NaCl, 2.7 mM KCl, 25 mM Tris, and 0.05% Tween 20) was used to wash the membranes to remove the extra methanol three times at room temperature. Then, the membranes were blocked with 5% nonfat milk in TBST for 2 h. After being washed in 1 × TBST three times, the membranes were cut, and the proteins were incubated with the indicated NRP1 and β-actin/HSP70 antibodies in 2% nonfat milk in 1 × TBST at 4 °C all night. The next day, 1 × TBST was used to wash the membranes to remove the extra primary antibodies three times, and then, the secondary antibodies were added with 2% nonfat milk in 1 × TBST for 2 h; then, 1 × TBST was washed for three times. Finally, the bands on the membranes were measured under the image scanner (Gene Company Limited, Gbox Chemi, DRXV4/1068, Hong Kong, China) after adding the Super Signal West Femto Maximum Sensitivity Substrate (Thermo Fish Scientific, XG346245, Boston, MA, USA) and BeyoECL Plus (P0018S, Shanghai, China). All experiments were repeated three times.

2.6. Semi-Quantitative RT-PCR

The CD-treated cells were extracted using RNA; then, the mRNA was reversely transcribed into cDNA with reverse transcriptase. A semi-quantitative RT-PCR was performed using NRP1 RT-PCR primers and ACTB RT-PCR primers using the above cDNA as a template. The RT-PCR primers for *NRP1* were as follows: RT-NRP1-5:5′-ccacagtggaacaggtgatg-3′ and RT-NRP1-3:5′-cgtactcctctggcttctgg-3′. The product size was 416 bp. The RT-PCR primers for *A2AR* (Genbank No. NM_000675.6) were as follows: RT-A2AR-L: 5′-tcaacagcaacctgcagaac-3′ and RT-A2AR-R: 5′-tccaacctagcatgggagtc-3′. The product size was 333 bp. *ACTB* was set up as an internal control with 510 bp in size. The *ACTB* was used as an internal control. All experiments were repeated three times. The primer sequences for other immuno-response genes and the amplified size for the RT-PCR are presented in Table 1.

Table 1. Immuno-response genes, primer sequences, and amplified size for RT-PCR in mice.

Gene Name	Primers	Sequence (from 5′-3′)	GenBank No.	Size (bp)
Cd28	RT-mCD28-L	acaacgagaggagcaatgga	NM_007642.4	401
	RT-mCD28-R	gcccagtagaggtccaaagt		
Cxcl12	RT-mCXCL12-L	ctttcactctcggtccacct	NM_001012477.2	258
	RT-mCXCL12-R	gcaacaatctgaagggcaca		
Csf1r	RT-mCSF1R-L	gcctcttcctctgttccctt	NM_001037859.2	372
	RT-mCSF1R-R	attcagggtccaaggtccag		
Kdr	RT-mKDR-L	ggagtctgtgcctgagaact	NM_010612.3	440
	RT-mKDR-R	acagaggcgatgaatggtga		
Ccr1	RT-mCCR1-L	ttggaaccagagagaagccg	NM_001295.3	259
	RT-mCCR1-R	agaaatggccaggttcagga		
Il2ra	RT-mIL2RA-L	acaagaacggcaccatccta	NM_008367.3	525
	RT-mIL2RA-R	agtctgtggtggttatggg		

2.7. Molecular Docking

The 3D structure files of the ligand CD (PubChem CID:6303), the protein NRP1(b1b2, the structure of b1b2 domains) (PDB ID:2QQI), and the RP1(b1, the structure of b1b2 domains) (PDB

ID:1KEX) were obtained from the PubChem database (https://pubchem.ncbi.nlm.nih.gov/, accessed on 1 January 2023) [50] and the Protein Data Bank (PDB, https://www.rcsb.org/, accessed on 1 January 2023), respectively. Default docking studies were attempted to explore the binding mode of the suggested CD onto the 3D model of NRP1 using AUTODOCK tools 1.5.7 [51]. The crystal structure of the center of the NRP1 was placed as the center of the molecular docking box. The Vina algorithm was applied in this research. The maximum number of binding modes was nine. Default settings were used for all other parameters. Output files for the docking were saved as both ligand_out.pdbqt and log.txt files. The PyMol (v2.0) and the BIOVIA Discovery Studio Visualizer (v21.1.020298) were employed to visualize the binding interactions between CD and NRP1.

2.8. Cell Transfection and Syncytial Formation

Syncytia formations were regarded as hallmark cellular events for SARS-CoV-2 invasion [52]. The SARS-CoV-2 spike plasmid, carrying green fluorescent protein (GFP) fluorescence pCDH-CMV-HnCoV-S-EF1-copGFP, was purchased from Shanghai Hedge-hogBio Science and Technology Ltd. (Shanghai, China) The 293T-hACE2 cell lines were transfected via the SARS-CoV-2 spike plasmid for 24 h, then 20 µM of CD was added for another 24 h. The syncytial formation was examined using a ZOE Fluorescent Cell Imager (Bio-Rad Laboratories, Inc., Hercules, CA, USA). The NRP1 protein level was monitored using Western blotting.

2.9. Statistical Analysis

The statistical analysis was conducted using a *t*-test (two groups), expressed as a mean $\pm$ standard deviation (mean $\pm$ SD). The mean grayscale values and fluorescence area of individual fluorescence images were monitored using Image J software (Java 1.8.0_322). $p < 0.05$ was considered to be different, whereas $p < 0.01$ to be significantly different.

3. Results

3.1. Cordycepin (CD) Inhibits NRP1 Expression in Various Cells

Some natural active components or small molecules could modulate gene expression. Cordycepin (CD) is an active gradient or natural product from traditional Chinese medicine. As an adenosine derivative, CD processes a diverse, broad spectrum of biological/pharmacological activities, such as anti-cancer, antimetastatic, anti-viral, antiprotozoal, antimalarial, antimicrobial, insecticidal, anti-inflammatory, antioxidant, and immunomodulatory/immunoregulatory [39]. Thus, the CD was used to test the impact on NRP1 expressions in human cancer cell lines. The results are shown in Figure 1, where CD inhibits the NRP1 expressions in both the protein and the mRNA in dosage-dependent manners in the H1975 cells (Figure 1A,B), the BT549 cancer cells (Figure 1C,D), the PC3 prostate cancer cells (Figure 1E,F), and the 22RV1 prostate cancer cells (Figure 1G,H), respectively.

3.2. Docking and Molecular Interaction Study of CD with NRP1

In silico analysis found that interfering with SARS-CoV-2 binds to NRP1 via small molecules seem to be potential candidates as novel anti-viral agents [31–34]. Folic acid, allleucovorin, and alimemazine may have the potential to prevent SARS-CoV-2 internalization by interacting with the S-protein/NRP1 complex [35,36]. Recently, Skrbic et al. used NRP1(b1b2), the structure of the b1b2 domains of NRP1, to perform a molecular docking study [35]. To this end, we also used NRP1(b1b2) for CD docking in silico, and the results are shown in Figure 2A and Table 2. The molecular docking results showed that the highest binding affinity between CD and NRP1 (b1b2) was −6.3 kcal/mol. CD can form a strong hydrogen bond with the residue of NRP1 (b1b2) Pro281 with a distance of 3.3 Å (Figure 2A, right upper). In addition, the five-membered aromatic ring of CD can form significant hydrophobic interactions with the residue Glu282 of NRP1 (b1b2) (Figure 2A). Through two-dimensional (2D) modeling, we observed that CD engages with NRP1(b1b2) via a variety of non-covalent bonds and interactions (Figure 2A, right bottom).

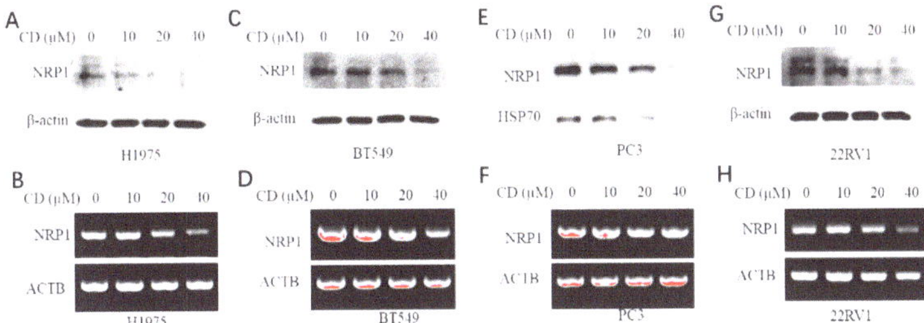

Figure 1. Cordycepin (CD) inhibits NRP1 expressions of both the mRNA and the protein in various cancer cell lines. (**A,B**) CD decreases NRP1 expressions in the H1975 lung cancer cells. (**C,D**) CD decreases NRP1 expressions in the BT549 breast cancer cells. (**E,F**) CD decreases NRP1 expressions in the PC3 prostate cancer cells. (**G,H**) CD decreases NRP1 expressions in the 22RV1 prostate cancer cells. (**A,C,E,G**) are for the NRP1 protein level of NRP1, and (**B,D,F,H**) are for the NRP1 mRNA level.

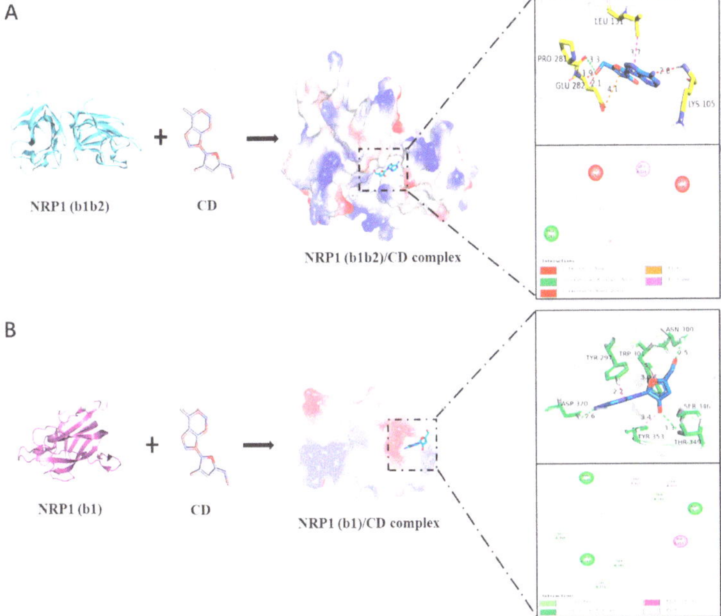

Figure 2. Binding mode of Cordycepin (CD) and NRP1 and two-dimensional illustration of interactions with NRP1 residues. (**A**) The left panel shows the three-dimensional structure for CD and NRP1(b1b2), respectively, the middle panel shows the three-dimensional conformational alignment for CD in the binding pocket, and the right panels show the binding mode of CD and the b1b2 domains of NRP1 (**upper**) and two-dimensional illustration of interactions with NRP1 b1b2 residues (**bottom**). (**B**) The left panel shows the three-dimensional structure for CD and NRP1 (b1), the middle panel shows the three-dimensional conformational alignment of CD in the binding pocket, and the right panels show the binding mode of CD and the b1 domains of NRP1 (**upper**) and two-dimensional illustration of interactions with NRP1 b1 residues (**bottom**). The image has been generated using PyMOL (v2.0) and BIOVIA Discovery Studio Visualizer software (v21.1.020298). In the binding pattern diagram, the red, orange, purple, pink, light pink, green and light green dashed lines represent unfavourable bump, unfavourable donor-donor, pi-sigma, pi-pi stacked, pi-alkyl, conventional hydrogen bond, van der waals and other interactions, respectively. Key binding residues of CD to NRP1(b1) and NRP1(b1b2) are indicated by yellow and green bars, respectively..

Table 2. The binding affinity of the CD-NRP1 complex and contacting residues of NRP1.

Protein−Ligand Complex	Binding Affinity (kcal/mol)	NRP-1-Contacting Residues
CD-NRP1(b1b2)	−6.3 #	Lys105, Leu131, Pro281 *, Glu282
CD-NRP1(b1)	−6.5 #	Tyr297, Asn300 *, Trp301, Asp320 *, Thr349 *, Tyr353

the highest biding affinity; * hydrogen bond interaction sites.

Recent studies have shown that the CendR sequence of the SARS-CoV-2 S-protein can bind to the NRP1 protein b1 domain to enhance virus entry into host cells [7,8]. However, when we used docking software (AUTODOCK tools 1.5.7) to analyze the interaction between the b1b2 domain of NRP1 and CD, we found that the position of CD docking was not located at the natural active site of the b1 domain as they reported. In order to further investigate this, we decided to dock the CD and the NRP1 b1 domain. The highest binding affinity of CD to NRP1 b1 was −6.5 kcal/mol (Table 2). Three hydrogen bonds of Asp 320, Asn 300, and Thr349 residues stabilized the target protein-binding molecule CD with distances of 2.6 Å, 2.5 Å, and 3.3 Å, respectively (Figure 2B, right upper). The benzene ring of CD has a Pi-Pi stacking with residue Tyr297 (Figure 2B, right upper). Further 2D modeling revealed diverse non-covalent bonds and interactions between CD and NRP1 (b1) (Figure 2B, right bottom).

3.3. CD Inhibits Syncytial Formation Likely through NRP1

A pathological hallmark for SARS-CoV-2 entry forms syncytia with multinucleated cells, evidenced in patients with COVID-19 [53]. Syncytium formation is required to participate in the S-protein of SARS-CoV-2 when host cells have the human *ACE2* gene [52]. First, we used 293T-hACE2 cells to treat with CD and found that CD decreased NRP1 protein expression in a dosage-dependent context (Figure 3A). After the CD treatment and transfection of SARS-CoV-2 spike plasmids with GFP fluorescence in 293T-hACE2 cells, the area of fluorescence of GFP-positive syncytia (Figure 3A, bottom panel) was significantly decreased when compared with the control cells, which indicate SARS-CoV-2 cell entry (Figure 3A, upper panel). The quantitative results are shown in Figure 3C. To investigate whether treatment with CD inhibited syncytia formation, at least partially, via NRP1, further Western blotting was performed, and the results in Figure 3D show that the level of the NRP1 protein is significantly downregulated in 293T-hACE2 cells treated with CD compared with control cells (Figure 3D). Therefore, the CD might inhibit the formation of syncytia via NRP1.

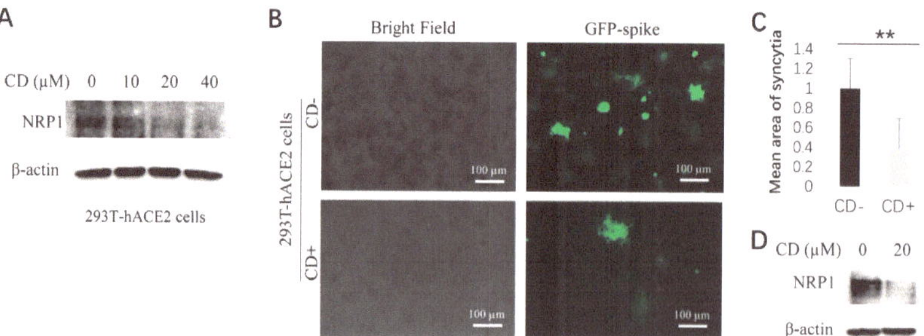

Figure 3. Cordycepin (CD) inhibits NRP1 expressions and syncytial formation in 293T-hACE2 cells. (**A**) NRP1 protein expressions in 293T-hACE2 cells with different amounts of CD treatment. (**B**) Representative images for syncytia formation in control without CD (CD−) and treated with CD (CD+) of 293T-hACE2 cells. (**C**) The quantitative results for (**B**). (**D**) NRP1 protein expression in 293T-hACE2 cells with CD treatment for (**B**). An unpaired student test was used for statistical analysis. "**", $p < 0.01$.

3.4. CD Roles in Immune Molecules and NRP1 Expression Analysis on Correlated Genes

We want to know the associations between the abundance of tumor-infiltrating lymphocytes (TILs) and expressions of NRP1 across human cancers, so an integrated repository portal for TISIDB was applied for the analysis. The results are shown in Figure 4, where we, interestingly, found significant associations between *NRP1* expressions and tumor–immune response in immune lymphocytes (Figure 4A), chemokines (Figure 4B), receptors (Figure 4C), immune inhibitors (Figure 4D), immunostimulators (Figure 4E), and major histocompatibility complex (MHC) molecules (Figure 4F) in most pan-cancers. Specifically, many immuno-response genes have been shown to be significantly changed, such as *CD28*, *CXCL12*, *CSF1R*, *KDR*, *CCR1*, *IL2RA*, etc. (Table 2).

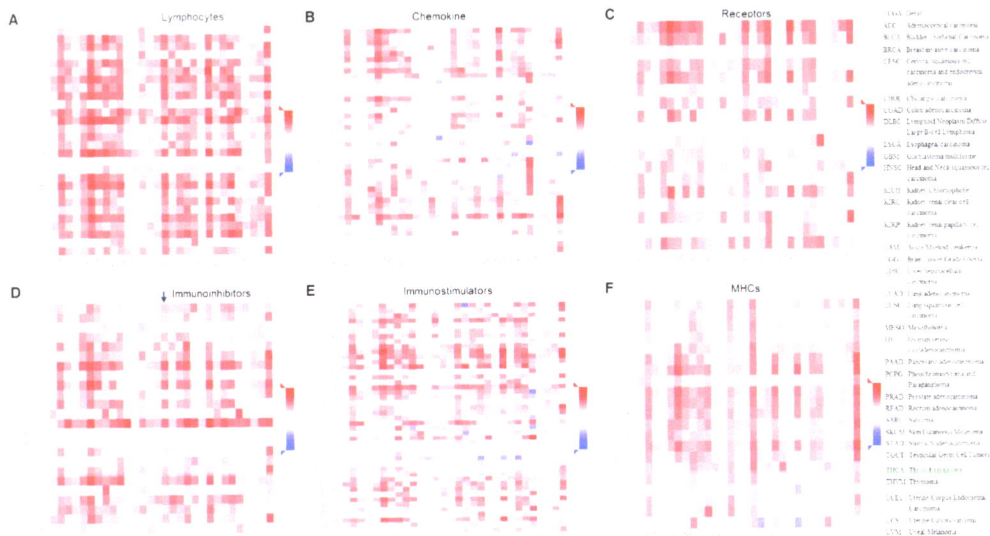

Figure 4. Associations of NRP1 expressions with a tumor–immune response in different cancers. (**A**) The associations between NRP1 expressions and lymphocyte response in cancers. (**B**) The associations between NRP1 expressions and chemokine response in cancers. (**C**) The associations between NRP1 expressions and receptor response in cancers. (**D**) The associations between NRP1 expressions and immunoinhibitor response in cancers. (**E**) The associations between NRP1 expressions and immunostimulator response in cancers. (**F**) The associations between NRP1 expressions and MHC response in cancers. Spearman associations between expressions of NRP1 and TILs (Y-axis) across human cancers (X-axis). The full names of cancer types are shown on the right.

Cancer cell lines treated with CD, an adenosine derivative, downregulated the NRP1 expression. The involvement of immune molecules from the adenosine/A2AR pathway has been described [54–57]. Our previous study showed that both adenosine derivatives, N6, N6-dimethyladenosine, CD, adenosine-inhibited DPP4/CD26 expression in cancer cells, and adenosine further revealed that it significantly suppresses the expression of the lymphocyte activating factor 3 (Lag3) in mice with AD injection. Thus, we wanted to know which immune molecules are influenced by CD and are correlated with a NRP1 downregulated expression. In mice treated with or without CD, isolated lymphocytes, Western blotting, and a semi-quantitative RT-PCR were performed to monitor the NRP1 expression. The results are shown in Figure 5, which shows that both protein (Figure 5A) and mRNA (Figure 5B) levels of NRP1 are significantly downregulated. Then, we further examined whether the above immuno-response genes were changed in those isolated lymphocytes from mice, and the results shown in Supplementary Figure S1 explain that the expressions for *Cd28*, *Cxcl12*, *Csf1r*, *Kdr*, *Ccr1*, and *Il2ra* are not significantly downregulated.

These data implied NRP1 roles and mechanisms in both anti-cancers and anti-SARS-CoV-2 entry, probably through immuno-response genes/pathways, other than Cd28, Cxcl12, Csf1r, Kdr, Ccr1, and Il2ra in mice.

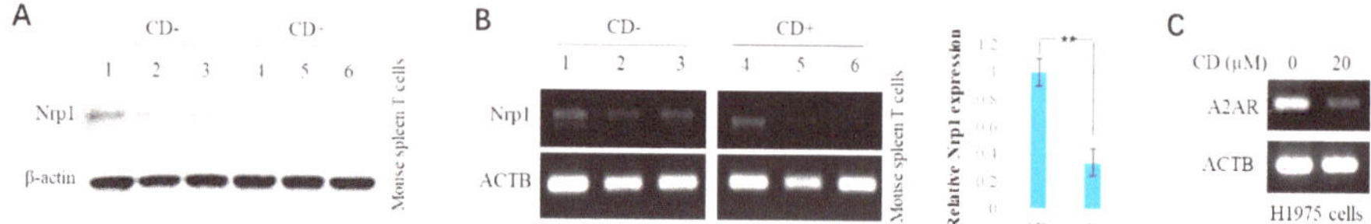

Figure 5. Cordycepin (CD) inhibits NRP1 expressions in lymphocytes in mice and cells. (**A**) CD inhibits NRP1 protein expressions in lymphocytes in vivo. (**B**) CD inhibits NRP1 mRNA expressions in lymphocytes in vivo. Quantitative data are shown in the right panel. **, $p < 0.01$. (**C**) CD inhibits A2AR mRNA expressions in the lung cancer cell line H1975.

Then, we carefully looked into adenosine-mediated genes and found that the *A2AR* (*ADORA2A*) gene is relatively highly upregulated in lung cancer (lung squamous cell carcinoma, LUSC) (Figure 4D, arrow). Thus, we treated an adenosine derivative, CD, as the above-tested lung cancer cell line H1975, and a RT-PCR found that CD significantly inhibited *A2AR* expression (Figure 5C).

4. Discussion

NRP1 can act as a co-receptor to fascinate SARS-CoV-2 invasion into host cells [7–9,19]. Thus, it is important to investigate NRP1 expression regulation via small molecules and the potential role of SARS-CoV-2-infected cancer patients. In current studies, we revealed that adenosine derivatives CD-suppressed NRP1 expression in cancer cells, implying the therapeutic potential for anti-cancer. Our previous study showed that CD has been reported to inhibit tumorigenesis and cancer metastasis/invasion both in vitro and in vivo [40,41].

Cordycepin (CD) is one of the main active gradients that was isolated from traditional Chinese medicine mushrooms *Ophiocordyceps* Sinensis (Berk.) [58] and *Cordyceps militaris* Link [59]. As a well-known natural adenosine analog of fungal origin, the CD can be synthesized, making it more possible for the study. CD processes a diverse, broad spectrum of biological/pharmacological activities, such as anti-cancer, antimetastatic, anti-viral, antiprotozoal, antimalarial, antimicrobial, insecticidal, anti-inflammatory, antioxidant, immunomodulatory/immunoregulatory, antileukemic, antiproliferative, apoptosis inducer, antifibrotic, antihyperglycemic/antidiabetic, antihyperlipidemic, antitachycardic, antihypercholesterolemic, antiarrhythmic, angiogenic, antihypertensive, antithrombotic/fibrinolytic/thrombolytic, anti-ischemic, reperfusion therapy, antistroke, hepatoprotective, renal functions improver/nephroprotective, chondrogenesis promoter, antiarthritic, antiosteoporotic, intervertebral disc regenerator, cystic fibrosis, acute lung inflammation/injury healer, chronic obstructive pulmonary disease (COPD), antihypoxic, cough/common cold suppressant, antidepressant, natural endurance booster, antifatigue, pain killer/analgesic, erythropoiesis stimulator, antiparkinsonian, neuronal regenerator, antisleep disorders, antiaging, aphrodisiac, sexual enhancer, spermatogenic, antiinfertility, some toxins antidote, and cosmeceutical [40,41,60–62]. These aforementioned activities make CD one of the most promising drugs with pharmacological and therapeutic potential [63–65]. Importantly, CD has recently discovered potent inhibitory activities on SARS-CoV-2 replication [60,66] that could contribute to treatments for COVID-19 [67]. This probable inhibitory affinity for CD against the principal protein targets of SARS-CoV-2 included the S-protein, enzymes of protease (Mpro), and the RNA-dependent RNA polymerase (RdRp) [62]. Our study found that CD inhibits the NRP1 expression of both protein and mRNA levels in a dosage-dependent manner in various cancer cell lines, implying the therapeutic potential for anti-SARS-CoV-2 and anti-cancers. This is the first study to identify that CD can inhibit NRP1 expression. Recently, we also showed that CD inhibited the expressions for CTSL, CD147, DPP4/CD26, furin, and SARS-CoV-2 entry proteins [38,48,68]. Moreover, CD might inhibit the formation of syncytia via NRP1, at least in part. Molecular docking results showed that there were multiple hydrogen bonds and hydrophobic interactions between CD and NRP1, with the highest binding affinity of CD to NRP1 b1 being −6.5 kcal/mol. Strikingly, CD binding exhibited strong similarity to the structure of the NRP1 b1 domain in the complex of the S1 Cend R peptide-NRP1 b1 and the known NRP1 inhibitors-NRP1 b1 [8,69]. This shows some common interactions, including the binding of the 320th aspartic acid (Asp) and the 300th asparagine (Asn) to the NRP1 b1 domain, which may be through different mechanisms, not interfering with NRP1-mediated SARS-CoV-2 S-protein initiation rather than inhibiting NRP1 expression via CD, thereby inhibiting the virus's subcellular entry.

Recently, Hou et al. [70] investigated interactions between NRP1 and the S-protein of SARS-CoV-2 under a custom-built atomic force microscopy (AFM) and found biophysical characteristics of interactions with various S-protein fragments, including the S-protein trimer and the receptor-binding domain (RBD). Predicting via AlphaFold2 and MD simulation in NRP1 a1a2b1b2 domains between residue 22 and 591 and the SARS-CoV-2 S-protein RBD between residue 319 and 537 revealed two models (models 2 and 3). Model 2 showed that the receptor-binding motif (RBM) was in close contact with the NRP1 b1 domain between residues 254 and 403. The representative interacting residue pairs of RBM (a crucial binding sequence of RBD) and NRP1 were K458-D320, F456-Y297, N501-K351, and T500-K350 (RBM-NRP1). However, in model 3, the interacting residues are slightly different from model 2, where the Q493 and Y505 (RBD-NRP1) of the RBD were involved in the interface interactions, Q493 showed a charge–charge interaction with K351 and Y297, and Y505 showed hydrophobic interactions with Y297. The residue Y297 of NRP1 also interacted with the N501 of the RBD, and F456 had close contact with the residue W411 of NRP1 via π–π interactions. The RBM-NRP1 interface is similar to those in the RBD-ACE2 interface. Nevertheless, based on the interaction overlapping for NRP1 b1 between CD and the S-protein of SARS-CoV-2, CD not only inhibits NRP1 expression but also interrupts the interaction of the SARS-CoV-2 S-protein, thereby inhibiting the virus's subcellular entry.

NRP1 expression is upregulated in many cancer types, including kidney renal clear cell carcinoma (KIRC) and kidney renal papillary cell carcinoma (KIRP), compared to the matched healthy tissues and is positively correlated with the survivability rate of KIRC patients [71]. The high-affinity binding between the SARS-CoV-2 S-protein and NRP1 suggested that this binding might play a role in COVID-19 severity since their binding promotes SARS-CoV-2 invasion through NRP1. It is well-known that NRP1 is expressed in normal kidney tubule tissue, KIRC, and KIRP, implying a possible target for budding therapeutics in cancers [72]. NRP1 is also highly expressed in neuronal cells and olfactory epithelium, thus contributing to the SARS-CoV-2 entering the central nervous system, causing a pathological complication, and enhancing the deterioration of glioblastoma or brain tumors [73].

Additionally, we interestingly reveal significant associations between *NRP1* expressions and the tumor–immune response in immune lymphocytes, chemokines, receptors, immunostimulators, immune inhibitors, and MHC molecules in almost all pan cancers. Specifically, many immuno-response genes are significantly changed, such as *CD28, CXCL12, CSF1R, KDR, CCR1, IL2RA*, etc. Thus, we further examined whether the above immuno-response genes were changed in those isolated lymphocytes from mice and found that the expressions for *Cd28, Cxcl12, Csf1r, Kdr, Ccr1,* and *Il2ra* are not significantly downregulated, implying NRP1 roles and mechanisms in both anti-cancers and anti-SARS-CoV-2 entry, probably through immuno-response genes/pathways, other than *CD28, CXCL12, CSF1R, KDR, CCR1,* and *IL2RA*.

Of course, we should note that we have analyzed those genes in mice, not humans; there may be differences between different species when treated with CD. With this regard, we carefully looked into adenosine-mediated genes and found that the *A2AR* gene is relatively highly upregulated in lung cancer. The A2AR is a novel immune checkpoint gene, and Fong et al. reported that A2AR antagonists can be used for immunotherapy for patients with refractory renal cell cancer [55]. Thus, we treated an adenosine derivative, CD, in the lung cancer cell line H1975 and found that CD significantly inhibited A2AR expression, highlighting the CD/A2AR/immunotherapy pathway in anti-cancer and anti-SARS-CoV-2.

Moreover, NRP1 also facilitated other viral infections, such as the (EBV) [26], the PRV [27], the mCMV [28], the HTLV-1 and HTLV-2 [29], and CD inhibited NRP1 expression and viral syncytial formation, highlighting therapeutic significances for anti-different viruses.

5. Conclusions

In conclusion, our study highlights the significance of NRP1 expression regulation, and the natural product CD downregulated the expressions not only in NRP1 but also in immune molecules such as A2AR, implying a NRP1 mechanism probably through immuno-response pathways, providing a potential CD therapy for anti-cancer and anti-viral diseases, including COVID-19.

Supplementary Materials: The following supporting information can be downloaded at: https://www.mdpi.com/article/10.3390/microorganisms11122953/s1, Figure S1: The mRNA expressions of *Cd28*, *Cxcl12*, *Csf1r*, *Kdr*, *Ccr1*, and *Il2ra* when treated with CD in mice.

Author Contributions: J.F. (Jiewen Fu), T.L., J.D., J.H., J.C., D.L., N.L., M.Z., Z.L. and Q.T. carried out experimental studies, data acquisition, and analysis. J.F. (Junjiang Fu) collected and analyzed the data. J.F. (Junjiang Fu) designed and supervised the project. J.F. (Junjiang Fu) wrote and edited the manuscript. All authors have read and agreed to the published version of the manuscript.

Funding: This work was supported by the Foundation of Science and Technology Department of Sichuan Province (grant nos. 2022NSFSC0737, 2023NSFSC0673, and 2022NSFSC1319) and in part by the National Natural Science Foundation of China (grant nos. 81672887 and 82073263).

Institutional Review Board Statement: The animal experiments followed the international, national, and institutional guidelines for the care and use of animal subjects. The study was approved by the Ethical Committee of Southwest Medical University (No.: 20210930-007).

Informed Consent Statement: Not applicable.

Data Availability Statement: Data are contained within the article.

Acknowledgments: The authors truly thank people from the Research Center for Preclinical Medicine, Southwest Medical University. We also thank Pengfei Zhang from the NHC Key Laboratory of Cancer Proteomics, Department of Oncology, Xiangya Hospital, Central South University.

Conflicts of Interest: The authors declare that they have no competing interest.

References

1. Takagi, S.; Tsuji, T.; Amagai, T.; Takamatsu, T.; Fujisawa, H. Specific cell surface labels in the visual centers of xenopus laevis tadpole identified using monoclonal antibodies. *Dev. Biol.* **1987**, *122*, 90–100. [CrossRef]
2. Fujisawa, H.; Ohtsuki, T.; Takagi, S.; Tsuji, T. An aberrant retinal pathway and visual centers in xenopus tadpoles share a common cell surface molecule, a5 antigen. *Dev. Biol.* **1989**, *135*, 231–240. [CrossRef] [PubMed]
3. Kolodkin, A.L.; Levengood, D.V.; Rowe, E.G.; Tai, Y.T.; Giger, R.J.; Ginty, D.D. Neuropilin is a semaphorin iii receptor. *Cell* **1997**, *90*, 753–762. [CrossRef] [PubMed]
4. He, Z.; Tessier-Lavigne, M. Neuropilin is a receptor for the axonal chemorepellent semaphorin iii. *Cell* **1997**, *90*, 739–751. [CrossRef]
5. Soker, S.; Takashima, S.; Miao, H.Q.; Neufeld, G.; Klagsbrun, M. Neuropilin-1 is expressed by endothelial and tumor cells as an isoform-specific receptor for vascular endothelial growth factor. *Cell* **1998**, *92*, 735–745. [CrossRef] [PubMed]
6. Al-Zeheimi, N.; Gao, Y.; Greer, P.A.; Adham, S.A. Neuropilin-1 knockout and rescue confirms its role to promote metastasis in MDA-MB-231 breast cancer cells. *Int. J. Mol. Sci.* **2023**, *24*, 7792. [CrossRef] [PubMed]
7. Cantuti-Castelvetri, L.; Ojha, R.; Pedro, L.D.; Djannatian, M.; Franz, J.; Kuivanen, S.; van der Meer, F.; Kallio, K.; Kaya, T.; Anastasina, M.; et al. Neuropilin-1 facilitates SARS-CoV-2 cell entry and infectivity. *Science* **2020**, *370*, 856–860. [CrossRef] [PubMed]
8. Daly, J.L.; Simonetti, B.; Klein, K.; Chen, K.E.; Williamson, M.K.; Anton-Plagaro, C.; Shoemark, D.K.; Simon-Gracia, L.; Bauer, M.; Hollandi, R.; et al. Neuropilin-1 is a host factor for SARS-CoV-2 infection. *Science* **2020**, *370*, 861–865. [CrossRef]

9.   Mayi, B.S.; Leibowitz, J.A.; Woods, A.T.; Ammon, K.A.; Liu, A.E.; Raja, A. The role of neuropilin-1 in COVID-19. *PLoS Pathog.* **2021**, *17*, e1009153. [CrossRef]
10.   Li, T.; Fu, J.; Cheng, J.; Elfiky, A.A.; Wei, C.; Fu, J. New progresses on cell surface protein HSPA5/BIP/GRP78 in cancers and COVID-19. *Front. Immunol.* **2023**, *14*, 1166680. [CrossRef]
11.   Fu, J.; Zhou, B.; Zhang, L.; Balaji, K.S.; Wei, C.; Liu, X.; Chen, H.; Peng, J.; Fu, J. Expressions and significances of the angiotensin-converting enzyme 2 gene, the receptor of SARS-CoV-2 for COVID-19. *Mol. Biol. Rep.* **2020**, *47*, 4383–4392. [CrossRef] [PubMed]
12.   Wang, C.; Horby, P.W.; Hayden, F.G.; Gao, G.F. A novel coronavirus outbreak of global health concern. *Lancet* **2020**, *395*, 470–473. [CrossRef] [PubMed]
13.   Coutard, B.; Valle, C.; de Lamballerie, X.; Canard, B.; Seidah, N.G.; Decroly, E. The spike glycoprotein of the new coronavirus 2019-nCoV contains a furin-like cleavage site absent in CoV of the same clade. *Antiviral. Res.* **2020**, *176*, 104742. [CrossRef]
14.   Katopodis, P.; Randeva, H.S.; Spandidos, D.A.; Saravi, S.; Kyrou, I.; Karteris, E. Host cell entry mediators implicated in the cellular tropism of SARSCoV2, the pathophysiology of COVID19 and the identification of microRNAs that can modulate the expression of these mediators (review). *Int. J. Mol. Med.* **2022**, *49*, 20. [CrossRef] [PubMed]
15.   Ishitoku, M.; Mokuda, S.; Araki, K.; Watanabe, H.; Kohno, H.; Sugimoto, T.; Yoshida, Y.; Sakaguchi, T.; Masumoto, J.; Hirata, S.; et al. Tumor necrosis factor and interleukin-1beta upregulate NRP2 expression and promote SARS-CoV-2 proliferation. *Viruses* **2023**, *15*, 1498. [CrossRef] [PubMed]
16.   Wang, S.; Zhao, L.; Zhang, X.; Zhang, J.; Shang, H.; Liang, G. Neuropilin-1, a myeloid cell-specific protein, is an inhibitor of hiv-1 infectivity. *Proc. Natl. Acad. Sci. USA* **2022**, *119*, e2114884119. [CrossRef] [PubMed]
17.   Adimulam, T.; Arumugam, T.; Naidoo, A.; Naidoo, K.; Ramsuran, V. Polymorphisms within the SARS-CoV-2 human receptor genes associate with variable disease outcomes across ethnicities. *Genes* **2023**, *14*, 1798. [CrossRef]
18.   Adimulam, T.; Arumugam, T.; Gokul, A.; Ramsuran, V. Genetic variants within SARS-CoV-2 human receptor genes may contribute to variable disease outcomes in different ethnicities. *Int. J. Mol. Sci.* **2023**, *24*, 8711. [CrossRef] [PubMed]
19.   Pal, D.; De, K.; Yates, T.B.; Kolape, J.; Muchero, W. Mutating novel interaction sites in nrp1 reduces SARS-CoV-2 spike protein internalization. *iScience* **2023**, *26*, 106274. [CrossRef]
20.   Ozkan Oktay, E.; Kaman, T.; Karasakal, O.F.; Enisoglu Atalay, V. In silico prediction and molecular docking of SNPs in nrp1 gene associated with SARS-CoV-2. *Biochem. Genet.* **2023**, 1–20. [CrossRef]
21.   Chapoval, S.P.; Keegan, A.D. Perspectives and potential approaches for targeting neuropilin 1 in SARS-CoV-2 infection. *Mol. Med.* **2021**, *27*, 162. [CrossRef]
22.   Ackermann, M.; Verleden, S.E.; Kuehnel, M.; Haverich, A.; Welte, T.; Laenger, F.; Vanstapel, A.; Werlein, C.; Stark, H.; Tzankov, A.; et al. Pulmonary vascular endothelialitis, thrombosis, and angiogenesis in COVID-19. *N. Engl. J. Med.* **2020**, *383*, 120–128. [CrossRef]
23.   Mercurio, A.M. Vegf/neuropilin signaling in cancer stem cells. *Int. J. Mol. Sci.* **2019**, *20*, 490. [CrossRef] [PubMed]
24.   Rachner, T.D.; Kasimir-Bauer, S.; Goebel, A.; Erdmann, K.; Hoffmann, O.; Rauner, M.; Hofbauer, L.C.; Kimmig, R.; Bittner, A.K. Soluble neuropilin-1 is an independent marker of poor prognosis in early breast cancer. *J. Cancer Res. Clin. Oncol.* **2021**, *147*, 2233–2238. [CrossRef] [PubMed]
25.   Nasarre, C.; Roth, M.; Jacob, L.; Roth, L.; Koncina, E.; Thien, A.; Labourdette, G.; Poulet, P.; Hubert, P.; Cremel, G.; et al. Peptide-based interference of the transmembrane domain of neuropilin-1 inhibits glioma growth in vivo. *Oncogene* **2010**, *29*, 2381–2392. [CrossRef] [PubMed]
26.   Wang, H.B.; Zhang, H.; Zhang, J.P.; Li, Y.; Zhao, B.; Feng, G.K.; Du, Y.; Xiong, D.; Zhong, Q.; Liu, W.L.; et al. Neuropilin 1 is an entry factor that promotes ebv infection of nasopharyngeal epithelial cells. *Nat. Commun.* **2015**, *6*, 6240. [CrossRef]
27.   Chen, M.; Wang, M.H.; Shen, X.G.; Liu, H.; Zhang, Y.Y.; Peng, J.M.; Meng, F.; Wang, T.Y.; Bai, Y.Z.; Sun, M.X.; et al. Neuropilin-1 facilitates pseudorabies virus replication and viral glycoprotein b promotes its degradation in a furin-dependent manner. *J. Virol.* **2022**, *96*, e0131822. [CrossRef]
28.   Lane, R.K.; Guo, H.; Fisher, A.D.; Diep, J.; Lai, Z.; Chen, Y.; Upton, J.W.; Carette, J.; Mocarski, E.S.; Kaiser, W.J. Necroptosis-based crispr knockout screen reveals neuropilin-1 as a critical host factor for early stages of murine cytomegalovirus infection. *Proc. Natl. Acad. Sci. USA* **2020**, *117*, 20109–20116. [CrossRef]
29.   Ghez, D.; Lepelletier, Y.; Lambert, S.; Fourneau, J.M.; Blot, V.; Janvier, S.; Arnulf, B.; van Endert, P.M.; Heveker, N.; Pique, C.; et al. Neuropilin-1 is involved in human t-cell lymphotropic virus type 1 entry. *J. Virol.* **2006**, *80*, 6844–6854. [CrossRef]
30.   Kolaric, A.; Jukic, M.; Bren, U. Novel small-molecule inhibitors of the SARS-CoV-2 spike protein binding to neuropilin 1. *Pharmaceuticals* **2022**, *15*, 165. [CrossRef]
31.   Charoute, H.; Elkarhat, Z.; Elkhattabi, L.; El Fahime, E.; Oukkache, N.; Rouba, H.; Barakat, A. Computational screening of potential drugs against COVID-19 disease: The neuropilin-1 receptor as molecular target. *Virusdisease* **2022**, *33*, 23–31. [CrossRef] [PubMed]
32.   Alshawaf, E.; Hammad, M.M.; Marafie, S.K.; Ali, H.; Al-Mulla, F.; Abubaker, J.; Mohammad, A. Discovery of natural products to block SARS-CoV-2 s-protein interaction with neuropilin-1 receptor: A molecular dynamics simulation approach. *Microb. Pathog.* **2022**, *170*, 105701. [CrossRef] [PubMed]
33.   Ganguly, A.; Mandi, M.; Dutta, A.; Rajak, P. In silico analysis reveals the inhibitory potential of madecassic acid against entry factors of SARS-CoV-2. *ACS Appl. Bio Mater.* **2023**, *6*, 652–662. [CrossRef]

34. Karkashan, A.; Attar, R. Computational screening of natural products to identify potential inhibitors for human neuropilin-1 (nrp1) receptor to abrogate the binding of SARS-CoV-2 and host cell. *J. Biomol. Struct. Dyn.* **2023**, *41*(19), 9987–9996. [CrossRef] [PubMed]

35. Skrbic, R.; Travar, M.; Stojiljkovic, M.P.; Djuric, D.M.; Surucic, R. Folic acid and leucovorin have potential to prevent SARS-CoV-2-virus internalization by interacting with s-glycoprotein/neuropilin-1 receptor complex. *Molecules* **2023**, *28*, 2294. [CrossRef]

36. Hashizume, M.; Takashima, A.; Ono, C.; Okamoto, T.; Iwasaki, M. Phenothiazines inhibit SARS-CoV-2 cell entry via a blockade of spike protein binding to neuropilin-1. *Antiviral Res.* **2023**, *209*, 105481. [CrossRef]

37. Perez-Miller, S.; Patek, M.; Moutal, A.; Duran, P.; Cabel, C.R.; Thorne, C.A.; Campos, S.K.; Khanna, R. Novel compounds targeting neuropilin receptor 1 with potential to interfere with SARS-CoV-2 virus entry. *ACS Chem. Neurosci.* **2021**, *12*, 1299–1312. [CrossRef]

38. Li, D.; Liu, X.; Zhang, L.; He, J.; Chen, X.; Liu, S.; Fu, J.; Fu, S.; Chen, H.; Fu, J.; et al. COVID-19 disease and malignant cancers: The impact for the furin gene expression in susceptibility to SARS-CoV-2. *Int. J. Biol. Sci.* **2021**, *17*, 3954–3967. [CrossRef] [PubMed]

39. Chen, M.; Luo, J.; Jiang, W.; Chen, L.; Miao, L.; Han, C. Cordycepin: A review of strategies to improve the bioavailability and efficacy. *Phytother. Res.* **2023**, *37*, 3839–3858. [CrossRef]

40. Wei, C.; Khan, M.A.; Du, J.; Cheng, J.; Tania, M.; Leung, E.L.; Fu, J. Cordycepin inhibits triple-negative breast cancer cell migration and invasion by regulating emt-tfs slug, twist1, snail1, and zeb1. *Front. Oncol.* **2022**, *12*, 898583. [CrossRef]

41. Wei, C.; Yao, X.; Jiang, Z.; Wang, Y.; Zhang, D.; Chen, X.; Fan, X.; Xie, C.; Cheng, J.; Fu, J.; et al. Cordycepin inhibits drug-resistance non-small cell lung cancer progression by activating ampk signaling pathway. *Pharmacol. Res.* **2019**, *144*, 79–89. [CrossRef]

42. He, J.; Liu, S.; Tan, Q.; Liu, Z.; Fu, J.; Li, T.; Wei, C.; Liu, X.; Mei, Z.; Cheng, J.; et al. Antiviral potential of small molecules cordycepin, thymoquinone, and n6, n6-dimethyladenosine targeting SARS-CoV-2 entry protein adam17. *Molecules* **2022**, *27*, 9044. [CrossRef] [PubMed]

43. Fu, J.; Liu, S.; Tan, Q.; Liu, Z.; Qian, J.; Li, T.; Du, J.; Song, B.; Li, D.; Zhang, L.; et al. Impact of tmprss2 expression, mutation prognostics, and small molecule (cd, ad, tq, and tqfl12) inhibition on pan-cancer tumors and susceptibility to SARS-CoV-2. *Molecules* **2022**, *27*, 7413. [CrossRef] [PubMed]

44. Ru, B.; Wong, C.N.; Tong, Y.; Zhong, J.Y.; Zhong, S.S.W.; Wu, W.C.; Chu, K.C.; Wong, C.Y.; Lau, C.Y.; Chen, I.; et al. Tisidb: An integrated repository portal for tumor-immune system interactions. *Bioinformatics* **2019**, *35*, 4200–4202. [CrossRef] [PubMed]

45. Untergasser, A.; Cutcutache, I.; Koressaar, T.; Ye, J.; Faircloth, B.C.; Remm, M.; Rozen, S.G. Primer3—New capabilities and interfaces. *Nucleic Acids Res.* **2012**, *40*, e115. [CrossRef]

46. Kubra, S.; Zhang, H.; Si, Y.; Gao, X.; Wang, T.; Pan, L.; Li, L.; Zhong, N.; Fu, J.; Zhang, B.; et al. Reggamma regulates circadian clock by modulating bmal1 protein stability. *Cell Death Discov.* **2021**, *7*, 335. [CrossRef]

47. Wei, C.; Liu, Y.; Liu, X.; Cheng, J.; Fu, J.; Xiao, X.; Moses, R.E.; Li, X.; Fu, J. The speckle-type poz protein (spop) inhibits breast cancer malignancy by destabilizing twist1. *Cell Death Discov.* **2022**, *8*, 389. [CrossRef]

48. Zhang, L.; Wei, C.; Li, D.; He, J.; Liu, S.; Deng, H.; Cheng, J.; Du, J.; Liu, X.; Chen, H.; et al. COVID-19 receptor and malignant cancers: Association of ctsl expression with susceptibility to SARS-CoV-2. *Int. J. Biol. Sci.* **2022**, *18*, 2362–2371. [CrossRef]

49. Liu, G.; Du, W.; Sang, X.; Tong, Q.; Wang, Y.; Chen, G.; Yuan, Y.; Jiang, L.; Cheng, W.; Liu, D.; et al. Rna g-quadruplex in tmprss2 reduces SARS-CoV-2 infection. *Nat. Commun.* **2022**, *13*, 1444. [CrossRef]

50. Kim, S.; Thiessen, P.A.; Bolton, E.E.; Chen, J.; Fu, G.; Gindulyte, A.; Han, L.; He, J.; He, S.; Shoemaker, B.A.; et al. Pubchem substance and compound databases. *Nucleic Acids Res.* **2016**, *44*, D1202–D1213. [CrossRef]

51. Goodsell, D.S.; Olson, A.J. Automated docking of substrates to proteins by simulated annealing. *Proteins* **1990**, *8*, 195–202. [CrossRef]

52. Jocher, G.; Grass, V.; Tschirner, S.K.; Riepler, L.; Breimann, S.; Kaya, T.; Oelsner, M.; Hamad, M.S.; Hofmann, L.I.; Blobel, C.P.; et al. Adam10 and adam17 promote SARS-CoV-2 cell entry and spike protein-mediated lung cell fusion. *EMBO Rep.* **2022**, *23*, e54305. [CrossRef] [PubMed]

53. Braga, L.; Ali, H.; Secco, I.; Chiavacci, E.; Neves, G.; Goldhill, D.; Penn, R.; Jimenez-Guardeno, J.M.; Ortega-Prieto, A.M.; Bussani, R.; et al. Drugs that inhibit tmem16 proteins block SARS-CoV-2 spike-induced syncytia. *Nature* **2021**, *594*, 88–93. [CrossRef] [PubMed]

54. Cekic, C.; Linden, J. Purinergic regulation of the immune system. *Nat. Rev. Immunol.* **2016**, *16*, 177–192. [CrossRef] [PubMed]

55. Fong, L.; Hotson, A.; Powderly, J.D.; Sznol, M.; Heist, R.S.; Choueiri, T.K.; George, S.; Hughes, B.G.M.; Hellmann, M.D.; Shepard, D.R.; et al. Adenosine 2a receptor blockade as an immunotherapy for treatment-refractory renal cell cancer. *Cancer Discov.* **2020**, *10*, 40–53. [CrossRef] [PubMed]

56. Novitskiy, S.V.; Ryzhov, S.; Zaynagetdinov, R.; Goldstein, A.E.; Huang, Y.; Tikhomirov, O.Y.; Blackburn, M.R.; Biaggioni, I.; Carbone, D.P.; Feoktistov, I.; et al. Adenosine receptors in regulation of dendritic cell differentiation and function. *Blood* **2008**, *112*, 1822–1831. [CrossRef]

57. Liu, J.; Shi, Y.; Liu, X.; Zhang, D.; Bai, Y.; Xu, Y.; Wang, M. Blocking adenosine/A2AR pathway for cancer therapy. *Zhongguo Fei Ai Za Zhi* **2022**, *25*, 460–467.

58. Zhou, X.; Luo, L.; Dressel, W.; Shadier, G.; Krumbiegel, D.; Schmidtke, P.; Zepp, F.; Meyer, C.U. Cordycepin is an immunoregulatory active ingredient of cordyceps sinensis. *Am. J. Chin. Med.* **2008**, *36*, 967–980. [CrossRef]

59. Cunningham, K.G.; Manson, W.; Spring, F.S.; Hutchinson, S.A. Cordycepin, a metabolic product isolated from cultures of *Cordyceps militaris* (linn.) link. *Nature* **1950**, *166*, 949. [CrossRef]

60. Rabie, A.M. Potent inhibitory activities of the adenosine analogue cordycepin on SARS-CoV-2 replication. *ACS Omega* **2022**, *7*, 2960–2969. [CrossRef]
61. Radhi, M.; Ashraf, S.; Lawrence, S.; Tranholm, A.A.; Wellham, P.A.D.; Hafeez, A.; Khamis, A.S.; Thomas, R.; McWilliams, D.; de Moor, C.H. A systematic review of the biological effects of cordycepin. *Molecules* **2021**, *26*, 5886. [CrossRef]
62. Shi, L.; Cao, H.; Fu, S.; Jia, Z.; Lu, X.; Cui, Z.; Yu, D. Cordycepin enhances hyperthermia-induced apoptosis and cell cycle arrest by modulating the mapk pathway in human lymphoma u937 cells. *Mol. Biol. Rep.* **2022**, *49*, 8673–8683. [CrossRef] [PubMed]
63. Tuli, H.S.; Sharma, A.K.; Sandhu, S.S.; Kashyap, D. Cordycepin: A bioactive metabolite with therapeutic potential. *Life Sci.* **2013**, *93*, 863–869. [CrossRef] [PubMed]
64. Qin, P.; Li, X.; Yang, H.; Wang, Z.Y.; Lu, D. Therapeutic potential and biological applications of cordycepin and metabolic mechanisms in cordycepin-producing fungi. *Molecules* **2019**, *24*, 2231. [CrossRef]
65. Tuli, H.S.; Sandhu, S.S.; Sharma, A.K. Pharmacological and therapeutic potential of cordyceps with special reference to cordycepin. *3 Biotech* **2014**, *4*, 1–12. [CrossRef]
66. Bibi, S.; Hasan, M.M.; Wang, Y.B.; Papadakos, S.P.; Yu, H. Cordycepin as a promising inhibitor of SARS-CoV-2 RNA dependent rna polymerase (rdrp). *Curr. Med. Chem.* **2022**, *29*, 152–162. [CrossRef]
67. Wang, Z.; Wang, N.; Yang, L.; Song, X.Q. Bioactive natural products in COVID-19 therapy. *Front. Pharmacol.* **2022**, *13*, 926507. [CrossRef]
68. Fu, J.; Song, B.; Du, J.; Liu, S.; He, J.; Xiao, T.; Zhou, B.; Li, D.; Liu, X.; He, T.; et al. Impact of bsg/cd147 gene expression on diagnostic, prognostic and therapeutic strategies towards malignant cancers and possible susceptibility to SARS-CoV-2. *Mol. Biol. Rep.* **2023**, *50*, 2269–2281. [CrossRef]
69. Powell, J.; Mota, F.; Steadman, D.; Soudy, C.; Miyauchi, J.T.; Crosby, S.; Jarvis, A.; Reisinger, T.; Winfield, N.; Evans, G.; et al. Small molecule neuropilin-1 antagonists combine antiangiogenic and antitumor activity with immune modulation through reduction of transforming growth factor beta (tgfbeta) production in regulatory t-cells. *J. Med. Chem.* **2018**, *61*, 4135–4154. [CrossRef]
70. Hou, D.; Cao, W.; Kim, S.; Cui, X.; Ziarnik, M.; Im, W.; Zhang, X.F. Biophysical investigation of interactions between SARS-CoV-2 spike protein and neuropilin-1. *Protein Sci.* **2023**, *32*, e4773. [CrossRef] [PubMed]
71. Hossain, M.G.; Akter, S.; Uddin, M.J. Emerging role of neuropilin-1 and angiotensin-converting enzyme-2 in renal carcinoma-associated COVID-19 pathogenesis. *Infect. Dis. Rep.* **2021**, *13*, 902–909. [CrossRef] [PubMed]
72. Gold, S.A.; Margulis, V. Uncovering a link between COVID-19 and renal cell carcinoma. *Nat. Rev. Urol.* **2023**, *20*, 330–331. [CrossRef] [PubMed]
73. Zalpoor, H.; Shapourian, H.; Akbari, A.; Shahveh, S.; Haghshenas, L. Increased neuropilin-1 expression by COVID-19: A possible cause of long-term neurological complications and progression of primary brain tumors. *Hum. Cell* **2022**, *35*, 1301–1303. [CrossRef] [PubMed]

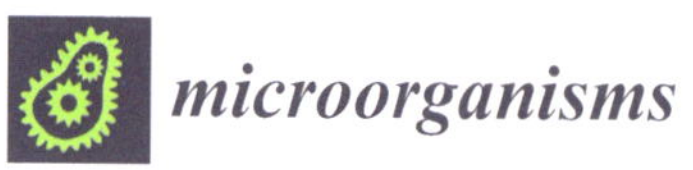

microorganisms

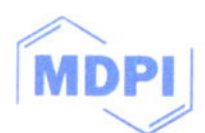

Review

Potential Beneficial Effects of Naringin and Naringenin on Long COVID—A Review of the Literature

Siqi Liu [1], Mengli Zhong [1], Hao Wu [1], Weiwei Su [1,2], Yonggang Wang [1] and Peibo Li [1,*]

[1] Guangdong Engineering and Technology Research Center for Quality and Efficacy Re-Evaluation of Post-Market Traditional Chinese Medicine, State Key Laboratory of Biocontrol, Guangdong Provincial Key Laboratory of Plant Resources, School of Life Sciences, Sun Yat-sen University, Guangzhou 510275, China; liusq67@mail2.sysu.edu.cn (S.L.); zhongmli@mail2.sysu.edu.cn (M.Z.); wuhao_cpu@126.com (H.W.); lssww@mail.sysu.edu.cn (W.S.); wangyg@mail.sysu.edu.cn (Y.W.)

[2] Maoming Branch, Guangdong Laboratory for Lingnan Modern Agriculture, Maoming 525000, China

[*] Correspondence: lipeibo@mail.sysu.edu.cn; Tel./Fax: +86-20-8411-2398

Abstract: Coronavirus disease 2019 (COVID-19) caused a severe epidemic due to severe acute respiratory syndrome coronavirus-2 (SARS-CoV-2). Recent studies have found that patients do not completely recover from acute infections, but instead, suffer from a variety of post-acute sequelae of SARS-CoV-2 infection, known as long COVID. The effects of long COVID can be far-reaching, with a duration of up to six months and a range of symptoms such as cognitive dysfunction, immune dysregulation, microbiota dysbiosis, myalgic encephalomyelitis/chronic fatigue syndrome, myocarditis, pulmonary fibrosis, cough, diabetes, pain, reproductive dysfunction, and thrombus formation. However, recent studies have shown that naringenin and naringin have palliative effects on various COVID-19 sequelae. Flavonoids such as naringin and naringenin, commonly found in fruits and vegetables, have various positive effects, including reducing inflammation, preventing viral infections, and providing antioxidants. This article discusses the molecular mechanisms and clinical effects of naringin and naringenin on treating the above diseases. It proposes them as potential drugs for the treatment of long COVID, and it can be inferred that naringin and naringenin exhibit potential as extended long COVID medications, in the future likely serving as nutraceuticals or clinical supplements for the comprehensive alleviation of the various manifestations of COVID-19 complications.

Keywords: long COVID; SARS-CoV-2; COVID-19; naringin; naringenin; beneficial effects

Citation: Liu, S.; Zhong, M.; Wu, H.; Su, W.; Wang, Y.; Li, P. Potential Beneficial Effects of Naringin and Naringenin on Long COVID—A Review of the Literature. *Microorganisms* **2024**, *12*, 332. https://doi.org/10.3390/microorganisms12020332

Academic Editor: Flor Helene Pujol

Received: 9 January 2024
Revised: 29 January 2024
Accepted: 31 January 2024
Published: 4 February 2024

1. Introduction

COVID-19 encompasses a range of illnesses resulting from the contraction of severe acute respiratory syndrome coronavirus 2 (SARS-CoV-2). It is spread in the population mainly through droplets, but also via aerosol transmission [1], contamination transmission [2], and the fecal–oral route of transmission [3]. SARS-CoV-2 binds to the angiotensin-converting enzyme II (ACE2) receptor in the body via the S protein, which then invades human tissues and releases RNA via cytotoxicity [4]. The ACE2 receptor is mainly found in type II alveolar cells and is also found in many tissues, such as the heart, esophagus, kidneys, and bladder [5]. Therefore, SARS-CoV-2 invades the human body and causes a multi-tissue disease, including respiratory symptoms. SARS-CoV-2 has a high rate of transmission. The majority of patients experience acute symptoms within a span of 2–14 days following viral exposure. The symptoms are primarily fever, cough, sore throat, myalgia, and an altered sense of smell/taste [6,7]. In addition to cardiac disease [8], neurologic disease [9] and gastrointestinal disease are also seen in critical patients [10]. Most acute symptoms subside within 2–3 weeks of being infected with the virus, although subsequent research has revealed that certain individuals do not completely recuperate from their ailment, but instead, experience post-acute consequences of SARS-CoV-2 infection (PASC), commonly referred to as long COVID [11].

Long COVID is characterized by the presence of persistent, relapsing, new symptoms, or other health effects that manifest following acute SARS-CoV-2 infection [12]. Approximately half of the infected individuals worldwide will develop long COVID, especially in Asia (51%), Europe (44%), and the United States of America (31%), and this figure could be higher due to insufficient statistics and a lack of standardized scoring [13,14]. The symptoms of long COVID are more widespread and have a greater impact on human health and working ability [15]. Statistical analysis of the symptoms of COVID-19 patients one year after infection found that the main symptoms of long COVID include dizziness, fatigue, sleep difficulties, memory loss, anxiety and depression, hair loss, smell and taste disorder, decreased appetite, thirst, chronic cough, pulmonary fibrosis, palpitations, chest pain, diarrhea or vomiting, gastrointestinal disorders, diabetes, changes in sexual desire or capacity, joint and muscle pain, post-exertional malaise, abnormal movements, and thrombus formation [12,16] (Figure 1). Among them, fatigue, memory loss, multiorgan abnormalities, pulmonary fibrosis, heart damage, sleep difficulties, and anxiety and depression will continue unimproved for four months up to two years [17,18]. Furthermore, women and individuals with chronic underlying conditions are more susceptible to the detrimental effects of long COVID, and the intensity of symptoms can be affected by vaccination and the mutated strains of the virus [19]. Current research suggests that the main pathogenic mechanisms of long COVID are the persistence of the SARS-CoV-2 virus [20], microthrombosis [21], immune dysregulation [22], the disruption of mitochondrial function [23], the activation of pathogens such as Epstein–Barr virus (EBV) and human herpesvirus 6 (HHV6) [24], changes in the body microbiota [25], persistent inflammation [26], the activation of autoimmunity [27], brainstem signal transduction, and vagal signaling dysfunction [28,29].

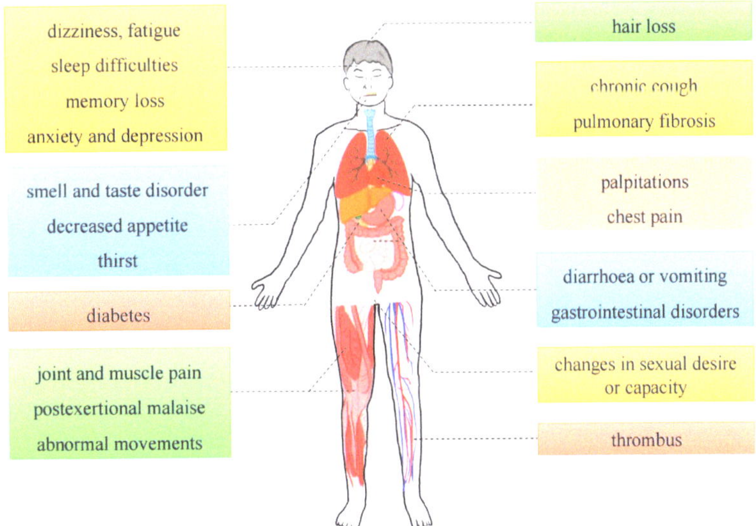

Figure 1. Long COVID symptoms.

At present, the primary treatment for long COVID is based on distinct symptoms, and there are no definitive medications and therapies for long COVID treatment [30]. However, a large number of studies have identified several potential therapeutic agents against long COVID in the natural constituents of medicinal plants, including the organic sulfur compound from garlic (*Allium sativum* L.) [31], curcumin from *Curcuma longa* [32], nigellone and α-hederin from *Nigella sativ* [33,34], phytocompound 6-gingerol from *Zingiber officinale* [35], and flavonoids from garlic, propolis, and honey [31,36]. In particular, natural and semi-synthetic flavonoids and neutrophil elastase inhibitors isolated from natural sources show great advantages in fighting SARS-CoV-2 or treating long COVID [37–39].

Naringin and naringenin are two of the most common flavanones found in citrus plants (Figure 2). They are known to cause bitterness in citrus fruits and have a wide range of biological functions. Naringin is the glycoside form of naringenin. After the oral ingestion of naringin or naringenin by the human body, naringin is converted to naringenin in the presence of intestinal microorganisms and absorbed in the intestinal epithelium [40]. The efficacy of naringin and naringenin is due to anti-inflammatory [41], anticancer [42], antioxidant properties [43,44], treatment of cardiovascular disease [45], antiviral [36] and immune-modulation effects [41], which may play an effective role in treating long COVID. The anti-inflammatory and antioxidant effects of naringenin can effectively counteract the cytokine storm induced by SARS-CoV-2, especially targeting and inhibiting interleukin(IL)-6, the main pro-inflammatory factor of COVID-19 [46]. Moreover, numerous molecular docking studies reveal that naringenin binds to viral spiking proteins, viral major proteases, host receptors, and host viral transport channels and has multiple antiviral effects against SARS-CoV-2 [47]. For instance, naringenin can influence the replication of the viral genome by attaching to SARS-CoV-2 macrodomain RNA polymerase (NSP3), SARS-CoV-2 RNA-dependent RNA polymerase (NSP12), and 3-chymotrypsin-like protease, as well as affect viral invasion by attaching to the ACE2 receptor to achieve an antiviral effect [48,49]. However, despite the abundance of evidence suggesting that naringin and naringenin can be more effective in treating various illnesses, there is yet to be a review of their combined potential in treating multiple coexisting conditions of long COVID. The purpose of this research was to assess the potential beneficial effects of naringin and naringenin in treating long COVID.

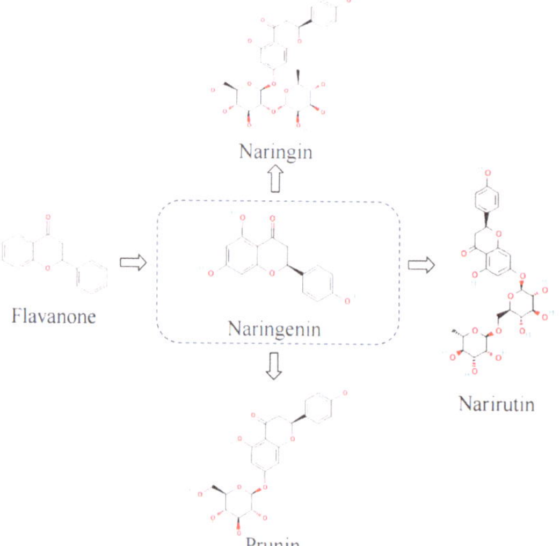

Figure 2. Chemical structures of flavanone, naringenin, and its derivatives. The 2D structure images were obtained from PubChem (https://pubchem.ncbi.nlm.nih.gov).

2. Therapeutic Potential of Naringin and Naringenin in Long COVID

In the following, we will discuss the pathogenesis of 11 common symptoms in patients with long COVID and make reasonable assumptions about the potential therapeutic role of naringin and naringenin in treating these symptoms (Figure 3).

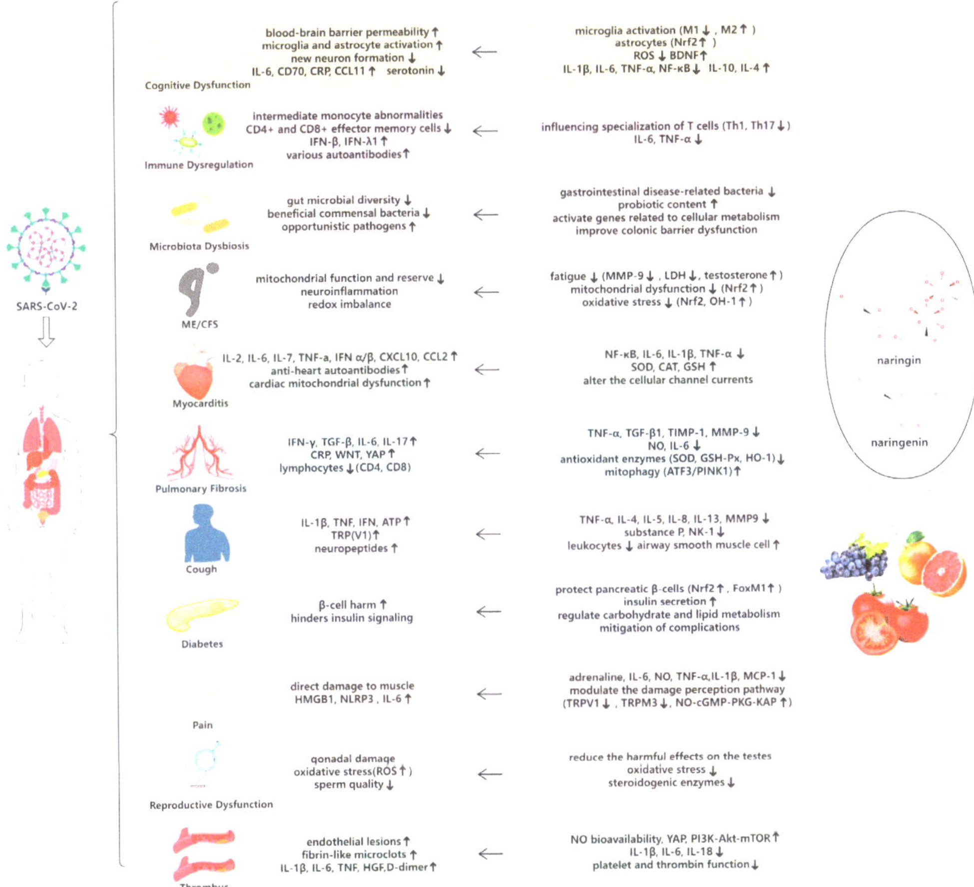

Figure 3. Summary of long COVID symptom pathogenesis (**left**) and potential therapeutic mechanisms (**right**). Upward arrows (↑) in the colored panels of the table indicate increases and downward arrows (↓) indicate decreases. Leftward arrows (←) between the panels indicate the palliative and therapeutic effects of naringin on long COVID symptoms.

2.1. Cognitive Dysfunction

Cognitive dysfunction is an extremely common persistent psychiatric manifestation after COVID-19 referred to as "brain fog". It is characterized by attention/processing speed deficits, mainly in memory and executive functioning [50]. Fatigue, sleep disturbances, language disorders, and loss of smell/taste accompany it [51,52]. According to meta-statistics, cognitive dysfunction was found to be present in 22% of COVID-19 patients 19 weeks after diagnosis, and the symptom was continued in 19.7% at 9 months after infection [53,54]. The condition is seen in both mildly and severely ill patients and persists for long periods without relief, and the longer the duration of symptoms, the greater the cognitive impairment [55]. The main way that COVID-19 survivors experience cognitive decline is through the extended inflammation caused by SARS-CoV-2, which can increase blood–brain barrier permeability and activate microglia and astrocyte subtypes, leading to cellular stress and neuronal damage [56,57]. The invasion of SARS-CoV-2 also causes midbrain dopamine neuron senescence, which has been implicated in Parkinson's disease [58]. The downregulation of new neuron formation caused by long-term inflammation leads to reduced synaptic plasticity in the hippocampus, resulting in memory loss in COVID-19 survivors [59]. Moreover, some of the pro-inflammatory factors are involved in mood regulation, leading to depression and other mood abnormalities in survivors [60]. In addition, SARS-CoV-2 directly infects the nervous system and causes neurological destruction mediated by neurological inflammation [61,62]. The virus directly damages the olfactory epithelium via neuropilin-1 and ACE2, thereby affecting the olfactory neural network and causing olfactory malfunction [63]. Patients have exhibited notable enhancements in IL-6, CD70, C-reactive protein (CRP), C-C Motif Chemokine Ligand 11 (CCL11), serotonin, and serum biomarkers of neuronal and gliotic degeneration in the blood, as well as alterations in the brain's microstructure and functional brain integrity, as indicated by neuropsychological tests, blood tests, and diagnostic brain imaging [64–66].

Naringin and naringenin have been shown to provide protection and potentially offer therapeutic benefits against cognitive decline in neurological disorders like Alzheimer's disease [67,68]. Therefore, they can be reasonably hypothesized to have an ameliorative effect on cognitive dysfunction after COVID-19. Naringin shows a protective effect on the nervous system, mainly through the modulation of glial cell activation and protection against nervous system stresses. Microglia and astrocytes are both essential for safeguarding neurons. Microglia have two activation phenotypes: the M1 type is pro-inflammatory and damages neurons, while the M2 phenotype exerts anti-inflammatory and neuronal-repair functions. Naringin can promote microglia activation toward the M2 type and inhibit its activation toward the M1 type by modulating the janus kinase/signal transd ucer and activator of transcription 3 (JAK/STAT3) signaling pathway [69]. Astrocytes are protective of neuronal cells [70]. Naringin regulates the expression of nuclear factor erythroid 2-related factor 2 (Nrf2), thereby enhancing neuronal protection by astrocytes [71]. Naringenin combination therapy attenuates the pro-inflammatory activation of astrocytes and significantly attenuates 3-nitro propionic acid-induced neuronal cell death [72]. Naringin and naringenin have been shown to protect the nervous system from oxidative stress and inflammation in various studies. Naringenin reduces the production of reactive oxygen species, modulates pro-inflammatory cytokines (IL-1β, IL-6, and (tumor necrosis factor)TNF-α) and anti-inflammatory cytokines (IL-10 and IL-4) to reduce inflammation, and enhances synaptic plasticity by increasing the expression of N-methyl-D-aspartate receptors associated with learning and memory [73]. Naringin significantly attenuates D-galactose, doxorubicin, and Bisphenol A-induced oxidative stress in the nervous system and improves cognitive performance after treatment [74–76]. Naringenin exerts a protective effect against lead damage to the nervous system by maintaining the antioxidant enzyme system (superoxide dismutase (SOD), catalase (CAT), and glutathione (GSH)) and inhibiting the elevation of inflammatory factors (NF-κB) and proapoptotic-related protein (Bcl-2 and caspase-3) [77].

Moreover, naringenin has depression-relieving effects. Depression disorders are linked to decreased levels of brain-derived neurotrophic factor (BDNF), which is controlled by the cyclic adenosine monophosphate (cAMP)-cAMP response element binding protein (CREB)-BDNF signaling pathway [78,79]. Naringenin reverses the reduction in BDNF expression induced by high cortisol levels and modulates the mitochondrial apoptotic pathway to inhibit hippocampal apoptosis [80]. Naringenin can potentially enhance the endocrine nervous system by controlling the levels of glucocorticoid receptors and monoamines in the hippocampus, resulting in an antidepressant impact [81]. Furthermore, naringenin and SARS-CoV-2 can cross the blood–brain barrier and enter brain tissue [73]. The combination of naringenin and naringin, which block primary viral proteases, decrease receptor activity, and attach to viral spiny proteins, could potentially lessen neurological harm [48,82].

2.2. Immune Dysregulation

SARS-CoV-2 invasion activates the body's innate and adaptive immunity to clear the invading pathogen [83]. Patients with long COVID have exhibited changes in immune cells, increased levels of autoantibodies, and the reactivation of dormant viruses [27,84,85]. The long-term effects of COVID-19 on the patient's immune system can be seen through alterations in the epigenetic and transcriptional makeup of monocytes, which can result in long-term inflammation, excessive autoimmune activity, and long-term consequences in the body [86]. Intermediate monocyte abnormalities and T-cell activation were found in recovering COVID-19 patients, which were associated with persistent endothelial cell activation and coagulation dysfunction [87,88]. Patients with long COVID exhibited a decline in cluster of differentiation (CD)4$^+$ and CD8$^+$ effector memory cells [22], and the expression of the pro-inflammatory cytokines interferon (IFN)-β and IFN-λ1 remained high during the 8 months after infection [89]. The persistence of SARS-CoV-2 also leads to a lack of dendritic cells in the host [90], along with a reduction in non-classical monocyte and lymphocyte subsets [91]. The persistent aberrant activation of immunity produces a broad spectrum of self-targeting antibodies and is hypothesized to be associated with different long COVID symptoms [92]. Long COVID patients exhibit abnormally high levels of functional autoantibodies targeting different G protein-coupled receptors, which are associated with persistent neurological and cardiovascular symptoms in patients [93]. SARS-CoV-2-induced autoimmunity causes immune blood disorders, antiphospholipid syndrome, systemic lupus erythematosus, vasculitis, acute arthritis, and Kawasaki-like syndromes [94].

Naringenin has a palliative effect on T cell-mediated autoimmune diseases [95,96]. Following antigen induction, CD4$^+$ T cells differentiate into distinct subpopulations, encompassing pro-inflammatory T cells and anti-inflammatory regulatory T cells, which maintain equilibrium within healthy organisms [97]. Naringenin modulates the immune system's response to autoantigens by influencing the growth and specialization of T cells, as well as cytokine signaling [98,99]. Naringenin effectively alleviates symptoms of rheumatoid arthritis in rats by modulating lymphocyte polarization, primarily through the reduction in T helper (Th)1 and Th17 cell differentiation and the reduction in IL-6 and TNF-α levels [99,100]. Similarly, naringenin alleviates symptoms of multiple sclerosis and systemic lupus erythematosus by inhibiting the growth and specialization of harmful pro-inflammatory T cells while maintaining the differentiation of anti-inflammatory subgroups [101,102]. Naringenin also modulates cellular inflammatory responses by regulating the transcription of inflammatory factors and enhancing the lysosomal degradation of cellular inflammatory factors [103,104].

2.3. Microbiota Dysbiosis

SARS-CoV-2 leads to long-term changes in the microbiota, with decreased gut microbial diversity, fewer beneficial commensal bacteria, and increased opportunistic pathogens in patients [105]. Viral invasion dysregulates gut ecology by activating immunity, deregulating ACE2 expression, disrupting the intestinal barrier, and directly infecting bacteria [106,107]. Moreover, the antibiotics administered during treatment can cause more harm to the patient's intestinal flora [108]. Furthermore, COVID-19 patients exhibited noteworthy alterations in the lung [109], oral [110], and nasopharyngeal microbiomes [111]. Changes in the microbiome persist for an extended period, and patients do not return to normal microbial abundance after 6 months of rehabilitation therapy [112]. Gut microbes remained significantly different from healthy controls after 3 months of recovery and showed a correlation with persistent symptoms of long COVID [113]. Changes in the composition and abundance of a patient's gut microbes also affect their susceptibility to long COVID and complication severity [25]. These changes can have a serious impact on the health of the survivor, causing an inflammatory immune response in the body, changes in the levels of basal metabolite levels (e.g., amino acids, carbohydrates, and neurotransmitters), and clinical gastrointestinal symptoms [114]. Gut microflora dysbiosis can have neurological and pulmonary effects through cytokines and metabolites [115], which are mediated through the gut–lung and brain–gut axes [116,117].

Naringin and naringenin have been found to have beneficial regulatory effects on the composition and metabolism of gut flora [118,119]. The dietary intake of naringin and naringenin helps to control the intestinal microenvironment [120]. Naringin and naringenin can directly regulate the intestinal microbiota and its metabolism. Naringin significantly reduces the abundance of gastrointestinal disease-related bacteria (e.g., *Lachnoclostridium* and *Bilophila*) and enhances probiotic content in experiments [121]. Naringenin can regulate the growth and gene expression pattern of intestinal commensal microorganisms through interaction and activate genes related to cellular metabolism [122]. In addition, gut barrier dysfunction caused by microbiota dysbiosis may increase bacterial ectopia and contribute to host immune destabilization [123]. Naringin has been shown to reduce inflammation-associated protein expression and colonic damage caused by dextran sulfate sodium, as well as improve colonic barrier dysfunction [124].

2.4. Myalgic Encephalomyelitis/Chronic Fatigue Syndrome (ME/CFS)

ME/CFS is a chronic multisystem disease that often follows infectious diseases and may be associated with chronic viral infections such as human herpesviruses, human parvovirus B19V, and enteroviruses [125]. Patients with long COVID often experience persistent fatigue, myalgia, post-exertional malaise, insomnia, and exercise intolerance, with symptoms resembling the diagnostic criteria for ME/CFS [126]. Although there are no studies directly proving that acute COVID-19 triggers ME/CFS, several studies have identified multiple overlapping or similar symptoms between long COVID and ME/CFS [127]. COVID-19 also greatly increases the number of patients with ME/CFS [128], and bioinformatics analysis has identified a common network of genetic interactions between the two [129]. According to the diagnostic criteria for ME/CFS, the overall prevalence of ME/CFS was as high as 43% among patients with long COVID, with fatigue, malaise on exertion, and insomnia representing the main symptoms [130]. The invasion of SARS-CoV-2 significantly impacts both mitochondrial function and reserves, and the SARS-CoV-2 membrane protein causes mitochondrial apoptosis in epithelial cells [131]. Virus-induced decreases in mitochondrial membrane potential [132] and the downregulation of nuclear-encoded mitochondrial genes [133] have been observed in patients. In addition, the infiltration of amyloid-containing deposits and skeletal muscle injuries have also been observed in patients with long COVID [134]. The pathogenesis of ME/CFS involves neuroinflammation, redox imbalance, mitochondrial dysfunction, autoantibodies, and autonomic dysfunction [135–137].

The treatment of ME/CFS is still unclear and there are no effective treatments. Most treatments are based on the clinical condition and include central nervous system drugs, antiviral drugs, immunomodulators, analgesics, and nutritional supplements [138]. Fatigue and post-exercise discomfort may be due to reduced energy sources, mitochondrial dysfunction, and redox imbalance. Serum matrix metalloproteinase 9 (MMP-9) and muscle damage-associated lactate dehydrogenase (LDH) are associated with muscle fatigue. By stabilizing redox and elevating blood glucose levels, naringin effectively diminishes MMP-9 and LDH concentrations, thereby augmenting energy sources. This prolongs the duration of fatigue-inducing exercise and relieves post-exercise discomfort [139,140]. Moreover, naringenin can exert anti-fatigue effects by participating in the promotion of testosterone secretion [141]. Additionally, naringin can help to stabilize mitochondrial membrane potential, preserve mitochondrial integrity, and sustain mitochondrial complex activity [142,143], all of which can help to reduce mitochondrial dysfunction. Naringenin also protects neuronal mitochondrial function by activating the transcription factor Nrf2 [144]. In addition, naringin and naringenin are important redox regulators. Naringin significantly attenuated antigen-induced oxidative stress and reduced TNF-α levels in fatigued mice [145] while reinstating oxidative stress markers in rodent brains [146].

2.5. Myocarditis

Certain individuals who have survived the initial stages of COVID-19 experience enduring cardiac impairment following their recovery, ultimately resulting in myocarditis [147]. The clinical signs of myocarditis are heterogeneous and non-specific, typically consisting of chest pain, arrhythmias, generalized fatigue, dyspnea, and tachycardia [148]. The analysis of cardiac symptoms among COVID-19 survivors revealed that 9.79 percent displayed indications of chest pain, whereas 8.22 percent presented with arrhythmias [149]. Within a span of 2–3 months following SARS-CoV-2 infection, 19% of patients developed persistent symptoms of myocarditis [150]. One year after rehabilitation, patients had a significant 4.16-fold increased risk of myocarditis [151] and poorer clinical outcomes, with a mortality rate of 1.36% to 5% [152]. The direct pathogenic mechanism of myocarditis in long COVID is the direct interaction of SARS-CoV-2 with ACE2 receptors in cardiomyocytes and pericytes, causing immune dysregulation. Subsequently, immune dysregulation leads to cardiomyocyte injury and the release of inflammatory factors, such as IL-2, IL-6, IL-7, TNF-a, IFN-α/β, C-X-C motif cytokine 10 (CXCL10), and C-C motif ligand 2 (CCL2), which, in turn, induces persistent low-level inflammation [153]. Indirect pathogenic mechanisms include hypoxemia caused by the cytokine storm [154], high levels of antiheart autoantibodies caused by $CD4^+$ T-lymphocytes [155], and cardiac mitochondrial dysfunction [156]. Myocardial injury can be identified by the presence of markers such as myoglobin, troponin, creatine kinase-MB, IL-6, LDH, and N-terminal pro-b-type natriuretic peptide [157].

Naringin and naringenin have been shown to have cardioprotective properties [45]. First, the anti-inflammatory properties of naringin can drastically reduce the inflammatory factors associated with cardiovascular injury, such as NF-κB, IL-6, IL-1β, and TNF-α, and suppress the inflammatory response [158]. Furthermore, the antioxidant effects of naringin can scavenge free radicals and increase the activity of antioxidant enzymes (superoxide dismutase and catalase) and GSH levels, effectively protecting the heart mitochondria from damage, thereby reducing DOX-induced apoptosis and vacuolization in cardiomyocytes [67]. In addition, naringin has the potential to alter the cellular channel currents in mouse ventricular myocytes, consequently exerting antiarrhythmic effects [159].

2.6. Pulmonary Fibrosis

Pulmonary fibrosis is one of the serious sequelae of COVID-19. It is estimated that 19% of patients recovering from COVID-19 have residual lung abnormalities [160]. The lungs are the primary target organ for viral invasion. SARS-CoV-2 causes severe lung damage, ultimately leading to post-COVID-19 pulmonary fibrosis (PCPF). Radiological manifestations of pulmonary fibrosis usually include bilateral lung infiltrates, "ground glass" opacity, and "honeycomb" lungs [161]. Its cellular and molecular characteristics include a decrease in lymphocytes and an increase in CRP and IL-6 [162]. Multiple studies have shown that the prevalence of PCPF among COVID-19 survivors is more than 9.3% [163]. Alveolar injury caused by SARS-CoV-2 leads to the secretion of pro-fibrotic and pro-inflammatory cytokines by alveolar macrophages and type 2 alveolar epithelial cells (AEC), including IFN-γ, transforming growth factor (TGF)-β, and IL-6 and IL-17. Cytokines induce myofibroblast differentiation by activating the WNT/β-catenin and YAP/TAZ pathways, ultimately leading to the combined effects of pulmonary fibrosis [164,165].

Naringin and naringenin are effective inhibitors of pulmonary fibrosis. The main target of current anti-pulmonary fibrosis therapy is the TGF-β/Smad pathway [166]. It has been shown that naringin inhibits cellular fibrosis by suppressing TGF-β overexpression and reducing downstream regulatory factor phosphorylation [167]. Moreover, the anti-inflammatory and antioxidant effects of naringin and naringenin can be used against pulmonary fibrosis [168]. Naringin has been shown to significantly reduce the infiltration of inflammatory cells induced by lipopolysaccharide and decrease the production of macrophage nitrogen monoxide (NO) and IL-6 [169]. In critically ill COVID-19 patients, naringenin also showed excellent IL-6 inhibition compared to synthetic monoclonal antibodies [46]. In a paraquat-induced acute lung injury model, naringin not only decreased the production of the inflammatory cytokines TNF-α and TNF-β1 but also inhibited oxidative stress by activating the expression of antioxidant enzymes (superoxide dismutase, glutathione peroxidase, and heme oxygenase 1) and regulated collagen formation by modulating the ratio of tissue inhibitors of metalloproteinases-1 (TIMP-1) to MMP-9, thereby preventing lung fibrosis [170]. Furthermore, naringin modulates the activating transcription factor 3/PTEN-induced kinase 1 (ATF3/PINK1) pathway and enhances mitophagy in lung tissues, resulting in the alleviation of bleomycin-induced idiopathic pulmonary fibrosis [171]. Naringenin also protects against cigarette-induced lung injury by regulating miRNAs in extracellular vesicles [172].

2.7. Cough

Coughing is the most common symptom of COVID-19 sequelae and is present in approximately 23% to 57% of COVID-19 survivors in all countries, and is highly prevalent in both mild and severe cases [173,174]. Cough can persist for months, with a prevalence of up to 2.5% even after one year of recovery [175], making it a major source of distress for patients. SARS-CoV-2 may induce chronic coughing through neuroinflammatory and neuroimmune mechanisms. Viral invasion causes the release of neuroinflammatory mediators (IL-1β, TNF, IFN, adenosine triphosphate (ATP)) and, in turn, activates vagal sensory neurons via transient receptor potential (TRP) channels. Sensory neurons release a variety of neuropeptides (calcitonin gene-related peptide, substance P, and neurokinin A), eventually leading to hypersensitivity of the cough pathway [176]. In addition, the underlying mechanisms of chronic cough may also be related to post-infectious lung abnormalities, cough underlying disease, upper airway cough syndrome, or cough-variant asthma (CVA) [177–179].

The current treatment of chronic coughing focuses on suppressing the cough reflex, reducing airway inflammation, drying and relieving coughing, and resolving phlegm to relieve coughing [180,181]. Naringin and naringenin have long been shown to have positive antitussive effects [182]. Naringenin can reduce inflammation caused by cigarette smoke in mice with chronic obstructive pulmonary disease by inhibiting the production of the pro-inflammatory factors IL-8, TNF-α, and MMP9, as well as the NF-κB pathway [183]. In an experimental CVA model, naringin has been shown to reduce irritation-induced cough and suppress the growth of airway-inflammatory factors (IL-4, IL-5, and IL-13) and leukocytes [184]. Moreover, naringin has been shown to significantly attenuate cigarette smoke-induced airway neurogenic inflammation by reducing substance P and NK-1 receptors [185]. Furthermore, naringin can be used in asthma treatment by promoting the proliferation of AECs through the bitter taste receptor (TAS2R)-related signal pathway, thereby inducing the relaxation of airway smooth muscle cells [186].

2.8. Diabetes

The occurrence of new-onset diabetes mellitus can be attributed to acute infection with SARS-CoV-2, and complications such as diabetic ketoacidosis (DKA) and hyperglycemic hyperosmolar syndrome are highly prevalent [187,188]. COVID-19 survivors have a 64–66% higher risk of developing diabetes than uninfected individuals [189]. The risk of developing diabetes in the first three months after COVID-19 infection was up to 95%, with a higher risk of developing type 2 diabetes (T2D) than type 1 diabetes (T1D) (70% and 48%, respectively) [190]. The data indicated that during the initial year of the COVID-19 outbreak, there was a notable surge of 9.5% and 25% in the occurrence of new pediatric T1Ds and DKAs, correspondingly, alongside a substantial rise in blood glucose levels [191]. A follow-up study found that most patients with new-onset T2D were cured 3 months after discharge from the hospital. In contrast, the remaining 37% of patients with T2D were diagnosed with persistent diabetes mellitus [192]. COVID-19-related abnormalities in glucose metabolism also recovered after one year [193]. On this bases, diabetes was also associated with serious illness, hospitalization, and death in COVID-19, so a bidirectional causal relationship between COVID-19 and diabetes was hypothesized [194]. Both COVID-19 patients and survivors exhibit insulin resistance and beta-cell dysfunction, which endure even after recuperation from the illness [195].

The pathogenesis of new-onset diabetes is mainly related to pancreatic autoimmunity, pancreatic injury, pro-inflammatory cytokine storms, the triggering of steroid drugs, and underlying diabetic activation of the body. T1D is an autoimmune disease, and the invasion of SARS-CoV-2 leads to autoimmune hyperactivation in the body [196]. Additionally, researchers have found pancreatic damage in some COVID-19 patients [197]. Thus there has been a hypothesis suggesting that ACE2 exhibits elevated expression levels in exocrine glands and pancreas islets [198] when SARS-CoV-2 enters them to induce pancreatic β-cell dysfunction or apoptosis, hindering insulin signaling [199]. T2D is mainly caused by short-term treatment and inflammation. Steroids, a widely prescribed medication for COVID-19, can potentially impact insulin sensitivity; nevertheless, the discontinuation of steroid therapy may lead to the recurrence of new-onset diabetes [200]. The inflammatory factor TNF has also been recognized as a common pathogenic target of COVID-19 and T2D [201].

Naringin and naringenin may exert antidiabetic potential by attenuating pancreatic β-cell damage or activating their proliferation. Naringenin protects pancreatic β-cells from streptozotocin (STZ)-induced immune stress by activating Nrf2, leading to a substantial decrease in blood glucose levels and restoring normal insulin levels [202]. Naringin inhibits mitochondria-mediated and death receptor-mediated apoptosis in pancreatic β cells [203]. Forkhead box M1 (FoxM1) transcription factor affects pancreatic adult beta cell proliferation, and naringin increases beta cell mass and treats diabetes by upregulating FoxM1 [204]. Naringin and naringenin also showed significant ameliorative effects on insulin resistance. In the an STZ- and a nicotinamide-induced T2D model, naringin and naringenin enhanced insulin secretory responses and the expression of insulin receptors and their sensitizers [205]. In T2D patients, naringin was found to improve glucose metabolism, increase residual insulin secretion, and stimulate glycogen synthesis; however, absolute insulin deficiency prevented it from regulating glucose levels in T1D patients, yet it could reverse T1D-induced DKA [206]. Furthermore, naringin and naringenin regulate carbohydrate and lipid metabolism. Naringin modulates the activity of glycolysis-related enzymes and regulates intestinal carbohydrate absorption [207]. Naringenin can reduce metabolic disorders by modulating immune-related inflammatory factors and inhibiting the infiltration of inflammatory cells into adipose tissue [208]. In addition, naringenin has a mitigating effect on the complications of diabetes. Naringenin, when used in conjunction with insulin, modulates matrix metalloproteinases to reduce neuropathic pain caused by diabetes [209]. Naringenin inhibits high-glucose-induced vasculopathy by downregulating the hyperproliferation and migration of vascular smooth muscle cells [210].

2.9. Pain

COVID-19 patients often have accompanying pain, including headache, musculoskeletal pain, and testicular pain, during the acute infection period and after rehabilitation [211,212]. Although the majority of pain symptoms subside two months after recovery, 10% of COVID-19 survivors still experience persistent musculoskeletal muscle pain, and the length of the pain does not correlate with the intensity of COVID-19 [213]. The post-infection follow-up of COVID-19 survivors unveiled a range of symptoms, encompassing general pain (13.40%), joint pain (28.25%), muscle pain (13.30%), headache (9.50%), and chest pain (12.12%) [214]. Pain development is mainly associated with direct action through ACE2 receptors [215], the inflammatory cytokine storm [216], and the driving effect of prostaglandins [217]. ACE2 receptors are abundant in skeletal muscle and other organs, resulting in viral harm to the muscles, and their neurophilicity can also lead to neuronal damage, resulting in pain [218]. The virus triggers an extended inflammatory reaction, resulting in heightened hyperexcitability of the central nervous system, thereby exacerbating pain [219]. COVID-19 patients experiencing headache symptoms exhibited elevated concentrations of inflammatory molecules and harmful molecules (high-mobility group protein B1 (HMGB1), NOD-like receptor thermal protein domain-associated protein 3 (NLRP3), and IL-6), potentially contributing to the initiation of trigeminal activation [220,221].

Naringin and naringenin have effective analgesic effects. Naringin and naringenin can attenuate neuronal stimulation directly by inhibiting the inflammatory response. Naringin attenuates iodoacetate-induced osteoarthritis pain by inhibiting the secretion of adrenaline and pro-inflammatory factors (IL-6, NO, and TNF-α) [222]. The administration of naringenin in a rat model of neuropathic pain resulted in the inhibition of glial cell activation caused by spinal nerve ligation injury, as well as a reduction in elevated levels of inflammatory factors (TNF-α, IL-1β, and monocyte chemotactic protein 1) [223]. Moreover, naringin and naringenin can directly modulate the damage perception pathway to achieve analgesic effects. Transient receptor potential vanilloid member 1 (TRPV1) is associated with noxious temperature sensation and inflammatory pain, and its antagonists have been considered potential analgesics [224–226]. By interacting with TRPV1, naringin suppresses nervous system hyperexcitability and potentially mitigates nerve pain by inhibiting oxidative stress [227]. Transient receptor potential melastatin-3 (TRPM3) ion channels are involved in organismal injury perception and are expressed on somatosensory neurons. Naringenin can effectively block TRPM3 channels in vivo and in vitro, thus supporting its analgesic effect [228]. Moreover, naringenin inhibits superoxide anion-induced inflammatory pain by activating the NO-cGMP-PKG-KAP signaling pathway and reducing nociceptive cytokine expression [229].

2.10. Reproductive Dysfunction

The acute infection phase of COVID-19 leads to reproductive dysfunction in both genders, including erectile dysfunction, orchitis, reduced testosterone levels, ovarian dysfunction, and menstrual changes [230,231]. After 3.8 months of recovery, 35.9% of men and 27.7% of women were found to have sexual dysfunction, with different mechanisms in both cases [232]. A continued high prevalence of erectile dysfunction in men was observed 3 months after COVID-19 recovery [233]. The impact of long COVID on women's reproductive health is mainly characterized by menstrual irregularities, gonadal dysfunction, and fertility problems [234]. Both ACE2 and transmembrane serine protease 2 (TMPRSS2) are highly expressed in the gonads, with higher expression in male gonads and detectable SARS-CoV-2 infection in the testis [235]. Therefore, it is hypothesized that the gonads, especially the testes, are susceptible to SARS-CoV-2 infection and damage. Male long COVID patients with coagulation abnormalities and endothelial damage also experience testicular inflammation [236]. Testicular injury, oxidative stress by reactive oxygen species [237], and decreased testosterone due to dysfunction of the hypothalamic–pituitary–gonadal axis [238] can lead to erectile dysfunction [239]. Moreover, the autoimmune inflammatory response of the body can also cause a decrease in sperm quality [240].

Naringenin also has an attenuating effect on testicular and sperm damage. Naringenin can reduce the harmful effects of bisphenol A on the testes by suppressing oxidative stress and mitochondrial apoptosis [241]. Naringenin has been shown to reduce the harmful effects of antiretroviral medication on the male reproductive system of rats while preserving the normal physical structure of the testes and sperm viability [242]. Furthermore, naringenin has a protective effect on the ovary and can alleviate polycystic ovary syndrome. In vivo naringin treatment in rats inhibits steroidogenic enzymes and consequently controls ovulation, thereby restoring ovarian morphology and cystic follicle levels in patients with polycystic ovary syndrome [243].

2.11. Thrombus Formation

Endothelial damage caused by SARS-CoV-2 can lead to coagulation dysfunction in certain patients, ultimately resulting in the development of long-term concomitant thrombosis [244]. Individuals afflicted with long COVID face an elevated likelihood of experiencing arterial thromboembolic events and venous thromboembolic events. They are susceptible to acute pulmonary embolism (PE), deep vein thrombosis (DVT), myocardial infarction, and acute respiratory distress syndrome (ARDS) [245,246]. COVID-19 survivors had a significantly higher incidence of thrombophilia, PE (2.5–6.3%), and DVT (1.2–6.4%), which was 2 to 3 times higher than in uninfected individuals [247]. Long COVID-induced thrombosis can be caused by various factors, such as damage to the endothelium, the abnormal production of fibrin during platelet aggregation, and dysregulation of the immune system [248]. SARS-CoV-2 invasion can promote endothelial damage and dysfunction through direct interaction with ACE2 receptors [244]. Its spiny proteins can also interact with platelets and fibrin, inducing the formation of fibrin-like microclots, which are difficult to hydrolyze [249]. Moreover, viral invasion inducing a storm of inflammatory factors (IL-1β, IL-6, and TNF) activates exogenous coagulation pathways and promotes the inhibition of anticoagulant routes [250]. In addition, the persistence of the virus in the outer vesicles, the formation of autoantibodies, and chronic hypoxia can lead to long-term coagulation disorders [251]. Patients with long COVID who displayed coagulation abnormalities exhibited increased levels of hepatocyte growth factor (HGF), IL-6, and D-dimer [252].

Naringin can exert its antithrombotic effect by protecting endothelial cells, inhibiting platelet activation, and inhibiting thrombin activity. Naringin has been shown to reduce inflammation and alter the permeability of endothelial cells, thus mitigating endothelial dysfunction [169]. Naringin protects endothelial cell function by upregulating NO bioavailability [253], decreasing levels of inflammatory factors (IL-1β, IL-6, and IL-18), and reversing YAP downregulation [254]. Naringin inhibits excessive autophagy in endothelial cells by activating the PI3K-Akt-mTOR pathway [255]. Moreover, naringenin can impede platelet aggregation. Naringenin has a structure-dependent inhibitory effect on platelet function in both whole blood and plasma [256], and can also inhibit platelet activation by targeting the PI3K/Akt pathway, preventing $FeCl_3$-induced carotid artery thrombosis and vascular occlusion and displaying effective antithrombotic properties [257]. In addition, research on molecular docking demonstrated that naringenin is strongly attracted to thrombin and can attach itself to the active core of thrombin, potentially impeding its activity [258]. Protein disulfide isomerase (PDI) in plasma is involved in the conformational formation of coagulation-associated proteins, and naringin can also affect thrombus formation and stabilization by binding to PDI and inducing conformational changes [259].

3. Conclusions and Prospects

This review addresses the pathogenesis and statistical status of eleven complications of long COVID and specifically addresses the therapeutic potential of naringin and naringenin in long COVID (Table 1). The clinical symptoms and biomarkers of long COVID have been widely reported, and long COVID can indeed have serious long-term effects on human health [260,261]. There are no definitive medications that directly treat multiple long COVID complications [262], and the treatment approach for long COVID is still based solely on clinical symptoms and the use of nutraceuticals and probiotics to improve symptoms [263]. Therefore, treating patients with multiple syndromes requires a combination of drugs. Naringin and naringenin, as important constituents of medicinal plants, are characterized by strong safety, multiple targets, and few side effects, with excellent performance in treating various diseases. They demonstrate protection against biotic stress by inducing a hormonal dose response in various cell models [264]. Moreover, it is worth noting that nano-preparations of natural products such as naringenin can improve their bioavailability and drug targeting after oral administration [265]. We enumerate the therapeutic and palliative effects of naringin and naringenin on conditions with symptoms or pathogenic mechanisms similar to those of long COVID, which are based on their anti-inflammatory, antimicrobial, antiviral, anti-free radical, cardiovascular-protection, microbiota-modulation, and neuron-protection effects. The purpose of this review is to provide a theoretical foundation for the use of naringin and naringenin as potential treatments for long COVID. Further research is necessary to ascertain the true efficacy and appropriate dosage of naringin and naringenin in treating long COVID, as well as conduct thorough follow-up clinical trials.

Table 1. Potential pathophysiological mechanisms of long COVID symptoms and the functions of naringin and/or naringenin.

Long COVID Symptoms	Potential Pathophysiological Mechanisms of Long COVID	Functions of Naringin and/or Naringenin
Cognitive Dysfunction	Interference with blood–brain barrier led to neuronal damage [56,57] Downregulation of new neuron formation [59] Pro-inflammatory factors led to depression [60] Direct damage to the olfactory epithelium [63]	Modulation of glial cell activation [69,71,72] Enhanced synaptic plasticity [73] Protected the nervous system from oxidative stress and inflammation [77] Inhibited hippocampal apoptosis [80] Enhanced the endocrine nervous system [81]
Immune Dysregulation	Intermediated monocyte abnormalities and T-cell activation [87,88] Decline in $CD4^+$ and $CD8^+$ effector memory cells [22] Lack of dendritic cells [90] Reduction in non-classical monocyte and lymphocyte subsets [91] Increased levels of autoantibodies [93]	Influenced growth and specialization of T cells [98–102] Regulated the transcription and lysosomal degradation of inflammatory factors [103,104]
Microbiota Dysbiosis	Changes in the composition and abundance of the gut [105], lung [109], oral [110], and nasopharyngeal microbiomes [111] Altered basal metabolite levels [114]	Controlled the intestinal microenvironment [120] and colonic barrier [124]. Regulated the intestinal microbiota [121] Regulated gene expression pattern of intestinal commensal microorganisms [122]
ME/CFS	Impacted both mitochondrial function and reserves [131–133] Infiltration of amyloid-containing deposits [134]	Stabilization of energy sources [139–141] Reduced mitochondrial dysfunction [142–144] Attenuated oxidative stress [145,146]
Myocarditis	Inflammation of cardiomyocytes through direct action of SARS-CoV-2 [153] Hypoxemia [154] High levels of antiheart autoantibodies [155] Cardiac mitochondrial dysfunction [156]	Reduced the inflammatory factors associated with cardiovascular injury [158] Protected cardiac mitochondria from oxidative damage [67] Altered the cellular channel currents [159]
Pulmonary Fibrosis	Alveolar injury led to secretion of pro-fibrotic and pro-inflammatory cytokines [164,165]	Inhibition of TGF-β overexpression [167] Reduced the infiltration of inflammatory cells [169] Regulated collagen formation [170] Enhanced mitophagy in lung tissues [171] Regulated miRNAs in extracellular vesicles [172]
Cough	Neuroinflammatory mediators led to hypersensitivity of the cough pathway [176]	Inhibited the production of pro-inflammatory factors [183,184] Attenuated airway neurogenic inflammation [185] Induced relaxation of airway smooth muscle cells [186]
Diabetes	Autoimmune hyperactivation in the body [196] β-cell harm and pancreatic damage [197,199] Steroids impacted insulin sensitivity [200]	Attenuated pancreatic β-cell damage or activated their proliferation [202–204] Ameliorative effect on insulin resistance [205,206] Regulated carbohydrate and lipid metabolism [207,208] Mitigated effect on the complications of diabetes [209,210]
Pain	Direct damage to muscle by the virus [218] Inflammation led to overstimulation of the nervous system [219–221]	Attenuated neuronal stimulation by inhibiting the inflammatory response [222,223] Modulated the damage perception pathway [227–229]
Reproductive Dysfunction	Virus-induced gonadal damage [235] Coagulation abnormalities and endothelial damage [236] Decreased testosterone [238] Decrease in sperm quality caused by inflammatory response [240]	Inhibition of oxidative stress and mitochondrial apoptosis in testes [241] Preserved the structure of the testes and sperm viability [242] Inhibited steroidogenic enzymes and controlled ovulation [243]
Thrombus Formation	Endothelial damage and dysfunction [244] Formation of fibrin-like microclots that are difficult to hydrolyze [249] Inflammatory factor storm activated exogenous coagulation pathways [250] Formation of autoantibodies and chronic hypoxia [251]	Upregulated NO bioavailability [253] Decreasing levels of inflammatory factors [254] Inhibited excessive autophagy in endothelial cells [255] Inhibited platelet activation [256,257] Inhibited thrombin activity [258,259]

Author Contributions: Conceptualization, S.L. and P.L.; methodology, M.Z.; validation, Y.W., P.L., and H.W.; investigation, S.L.; resources, P.L.; writing—original draft preparation, S.L.; writing—review and editing, M.Z.; visualization, H.W.; supervision, W.S.; project administration, P.L.; funding acquisition, W.S. All authors have read and agreed to the published version of the manuscript.

Funding: This research was funded by the Natural Science Foundation of Guangdong Province, grant number 2023A1515011953, the Open Competition Program of Ten Major Directions of Agricultural Science and Technology Innovation for the 14th Five-Year Plan of Guangdong Province, grant number 2022SDZG07, and the Research Fund of Maoming Branch, Guangdong Laboratory for Lingnan Modern Agriculture, grant number 2022ZD006.

Institutional Review Board Statement: Not applicable.

Informed Consent Statement: Not applicable.

Data Availability Statement: Not applicable.

Conflicts of Interest: The authors declare no conflicts of interest.

References

1. Yu, I.T.S.; Li, Y.; Wong, T.W.; Tam, W.; Chan, A.T.; Lee, J.H.W.; Leung, D.Y.C.; Ho, T. Evidence of Airborne Transmission of the Severe Acute Respiratory Syndrome Virus. *N. Engl. J. Med.* **2004**, *350*, 1731–1739. [CrossRef]
2. Cai, J.; Sun, W.; Huang, J.; Gamber, M.; Wu, J.; He, G. Indirect Virus Transmission in Cluster of COVID-19 Cases, Wenzhou, China, 2020. *Emerg. Infect. Dis.* **2020**, *26*, 1343–1345. [CrossRef] [PubMed]
3. da Silva, F.A.F.; de Brito, B.B.; Santos, M.L.C.; Marques, H.S.; da Silva Junior, R.T.; de Carvalho, L.S.; de Sousa Cruz, S.; Rocha, G.R.; Santos, G.L.C.; de Souza, K.C.; et al. Transmission of Severe Acute Respiratory Syndrome Coronavirus 2 via Fecal-Oral: Current Knowledge. *World J. Clin. Cases* **2021**, *9*, 8280–8294. [CrossRef]
4. Zhou, P.; Yang, X.-L.; Wang, X.-G.; Hu, B.; Zhang, L.; Zhang, W.; Si, H.-R.; Zhu, Y.; Li, B.; Huang, C.-L.; et al. A Pneumonia Outbreak Associated with a New Coronavirus of Probable Bat Origin. *Nature* **2020**, *579*, 270–273. [CrossRef]
5. Beyerstedt, S.; Casaro, E.B.; Rangel, É.B. COVID-19: Angiotensin-Converting Enzyme 2 (ACE2) Expression and Tissue Susceptibility to SARS-CoV-2 Infection. *Eur. J. Clin. Microbiol. Infect. Dis.* **2021**, *40*, 905–919. [CrossRef] [PubMed]
6. Sharma, A.; Ahmad Farouk, I.; Lal, S.K. COVID-19: A Review on the Novel Coronavirus Disease Evolution, Transmission, Detection, Control and Prevention. *Viruses* **2021**, *13*, 202. [CrossRef]
7. World Health Organization. Operational Planning Guidance to Support Country Preparedness and Response. Available online: https://www.who.int/publications-detail-redirect/draft-operational-planning-guidance-for-un-country-teams (accessed on 20 December 2023).
8. Wang, D.; Hu, B.; Hu, C.; Zhu, F.; Liu, X.; Zhang, J.; Wang, B.; Xiang, H.; Cheng, Z.; Xiong, Y.; et al. Clinical Characteristics of 138 Hospitalized Patients with 2019 Novel Coronavirus–Infected Pneumonia in Wuhan, China. *JAMA* **2020**, *323*, 1061–1069. [CrossRef] [PubMed]
9. Liotta, E.M.; Batra, A.; Clark, J.R.; Shlobin, N.A.; Hoffman, S.C.; Orban, Z.S.; Koralnik, I.J. Frequent Neurologic Manifestations and Encephalopathy-associated Morbidity in COVID-19 Patients. *Ann. Clin. Transl. Neurol.* **2020**, *7*, 2221–2230. [CrossRef]
10. Tian, Y.; Rong, L.; Nian, W.; He, Y. Review Article: Gastrointestinal Features in COVID-19 and the Possibility of Faecal Transmission. *Aliment. Pharmacol. Ther.* **2020**, *51*, 843–851. [CrossRef]
11. Chen, B.; Julg, B.; Mohandas, S.; Bradfute, S.B. Viral Persistence, Reactivation, and Mechanisms of Long COVID. *eLife* **2023**, *12*, e86015. [CrossRef]
12. Thaweethai, T.; Jolley, S.E.; Karlson, E.W.; Levitan, E.B.; Levy, B.; McComsey, G.A.; McCorkell, L.; Nadkarni, G.N.; Parthasarathy, S.; Singh, U.; et al. Development of a Definition of Postacute Sequelae of SARS-CoV-2 Infection. *JAMA* **2023**, *329*, 1934–1946. [CrossRef]
13. Chen, C.; Haupert, S.R.; Zimmermann, L.; Shi, X.; Fritsche, L.G.; Mukherjee, B. Global Prevalence of Post-Coronavirus Disease 2019 (COVID-19) Condition or Long COVID: A Meta-Analysis and Systematic Review. *J. Infect. Dis.* **2022**, *226*, 1593–1607. [CrossRef]
14. Kingery, J.R.; Safford, M.M.; Martin, P.; Lau, J.D.; Rajan, M.; Wehmeyer, G.T.; Li, H.A.; Alshak, M.N.; Jabri, A.; Kofman, A.; et al. Health Status, Persistent Symptoms, and Effort Intolerance One Year after Acute COVID-19 Infection. *J. Gen. Intern. Med.* **2022**, *37*, 1218–1225. [CrossRef] [PubMed]
15. Kerksieck, P.; Ballouz, T.; Haile, S.R.; Schumacher, C.; Lacy, J.; Domenghino, A.; Fehr, J.S.; Bauer, G.F.; Dressel, H.; Puhan, M.A.; et al. Post COVID-19 Condition, Work Ability and Occupational Changes in a Population-Based Cohort. *Lancet Reg. Health-Eur.* **2023**, *31*, 100671. [CrossRef] [PubMed]
16. Huang, C.; Huang, L.; Wang, Y.; Li, X.; Ren, L.; Gu, X.; Kang, L.; Guo, L.; Liu, M.; Zhou, X.; et al. 6-Month Consequences of COVID-19 in Patients Discharged from Hospital: A Cohort Study. *Lancet* **2023**, *401*, e21–e33. [CrossRef]
17. Yong, S.J. Long COVID or Post-COVID-19 Syndrome: Putative Pathophysiology, Risk Factors, and Treatments. *Infect. Dis.* **2021**, *53*, 737–754. [CrossRef] [PubMed]

18. Ballouz, T.; Menges, D.; Anagnostopoulos, A.; Domenghino, A.; Aschmann, H.E.; Frei, A.; Fehr, J.S.; Puhan, M.A. Recovery and Symptom Trajectories up to Two Years after SARS-CoV-2 Infection: Population Based, Longitudinal Cohort Study. *BMJ* **2023**, *381*, e074425. [CrossRef]

19. Bostanci, A.; Gazi, U.; Tosun, O.; Suer, K.; Unal Evren, E.; Evren, H.; Sanlidag, T. Long-COVID-19 in Asymptomatic, Non-Hospitalized, and Hospitalized Populations: A Cross-Sectional Study. *J. Clin. Med.* **2023**, *12*, 2613. [CrossRef] [PubMed]

20. Vibholm, L.K.; Nielsen, S.S.F.; Pahus, M.H.; Frattari, G.S.; Olesen, R.; Andersen, R.; Monrad, I.; Andersen, A.H.F.; Thomsen, M.M.; Konrad, C.V.; et al. SARS-CoV-2 Persistence Is Associated with Antigen-Specific CD8 T-Cell Responses. *EBioMedicine* **2021**, *64*, 103230. [CrossRef] [PubMed]

21. Ahamed, J.; Laurence, J. Long COVID Endotheliopathy: Hypothesized Mechanisms and Potential Therapeutic Approaches. *J. Clin. Investig.* **2022**, *132*, e161167. [CrossRef]

22. Glynne, P.; Tahmasebi, N.; Gant, V.; Gupta, R. Long COVID Following Mild SARS-CoV-2 Infection: Characteristic T Cell Alterations and Response to Antihistamines. *J. Investig. Med. Off. Publ. Am. Fed. Clin. Res.* **2022**, *70*, 61–67. [CrossRef]

23. Noonong, K.; Chatatikun, M.; Surinkaew, S.; Kotepui, M.; Hossain, R.; Bunluepuech, K.; Noothong, C.; Tedasen, A.; Klangbud, W.K.; Imai, M.; et al. Mitochondrial Oxidative Stress, Mitochondrial ROS Storms in Long COVID Pathogenesis. *Front. Immunol.* **2023**, *14*, 1275001. [CrossRef]

24. Zubchenko, S.; Kril, I.; Nadizhko, O.; Matsyura, O.; Chopyak, V. Herpesvirus Infections and Post-COVID-19 Manifestations: A Pilot Observational Study. *Rheumatol. Int.* **2022**, *42*, 1523–1530. [CrossRef] [PubMed]

25. Álvarez-Santacruz, C.; Tyrkalska, S.D.; Candel, S. The Microbiota in Long COVID. *Int. J. Mol. Sci.* **2024**, *25*, 1330. [CrossRef]

26. Talla, A.; Vasaikar, S.V.; Szeto, G.L.; Lemos, M.P.; Czartoski, J.L.; MacMillan, H.; Moodie, Z.; Cohen, K.W.; Fleming, L.B.; Thomson, Z.; et al. Persistent Serum Protein Signatures Define an Inflammatory Subcategory of Long COVID. *Nat. Commun.* **2023**, *14*, 3417. [CrossRef] [PubMed]

27. Su, Y.; Yuan, D.; Chen, D.G.; Ng, R.H.; Wang, K.; Choi, J.; Li, S.; Hong, S.; Zhang, R.; Xie, J.; et al. Multiple Early Factors Anticipate Post-Acute COVID-19 Sequelae. *Cell* **2022**, *185*, 881–895. [CrossRef]

28. Matschke, J.; Lütgehetmann, M.; Hagel, C.; Sperhake, J.P.; Schröder, A.S.; Edler, C.; Mushumba, H.; Fitzek, A.; Allweiss, L.; Dandri, M.; et al. Neuropathology of Patients with COVID-19 in Germany: A Post-Mortem Case Series. *Lancet Neurol.* **2020**, *19*, 919–929. [CrossRef] [PubMed]

29. Spudich, S.; Nath, A. Nervous System Consequences of COVID-19. *Science* **2022**, *375*, 267–269. [CrossRef] [PubMed]

30. Yong, S.J.; Halim, A.; Halim, M.; Ming, L.C.; Goh, K.W.; Alfaresi, M.; AlShehail, B.M.; Al Fares, M.A.; Alissa, M.; Sulaiman, T.; et al. Experimental Drugs in Randomized Controlled Trials for Long-COVID: What's in the Pipeline? A Systematic and Critical Review. *Expert Opin. Investig. Drugs* **2023**, *32*, 655–667. [CrossRef] [PubMed]

31. Khubber, S.; Hashemifesharaki, R.; Mohammadi, M.; Gharibzahedi, S.M.T. Garlic (*Allium Sativum* L.): A Potential Unique Therapeutic Food Rich in Organosulfur and Flavonoid Compounds to Fight with COVID-19. *Nutr. J.* **2020**, *19*, 124. [CrossRef]

32. Suresh, M.V.; Francis, S.; Aktay, S.; Kralovich, G.; Raghavendran, K. Therapeutic Potential of Curcumin in ARDS and COVID-19. *Clin. Exp. Pharmacol. Physiol.* **2023**, *50*, 267–276. [CrossRef]

33. Imran, M.; Khan, S.A.; Abida; Alshammari, M.K.; Alkhaldi, S.M.; Alshammari, F.N.; Kamal, M.; Alam, O.; Asdaq, S.M.B.; Alzahrani, A.K.; et al. *Nigella sativa* L. and COVID-19: A Glance at The Anti-COVID-19 Chemical Constituents, Clinical Trials, Inventions, and Patent Literature. *Molecules* **2022**, *27*, 2750. [CrossRef]

34. Pakkir Maideen, N.M.; Hassan Jumale, A.; Ramadan Barakat, I.; Khalifa Albasti, A. Potential of Black Seeds (*Nigella Sativa*) in the Management of Long COVID or Post-Acute Sequelae of COVID-19 (PASC) and Persistent COVID-19 Symptoms—An Insight. *Infect. Disord. Drug Targets* **2023**, *23*, e230223213955. [CrossRef]

35. Rathinavel, T.; Palanisamy, M.; Srinivasan, P.; Subramanian, A.; Thangaswamy, S. Phytochemical 6-Gingerol-A Promising Drug of Choice for COVID-19. *Int. J. Adv. Sci. Eng.* **2020**, *6*, 1482–1489. [CrossRef]

36. Ali, A.M.; Kunugi, H. Propolis, Bee Honey, and Their Components Protect against Coronavirus Disease 2019 (COVID-19): A Review of in Silico, in Vitro, and Clinical Studies. *Molecules* **2021**, *26*, 1232. [CrossRef] [PubMed]

37. Melrose, J.; Smith, M.M. Natural and Semi-Synthetic Flavonoid Anti-SARS-CoV-2 Agents for the Treatment of Long COVID-19 Disease and Neurodegenerative Disorders of Cognitive Decline. *Front. Biosci.* **2022**, *14*, 27. [CrossRef] [PubMed]

38. Rizzuti, B.; Ceballos-Laita, L.; Ortega-Alarcon, D.; Jimenez-Alesanco, A.; Vega, S.; Grande, F.; Conforti, F.; Abian, O.; Velazquez-Campoy, A. Sub-Micromolar Inhibition of SARS-CoV-2 3CLpro by Natural Compounds. *Pharmaceuticals* **2021**, *14*, 892. [CrossRef] [PubMed]

39. Marinaccio, L.; Stefanucci, A.; Scioli, G.; Della Valle, A.; Zengin, G.; Cichelli, A.; Mollica, A. Peptide Human Neutrophil Elastase Inhibitors from Natural Sources: An Overview. *Int. J. Mol. Sci.* **2022**, *23*, 2924. [CrossRef]

40. Bai, Y.; Peng, W.; Yang, C.; Zou, W.; Liu, M.; Wu, H.; Fan, L.; Li, P.; Zeng, X.; Su, W. Pharmacokinetics and Metabolism of Naringin and Active Metabolite Naringenin in Rats, Dogs, Humans, and the Differences between Species. *Front. Pharmacol.* **2020**, *11*, 364. [CrossRef] [PubMed]

41. Miles, E.A.; Calder, P.C. Effects of Citrus Fruit Juices and Their Bioactive Components on Inflammation and Immunity: A Narrative Review. *Front. Immunol.* **2021**, *12*, 712608. [CrossRef]

42. Stabrauskiene, J.; Kopustinskiene, D.M.; Lazauskas, R.; Bernatoniene, J. Naringin and Naringenin: Their Mechanisms of Action and the Potential Anticancer Activities. *Biomedicines* **2022**, *10*, 1686. [CrossRef]

43. Chen, X.; Xue, Y.; Jia, G.; Zhao, H.; Liu, G.; Huang, Z. Antifatigue Effect of Naringin on Improving Antioxidant Capacity and Mitochondrial Function and Preventing Muscle Damage. *Exp. Biol. Med.* **2022**, *247*, 1776–1784. [CrossRef] [PubMed]
44. Casacchia, T.; Occhiuzzi, M.A.; Grande, F.; Rizzuti, B.; Granieri, M.C.; Rocca, C.; Gattuso, A.; Garofalo, A.; Angelone, T.; Statti, G. A Pilot Study on the Nutraceutical Properties of the *Citrus* Hybrid Tacle® as a Dietary Source of Polyphenols for Supplementation in Metabolic Disorders. *J. Funct. Foods* **2019**, *52*, 370–381. [CrossRef]
45. Heidary Moghaddam, R.; Samimi, Z.; Moradi, S.Z.; Little, P.J.; Xu, S.; Farzaei, M.H. Naringenin and Naringin in Cardiovascular Disease Prevention: A Preclinical Review. *Eur. J. Pharmacol.* **2020**, *887*, 173535. [CrossRef] [PubMed]
46. AmeliMojarad, M.; AmeliMojarad, M. Interleukin-6 Inhibitory Effect of Natural Product Naringenin Compared to a Synthesised Monoclonal Antibody against Life-Threatening COVID-19. *Rev. Med. Virol.* **2023**, *33*, e2445. [CrossRef]
47. Agrawal, P.K.; Agrawal, C.; Blunden, G. Naringenin as a Possible Candidate against SARS-CoV-2 Infection and in the Pathogenesis of COVID-19. *Nat. Prod. Commun.* **2021**, *16*, 1934578X211066723. [CrossRef]
48. Tutunchi, H.; Naeini, F.; Ostadrahimi, A.; Hosseinzadeh-Attar, M.J. Naringenin, a Flavanone with Antiviral and Anti-inflammatory Effects: A Promising Treatment Strategy against COVID-19. *Phytother. Res.* **2020**, *34*, 3137–3147. [CrossRef] [PubMed]
49. Aleebrahim-Dehkordi, E.; Ghoshouni, H.; Koochaki, P.; Esmaili-Dehkordi, M.; Aleebrahim, E.; Chichagi, F.; Jafari, A.; Hanaei, S.; Heidari-Soureshjani, E.; Rezaei, N. Targeting the Vital Non-Structural Proteins (NSP12, NSP7, NSP8 and NSP3) from SARS-CoV-2 and Inhibition of RNA Polymerase by Natural Bioactive Compound Naringenin as a Promising Drug Candidate against COVID-19. *J. Mol. Struct.* **2023**, *1287*, 135642. [CrossRef]
50. Matias-Guiu, J.A.; Herrera, E.; González-Nosti, M.; Krishnan, K.; Delgado-Alonso, C.; Díez-Cirarda, M.; Yus, M.; Martínez-Petit, Á.; Pagán, J.; Matías-Guiu, J.; et al. Development of Criteria for Cognitive Dysfunction in Post-COVID Syndrome: The IC-CoDi-COVID Approach. *Psychiatry Res.* **2023**, *319*, 115006. [CrossRef]
51. Premraj, L.; Kannapadi, N.V.; Briggs, J.; Seal, S.M.; Battaglini, D.; Fanning, J.; Suen, J.; Robba, C.; Fraser, J.; Cho, S.-M. Mid and Long-Term Neurological and Neuropsychiatric Manifestations of Post-COVID-19 Syndrome: A Meta-Analysis. *J. Neurol. Sci.* **2022**, *434*, 120162. [CrossRef]
52. Reiss, A.B.; Greene, C.; Dayaramani, C.; Rauchman, S.H.; Stecker, M.M.; De Leon, J.; Pinkhasov, A. Long COVID, the Brain, Nerves, and Cognitive Function. *Neurol. Int.* **2023**, *15*, 821–841. [CrossRef]
53. Ceban, F.; Ling, S.; Lui, L.M.W.; Lee, Y.; Gill, H.; Teopiz, K.M.; Rodrigues, N.B.; Subramaniapillai, M.; Di Vincenzo, J.D.; Cao, B.; et al. Fatigue and Cognitive Impairment in Post-COVID-19 Syndrome: A Systematic Review and Meta-Analysis. *Brain Behav. Immun.* **2022**, *101*, 93–135. [CrossRef] [PubMed]
54. Zeng, N.; Zhao, Y.-M.; Yan, W.; Li, C.; Lu, Q.-D.; Liu, L.; Ni, S.-Y.; Mei, H.; Yuan, K.; Shi, L.; et al. A Systematic Review and Meta-Analysis of Long Term Physical and Mental Sequelae of COVID-19 Pandemic: Call for Research Priority and Action. *Mol. Psychiatry* **2023**, *28*, 423–433. [CrossRef] [PubMed]
55. Cheetham, N.J.; Penfold, R.; Giunchiglia, V.; Bowyer, V.; Sudre, C.H.; Canas, L.S.; Deng, J.; Murray, B.; Kerfoot, E.; Antonelli, M.; et al. The Effects of COVID-19 on Cognitive Performance in a Community-Based Cohort: A COVID Symptom Study Biobank Prospective Cohort Study. *EClinicalMedicine* **2023**, *62*, 102086. [CrossRef] [PubMed]
56. Wang, P.; Jin, L.; Zhang, M.; Wu, Y.; Duan, Z.; Guo, Y.; Wang, C.; Guo, Y.; Chen, W.; Liao, Z.; et al. Blood–Brain Barrier Injury and Neuroinflammation Induced by SARS-CoV-2 in a Lung–Brain Microphysiological System. *Nat. Biomed. Eng.* **2023**, 1–16. [CrossRef]
57. Soung, A.L.; Vanderheiden, A.; Nordvig, A.S.; Sissoko, C.A.; Canoll, P.; Mariani, M.B.; Jiang, X.; Bricker, T.; Rosoklija, G.B.; Arango, V.; et al. COVID-19 Induces CNS Cytokine Expression and Loss of Hippocampal Neurogenesis. *Brain* **2022**, *145*, 4193–4201. [CrossRef]
58. Yang, L.; Kim, T.W.; Han, Y.; Nair, M.S.; Harschnitz, O.; Zhu, J.; Wang, P.; Koo, S.Y.; Lacko, L.A.; Chandar, V.; et al. SARS-CoV-2 Infection Causes Dopaminergic Neuron Senescence. *Cell Stem Cell* **2024**, S1934590923004423. [CrossRef]
59. Kavanagh, E. Long COVID Brain Fog: A Neuroinflammation Phenomenon? *Oxf. Open Immunol.* **2022**, *3*, iqac007. [CrossRef]
60. Beurel, E.; Toups, M.; Nemeroff, C.B. The Bidirectional Relationship of Depression and Inflammation: Double Trouble. *Neuron* **2020**, *107*, 234–256. [CrossRef]
61. Leng, A.; Shah, M.; Ahmad, S.A.; Premraj, L.; Wildi, K.; Li Bassi, G.; Pardo, C.A.; Choi, A.; Cho, S.-M. Pathogenesis Underlying Neurological Manifestations of Long COVID Syndrome and Potential Therapeutics. *Cells* **2023**, *12*, 816. [CrossRef]
62. Pröbstel, A.-K.; Schirmer, L. SARS-CoV-2-Specific Neuropathology: Fact or Fiction? *Trends Neurosci.* **2021**, *44*, 933–935. [CrossRef]
63. Cantuti-Castelvetri, L.; Ojha, R.; Pedro, L.D.; Djannatian, M.; Franz, J.; Kuivanen, S.; van der Meer, F.; Kallio, K.; Kaya, T.; Anastasina, M.; et al. Neuropilin-1 Facilitates SARS-CoV-2 Cell Entry and Infectivity. *Science* **2020**, *370*, 856–860. [CrossRef] [PubMed]
64. Quan, M.; Wang, X.; Gong, M.; Wang, Q.; Li, Y.; Jia, J. Post-COVID Cognitive Dysfunction: Current Status and Research Recommendations for High Risk Population. *Lancet Reg. Health West. Pac.* **2023**, *38*, 100836. [CrossRef] [PubMed]
65. Hugon, J.; Msika, E.-F.; Queneau, M.; Farid, K.; Paquet, C. Long COVID: Cognitive Complaints (Brain Fog) and Dysfunction of the Cingulate Cortex. *J. Neurol.* **2022**, *269*, 44–46. [CrossRef] [PubMed]
66. Wong, A.C.; Devason, A.S.; Umana, I.C.; Cox, T.O.; Dohnalová, L.; Litichevskiy, L.; Perla, J.; Lundgren, P.; Etwebi, Z.; Izzo, L.T.; et al. Serotonin Reduction in Post-Acute Sequelae of Viral Infection. *Cell* **2023**, *186*, 4851–4867. [CrossRef] [PubMed]
67. Kwatra, M.; Kumar, V.; Jangra, A.; Mishra, M.; Ahmed, S.; Ghosh, P.; Vohora, D.; Khanam, R. Ameliorative Effect of Naringin against Doxorubicin-Induced Acute Cardiac Toxicity in Rats. *Pharm. Biol.* **2016**, *54*, 637–647. [CrossRef] [PubMed]

68. Nouri, Z.; Fakhri, S.; El-Senduny, F.F.; Sanadgol, N.; Abd-ElGhani, G.E.; Farzaei, M.H.; Chen, J.-T. On the Neuroprotective Effects of Naringenin: Pharmacological Targets, Signaling Pathways, Molecular Mechanisms, and Clinical Perspective. *Biomolecules* **2019**, *9*, 690. [CrossRef] [PubMed]

69. Li, L.; Liu, R.; He, J.; Li, J.; Guo, J.; Chen, Y.; Ji, K. Naringin Regulates Microglia BV-2 Activation and Inflammation via the JAK/STAT3 Pathway. *Evid.-Based Complement. Altern. Med.* **2022**, *2022*, 3492058. [CrossRef] [PubMed]

70. Liddell, J.R. Are Astrocytes the Predominant Cell Type for Activation of Nrf2 in Aging and Neurodegeneration? *Antioxidants* **2017**, *6*, 65. [CrossRef]

71. Wang, G.-Q.; Zhang, B.; He, X.-M.; Li, D.-D.; Shi, J.-S.; Zhang, F. Naringenin Targets on Astroglial Nrf2 to Support Dopaminergic Neurons. *Pharmacol. Res.* **2019**, *139*, 452–459. [CrossRef]

72. Salman, M.; Sharma, P.; Alam, M.d.I.; Tabassum, H.; Parvez, S. Naringenin Mitigates Behavioral Alterations and Provides Neuroprotection against 3-Nitropropinoic Acid-Induced Huntington's Disease like Symptoms in Rats. *Nutr. Neurosci.* **2022**, *25*, 1898–1908. [CrossRef]

73. Zhang, J.; Zhang, Y.; Liu, Y.; Niu, X. Naringenin Attenuates Cognitive Impairment in a Rat Model of Vascular Dementia by Inhibiting Hippocampal Oxidative Stress and Inflammatory Response and Promoting N-Methyl-D-Aspartate Receptor Signaling Pathway. *Neurochem. Res.* **2022**, *47*, 3402–3413. [CrossRef] [PubMed]

74. Kumar, A.; Prakash, A.; Dogra, S. Naringin Alleviates Cognitive Impairment, Mitochondrial Dysfunction and Oxidative Stress Induced by D-Galactose in Mice. *Food Chem. Toxicol. Int. J. Publ. Br. Ind. Biol. Res. Assoc.* **2010**, *48*, 626–632. [CrossRef] [PubMed]

75. Kwatra, M.; Jangra, A.; Mishra, M.; Sharma, Y.; Ahmed, S.; Ghosh, P.; Kumar, V.; Vohora, D.; Khanam, R. Naringin and Sertraline Ameliorate Doxorubicin-Induced Behavioral Deficits through Modulation of Serotonin Level and Mitochondrial Complexes Protection Pathway in Rat Hippocampus. *Neurochem. Res.* **2016**, *41*, 2352–2366. [CrossRef] [PubMed]

76. Mahdavinia, M.; Ahangarpour, A.; Zeidooni, L.; Samimi, A.; Alizadeh, S.; Dehghani, M.A.; Alboghobeish, S. Protective Effect of Naringin on Bisphenol A-Induced Cognitive Dysfunction and Oxidative Damage in Rats. *Int. J. Mol. Cell. Med.* **2019**, *8*, 141–153. [CrossRef] [PubMed]

77. Mansour, L.A.H.; Elshopakey, G.E.; Abdelhamid, F.M.; Albukhari, T.A.; Almehmadi, S.J.; Refaat, B.; El-Boshy, M.; Risha, E.F. Hepatoprotective and Neuroprotective Effects of Naringenin against Lead-Induced Oxidative Stress, Inflammation, and Apoptosis in Rats. *Biomedicines* **2023**, *11*, 1080. [CrossRef] [PubMed]

78. Phillips, C. Brain-Derived Neurotrophic Factor, Depression, and Physical Activity: Making the Neuroplastic Connection. *Neural. Plast.* **2017**, *2017*, 7260130. [CrossRef]

79. Esvald, E.-E.; Tuvikene, J.; Sirp, A.; Patil, S.; Bramham, C.R.; Timmusk, T. CREB Family Transcription Factors Are Major Mediators of BDNF Transcriptional Autoregulation in Cortical Neurons. *J. Neurosci.* **2020**, *40*, 1405–1426. [CrossRef] [PubMed]

80. Zhang, L.; Lu, R.-R.; Xu, R.-H.; Wang, H.-H.; Feng, W.-S.; Zheng, X.-K. Naringenin and Apigenin Ameliorates Corticosterone-Induced Depressive Behaviors. *Heliyon* **2023**, *9*, e15618. [CrossRef]

81. Yi, L.-T.; Li, J.; Li, H.-C.; Su, D.-X.; Quan, X.-B.; He, X.-C.; Wang, X.-H. Antidepressant-like Behavioral, Neurochemical and Neuroendocrine Effects of Naringenin in the Mouse Repeated Tail Suspension Test. *Prog. Neuropsychopharmacol. Biol. Psychiatry* **2012**, *39*, 175–181. [CrossRef]

82. Jain, A.S.; Sushma, P.; Dharmashekar, C.; Beelagi, M.S.; Prasad, S.K.; Shivamallu, C.; Prasad, A.; Syed, A.; Marraiki, N.; Prasad, K.S. In Silico Evaluation of Flavonoids as Effective Antiviral Agents on the Spike Glycoprotein of SARS-CoV-2. *Saudi J. Biol. Sci.* **2021**, *28*, 1040–1051. [CrossRef]

83. Sette, A.; Crotty, S. Adaptive Immunity to SARS-CoV-2 and COVID-19. *Cell* **2021**, *184*, 861–880. [CrossRef]

84. Davis, H.E.; McCorkell, L.; Vogel, J.M.; Topol, E.J. Long COVID: Major Findings, Mechanisms and Recommendations. *Nat. Rev. Microbiol.* **2023**, *21*, 133–146. [CrossRef] [PubMed]

85. Klein, J.; Wood, J.; Jaycox, J.R.; Dhodapkar, R.M.; Lu, P.; Gehlhausen, J.R.; Tabachnikova, A.; Greene, K.; Tabacof, L.; Malik, A.A.; et al. Distinguishing Features of Long COVID Identified through Immune Profiling. *Nature* **2023**, *623*, 139–148. [CrossRef] [PubMed]

86. Cheong, J.-G.; Ravishankar, A.; Sharma, S.; Parkhurst, C.N.; Grassmann, S.A.; Wingert, C.K.; Laurent, P.; Ma, S.; Paddock, L.; Miranda, I.C.; et al. Epigenetic Memory of Coronavirus Infection in Innate Immune Cells and Their Progenitors. *Cell* **2023**, *186*, 3882–3902.e24. [CrossRef] [PubMed]

87. Fogarty, H.; Ward, S.E.; Townsend, L.; Karampini, E.; Elliott, S.; Conlon, N.; Dunne, J.; Kiersey, R.; Naughton, A.; Gardiner, M.; et al. Sustained VWF-ADAMTS-13 Axis Imbalance and Endotheliopathy in Long COVID Syndrome Is Related to Immune Dysfunction. *J. Thromb. Haemost.* **2022**, *20*, 2429–2438. [CrossRef] [PubMed]

88. Townsend, L.; Dyer, A.H.; Naughton, A.; Kiersey, R.; Holden, D.; Gardiner, M.; Dowds, J.; O'Brien, K.; Bannan, C.; Nadarajan, P.; et al. Longitudinal Analysis of COVID-19 Patients Shows Age-Associated T Cell Changes Independent of Ongoing Ill-Health. *Front. Immunol.* **2021**, *12*, 676932. [CrossRef] [PubMed]

89. Phetsouphanh, C.; Darley, D.R.; Wilson, D.B.; Howe, A.; Munier, C.M.L.; Patel, S.K.; Juno, J.A.; Burrell, L.M.; Kent, S.J.; Dore, G.J.; et al. Immunological Dysfunction Persists for 8 Months Following Initial Mild-to-Moderate SARS-CoV-2 Infection. *Nat. Immunol.* **2022**, *23*, 210–216. [CrossRef] [PubMed]

90. Sumi, T.; Harada, K. Immune Response to SARS-CoV-2 in Severe Disease and Long COVID-19. *iScience* **2022**, *25*, 104723. [CrossRef] [PubMed]

91. Gruber, C.N.; Patel, R.S.; Trachtman, R.; Lepow, L.; Amanat, F.; Krammer, F.; Wilson, K.M.; Onel, K.; Geanon, D.; Tuballes, K.; et al. Mapping Systemic Inflammation and Antibody Responses in Multisystem Inflammatory Syndrome in Children (Mis-c). *Cell* **2020**, *183*, 982–995. [CrossRef]

92. Wang, E.Y.; Mao, T.; Klein, J.; Dai, Y.; Huck, J.D.; Jaycox, J.R.; Liu, F.; Zhou, T.; Israelow, B.; Wong, P.; et al. Diverse Functional Autoantibodies in Patients with COVID-19. *Nature* **2021**, *595*, 283–288. [CrossRef] [PubMed]

93. Wallukat, G.; Hohberger, B.; Wenzel, K.; Fürst, J.; Schulze-Rothe, S.; Wallukat, A.; Hönicke, A.-S.; Müller, J. Functional Autoantibodies against G-Protein Coupled Receptors in Patients with Persistent Long-COVID-19 Symptoms. *J. Transl. Autoimmun.* **2021**, *4*, 100100. [CrossRef]

94. Novelli, L.; Motta, F.; De Santis, M.; Ansari, A.A.; Gershwin, M.E.; Selmi, C. The JANUS of Chronic Inflammatory and Autoimmune Diseases Onset during COVID-19—A Systematic Review of the Literature. *J. Autoimmun.* **2021**, *117*, 102592. [CrossRef]

95. Liu, Z.; Niu, X.; Wang, J. Naringenin as a Natural Immunomodulator against T Cell-Mediated Autoimmune Diseases: Literature Review and Network-Based Pharmacology Study. *Crit. Rev. Food Sci. Nutr.* **2022**, *63*, 11026–11043. [CrossRef]

96. Wang, H.-K.; Yeh, C.-H.; Iwamoto, T.; Satsu, H.; Shimizu, M.; Totsuka, M. Dietary Flavonoid Naringenin Induces Regulatory T Cells via an Aryl Hydrocarbon Receptor Mediated Pathway. *J. Agric. Food Chem.* **2012**, *60*, 2171–2178. [CrossRef]

97. Zhu, J.; Yamane, H.; Paul, W.E. Differentiation of Effector CD4 T Cell Populations. *Annu. Rev. Immunol.* **2010**, *28*, 445–489. [CrossRef] [PubMed]

98. Niu, X.; Wu, C.; Li, M.; Zhao, Q.; Meydani, S.N.; Wang, J.; Wu, D. Naringenin Is an Inhibitor of T Cell Effector Functions. *J. Nutr. Biochem.* **2018**, *58*, 71–79. [CrossRef] [PubMed]

99. Wang, J.; Niu, X.; Wu, C.; Wu, D. Naringenin Modifies the Development of Lineage-Specific Effector CD4+ t Cells. *Front. Immunol.* **2018**, *9*, 2267. [CrossRef]

100. Jiang, Y.-P.; Wen, J.-J.; Zhao, X.-X.; Gao, Y.-C.; Ma, X.; Song, S.-Y.; Jin, Y.; Shao, T.-J.; Yu, J.; Wen, C.-P. The Flavonoid Naringenin Alleviates Collagen-Induced Arthritis through Curbing the Migration and Polarization of Cd4+ t Lymphocyte Driven by Regulating Mitochondrial Fission. *Int. J. Mol. Sci.* **2022**, *24*, 279. [CrossRef]

101. Abrego-Peredo, A.; Romero-Ramírez, H.; Espinosa, E.; López-Herrera, G.; García-García, F.; Flores-Muñoz, M.; Sandoval-Montes, C.; Rodríguez-Alba, J.C. Naringenin Mitigates Autoimmune Features in Lupus-Prone Mice by Modulation of T-Cell Subsets and Cytokines Profile. *PLoS ONE* **2020**, *15*, e0233138. [CrossRef]

102. Wang, J.; Qi, Y.; Niu, X.; Tang, H.; Meydani, S.N.; Wu, D. Dietary Naringenin Supplementation Attenuates Experimental Autoimmune Encephalomyelitis by Modulating Autoimmune Inflammatory Responses in Mice. *J. Nutr. Biochem.* **2018**, *54*, 130–139. [CrossRef] [PubMed]

103. Zeng, W.; Jin, L.; Zhang, F.; Zhang, C.; Liang, W. Naringenin as a Potential Immunomodulator in Therapeutics. *Pharmacol. Res.* **2018**, *135*, 122–126. [CrossRef] [PubMed]

104. Jin, L.; Zeng, W.; Zhang, F.; Zhang, C.; Liang, W. Naringenin Ameliorates Acute Inflammation by Regulating Intracellular Cytokine Degradation. *J. Immunol.* **2017**, *199*, 3466–3477. [CrossRef] [PubMed]

105. Yeoh, Y.K.; Zuo, T.; Lui, G.C.-Y.; Zhang, F.; Liu, Q.; Li, A.Y.; Chung, A.C.; Cheung, C.P.; Tso, E.Y.; Fung, K.S.; et al. Gut Microbiota Composition Reflects Disease Severity and Dysfunctional Immune Responses in Patients with COVID-19. *Gut* **2021**, *70*, 698–706. [CrossRef] [PubMed]

106. Zhang, F.; Lau, R.I.; Liu, Q.; Su, Q.; Chan, F.K.L.; Ng, S.C. Gut Microbiota in COVID-19: Key Microbial Changes, Potential Mechanisms and Clinical Applications. *Nat. Rev. Gastroenterol. Hepatol.* **2023**, *20*, 323–337. [CrossRef] [PubMed]

107. de Ana Patrícia, O.; Lopes, A.L.F.; Pacheco, G.; de Sá Guimarães Nolêto, I.R.; Nicolau, L.A.D.; Medeiros, J.V.R. Premises among SARS-CoV-2, Dysbiosis and Diarrhea: Walking through the ACE2/mTOR/Autophagy Route. *Med. Hypotheses* **2020**, *144*, 110243. [CrossRef]

108. Gu, S.; Chen, Y.; Wu, Z.; Chen, Y.; Gao, H.; Lv, L.; Guo, F.; Zhang, X.; Luo, R.; Huang, C.; et al. Alterations of the Gut Microbiota in Patients with COVID-19 or H1n1 Influenza. *Clin. Infect. Dis. Off. Publ. Infect. Dis. Soc. Am.* **2020**, *71*, ciaa709. [CrossRef]

109. Zhong, H.; Wang, Y.; Shi, Z.; Zhang, L.; Ren, H.; He, W.; Zhang, Z.; Zhu, A.; Zhao, J.; Xiao, F.; et al. Characterization of Respiratory Microbial Dysbiosis in Hospitalized COVID-19 Patients. *Cell Discov.* **2021**, *7*, 23. [CrossRef]

110. Soffritti, I.; D'Accolti, M.; Fabbri, C.; Passaro, A.; Manfredini, R.; Zuliani, G.; Libanore, M.; Franchi, M.; Contini, C.; Caselli, E. Oral Microbiome Dysbiosis Is Associated with Symptoms Severity and Local Immune/Inflammatory Response in COVID-19 Patients: A Cross-Sectional Study. *Front. Microbiol.* **2021**, *12*, 687513. [CrossRef]

111. Nardelli, C.; Gentile, I.; Setaro, M.; Di Domenico, C.; Pinchera, B.; Buonomo, A.R.; Zappulo, E.; Scotto, R.; Scaglione, G.L.; Castaldo, G.; et al. Nasopharyngeal Microbiome Signature in COVID-19 Positive Patients: Can We Definitively Get a Role to *Fusobacterium Periodonticum*? *Front. Cell. Infect. Microbiol.* **2021**, *11*, 625581. [CrossRef]

112. Chen, Y.; Gu, S.; Chen, Y.; Lu, H.; Shi, D.; Guo, J.; Wu, W.-R.; Yang, Y.; Li, Y.; Xu, K.-J.; et al. Six-Month Follow-up of Gut Microbiota Richness in Patients with COVID-19. *Gut* **2022**, *71*, 222–225. [CrossRef] [PubMed]

113. Zhou, Y.; Zhang, J.; Zhang, D.; Ma, W.-L.; Wang, X. Linking the Gut Microbiota to Persistent Symptoms in Survivors of COVID-19 after Discharge. *J. Microbiol.* **2021**, *59*, 941–948. [CrossRef] [PubMed]

114. Nagata, N.; Takeuchi, T.; Masuoka, H.; Aoki, R.; Ishikane, M.; Iwamoto, N.; Sugiyama, M.; Suda, W.; Nakanishi, Y.; Terada-Hirashima, J.; et al. Human Gut Microbiota and Its Metabolites Impact Immune Responses in COVID-19 and Its Complications. *Gastroenterology* **2023**, *164*, 272–288. [CrossRef] [PubMed]

115. de Gislane Lelis Vilela, O.; Oliveira, C.N.S.; Pinzan, C.F.; de Salis, L.V.V.; Cardoso, C.R.d.B. Microbiota Modulation of the Gut-Lung Axis in COVID-19. *Front. Immunol.* **2021**, *12*, 635471. [CrossRef]
116. Chen, J.; Vitetta, L. The Role of the Gut-Lung Axis in COVID-19 Infections and Its Modulation to Improve Clinical Outcomes. *Front. Biosci. Sch. Ed.* **2022**, *14*, 23. [CrossRef] [PubMed]
117. Carloni, S.; Bertocchi, A.; Mancinelli, S.; Bellini, M.; Erreni, M.; Borreca, A.; Braga, D.; Giugliano, S.; Mozzarelli, A.M.; Manganaro, D.; et al. Identification of a Choroid Plexus Vascular Barrier Closing during Intestinal Inflammation. *Science* **2021**, *374*, 439–448. [CrossRef] [PubMed]
118. Feng, W.; Ao, H.; Peng, C.; Yan, D. Gut Microbiota, a New Frontier to Understand Traditional Chinese Medicines. *Pharmacol. Res.* **2019**, *142*, 176–191. [CrossRef] [PubMed]
119. Cheng, H.; Zhang, D.; Wu, J.; Liu, J.; Zhou, Y.; Tan, Y.; Feng, W.; Peng, C. Interactions between Gut Microbiota and Polyphenols: A Mechanistic and Metabolomic Review. *Phytomedicine Int. J. Phytother. Phytopharm.* **2023**, *119*, 154979. [CrossRef]
120. Li, P.; Yao, X.; Zhou, Q.; Meng, X.; Zhou, T.; Gu, Q. Citrus Peel Flavonoid Extracts: Health-Beneficial Bioactivities and Regulation of Intestinal Microecology in Vitro. *Front. Nutr.* **2022**, *9*, 888745. [CrossRef]
121. Pan, L.; Ye, H.; Pi, X.; Liu, W.; Wang, Z.; Zhang, Y.; Zheng, J. Effects of Several Flavonoids on Human Gut Microbiota and Its Metabolism by in Vitro Simulated Fermentation. *Front. Microbiol.* **2023**, *14*, 1092729. [CrossRef]
122. Firrman, J.; Liu, L.; Argoty, G.A.; Zhang, L.; Tomasula, P.; Wang, M.; Pontious, S.; Kobori, M.; Xiao, W. Analysis of Temporal Changes in Growth and Gene Expression for Commensal Gut Microbes in Response to the Polyphenol Naringenin. *Microbiol. Insights* **2018**, *11*, 1178636118775100. [CrossRef]
123. Sun, Z.; Song, Z.-G.; Liu, C.; Tan, S.; Lin, S.; Zhu, J.; Dai, F.-H.; Gao, J.; She, J.-L.; Mei, Z.; et al. Gut Microbiome Alterations and Gut Barrier Dysfunction Are Associated with Host Immune Homeostasis in COVID-19 Patients. *BMC Med.* **2022**, *20*, 24. [CrossRef]
124. Wu, X.; Guo, H.; Pan, X.; Huang, R.; Wang, G.; Liu, J. Naringin Exhibited Therapeutic Effects against DSS-Induced Mice Ulcerative Colitis in Intestinal Barrier–Dependent Manner. *Molecules* **2021**, *26*, 6604. [CrossRef]
125. Rasa, S.; Nora-Krukle, Z.; Henning, N.; Eliassen, E.; Shikova, E.; Harrer, T.; Scheibenbogen, C.; Murovska, M.; Prusty, B.K. Chronic Viral Infections in Myalgic Encephalomyelitis/Chronic Fatigue Syndrome (ME/CFS). *J. Transl. Med.* **2018**, *16*, 268. [CrossRef]
126. Renz-Polster, H.; Scheibenbogen, C. Post-COVID-Syndrom Mit Fatigue Und Belastungsintoleranz: Myalgische Enzephalomyelitis Bzw. Chronisches Fatigue-Syndrom. *Inn. Med.* **2022**, *63*, 830–839. [CrossRef]
127. Komaroff, A.L.; Lipkin, W.I. ME/CFS and Long COVID Share Similar Symptoms and Biological Abnormalities: Road Map to the Literature. *Front. Med.* **2023**, *10*, 1187163. [CrossRef] [PubMed]
128. Komaroff, A.L.; Bateman, L. Will COVID-19 Lead to Myalgic Encephalomyelitis/Chronic Fatigue Syndrome? *Front. Med.* **2021**, *7*, 606824. [CrossRef] [PubMed]
129. Lv, Y.; Zhang, T.; Cai, J.; Huang, C.; Zhan, S.; Liu, J. Bioinformatics and Systems Biology Approach to Identify the Pathogenetic Link of Long COVID and Myalgic Encephalomyelitis/Chronic Fatigue Syndrome. *Front. Immunol.* **2022**, *13*, 952987. [CrossRef]
130. Bonilla, H.; Quach, T.C.; Tiwari, A.; Bonilla, A.E.; Miglis, M.; Yang, P.C.; Eggert, L.E.; Sharifi, H.; Horomanski, A.; Subramanian, A.; et al. Myalgic Encephalomyelitis/Chronic Fatigue Syndrome Is Common in Post-Acute Sequelae of SARS-CoV-2 Infection (PASC): Results from a Post-COVID-19 Multidisciplinary Clinic. *Front. Neurol.* **2023**, *14*, 1090747. [CrossRef]
131. Yang, Y.; Wu, Y.; Meng, X.; Wang, Z.; Younis, M.; Liu, Y.; Wang, P.; Huang, X. SARS-CoV-2 Membrane Protein Causes the Mitochondrial Apoptosis and Pulmonary Edema via Targeting BOK. *Cell Death Differ.* **2022**, *29*, 1395–1408. [CrossRef]
132. Díaz-Resendiz, K.J.G.; Benitez-Trinidad, A.B.; Covantes-Rosales, C.E.; Toledo-Ibarra, G.A.; Ortiz-Lazareno, P.C.; Girón-Pérez, D.A.; Bueno-Durán, A.Y.; Pérez-Díaz, D.A.; Barcelos-García, R.G.; Girón-Pérez, M.I. Loss of Mitochondrial Membrane Potential ($\Delta\Psi$ m) in Leucocytes as post-COVID-19 Sequelae. *J. Leukoc. Biol.* **2022**, *112*, 23–29. [CrossRef]
133. Miller, B.; Silverstein, A.; Flores, M.; Cao, K.; Kumagai, H.; Mehta, H.H.; Yen, K.; Kim, S.-J.; Cohen, P. Host Mitochondrial Transcriptome Response to SARS-CoV-2 in Multiple Cell Models and Clinical Samples. *Sci. Rep.* **2021**, *11*, 3. [CrossRef]
134. Appelman, B.; Charlton, B.T.; Goulding, R.P.; Kerkhoff, T.J.; Breedveld, E.A.; Noort, W.; Offringa, C.; Bloemers, F.W.; Van Weeghel, M.; Schomakers, B.V.; et al. Muscle Abnormalities Worsen after Post-Exertional Malaise in Long COVID. *Nat. Commun.* **2024**, *15*, 17. [CrossRef]
135. Chaves-Filho, A.M.; Braniff, O.; Angelova, A.; Deng, Y.; Tremblay, M.-È. Chronic Inflammation, Neuroglial Dysfunction, and Plasmalogen Deficiency as a New Pathobiological Hypothesis Addressing the Overlap between Post-COVID-19 Symptoms and Myalgic Encephalomyelitis/Chronic Fatigue Syndrome. *Brain Res. Bull.* **2023**, *201*, 110702. [CrossRef]
136. Komaroff, A.L.; Lipkin, W.I. Insights from Myalgic Encephalomyelitis/Chronic Fatigue Syndrome May Help Unravel the Pathogenesis of Postacute COVID-19 Syndrome. *Trends Mol. Med.* **2021**, *27*, 895–906. [CrossRef] [PubMed]
137. Paul, B.D.; Lemle, M.D.; Komaroff, A.L.; Snyder, S.H. Redox Imbalance Links COVID-19 and Myalgic Encephalomyelitis/Chronic Fatigue Syndrome. *Proc. Natl. Acad. Sci. USA* **2021**, *118*, e2024358118. [CrossRef] [PubMed]
138. Toogood, P.L.; Clauw, D.J.; Phadke, S.; Hoffman, D. Myalgic Encephalomyelitis/Chronic Fatigue Syndrome (ME/CFS): Where Will the Drugs Come From? *Pharmacol. Res.* **2021**, *165*, 105465. [CrossRef] [PubMed]
139. Zamanian, M.; Hajizadeh, M.; Shamsizadeh, A.; Moemenzadeh, M.; Amirteimouri, M.; Elshiekh, M.; Allahtavakoli, M. Effects of Naringin on Physical Fatigue and Serum MMP-9 Concentration in Female Rats. *Pharm. Biol.* **2016**, *55*, 423–427. [CrossRef] [PubMed]

140. Balachandran, A.; Choi, S.B.; Beata, M.-M.; Małgorzata, J.; Froemming, G.R.A.; Lavilla, C.A.; Billacura, M.P.; Siyumbwa, S.N.; Okechukwu, P.N. Antioxidant, Wound Healing Potential and in Silico Assessment of Naringin, Eicosane and Octacosane. *Molecules* **2023**, *28*, 1043. [CrossRef] [PubMed]

141. Li, X.; Deng, S.; Li, J.; Gong, S.; Song, T.; Ge, J.; Zhao, Y.; Zhang, J.; Ma, L.; Zheng, Y.; et al. UPLC-MS Analysis and Network Pharmacology-Based Investigation into the Active Ingredients and Molecular Mechanisms of Anti-Fatigue of Male Flowers with Eucommia Ulmoides Oliv. *Fundam. Clin. Pharmacol.* **2022**, *36*, 1083–1098. [CrossRef] [PubMed]

142. Kulasekaran, G.; Ganapasam, S. Neuroprotective Efficacy of Naringin on 3-Nitropropionic Acid-Induced Mitochondrial Dysfunction through the Modulation of Nrf2 Signaling Pathway in PC12 Cells. *Mol. Cell. Biochem.* **2015**, *409*, 199–211. [CrossRef] [PubMed]

143. Varshney, V.; Garabadu, D. Naringin Exhibits Mas Receptor–Mediated Neuroprotection against Amyloid Beta–Induced Cognitive Deficits and Mitochondrial Toxicity in Rat Brain. *Neurotox. Res.* **2021**, *39*, 1023–1043. [CrossRef] [PubMed]

144. Wang, K.; Chen, Z.; Huang, L.; Meng, B.; Zhou, X.; Wen, X.; Ren, D. Naringenin Reduces Oxidative Stress and Improves Mitochondrial Dysfunction via Activation of the Nrf2/ARE Signaling Pathway in Neurons. *Int. J. Mol. Med.* **2017**, *40*, 1582–1590. [CrossRef] [PubMed]

145. Vij, G.; Gupta, A.; Chopra, K. Modulation of Antigen-Induced Chronic Fatigue in Mouse Model of Water Immersion Stress by Naringin, a Polyphenolic Antioxidant. *Fundam. Clin. Pharmacol.* **2009**, *23*, 331–337. [CrossRef] [PubMed]

146. Viswanatha, G.L.; Shylaja, H.; Moolemath, Y. The Beneficial Role of Naringin- a Citrus Bioflavonoid, against Oxidative Stress-Induced Neurobehavioral Disorders and Cognitive Dysfunction in Rodents: A Systematic Review and Meta-Analysis. *Biomed. Pharmacother.* **2017**, *94*, 909–929. [CrossRef] [PubMed]

147. Xie, Y.; Xu, E.; Bowe, B.; Al-Aly, Z. Long-Term Cardiovascular Outcomes of COVID-19. *Nat. Med.* **2022**, *28*, 583–590. [CrossRef]

148. Huseynov, A.; Akin, I.; Duerschmied, D.; Scharf, R.E. Cardiac Arrhythmias in Post-COVID Syndrome: Prevalence, Pathology, Diagnosis, and Treatment. *Viruses* **2023**, *15*, 389. [CrossRef]

149. Guo, B.; Zhao, C.; He, M.Z.; Senter, C.; Zhou, Z.; Peng, J.; Li, S.; Fitzpatrick, A.L.; Lindström, S.; Stebbins, R.C.; et al. Identifying Patterns of Reported Findings on Long-Term Cardiac Complications of COVID-19: A Systematic Review and Meta-Analysis. *BMC Med.* **2023**, *21*, 468. [CrossRef]

150. Szarpak, L.; Pruc, M.; Filipiak, K.J.; Popieluch, J.; Bielski, A.; Jaguszewski, M.J.; Gilis-Malinowska, N.; Chirico, F.; Afique, Z.R.; Peacock, F.W. Myocarditis: A Complication of COVID-19 and Long-COVID-19 Syndrome as a Serious Threat in Modern Cardiology. *Cardiol. J.* **2022**, *29*, 178–179. [CrossRef]

151. Zuin, M.; Rigatelli, G.; Bilato, C.; Porcari, A.; Merlo, M.; Roncon, L.; Sinagra, G. One-Year Risk of Myocarditis after COVID-19 Infection: A Systematic Review and Meta-Analysis. *Can. J. Cardiol.* **2023**, *39*, 839–844. [CrossRef] [PubMed]

152. Sattar, Y.; Sandhyavenu, H.; Patel, N.; Victor, V.; Patel, D.; Hussain, B.; Titus, A.; Thyagaturu, H.; Alraiyes, M.; Atti, L.; et al. In-Hospital Outcomes of COVID-19 Associated Myocarditis (from a Nationwide Inpatient Sample Database Study). *Am. J. Cardiol.* **2023**, *192*, 39–44. [CrossRef]

153. Okor, I.; Bob-Manuel, T.; Price, J.; Sleem, A.; Amoran, O.; Kelly, J.; Ekerete, M.F.; Bamghose, M.O.; Bolaji, O.A.; Krim, S.R. COVID-19 Myocarditis: An Emerging Clinical Conundrum. *Curr. Probl. Cardiol.* **2022**, *47*, 101268. [CrossRef]

154. Elseidy, S.A.; Awad, A.K.; Vorla, M.; Fatima, A.; Elbadawy, M.A.; Mandal, D.; Mohamad, T. Cardiovascular Complications in the Post-Acute COVID-19 Syndrome (Pacs). *Int. J. Cardiol. Heart Vasc.* **2022**, *40*, 101012. [CrossRef] [PubMed]

155. Silva, L.S.; Boldrini, V.O.; Marques, A.M.; Yasuda, C.L. Post-COVID Myocarditis with Antiheart Antibodies Persistence: Clues for Autoimmunity? *Clin. Cardiol.* **2023**, *46*, 350–351. [CrossRef] [PubMed]

156. Chang, X.; Ismail, N.I.; Rahman, A.; Xu, D.; Chan, R.W.Y.; Ong, S.-G.; Ong, S.-B. Long COVID-19 and the Heart: Is Cardiac Mitochondria the Missing Link? *Antioxid. Redox Signal.* **2023**, *38*, 599–618. [CrossRef]

157. Naeem, A.; Tabassum, S.; Gill, S.; Khan, M.Z.; Mumtaz, N.; Qaiser, Q.; Karamat, M.; Arif, M.; Naeem, F.; Afifi, A.; et al. COVID-19 and Cardiovascular Diseases: A Literature Review from Pathogenesis to Diagnosis. *Cureus* **2023**, *15*, e35658. [CrossRef]

158. Sun, L.-J.; Qiao, W.; Xiao, Y.-J.; Cui, L.; Wang, X.; Ren, W.-D. Naringin Mitigates Myocardial Strain and the Inflammatory Response in Sepsis-Induced Myocardial Dysfunction through Regulation of PI3K/AKT/NF-κB Pathway. *Int. Immunopharmacol.* **2019**, *75*, 105782. [CrossRef]

159. Li, S.-H.; Ma, G.-L.; Zhang, S.-L.; Yang, Y.-Y.; Liu, H.-F.; Luo, A.; Wen, J.; Cao, Z.-Z.; Jia, Y.-Z. Naringin Exerts Antiarrhythmic Effects by Inhibiting Channel Currents in Mouse Cardiomyocytes. *J. Electrocardiol.* **2023**, *80*, 69–80. [CrossRef]

160. Stewart, I.; Jacob, J.; George, P.M.; Molyneaux, P.L.; Porter, J.C.; Allen, R.J.; Aslani, S.; Baillie, J.K.; Barratt, S.L.; Beirne, P.; et al. Residual Lung Abnormalities after COVID-19 Hospitalization: Interim Analysis of the UKILD Post–COVID-19 Study. *Am. J. Respir. Crit. Care Med.* **2023**, *207*, 693–703. [CrossRef]

161. Farghaly, S.; Badedi, M.; Ibrahim, R.; Sadhan, M.H.; Alamoudi, A.; Alnami, A.; Muhajir, A. Clinical Characteristics and Outcomes of Post-COVID-19 Pulmonary Fibrosis. *Medicine* **2022**, *101*, e28639. [CrossRef]

162. Espín, E.; Yang, C.; Shannon, C.P.; Assadian, S.; He, D.; Tebbutt, S.J. Cellular and Molecular Biomarkers of Long COVID: A Scoping Review. *EBioMedicine* **2023**, *91*, 104552. [CrossRef]

163. Hama Amin, B.J.; Kakamad, F.H.; Ahmed, G.S.; Ahmed, S.F.; Abdulla, B.A.; Mohammed, S.H.; Mikael, T.M.; Salih, R.Q.; Ali, R.k.; Salh, A.M.; et al. Post COVID-19 Pulmonary Fibrosis; a Meta-Analysis Study. *Ann. Med. Surg.* **2022**, *77*, 103590. [CrossRef]

164. Hirawat, R.; Jain, N.; Aslam Saifi, M.; Rachamalla, M.; Godugu, C. Lung Fibrosis: Post-COVID-19 Complications and Evidences. *Int. Immunopharmacol.* **2023**, *116*, 109418. [CrossRef]

165. Patrucco, F.; Solidoro, P.; Gavelli, F.; Apostolo, D.; Bellan, M. Idiopathic Pulmonary Fibrosis and Post-COVID-19 Lung Fibrosis: Links and Risks. *Microorganisms* **2023**, *11*, 895. [CrossRef]
166. George, P.M.; Wells, A.U.; Jenkins, R.G. Pulmonary Fibrosis and COVID-19: The Potential Role for Antifibrotic Therapy. *Lancet Respir. Med.* **2020**, *8*, 807–815. [CrossRef]
167. Wang, R.; Wu, G.; Dai, T.; Lang, Y.; Chi, Z.; Yang, S.; Dong, D. Naringin Attenuates Renal Interstitial Fibrosis by Regulating the TGF-β/Smad Signaling Pathway and Inflammation. *Exp. Ther. Med.* **2021**, *21*, 66. [CrossRef]
168. Wang, Q.; Li, W.; Hu, H.; Lu, X.; Qin, S. Monomeric Compounds from Traditional Chinese Medicine: New Hopes for Drug Discovery in Pulmonary Fibrosis. *Biomed. Pharmacother.* **2023**, *159*, 114226. [CrossRef]
169. Zhang, H.; Zhou, X.; Zhong, Y.; Ji, L.; Yu, W.; Fang, J.; Ying, H.; Li, C. Naringin Suppressed Airway Inflammation and Ameliorated Pulmonary Endothelial Hyperpermeability by Upregulating Aquaporin1 in Lipopolysaccharide/Cigarette Smoke-Induced Mice. *Biomed. Pharmacother.* **2022**, *150*, 113035. [CrossRef]
170. Chen, Y.; Nie, Y.; Luo, Y.; Lin, F.; Zheng, Y.; Cheng, G.; Wu, H.; Zhang, K.; Su, W.; Shen, J.; et al. Protective Effects of Naringin against Paraquat-Induced Acute Lung Injury and Pulmonary Fibrosis in Mice. *Food Chem. Toxicol.* **2013**, *58*, 133–140. [CrossRef]
171. Wei, Y.; Sun, L.; Liu, C.; Li, L. Naringin Regulates Endoplasmic Reticulum Stress and Mitophagy through the ATF3/PINK1 Signaling Axis to Alleviate Pulmonary Fibrosis. *Naunyn. Schmiedebergs Arch. Pharmacol.* **2023**, *396*, 1155–1169. [CrossRef]
172. Fan, W.; Xu, Z.; Zhang, J.; Guan, M.; Zheng, Y.; Wang, Y.; Wu, H.; Su, W.; Li, P. Naringenin Regulates Cigarette Smoke Extract-Induced Extracellular Vesicles from Alveolar Macrophage to Attenuate the Mouse Lung Epithelial Ferroptosis through Activating EV miR-23a-3p/ACSL4 Axis. *Phytomedicine* **2024**, *124*, 155256. [CrossRef] [PubMed]
173. Mahmoud, N.; Radwan, N.; Alkattan, A.; Hassanien, M.; Elkajam, E.; Alqahtani, S.; Haji, A.; Alfaifi, A.; Alfaleh, A.; Alabdulkareem, K. Post-COVID-19 Syndrome: Nature of Symptoms and Associated Factors. *Z. Cesundh. Wiss.* **2023**, *32*, 207–212. [CrossRef] [PubMed]
174. Chudzik, M.; Babicki, M.; Kapusta, J.; Kałuzińska-Kołat, Ż.; Kołat, D.; Jankowski, P.; Mastalerz-Migas, A. Long-COVID Clinical Features and Risk Factors: A Retrospective Analysis of Patients from the STOP-COVID Registry of the poLoCOV Study. *Viruses* **2022**, *14*, 1755. [CrossRef] [PubMed]
175. Fernández-de-las-Peñas, C.; Guijarro, C.; Plaza-Canteli, S.; Hernández-Barrera, V.; Torres-Macho, J. Prevalence of Post-COVID-19 Cough One Year after SARS-CoV-2 Infection: A Multicenter Study. *Lung* **2021**, *199*, 249–253. [CrossRef] [PubMed]
176. Song, W.-J.; Hui, C.K.M.; Hull, J.H.; Birring, S.S.; McGarvey, L.; Mazzone, S.B.; Chung, K.F. Confronting COVID-19-Associated Cough and the Post-COVID Syndrome: Role of Viral Neurotropism, Neuroinflammation, and Neuroimmune Responses. *Lancet Respir. Med.* **2021**, *9*, 533–544. [CrossRef] [PubMed]
177. Nguyen-Ho, L.; Nguyen-Nhu, V.; Tran-Thi, T.-T.; Solomon, J.J. Severe Chronic Cough Relating to Post-COVID-19 Interstitial Lung Disease: A Case Report. *Asia Pac. Allergy* **2022**, *12*, e42. [CrossRef] [PubMed]
178. Rouadi, P.W.; Idriss, S.A.; Bousquet, J.; Laidlaw, T.M.; Azar, C.R.; Al-Ahmad, M.S.; Yañez, A.; Al-Nesf, M.A.Y.; Nsouli, T.M.; Bahna, S.L.; et al. WAO-ARIA Consensus on Chronic Cough—Part II: Phenotypes and Mechanisms of Abnormal Cough Presentation—Updates in COVID-19. *World Allergy Organ. J.* **2021**, *14*, 100618. [CrossRef] [PubMed]
179. Gencer, A.; Caliskaner Ozturk, B.; Borekci, S.; Gemicioglu, B. Bronchodilator Reversibility Testing in Long-Term Cough and Dyspnea after COVID-19 Viral Infection: A Trigger for Asthma? *J. Asthma Off. J. Assoc. Care Asthma* **2023**, *60*, 1221–1226. [CrossRef]
180. Rai, D.K.; Sharma, P.; Karmakar, S.; Thakur, S.; Ameet, H.; Yadav, R.; Gupta, V.B. Approach to Post COVID-19 Persistent Cough: A Narrative Review. *Lung India* **2023**, *40*, 149–154. [CrossRef]
181. Zanasi, A.; Fontana, G.A.; Mutolo, D. *Cough: Pathophysiology, Diagnosis and Treatment*, 1st ed.; Springer International Publishing: Cham, Switzerland, 2020; ISBN 10:3030485714. [CrossRef]
182. Gupta, G.; Almalki, W.H.; Kazmi, I.; Fuloria, N.K.; Fuloria, S.; Subramaniyan, V.; Sekar, M.; Singh, S.K.; Chellappan, D.K.; Dua, K. Current Update on the Protective Effect of Naringin in Inflammatory Lung Diseases. *EXCLI J.* **2022**, *21*, 573–579. [CrossRef]
183. Liu, J.; Yao, J.; Zhang, J. Naringenin Attenuates Inflammation in Chronic Obstructive Pulmonary Disease in Cigarette Smoke Induced Mouse Model and Involves Suppression of NF-κB. *J. Microbiol. Biotechnol.* **2018**. [CrossRef]
184. Jiao, H.; Su, W.; Li, P.; Liao, Y.; Zhou, Q.; Zhu, N.; He, L. Therapeutic Effects of Naringin in a Guinea Pig Model of Ovalbumin-Induced Cough-Variant Asthma. *Pulm. Pharmacol. Ther.* **2015**, *33*, 59–65. [CrossRef]
185. Luo, Y.; Li, P.; Zhang, C.; Zheng, Y.; Wang, S.; Nie, Y.; Zhang, K.; Su, W. Effects of Four Antitussives on Airway Neurogenic Inflammation in a Guinea Pig Model of Chronic Cough Induced by Cigarette Smoke Exposure. *Inflamm. Res.* **2013**, *62*, 1053–1061. [CrossRef]
186. Ni, K.; Guo, J.; Bu, B.; Pan, Y.; Li, J.; Liu, L.; Luo, M.; Deng, L. Naringin as a Plant-Derived Bitter Tastant Promotes Proliferation of Cultured Human Airway Epithelial Cells via Activation of TAS2R Signaling. *Phytomedicine* **2021**, *84*, 153491. [CrossRef]
187. Khunti, K.; Valabhji, J.; Misra, S. Diabetes and the COVID-19 Pandemic. *Diabetologia* **2023**, *66*, 255–266. [CrossRef]
188. Suwanwongse, K.; Shabarek, N. Newly Diagnosed Diabetes Mellitus, DKA, and COVID-19: Causality or Coincidence? A Report of Three Cases. *J. Med. Virol.* **2021**, *93*, 1150–1153. [CrossRef] [PubMed]
189. Ssentongo, P.; Zhang, Y.; Witmer, L.; Chinchilli, V.M.; Ba, D.M. Association of COVID-19 with Diabetes: A Systematic Review and Meta-Analysis. *Sci. Rep.* **2022**, *12*, 20191. [CrossRef]
190. Zhang, T.; Mei, Q.; Zhang, Z.; Walline, J.H.; Liu, Y.; Zhu, H.; Zhang, S. Risk for Newly Diagnosed Diabetes after COVID-19: A Systematic Review and Meta-Analysis. *BMC Med.* **2022**, *20*, 444. [CrossRef]

191. Rahmati, M.; Keshvari, M.; Mirnasuri, S.; Yon, D.K.; Lee, S.W.; Il Shin, J.; Smith, L. The Global Impact of COVID-19 Pandemic on the Incidence of Pediatric New-onset Type 1 Diabetes and Ketoacidosis: A Systematic Review and Meta-analysis. *J. Med. Virol.* **2022**, *94*, 5112–5127. [CrossRef]

192. Lu, J.Y.; Wilson, J.; Hou, W.; Fleysher, R.; Herold, B.C.; Herold, K.C.; Duong, T.Q. Incidence of New-Onset in-Hospital and Persistent Diabetes in COVID-19 Patients: Comparison with Influenza. *EBioMedicine* **2023**, *90*, 104487. [CrossRef]

193. Laurenzi, A.; Caretto, A.; Molinari, C.; Mercalli, A.; Melzi, R.; Nano, R.; Tresoldi, C.; Rovere Querini, P.; Ciceri, F.; Lampasona, V.; et al. No Evidence of Long-Term Disruption of Glycometabolic Control after SARS-CoV-2 Infection. *J. Clin. Endocrinol. Metab.* **2021**, *107*, e1009–e1019. [CrossRef]

194. Cao, H.; Baranova, A.; Wei, X.; Wang, C.; Zhang, F. Bidirectional Causal Associations between Type 2 Diabetes and COVID-19. *J. Med. Virol.* **2023**, *95*, e28100. [CrossRef] [PubMed]

195. Montefusco, L.; Ben Nasr, M.; D'Addio, F.; Loretelli, C.; Rossi, A.; Pastore, I.; Daniele, G.; Abdelsalam, A.; Maestroni, A.; Dell'Acqua, M.; et al. Acute and Long-Term Disruption of Glycometabolic Control after SARS-CoV-2 Infection. *Nat. Metab.* **2021**, *3*, 774–785. [CrossRef]

196. Fotea, S.; Ghiciuc, C.M.; Stefanescu, G.; Cianga, A.L.; Mihai, C.M.; Lupu, A.; Butnariu, L.I.; Starcea, I.M.; Salaru, D.L.; Mocanu, A.; et al. Pediatric COVID-19 and Diabetes: An Investigation into the Intersection of Two Pandemics. *Diagnostics* **2023**, *13*, 2436. [CrossRef]

197. Liu, F.; Long, X.; Zhang, B.; Zhang, W.; Chen, X.; Zhang, Z. ACE2 Expression in Pancreas May Cause Pancreatic Damage after SARS-CoV-2 Infection. *Clin. Gastroenterol. Hepatol.* **2020**, *18*, 2128–2130. [CrossRef]

198. Kusmartseva, I.; Wu, W.; Syed, F.; Van Der Heide, V.; Jorgensen, M.; Joseph, P.; Tang, X.; Candelario-Jalil, E.; Yang, C.; Nick, H.; et al. Expression of SARS-CoV-2 Entry Factors in the Pancreas of Normal Organ Donors and Individuals with COVID-19. *Cell Metab.* **2020**, *32*, 1041–1051. [CrossRef] [PubMed]

199. Hayden, M.R. An Immediate and Long-Term Complication of COVID-19 May Be Type 2 Diabetes Mellitus: The Central Role of β-Cell Dysfunction, Apoptosis and Exploration of Possible Mechanisms. *Cells* **2020**, *9*, 2475. [CrossRef]

200. Birabaharan, M.; Kaelber, D.C.; Pettus, J.H.; Smith, D.M. Risk of New-Onset Type 2 Diabetes Mellitus in 600,055 Persons after COVID-19: A Cohort Study. *Diabetes Obes. Metab.* **2022**, *24*, 1176–1179. [CrossRef]

201. Zhao, T.; Ding, J.; Liang, Z.; Cui, X.; He, K.; Chen, L.; Li, J. When Type II Diabetes Mellitus Meets COVID-19—Identification of the Shared Gene Signatures and Biological Mechanism between the Two Diseases. *Eur. J. Clin. Investig.* **2023**, *53*, e13955. [CrossRef]

202. Rajappa, R.; Sireesh, D.; Salai, M.B.; Ramkumar, K.M.; Sarvajayakesavulu, S.; Madhunapantula, S.V. Treatment with Naringenin Elevates the Activity of Transcription Factor Nrf2 to Protect Pancreatic β-Cells from Streptozotocin-Induced Diabetes in Vitro and in Vivo. *Front. Pharmacol.* **2018**, *9*, 1562. [CrossRef]

203. Lim, Y.J.; Kim, J.H.; Pan, J.H.; Kim, J.K.; Park, T.-S.; Kim, Y.J.; Lee, J.H.; Kim, J.H. Naringin Protects Pancreatic β-Cells against Oxidative Stress-Induced Apoptosis by Inhibiting Both Intrinsic and Extrinsic Pathways in Insulin-Deficient Diabetic Mice. *Mol. Nutr. Food Res.* **2018**, *62*, 1700810. [CrossRef] [PubMed]

204. Subramanian, M.; Thotakura, B.; Chandra Sekaran, S.P.; Jyothi, A.K.; Sundaramurthi, I. Naringin Ameliorates Streptozotocin-Induced Diabetes through Forkhead Box M1-Mediated Beta Cell Proliferation. *Cells Tissues Organs* **2019**, *206*, 242–253. [CrossRef] [PubMed]

205. Ahmed, O.M.; Hassan, M.A.; Abdel-Twab, S.M.; Abdel Azeem, M.N. Navel Orange Peel Hydroethanolic Extract, Naringin and Naringenin Have Anti-Diabetic Potentials in Type 2 Diabetic Rats. *Biomed. Pharmacother.* **2017**, *94*, 197–205. [CrossRef] [PubMed]

206. Murunga, A.N.; Miruka, D.O.; Driver, C.; Nkomo, F.S.; Cobongela, S.Z.Z.; Owira, P.M.O. Grapefruit Derived Flavonoid Naringin Improves Ketoacidosis and Lipid Peroxidation in Type 1 Diabetes Rat Model. *PLoS ONE* **2016**, *11*, e0153241. [CrossRef] [PubMed]

207. Mahmoud, A.M.; Ahmed, O.M.; Ashour, M.B.; Abdel-Moneim, A. In Vivo and in Vitro Antidiabetic Effects of Citrus Flavonoids; a Study on the Mechanism of Action. *Int. J. Diabetes Dev. Ctries.* **2015**, *35*, 250–263. [CrossRef]

208. Yoshida, H.; Watanabe, H.; Ishida, A.; Watanabe, W.; Narumi, K.; Atsumi, T.; Sugita, C.; Kurokawa, M. Naringenin Suppresses Macrophage Infiltration into Adipose Tissue in an Early Phase of High-Fat Diet-Induced Obesity. *Biochem. Biophys. Res. Commun.* **2014**, *454*, 95–101. [CrossRef] [PubMed]

209. Singh, P.; Bansal, S.; Kuhad, A.; Kumar, A.; Chopra, K. Naringenin Ameliorates Diabetic Neuropathic Pain by Modulation of Oxidative-Nitrosative Stress, Cytokines and MMP-9 Levels. *Food Funct.* **2020**, *11*, 4548–4560. [CrossRef] [PubMed]

210. He, W.; Wang, Y.; Yang, R.; Ma, H.; Qin, X.; Yan, M.; Rong, Y.; Xie, Y.; Li, L.; Si, J.; et al. Molecular Mechanism of Naringenin against High-Glucose-Induced Vascular Smooth Muscle Cells Proliferation and Migration Based on Network Pharmacology and Transcriptomic Analyses. *Front. Pharmacol.* **2022**, *13*, 862709. [CrossRef]

211. Fiala, K.; Martens, J.; Abd-Elsayed, A. Post-COVID Pain Syndromes. *Curr. Pain Headache Rep.* **2022**, *26*, 379–383. [CrossRef]

212. Malik, P.; Patel, K.; Pinto, C.; Jaiswal, R.; Tirupathi, R.; Pillai, S.; Patel, U. Post-acute COVID-19 Syndrome (PCS) and Health-related Quality of Life (HRQoL)—A Systematic Review and Meta-analysis. *J. Med. Virol.* **2022**, *94*, 253–262. [CrossRef]

213. Fernández-de-las-Peñas, C.; Navarro-Santana, M.; Plaza-Manzano, G.; Palacios-Ceña, D.; Arendt-Nielsen, L. Time Course Prevalence of Post-COVID Pain Symptoms of Musculoskeletal Origin in Patients Who Had Survived Severe Acute Respiratory Syndrome Coronavirus 2 Infection: A Systematic Review and Meta-Analysis. *Pain* **2022**, *163*, 1220. [CrossRef]

214. Natarajan, A.; Shetty, A.; Delanerolle, G.; Zeng, Y.; Zhang, Y.; Raymont, V.; Rathod, S.; Halabi, S.; Elliot, K.; Shi, J.Q.; et al. A Systematic Review and Meta-Analysis of Long COVID Symptoms. *Syst. Rev.* **2023**, *12*, 88. [CrossRef]

215. Wu, Y.; Xu, X.; Chen, Z.; Duan, J.; Hashimoto, K.; Yang, L.; Liu, C.; Yang, C. Nervous System Involvement after Infection with COVID-19 and Other Coronaviruses. *Brain Behav. Immun.* **2020**, *87*, 18–22. [CrossRef] [PubMed]
216. Bussmann, A.J.C.; Ferraz, C.R.; Lima, A.V.A.; Castro, J.G.S.; Ritter, P.D.; Zaninelli, T.H.; Saraiva-Santos, T.; Verri, W.A.; Borghi, S.M. Association between IL-10 Systemic Low Level and Highest Pain Score in Patients during Symptomatic SARS-CoV-2 Infection. *Pain Pract. Pain* **2022**, *22*, 453–462. [CrossRef] [PubMed]
217. Rani, M.; Uniyal, A.; Akhilesh; Tiwari, V. Decrypting the Cellular and Molecular Intricacies Associated with COVID-19-Induced Chronic Pain. *Metab. Brain Dis.* **2022**, *37*, 2629–2642. [CrossRef] [PubMed]
218. Takeshita, H.; Yamamoto, K. Tryptophan Metabolism and COVID-19-Induced Skeletal Muscle Damage: Is ACE2 a Key Regulator? *Front. Nutr.* **2022**, *9*, 868845. [CrossRef] [PubMed]
219. Tana, C.; Bentivegna, E.; Cho, S.-J.; Harriott, A.M.; García-Azorín, D.; Labastida-Ramirez, A.; Ornello, R.; Raffaelli, B.; Beltrán, E.R.; Ruscheweyh, R.; et al. Long COVID Headache. *J. Headache Pain* **2022**, *23*, 93. [CrossRef] [PubMed]
220. Bolay, H.; Karadas, Ö.; Oztürk, B.; Sonkaya, R.; Tasdelen, B.; Bulut, T.D.S.; Gülbahar, Ö.; Özge, A.; Baykan, B. HMGB1, NLRP3, IL-6 and ACE2 Levels Are Elevated in COVID-19 with Headache: A Window to the Infection-Related Headache Mechanism. *J. Headache Pain* **2021**, *22*, 94. [CrossRef] [PubMed]
221. Caronna, E.; Ballvé, A.; Llauradó, A.; Gallardo, V.J.; Ariton, D.M.; Lallana, S.; López Maza, S.; Olivé Gadea, M.; Quibus, L.; Restrepo, J.L.; et al. Headache: A Striking Prodromal and Persistent Symptom, Predictive of COVID-19 Clinical Evolution. *Cephalalgia* **2020**, *40*, 1410–1421. [CrossRef]
222. Xu, Q.; Zhang, Z.; Sun, W. Effect of Naringin on Monosodium Iodoacetate-Induced Osteoarthritis Pain in Rats. *Med. Sci. Monit.* **2017**, *23*, 3746–3751. [CrossRef]
223. Hu, C.; Zhao, Y.-T. Analgesic Effects of Naringenin in Rats with Spinal Nerve Ligation-Induced Neuropathic Pain. *Biomed. Rep.* **2014**, *2*, 569–573. [CrossRef]
224. Aghazadeh Tabrizi, M.; Baraldi, P.G.; Baraldi, S.; Gessi, S.; Merighi, S.; Borea, P.A. Medicinal Chemistry, Pharmacology, and Clinical Implications of TRPV1 Receptor Antagonists. *Med. Res. Rev.* **2017**, *37*, 936–983. [CrossRef]
225. Katz, B.; Zaguri, R.; Edvardson, S.; Maayan, C.; Elpeleg, O.; Lev, S.; Davidson, E.; Peters, M.; Kfir-Erenfeld, S.; Berger, E.; et al. Nociception and Pain in Humans Lacking a Functional TRPV1 Channel. *J. Clin. Investig.* **2023**, *133*, e153558. [CrossRef]
226. Gouin, O.; L'Herondelle, K.; Lebonvallet, N.; Le Gall-Ianotto, C.; Sakka, M.; Buhé, V.; Plée-Gautier, E.; Carré, J.-L.; Lefeuvre, L.; Misery, L.; et al. TRPV1 and TRPA1 in Cutaneous Neurogenic and Chronic Inflammation: Pro-Inflammatory Response Induced by Their Activation and Their Sensitization. *Protein Cell* **2017**, *8*, 644–661. [CrossRef]
227. Eom, S.; Lee, B.-B.; Lee, S.; Park, Y.; Yeom, H.D.; Kim, T.-H.; Nam, S.-H.; Lee, J.H. Antioxidative and Analgesic Effects of Naringin through Selective Inhibition of Transient Receptor Potential Vanilloid Member 1. *Antioxidants* **2021**, *11*, 64. [CrossRef] [PubMed]
228. Straub, I.; Mohr, F.; Stab, J.; Konrad, M.; Philipp, S.; Oberwinkler, J.; Schaefer, M. Citrus Fruit and Fabacea Secondary Metabolites Potently and Selectively Block TRPM3. *Br. J. Pharmacol.* **2013**, *168*, 1835–1850. [CrossRef] [PubMed]
229. Manchope, M.F.; Calixto-Campos, C.; Coelho-Silva, L.; Zarpelon, A.C.; Pinho-Ribeiro, F.A.; Georgetti, S.R.; Baracat, M.M.; Casagrande, R.; Verri, W.A. Naringenin Inhibits Superoxide Anion-Induced Inflammatory Pain: Role of Oxidative Stress, Cytokines, Nrf-2 and the NO−cGMP−PKG−KATP Channel Signaling Pathway. *PLoS ONE* **2016**, *11*, e0153015. [CrossRef] [PubMed]
230. Pourmasumi, S.; Kounis, N.G.; Naderi, M.; Hosseinisadat, R.; Khoradmehr, A.; Fagheirelahee, N.; Kouni, S.N.; de Gregorio, C.; Dousdampanis, P.; Mplani, V.; et al. Effects of COVID-19 Infection and Vaccination on the Female Reproductive System: A Narrative Review. *Balk. Med. J.* **2023**, *40*, 153–164. [CrossRef] [PubMed]
231. Nassau, D.E.; Best, J.C.; Kresch, E.; Gonzalez, D.C.; Khodamoradi, K.; Ramasamy, R. Impact of the SARS-CoV-2 Virus on Male Reproductive Health. *Bju Int.* **2022**, *129*, 143–150. [CrossRef] [PubMed]
232. Yelin, D.; Daitch, V.; Kalfon, T.; Mor, M.; Buchrits, S.; Shafir, Y.; Awwad, M.; Ghantous, N.; Shapira-Lichter, I.; Leibovici, L.; et al. Long COVID Sexual Dysfunction among Both Genders: Evaluation of a Cohort of COVID-19 Recoverees. *Infect. Dis. Now* **2023**, *53*, 104750. [CrossRef] [PubMed]
233. Harirugsakul, K.; Wainipitapong, S.; Phannajit, J.; Paitoonpong, L.; Tantiwongse, K. Erectile Dysfunction after COVID-19 Recovery: A Follow-up Study. *PLoS ONE* **2022**, *17*, e0276429. [CrossRef] [PubMed]
234. Pollack, B.; Von Saltza, E.; McCorkell, L.; Santos, L.; Hultman, A.; Cohen, A.K.; Soares, L. Female Reproductive Health Impacts of Long COVID and Associated Illnesses Including ME/CFS, POTS, and Connective Tissue Disorders: A Literature Review. *Front. Rehabil. Sci.* **2023**, *4*, 1122673. [CrossRef] [PubMed]
235. Bechmann, N.; Maccio, U.; Kotb, R.; Dweik, R.A.; Cherfane, M.; Moch, H.; Bornstein, S.R.; Varga, Z. COVID-19 Infections in Gonads: Consequences on Fertility? *Horm. Metab. Res.* **2022**, *54*, 549–555. [CrossRef] [PubMed]
236. Corona, G.; Baldi, E.; Isidori, A.M.; Paoli, D.; Pallotti, F.; De Santis, L.; Francavilla, F.; La Vignera, S.; Selice, R.; Caponecchia, L.; et al. SARS-CoV-2 Infection, Male Fertility and Sperm Cryopreservation: A Position Statement of the Italian Society of Andrology and Sexual Medicine (SIAMS) (Società Italiana Di Andrologia e Medicina Della Sessualità). *J. Endocrinol. Investig.* **2020**, *43*, 1153–1157. [CrossRef] [PubMed]
237. Sengupta, P.; Dutta, S.; Roychoudhury, S.; D'Souza, U.J.A.; Govindasamy, K.; Kolesarova, A. COVID-19, Oxidative Stress and Male Reproduction: Possible Role of Antioxidants. *Antioxidants* **2022**, *11*, 548. [CrossRef] [PubMed]

238. Sauve, F.; Nampoothiri, S.; Clarke, S.A.; Fernandois, D.; Ferreira Coêlho, C.F.; Dewisme, J.; Mills, E.G.; Ternier, G.; Cotellessa, L.; Iglesias-Garcia, C.; et al. Long-COVID Cognitive Impairments and Reproductive Hormone Deficits in Men May Stem from GnRH Neuronal Death. *EBioMedicine* **2023**, *96*, 104784. [CrossRef]

239. Al-kuraishy, H.M.; Al-Gareeb, A.I.; Alarfaj, S.J.; Al-Akeel, R.K.; Faidah, H.; El-Bouseary, M.M.; Sabatier, J.-M.; De Waard, M.; El-Masry, T.A.; Batiha, G.E.-S. Long COVID and Risk of Erectile Dysfunction in Recovered Patients from Mild to Moderate COVID-19. *Sci. Rep.* **2023**, *13*, 5977. [CrossRef]

240. Li, H.; Xiao, X.; Zhang, J.; Zafar, M.I.; Wu, C.; Long, Y.; Lu, W.; Pan, F.; Meng, T.; Zhao, K.; et al. Impaired Spermatogenesis in COVID-19 Patients. *EClinicalMedicine* **2020**, *28*, 100604. [CrossRef]

241. Chen, H.; Chen, J.; Shi, X.; Li, L.; Xu, S. Naringenin Protects Swine Testis Cells from Bisphenol A-Induced Apoptosis via Keap1/Nrf2 Signaling Pathway. *BioFactors* **2022**, *48*, 190–203. [CrossRef]

242. Adana, M.Y.; Akang, E.N.; Peter, A.I.; Jegede, A.I.; Naidu, E.C.S.; Tiloke, C.; Chuturgoon, A.A.; Azu, O.O. Naringenin Attenuates Highly Active Antiretroviral Therapy-Induced Sperm DNA Fragmentations and Testicular Toxicity in Sprague-Dawley Rats. *Andrology* **2018**, *6*, 166–175. [CrossRef]

243. Rashid, R.; Tripathi, R.; Singh, A.; Sarkar, S.; Kawale, A.; Bader, G.N.; Gupta, S.; Gupta, R.K.; Jha, R.K. Naringenin Improves Ovarian Health by Reducing the Serum Androgen and Eliminating Follicular Cysts in Letrozole-Induced Polycystic Ovary Syndrome in the Sprague Dawley Rats. *Phytother. Res.* **2023**, *37*, 4018–4041. [CrossRef] [PubMed]

244. Wu, X.; Xiang, M.; Jing, H.; Wang, C.; Novakovic, V.A.; Shi, J. Damage to Endothelial Barriers and Its Contribution to Long COVID. *Angiogenesis* **2023**, 1–18. [CrossRef] [PubMed]

245. Candeloro, M.; Schulman, S. Arterial Thrombotic Events in Hospitalized COVID-19 Patients: A Short Review and Meta-Analysis. *Semin. Thromb. Hemost.* **2023**, *49*, 47–54. [CrossRef] [PubMed]

246. Di Minno, A.; Ambrosino, P.; Calcaterra, I.; Di Minno, M.N.D. COVID-19 and Venous Thromboembolism: A Meta-Analysis of Literature Studies. *Semin. Thromb. Hemost.* **2020**, *46*, 763–771. [CrossRef] [PubMed]

247. Zuin, M.; Engelen, M.M.; Barco, S.; Spyropoulos, A.C.; Vanassche, T.; Hunt, B.J.; Vandenbriele, C.; Verhamme, P.; Kucher, N.; Rashidi, F.; et al. Incidence of Venous Thromboembolic Events in COVID-19 Patients after Hospital Discharge: A Systematic Review and Meta-Analysis. *Thromb. Res.* **2022**, *209*, 94–98. [CrossRef]

248. Martins-Gonçalves, R.; Hottz, E.D.; Bozza, P.T. Acute to Post-Acute COVID-19 Thromboinflammation Persistence: Mechanisms and Potential Consequences. *Curr. Res. Immunol.* **2023**, *4*, 100058. [CrossRef]

249. Grobbelaar, L.M.; Venter, C.; Vlok, M.; Ngoepe, M.; Laubscher, G.J.; Lourens, P.J.; Steenkamp, J.; Kell, D.B.; Pretorius, E. SARS-CoV-2 Spike Protein S1 Induces Fibrin(Ogen) Resistant to Fibrinolysis: Implications for Microclot Formation in COVID-19. *Biosci. Rep.* **2021**, *41*, BSR20210611. [CrossRef]

250. Schultheiß, C.; Willscher, E.; Paschold, L.; Gottschick, C.; Klee, B.; Henkes, S.-S.; Bosurgi, L.; Dutzmann, J.; Sedding, D.; Frese, T.; et al. The IL-1β, IL-6, and TNF Cytokine Triad Is Associated with Post-Acute Sequelae of COVID-19. *Cell Rep. Med.* **2022**, *3*, 100663. [CrossRef]

251. Turner, S.; Khan, M.A.; Putrino, D.; Woodcock, A.; Kell, D.B.; Pretorius, E. Long COVID: Pathophysiological Factors and Abnormalities of Coagulation. *Trends Endocrinol. Metab.* **2023**, *34*, 321. [CrossRef]

252. Zaira, B.; Yulianti, T.; Levita, J. Correlation between Hepatocyte Growth Factor (HGF) with D-Dimer and Interleukin-6 as Prognostic Markers of Coagulation and Inflammation in Long COVID-19 Survivors. *Curr. Issues Mol. Biol.* **2023**, *45*, 5725–5740. [CrossRef]

253. Malakul, W.; Pengnet, S.; Kumchoom, C.; Tunsophon, S. Naringin Ameliorates Endothelial Dysfunction in Fructose-Fed Rats. *Exp. Ther. Med.* **2018**, *15*, 3140–3146. [CrossRef]

254. Zhao, H.; Liu, M.; Liu, H.; Suo, R.; Lu, C. Naringin Protects Endothelial Cells from Apoptosis and Inflammation by Regulating the Hippo-YAP Pathway. *Biosci. Rep.* **2020**, *40*, BSR20193431. [CrossRef]

255. Wang, K.; Peng, S.; Xiong, S.; Niu, A.; Xia, M.; Xiong, X.; Zeng, G.; Huang, Q. Naringin Inhibits Autophagy Mediated by PI3K-Akt-mTOR Pathway to Ameliorate Endothelial Cell Dysfunction Induced by High Glucose/High Fat Stress. *Eur. J. Pharmacol.* **2020**, *874*, 173003. [CrossRef]

256. Wright, B.; Spencer, J.P.E.; Lovegrove, J.A.; Gibbins, J.M. Flavonoid Inhibitory Pharmacodynamics on Platelet Function in Physiological Environments. *Food Funct.* **2013**, *4*, 1803–1810. [CrossRef]

257. Huang, M.; Deng, M.; Nie, W.; Zou, D.; Wu, H.; Xu, D. Naringenin Inhibits Platelet Activation and Arterial Thrombosis through Inhibition of Phosphoinositide 3-Kinase and Cyclic Nucleotide Signaling. *Front. Pharmacol.* **2021**, *12*, 722257. [CrossRef]

258. Li, Q.-Q.; Yang, Y.-X.; Qv, J.-W.; Hu, G.; Hu, Y.-J.; Xia, Z.-N.; Yang, F.-Q. Investigation of Interactions between Thrombin and Ten Phenolic Compounds by Affinity Capillary Electrophoresis and Molecular Docking. *J. Anal. Methods Chem.* **2018**, *2018*, 4707609. [CrossRef] [PubMed]

259. Khan, A.B.; Siddiqui, U.; Fatima, S.; Rehman, A.A.; Jairajpuri, M.A. Naringin Binds to Protein Disulfide Isomerase to Inhibit Its Activity and Modulate the Blood Coagulation Rates: Implications in Controlling Thrombosis. *Int. J. Biol. Macromol.* **2023**, *252*, 126241. [CrossRef] [PubMed]

260. Tsilingiris, D.; Vallianou, N.G.; Karampela, I.; Christodoulatos, G.S.; Papavasileiou, G.; Petropoulou, D.; Magkos, F.; Dalamaga, M. Laboratory Findings and Biomarkers in Long COVID: What Do We Know so Far? Insights into Epidemiology, Pathogenesis, Therapeutic Perspectives and Challenges. *Int. J. Mol. Sci.* **2023**, *24*, 10458. [CrossRef] [PubMed]

261. Kenny, G.; Townsend, L.; Savinelli, S.; Mallon, P.W.G. Long COVID: Clinical Characteristics, Proposed Pathogenesis and Potential Therapeutic Targets. *Front. Mol. Biosci.* **2023**, *10*, 1157651. [CrossRef] [PubMed]
262. Bonilla, H.; Peluso, M.J.; Rodgers, K.; Aberg, J.A.; Patterson, T.F.; Tamburro, R.; Baizer, L.; Goldman, J.D.; Rouphael, N.; Deitchman, A.; et al. Therapeutic Trials for Long COVID-19: A Call to Action from the Interventions Taskforce of the RECOVER Initiative. *Front. Immunol.* **2023**, *14*, 1129459. [CrossRef] [PubMed]
263. Chee, Y.J.; Fan, B.E.; Young, B.E.; Dalan, R.; Lye, D.C. Clinical Trials on the Pharmacological Treatment of Long COVID: A Systematic Review. *J. Med. Virol.* **2023**, *95*, e28289. [CrossRef] [PubMed]
264. Calabrese, E.J.; Pressman, P.; Hayes, A.W.; Dhawan, G.; Kapoor, R.; Agathokleous, E.; Manes, P.; Calabrese, V. Naringin Commonly Acts via Hormesis. *Sci. Total Environ.* **2023**, *896*, 164728. [CrossRef] [PubMed]
265. Davatgaran Taghipour, Y.; Hajialyani, M.; Naseri, R.; Hesari, M.; Mohammadi, P.; Stefanucci, A.; Mollica, A.; Farzaei, M.H.; Abdollahi, M. Nanoformulations of Natural Products for Management of Metabolic Syndrome. *Int. J. Nanomed.* **2019**, *14*, 5303–5321. [CrossRef] [PubMed]

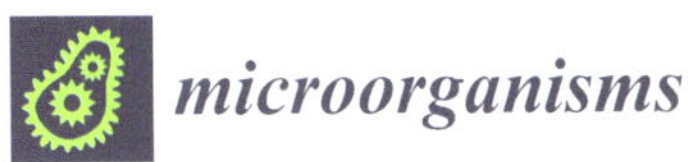

Review

Vaccinating against a Novel Pathogen: A Critical Review of COVID-19 Vaccine Effectiveness Evidence

Bernard Black [1,*] and David B. Thaw [2]

[1] Pritzker School of Law and Kellogg School of Management, Northwestern University, Chicago, IL 60201, USA
[2] School of Computing & Information and School of Law, University of Pittsburgh, Pittsburgh, PA 15260, USA
* Correspondence: bblack@northwestern.edu; Tel.: +1-(312)-503-2784

Abstract: We study the experience with COVID-19 vaccination of an initially naïve population, which can inform planning for vaccination against the next novel, highly transmissible pathogen. We focus on the first two pandemic years (wild strain through Delta), because after the Omicron wave in early 2022, very few people were still SARS-CoV-2-naïve. Almost all were vaccinated, infected, or often both. We review the evidence on COVID-19 vaccine effectiveness (VE) and waning effectiveness over time and the relative effectiveness of the four principal vaccines used in developed Western countries: BNT162b2 (Pfizer-BioNTech), mRNA1273 (Moderna), Ad26.CoV2.S (Johnson&Johnson), and ChAdOx1-S (AstraZeneca). As a basis for our analysis, we conducted a PRISMA-compliant review of all studies on PubMed through 15 August 2022, reporting VE against four endpoints for these four vaccines: any infection, symptomatic infection, hospitalization, and death. The mRNA vaccines (BNT162b2, mRNA1273) had high initial VE against all endpoints but protection waned after approximately six months, with BNT162b2 declining faster than mRNA1273. Both mRNA vaccines outperformed the viral vector vaccines (Ad26.CoV2.S and ChAdOx1-S). A third "booster" dose, roughly six months after the initial doses, substantially reduced symptomatic infection, hospitalization, and death. In hindsight, a third dose should be seen as part of the normal vaccination schedule. Our analysis highlights the importance of the real-time population-level surveillance needed to assess evidence for waning, and the need for rapid regulatory response to this evidence.

Keywords. COVID-19; SARS-CoV-2; vaccine; vaccine efficacy; vaccine effectiveness; vaccine booster; BNT162b2; mRNA1273; Ad26.COV2.S; ChAdOx1-S; SARS-CoV-2 variants

Citation: Black, B.; Thaw, D.B. Vaccinating against a Novel Pathogen: A Critical Review of COVID-19 Vaccine Effectiveness Evidence. *Microorganisms* **2024**, *12*, 89. https://doi.org/10.3390/microorganisms12010089

Academic Editors: Qibin Geng and Ahmed Atef Mesalam

Received: 25 November 2023
Revised: 18 December 2023
Accepted: 22 December 2023
Published: 31 December 2023

1. Introduction

The COVID-19 pandemic was the first global pandemic in the era of modern air travel, involving a novel, highly transmissible respiratory pathogen, with significant rates of severe disease and death. Vaccines, developed in record time, became a crucial means of preventing severe disease. Masking, lockdowns, remote work, and other mitigation measures slowed the spread of infections and reduced mortality rates, but in the end, these measures were only stopgaps. While the origins of SARS-CoV-2 remain debated, the risk from future respiratory pathogens remains high. A future pathogen could have some or all of the features that made COVID-19 so difficult to control, including asymptomatic spread, aerosol spread, high transmissibility, and rapid evolution to evade immune response even when the immune system has been primed by vaccination or prior infection.

Thus, it is critical to use the experience with COVID-19 to study vaccine effectiveness and the timing of vaccine doses, as a guide to planning for the next major respiratory pathogen. With that goal in mind, we review the COVID-19 vaccination campaign, including both the initial, primary vaccination and a booster dose. The extensive research on the COVID-19 vaccines provides a unique opportunity to study vaccination practices against a novel respiratory pathogen, including vaccine dosage and timing, vaccine waning over time, and how to measure vaccine effectiveness (VE), including against which endpoints.

Here, we provide an installment on the broader project of learning lessons from this pandemic, to guide planning for the next one. We focus on what is known about initial and longer-term VE for four leading COVID-19 vaccines against four different endpoints (infection, symptomatic infection, hospitalization, and death). We study and compare the four COVID-19 vaccines that were widely used in the United States (US), Canada, Israel, the United Kingdom (UK), and the European Union. Two were mRNA-based: BNT162b2 (Pfizer-BioNTech) and mRNA1273 (Moderna). Two used an adenovirus vector: Ad26.COV2.S (Johnson&Johnson, below, J&J) and ChAdOx1-S (AstraZeneca). BNT162b2, mRNA1273, and ChAdOx1-S are two-dose vaccines; Ad26.CoV2.S is single-dose.

The first U.S. vaccine authorizations were on 11 December 2020, for BNT162b2 and a week later for mRNA1273 [1,2]. Both vaccines were widely used in many countries. Ad26.CoV2 received U.S. authorization in February 2021 [3] and was used primarily in the U.S. ChAdOx1-S was authorized in the UK on 30 December 2020 [4] and soon thereafter in the European Union. It was not authorized in the U.S. but was widely used in other countries.

We focus on the period from initial vaccine authorization through the end of 2021, during which SARS-CoV-2 infection came primarily from early virus variants through roughly February 2021, then primarily from the Alpha variant through June 2021, and primarily from the Delta variant for the rest of 2021. We do not study the Omicron-dominant period that began at the very end of 2021, both because after 2021, there is limited information about infection rates due to widespread at-home testing, and because by early 2022, almost the entire population was vaccinated, infected, or both, and thus no longer naïve to the SARS-CoV-2 virus [for U.S. evidence, see [5–7]].

This review reports vaccine-specific evidence from studies known to us or available on PubMed through 15 August 2022, from both clinical trials and observational studies; including evidence on waning VE following initial vaccination and the value of a third, booster dose against the Delta (VoC B.1.617.2) variant.

The use and timing of booster doses was initially controversial, partly reflecting disagreement on the goals of vaccination [8]. Booster skeptics asserted that the principal goal of vaccination should be to prevent severe disease and death, and wanted to wait for strong evidence of waning against severe disease before authorizing boosters. Proponents of faster booster rollout were willing to accept imperfect evidence on waning in the middle of an ongoing pandemic. The booster proponents were also more willing to provide boosters to younger people, not at high risk of severe disease, to limit the spread of infection to older, higher risk people (see [9] for evidence supporting this strategy). Neither side could draw on experience with a prior, novel, highly transmissible respiratory pathogen with significant mortality. The most relevant prior pandemic, the 1918 influenza pandemic, predated modern air travel and vaccine development. This review provides such evidence by examining COVID-19 vaccine effectiveness from widespread deployment of vaccines in early 2021 through the emergence of the Omicron variant at the end of 2021.

The main contributions of this review, relative to the principal prior review [10], are that (i) this review covers many more studies over a longer period; (ii) the prior review reported only "minimal" waning against severe disease (thus supporting booster skeptics) and did not study death as an endpoint; and (iii) the prior review did not compare vaccines. This review provides strong evidence of progressive waning of VE against all endpoints, including hospitalization and death. VE for BNT162b2 shows a noticeable decline beginning at 4–5 months after initial vaccination; mRNA1273 wanes somewhat more slowly. ChAdOx1-S has both lower initial VE than the mRNA vaccines and substantial waning; Ad26.COV2.S has much lower initial VE than ChAdOx1-S but less evidence of waning. Our data thus support a ranking of vaccines based on near and medium-term VE hierarchy: mRNA1273 > BNT162b2 VE > ChAdOx1-S > Ad26.COV2.S; and 2 initial doses > 1 dose.

We also report evidence for booster value. As we show below (Table 5), an mRNA booster substantially increases VE for symptomatic infection for all ages and for hospitalization and death for ages 60+. This supports the value of a booster dose, especially for older adults, starting 5–6 months after vaccination. Less definitive evidence suggests booster waning and the value of a fourth dose for ages 60+ (e.g., [11,12]).

An innovation in this review is to use remaining risk instead of VE (RR is defined as $1 - $ VE) as a core measure of interest, especially against severe disease [13]. For highly effective vaccines, a small drop in VE can imply a large percentage increase in RR. For example, a drop in VE against death from 95% to 90% implies a doubling in RR from 5% to 10%, and thus a doubling in mortality risk for among vaccinated people. It is easier to observe evidence for waning in the data and understand its significance for severe disease, by studying RR rather than VE. RRs can also provide a basis for comparing vaccines that is more sensitive than VE to moderate differences in remaining risk. We speculate that a focus on VE could explain why both individual studies (e.g., [14,15]) and the principal prior review [10] downplayed the evidence on waning and the differences between vaccines, which this review finds and highlights.

The prior reviews [16–18], other than [10], are narrow in scope; none of them address waning. The review in [16] does not address waning; the review in [17] covers only early 2021 studies, before waning had occurred; and the review in [18] covers only randomized trials.

2. Materials and Methods

2.1. Scope of Review and Literature Search

To be included in this review, a study needed to (i) report vaccine efficacy (for a randomized trial) or VE (for an observational study) for full primary vaccination (two doses for mRNA1273, BNT162b2 VE, and ChAdOx1-S; one dose for Ad26.COV2); (ii) use standard timing between doses (4 weeks for mRNA1273 and ChAdOx1-S; 3 weeks for BNT162b2; not applicable for Ad26.COV2); and (iii) report evidence for one or more of the four endpoints. The requirement for standard timing of initial doses excluded some studies in countries, notably the U.K. and Canada, which in early 2021 spaced out the time between the first and second dose in order to reach more people sooner with a first dose. We accepted studies using a test-negative design, including retrospective studies, despite the known potential bias in this design [19], because the test-negative design is the dominant design used in observational studies.

The exclusion criteria were (i) the source reported vaccine-specific results; (ii) the source reported time since vaccination with enough granularity so that we could assess evidence for waning; (iii) the sample was large enough to provide reasonable precision for the reported endpoint(s) (we generally required at least 5000 vaccinated people and 5000 controls); (iv) the sample did not have apparent biases that could affect generalization (as would be the case for studies of specific populations such as healthcare workers, military veterans, nursing home residents, children, prisoners, and people who visited the emergency department or who were already hospitalized); and (v) the study included a control group without obvious bias, relative to the treatment group. See Supplementary Materials for additional inclusion and exclusion details.

Since early 2021, the authors manually tracked COVID-19 studies. The studies identified in this way were combined with a PRISMA-compliant review of all papers indexed by PubMed (including preprints) from 1 December 2020 through 15 August 2022, using search criteria which required the title, abstract, or keywords to refer to (1) disease or pathogen name; (2) one or more of the studied vaccines; and (3) vaccine efficacy or vaccine effectiveness. This initial search returned >10,000 papers; it was therefore modified to exclude papers with titles referring to adverse effects, specific populations, high-risk conditions such as obesity, diabetes, and immune-compromised, and antibody levels, which are outside of the scope of this review. Comments, responses, and reviews were excluded as not providing primary evidence. See Supplementary Materials for search details.

The revised PubMed search returned 1169 results, which were screened based on title and abstract. This screening produced 183 candidates (89 new, 94 previously identified in our manual review), which were retrieved and evaluated against the inclusion and exclusion criteria. Sixty-three papers passed this assessment (27 new, 36 previously identified). Of the 18 studies included in the prior review in [10], 12 are included here; the other 6 did not meet our criteria. The Supplementary Materials include a PRISMA flowchart.

2.2. Data Limitations, Implications for Inclusion, and Presentation of Results

An ideal VE study would (i) report vaccine-specific and ideally variant-specific evidence; (ii) report the time of both full initial vaccination (below, simply "vaccination") and the relevant endpoint; (iii) include a matched, unvaccinated control group; (iv) cover a population-representative sample, large enough to provide reasonably tight confidence intervals (CIs); (v) report VE or RR for standard, well-defined endpoint(s); (vi) report results within age ranges; and (vii) study a post-vaccination period long enough to allow more severe endpoints to be reached. For example, studying post vaccination mortality only for 30–40 days after vaccination or after a booster, as some studies do (e.g., [11,20]) is insufficient), given the typical lags from vaccination to when the vaccine is fully effective and from infection to death [21]. Even the best available studies do not achieve all of this. Therefore, compromises are needed in assessing which studies to rely on and which questions they can answer.

The principal analysis addresses the limited granularity of data on the time since vaccination by grouping "early" evidence (up to 120 days since vaccination) and "late" evidence (after 120 days). We do not report results by gender or age range. The included studies are consistent with gender having only modest effects on VE and age having only modest effects on VE against the infection endpoints (e.g., [22,23]). More recent studies provide evidence that waning VE against hospitalization and death occurred principally for ages 60+ [11,24,25]. Most studies report VE for the whole adult population, without controlling for prior infection. When VE was reported with-versus-without prior infection, we used the without-prior-infection data. When multiple protocols were used, the lower VE rate is reported.

3. Results

Our review includes the initial clinical trials, as well as observational studies covering the period through for end of 2021. It includes data from late 2021 on booster VE against the Delta variant.

3.1. Empirical Challenges and Choice of Endpoints

A major challenge in analyzing data across countries, trials, and observational studies is varying definitions of illness severity. These include asymptomatic, symptomatic, mild, requiring medical intervention, moderate, mild to moderate, serious, severe, moderate to severe, hospitalization, admission to an intensive care unit (ICU), critical, and death, among others. Definitions of the same term can vary across nations and studies. Four severity categories emerged from our review of the available studies as the most feasible to examine: (1) any infection (identified through a positive SARS-CoV-2 test); (2) symptomatic infection (infection plus presence of COVID-19 symptoms); (3) hospitalization, defined as symptomatic infection plus inpatient admittance; and (4) death with COVID-19 as a primary cause. For studies which report data for "severe disease" but not hospitalization, we generally assume VE for hospitalization equals reported VE for severe disease. It often required judgment to assess whether reported VE against infection was better understood as being against any infection or against symptomatic infection.

3.2. Evidence from Phase 3 Clinical Trials

The Phase 3 vaccine trials, summarized in Table 1, provide evidence for VE against symptomatic infection against the then-prevalent variants, principally the original "wild" variant and immediate descendants. The primary endpoint for the trials of all four vaccines was symptomatic infection. There were too few hospitalizations and deaths to permit more than a rough assessment of efficacy for these outcomes. The trials were not sized and could not feasibly have been sized to have reasonable power to assess efficacy against these less-common events.

Table 1. Vaccine efficacy rates against harmonized endpoints in Phase 3 trials.

	Efficacy vs.			
Vaccine	**Any Infection**	**Symptomatic Infection**	**Hospitalization**	**Death**
BNT162b2 (Pfizer-BioNTech)	NR	95%	100% [b, c, d]	100% [b, c]
mRNA1273 (Moderna)	NR	94.5%	100% [b, c]	100% [b, c]
Ad26.COV2.S (J&J)	59.7%	66.5%	76.7–83.5% [a]	100% [b]
ChAdOx1-S (AstraZeneca)	27.3–64.3% [e]	70.4–74.0%	94.2–100% [b, c]	100% [b, c]

Table sources. NR = not reported or not computable from the reported data. Data for BNT162b2 [26], mRNA1273 [27], and Ad26.CoV2.S [28] are from documents provided by the U.S. Food and Drug Administration (FDA) to Vaccines and Related Biological Products Advisory Committee meetings. Additional data for Ad26.COV2.S are from [29,30], which report lower efficacy against hospitalization than the FDA submission. Data for ChAdOx1-S are from [31,32]. [a] The Ad26.CoV2.S protocol did not distinguish between actual hospitalizations and people who came to the emergency department but were not hospitalized. [b] Results reported as "100%" indicate no qualifying events in the treatment group, and do not imply that the vaccine would achieve actual efficacy of 100% in a larger population. [c] Inferred from no adjudicated cases in the treatment group requiring hospitalization. [d] The formal Pfizer submission to the FDA reported no hospitalizations among vaccinated people, but 4 individuals with "severe illness", of whom 1 was in the vaccine group (not hospitalized). The related academic article [33] reported 6 severe cases between 14 and 112 days after receiving vaccine or placebo, of whom 1 was in the vaccine group. [e] Protocols for defining asymptomatic infection varied across the countries in the ChAdOx1-S trial, which limits the reliability of these point estimates.

This and later tables report point estimates from the indicated studies. Where there are multiple estimates from a single study, or from multiple studies, we report the range of the point estimates.

The Phase 3 trial results were highly promising, especially for the mRNA vaccines. Efficacy against symptomatic disease was high, as was the apparent efficacy against hospitalization or death. The viral vector vaccines (Ad26.CoV2.S and ChAdOx1-S) showed lower efficacy against symptomatic disease, but performed strongly against hospitalization or death, especially ChAdOx1-S.

3.3. Evidence from Observational Studies on VE Soon within 120 Days after Vaccination

Table 2 summarizes evidence from observational studies of VE in the general population within 120 days after vaccination. The data from Israel on BNT162b2 is particularly compelling, given high-quality, population-level data, and several excellent research groups. Qatar also vaccinated principally with BNT162b2. It has similar data quality but a much younger population (91% under age 50), so may be less representative of outcomes for older adults. Data on ChAdOx1-S are limited because many UK studies did not report vaccine-specific results and the UK used an extended time interval between doses, so some UK studies did not satisfy the inclusion criteria.

The principal relevant variants for these studies were the late-2020, Alpha, and Beta variants.

Overall, the evidence for the mRNA vaccines and ChAdOx1-S was consistent with the clinical trials for any infection and symptomatic infection, although some observational studies reported a lower VE than found in the trials. The early studies confirmed the superior performance for the mRNA vaccines against symptomatic infection, compared to the viral vector vaccines.

The early observational studies also provided large-sample evidence, not available from the initial trials, of strong performance for all four vaccines against hospitalization and death. Anecdotal evidence suggested that most vaccinated persons who required hospitalization were very old or had major comorbidities. The mRNA vaccines were more protective than the viral vector vaccines, and VE for the one-dose Ad26.CoV2.S vaccine against hospitalization and death was below the levels seen for the other vaccines.

Table 2. Early observational evidence on vaccine effectiveness (pre-Delta).

	Efficacy vs.			
	Any Infection	**Symptomatic Infection**	**Hospitalization [b]**	**Death [b]**
Vaccine				
BNT162b2	65.1–93.8% [a]	86.0–97.7%	87.0–100.0%	91.1–100.0%
mRNA1273	65.1–96.4%	84.9–96.3%	90.6–100.0%	96.0–99.0%
Ad26.CoV2.S	64.0–74.2%	NR	71.0–83.5%	78.0–82.8%
ChAdOx1-S	63.1–67.0%	44.5–74.5%	75.7–95.2%	93.0–94.1%

Table sources: [14,23,34–50]. NR = not reported or not computable from the reported data. The samples in [37,38] overlap. [a] The value for [36] is an average of estimates for shorter time periods after second dose. [b] Results reported as "100%" indicate no qualifying events in the treatment group and do not imply that the vaccine would achieve actual VE of 100% in a larger population.

3.4. Evidence on Waning, Principally against Delta Variant

By July 2021, the COVID-19 situation had greatly changed. The Delta variant had become dominant, and Israeli data provided evidence that VE for BNT162b2 had declined substantially against all outcomes by 5–6 months post-vaccination. Table 3 summarizes the evidence on VE more than 120 days after vaccination. Delta became dominant over the same period in which VE was waning. From the available data, it is not feasible to separate waning into the waning that would have occurred against earlier variants, additional or more rapid waning against Delta, and lower VE against Delta than against earlier variants. The limited available evidence supports waning against both Delta and earlier variants, as well as lower VE against Delta, for both symptomatic infection and hospitalization [22,50–53].

Table 3. VE against harmonized endpoints at last 120 days after vaccination, principally against Delta variant.

	Efficacy vs.			
	Any Infection	**Symptomatic Infection**	**Hospitalization**	**Death**
Vaccine				
BNT162b2	0.0–54·0% [a, b]	0.0–70.1% [a, b]	71.5–90.7%	83.0–90.4%
mRNA1273	0.0–80.0% [b]	52.1–81.9%	61.0–92.3%	88.0–93.7%
Ad26.CoV2.S	36.0%	37.5–64.3%	65.0–80.0%	73.0–80.0%
ChAdOx1-S	NR	0.0–59.0% [b]	52.3–77.0%	78.7–82.0%

Table sources: [23,36,39,41,43–45,53–60]. NR = not reported or not computable from the reported data. [a] For BNT162b2, [36] reports negative point estimates for any infection and symptomatic infection as 0.0. Post-authorization clinical trial results for BNT162b2, not included in Table 3 because they predated the Delta variant, found waning against symptomatic infection [61]. [b] Insignificant negative point estimates reported in a few studies are reported in this table as 0%.

The 120-day lower bound was chosen based on evidence of clinically important waning beginning around then, our assessment of the time periods since vaccination for which the included studies reported data, and the small number of studies presenting data for a longer period since vaccination or permitting finer decomposition. Waning was progressive, and the Supplementary Materials includes several graphs from individual studies that show this (e.g., [22,51]). Since waning is progressive, the point estimates in Table 3 will overstate VE for periods substantially longer than 120 days after initial vaccination.

Table 3 provides evidence of waning for all vaccines across all outcomes. It also provides further evidence for a comparative ranking of vaccines. mRNA1273 wanes more slowly than BNT162b2, and the mRNA vaccines continue to have higher VE than the viral vector vaccines against hospitalization and death.

3.5. Evidence for Important Waning against Severe Disease and Death

In the summer and fall of 2021, booster skeptics argued against the need for boosters, citing studies, including those reported in Table 3, that showed substantial VE against severe disease and death and modest percentage declines from the initial VE percentages shown in Table 2. Indeed, the VE declines against hospitalization and death may appear small. However, Tables 1–3 adopt the standard practice of reporting VE as a percent reduction in risk, relative to no vaccination. An alternative view, adopted in Table 4, focuses instead on the remaining risk of an outcome (RR = 100% − VE). As Table 4 shows, RR levels are sharply higher after waning, including against hospitalization and death, for BNT162b2, mRNA1273, and ChAdOx1-S. Ad26.CoV2.S does not wane as strongly, but this is from much higher RR levels soon after vaccination.

Table 4. Remaining risk (RR): <120 days (Panel A) vs. >120 days (Panel B) after vaccination.

	Remaining Risk (RR) vs.			
	Any Infection	Symptomatic Infection	Hospitalization [b]	Death [b]
Panel A: Evidence within 120 days after Initial Vaccination				
BNT162b2	6.2–34.9%	2.3–14.0%	0.0–13.0%	0.0–8.9%
mRNA1273	6.3–34.9%	3.7–15.2%	0.0–9.4%	1.0–4.0%
Ad26.CoV2.S	25.8–36%	NR	15.6–29.0%	17.2–220%
ChAdOx1-S	33.0–36.9%	25.5–55.5%	4.8–24.3%	5.9–7.0%
Panel B. Evidence Over 120 days after Initial Vaccination				
BNT162b2	46.0–100%	29.9–100%	9.3–28.5%	9.6–17.0%
mRNA1273	20.0–100%	18.1–48.8%	7.7–39.0%	6.3–12.0%
Ad26.CoV2.S	64.0%	35.7–62.5%	20.0–35.0%	20.0–27.0%
ChAdOx1-S	NR	41.1–100%	23.0–47.7%	18.0–21.3%

Panel A reports point estimates for remaining risk (RR) within 120 days after initial vaccination, based on the VE estimates in Table 2. Panel B reports point estimates for RR more than 120 days after initial vaccination, thus allowing for waning, based on the VE estimates in Table 3. RR = 100% − VE. NR = not reported or not computable from the reported data. [b] Insignificant negative point estimates reported in a few studies are reported in this table as 0%.

Consider the death outcome and the midpoints of the ranges in Table 4. For BNT162b2, RR against death increases from 4.5% to 13.3% (roughly tripling). For mRNA1273, RR against death increases from 2.5% to 9.2% (more than tripling, but from a lower base). For ChAdOx1-S, RR against death increases from 6.5% to 19.7% (tripling, from a higher base). These RR increases have major implications for the mortality of vaccinated persons, and thus for the value of a booster dose. Remaining hospitalization risk also rises sharply for all three vaccines.

In Panel B, the mRNA vaccines have a smaller advantage over the viral vector vaccines and perhaps no remaining advantage against infection or symptomatic infection. However, the mRNA vaccines retain a strong advantage over viral vector vaccines against hospitalization and death. When comparing the viral vector vaccines, Ad26.CoV2.S catches up to ChAdOx1-S against hospitalization and death.

The waning effectiveness of vaccines against hospitalization and death was observed in a real-world setting for BNT162b2 in Israel in mid-2021. Israel was one of the first countries to vaccinate its population, almost exclusively with BNT162b2, and thus one of the first to experience waning. Israel responded with a booster campaign, discussed in the next section.

3.6. Evidence on Booster Effectiveness against Delta Variant

Data on booster VE are limited to boosters for the mRNA vaccines and VE against to the Delta variant, which became dominant in mid-2021 before boosters were used. ChAdOx1-S was not often used as a booster during the period we studied, and J&J was rarely used as a booster due to its inferior performance for initial vaccination. The most complete data are for BNT162b2 from Israel, which responded to evidence on waning by launching an aggressive booster vaccination campaign, beginning in July 2021, with eligibility starting 5 months after the initial vaccination [9,62]. Studies in countries with later booster rollouts, including the U.S., cannot separate the effects of the booster dose from the large differences in infectiousness and immune evasion between the Delta and Omicron variants.

Table 5 reports evidence on VE for persons receiving a booster relative to vaccinated but unboosted persons (Panel A), as well as more limited evidence on VE for persons receiving a booster relative to unvaccinated people (Panel B).

Table 5. Booster effectiveness.

	Any Infection	Symptomatic Infection	Hospitalization	Death
Panel A. Risk Reduction (Booster vs. Vaccinated)				
Vaccine				
BNT162b2	86–91%	75–95%	70–95%	81–97%
mRNA1273		86–89%	82%	
Panel B. VE vs. Unvaccinated				
BNT162b2		90–93%	88–99%	93–99%
mRNA1273		89%	86%	87%

Table sources: Panel A [63–70]. Panel B [24,66,69,71,72]. Panel A reports point estimates for risk reduction for vaccinated plus boosted people versus people vaccinated without booster, to nearest percent, for endpoints with available data. Panel B reports VE for people with initial vaccination plus booster versus. unvaccinated persons.

The estimates of booster effectiveness from Table 5 suggest that the booster dose was able to substantially restore, against the Delta variant, the high protection against hospitalization and death seen for earlier variants soon after vaccination. However, the booster dose was itself subject to waning VE against infection by the Omicron variant [73]. The extent to which the booster would have waned against the Delta variant is not knowable, due to the short time between when boosters became available and the early 2022 emergence of Omicron as the dominant variant.

4. Discussion
4.1. Developing Vaccines for a Novel Pathogen

The vaccines against COVID-19 were developed, tested in randomized trials for efficacy against symptomatic infection and for safety, and authorized by regulators in record time. The rapid authorization of several vaccines in late 2020 surely saved millions of lives worldwide. However, the speed with which these vaccines were developed, tested, and authorized involved tradeoffs. The short interval between the first and second doses for the two-dose vaccines was established by the manufacturers with an eye to the minimum spacing needed to establish near-term efficacy, rather than with a view toward optimal dose spacing for longer-lasting protection. Based on experience with other vaccines [74], there was always a likelihood that the initial protection would wane and a booster would be needed, even if the extent and speed of waning was yet to be determined. Moreover, the initial trials were not sized to study efficacy against hospitalization and death, given the low population rates for those endpoints.

The initial speed was wonderful and provides a model to build on. But both vaccine manufacturers and public health authorities fell short in planning for the evaluation of potential waning of VE, and in failing to use RR as a metric for evaluating vaccine performance, especially against severe disease. Observational data to assess waning was potentially available on a massive scale, but in most countries, these data were not systematically collected and analyzed.

This review offers evidence on VE and RR against severe disease and on the waning that was actually experienced, against both infection and severe disease. It can guide the response to a future novel pathogen.

4.2. Overall Evidence on Booster Value

There is strong evidence of both (i) vaccine waning beginning 4–5 months after initial vaccination and (ii) significantly higher VE (lower RR) following a booster. Waning began before the mid-2021 emergence of the Delta variant, continued during the Delta-dominant period, and may have been accelerated by the transition from Alpha to Delta as the dominant SARS-CoV-2 strain. After initial caution, e.g., [58], the FDA strongly supports the value of a booster dose, with the FDA commissioner and head of vaccines unit writing in May 2022 that "it is critical that patients and caregivers understand the profound benefit of a booster dose of the mRNA vaccines" [75].

The value of a booster against hospitalization and death is seen primarily for ages 60+ (e.g., [62,64]). But older people account for the vast majority of COVID-19 deaths. The real-world implications of booster doses in reducing mortality are large. A recent study uses Israel as a counterfactual for the U.S. and concludes that if the U.S. had matched Israel's timing for booster authorization, uptake speed, and eventual uptake rates, this would have saved the lives of 29,000 people aged 55+, versus the actual U.S. booster experience. Conversely, never authorizing a booster dose would have cost an additional 41,000 lives [62]. These amounts are substantial fractions of the 106,000 deaths among vaccinated people during the study period. Giving greater weight to RR as a metric, rather than VE, might have led to faster recognition of waning and booster approval.

4.3. Re-Examining Vaccine Dose Timing

The evidence for waning VE suggests that, at least for older people, vaccination for SARS-CoV-2 should include an initial two-dose primary series plus at least one booster, 6 months or so after the first two doses. The vaccination pattern of an initial dose or doses and then a gap before an additional dose, is familiar from recommended schedules for other vaccines [76]. The mRNA vaccines were more effective than the viral vector vaccines, at least in developed countries where the cold-chain requirements for these vaccines could be met. Additional booster doses may be appropriate, at least for ages 60+ [12,20,73], but waning VE for a first booster and thus the potential value of a second or subsequent booster cannot be reliably assessed within the time period of this study.

The interval between primary doses and subsequent (booster) dose(s), and whether that interval depends on vaccine type or patient age, are topics for future research. So is the value of mixing and matching vaccines, either across vaccine types (mRNA versus viral vector or other types, such as the Novavax spike-protein based vaccine [77]) or within types (e.g., mRNA1273 vs. BNT162b2). One UK study finds similar VE against infection for ChAdOx1-S boosted with BNT162b2 versus homologous BNT162b2 vaccination plus a booster dose [78]. A further factor is the risk, illustrated by the emergence of Omicron, of the emergence of more infectious or immune-evasive virus variants. Regulatory decisions on when to allow or recommend additional doses also need to take into account the time needed for population rollout. Thus, even if boosting at 6 months was optimal spacing for individuals, earlier *availability* (perhaps at 5 months as Israel decided) would likely be preferable. The optimal number and timing of vaccine doses might be different for the previously infected, who face a lower risk of severe disease [42,79,80].

4.4. Comparing across Vaccines: RR for Hospitalization and Death

For both initial vaccination and a booster dose, RR against hospitalization or death provides a valuable, underused metric for comparing vaccines. Using RR as the metric, a clear preference order emerges for both of these endpoints, both before and after waning: mRNA1273 > BNT162b2 > ChAdOx1-S > Ad26.CoV2.S. The RRs for death, measured at midpoints after waning, are 9.2% for mRNA1273; 13.3% for BNT162b2; 19.7% for ChAdOx1-S; and 23.5% for Ad26.CoV2.S. A similar gradient is seen for hospitalization.

When comparing vaccines, the endpoint matters and so does the time since initial vaccination. Ad26.CoV2.S is initially inferior for all endpoints (Table 2) but wanes more slowly and after 120 days is comparable to ChAdOx1-S for infection (Table 3) and only modestly inferior to ChAdOx1-S against hospitalization and death.

However, differences between vaccines seen for primary vaccination may diminish after a booster. A U.S. study compares BNT162b2 and mRNA1273 and finds a BNT162b2/mRNA1273 odds ratio for death of 2.40 (z = 4.26) after waning for primary vaccination, but only 1.25 (insignificant, z = 0.50) after a booster dose [24]. Whether larger differences between vaccines after a booster dose would emerge over a longer time period is unknown.

4.5. Population Implications of Booster Use

Our analysis focused on the benefit of a booster dose for those receiving it. But there can also be benefits to others. One benefit is reduced infection spread. If R_t (the time-varying mean number of people infected by each initially infected person) exceeds 1, a single infection can lead to a large number of follow-on infections. Even if R_t is modestly below 1, a single infection predicts multiple follow-on infections. For example, for an R_t of 0.9, each infection predicts roughly five additional infections $(0.9 + 0.9^2 + 0.9^3 + \ldots)$. The young, who generally experience less severe illness, can infect the old, who are more likely to experience severe illness [9]. The vaccinated can infect the unvaccinated. The relevant R_t is time-varying and unknown, but greater booster uptake should imply lower transmission. Also, at various times during the pandemic, including early 2022, many hospitals were at or beyond normal capacity, leading to higher mortality for both COVID-19 and other conditions. Reducing infections during peak periods can also reduce demand for treatments that are in short supply.

4.6. Value of Harmonized Endpoints

There are no generally accepted, -standardized protocols for clinical endpoints for measuring VE. A lesson from this project is the difficulty of reporting data for harmonized endpoints across studies and countries. We propose that useful categories, which researchers should report where feasible, should include any infection, symptomatic infection, hospitalization, death, and ideally a category between hospitalization and death (perhaps admission to intensive care). Even here, there will be uncertainty—deciding which symptoms count as symptomatic infection, the challenge of measuring asymptomatic infection reliably, and different criteria used in different countries for which patients need hospitalization or intensive care. But these categories are more manageable than categories such as "severe" or "critical" disease, which may be feasible to use in a formal trial or a single country [81] but translate poorly across countries and health systems.

4.7. Healthy Vaccinee Bias and Behavioral Differences between the Vaccinated and Unvaccinated

The observational studies we rely on generally cannot address differences between vaccinated and unvaccinated people in behavior or underlying health. For example, test-negative designs, which were the principal designs used in the observational studies that we reviewed, suffer from healthy vaccinee bias [82,83], in which healthier people, who face lower background risk of severe disease, are more likely to become vaccinated or boosted.

This bias can be substantial, especially for VE against hospitalization or death [13,24]. The implication is that many studies overestimate VE (underestimate RR). Most studies do not match vaccinated to unvaccinated (beyond age and gender), and those that do often do not control for prior infection. Underestimates of RR need not change the relative ranking of vaccines. However, higher RR for initial vaccination implies a greater value for a booster dose [13].

A separate concern is behavioral differences between the vaccinated and unvaccinated, based on their knowledge of their own status. The negative VE point estimates against infection after waning, found in some studies [36,39], could reflect the vaccinated relaxing their guard against infection. Even careful matching cannot address behavior differences between the vaccinated and unvaccinated. However, another possible explanation for negative point estimates is immune imprinting, a hypothesis still under study in which initial (naïve) exposure (whether to the pathogen or through immunization), and possibly subsequent exposure to the same pathogen/vaccine, causes the body's immune system to "imprint" the virus variant from initial exposure(s) and to under-react to a newer immune-evasive variant by developing fewer new antibodies that target the new variant, and instead continuing to produce antibodies targeted to the initial exposure(s) [84].

4.8. The Need for Data Collection Infrastructure

The COVID-19 pandemic was worldwide as was vaccination. Yet the studies that met our inclusion and exclusion criteria generally fell into several limited groups: (i) the initial, multicountry randomized trials and followup studies, which were not sized to have power to measure VE against hospitalization and death; (ii) studies from Israel, Qatar, and the U.K., which have national public health data infrastructure and strong research teams that could exploit this data; (iii) the U.S., which has fragmented data but good research teams who were able to obtain data from individual health systems or individual states; and (iv) other single-country studies, usually from smaller countries with national data, which often was less effectively exploited. These limits on the available studies affect the generalizability of this review.

The limits on available data also underscore the value of data infrastructure and the need to take steps to improve this infrastructure worldwide before the next pandemic. To respond promptly to emerging evidence—for COVID-19, the evidence on waning that emerged beginning in mid-2021—regulators need access to population-level data in real time, including linkages across datasets (e.g., vaccination, infection, hospitalization, death). They also need the willingness to act on initial evidence, that is less complete or definitive than they might want in a non-crisis situation.

5. Conclusions

The mRNA-based COVID-19 vaccines were initially highly effective against all endpoints. The viral vector vaccines were also effective but less so, especially Ad26.CoV2.S (Tables 1 and 2). However, all vaccines waned substantially against all endpoints, over a limited time period after primary vaccination. This is easier to see using RR as the metric instead of VE (Table 4). Data for booster doses of the mRNA vaccines show substantial reduction in RR, which translates into many lives saved among older people who obtained booster doses. Vaccine development and VE assessment could have, but did not, included explicit assessment of waning, using the observational data generated by the worldwide rollout of primary vaccination.

The experience with COVID-19 suggests that even with two-dose primary vaccination, initial vaccination planning for a novel, highly transmissible respiratory pathogen should reflect the potential value of at least one additional dose and should include population-level surveillance plans sufficient to identify, in close to real time, the timing and need for such a dose. Public health authorities also should prepare the ground for a possible additional dose, and not overpromise with regard to the duration of protection from initial vaccination.

Supplementary Materials: Supplementary materials for this article can be downloaded at: https://www.mdpi.com/article/10.3390/microorganisms12010089/s1, They include textual material, as well as the following tables and figures: PRISMA Flowchart; PRISMA Checklist; PRISMA-S Checklist; Table S2.1. Data Sources Satisfying Inclusion Criteria for Table 2—BNT162b2 (Pfizer); Table S2.2: Data Sources Satisfying Inclusion Criteria for Table 2—mRNA1273 (Moderna); Table S2.3: Data Sources Satisfying Inclusion Criteria for Table 2—Ad26.CoV2.S (J&J); Table S2.4 Data Sources Satisfying Inclusion Criteria for Table 2—ChAdOxS-1 (AstraZeneca); Table S3.1 Data Sources Satisfying Inclusion Criteria for Table 3—BNT162b2 (Pfizer); Table S3.2 Data Sources Satisfying Inclusion Criteria for Table 3—mRNA1273 (Moderna); Table S3.3 Data Sources Satisfying Inclusion Criteria for Table 3—Ad26.CoV2.S (J&J); Table S3.4 Data Sources Satisfying Inclusion Criteria for Table 3—ChAdOx1-S (AstraZeneca).

Author Contributions: Both authors contributed to all aspects of the research. All authors have read and agreed to the published version of the manuscript.

Funding: Black received funding for related work from the National Institutes of Health, Award Number UL1TR001436. Thaw reports no funding.

Data Availability Statement: Not applicable because this review does not rely on original data.

Conflicts of Interest: The authors declare no conflicts of interest.

References

1. FDA News Release (11 December 2020): FDA Takes Key Action in Fight against COVID-19 by Issuing Emergency Use Authorization for First COVID-19 Vaccine. Available online: https://www.fda.gov/news-events/press-announcements/fda-takes-key-action-fight-against-covid-19-issuing-emergency-use-authorization-first-covid-19 (accessed on 17 December 2023).

2. FDA News Release (18 December 2020), FDA Takes Additional Action in Fight Against COVID-19 by Issuing Emergency Use Authorization for Second COVID-19 Vaccine. Available online: https://www.fda.gov/news-events/press-announcements/fda-takes-additional-action-fight-against-covid-19-issuing-emergency-use-authorization-second-covid (accessed on 17 December 2023).

3. Burton, T.; Loftus, P. J&J Single-Dose COVID-19 Vaccine Gains Backing from FDA Advisory Panel. *Wall Str. J.* 26 February 2021.

4. AstraZeneca Press Release (30 December 2020). AstraZeneca's COVID-19 Vaccine Authorised for Emergency Supply in the UK. Available online: https://www.astrazeneca.com/media-centre/press-releases/2020/astrazenecas-covid-19-vaccine-authorised-in-uk.html# (accessed on 17 December 2023).

5. Franchi; Lorenzo; Bates, G.; Stake, M.; Osinski, K.; Ahn, K.-W.; Meurer, J.R.; Black, B. The Disappearing COVID-Naïve Population: Evidence from Antibody Seroprevalence in Milwaukee County, Wisconsin (working paper, December 2023).

6. Wiegand, R.E.; Deng, Y.; Deng, X.; Lee, A.; Meyer, W.A.; Letovsky, S.; Charles, M.D.; Gundlapalli, A.V.; MacNeil, A.; Hall, A.J.; et al. Estimated SARS-CoV-2 antibody seroprevalence trends and relationship to reported case prevalence from a repeated, cross-sectional study in the 50 states and the District of Columbia, United States—October 25, 2020–February 26, 2022. *Lancet Reg. Health Am.* **2023**, *18*, 100403. [CrossRef]

7. Jones, J.M.; Manrique, I.M.; Stone, M.S.; Grebe, E.; Saa, P.; Germanio, C.D.; Spencer, B.R.; Notari, E.; Bravo, M.; Lanteri, M.C.; et al. Estimates of SARS-CoV-2 Seroprevalence and Incidence of Primary SARS-CoV-2 Infections Among Blood Donors, by COVID-19 Vaccination Status—United States, April 2021–September 2022. *Morb. Mortal. Wkly. Rep.* **2023**, *72*, 601–605. [CrossRef]

8. Krause, P.R.; Fleming, T.R.; Peto, R.; Longini, I.M.; Figueroa, J.P.; Sterne, J.A.; Henao-Restrepo, A.M. Considerations in Boosting COVID-19 Immune Response. *Lancet* **2021**, *398*, 1377–1380. [CrossRef]

9. Gavish, N.; Yaari, R.; Huppert, A.; Katriel, G. Population-level implications of the Israeli booster campaign to curtail COVID-19 resurgence. *Sci. Transl. Med.* **2022**, *14*, eabn9836. [CrossRef]

10. Feikin, D.R.; Higdon, M.M.; Abu-Raddad, L.J.; Andrews, N.; Araos, R.; Goldberg, Y.; Patel, M.K. Duration of effectiveness of vaccines against SARS-CoV-2 infection and COVID-19 disease: Results of a systematic review and meta-regression. *Lancet* **2022**, *399*, 924–944. [CrossRef]

11. Magen, O.; Waxman, J.G.; Makov-Assif, M.; Vered, R.; Dicker, D.; Hernán, M.A.; Lipsitch, M.; Reis, B.Y.; Balicer, R.D.; Dagan, N. Fourth Dose of BNT162b2 mRNA COVID-19 Vaccine in a Nationwide Setting. *N. Engl. J. Med.* **2022**, *386*, 1603–1614. [CrossRef]

12. Bar-On, Y.M.; Goldberg, Y.; Mandel, M.; Bodenheimer, O.; Amir, O.; Freedman, L.; Alroy-Preis, S.; Ash, N.; Huppert, A.; Milo, R. Protection by a Fourth Dose of BNT162b2 against Omicron in Israel. *N. Engl. J. Med.* **2022**, *386*, 1712–1720. [CrossRef]

13. Atanasov, V.; Barreto, N.; Whittle, J.; Meurer, J.; Weston, B.W.; Luo, Q.; Franchi, L.; Yuan, A.Y.; Zhang, R.; Black, B. Understanding COVID-19 Vaccine Effectiveness against Death Using a Novel Measure: COVID Excess Mortality Percentage. *Vaccines* **2023**, *11*, 379. [CrossRef]

14. Robles-Fontan, M.M.; Nieves, E.G.; Cardona-Gerena, I.; Izirarry, R.A. Effectiveness Estimates of Three COVID-19 Vaccines Based on Observational Data from Puerto Rico. *Lancet Reg. Health-Am.* **2022**, *9*, 100212. [CrossRef]

15. Lytras, T.; Kontopidou, F.; Lambrou, A.; Tsiodras, S. Comparative effectiveness and durability of COVID-19 vaccination against death and severe disease in an ongoing nationwide mass vaccination campaign. *J. Med Virol.* **2022**, *94*, 5044–5050. [CrossRef]
16. Zeng, B.; Gao, L.; Zhou, Q.; Yu, K.; Sun, F. Effectiveness of COVID-19 vaccines against SARS-CoV-2 variants of concern: A systematic review and meta-analysis. *BMC Med.* **2022**, *20*, 200. [CrossRef]
17. Mohammed, I.; Nauman, A.; Paul, P.; Ganesan, S.; Chen, K.-H.; Jalil, S.M.S.; Jaouni, S.H.; Kawas, H.; Khan, W.A.; Vattoth, A.L.; et al. The efficacy and effectiveness of the COVID-19 vaccines in reducing infection, severity, hospitalization, and mortality: A systematic review. *Hum. Vaccines Immunother.* **2022**, *18*, 2027160. [CrossRef]
18. Graña, C.; Ghosn, L.; Evrenoglou, T.; Jarde, A.; Minozzi, S.; Bergman, H.; Buckley, B.S.; Probyn, K.; Villanueva, G.; Henschke, N.; et al. Efficacy and safety of COVID-19 vaccines. *Cochrane Database Syst. Rev.* **2022**, *2023*, CD015477. [CrossRef]
19. Dean, N.E.; Hogan, J.W.; Schnitzer, M.E. COVID-19 Vaccine Effectiveness and the Test-Negative Design. *N. Engl. J. Med.* **2021**, *385*, 1431–1433. [CrossRef]
20. Arbel, R.; Sergienko, R.; Friger, M.; Peretz, A.; Beckenstein, T.; Yaron, S.; Netzer, D.; Hammerman, A. Effectiveness of a second BNT162b2 booster vaccine against hospitalization and death from COVID-19 in adults aged over 60 years. *Nat. Med.* **2022**, *28*, 1486–1490. [CrossRef]
21. Glatman-Freedman, A.; Bromberg, M.; Dichtiar, R.; Hershkovitz, Y.; Keinan-Boker, L. The BNT162b2 vaccine effectiveness against new COVID-19 cases and complications of breakthrough cases: A nation-wide retrospective longitudinal multiple cohort analysis using individualised data. *EBioMedicine* **2021**, *72*, 103574. [CrossRef]
22. Goldberg, Y.; Mandel, M.; Bar-On, Y.M.; Bodenheimer, O.; Freedman, L.; Haas, E.J.; Milo, R.; Alroy-Preis, S.; Ash, N.; Huppert, A. Waning Immunity after the BNT162b2 Vaccine in Israel. *N. Engl. J. Med.* **2021**, *385*, e85. [CrossRef]
23. Berec, L.; Šmíd, M.; Přibylová, L.; Májek, O.; Pavlík, T.; Jarkovský, J.; Zajíček, M.; Weiner, J.; Barusová, T.; Trnka, J. Protection provided by vaccination, booster doses and previous infection against COVID-19 infection, hospitalisation or death over time in Czechia. *PLoS ONE* **2022**, *17*, e0270801. [CrossRef]
24. Atanasov, V.; Barreto, N.; Whittle, J.; Meurer, J.; Weston, B.W.; Luo, Q.; Yuan, A.Y.; Franchi, L.; Zhang, R.; Black, B. Selection Effects and COVID-19 Mortality Risk after Pfizer vs. Moderna Vaccination: Evidence from Linked Mortality and Vaccination Records. *Vaccines* **2023**, *11*, 971. [CrossRef]
25. Schaffer, A.L.; Hulme, W.J.; Horne, E.M.; Parker, E.P.; Walker, V.; Stables, C.; Sterne, J.A. Effect of the 2022 COVID-19 booster vaccination campaign on 50-year-olds in England: Regression discontinuity analysis in OpenSAFELY. *medRxiv* **2023**. [CrossRef]
26. U.S. Food and Drug Administration Briefing Document, Pfizer-BioNTech COVID-19 Vaccine, Vaccines and Related Biological Products Advisory Committee Meeting. 10 December 2020. Available online: https://www.fda.gov/media/144245/download (accessed on 17 December 2023).
27. U.S. Food and Drug Administration Briefing Document, Moderna COVID-19 Vaccine, Vaccines and Related Biological Products Advisory Committee Meeting. 17 December 2020. Available online: https://www.fda.gov/media/144434/download (accessed on 17 December 2023).
28. U.S. Food and Drug Administration Briefing Document, Janssen Ad26.COV2.S Vaccine for the Prevention of COVID-19, Vaccines and Related Biological Products Advisory Committee Meeting. 26 February 2021. Available online: https://www.fda.gov/media/146217/download (accessed on 17 December 2023).
29. Sadoff, J.; Gray, G.; Vandebosch, A.; Cárdenas, V.; Shukarev, G.; Grinsztejn, B.; Goepfert, P.A.; Truyers, C.; Fennema, H.; Spiessens, B.; et al. Safety and Efficacy of Single-Dose Ad26.COV2.S Vaccine against COVID-19. *N. Engl. J. Med.* **2021**, *384*, 2187–2201. [CrossRef] [PubMed]
30. Sadoff, J.; Gray, G.; Vandebosch, A.; Cárdenas, V.; Shukarev, G.; Grinsztejn, B.; Goepfert, P.A.; Truyers, C.; Van Dromme, I.; Spiessens, B.; et al. Final Analysis of Efficacy and Safety of Single-Dose Ad26.COV2.S. *N. Engl. J. Med.* **2022**, *386*, 847–860. [CrossRef] [PubMed]
31. Voysey, M.; Clemens SA, C.; Madhi, S.A.; Weckx, L.Y.; Folegatti, P.M.; Aley, P.K.; Bijker, E. Safety and Efficacy of the ChAdOx1 nCoV-19 Vaccine Against SARS-CoV-2: An Interim Analysis of Four Randomized Controlled Trials in Brazil, South Africa, and the UK. *Lancet* **2021**, *397*, 99–111. [CrossRef] [PubMed]
32. Falsey, A.R.; Sobieszczyk, M.E.; Hirsch, I.; Villafana, T.; Gonzalez-Lopez, A. Phase 3 Safety and Efficacy of AZD1222 (ChAdOx1 Ncov-10) COVID-19 Vaccine. *N. Engl. J. Med.* **2021**, *385*, 2348–2360. [CrossRef] [PubMed]
33. Polack, F.P.; Thomas, S.J.; Kitchin, N.; Jansen, K.U.; Gruber, W.C. Safety and Efficacy of the BNT162b2 mRNA COVID-19 Vaccine. *N. Engl. J. Med.* **2020**, *383*, 2603–2615. [CrossRef]
34. Abu-Raddad, L.J.; Chemaitelly, H.; Butt, A.A. Effectiveness of the BNT162b2 COVID-19 Vaccine against the B.1.1.7 and B.1.351 Variants. *N. Engl. J. Med.* **2021**, *385*, 187–189. [CrossRef]
35. Lopez Bernal, J.; Andrews, N.; Gower, C.; Chand, M.; Ramsay, M. Effectiveness of COVID-19 Vaccines against the B.1.617.2 (Delta) Variant. *N. Engl. J. Med.* **2021**, *385*, 585–594. [CrossRef]
36. Chemaitelly, H.; Tang, P.; Hasan, M.R.; AlMukdad, S.; Yassine, H.M.; Benslimane, F.M.; Abu-Raddad, L.J. Waning of BNT162b2 vaccine protection against SARS-CoV-2 infection in Qatar. *N. Engl. J. Med.* **2021**, *385*, e83. [CrossRef]
37. Dagan, N.; Barda, N.; Kepten, E.; Miron, O.; Perchik, S.; Katz, M.A.; Balicer, R.D. BNT162b2 mRNA COVID-19 Vaccine in a Nationwide Mass Vaccination Setting. *N. Engl. J. Med.* **2021**, *384*, 1412–1423. [CrossRef]

38. Haas, E.J.; Angulo, F.J.; McLaughlin, J.M.; Anis, E.; Singer, S.R.; Khan, F.; Books, N.; Smaja, M.; Mircus, G.; Pan, K.; et al. Impact and effectiveness of mRNA BNT162b2 vaccine against SARS-CoV-2 infections and COVID-19 cases, hospitalisations, and deaths following a nationwide vaccination campaign in Israel: An observational study using national surveillance data. *Lancet* **2021**, *397*, 1819–1829. [CrossRef]

39. Nordstrom, P.; Ballin, M.; Nordstrom, A. Risk of infection, hospitalisation, and death up to 9 months after a second dose of COVID-19 vaccine: A retrospective, total population cohort study in Sweden. *Lancet* **2022**, *399*, 814–823. [CrossRef] [PubMed]

40. Pilishvili, T.; Gierke, R.; Fleming-Dutra, K.E.; Farrar, J.L.; Mohr, N.M.; Talan, D.A.; Krishnadasan, A.; Harland, K.K.; Smithline, H.A.; Hou, P.C.; et al. Effectiveness of mRNA COVID-19 Vaccine among U.S. Health Care Personnel. *N. Engl. J. Med.* **2021**, *385*, e90. [CrossRef] [PubMed]

41. Self, W.H.; Tenforde, M.W.; Rhoads, J.P.; Gaglani, M.; Ginde, A.A.; Douin, D.J.; Cass, C. Comparative Effectiveness of Moderna, Pfizer-BioNTech, and Janssen (Johnson & Johnson) Vaccines in Preventing COVID-19 Hospitalizations Among Adults Without Immunocompromising Conditions—United States, March–August 2021. *Morb. Mortal. Wkly. Rep.* **2021**, *70*, 1337–1343.

42. Bruxvoort, K.J.; Sy, L.S.; Qian, L.; Ackerson, B.K.; Luo, Y.; Lee, G.S.; Tian, Y.; Florea, A.; Takhar, H.S.; Tubert, J.E.; et al. Real-world effectiveness of the mRNA-1273 vaccine against COVID-19: Interim results from a prospective observational cohort study. *Lancet Reg. Health-Am.* **2022**, *6*, 100134. [CrossRef] [PubMed]

43. Katikireddi, S.F.; Cerqueira-Silva, T.; Sheikh, A. Two-dose ChAdOx1 nCoV-19 vaccine protection against COVID-19 hospital admissions and deaths over time: A retrospective, population-based cohort study in Scotland and Brazil. *Lancet* **2022**, *399*, 25–35. [CrossRef] [PubMed]

44. Andrews, N.; Tessler, E.; Lopez Bernal, J. Duration of Protection against Mild and Severe Disease by COVID-19 Vaccines. *N. Engl. J. Med.* **2022**, *386*, 340–350. [CrossRef] [PubMed]

45. Thompson, M.G.; Burgess, J.L.; Naleway, A.L.; Tyner, H.; Yoon, S.K.; Meece, J.; Olsho, L.E.W.; Caban-Martinez, A.J.; Fowlkes, A.L.; Lutrick, K.; et al. Prevention and Attenuation of COVID-19 with the BNT162b2 and mRNA-1273 Vaccines. *N. Engl. J. Med.* **2021**, *385*, 320–329. [CrossRef] [PubMed]

46. Chemaitelly, H.; Yassine, H.M.; Benslimane, F.M.; Al Khatib, H.A.; Tang, P.; Hasan, M.R.; Malek, J.A.; Coyle, P.; Ayoub, H.H.; Al Kanaani, Z.; et al. mRNA-1273 COVID-19 vaccine effectiveness against the B.1.1.7 and B.1.351 variants and severe COVID-19 disease in Qatar. *Nat. Med.* **2021**, *27*, 1614–1621. [CrossRef]

47. Saciuk, Y.; Kertes, J.; Stein, N.S.; Zohar, A.E. Effectiveness of a Third Dose of BNT162b2 mRNA Vaccine. *J. Infect. Dis.* **2021**, *225*, 30–33. [CrossRef]

48. Thiruvengadam, R.; Awasthi, A.; Medigeshi, G.; Bhattacharya, S.; Mani, S.; Sivasubbu, S.; Garg, P.K. Effectiveness of ChAdOx1 nCoV-19 vaccine against SARS-CoV-2 infection during the delta (B.1.617.2) variant surge in India: A test-negative, case-control study and a mechanistic study of post-vaccination immune responses. *Lancet Infect. Dis.* **2022**, *22*, 473–482. [CrossRef]

49. Chung, H.; He, S.; Nasreen, S.; Sundaram, M.E.; Buchan, S.A.; Wilson, S.E.; Chen, B.; Calzavara, A.; Fell, D.B.; Austin, P.C.; et al. Effectiveness of BNT162b2 and mRNA-1273 COVID-19 vaccines against symptomatic SARS-CoV-2 infection and severe COVID-19 outcomes in Ontario, Canada: Test negative design study. *BMJ* **2021**, *374*, n1943. [CrossRef] [PubMed]

50. Pouwels, K.B.; Pritchard, E.; Matthews, P.C.; Stoesser, N.; Eyre, D.W.; Vihta, K.D.; House, T.; Hay, J.; Bell, J.I.; Newton, J.N.; et al. Effect of Delta variant on viral burden and vaccine effectiveness against new SARS-CoV-2 infections in the UK. *Nat. Med.* **2021**, *27*, 2127–2135. [CrossRef] [PubMed]

51. Israel, A.; Merzon, E.; Schäffer, A.A.; Shenhar, Y.; Green, I.; Golan-Cohen, A.; Ruppin, E.; Magen, E.; Vinker, S. Elapsed time since BNT162b2 vaccine and risk of SARS-CoV-2 infection: Test negative design study. *BMJ* **2021**, *375*, e067873. [CrossRef] [PubMed]

52. Mizrahi, B.; Lotan, R.; Kalkstein, N.; Peretz, A.; Perez, G.; Ben-Tov, A.; Chodick, G.; Gazit, S.; Patalon, T. Correlation of SARS-CoV-2 Breakthrough Infections to Time-from-Vaccine; Preliminary Study. 31 July 2021. Working Paper. Available online: https://www.medrxiv.org/content/10.1101/2021.07.29.21261317v1 (accessed on 17 December 2023).

53. Keegan, L.T.; Truelove, S.; Lessler, J. Analysis of Vaccine Effectiveness Against COVID-19 and the Emergence of Delta and Other Variants of Concern in Utah. *JAMA Netw. Open* **2021**, *4*, e2140906. [CrossRef] [PubMed]

54. Britton, A.; Fleming-Dutra, K.E.; Shang, N.; Smith, Z.R.; Dorji, T.; Derado, G.; Accorsi, E.K.; Ajani, U.A.; Miller, J.; Schrag, S.J.; et al. Association of COVID-19 Vaccination With Symptomatic SARS-CoV-2 Infection by Time Since Vaccination and Delta Variant Predominance. *JAMA* **2022**, *327*, 1032–1041. [CrossRef] [PubMed]

55. Gray, G.; Bekker, L. Update on the Janssen (JNJ) Ad26.COV2.S vaccine. *Rep. S. Afr. Dept Health* **2021**. Available online: https://sacoronavirus.co.za/2021/08/06/update-on-the-janssenjnj-ad26-cov2-s-vaccine-professors-glenda-gray-linda-gail-bekker/ (accessed on 17 December 2023).

56. Lin, D.-Y.; Gu, Y.; Wheeler, B.; Young, H.; Holloway, S.; Sunny, S.-K.; Moore, Z.; Zeng, D. Effectiveness of COVID-19 Vaccines over a 9-Month Period in North Carolina. *N. Engl. J. Med.* **2022**, *386*, 933–941. [CrossRef]

57. Tartof, S.Y.; Slezak, J.M.; Fischer, H.; Hong, V.; Ackerson, B.K.; Ranasinghe, O.N.; Frankland, T.B.; Ogun, O.A.; Zamparo, J.M.; Gray, S.; et al. Effectiveness of mRNA BNT162b2 COVID-19 vaccine up to 6 months in a large integrated health system in the USA: A retrospective cohort study. *Lancet* **2021**, *398*, 1407–1416. [CrossRef]

58. U.S. Food and Drug Administration Briefing Document, Emergency Use Authorization Amendment for a Booster Dose for the Janssen COVID-19 Vaccine (Ad26.COV2.S), Vaccines and Related Biological Products Advisory Committee Meeting. 15 October 2021. Available online: https://www.fda.gov/media/153129/download (accessed on 17 December 2023).

59. Bruxvoort, K.J.; Sy, L.S.; Qian, L.; Ackerson, B.K.; Luo, Y.; Lee, G.S.; Tian, Y.; Florea, A.; Aragones, M.; Tubert, J.E.; et al. Effectiveness of mRNA-1273 against delta, mu, and other emerging variants of SARS-CoV-2: Test negative case-control study. *BMJ* **2021**, *375*, e068848. [CrossRef]

60. Abu-Raddad, L.J.; Chemaitelly, H.; Bertollini, R. Waning mRNA-1273 Vaccine Effectiveness against SARS-CoV-2 Infection in Qatar. *N. Engl. J. Med.* **2022**, *386*, 1091–1093. [CrossRef]

61. Thomas, S.J.; Moreira, E.D., Jr.; Kitchin, N.; Absalon, J.; Gurtman, A.; Lockhart, S.; Perez, J.L.; Pérez Marc, G.; Polack, F.P.; Zerbini, C.; et al. Safety and Efficacy of the BNT162b2 mRNA COVID-19 Vaccine through 6 Months. *N. Engl. J. Med.* **2021**, *385*, 1761–1773. [CrossRef] [PubMed]

62. Bernard, B.; Atanasov, V.; Glatman-Freedman, A.; Keinan-Boker, L.; Reichman, A.; Franchi, L.; Meurer, J.R.; Luo, Q.; Thaw, D.B.; Moghtaderi, A. COVID-19 Boosters: If The US Had Matched Israel's Speed And Take-Up, An Estimated 29,000 US Lives Would Have Been Saved. *Health Aff.* **2023**, *42*, 1747–1757.

63. Arbel, R.; Hammerman, A.; Sergienko, R.; Friger, M.; Peretz, A.; Netzer, D.; Yaron, S. BNT162b2 Vaccine Booster and Mortality Due to COVID-19. *N. Engl. J. Med.* **2021**, *385*, 2413–2420. [CrossRef] [PubMed]

64. Bar-On, Y.M.; Goldberg, Y.; Mandel, M.; Bodenheimer, O.; Freedman, L.; Alroy-Preis, S.; Ash, N.; Huppert, A.; Milo, R. Protection against COVID-19 by BNT162b2 Booster across Age Groups. *N. Engl. J. Med.* **2021**, *385*, 2421–2430. [CrossRef] [PubMed]

65. Bar-On, Y.M.; Goldberg, Y.; Mandel, M.; Bodenheimer, O.; Freedman, L.; Kalkstein, N.; Mizrahi, B.; Alroy-Preis, S.; Ash, N.; Milo, R.; et al. Protection of BNT162b2 Vaccine Booster against COVID-19 in Israel. *N. Engl. J. Med.* **2021**, *385*, 1393–1400. [CrossRef] [PubMed]

66. Barda, N.; Dagan, N.; Cohen, C.; Hernán, M.A.; Lipsitch, M.; Kohane, I.S.; Reis, B.Y.; Balicer, R.D. Effectiveness of a third dose of the BNT162b2 mRNA COVID-19 vaccine for preventing severe outcomes in Israel: An observational study. *Lancet* **2021**, *398*, 2093–2100. [CrossRef]

67. Patalon, T.; Gazit, S.; Pitzer, V.E.; Prunas, O.; Warren, J.L.; Weinberger, D.M. Odds of Testing Positive for SARS-CoV-2 Following Receipt of 3 vs 2 Doses of the BNT162b2 mRNA Vaccine. *JAMA Intern. Med.* **2021**, *182*, 179–184. [CrossRef]

68. Drawz, P.E.; DeSilva, M.; Bodurtha, P.; Benitez, G.V.; Murray, A.; Chamberlain, A.M.; Dudley, R.A.; Waring, S.; Kharbanda, A.B.; Murphy, D.; et al. Effectiveness of BNT162b2 and mRNA-1273 Second Doses and Boosters for Severe Acute Respiratory Syndrome Coronavirus 2 (SARS-CoV-2) Infection and SARS-CoV-2–Related Hospitalizations: A Statewide Report From the Minnesota Electronic Health Record Consortium. *Clin. Infect. Dis.* **2022**, *75*, 890–892. [CrossRef]

69. Tartof, S.Y.; Slezak, J.M.; Puzniak, L.; Hong, V.; Frankland, T.B.; Ackerson, B.K.; Takhar, H.S.; Ogun, O.A.; Simmons, S.R.; Zamparo, J.M.; et al. Effectiveness of a third dose of BNT162b2 mRNA COVID-19 vaccine in a large US health system: A retrospective cohort study. *Lancet Reg. Health-Am.* **2022**, *9*, 100198. [CrossRef]

70. Moreira, E.D.; Kitchin, N.; Xu, X.; Dychter, S.S.; Lockhart, S.; Gurtman, A.; Perez, J.L.; Zerbini, C.; Dever, M.E.; Jennings, T.W.; et al. Safety and Efficacy of a Third Dose of BNT162b2 COVID-19 Vaccine. *N. Engl. J. Med.* **2022**, *386*, 1910–1921. [CrossRef]

71. Niesen, M.J.M.; Matson, R.; Puranik, A.; O'Horo, J.C.; Pawlowski, C.; Vachon, C.; Challener, D.; Virk, A.; Swift, M.; Speicher, L.; et al. Third dose vaccination with mRNA-1273 or BNT162b2 vaccines improves protection against SARS-CoV-2 infection. *PNAS Nexus* **2022**, *1*, pgac042. [CrossRef] [PubMed]

72. Andrews, N.; Stowe, J.; Kirsebom, F.; Toffa, S.; Sachdeva, R.; Gower, C.; Ramsay, M.; Bernal, J.L. Effectiveness of COVID-19 booster vaccines against COVID-19-related symptoms, hospitalization and death in England. *Nat. Med.* **2022**, *28*, 831–837. [CrossRef] [PubMed]

73. Patalon, T.; Saciuk, Y.; Peretz, A.; Perez, G.; Lurie, Y.; Maor, Y.; Gazit, S. Waning effectiveness of the third dose of the BNT162b2 mRNA COVID-19 vaccine. *Nat. Commun.* **2022**, *13*, 1–7. [CrossRef] [PubMed]

74. U.S. Centers for Disease Control and Prevention, Recommended Child and Adolescent Immunization Schedule for ages 18 years or younger, United States, 2021. Table 1. Available online: https://www.cdc.gov/vaccines/schedules/hcp/imz/child-adolescent.html (accessed on 17 December 2023).

75. Marks, P.; Woodcock, J.; Califf, R. COVID-19 Vaccination—Becoming Part of the New Normal. *JAMA* **2022**, *327*, 1863–1864. [CrossRef] [PubMed]

76. Jara, A.; Cuadrado, C.; Undurraga, E.A.; García, C.; Nájera, M.; Bertoglia, M.P.; Vergara, V.; Fernández, J.; García-Escorza, H.; Araos, R. Effectiveness of the second COVID-19 booster against Omicron: A large-scale cohort study in Chile. *Nat. Commun.* **2023**, *14*, 1–7. [CrossRef] [PubMed]

77. Branswell, H. FDA Authorized Novavax's Updated COVID-19 Vaccine. *Stat News.* 3 October 2023. Available online: https://www.statnews.com/2023/10/03/fda-authorizes-novavaxs-updated-covid-19-vaccine/ (accessed on 17 December 2023).

78. UK Health Security Agency, SARS-CoV-2 Variants of Concern and Variants under Investigation in England, Technical briefing:33 (update) (31 December 2021), Update on Hospitalization and Vaccine Effectiveness for Omicron, VOC-21NOV-01 (B.1.1.529). Available online: https://assets.publishing.service.gov.uk/government/uploads/system/uploads/attachment_data/file/1045619/Technical-Briefing-31-Dec-2021-Omicron_severity_update.pdf (accessed on 17 December 2023).

79. Andrews, N.; Stowe, J.; Kirsebom, F.; Toffa, S.; Rickeard, T.; Gallagher, E.; Gower, C.; Kall, M.; Groves, N.; O'Connell, A.-M.; et al. COVID-19 Vaccine Effectiveness against the Omicron (B.1.1.529) Variant. *N. Engl. J. Med.* **2022**, *386*, 1532–1546. [CrossRef] [PubMed]

80. Waxman, J.G.; Makov-Assif, M.; Reis, B.Y.; Netzer, D.; Balicer, R.D.; Dagan, N.; Barda, N. Comparing COVID-19-related hospitalization rates among individuals with infection-induced and vaccine-induced immunity in Israel. *Nat. Commun.* **2022**, *13*, 1–6. [CrossRef] [PubMed]

81. Mehrotra, D.V.; Janes, H.E.; Gilbert, P.B. Clinical Endpoints for Evaluating Efficacy in COVID-19 Vaccine Trials. *Ann. Intern. Med.* **2021**, *174*, 221–228. [CrossRef]

82. Høeg, T.B.; Duriseti, R.; Prasad, V. Potential "Healthy Vaccinee Bias" in a Study of BNT162b2 Vaccine against COVID-19. *N. Engl. J. Med.* **2023**, *389*, 284–285.

83. Shrank, W.H.; Patrick, A.R.; Brookhart, M.A. Healthy User and Related Biases in Observational Studies of Preventive Interventions: A Primer for Physicians. *J. Gen. Intern. Med.* **2011**, *26*, 546–550. [CrossRef]

84. Chemaitelly, H.; Ayoub, H.H.; Tang, P.; Coyle, P.; Yassine, H.M.; Al Thani, A.A.; Al-Khatib, H.A.; Hasan, M.R.; Al-Kanaani, Z.; Al-Kuwari, E.; et al. Long-term COVID-19 booster effectiveness by infection history and clinical vulnerability and immune imprinting: A retrospective population-based cohort study. *Lancet Infect. Dis.* **2023**, *23*, 816–827. [CrossRef] [PubMed]

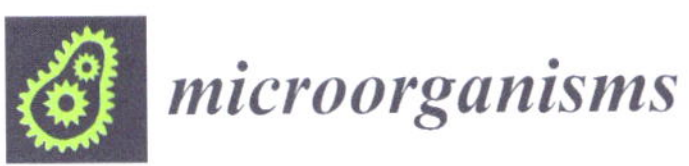

microorganisms

MDPI

Article

T Cell Response in Tuberculosis-Infected Patients Vaccinated against COVID-19

Luiz Henrique Agra Cavalcante-Silva [1], Ericka Garcia Leite [1], Fernanda Silva Almeida [1], Arthur Gomes de Andrade [1], Fernando Cézar Comberlang [1], Cintya Karina Rolim Lucena [2], Anna Stella Cysneiros Pachá [3], Bárbara Guimarães Csordas [1] and Tatjana S. L. Keesen [1,*]

[1] Immunology of Infectious Diseases Laboratory, Department of Cellular and Molecular Biology, Federal University of Paraíba, João Pessoa 58051-900, PB, Brazil; luiz0710@gmail.com (L.H.A.C.-S.); erickacg7@hotmail.com (E.G.L.); fernandaalmeida.ufpb@gmail.com (F.S.A.); arthurg.hit@gmail.com (A.G.d.A.); fcezar14@gmail.com (F.C.C.); barbara.guima.csordas@gmail.com (B.G.C.)
[2] Infectious and Contagious Disease Complex Dr. Clementino Fraga, João Pessoa 58015-270, PB, Brazil; cintyabeatriz@hotmail.com
[3] Health Secretary of the Paraíba State, João Pessoa 58040-440, PB, Brazil; anna.vigsaude@gmail.com
* Correspondence: tat.keesen@cbiotec.ufpb.br

Abstract: Many studies have focused on SARS-CoV-2 and *Mycobacterium tuberculosis* (*Mtb*) co-infection consequences. However, after a vaccination plan against COVID-19, the cases of severe disease and death are consistently controlled, although cases of asymptomatic and mild COVID-19 still happen together with tuberculosis (TB) cases. Thus, in this context, we sought to compare the T cell response of COVID-19-non-vaccinated and -vaccinated patients with active tuberculosis exposed to SARS-CoV-2 antigens. Flow cytometry was used to analyze activation markers (i.e., CD69 and CD137) and cytokines (IFN-γ, TNFα, IL-17, and IL-10) levels in CD4$^+$ and CD8$^+$ T cells upon exposure to SARS-CoV-2 peptides. The data obtained showed that CD8$^+$ T cells from non-vaccinated TB patients present a high frequency of CD69 and TNF-α after viral challenge compared to vaccinated TB donors. Conversely, CD4$^+$ T cells from vaccinated TB patients show a high frequency of IL-10 after spike peptide stimulus compared to non-vaccinated patients. No differences were observed in the other parameters analyzed. The results suggest that this reduced immune balance in coinfected individuals may have consequences for pathogen control, necessitating further research to understand its impact on clinical outcomes after COVID-19 vaccination in those with concurrent SARS-CoV-2 and *Mtb* infections.

Keywords: infection; immune response; vaccines; lymphocytes

Citation: Cavalcante-Silva, L.H.A.; Leite, E.G.; Almeida, F.S.; Andrade, A.G.d.; Comberlang, F.C.; Lucena, C.K.R.; Pachá, A.S.C.; Csordas, B.G.; Keesen, T.S.L. T Cell Response in Tuberculosis-Infected Patients Vaccinated against COVID-19. *Microorganisms* **2023**, *11*, 2810. https://doi.org/10.3390/microorganisms11112810

Academic Editor: Qibin Geng

Received: 28 September 2023
Revised: 1 November 2023
Accepted: 10 November 2023
Published: 19 November 2023

1. Introduction

In the context of respiratory infections, the COVID-19 pandemic has generated new challenges for patients with pre-existing conditions. The interaction between COVID-19 and tuberculosis (TB) is particularly concerning, a combination that presents a complex clinical landscape [1]. Both respiratory infections exhibit hyperinflammatory patterns characterized by prominent pro-inflammatory cytokines, including TNF-a, IL-6, and IL-1. These released cytokines and chemokines attract immune cells that intensify the pro-inflammatory reactions, thereby contributing to tissue damage [2–4]. These findings underscore the gravity of this interaction, revealing that concurrent or sequential pulmonary infections involving COVID-19 and TB lead to exacerbated respiratory symptoms and a pronounced decline in lung function [5,6].

Some studies suggest that tuberculosis may impact the severity of COVID-19 due to compromised immunity and chronic lung inflammation [7,8]. Patients with active tuberculosis exhibit a dysregulated immune response that could impair the immune response to COVID-19, resulting in increased disease severity. Furthermore, COVID-19 can reactivate latent tuberculosis in patients with a history of the disease, further escalating symptom severity [9,10]. It has been demonstrated that *Mycobacterium tuberculosis* (*Mtb*) infection in patients with COVID-19 was more common than other comorbidities such as diabetes, hypertension, and coronary disease. When comparing patients with both TB and COVID-19 to those with pneumonia, 22% of the evaluated TB patients presented with mild/moderate clinical forms of the disease, while the remaining 78% developed more severe forms of COVID [11].

In individuals with latent tuberculosis infection (LTBI), previous contact with and containment of *Mtb* resulted in primed innate immunity. This then triggers the prompt emergence of T cell immunity. This process is accompanied by the formation of cross-reactive heterologous immunity, causing memory T lymphocytes to activate upon exposure to SARS-CoV-2 peptides [12].

An in-depth analysis of transcriptomic patterns drawn from single-cell RNA sequencing in individuals spanning the spectrum of TB infections has revealed heightened signatures linked to COVID-19 risk. These signatures were notably prominent in active TB patients and individuals progressing from latent to active TB [13]. Moreover, monocyte-derived macrophages (MDM) infection with *Mtb* revealed a heightened expression of ACE2 and TMPRSS2. Intriguingly, when MDMs were exposed to conditioned media from *Mtb*-infected MDMs, this exposure not only promoted SARS-CoV-2 infection but also triggered the expression of pro-inflammatory cytokines [13]. These findings align with clinical reports that propose specific responses in TB patients that elevate the susceptibility to severe COVID-19 [14,15].

Recent studies indicate a potential connection between SARS-CoV-2 infection and latent tuberculosis (TB) progression to an active state. This could be influenced by factors like host CD4$^+$ T cell depletion, lung inflammation, and the activation of stem cell-mediated defenses [16,17]. On the other hand, while the impact of SARS-CoV-2 infection on TB resolution is debated, studies on mice suggest prior *Mtb* infection might protect against SARS-CoV-2-related disease [18]. Also, *Mtb* infection-mediated protection against viruses, such as SARS-CoV-2, has been demonstrated in BCG vaccination and immunity studies, suggesting a potential protection against COVID-19 [19–21]. Such findings hint at pathogen interplay, though mechanisms are unclear, underscoring the necessity for further in-depth investigations.

Following the implementation of the COVID-19 vaccination program, there has been consistent control over severe disease and mortality associated with COVID-19. Nevertheless, instances of asymptomatic and mild COVID-19 cases continue to occur in conjunction with cases of TB. Therefore, this study aims to compare the T cell response of COVID-19 non-vaccinated and vaccinated patients with active tuberculosis upon stimulation with SARS-CoV-2 antigens.

2. Materials and Methods

2.1. Ethics Statement

This study was approved by the National Commission of Ethics in Research (Approval Number: 4.101.879 and certificate CAAE: 31354720.0.0000.5188). All experiments complied with the Declaration of Helsinki's relevant regulations, institutional guidelines, and ethical standards. Informed consent was obtained from all the enrolled volunteers.

2.2. Patient Recruitment

The recruitment of volunteers took place between May 2020 and July 2023. The study was conducted by 20 volunteers divided into 3 groups: The first group was the control group (CTL, *n* = 9), consisting of healthy volunteers who were not previously vaccinated against COVID-19, were reportedly asymptomatic for the last 10 weeks, were negative via a certified SARS-CoV-2 antibody test (Euroimmun Anti-SARS-CoV-2 assay Perkin Elmer Company, Waltham, MA, USA) and had a negative RT-qPCR test for SARS-CoV-2. They were recruited between May 2020 in Brazil, when the original lineage and gamma variants of SARS-CoV-2 were present, and April 2021. The second group was individuals diagnosed with active pulmonary TB caused by *Mycobacterium tuberculosis* and not vaccinated against COVID-19 (NTB group) (n = 3). Finally, the third group was the volunteers who had a previous COVID-19 vaccination and were diagnosed with active pulmonary tuberculosis (VTB group) (n = 8). TB diagnostics were made through a real-time polymerase chain reaction (PCR) test, known as TRM-TB. Peripheral blood mononuclear cells (PBMCs) were collected in heparinized tubes.

2.3. Isolation of PBMCs

Peripheral blood mononuclear cells (PBMCs) collected from the volunteer groups were obtained from heparinized venous blood using density gradient centrifugation (Ficoll-Paque™ Plus, GE Healthcare, Life Sciences, Pittsburgh, PA, USA); the PBMCs were centrifuged for 40 min at $400\times g$ and washed three times ($200\times g$, 8 min, 4 °C) with phosphate-buffered saline (PBS) (Gibco™, Grand Island, NY, USA) before counting. The cells obtained were resuspended in RPMI 1640 medium, supplemented with 1% antibiotic solution (penicillin, 200 U/mL; streptomycin), 1 mM L-glutamine (1 mM), and 10% fetal bovine serum (Gibco™, Grand Island, NY, USA). Cultures were set up at a concentration of 2.5×10^5 cells/well in 96-well plates in the presence or absence of SARS-CoV-2 antigens (Pool CoV-2, which contained peptides from the spike protein and non-spike proteins, and Pool Spike Cov-2, which had peptides from the spike protein only) and Staphylococcal enterotoxin B from *Staphylococcus aureus* (SEB, Sigma-Aldrich, Saint Louis, MO, USA). The PBMCs were subjected to four different conditions: unstimulated (medium), stimulated with SARS-CoV-2 antigens (Pool Spike Cov-2 and Pool Cov-2, each at 1 µg/well), and stimulated with SEB (1 µg/well). The cells were incubated at 37 °C, 5% CO_2, for 16 h. Next, brefeldin-A (1 mg/mL, Sigma-Aldrich) was added, and the samples were incubated at 37 °C for 4 h.

2.4. Monoclonal Antibodies (mAbs)

The antibodies used for staining were anti-CD4 (APC-Cy7—Clone RPA-T4, cat. 557871), anti-CD8 (APC—Clone RPA-T8, cat. 555369), anti-CD137 (APC—clone 4B4-1, cat. 561702), anti-CD8 (PerCP-Cy5—clone RPA-T8, cat. 555368), anti-CD137 (APC—clone 4B4-1, cat. 561702), anti-CD69 (FITC—clone FN50, cat. 555530), anti-IL10 (APC—clone JES3-19F1, cat. 554707), anti-IL-6 (PE—clone MQ2-6A3, cat. 559331) anti-TNF (PE—clone Mab11, cat. 559321), and anti-IL-17A (PE—clone N49-653, cat. 560486) obtained from BD Biosciences (Franklin Lakes, NJ, USA), along with antibody anti-IFN-γ (PE-Cy5—clone 4S.B3, cat. 25731982) (Invitrogen, Thermo Fisher Scientific, Carlsbad, CA, USA).

2.5. Flow Cytometry Assay

Isolated PBMCs were plated at a concentration of 2.5×10^5 cells per well in a 96-well U-bottom plate. For the extracellular staining, cocktails of mAbs were added and incubated for 30 min at 4 °C. After incubation, the cells were washed with 150 µL of PBS. The plate was centrifuged (8 min, $244\times g$, 4 °C), the supernatant was removed, and 100 µL of 4% formaldehyde and 100 µL of PBS were added to the wells. The plate was incubated at room temperature (25 °C) for 20 min to fix the extracellular staining. After centrifugation (8 min, $244\times g$, 4 °C), the supernatant was removed, and the samples were washed with 150 µL of PBS. The cells were centrifuged again (8 min, $244\times g$, 4 °C) to perform intracellular staining, and the supernatant was discarded. For intracellular staining, the cells were permeabilized with 150 µL of permeabilization buffer (0.5% bovine serum albumin (BSA), w/v and 0.5% saponin, w/v in PBS) for 10 min at room temperature (25 °C). After centrifugation (8 min, $244\times g$, 4 °C), the supernatant was removed, and intracellular antibodies were added at a volume suggested by the manufacturer (BD Bioscience, San Jose, CA, USA). Then, the plate was incubated for 30 min at room temperature (25 °C), and after this, 150 µL/well of permeabilization buffer was added. The supernatant was removed after centrifugation (8 min, $577\times g$, 4 °C). Finally, 200 µL/well of Wash B (PBS/BSA) was added, and the samples were transferred to FACS tubes and stored at 4 °C. At least 30,000 gated events were acquired using FACS CANTO II (BD Biosciences, USA) and analyzed using FlowJo v. 10.8 software (BD, Ashland, CA, USA). The BD™ CompBeads Set Anti-Mouse Ig (BD Biosciences, USA) were used as compensation settings during the flow cytometric analyses.

2.6. Flow Cytometry Data Analysis

All parameters evaluated on CD4$^+$ and CD8$^+$ T cells were analyzed using FlowJo software v. 10.8 (BD, Ashland, CA, USA). Limits for the quadrant markers were set based on negative populations (cells) and Fluorescence Minus One (FMO) control. The strategy of the gate is described in Supplementary Figure S1.

2.7. Statistical Analysis

The statistical analyses were performed using GraphPad Prism software version 9. The Shapiro–Wilk test for normality was applied. Two-way ANOVA (followed by Tukey's post-test) was used for multiple group comparisons. The results were presented as the mean ± standard error of the mean (SEM). The confidence interval was 95%, and values were considered significant when $p < 0.05$.

3. Results

3.1. Demographical Characteristics

We recruited 20 volunteers for this study and distributed them into three groups. The non-vaccinated patients with active TB (NTB) group included three volunteers (three male) with a mean age of 26 (±1.00). Eight volunteers were enrolled in the vaccinated patients with active TB (VTB) group (four males and four females) with a mean age of 34.69 (±3.01). The healthy control was formed of nine donors (five females and four males) with a mean age of 35.63 (±3.05). No significant differences in age were found between the groups. All demographic characteristics are presented in Supplementary Figure S1.

3.2. NTB Patients Express Higher CD69$^+$CD4$^+$ T Cells than the VTB Group after Viral Antigen Stimulation

Initially, activation marker expression was evaluated in both CD4$^+$ and CD8$^+$ T cells. In CD4$^+$ T cells, there was no difference in CD69 expression between the HC, NTB, and VTB groups when assessed at the base level and after viral stimuli. Conversely, when subjected to SEB stimulation, HC donors exhibited markedly higher levels of CD69$^+$CD4$^+$ T cells (24.83 ± 6.75) when compared to the NTB (14.20 ± 2.71) and VTB (8.81 ± 1.67) groups. Furthermore, SEB induced greater CD69 expression within all three groups than its corresponding medium condition (Figure 1a). Concerning the evaluation of the CD137 marker, there was no difference between the NTB and VTB groups. However, the HC group consistently exhibited lower levels of CD137$^+$CD4$^+$ T cells compared to NTB in all conditions (Figure 1b).

Amid CD8$^+$ T cells, NTB patients exhibited a notably higher frequency of CD69 expression (PS = 18.53 ± 4.24; PT= 14.13 ± 3.79) compared to patients in the VTB group following viral challenge (PS = 8.17 ± 1.35; PT = 4.79 ± 0.67). In the HC group, SEB stimulation induced a heightened frequency of CD69$^+$CD8$^+$ T cell (18.84 ± 3.83) compared to unstimulated conditions (Figure 1c). In contrast, no significant differences were observed between the HC, NTB, and VTB groups when CD137 expression was assessed in different conditions (Figure 1d).

3.3. CD8$^+$ T Cells from TB Patients Vaccinated against COVID-19 Have Lower Frequencies of TNF-α, While CD4$^+$ T Cells Express Higher IL-10 Levels

Furthermore, pro- and anti-inflammatory cytokine levels in T cells were assessed. As expected, CD4$^+$ T cells from the HC donors exhibited diminished expression levels of pro-inflammatory cytokines, specifically TNF-α, IFN-γ, and IL-17, compared to NTB patients at baseline and following viral antigen stimuli (Figure 2a–c). On the other hand, the frequency of IL-10$^+$CD4$^+$ T cells was higher in the VTB group (5.88 $\pm$ 0.83) compared to the NTB group (3.12 $\pm$ 0.17) following the PS stimulus (Figure 2d).

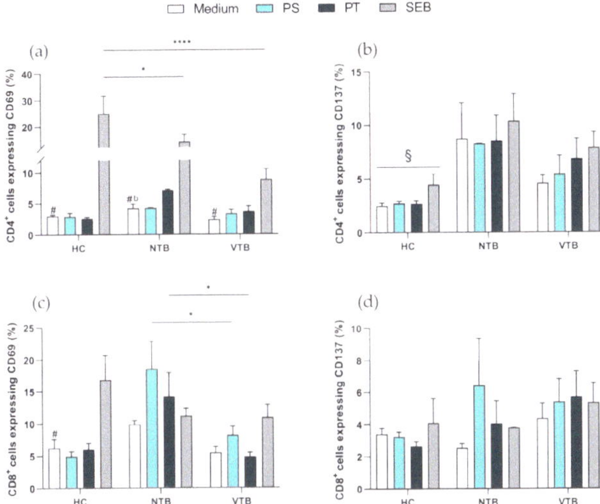

Figure 1. Profile of activation markers in T cells. (**a**) CD69 and (**b**) CD137 expression in CD4$^+$ T cells. (**c**) CD69 and (**d**) CD137 expression in CD8$^+$ T cells. Graphs are expressed as mean $\pm$ standard error (SEM). * $p < 0.05$, **** $p < 0.0001$, # $p < 0.05$ medium vs. SEB within each group, b $p < 0.05$ NTB medium vs. HC medium, § $p < 0.05$ HC vs. NTB; HC = healthy control ($n = 9$); NTB = non-vaccinated with active tuberculosis ($n = 3$); VTB = vaccinated with active tuberculosis ($n = 8$). PS = Pool Spike Cov-2; PT = Pool CoV-2; SEB = staphylococcal enterotoxin B.

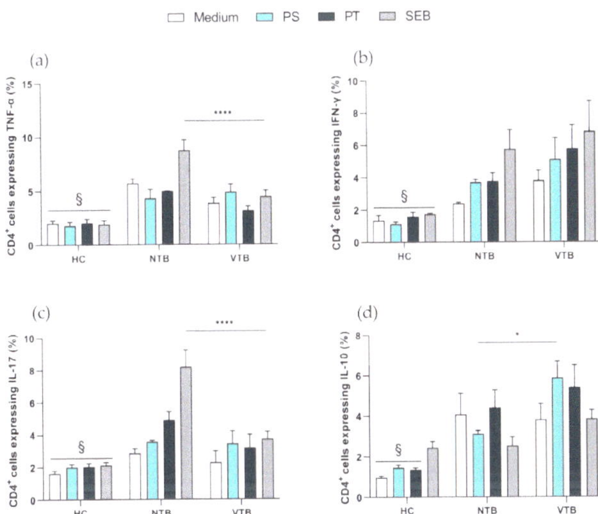

Figure 2. Profile of cytokines in CD4$^+$ T cells. (**a**) TNF-α, (**b**) IFN-γ, (**c**) IL-17, and (**d**) IL-10. Graphs are expressed as mean $\pm$ standard error (SEM). * $p < 0.05$, **** $p < 0.0001$, § $p < 0.05$ HC vs. NTB; HC = healthy control ($n = 9$); NTB = non-vaccinated with active tuberculosis ($n = 3$); VTB = vaccinated with active tuberculosis ($n = 8$). PS = Pool Spike Cov-2; PT = Pool CoV-2; SEB = staphylococcal enterotoxin B.

In the context of the CD8$^+$ T cell findings, it is noteworthy that NTB patients displayed an elevated frequency of TNF-α (PS = 11.94 ± 5.11; PT = 15.03 ± 0.03) in response to viral stimuli, as opposed to the VTB group (PS = 5.09 ± 0.64; PT = 7.47 ± 1.71) (Figure 3a). Similar to what was observed in CD4$^+$ T cells, the HC group demonstrated reduced frequencies of IFN-γ and IL-17 expression in CD8$^+$ T cells when compared to NTB donors (Figure 3b,c). However, no significant differences were observed across all groups regarding IL-10 expression (Figure 3d).

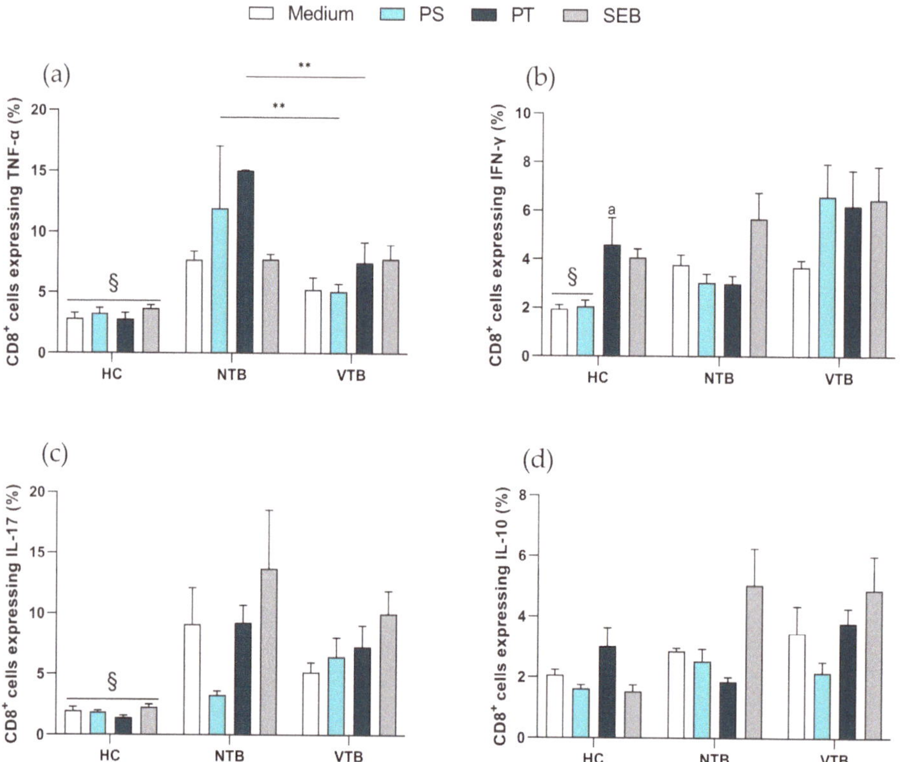

Figure 3. Profile of cytokines in CD8$^+$ T cells. (**a**) TNF-α, (**b**) IFN-γ, (**c**) IL-17, (**d**) IL-10. Graphs are expressed as mean ± standard error (SEM). ** $p < 0.01$, [a] $p < 0.05$ HC PT vs. HC medium, [§] $p < 0.05$ HC vs. NTB; HC = healthy control ($n = 9$); NTB = non-vaccinated with active tuberculosis ($n = 3$); VTB = vaccinated with active tuberculosis ($n = 8$). PS = Pool Spike Cov-2; PT = Pool CoV-2; SEB = staphylococcal enterotoxin B.

The immune profiles of healthy donors and non-vaccinated and vaccinated against COVID-19 patients with active tuberculosis are shown in Figure 4. In addition, all the means ± standard error (SEM) of all parameters analyzed are expressed in Supplementary Tables S2 and S3.

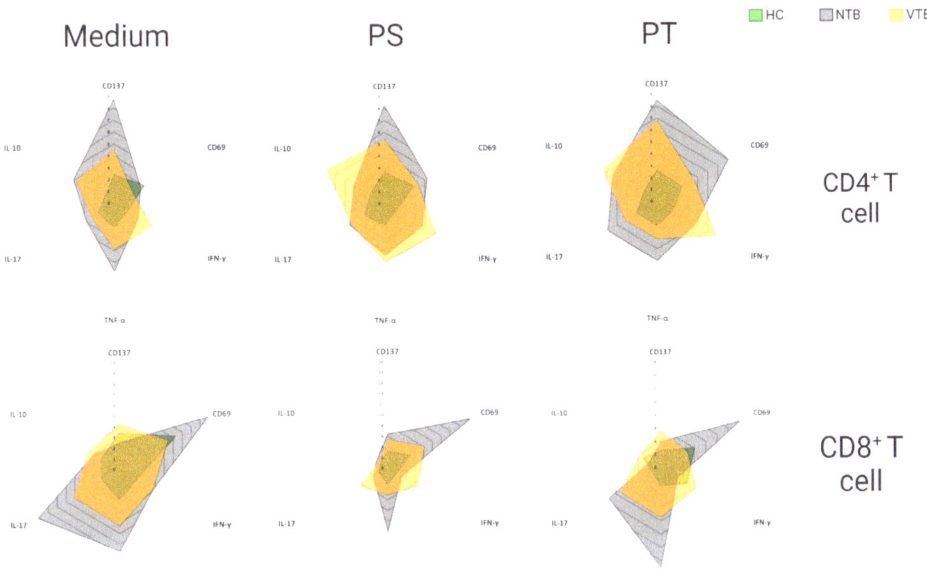

Figure 4. Radar charts of immune profile of CD4$^+$ and CD8$^+$ T cells. HC = healthy control ($n = 9$); NTB = non-vaccinated with active tuberculosis ($n = 3$); VTB = vaccinated with active tuberculosis ($n = 8$). PS = Pool Spike Cov-2; PT = Pool CoV-2.

4. Discussion

The relationship between COVID-19 and TB has been extensively studied, focusing on co-infection and the effects of SARS-CoV-2 infection on latent TB. This study investigated how COVID-19 vaccination influences TB progression when exposed to viral antigens. Our results indicate a potential decrease in the effector response and an enhancement of regulatory mechanisms upon re-exposure to SARS-CoV-2 peptides.

T cells undergo dynamic alterations in functional and phenotypic characteristics following antigenic stimulation. Notably, they exhibit increased surface expression of activation biomarkers and cytokine production [22,23]. In TB infection, CD69 and CD137 markers were employed to elucidate the state of T cell activation [23–26]. As described in our findings, CD4$^+$ T cells of NTB patients exhibited activation levels comparable to those in individuals of the VTB group. This similarity was evident in the CD69 and CD137 expression levels at baseline and following viral stimulation. These observations suggest that prior COVID-19 vaccination does not significantly influence the activation pattern of CD4$^+$ T cells in tuberculosis patients upon re-exposure to the SARS-CoV-2 virus. Furthermore, the CD8$^+$ T cells of VTB patients exhibited diminished CD69 expression levels after the viral antigen challenge compared to the NTB patients.

These results potentially indicate a protective effect for these TB patients in the event of a subsequent SARS-CoV-2 infection. This protective mechanism may arise from avoiding excessive T cell activation, as excessively elevated levels of T cell activation have been linked with unfavorable clinical outcomes [27,28]. Previous studies showed that TB-COVID-19 co-infection reduces the ability to respond to SARS-CoV-2 in vitro [14,29]. Since vaccination against COVID-19 elicits a memory T cell response, the new encounter with SARS-CoV-2 could be more controlled with diminished effects on TB progression.

CD137 is a compelling biomolecular indicator of antigen-activated T cells [23]. Notably, in contrast to the observed outcomes with the CD69 marker, no discernible differences were observed in the CD137 marker expression within the CD4$^+$ and CD8$^+$ T cell populations. CD69 operates as an early-phase biomarker, manifesting promptly after T cell activation.

However, it has an immunoregulatory complex role [30], whereas CD137, a TNFR superfamily member, assumes the role of a co-stimulatory receptor (4-1BB or TNFRS9), attaining functional activity during subsequent phases of T cell activation [31]. In our experimental conditions, the absence of a diminishment in CD137 levels within T cells following viral challenge holds particular significance. This observation is noteworthy as this molecule's expression is associated with defense against tuberculosis through the modulation of IFN-γ and TNF-α [32].

As CD137 and CD69 markers are closely associated with cytokine production [22,30], the expression of different cytokines in T cells was subsequently evaluated. The interferon response is fundamental to restrain and abrogate viral and bacterial infection [33–35], especially IFN-γ, a cytokine associated with the Th1 immune response [36]. The data obtained in this study indicate that a new exposure to SARS-CoV-2 antigens does not modulate the IFN-γ levels in COVID-19-vaccinated patients with active tuberculosis and their non-vaccinated counterparts. It is worth noting that stimulation with the PT antigens within the healthy group increased IFN-γ levels in CD8$^+$ T cells compared to their baseline levels. This may have happened due to cross-immunity between SARS-CoV-2 and other coronaviruses, as previously reported [37].

When IFN-γ levels are insufficient due to genetic predisposition, immunosuppression, or immune evasion mechanisms employed by the pathogens, the immune system may fail to control COVID-19 and tuberculosis [38]. In COVID-19, reduced IFN-γ levels may contribute to the persistence of viral replication and an increased risk of severe disease, while in tuberculosis, it may result in uncontrolled bacterial growth, dissemination, and the development of active disease [9]. Therefore, the observed persistence of IFN-γ in T cells in our data appears to be a favorable response to new exposure to SARS-CoV-2 antigens in TB patients.

As with IFN-γ, TNF-α is known to be a critical component of the immune response against both tuberculosis and COVID-19. However, elevated TNF-α levels have been linked with immunopathology in severe COVID-19 cases, while in TB, TNF-α is essential for granuloma formation and the containment of the infection [13,15]. Patients diagnosed with pulmonary active tuberculosis develop diverse granulomatous lesions, reflecting a robust inflammatory process primarily driven by cell-mediated immunity [39]. This immunity involves the production of crucial cytokines such as TNF-α, IFN-γ, and IL-12 to combat the *Mtb* infection [40]. When coupled with a coexisting COVID-19 infection, this setting can inflict additional harm to the pulmonary tissue [41].

The reduction in TNF-α levels in CD8$^+$ T cells following viral stimuli in COVID-19-vaccinated patients with active tuberculosis suggests a potential negative immunomodulatory effect of the combined immune response of vaccination and against *Mtb*. This effect may have protective implications by preventing excessive inflammation and immunopathology during these concurrent infections. Conversely, no significant alteration in IL-17 levels in active TB was observed in CD4$^+$ and CD8$^+$ T cells. Tuberculosis is associated with a decline in Th17 cell level [42], while COVID-19 immunopathogenesis seems related to elevated levels of IL-17A [43]. The maintenance of IL-17 levels at similar levels in both groups suggests that the impact of the vaccine in active TB patients may not extend to altering the proinflammatory response driven by IL-17.

To ensure an effective immune response, different regulatory mechanisms must be performed. This phenomenon may happen through several mechanisms, including inhibitory co-stimuli (e.g., CTLA-4) and soluble mediators (e.g., TGF-β and IL-10) [44]. The increase in IL-10 levels in CD4$^+$ T cells following spike peptide stimuli in VTB patients may correlate with the reduction in TNF-α. Besides immunoregulatory activity, IL-10 can also trigger antiviral immunity [45]. This antiviral effect of IL-10 is partially associated with its ability to enhance NK cell activity, modifying surface receptors, cytotoxicity [46], and cytokine production [47].

A prior investigation conducted by Andrade and his colleagues [48] revealed that the spike peptides employed in our study induce the activation of CD4$^+$ and CD8$^+$ T cells, as evidenced by an increased frequency of CD69 expression. Furthermore, it was observed that CD8$^+$ T cells exhibit heightened responsiveness to spike-related stimuli when compared to CD4$^+$ T cells. The authors also presented evidence of a robust T cell response directed against peptides derived from ORF proteins and the nucleocapsid protein. These observations suggest that healthy individuals previously vaccinated against COVID-19, who are subsequently re-exposed to SARS-CoV-2 antigens, manifest both antiviral and regulatory immune responses.

Rosas Mejia et al. demonstrated that TB-infected mice exposed to a secondary infection with SARS-CoV-2 are resistant to the pathological consequences of secondary viral infection [18]. The authors claim that tuberculosis-infected lungs already host a variety of innate immune cell types that limit the replication of both SARS-CoV-2 or *Mtb* infection and can trigger an adaptive immune response that recognizes SARS-CoV-2 antigens, providing a form of cross-reactive immunity [18]. If we extrapolate these data from mice to humans, we can draw a parallel to what was observed in this study. Vaccination against COVID-19, before *Mtb* infection, generates a cellular memory response that can contain the re-exposure to SARS-CoV-2. Furthermore, as mentioned by the authors, the immune response against *Mtb* itself can reduce the damage caused by COVID-19.

In summary, the reduced presence of CD69$^+$CD8$^+$ T cells and TNF$^+$CD8$^+$ T cells and elevated IL-10$^+$CD4$^+$ T cells in coinfected individuals may reduce inflammation and immunopathological responses. However, this fact prompts inquiries regarding its potential effects on pathogen containment and elimination. To better understand these dynamics, further research is needed to elucidate the mechanisms underlying this phenomenon and to assess its consequences on clinical outcomes in individuals with concurrent SARS-CoV-2 and *Mtb* infections after COVID-19 vaccination.

Our study possesses certain limitations, notably the relatively small sample size within the non-vaccinated group afflicted with active tuberculosis. Additionally, some patients could not recall the specific type of vaccine they received. However, notwithstanding these constraints, our research yields valuable insights into the interplay between COVID-19 and tuberculosis, elucidating the potential impact of vaccination on immune responses in cases of co-infection.

Supplementary Materials: The following supporting information can be downloaded at: https://www.mdpi.com/article/10.3390/microorganisms11112810/s1, Figure S1: Flow cytometry data analysis. It was first selected the total lymphocyte gate through SSC and FSC-A profiles, followed by singlet separation using the FSC-A × FSC-H parameters. Next, it was set the CD4$^+$ or CD8$^+$ T cells using FSC-A x CD8/CD4 parameters. Finally, it was set the markers/CD4 (e.g., IL-17/CD4) or CD8 (e.g., TNF-α/CD8); Table S1: Gender, age, and ethnic-racial self-classification, comorbidities of donors; Table S2: Means $\pm$ standard error (SEM) of all parameters analyzed in CD4$^+$ T cells.; Table S3: Means $\pm$ standard error (SEM) of all parameters analyzed in CD8$^+$ T cells.

Author Contributions: Conceptualization, T.S.L.K., L.H.A.C.-S., F.S.A. and B.G.C.; experiment design and performance, L.H.A.C.-S., A.G.d.A., F.C.C., E.G.L., F.S.A., C.K.R.L., A.S.C.P. and B.G.C.; writing—original draft preparation, L.H.A.C.-S., A.G.d.A. and F.S.A.; writing—review, editing and supervision, T.S.L.K. All authors have read and agreed to the published version of the manuscript.

Funding: This research was funded by "Conselho Nacional de Desenvolvimento Científico e Tecnológico (CNPq) (Number: 440939/2020-8)" and "Fundação de Apoio à Pesquisa do Estado da Paraíba- FAPESQ-PB/CNPq (Number: 150848/2023-4)". The funding sources were not involved in the study design, collection, analysis, interpretation of data, writing of the report, or submitting the article for publication.

Data Availability Statement: Data are available on request from the authors.

Acknowledgments: The authors are grateful to all the volunteers who enrolled in this study and the Federal University of Paraiba, Brazil, for providing the structure to perform this work.

Conflicts of Interest: The authors declare no conflict of interest.

References

1.   Shah, T.; Shah, Z.; Yasmeen, N.; Baloch, Z.; Xia, X. Pathogenesis of SARS-CoV-2 and Mycobacterium tuberculosis Coinfection. *Front. Immunol.* **2022**, *13*, 909011. [CrossRef] [PubMed]
2.   Tan, L.Y.; Komarasamy, T.V.; RMT Balasubramaniam, V. Hyperinflammatory Immune Response and COVID-19: A Double Edged Sword. *Front. Immunol.* **2021**, *12*, 742941. [CrossRef] [PubMed]
3.   Ravimohan, S.; Kornfeld, H.; Weissman, D.; Bisson, G.P. Tuberculosis and lung damage: From epidemiology to pathophysiology. *Eur. Respir. Rev.* **2018**, *27*, 170077. [CrossRef] [PubMed]
4.   Muefong, C.N.; Sutherland, J.S. Neutrophils in Tuberculosis-Associated Inflammation and Lung Pathology. *Front. Immunol.* **2020**, *11*, 539802. [CrossRef] [PubMed]
5.   Kang, T.G.; Kwon, K.W.; Kim, K.; Lee, I.; Kim, M.J.; Ha, S.J.; Shin, S.J. Viral coinfection promotes tuberculosis immunopathogenesis by type I IFN signaling-dependent impediment of Th1 cell pulmonary influx. *Nat. Commun.* **2022**, *13*, 3155. [CrossRef] [PubMed]
6.   Singh, D.D.; Han, I.; Choi, E.H.; Yadav, D.K. A Clinical Update on SARS-CoV-2: Pathology and Development of Potential Inhibitors. *Curr. Issues Mol. Biol.* **2023**, *45*, 400–433. [CrossRef] [PubMed]
7.   Mousquer, G.T.; Peres, A.; Fiegenbaum, M. Pathology of TB/COVID-19 Co-Infection: The phantom menace. *Tuberculosis* **2021**, *126*, 102020. [CrossRef]
8.   Wells, G.; Glasgow, J.N.; Nargan, K.; Lumamba, K.; Madansein, R.; Maharaj, K.; Perumal, L.Y.; Matthew, M.; Hunter, R.L.; Pacl, H.; et al. A high-resolution 3D atlas of the spectrum of tuberculous and COVID-19 lung lesions. *EMBO Mol. Med.* **2022**, *14*, e16283. [CrossRef]
9.   Flores-Lovon, K.; Ortiz-Saavedra, B.; Cueva-Chicaña, L.A.; Aperrigue-Lira, S.; Montes-Madariaga, E.S.; Soriano-Moreno, D.R.; Bell, B.; Macedo, R. Immune responses in COVID-19 and tuberculosis coinfection: A scoping review. *Front. Immunol.* **2022**, *13*, 992743. [CrossRef]
10.   du Bruyn, E.; Stek, C.; Daroowala, R.; Said-Hartley, Q.; Hsiao, M.; Schafer, G.; Goliath, R.T.; Abrahams, F.; Jackson, A.; Wasserman, S.; et al. Effects of tuberculosis and/or HIV-1 infection on COVID-19 presentation and immune response in Africa. *Nat. Commun.* **2023**, *14*, 188. [CrossRef]
11.   Chen, Y.; Wang, Y.; Fleming, J.; Yu, Y.; Gu, Y.; Liu, C.; Fan, L.; Wang, X.; Cheng, M.; Bi, L.; et al. Active or latent tuberculosis increases susceptibility to COVID-19 and disease severity. *medRxiv* **2020**. [CrossRef]
12.   Gonzalez-Perez, M.; Sanchez-Tarjuelo, R.; Shor, B.; Nistal-Villan, E.; Ochando, J. The BCG Vaccine for COVID-19: First Verdict and Future Directions. *Front. Immunol.* **2021**, *12*, 632478. [CrossRef] [PubMed]
13.   Sheerin, D.; Abhimanyu; Peton, N.; Vo, W.; Allison, C.C.; Wang, X.; Johnson, W.E.; Coussens, A.K. Immunopathogenic overlap between COVID-19 and tuberculosis identified from transcriptomic meta-analysis and human macrophage infection. *iScience* **2022**, *25*, 104464. [CrossRef] [PubMed]
14.   Petrone, L.; Petruccioli, E.; Vanini, V.; Cuzzi, G.; Gualano, G.; Vittozzi, P.; Nicastri, E.; Maffongelli, G.; Grifoni, A.; Sette, A.; et al. Coinfection of tuberculosis and COVID-19 limits the ability to in vitro respond to SARS-CoV-2. *Int. J. Infect. Dis.* **2021**, *113* (Suppl. S1), S82–S87. [CrossRef] [PubMed]
15.   Chiok, K.R.; Dhar, N.; Banerjee, A. Mycobacterium tuberculosis and SARS-CoV-2 co-infections: The knowns and unknowns. *iScience* **2023**, *26*, 106629. [CrossRef]
16.   Riou, C.; du Bruyn, E.; Stek, C.; Daroowala, R.; Goliath, R.T.; Abrahams, F.; Said-Hartley, Q.; Allwood, B.W.; Hsiao, N.Y.; Wilkinson, K.A.; et al. Relationship of SARS-CoV-2-specific CD4 response to COVID-19 severity and impact of HIV-1 and tuberculosis coinfection. *J. Clin. Investig.* **2021**, *131*, e149125. [CrossRef]
17.   Pathak, L.; Gayan, S.; Pal, B.; Talukdar, J.; Bhuyan, S.; Sandhya, S.; Yeger, H.; Baishya, D.; Das, B. Coronavirus Activates an Altruistic Stem Cell-Mediated Defense Mechanism that Reactivates Dormant Tuberculosis: Implications in Coronavirus Disease 2019 Pandemic. *Am. J. Pathol.* **2021**, *191*, 1255–1268. [CrossRef]
18.   Mejia, O.R.; Gloag, E.S.; Li, J.; Ruane-Foster, M.; Claeys, T.A.; Farkas, D.; Wang, S.H.; Farkas, L.; Xin, G.; Robinson, R.T. Mice infected with Mycobacterium tuberculosis are resistant to acute disease caused by secondary infection with SARS-CoV-2. *PLoS Pathog.* **2022**, *18*, e1010093. [CrossRef]
19.   Wang, J.; Zhang, Q.; Wang, H.; Gong, W. The Potential Roles of BCG Vaccine in the Prevention or Treatment of COVID-19. *Front. Biosci.* **2022**, *27*, 157. [CrossRef]
20.   Pittet, L.F.; Messina, N.L.; Orsini, F.; Moore, C.L.; Abruzzo, V.; Barry, S.; Bonnici, R.; Bonten, M.; Campbell, J.; Croda, J.; et al. Randomized Trial of BCG Vaccine to Protect against COVID-19 in Health Care Workers. *N. Engl. J. Med.* **2023**, *388*, 1582–1596. [CrossRef]
21.   Zhang, B.Z.; Shuai, H.; Gong, H.R.; Hu, J.C.; Yan, B.; Yuen, T.T.T.; Hu, Y.F.; Yoon, C.; Wang, X.L.; Hou, Y.; et al. Bacillus Calmette-Guérin-induced trained immunity protects against SARS-CoV-2 challenge in K18-hACE2 mice. *JCI Insight* **2022**, *7*, e157393. [CrossRef] [PubMed]
22.   Yan, Z.H.; Zheng, X.F.; Yi, L.; Wang, J.; Wang, X.J.; Wei, P.J.; Jia, H.Y.; Zhou, L.J.; Zhao, Y.L.; Zhang, H.T. CD137 is a Useful Marker for Identifying CD4+ T Cell Responses to Mycobacterium tuberculosis. *Scand. J. Immunol.* **2017**, *85*, 372–380. [CrossRef] [PubMed]
23.   Smith-Garvin, J.E.; Koretzky, G.A.; Jordan, M.S. T Cell Activation. *Annu. Rev. Immunol.* **2009**, *27*, 591. [CrossRef] [PubMed]
24.   Chen, Z.Y.; Wang, L.; Gu, L.; Qu, R.; Lowrie, D.B.; Hu, Z.; Sha, W.; Fan, X.Y. Decreased Expression of CD69 on T Cells in Tuberculosis Infection Resisters. *Front. Microbiol.* **2020**, *11*, 557348. [CrossRef] [PubMed]

25. Luo, Y.; Xue, Y.; Mao, L.; Lin, Q.; Tang, G.; Song, H.; Liu, W.; Tong, S.; Hou, H.; Huang, M.; et al. Activation Phenotype of Mycobacterium tuberculosis-Specific CD4+ T Cells Promoting the Discrimination Between Active Tuberculosis and Latent Tuberculosis Infection. *Front. Immunol.* **2021**, *12*, 721013. [CrossRef]
26. Musvosvi, M.; Huang, H.; Wang, C.; Xia, Q.; Rozot, V.; Krishnan, A.; Acs, P.; Cheruku, A.; Obermoser, G.; Leslie, A.; et al. T cell receptor repertoires associated with control and disease progression following Mycobacterium tuberculosis infection. *Nat. Med.* **2023**, *29*, 258–269. [CrossRef]
27. Ueland, T.; Heggelund, L.; Lind, A.; Holten, A.R.; Tonby, K.; Michelsen, A.E.; Jenum, S.; Jørgensen, M.J.; Barratt-Due, A.; Skeie, L.G.; et al. Elevated plasma sTIM-3 levels in patients with severe COVID-19. *J. Allergy Clin. Immunol.* **2021**, *147*, 92–98. [CrossRef]
28. Kalfaoglu, B.; Almeida-Santos, J.; Tye, C.A.; Satou, Y.; Ono, M. T-cell dysregulation in COVID-19. *Biochem. Biophys. Res. Commun.* **2021**, *538*, 204–210. [CrossRef]
29. Najafi-Fard, S.; Aiello, A.; Navarra, A.; Cuzzi, G.; Vanini, V.; Migliori, G.B.; Gualano, G.; Cerva, C.; Grifoni, A.; Sette, A.; et al. Characterization of the immune impairment of patients with tuberculosis and COVID-19 coinfection. *Int. J. Infect. Dis.* **2023**, *130* (Suppl. S1), S34–S42. [CrossRef]
30. Sancho, D.; Gómez, M.; Sánchez-Madrid, F. CD69 is an immunoregulatory molecule induced following activation. *Trends Immunol.* **2005**, *26*, 136–140. [CrossRef]
31. Watts, T.H. TNF/TNFR family members in costimulation of T cell responses. *Annu. Rev. Immunol.* **2005**, *23*, 23–68. [CrossRef] [PubMed]
32. Fernández Do Porto, D.A.; Jurado, J.O.; Pasquinelli, V.; Alvarez, I.B.; Aspera, R.H.; Musella, R.M.; García, V.E. CD137 differentially regulates innate and adaptive immunity against Mycobacterium tuberculosis. *Immunol. Cell Biol.* **2012**, *90*, 449–456. [CrossRef] [PubMed]
33. Lee, A.J.; Ashkar, A.A. The Dual Nature of Type I and Type II Interferons. *Front. Immunol.* **2018**, *9*, 2061. [CrossRef] [PubMed]
34. Mertowska, P.; Smolak, K.; Mertowski, S.; Grywalska, E. Immunomodulatory Role of Interferons in Viral and Bacterial Infections. *Int. J. Mol. Sci.* **2023**, *24*, 10115. [CrossRef] [PubMed]
35. Bergeron, H.C.; Hansen, M.R.; Tripp, R.A. Interferons—Implications in the Immune Response to Respiratory Viruses. *Microorganisms* **2023**, *11*, 2179. [CrossRef]
36. Aiello, A.; Najafi-Fard, S.; Goletti, D. Initial immune response after exposure to Mycobacterium tuberculosis or to SARS-COV-2: Similarities and differences. *Front. Immunol.* **2023**, *14*, 1244556. [CrossRef]
37. Grifoni, A.; Weiskopf, D.; Ramirez, S.I.; Mateus, J.; Dan, J.M.; Moderbacher, C.R.; Rawlings, S.A.; Sutherland, A.; Premkumar, L.; Jadi, R.S.; et al. Targets of T Cell Responses to SARS-CoV-2 Coronavirus in Humans with COVID-19 Disease and Unexposed Individuals. *Cell* **2020**, *181*, 1489–1501.e15. [CrossRef]
38. Baker, P.J.; Amaral, E.P.; Castro, E.; Bohrer, A.C.; Torres-Juárez, F.; Jordan, C.M.; Nelson, C.E.; Barber, D.L.; Johnson, R.F.; Hilligan, K.L.; et al. Co-infection of mice with SARS-CoV-2 and Mycobacterium tuberculosis limits early viral replication but does not affect mycobacterial loads. *Front. Immunol.* **2023**, *14*, 1240419. [CrossRef]
39. Cronan, M.R. In the Thick of It: Formation of the Tuberculous Granuloma and Its Effects on Host and Therapeutic Responses. *Front. Immunol.* **2022**, *13*, 820134. [CrossRef]
40. Brighenti, S.; Andersson, J. Local Immune Responses in Human Tuberculosis: Learning from the Site of Infection. *J. Infect. Dis.* **2012**, *205*, S316–S324. [CrossRef]
41. Koupaei, M.; Naimi, A.; Moafi, N.; Mohammadi, P.; Tabatabaei, F.S.; Ghazizadeh, S.; Heidary, M.; Khoshnood, S. Clinical Characteristics, Diagnosis, Treatment, and Mortality Rate of TB/COVID-19 Coinfectetd Patients: A Systematic Review. *Front. Med.* **2021**, *8*, 740593. [CrossRef] [PubMed]
42. Starshinova, A.; Kudryavtsev, I.; Rubinstein, A.; Malkova, A.; Dovgaluk, I.; Kudlay, D. Tuberculosis and COVID-19 Dually Affect Human Th17 Cell Immune Response. *Biomedicines* **2023**, *11*, 2123. [CrossRef] [PubMed]
43. Majeed, A.Y.; Zulkafli, N.E.S.; Ad'hiah, A.H. Serum profiles of pro-inflammatory and anti-inflammatory cytokines in non-hospitalized patients with mild/moderate COVID-19 infection. *Immunol. Lett.* **2023**, *260*, 24–34. [CrossRef] [PubMed]
44. Jiang, H.; Chess, L. Regulation of immune responses by T cells. *N. Engl. J. Med.* **2006**, *354*, 1166–1176. [CrossRef] [PubMed]
45. Mocellin, S.; Panelli, M.C.; Wang, E.; Nagorsen, D.; Marincola, F.M. The dual role of IL-10. *Trends Immunol.* **2003**, *24*, 36–43. [CrossRef] [PubMed]
46. Parato, K.G.; Kumar, A.; Badley, A.D.; Sanchez-Dardon, J.L.; Chambers, K.A.; Young, C.D.; Lim, W.T.; Kravcik, S.; Cameron, D.W.; Angel, J.B. Normalization of natural killer cell function and phenotype with effective anti-HIV therapy and the role of IL-10. *AIDS* **2002**, *16*, 1251–1256. [CrossRef]
47. Cai, G.; Kastelein, R.A.; Hunter, C.A. IL-10 enhances NK cell proliferation, cytotoxicity and production of IFN-q when combined with IL-18. *Eur. J. Immunol.* **1999**, *29*, 2658–2665. [CrossRef]
48. de Andrade, A.G.; Comberlang, F.C.; Cavalcante-Silva, L.H.A.; Kessen, T.S.L. COVID-19 vaccination: Effects of immunodominant peptides of SARS-CoV-2. *Cytokine* **2023**, *170*, 156339. [CrossRef]

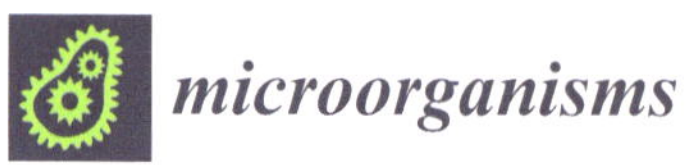
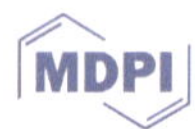

Article

Analyzing the Interplay between COVID-19 Viral Load, Inflammatory Markers, and Lymphocyte Subpopulations on the Development of Long COVID

Andrea Rivera-Cavazos [1,2], José Antonio Luviano-García [1,3], Arnulfo Garza-Silva [1,2], Devany Paola Morales-Rodríguez [1,2], Mauricio Kuri-Ayache [4], Miguel Ángel Sanz-Sánchez [1,2], Juan Enrique Santos-Macías [1,3], Maria Elena Romero-Ibarguengoitia [1,2,*] and Arnulfo González-Cantú [2,3]

[1] Vicerrectoría de Ciencias de la Salud, Escuela de Medicina, Universidad de Monterrey,
     San Pedro Garza García 66238, Nuevo León, Mexico; andrea.riverac@udem.edu (A.R.-C.)
[2] Research Department, Hospital Clínica Nova de Monterrey,
     San Nicolás de los Garza 66450, Nuevo León, Mexico; drgzzcantu@gmail.com
[3] Internal Medicine Department, Hospital Clínica Nova de Monterrey,
     San Nicolás de los Garza 66450, Nuevo León, Mexico
[4] Cardiology Department, Hospital Clínica Nova de Monterrey,
     San Nicolás de los Garza 66450, Nuevo León, Mexico
*   Correspondence: mromeroi@novaservicios.com.mx; Tel.: +52-81-8865-5700

Abstract: The global impact of the SARS-CoV-2 infection has been substantial, affecting millions of people. Long COVID, characterized by persistent or recurrent symptoms after acute infection, has been reported in over 40% of patients. Risk factors include age and female gender, and various mechanisms, including chronic inflammation and viral persistence, have been implicated in long COVID's pathogenesis. However, there are scarce studies in which multiple inflammatory markers and viral load are analyzed simultaneously in acute infection to determine how they predict for long COVID at long-term follow-up. This study explores the association between long COVID and inflammatory markers, viral load, and lymphocyte subpopulation during acute infection in hospitalized patients to better understand the risk factors of this disease. This longitudinal retrospective study was conducted in patients hospitalized with COVID-19 in northern Mexico. Inflammatory parameters, viral load, and lymphocyte subpopulation during the acute infection phase were analyzed, and long COVID symptoms were followed up depending on severity and persistence (weekly or monthly) and assessed 1.5 years after the acute infection. This study analyzed 79 patients, among them, 41.8% presented long COVID symptoms, with fatigue being the most common (45.5%). Patients with long COVID had higher lymphocyte levels during hospitalization, and NK cell subpopulation levels were also associated with long COVID. ICU admission during acute COVID-19 was also linked to the development of long COVID symptoms.

Keywords: COVID-19; SARS-CoV-2 infection; long COVID; natural killer cells; lymphocytes

Citation: Rivera-Cavazos, A.; Luviano-García, J.A.; Garza-Silva, A.; Morales-Rodríguez, D.P.; Kuri-Ayache, M.; Sanz-Sánchez, M.Á.; Santos-Macías, J.E.; Romero-Ibarguengoitia, M.E.; González-Cantú, A. Analyzing the Interplay between COVID-19 Viral Load, Inflammatory Markers, and Lymphocyte Subpopulations on the Development of Long COVID. *Microorganisms* **2023**, *11*, 2241. https://doi.org/10.3390/microorganisms11092241

Academic Editor: Qibin Geng

Received: 25 July 2023
Revised: 30 August 2023
Accepted: 31 August 2023
Published: 6 September 2023

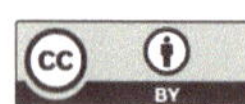

1. Introduction

The infection caused by SARS-CoV-2, which originated in Wuhan, China, in December 2019, has had a significant impact globally. To date, it is estimated to have infected more than 767 million people and has been responsible for nearly 7 million deaths [1].

The term "Long-COVID" is used to describe the presence of prolonged or recurrent symptoms that persist for at least four weeks after an acute infection with the SARS-CoV-2 virus and that cannot be attributed to any other disease, according to the US Centers for Disease Control and Prevention (CDC) [2–5]. Long COVID has been reported to affect more than 40% of patients who experienced acute COVID-19 infection, and there are even investigations that found its presence in up to 60% of patients [6,7]. The associated symptoms are diverse, although fatigue is one of the most frequent, and all of them have in common the negative impact they have on the quality of life of patients [3,8–10]. Patient age, body mass index, and female gender were found to be risk factors associated with the occurrence of long COVID [11–13].

There are several mechanisms that contribute to the pathogenesis of COVID-19 that have also been implicated in the development of long COVID. It was observed that after acute infection, some patients experience the persistence of SARS-CoV-2 in various organs, leading to chronic stimulation of the adaptive immune system and subsequent generation of cellular damage due to chronic hyperinflammation. In addition, this hyperinflammatory state can trigger hemostatic changes, such as coagulopathies [5,14–16]. Although some studies suggest that the inflammatory response plays an important role in the development of long COVID, information varies depending on the type of biomarker and its timeline of measurement, for example, if it is measured during acute infection or months/years after infection [3,6,17]. In addition, a possible association between the severity of acute COVID-19 infection and the development of long COVID has been observed in other studies, although the results are inconsistent. Most studies focused on taking laboratory samples when patients already have long COVID, and few studies focused on baseline laboratory parameters during the acute phase of infection like lymphocyte subpopulation, viral load, blood count, D-dimer, lactate dehydrogenase, interleukin 6, ferritin, and C-reactive protein. It was observed that patients with long COVID show elevated levels of inflammatory parameters and chemotactic and angiogenic cytokines in contrast to those patients who do not experience persistent symptoms. However, the clinical significance of these parameters has not yet been conclusively established [6,14]. While there is information available regarding viral load during the acute stage of infection and its relation to what was previously referred to as post-acute COVID-19 syndrome, various studies have yet to reach a consensus on a definitive outcome; however, they point toward a relationship between viral load and long COVID [18–20]. A research study conducted by Giron-Perez et al. proposed a positive correlation between viral load and the number of symptoms experienced during long COVID, implying that a higher viral load might result in a lower probability of experiencing long-term COVID symptoms [21]. A study conducted also during the early stages of the pandemic asserted that viral load can serve as a predictor for long COVID [22].

There is little information on the interrelationship between inflammatory parameters, such as C-reactive protein, lactate dehydrogenase, leukocyte count, lymphocyte count, procalcitonin, ferritin, D-dimer, interleukin-6 (IL-6), viral load level, and lymphocyte subpopulation, in the development of long COVID on a long-term follow-up. Therefore, an analysis of these parameters during the acute infection phase in hospitalized patients with COVID-19 was carried out in order to identify possible relationships between these parameters and the subsequent development of long COVID.

2. Materials and Methods

2.1. Study Population and Study Design

This study was carried out in May 2023 on patients who were hospitalized from April 2021 to January 2022 with a diagnosis of COVID-19 at Hospital Clinica Nova, a private hospital in northern Mexico. A longitudinal retrospective study was conducted following the STROBE reporting guidelines [23]. The study protocol was reviewed and approved by the Research Committee of the University of Monterrey, with registration number 25052023-CN-ENM3-CI. Since it was a retrolective study, it was not necessary to obtain informed consent from the participants.

The inclusion criteria were patients with COVID-19 confirmed with nasopharyngeal PCR who were hospitalized for severe symptoms involving decreased oxygen saturation (<94%), respiratory rate over 30 breaths/minute, and lung infiltrates > 50%. Patients from both genders, adults (18+), and those who, subsequently to the acute disease, attended COVID-19 follow-up appointments with an internist, were also included. Individuals who had previously received treatment with antivirals, steroids, convalescent plasma, or immunosuppressants prior to hospitalization as well as patients who did not have their COVID-19 variant, lymphocyte subpopulation, and viral load registered in medical history were excluded.

Various medical history data were collected, such as age, history of diabetes, systemic arterial hypertension, renal disease, chronic obstructive pulmonary disease, heart disease, among others, at the time of patient admission. Likewise, gender, oxygen requirements at admission, and vital signs were recorded.

On admission, the COVID-19 variant and lymphocyte subpopulation were measured. The time from symptoms on-set until sample collection had a median (IQR) of 8 (3) days. At admission and during hospitalization, multiple measurements were taken every 24 to 48 h including blood viral load, blood count (Sysmex XN-10, Kobe, Japan), and inflammatory parameters such as D-dimer, lactate dehydrogenase, interleukin 6, ferritin, and C-reactive protein (Roche-Cobas 6000 Module 501 & 601, Rotkreuz, Switzerland). Procalcitonin was taken on admission and in case of suspected secondary bacterial infection (DiaSorin-Liaison XL, Saluggia, Italy). Blood samples were peripheral venous punctures taken by the nursing staff. Samples regarding viral load and lymphocyte subpopulation were analyzed in the PGM Laboratory (Clinical Pathology and Genetics Laboratory), an external laboratory, which took one hour to arrive and were processed in the following two hours. The rest of the markers were analyzed in the hospital's own laboratory during the first hour after sample collection. Results were available in the medical record within the following eight hours.

Each patient diagnosed with COVID-19 was assigned an internal medicine doctor in charge of post-disease follow-up. Depending on the severity of symptoms, patients were followed each week, every two weeks, or every month until resolution. We defined long COVID as the ongoing, relapsing, or new symptoms or conditions present 30 or more days after infection [24]. The presence and duration of long COVID symptoms were recorded in the medical history and reassessed 1.5 years after the acute infection.

2.2. Sample Processing Method

For the analysis of viral load, each patient had a peripheral venous blood sample collected using a tube containing a stabilizer for circulating nucleic acids (PAXGENE®, Mexico City, Mexico). These samples were then transported at room temperature to an external laboratory, PGM Laboratory (Clinical Pathology and Genetics Laboratory), taking on average 1 h to arrive at the PGM Laboratory from the samples' collection [25]. At the laboratory, the samples were processed using a circulating nucleic acid extraction kit (QIAGEN® Mexico City, Mexico) designed for liquid biopsy, along with a TaqPath® COVID-19 kit (ThermoFisher Scientific®, Waltham, MA, USA) [19]. The extraction and amplification were performed using QuantStudio 5 thermal cyclers (Applied Biosystems® Waltham, MA, USA). The results were subsequently transmitted to our hospital facility and uploaded into the laboratory computer system. The minimum detectable concentration of the assay was 10 copies/mL, while the maximum was 100,000 copies/mL. Based on these findings and previous reports in the literature, the following reference intervals were established for plasma results: low (<100 copies/mL), moderate (>100 to 1000 copies/mL), and high (>1000 copies/mL) [20].

For the analysis of SARS-CoV-2 variants, the samples underwent a series of procedures. Firstly, nucleic acid extraction is performed on the samples. Subsequently, retrotranscription took place, followed by a PCR reaction using a ThermoFisher Veriti endpoint thermal cycler.

The lymphocyte subpopulation was assessed using flow cytometry (BD FACS CANTO II IVD, Becton Dickinson, East Rutherford, NJ, USA). This technique allows for the extraction of lymphocytes and the analysis of various subpopulations. The parameters examined included leukocyte count, total lymphocytes, T lymphocytes (CD4 and CD8), B lymphocytes (CD19), NK cells (CD16 and CD56), and the CD4/CD8 ratio. Becton Dickinson brand antibodies were utilized in the analysis, specifically: PerCP-Cy5.5 anti-human CD45, FITC anti-human CD3, PE-Cy7 anti-human CD4, APC Cy7 anti-human CD8, APC anti-human CD19, PE anti-human CD16, and PE anti-human CD56.

2.3. Statistical Analysis

The distribution of the variables was assessed using the Shapiro–Wilk test and Kolmogorov test, and appropriate transformations were applied to achieve normalization when necessary. A descriptive analysis of the variables and covariates was conducted using parametric statistics, presenting means and standard deviations for variables conforming to normality, or medians and interquartile ranges for variables deviating from normality. Qualitative variables are explored using frequencies. For the continuous quantitative variables, the unpaired samples *t*-test was used to analyze variables with normal distribution, while the Mann–Whitney test was used for variables with non-normal distribution. The chi-square test was used to compare long COVID patients and non-long COVID patients. If fewer than 5 patients were in the group, Fischer's exact test was used for univariate analysis. In addition, for a more robust model, a binary logistic regression analysis was performed to determine the association between long COVID symptoms and gender, age, inflammatory markers, ICU, and systematic arterial hypertension. A complete case analysis was conducted for missing values assumed to be missing completely at random. A value of $p < 0.05$ was considered significant. Statistical data were analyzed with SPSS vs. 25 and R v.4.0.3.

3. Results

Out of the cohort of 105 admitted patients with comprehensive laboratory results, a subset of 79 individuals qualified for inclusion in this study due to their adherence to follow-up appointments with the Internal Medicine Department. All had pneumonia during the acute phase. The follow-up lasted a period with a median (IQR) of 648 (68) days after the initial acute COVID-19 infection. Among the selected group of 79 participants, the median (IQR) age was 49 (22) years. A proportion of 33 individuals (41.8%) exhibited the presence of long COVID. In the long COVID group, it was observed that 22 (66.7%) were males. On the other hand, in the group without long COVID, it was found that 34 (73.9%) were males. The chi-square analysis was not significant for gender. Notably, fatigue emerged as the most recurrent symptom, shown in 15 (45.5%) patients, followed closely by tiredness, reported by another 15 (45.5%) patients. Moreover, difficulty breathing was documented among eight patients (24.2%). The patients' medical charts did not have any psychological disturbances, even though the physician asked about them. The finer specifics of additional symptomatology data are listed in Table 1.

Table 1. Long COVID symptoms.

Variable $n = 79$	Frequency (%)
Long COVID	33 (41.8)
Fatigue	15 (45.5)
Tiredness	14 (42.4)
Difficulty breathing	8 (24.2)
Paresthesia	3 (9.1)
Palpitations	2 (6.1)
Cough	2 (6.1)
Muscle pain	2 (6.1)
Chest pain	2 (6.1)
Dysgeusia	1 (3)
Difficulty swallowing	1 (3)
Alopecia	1 (3)
Insomnia	1 (3)

We observed that there was no significant difference between the variants of COVID-19 and the presence of long COVID using the chi-square test ($p = 0.631$). The variants in patients with long COVID were Delta in 19 (59.4%) patients, Alpha in 5 (15.6%) patients, Omicron in 4 (12.5%) patients, Gamma in 2 (6.1%) patients, and Beta and Epsilon in 1 (3%) patient each.

Regarding medical history, 7 (21.2%) patients with long COVID were vaccinated, while in patients without long COVID, 19 (42.2%) were vaccinated. Similarly, a chi-square analysis was performed, but no significant differences were found. The most common condition in both groups was obesity, with 23 patients (69.7%) having long COVID and 27 patients (58.7%) not having long COVID. However, no significant differences were found between the two groups in terms of obesity based on the chi-square analysis (Table 2).

Table 2. Personal history of patients.

Variable	Long COVID *n* = 33	No Long COVID *n* = 39	*p*-Value
Age	45.67 (15.95) [a]	52.43 (17.33) [a]	0.081 [a]
Males	22 (66.7)	34 (73.9)	0.484
Vaccination	2 (21.2)	19 (42.2)	0.128
Obesity	23 (69.7)	27 (58.7)	0.317
Diabetes mellitus type 2	10 (30.3)	15 (32.6)	0.828
Systematic arterial hypertension	6 (18.2)	17 (37)	0.070
Asthma	5 (15.2)	2 (4.3)	0.096
Smoking	4 (8.7)	4 (12.1)	0.619
Ischemic heart failure	3 (9.1)	4 (8.7)	0.951

[a] Data are presented as mean and standard deviation. The unpaired *t*-test was used for comparison. The remaining data are presented as frequencies and percentages. The chi-square test was used for comparison. A *p*-value < 0.05 was considered statistically significant.

Regarding respiratory treatment received in the hospital, it was observed that out of the patients with long COVID, four (12.5%) were admitted to the intensive care unit (ICU), while among the patients without long COVID, only two (4.3%) had a history of ICU admission. This difference was not statistically significant according to Fisher's exact test. The respiratory treatment required by the patients was also compared, and the most common method was the use of nasal cannulas. Among the patients with long COVID, 26 (78.8%) required nasal cannulas, while 28 (60.9%) of the patients without long COVID used nasal cannulas. The difference in the use of nasal cannulas was not statistically significant based on the chi-square test. The remaining variables concerning respiratory support and severity disease are listed in Table 3.

Table 3. Respiratory support and severity of disease.

Variable	Long COVID *n* = 33	No Long COVID *n* = 46	*p*-Value
ICU	4 (12.5) *	2 (4.3)	0.184 [a]
Low flow oxygenation	26 (78.8)	28 (60.9)	0.091 [b]
High flow oxygenation	10 (30.3)	8 (17.4)	0.177 [b]
Mechanical ventilation	4 (12.1)	2 (4.3)	0.198 [a]
Reservoir mask	1 (3)	4 (8.7)	0.394 [a]
Tracheostomy	2 (6.1)	0 (0)	0.910 [a]

Data are presented as frequencies and percentages. * There was a total number of 32 patients for the ICU variable. [a] Fischer's exact test was used for the comparison. [b] The chi-square test was used for the comparison.

The maximum peak of viral load presentation had a mean (SD) of 10 (2.64) days after the presentation of symptoms and had a non-significant median (IQR) between the long COVID and non-long COVID groups (462 (1155.82) vs. 259.0 (707.42), *p* = 0.067). Concerning the analyzed inflammatory markers, it was found that patients who developed long COVID had a higher peak of maximum lymphocytes mean (SD) during their hospitalization compared with patients without long COVID (2419.24 (1080.72) vs. 1967.15 (574.93), respectively), which was significant according to the unpaired *t*-test (*p* = 0.034). The peak of maximum leukocytes during hospitalization did not show a significant difference in median (IQR) between groups (8770 (3630) vs. 7655 (3700), $p = 0.173$). The peak of maximum lactate dehydrogenase during hospitalization did not show a significant difference in median (IQR) between groups (447.2 (224.7) vs. 399 (174.25), $p = 0.280$). The peak of maximum IL-6 during hospitalization did not show a significant difference in median (IQR) between groups (98 (434.2) vs. 89.15 (109.95), $p = 0.846$). The peak of maximum C-reactive protein during hospitalization did not show a significant difference in median (IQR) between groups (14.36 (11.84) vs. 13.79 (10.27), $p = 0.846$). The remaining inflammatory parameters during the hospital stay are listed in Table 4.

Table 4. Inflammatory parameters during the hospital stay.

Variable	Long COVID	No Long COVID	*p*-Value
Hemoglobin A1c ($n = 62$)	6.005 (0.6) [b]	6.2 (1.53) [b]	0.701
Max. peak leukocytes ($n = 79$)	8770 (3630) [b]	7655 (3700) [b]	0.173
Max. peak lymphocytes ($n = 79$)	2419.24 (1080.72) [a]	1967.15 (574.93) [a]	0.034
Max. peak neutrophils ($n = 79$)	6920 (3170) [b]	5550 (3773) [b]	0.340
Max. peak lactate dehydrogenase ($n = 75$)	447.2 (224.7) [b]	399 (174.25) [b]	0.280
Max. peak IL-6 ($n = 79$)	98 (434.2) [b]	89.15 (109.95) [b]	0.846
Max. peak C-reactive protein ($n = 79$)	14.36 (11.84) [b]	13.79 (10.27) [b]	0.846
Max. peak D-dimer ($n = 79$)	680 (1090) [b]	595 (455) [b]	0.178
Max. peak ferritin ($n = 79$)	1558 (2390.5) [b]	1468.53 (1732) [b]	0.811
Max. peak procalcitonin ($n = 70$)	0.11 (0.2) [b]	0.14 (0.36) [b]	0.775
Max. peak viral load ($n = 79$)	462 (1155.82) [b]	259.0 (707.42) [b]	0.067

[a] Data are presented as mean and standard deviation. The unpaired *t*-test was used for the comparison. [b] Data are presented as median and interquartile ranges. The Mann–Whitney U test was used for the comparison.

Regarding the analyzed lymphocyte subpopulation, individuals who subsequently experienced long COVID displayed an elevated count of total lymphocytes at the time of admission (1510.74 (1304.57) vs. 1133.77 (483.08), $p = 0.025$). Likewise, NK cells (CD16 and CD56) exhibited a higher presence among long COVID affected patients (224.79 (186.17) vs. 156.64 (129.72), $p = 0.027$). A comprehensive breakdown of the remaining lymphocyte subpopulations observed upon admission is listed in Table 5.

Table 5. Lymphocyte subpopulation at admission.

Variable	Long COVID ($n = 33$)	No Long COVID ($n = 46$)	*p*-Value
Total leukocyte subpopulation	7084.77 (2884.83) [a]	6067.31 (2360.05) [a]	0.089
Total lymphocyte subpopulation	1510.74 (1304.57) [a]	1133.77 (483.08) [a]	0.025
CD3+ T lymphocytes subpopulation	859.81 (882.7) [b]	685.7 (550.16) [b]	0.128
Subpopulation of helper T lymphocytes	498.53 (524.89) [b]	408.11 (333.53) [b]	0.223
CD8+ suppressor T lymphocyte subpopulation	255.62 (277.26) [b]	263.74 (277.96) [b]	0.382
B lymphocyte subpopulation CD19	164.90 (200.26) [b]	149.96 (115.53) [b]	0.551
Subpopulation of NK cells (CD16 and CD56)	224.79 (186.17) [b]	156.64 (129.72) [b]	0.027
Subpopulations CD4/CD8 ratio	2.34 (1.89) [b]	1.81 (1.18) [b]	0.937

[a] Data are presented as mean and standard deviation. The unpaired *t*-test was used for the comparison. [b] Data are presented as median and interquartile ranges. The Mann–Whitney U test was used for the comparison.

The outcomes regarding the logistic regression analysis of the risk factors and the presence of long COVID identified a positive correlation with increased levels of specific NK cell subpopulations (CD16 and CD56) (odds ratio (OR) = 1.006, $p = 0.009$). Notably, a significant positive link was also identified between the occurrence of long COVID and a prior history of ICU admission during hospitalization for acute COVID-19 (OR = 7.649, $p = 0.045$). For comprehensive further information, refer to Table 6, which provides a detailed breakdown of these findings and the non-significant variables.

Table 6. Binary logistic regression for prediction of long COVID.

Variable	β	Std Error	OR	*p*-Value	95%CI
Constant	−0.243	1.090	0.784	0.823	
Age	−0.016	0.021	0.984	0.450	0.945–0.025
Gender	−0.788	0.601	0.455	0.190	0.140–1.477
Subpopulation of NK cells (CD16 and CD56)	0.006	0.002	1.006	0.009	1.002–1.011
ICU	2.035	1.015	7.649	0.045	1.045–55.972
Systematic arterial hypertension	−1.075	0.753	2.042	0.153	0.078–1.491

Adjusted R-squared = 0.273. Dependent variable: long COVID symptoms. CI, confidence interval. Std, standard.

4. Discussion

In this study, we examined the association between long COVID 1.5 years after acute infection and various parameters recorded at the time of a patient's hospitalization. These included inflammatory markers, clinical parameters, viral load, and lymphocyte subpopulation. Among the 79 patients studied, 41.8% of them reported experiencing long COVID symptoms, with fatigue being the most common symptom in 45.5% of cases. These findings are consistent with results from other studies reporting a long COVID prevalence of approximately 40%, although some studies reported rates as high as 85% [13,26,27]. The frequency of fatigue is approximately 40% [26]. Dyspnea has also been reported at a frequency of approximately 20%, which aligns with our results [5]. In contrast to other studies, the frequency of other symptoms such as headache and sleep disorders was not as high [4].

In the literature, it is described that the main risk factors for presenting long COVID are being female, a history of hypertension, obesity, having a psychiatric condition, and being immunosuppressed, while age was reported not to be totally related with the presence of long COVID [2,28,29]. Regarding gender, our population did not show significant differences, which could be due the sample being limited to hospitalized patients, who were predominantly male. We did not find an association with hypertension or obesity, probably due to sample size. Also, psychiatric conditions and immunosuppressed patients were not studied since there were no patients presenting these conditions. In accordance with previous studies, we did not find any association with age.

Regarding severity, our regression model revealed that admission to the intensive care unit (ICU) was a significant risk factor associated with the onset of long COVID. This finding is consistent with results from other studies, where patients who required ICU care for COVID-19 treatment exhibited subsequent symptoms encompassing physical, mental, and cognitive aspects. Notably, a study conducted by Heesakkers et al. identified weakened physical condition as the most prevalent outcome, which aligns with our investigation where chronic fatigue emerged as the predominant symptom [30,31].

Although previous studies have indicated that the amount of SARS-CoV-2 viral load correlates with the presence of long COVID and the extent of its symptoms, the current study did not find this correlation [21,22]. What sets this study apart from its predecessors is its exclusive focus on hospitalized patients, its assessment of long-term COVID symptoms extending beyond three months post-illness, and its measurement of viral load using blood samples instead of nasal swabs, which were used in previous studies. Furthermore, the current study included a smaller cohort.

It was observed that lymphocytes and specific subsets of lymphocytes, such as CD4+T cells, CD8+T cells, and natural killer cells, play an important role in maintaining the immune system function. During the COVID-19 pandemic, there has been increasing recognition of the important role that lymphocytes and their subsets play in both the clinical characteristics and treatment efficacy of the disease [32,33]. Patients with severe COVID-19 have shown a significant reduction in levels of lymphocytes, monocytes, CD4+T cells, CD8+T cells, CD3 cells, CD19 cells, and natural killer cells. These alterations were also observed in patients with long COVID [34]. Contrary to this information, our patients did not present with lymphopenia during their hospital stay. One of the main rolls of natural killer cells is to provide early defense against viral infections. In this study, we found that the patients who developed long COVID had higher levels of NK cells during their hospitalization. This could be due to the persistent immune response required to control the viral infection. However, over time, these persistent immune responses may lead to dysfunction and exhaustion of NK cells. This depletion of NK cells, along with other lymphocyte subsets, may contribute to the development and persistence of long COVID symptoms [35]. Although there is limited research on the specific role of lymphocytes and NK cells in long COVID, several studies have shown that these cells are substantially depleted in patients with long COVID [32]. The pathophysiology of long COVID is a subject that continues to be studied because it has been shown to involve not only inflammatory response influences but also many other factors. The potential increase in NK cells during acute infection followed by a decrease during long COVID could be a sign of the known redistribution and sequestration during acute infection, which leads to an increased number of NK cells in the lungs and lower levels in the blood. These sequestered cells are known to have impaired expansion and cross-talk with other immune cells [36]. This suggests the presence of immune dysregulation and probable persistent viral replication, and further explains the potential long-term effects on lymphocyte dysfunction [37–39].

In the multivariate model that was performed to analyze age, gender, NK lymphocyte subpopulation, ICU and arterial hypertension, ICU and the amount of NK lymphocyte subpopulation at admission were associated with long COVID. These results are similar to those obtained in other studies. For example, in a study of 89 patients, it was also found that patients who were in the ICU during acute COVID infection had a higher risk of presenting long COVID when analyzed individually. The ICU environment is associated with a higher viral load, prolonged hospital stay, and increased exposure to inflammatory biomarkers that can further contribute to immune dysregulation and depletion of lymphocytes, including NK cells [40,41]. Regarding the viral load, in our population, it was not a significant factor in the subsequent development of long COVID. In other research studies, there is little information on viral load. Some studies found that there is an association, but in other studies, no such relationship with viral load was found. The relationship between long-COVID and COVID-19 viral load is a topic of ongoing research and debate [21,41,42].

One of the main limitations of the present study is that the laboratory samples were taken only during the hospitalization of the patients. No laboratory studies were performed after that. Therefore, future research should take additional samples so that it will be possible to compare the laboratory results during the hospitalization period with laboratory results during long COVID in order to observe changes over time in lymphocytes and inflammatory markers. Also, another important aspect to consider when interpreting the results is the sample size and gender. This study was conducted in a hospitalization context, and most of the subjects were males. Therefore, the sample does not represent the whole population with long COVID. In larger investigations, more COVID-19 symptoms can be included to perform a cluster study to determine if a group of symptoms is related to a more specific parameter.

The strengths of this study are that we included patients with very complete lab tests during their hospital stay and a very long-term follow of long COVID.

5. Conclusions

This study showed the interrelationship between inflammatory markers, such as NK cells, and the peak of lymphocytes during acute infection of COVID-19 and the presence of long COVID during a long-term follow-up of 1.5 years in hospitalized patients. The severity of the disease in our study evaluated through admittance to the ICU also was related to the presence of long COVID.

Author Contributions: Conceptualization, A.R.-C. and M.E.R.-I.; methodology, A.R.-C. and J.A.L.-G.; software, A.R.-C., A.G.-S. and A.G.-C.; validation, M.Á.S.-S. and M.E.R.-I.; formal analysis, A.R.-C., A.G.-S. and A.G.-C.; investigation, A.R.-C. and D.P.M.-R.; resources, J.A.L.-G.; data curation, A.R.-C. and J.A.L.-G.; writing—original draft preparation, A.R.-C., M.K.-A. and M.E.R.-I.; writing—review and editing, A.R.-C., J.A.L.-G., A.G.-S., D.P.M.-R., M.K.-A., M.Á.S.-S., J.E.S.-M., M.E.R.-I. and A.G.-C.; visualization, A.R.-C.; supervision, M.E.R.-I.; project administration, M.E.R.-I.; funding acquisition, M.Á.S.-S. All authors have read and agreed to the published version of the manuscript.

Funding: This research was conducted using private funding from Hospital Clinica Nova. The funders had no role in study design, data collection, analysis, or decision to publish.

Data Availability Statement: The database used and analyzed in this study is available from the corresponding author upon reasonable request.

Conflicts of Interest: The authors declare no conflict of interest.

References

1. World Health Organization. Coronavirus Disease (COVID-19). Available online: https://www.who.int/emergencies/diseases/novel-coronavirus-2019 (accessed on 3 July 2023).
2. Crook, H.; Raza, S.; Nowell, J.; Young, M.; Edison, P. Long Covid—Mechanisms, Risk Factors, and Management. *BMJ* **2021**, *374*, n1648. [CrossRef] [PubMed]
3. Greenhalgh, T.; Sivan, M.; Delaney, B.; Evans, R.; Milne, R. Long Covid—An Update for Primary Care. *BMJ* **2022**, *378*, e072117. [CrossRef]
4. Ziauddeen, N.; Gurdasani, D.; O'Hara, M.E.; Hastie, C.; Roderick, P.; Yao, G.; Alwan, N.A. Characteristics and Impact of Long Covid: Findings from an Online Survey. *PLoS ONE* **2022**, *17*, e0264331. [CrossRef] [PubMed]
5. Scharf, R.E.; Anaya, J.-M. Post-COVID Syndrome in Adults—An Overview. *Viruses* **2023**, *15*, 675. [CrossRef] [PubMed]
6. Alfadda, A.A.; Rafiullah, M.; Alkhowaiter, M.; Alotaibi, N.; Alzahrani, M.; Binkhamis, K.; Siddiqui, K.; Youssef, A.; Altalhi, H.; Almaghlouth, I.; et al. Clinical and Biochemical Characteristics of People Experiencing Post-Coronavirus Disease 2019-Related Symptoms: A Prospective Follow-up Investigation. *Front. Med.* **2022**, *9*, 1067082. [CrossRef]
7. Nair, C.V.; Moni, M.; Edathadathil, F.A.A.; Prasanna, P.; Pushpa Raghavan, R.; Sathyapalan, D.T.; Jayant, A. Incidence and Characterization of Post-COVID-19 Symptoms in Hospitalized COVID-19 Survivors to Recognize Syndemic Connotations in India: Single-Center Prospective Observational Cohort Study. *JMIR Form. Res.* **2023**, *7*, e40028. [CrossRef] [PubMed]
8. Taquet, M.; Dercon, Q.; Luciano, S.; Geddes, J.R.; Husain, M.; Harrison, P.J. Incidence, Co-Occurrence, and Evolution of Long-COVID Features: A 6-Month Retrospective Cohort Study of 273,618 Survivors of COVID-19. *PLoS Med.* **2021**, *18*, e1003773. [CrossRef]
9. Ji, G.; Chen, C.; Zhou, M.; Wen, W.; Wang, C.; Tang, J.; Cheng, Y.; Wu, Q.; Zhang, X.; Wang, M.; et al. Post-COVID-19 Fatigue among COVID-19 in Patients Discharged from Hospital: A Meta-Analysis. *J. Infect.* **2022**, *84*, 722–746. [CrossRef]
10. Sukocheva, O.A.; Maksoud, R.; Beeraka, N.M.; Madhunapantula, S.V.; Sinelnikov, M.; Nikolenko, V.N.; Neganova, M.E.; Klochkov, S.G.; Amjad Kamal, M.; Staines, D.R.; et al. Analysis of Post COVID-19 Condition and Its Overlap with Myalgic Encephalomyelitis/Chronic Fatigue Syndrome. *J. Adv. Res.* **2022**, *40*, 179–196. [CrossRef]
11. Sudre, C.H.; Murray, B.; Varsavsky, T.; Graham, M.S.; Penfold, R.S.; Bowyer, R.C.; Pujol, J.C.; Klaser, K.; Antonelli, M.; Canas, L.S.; et al. Attributes and Predictors of Long COVID. *Nat. Med.* **2021**, *27*, 626–631. [CrossRef]
12. Freidin, M.B.; Cheetham, N.; Duncan, E.L.; Steves, C.J.; Doores, K.J.; Malim, M.H.; Rossi, N.; Lord, J.M.; Franks, P.W.; Borsini, A.; et al. Long-COVID Fatigue Is Not Predicted by Pre-Pandemic Plasma IL-6 Levels in Mild COVID-19. *Inflamm. Res.* **2023**, *72*, 947–953. [CrossRef] [PubMed]
13. Çil, B.; Kabak, M. Department of Chest Diseases, Mardin Training and Research Hospital, Mardin, Turkey Persistent Post-COVID Symptoms and the Related Factors. *Turk. Thorac. J.* **2022**, *23*, 6–10. [CrossRef]
14. Yong, S.J. Long COVID or Post-COVID-19 Syndrome: Putative Pathophysiology, Risk Factors, and Treatments. *Infect. Dis.* **2021**, *53*, 737–754. [CrossRef] [PubMed]
15. Queiroz, M.A.F.; das Neves, P.F.M.; Lima, S.S.; Lopes, J.d.C.; Torres, M.K.d.S.; Vallinoto, I.M.V.C.; Bichara, C.D.A.; dos Santos, E.F.; de Brito, M.T.F.M.; da Silva, A.L.S.; et al. Cytokine Profiles Associated with Acute COVID-19 and Long COVID-19 Syndrome. *Front. Cell. Infect. Microbiol.* **2022**, *12*, 922422. [CrossRef] [PubMed]
16. Savchenko, A.A.; Kudryavtsev, I.V.; Isakov, D.V.; Sadowski, I.S.; Belenyuk, V.D.; Borisov, A.G. Recombinant Human Interleukin-2 Corrects NK Cell Phenotype and Functional Activity in Patients with Post-COVID Syndrome. *Pharmaceuticals* **2023**, *16*, 537. [CrossRef]
17. Fernández-de-las-Peñas, C.; Ryan-Murua, P.; Rodríguez-Jiménez, J.; Palacios-Ceña, M.; Arendt-Nielsen, L.; Torres-Macho, J. Serological Biomarkers at Hospital Admission Are Not Related to Long-Term Post-COVID Fatigue and Dyspnea in COVID-19 Survivors. *Respiration* **2022**, *101*, 658–665. [CrossRef]
18. Rao, S.N.; Manissero, D.; Steele, V.R.; Pareja, J. A Systematic Review of the Clinical Utility of Cycle Threshold Values in the Context of COVID-19. *Infect. Dis. Ther.* **2020**, *9*, 573–586. [CrossRef]

19. Abdulrahman, A.; Mallah, S.I.; Alqahtani, M. COVID-19 Viral Load Not Associated with Disease Severity: Findings from a Retrospective Cohort Study. *BMC Infect. Dis.* **2021**, *21*, 688. [CrossRef]
20. Kuri-Ayache, M.; Rivera-Cavazos, A.; Pérez-Castillo, M.F.; Santos-Macías, J.E.; González-Cantú, A.; Luviano-García, J.A.; Jaime-Villalón, D.; Gutierrez-González, D.; Romero-Ibarguengoitia, M.E. Viral Load and Its Relationship with the Inflammatory Response and Clinical Outcomes in Hospitalization of Patients with COVID-19. *Front. Immunol.* **2023**, *13*, 1060840. [CrossRef]
21. Girón Pérez, D.A.; Fonseca-Agüero, A.; Toledo-Ibarra, G.A.; Gomez-Valdivia, J.d.J.; Díaz-Resendiz, K.J.G.; Benitez-Trinidad, A.B.; Razura-Carmona, F.F.; Navidad-Murrieta, M.S.; Covantes-Rosales, C.E.; Giron-Pérez, M.I. Post-COVID-19 Syndrome in Outpatients and Its Association with Viral Load. *Int. J. Environ. Res. Public Health* **2022**, *19*, 15145. [CrossRef]
22. Su, Y.; Yuan, D.; Chen, D.G.; Ng, R.H.; Wang, K.; Choi, J.; Li, S.; Hong, S.; Zhang, R.; Xie, J.; et al. Multiple Early Factors Anticipate Post-Acute COVID-19 Sequelae. *Cell* **2022**, *185*, 881–895.e20. [CrossRef] [PubMed]
23. Cuschieri, S. The STROBE Guidelines. *Saudi J. Anaesth.* **2019**, *13*, 31. [CrossRef] [PubMed]
24. Thaweethai, T.; Jolley, S.E.; Karlson, E.W.; Levitan, E.B.; Levy, B.; McComsey, G.A.; McCorkell, L.; Nadkarni, G.N.; Parthasarathy, S.; Singh, U.; et al. Development of a Definition of Postacute Sequelae of SARS-CoV-2 Infection. *JAMA* **2023**, *329*, 1934. [CrossRef] [PubMed]
25. PAXgene Blood RNA Tubes (IVD). Available online: https://www.qiagen.com/gb/products/discovery-and-translational-research/sample-collection-stabilization/rna/paxgene-blood-rna-tubes?cmpid=PC_NON_NON_paxgene-traffic_0421_SEA_GA&gclid=Cj0KCQjwldKmBhCCARIsAP-0rfznNNnjmK5B31lxRS3paK_1622wvUvvQxcLvM6liSL2oQ2tRrUUhnYaAj5nEALw_wcB#orderinginformation (accessed on 1 June 2023).
26. Sisó-Almirall, A.; Brito-Zerón, P.; Conangla Ferrín, L.; Kostov, B.; Moragas Moreno, A.; Mestres, J.; Sellarès, J.; Galindo, G.; Morera, R.; Basora, J.; et al. Long COVID-19: Proposed Primary Care Clinical Guidelines for Diagnosis and Disease Management. *Int. J. Environ. Res. Public Health* **2021**, *18*, 4350. [CrossRef]
27. Peghin, M.; Palese, A.; Venturini, M.; De Martino, M.; Gerussi, V.; Graziano, E.; Bontempo, G.; Marrella, F.; Tommasini, A.; Fabris, M.; et al. Post-COVID-19 Symptoms 6 Months after Acute Infection among Hospitalized and Non-Hospitalized Patients. *Clin. Microbiol. Infect.* **2021**, *27*, 1507–1513. [CrossRef]
28. Notarte, K.I.; De Oliveira, M.H.S.; Peligro, P.J.; Velasco, J.V.; Macaranas, I.; Ver, A.T.; Pangilinan, F.C.; Pastrana, A.; Goldrich, N.; Kavteladze, D.; et al. Age, Sex and Previous Comorbidities as Risk Factors Not Associated with SARS-CoV-2 Infection for Long COVID-19: A Systematic Review and Meta-Analysis. *J. Clin. Med.* **2022**, *11*, 7314. [CrossRef]
29. Asadi-Pooya, A.A.; Akbari, A.; Emami, A.; Lotfi, M.; Rostamihosseinkhani, M.; Nemati, H.; Barzegar, Z.; Kabiri, M.; Zeraatpisheh, Z.; Farjoud-Kouhanjani, M.; et al. Risk Factors Associated with Long COVID Syndrome: A Retrospective Study. *Iran. J. Med. Sci.* **2021**, *46*, 428–436. [CrossRef]
30. Heesakkers, H.; Van Der Hoeven, J.G.; Corsten, S.; Janssen, I.; Ewalds, E.; Simons, K.S.; Westerhof, B.; Rettig, T.C.D.; Jacobs, C.; Van Santen, S.; et al. Clinical Outcomes Among Patients With 1-Year Survival Following Intensive Care Unit Treatment for COVID-19. *JAMA* **2022**, *327*, 559. [CrossRef]
31. Rousseau, A.-F.; Minguet, P.; Colson, C.; Kellens, I.; Chaabane, S.; Delanaye, P.; Cavalier, E.; Chase, J.G.; Lambermont, B.; Misset, B. Post-Intensive Care Syndrome after a Critical COVID-19: Cohort Study from a Belgian Follow-up Clinic. *Ann. Intensive Care* **2021**, *11*, 118. [CrossRef]
32. Karlsson, A.C.; Humbert, M.; Buggert, M. The Known Unknowns of T Cell Immunity to COVID-19. *Sci. Immunol.* **2020**, *5*, eabe8063. [CrossRef]
33. Ryan, F.J.; Hope, C.M.; Masavuli, M.G.; Lynn, M.A.; Mekonnen, Z.A.; Yeow, A.E.L.; Garcia-Valtanen, P.; Al-Delfi, Z.; Gummow, J.; Ferguson, C.; et al. Long-Term Perturbation of the Peripheral Immune System Months after SARS-CoV-2 Infection. *BMC Med.* **2022**, *20*, 26. [CrossRef] [PubMed]
34. Yang, H.; Xi, X.; Wang, W.; Gu, B. Immune Response, Viral Shedding Time, and Clinical Characterization in COVID-19 Patients with Gastrointestinal Symptoms. *Front. Med.* **2021**, *8*, 593623. [CrossRef] [PubMed]
35. Scalia, G.; Raia, M.; Gelzo, M.; Cacciapuoti, S.; Rosa, A.D.; Pinchera, B.; Scotto, R.; Tripodi, L.; Mormile, M.; Fabbrocini, G.; et al. Lymphocyte Population Changes at Two Time Points during the Acute Period of COVID-19 Infection. *J. Clin. Med.* **2022**, *11*, 4306. [CrossRef] [PubMed]
36. Di Vito, C.; Calcaterra, F.; Coianiz, N.; Terzoli, S.; Voza, A.; Mikulak, J.; Della Bella, S.; Mavilio, D. Natural Killer Cells in SARS-CoV-2 Infection: Pathophysiology and Therapeutic Implications. *Front. Immunol.* **2022**, *13*, 888248. [CrossRef]
37. Malengier-Devlies, B.; Filtjens, J.; Ahmadzadeh, K.; Boeckx, B.; Vandenhaute, J.; De Visscher, A.; Bernaerts, E.; Mitera, T.; Jacobs, C.; Vanderbeke, L.; et al. Severe COVID-19 Patients Display Hyper-Activated NK Cells and NK Cell-Platelet Aggregates. *Front. Immunol.* **2022**, *13*, 861251. [CrossRef] [PubMed]
38. Galán, M.; Vigón, L.; Fuertes, D.; Murciano-Antón, M.A.; Casado-Fernández, G.; Domínguez-Mateos, S.; Mateos, E.; Ramos-Martín, F.; Planelles, V.; Torres, M.; et al. Persistent Overactive Cytotoxic Immune Response in a Spanish Cohort of Individuals with Long-COVID: Identification of Diagnostic Biomarkers. *Front. Immunol.* **2022**, *13*, 848886. [CrossRef]
39. Mitsuyama, Y.; Yamakawa, K.; Kayano, K.; Maruyama, M.; Umemura, Y.; Wada, T.; Fujimi, S. Residual Persistence of Cytotoxicity Lymphocytes and Regulatory T Cells in Patients with Severe CORONAVIRUS DISEASE 2019 over a 1-year Recovery Process. *Acute Med. Surg.* **2022**, *9*, e803. [CrossRef]
40. Nune, A.; Durkowski, V.; Titman, A.; Gupta, L.; Hadzhiivanov, M.; Ahmed, A.; Musat, C.; Sapkota, H.R. Incidence and Risk Factors of Long Covid in the Uk: A Single-Centre Observational Study. *J. R. Coll. Physicians Edinb.* **2021**, *51*, 338–343. [CrossRef]

41. Baig, A.M. Chronic Long-COVID Syndrome: A Protracted COVID-19 Illness with Neurological Dysfunctions. *CNS Neurosci. Ther.*
     2021, *27*, 1433–1436. [CrossRef]
42. Lui, D.T.W.; Lee, C.H.; Chow, W.S.; Lee, A.C.H.; Tam, A.R.; Pang, P.; Ho, T.Y.; Fong, C.H.Y.; Law, C.Y.; Leung, E.K.H.; et al. Long
     COVID in Patients with Mild to Moderate Disease: Do Thyroid Function and Autoimmunity Play a Role? *Endocr. Pract.* **2021**, *27*,
     894–902. [CrossRef]

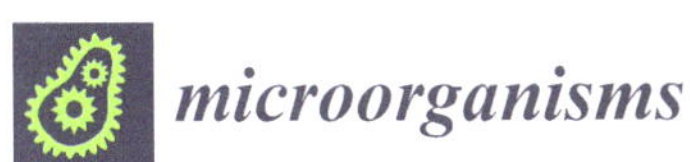 *microorganisms*

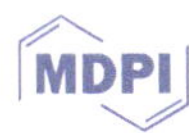

Review

Long COVID or Post-COVID-19 Condition: Past, Present and Future Research Directions

César Fernández-de-las-Peñas [1,2,*], Arkiath Veettil Raveendran [3], Rocco Giordano [2] and Lars Arendt-Nielsen [2,4,5]

[1] Department of Physical Therapy, Occupational Therapy, Physical Medicine and Rehabilitation, Universidad Rey Juan Carlos, 28922 Madrid, Spain

[2] Center for Neuroplasticity and Pain (CNAP), Center for Sensory-Motor Interaction (SMI), Department of Health Science and Technology, Faculty of Medicine, Aalborg University, DK-9220 Aalborg, Denmark; rg@hst.aau.dk (R.G.); lan@hst.aau.dk (L.A.-N.)

[3] Govt. Medical College, Kozhikode 676121, Kerala, India; raveendranav@yahoo.co.in

[4] Department of Medical Gastroenterology, Mech-Sense, Aalborg University Hospital, DK-9000 Aalborg, Denmark

[5] Steno Diabetes Center North Denmark, Clinical Institute, Aalborg University Hospital, DK-9000 Aalborg, Denmark

* Correspondence: cesar.fernandez@urjc.es; Tel.: +34-91-488-88-84

Abstract: The presence of symptoms after an acute SARS-CoV-2 infection (long-COVID) has become a worldwide healthcare emergency but remains underestimated and undertreated due to a lack of recognition of the condition and knowledge of the underlying mechanisms. In fact, the prevalence of post-COVID symptoms ranges from 50% during the first months after the infection up to 20% two-years after. This perspective review aimed to map the existing literature on post-COVID symptoms and to identify gaps in the literature to guide the global effort toward an improved understanding of long-COVID and suggest future research directions. There is a plethora of symptomatology that can be due to COVID-19; however, today, there is no clear classification and definition of this condition, termed long-COVID or post-COVID-19 condition. The heterogeneity in the symptomatology has led to the presence of groups/clusters of patients, which could exhibit different risk factors and different mechanisms. Viral persistence, long-lasting inflammation, immune dysregulation, autoimmune reactions, reactivation of latent infections, endothelial dysfunction and alteration in gut microbiota have been proposed as potential mechanisms explaining the complexity of long-COVID. In such an equation, viral biology (e.g., re-infections, SARS-CoV-2 variants), host biology (e.g., genetics, epigenetics) and external factors (e.g., vaccination) should be also considered. These various factors will be discussed in the current perspective review and future directions suggested.

Keywords: COVID-19; post-COVID; long-COVID; mechanisms; vaccine; reinfections; genetics

Citation: Fernández-de-las-Peñas, C.; Raveendran, A.V.; Giordano, R.; Arendt-Nielsen, L. Long COVID or Post-COVID-19 Condition: Past, Present and Future Research Directions. *Microorganisms* **2023**, *11*, 2959. https://doi.org/10.3390/microorganisms11122959

Academic Editor: Qibin Geng

Received: 11 November 2023
Revised: 2 December 2023
Accepted: 9 December 2023
Published: 11 December 2023

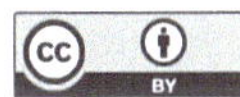

1. Introduction

The Severe Acute Respiratory Syndrome Coronavirus 2 (SARS-CoV-2), the pathogen responsible for the worldwide spread of coronavirus disease 2019 (COVID-19), has provoked one of the most important health crises of the current century. Over the course of the last three years, since the onset of the outbreak, the emergence of new several SARS-CoV-2 variants has perpetuated its relentless transmission, resulting in a staggering 768 million confirmed cases and nearly 7 million reported deaths globally [1]. Substantial efforts have been focused on managing COVID-19 symptoms at the acute phase [2,3], the introduction of vaccines for preventing the severe form of the disease and for decreasing mortality rates [4] and for preventing the spreading of SARS-CoV-2 variants [5].

A growing concern from the beginning of the pandemic has been also the development of long-lasting symptomatology once the acute phase of the infection has surpassed. From the beginning of the pandemic, more than 100 post-COVID symptoms affecting multiple systems, e.g., cardiovascular, neurological, respiratory and musculoskeletal, have been described [6]. The presence of long-lasting post-COVID symptoms is associated with reduced health-related quality of life [7], a substantial increase in healthcare utilization and increased direct and indirect medical costs [8]. In fact, the health-related quality of life of patients with long-lasting post-COVID symptoms is severely impacted and can be compared with that of people with chronic pain after spinal surgery [9].

Several meta-analyses have reported that up to 50% of individuals who had survived a SARS-CoV-2 acute infection exhibit a plethora of long-lasting symptoms from several weeks or months [10–12] up to one year after [13–15]. Thus, the Global Burden of Disease Long COVID study, which included 1.2 million subjects who had experienced an acute SARS-CoV-2 infection, reported that 51% of COVID-19 survivors suffered from at least one long-lasting post-COVID symptom the first three months after and that to up to 15.1% of subjects experience symptoms 12 months after [16]. A PubMed search conducted on 10 November 2023 revealed more than 2500 papers describing different post-COVID symptoms. Rahmati et al. observed that around 40% of COVID-19 survivors still experience at least one post-COVID symptom two years after the infection [17]. Fatigue (51%) [18], cognitive problems (25%) [19] and pain (20%) [20] are the most prevalent post-COVID symptoms. Overall, SARS-CoV-2 infection has been associated with a higher risk of developing post-COVID fatigue (RR 1.72, 95%CI 1.41, 2.10), dyspnea (RR 2.60, 95%CI 1.96, 3.44), memory difficulties (RR2.53, 95% CI 1.30, 4.93) and concentration difficulties (RR2.14, 95%CI 1.25, 3.67) [21].

It is important to consider the complex pathways that link SARS-CoV-2 acute infection, the putative biological mechanisms of the host and the heterogeneous phenotypes of post-COVID symptomatology [22]. The current perspective review aimed to map the existing literature on post-COVID symptomatology (from the definition of the condition to the underlying mechanisms (including genetics) and to identify gaps in the current literature to guide the global effort toward an improved understanding of long-COVID [23]. Each section reviews current literature and includes questions for future research.

2. How Should Post-COVID Symptoms Be Defined

Different terms have been used for defining the presence of symptoms persisting after the acute phase of a SARS-CoV-2 infection being post-COVID, long-COVID, post-COVID-19 condition, or post-acute sequelae of SARS-CoV-2 infection (PASC) are the most commonly used [24,25].

The World Health Organization (WHO) adopted the term post-COVID-19 condition: "post-COVID-19 condition occurs in people with a history of probable or confirmed SARS-CoV-2 infection, usually three months from the onset of infection, with symptoms that last for at least two months and cannot be explained by an alternative diagnosis. Common symptoms include, but are not limited to, fatigue, shortness of breath (dyspnea), and cognitive dysfunction, and generally have an impact on everyday functioning. Symptoms might be new onset following initial recovery from an acute COVID-19 episode or persist from the initial illness. Symptoms might also fluctuate or relapse over time" [26]. Several aspects of this definition should be considered.

First, the definition is focused on three symptoms, and although it includes "not limited to", it does not consider bothersome and prevalent symptoms such as pain. We believe that the presence of any symptom showing a temporal relationship with the SARS-CoV-2 infection (another aspect for clarification) should be included in the definition, independently of its prevalence. Although fatigue is by far the major post-COVID symptom, combined or as a singleton symptom [27], other post-COVID symptoms, e.g., dyspnea, have shown prevalence rates up to 26% [28]. Thus, one particular post-COVID symptom could have different repercussions in daily life activities depending on each particular patient, accordingly, personalized application of this definition must be provided.

Second, this definition did not consider the presence of previous symptoms or medical co-morbidities before the acute infection. This is an important topic because COVID-19 can promote the development of new symptoms (new-onset post-COVID symptom, a symptom not experienced before the infection and appearing after) or can also worsen previous symptoms (exacerbated post-COVID symptom) [29]. The definition of post-COVID-19 condition includes "symptoms might be new-onset after initial recovery from an acute COVID-19 episode or persist from the initial illness (persistent post-COVID symptom, a symptom experienced by a patient at the acute phase and persisting after without remission periods)". This aspect is related to the relapsing/remitting nature of post-COVID symptoms and the time existing between the appearance of the symptom in relation to the infection [30]. These two post-COVID symptoms are included in the main definition; however, a third type, delayed-onset post-COVID symptom (a symptom not experienced at the acute phase of the infection and appearing after a latency period in relation to the infection) has been also described, although questioned [30]. An explanation for a delayed-onset post-COVID symptom is that SARS-COV-2 can trigger latent neurodegenerative processes with residual damage on persistent immune activation or unmasking of underlying co-morbidities [31].

Third, the temporal relationship with the SARS-CoV-2 infection is one of the hottest topics for the diagnosis of post-COVID-19 condition, and most definitions have focused on this aspect. The National Institute for Health and Care Excellence (NICE) Guideline, the Scottish Intercollegiate Guidelines Network, and the Royal College of General Practitioners proposed a time four weeks after the infection [32], Baig proposed three weeks after [33], and Halpin et al. proposed 12 weeks after [34] for the diagnosis of post-COVID-19 condition. The WHO proposed a 12-week timeframe [26]. Determining the timeframe for the diagnosis of post-COVID-19 condition is critical for clinically identifying if the symptoms can or cannot be attributed to SARS-CoV-2 infection, but it is highly difficult from a clinical point of view due to the latency nature of some post-COVID symptoms and the neurotropism of SARS-CoV-2.

Finally, the term long-COVID (which was the term proposed by the patients themselves in Spring 2020 as well as the term long-haulers [35]) was proposed for the presence, overall, of any post-COVID symptom after surpassing the SARS-CoV-2 infection [36]. In this definition, all potential situations associated with pre-existing symptomatology or medical conditions before the infection and different time frames are considered [36].

Figure 1 graphs the proposed development of post-COVID symptoms considering all these discussion points. First, if the patient reports the presence of a previous symptom, clinicians should differentiate if a particular post-COVID symptom is "new" or "exacerbated". Similarly, the presence of a pre-existing medical co-morbidity who shares symptoms with COVID-19 should be also considered. In such a scenario, the temporality between the appearance of the symptom in relation to the acute infection should be investigated. If a symptom appears several months after the infection and is reasonably related (caused) by SARS-CoV-2, it should be considered as a post-COVID "delayed-onset" symptom. Second, the presence of a long-lasting post-COVID symptom that was also experienced at the acute phase of SARS-CoV-2 infection would lead to a "persistent" post-COVID symptom since this symptom started at the beginning of acute phase of infection and continue at post-infection without interruption.

<u>Future research direction</u>: We do not currently know if this proposal would lead to different treatment outcomes or to a better classification of post-COVID symptomatology.

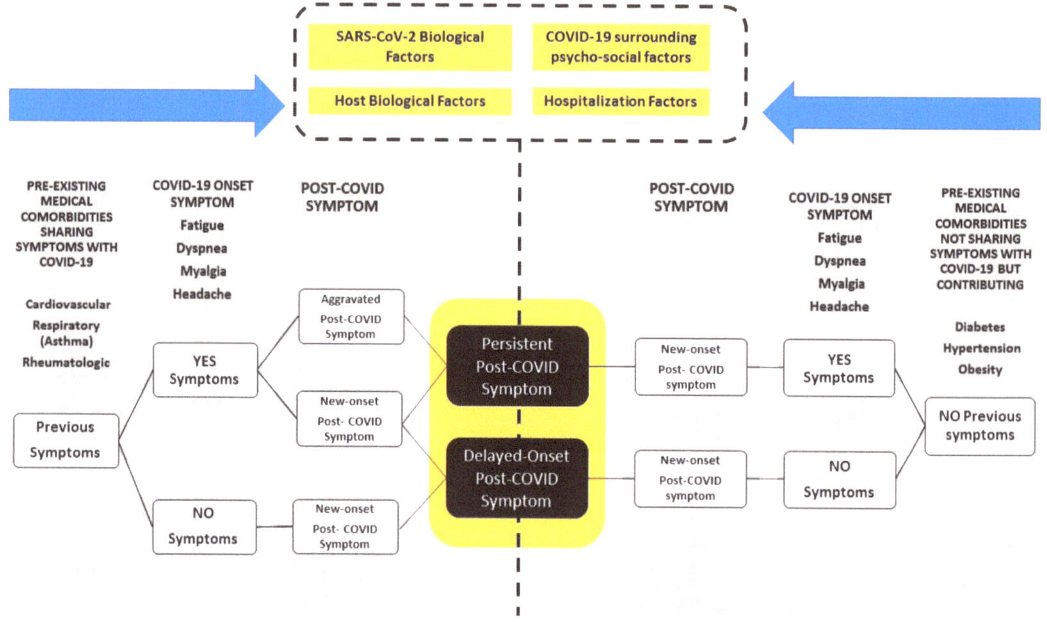

Figure 1. Proposal model for long-COVID symptomatology.

3. Subclassification (Clustering) and Phenotyping of Long-COVID

More than 100 symptoms could be attributed to SARs-CoV-2 infection [6]. It is clear that SARS-CoV-2 can affect all human systems: cardiorespiratory, gastrointestinal, neurological, dermatological, musculoskeletal, endocrine, visual and reproductive. Interestingly, research shows that patients with long-COVID tend to report post-COVID symptoms mostly associated with a particular system, leading to the hypothesis of the presence of clusters or subgroups. In fact, post-COVID clustering suggests different etiologies and mechanisms for each cluster.

The Global Burden of Disease Long-COVID study identified three clusters according to the most prevalent post-COVID symptoms: fatigue with pain in 51% of patients, respiratory symptoms in 60.4% of patients and cognitive problems in 35.4% of patients [16]. As it can be observed, the same patient could exhibit the combination of two clusters. Peter et al. found that the fatigue (37.2% of patients) and neurocognitive disturbances (31.3% of patients) groups were those mostly contributing to decreased health recovery whereas the musculoskeletal pain (16% of patients) group was the most disabled for working activities [37].

A recent meta-analysis has identified the following three clusters: (1) the cardiorespiratory cluster including fatigue, dyspnea, chest pain, muscle pain, headache, palpitations; (2) the systemic inflammatory cluster including dizziness, gastrointestinal symptoms, muscle pain, hair loss, muscle weakness and sleep disorders; or (3) the neurological cluster including headache, anosmia, paresthesia, neuropathies, dizziness, vision and balance problems, memory problems and poor concentration [15]. The estimated prevalence rates for the clusters were 36% (95%CI 32% to 40%) for the cardiorespiratory cluster (7 studies), 72% (95%CI 45% to 92%) for the neurological cluster (3 studies) and 46% (95%CI 17–77%) for the systemic inflammatory cluster (4 studies) [15]. As can be observed, pain symptomatology is present in all clusters identified by Kuodi et al. [15]. In fact, pain symptomatology is commonly found to be associated with the presence of fatigue or gastrointestinal problems in several chronic pain conditions; however, some authors have found that pain and fatigue can be also separated into two different clusters in individuals with post-COVID symptoms [38].

Future research direction: It is hypothesized that the different clusters/groups of patients with long-COVID could be associated with different underlying mechanisms; however, this has not yet been investigated. Future studies should "validate" the identified clusters by associating their symptoms with etiopathogenic mechanisms and treatment responses.

4. Risk Factors Associated with Long-COVID

Due to the catastrophic consequences of the COVID-19 outbreak, several attempts have been made to identify potential risk factors associated with the development of long-COVID. Initial evidence suggested that female sex, older age, a higher number of previous comorbidities, longer hospital stance, higher viral load, COVID-19 severity and a greater number of onset symptoms at the acute phase of the infection seem to be potential risk factors associated with long-COVID [39–41].

Different meta-analyses investigating risk factors associated with long-COVID have reported conflicting results. Maglietta et al. identified that the female sex was a risk factor for long-COVID whereas more severe SARS-CoV-2 infection was associated just with post-COVID respiratory symptoms [42]. Thompson et al. found that older age, female sex, white ethnicity, poor pre-infection health, obesity and asthma were associated with long-COVID [43]. Notarte et al. identified that the female sex and some specific comorbidities such as obesity were associated with long-COVID [44]. These authors observed that single studies reported that older age seems to be associated with long-COVID, but this association was not significant when they pooled data into their meta-analysis [44]. The most recent meta-analysis, conducted by Tsampasian et al. confirmed that female sex and obesity (higher body mass index) were associated with a higher risk of developing long-COVID [45]. This meta-analysis observed that older age, ICU admission and hospitalization were also associated with long-COVID [45].

To date, the only factor clearly associated with a higher risk of developing long-COVID is female sex [42–45]. Several biological and social factors can explain these sex differences. Interestingly, biological sex differences in the expression of angiotensin-converting enzyme 2 (ACE2) and transmembrane protease serine 2 (TMPRSS2) receptors can explain the higher survivor rate but a higher prevalence of long-COVID in female sex [46]. Thus, differences in physical capacity could also be involved. For instance, it has been recently observed that females who had been infected by SARS-CoV-2 exhibit a more reduced alveolar diffusion capacity or exercise tolerance than males [47]. In fact, although males and females have the same probability of being infected by SARS-CoV-2; males had higher rates of the severe form of COVID-19 and mortality than females [48–51]. Similarly, sex-dependent self-reporting bias should also be taken into account, considering the sex-dependent discrepancy in medical care already in place before the COVID-19 outbreak [27,52]. Accordingly, sex differences should be considered by clinicians when designing therapeutic strategies for a patient with long-COVID.

We could classify risk factors into: (1) host biological factors (those pre-infection features e.g., age, sex, pre-existing medical co-morbidities, previous health status, genetic predisposition); (2) SARS-CoV-2 biological factors (those associated with the infection e.g., disease severity, symptoms at onset, viral load, inflammatory response); (3) hospitalization factors (e.g., hospital stay, ICU admission, treatment received); and (4) surrounding psychosocial factors (e.g., stigmatization, sleep disorders, stressful situations, social influence, familiar problems).

Future research direction: It is possible that with the rapid increase in the number of long-COVID studies, all the risk factors have not yet been identified and further research is needed. For instance, the presence of depressive symptoms before the infection has been found to be a major risk factor for specific post-COVID symptomatology such as long-term dysautonomia as well as psychiatric symptoms in a single study [52].

5. Current Pathophysiology Theories of Long-COVID

Long-COVID denotes symptoms and signs affecting multiple tissues and organ systems in the body. Thus, symptoms vary depending on the organ systems involved and the predominant pathophysiological mechanisms operating, making the diagnosis a challenge for clinicians [53]. In fact, pathophysiological mechanisms of long-COVID are not fully understood and different mechanisms are proposed and summarized in Figure 2 [54,55].

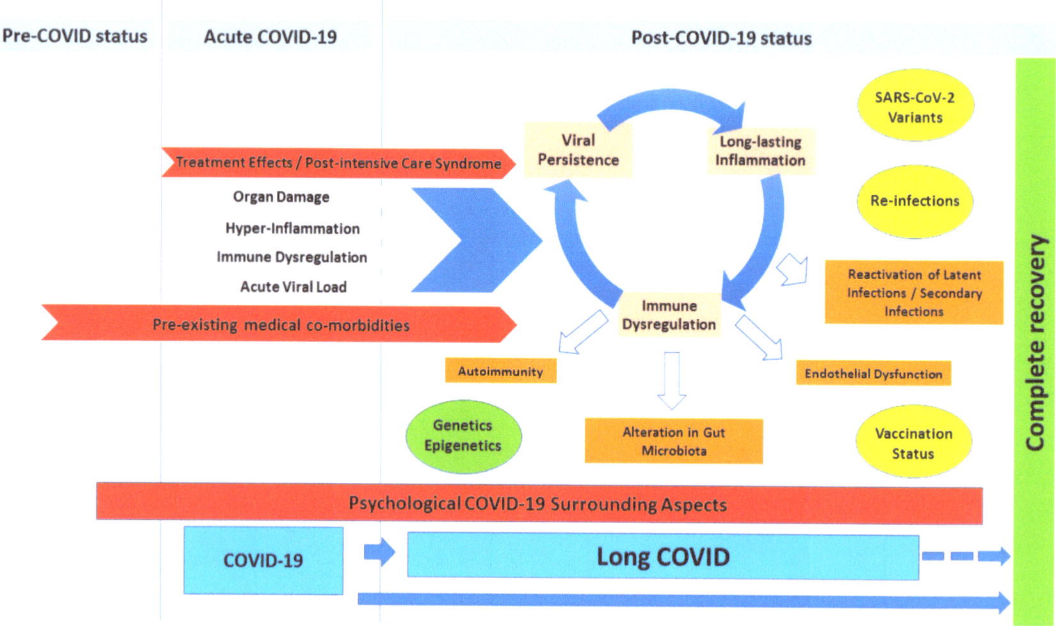

Figure 2. Potential pathophysiological mechanisms of long-COVID.

5.1. Viral Persistence

Viral persistence is postulated as one of the most robust hypotheses for long-COVID [56]. It is possible that the SARS-CoV-2 pathogen may establish a persistent infection or leave non-infectious remnants in deep human tissues. Such a persistent reservoir or remnants will be able to generate pathogen-associated molecular patterns (PAMPs), such as viral RNA or bacterial cell wall and could engage host pattern recognition receptors (PRRs) triggering innate immune activation [57].

Several studies have investigated the presence of viral persistence or laboratory signs of persistent infection in people with long-COVID; nevertheless, heterogeneous results have been found [58]. It seems that persisting SARS-CoV-2 RNA is present in different human tissues but this persistence is time-dependent, i.e., there is a tendency to disappear with time from the infection, and also symptom-dependent, i.e., the virus is still present in the tissue associated with a specific post-COVID symptom. In fact, evidence supports that genes and proteins of the SARS-CoV-2 virus persist in the human body for variable periods (2–9 months) after the acute infection; however, data on viral persistence in follow-ups longer than one year are scarce [58]. Thus, SARS-CoV-2 RNA has been found in different human tissues such as the lungs [59], brain [60] or gastrointestinal tract [61], which could explain the presence of post-COVID dyspnea, brain fog and gastrointestinal symptoms, respectively. In addition, the presence of persistent SARS-CoV-2 spikes in plasma could lead to more systemic post-COVID symptoms such as chronic fatigue [62]. However, not all individuals experiencing post-COVID symptoms exhibit persistent SARS-CoV-2 RNA.

It is possible that viral persistence is present in a range of 60% to 70% of individuals with long-COVID, but not in all. In fact, most published studies to date have not included a control (comparison) group of individuals who had been infected but did not develop persistent symptoms after SARS-CoV-2 acute infection [58]. Most studies have identified the presence of viral persistence in different tissues in small samples of patients with long-COVID but it has not been demonstrated yet if the same results would be observed in individuals without symptoms.

<u>Future research direction:</u> If viral persistence is observed in a significant proportion of patients with long-COVID, it would justify the application of antivirals for the management of post-COVID symptomatology. Evidence supports the use of antivirals such as Nirmatrelvir-Ritonavir during the COVID-19 acute phase [63]. However, no published study has investigated the effect of antivirals in the management of patients with long-COVID, although several trials are currently being conducted: https://clinicaltrials.gov/ct2/results?cond=Long+COVID&term=nirmatrelvir/ritonavir+&cntry=&state=&city=&dist= (accessed on 15 October 2023).

5.2. Long-Lasting Inflammation

Different types of inflammatory responses (e.g., specific SARS-CoV-2 responses, new-onset autoimmune responses or a loss of normal immunoregulation) play an important role in the pathophysiology of acute COVID-19 [64]. In fact, long-lasting inflammation (systemic and tissue-specific) has been also found to be an important factor contributing to the development of long-COVID [65]. However, data about the level of inflammatory biomarkers, e.g., interleukins (IL) are conflicting, probably because inflammatory biomarkers were evaluated at two different moments, at hospital admission during the acute infection or months after the infection. Yin et al. reported that the levels of IL-6 are increased in individuals with long-COVID several months after the infection [66]. Similarly, a meta-analysis including up to 110 biomarkers also observed up-regulated IL-6, C-reactive protein and tumor necrosis factor-alpha levels in individuals with long-COVID [67]. This meta-analysis included studies evaluating the levels of these biomarkers at both the acute phase and the post-acute phase of the infection [67]. On the contrary, Williams et al. reported significant reductions in levels of different interleukins (IL-6, IL-2, IL-17, IL-13 and IL-4) in people with long-COVID, although the moment of extraction was not specified [68].

Other potential mechanisms can contribute to and perpetuate a long-lasting inflammatory state. For instance, since lymphocytes usually participate in inflammation resolution following an acute infection, lymphopenia associated with COVID-19 may promote this inflammation [69]. In addition, chronic inflammation can lead to the uncoupling of endothelial nitric oxide synthetase and reactivation of oxygen species production, which results in the endothelial dysfunction observed in individuals with long-COVID [70].

<u>Future research direction:</u> Identification of inflammatory biomarkers at a specific moment of the infection could be crucial for preventing (in the acute phase) or treating (in the post-COVID phase) long-COVID symptoms. The association of long-COVID symptoms with higher inflammation either in the acute phase of the infection or in the post-COVID phase would support the use of anti-inflammatory medications. Thus, the use of corticoids in the COVID-19 phase is supported by the current literature [71,72]; however, data on post-COVID are still lacking. Badenes Bonet et al. found that administrating Dexamethasone during the acute COVID-19 phase led to a shorter duration of long-COVID symptomatology in individuals with moderate or severe COVID-19 one year after infection [73]. Surprisingly, no trial investigating the effect of dexamethasone or corticoids for the management of long-COVID is registered: https://clinicaltrials.gov/search?cond=Long%20COVID&intr=DEXAMETHASONE, https://clinicaltrials.gov/search?cond=Long%20COVID&intr=Corticosteroids (accessed on 15 October 2023).

5.3. Immune Dysregulation and Autoimmunity

During the acute COVID-19 phase, B cell function is altered resulting in the production of autoantibodies against interferon, neutrophils, connective tissue, cyclic citrullinated peptides and cell nucleus [74]. Further, acute SARS-CoV-2 infection leads to T cell dysfunction and antigen-presenting cells present antigens to autoreactive T cells by bystander activation, resulting in the infiltration of CD8+ T cells in various organs similar to that seen in autoimmune conditions [75]. Autoimmune response to various self-antigens through molecular mimicry will result in various organ damage [76].

The specific and autoreactive immune response induced by SARS-CoV-2 could persist in some individuals even after recovery from the acute infection and contribute to long-COVID [77]. In fact, elevated CD4+ T cell response and exhausted CD8+ T cell response with a dysregulation between humeral and cellular immunity is found in people with long-COVID [78].

<u>Future research direction:</u> Since immune response is intrinsically linked to the host, identification of predisposing individuals who exhibit a reduced or excessive response against SARS-CoV-2 could lead to early identification of potential long-lasting immune dysregulation or autoimmunity. No study has investigated this hypothesis.

5.4. Reactivation of Latent Infections

Reactivation of underlying pathogens in the body, e.g., herpes viruses such as Epstein–Barr virus (EBV) and human herpesvirus 6 (HHV-6) results in the development of various symptoms and has been observed in people infected by SARS-CoV-2 [57]. In fact, reactivation of EBV in patients with long-COVID is associated with fatigue and cognitive dysfunction [79]. A recent meta-analysis has found that the prevalence of different active herpes viruses ranges from 18% to 41% in COVID-19 survivors and that this prevalence is higher in individuals who have suffered from severe COVID-19 [80]. However, the prevalence of all evaluated active herpesvirus infections was not significantly different between infected and non-infected individuals [80]. Based on current data, the reactivation of latent infection in predisposing individuals can be another factor contributing to the development of some post-COVID symptoms.

<u>Future research direction:</u> Future studies should investigate the risk factors associated with the reactivation of latent infections in predisposing patients who have been infected with COVID-19. Thus, the time of reactivation, i.e., at the acute COVID-19 phase or at a post-acute phase, could be also relevant to identify the underlying mechanisms of this process.

5.5. Endothelial Dysfunction

Endotheliitis and thrombo-inflammation can occur at the acute COVID-19 phase and could persist even after recovery [81]. This is related to the fact that SARS-CoV-2 is able to penetrate the endothelial barrier, causing potential endothelial cell injury, hyper-inflammation cytokine storm syndrome, glycocalyx disruption, hypercoagulability and thrombosis [82]. In fact, oxidative stress, another process commonly observed during COVID-19 illness, also promotes endothelial damage, which increases the risk of long-COVID symptoms [83]. Thus, endothelial dysfunction and vascular damage of the brain could explain long-term post-COVID cognitive symptoms [84]. Based on current data, endothelial dysfunction can explain the heterogeneous cardiovascular post-COVID symptomatology experienced by patients, a condition called "vascular long-COVID" [85].

<u>Future research direction:</u> Future studies investigating if endothelial dysfunction in specific organs could be associated with a higher risk of developing particular post-COVID symptoms. Thus, early identification (in the acute COVID-19 phase if possible) of patients developing endothelial dysfunction could lead to better therapeutic strategies for preventing long-lasting symptoms.

5.6. Alteration in Gut Microbiota

Microbiota dysbiosis contributes to the onset and progression of several viral diseases, including COVID-19, which could serve as potential diagnostic and prognostic biomarkers [86]. Gut dysbiosis or alteration in the gut microbiome during the acute COVID-19 phase results in increased inflammation, prolonged fecal shedding of SARS-COV-2 and dysfunction of the microbiota-gut-brain axis, which can degrade the intestinal barrier and increase the permeability to harmful substances [87]. This gut dysbiosis can explain, not only gastrointestinal symptoms seen at the post-COVID phase but also post-COVID cognitive symptoms [87]. In fact, Liu et al. observed that gut pathogens such as Clostridium innocuum or Actinomyces naeslundii were also correlated with respiratory long-lasting post-COVID symptoms [88].

<u>Future research direction:</u> As with previous underlying mechanisms associated with long-COVID, early identification (at the acute COVID-19 phase if possible) of patients developing gut dysbiosis could lead to better therapeutic strategies for preventing long-lasting symptoms. For instance, it seems that COVID-19 can trigger irritable bowel syndrome [89]. In such a scenario, it is also possible that predisposing subjects with previous irritable bowel syndrome who are infected by SARS-CoV-2 can develop more long-lasting gut dysbiosis and, thus, more long-COVID symptomatology.

5.7. Psychological COVID-19 Surrounding Aspects

Stress events associated with the COVID-19 pandemic such as quarantine, social isolation, loss of friends or family, psychological disorders such as anxiety and depression, work stress, financial stress and post-traumatic stress disorders can promote or exacerbate long-COVID symptoms.

The presence of emotional aspects in people with long-COVID supports that biological and psychosocial factors interact in this complex condition [90]. The presence of mood disorders such as anxiety and depressive symptoms as well as sleep disturbances in individuals with long-COVID is supported by the current literature [41,91]. It has been found that depressive symptoms are associated with a higher risk of post-COVID fatigue [92] or dyspnea [93]. It has been hypothesized that sleep problems can perpetuate long-COVID symptomatology [94]. Thus, it is clinically seen that the interaction between anxiety, depression and sleep problems is complex in people with long-COVID [95]. Accordingly, the presence of associated psychological factors could promote or perpetuate long-COVID symptomatology.

<u>Future research direction:</u> It is possible that the personality traits of the patient could be risk factors for developing long-COVID symptomatology. We do not currently know the role of previous psychological disturbances due to the rapid spread of the main outbreak.

6. Genetic Influence on Long-COVID

With the introduction of high-throughput innovations such as genome-wide DNA-sequencing, imaging and bid data, it is accepted that the heterogeneity of many diseases requires treatment strategies targeting specific mechanisms—what has been called precision medicine [96]. Precision medicine refers to the ability to classify patients into subgroups that differ in their susceptibility to, biology, or prognosis of a particular disease or in their response to a specific treatment [97]. In such a scenario, genetic and epigenetic advances play a relevant role in precision treatment. For instance, since SARS-CoV-2 binds to human cells via ACE2 receptors, this receptor should be considered a vital medication target for managing COVID-19 [98]. At the beginning of the pandemic, early administration of non-steroidal anti-inflammatory drugs (NSAIDs) at the acute COVID-19 phase was contraindicated, since it was hypothesized that NSAIDs could interact with ACE2 receptors. Current research reveals that several NSAIDs do not exhibit any effects on ACE2 expression or activity [99].

Several studies have investigated long-COVID putting forth evidence that genetic elements may contribute significantly to this phenomenon, opening further comprehensive research into underlying mechanisms. Previous research has extensively looked into the potential role of genetics and epigenetics in determining an individual's predisposition to viral infections, as well as the severity and aggressiveness of such infections [100]. Genetic variations, including single nucleotide polymorphisms (SNPs), have demonstrated their involvement at various levels in viral infection processes [101]. These variations in SNPs influence diverse genes implicated in the regulation of viral pathogenesis and the initiation of immune response pathways within the infected host [101]. In the context of SARS-CoV-2 infection, multiple studies have evaluated the effects of variations in several genes concerning viral activity, increased infection risk and protective effects against its actions. The most investigated genes related to COVID-19 include ACE1, ACE2 and TPRSSM2 due to the functions of their products, which have been proven to be involved in the cell invasion process and cleavage and activation of the SARS-CoV-2 virus spike protein [102]. The genetic modification of ACE1, ACE2, or TMPRSS2 can elicit beneficial or protective outcomes against SARS-CoV-2 [103,104].

Extensive research has been also conducted on genetic variations of genes implicated in inflammatory and immune responses. Particular attention has been given to evaluating gene variations of interferons, a specialized family of cytokines crucial for initiating antiviral responses and activating the host's defense mechanisms against external viral infections [105]. These investigations revealed that certain gene variants of interferon-induced transmembrane protein SNPs were identified in subjects suffering from severe SARS-CoV-2 pneumonia, showing an association with COVID-19 severity [106]. Thus, genotyping of cytokine-related polymorphisms, such as IL-6, in the context of COVID-19 has also been conducted, although the association between IL-6 polymorphisms and SARS-CoV-2 pathogenesis and severity has not been firmly established [107]. It has been suggested that IL-6 polymorphisms should be considered as a critical factor in the development of targeted therapies against COVID-19 [107].

Our research group aimed to identify an association between some candidate genes and the development of long-COVID symptoms. The results did not reveal an association between SNPs of ACE2 and TMPRSS2 genes (involved in SARS-CoV-2 pathogenesis) and the development of long-COVID symptomatology [108]. Similarly, no association has been identified between SNPs of genes regulating the inflammatory (e.g., IL-6) [109] or the pain (e.g., COMT) [110] response and post-COVID pain. It is important to highlight that the reported results are based on an individual cohort.

<u>Future research direction:</u> A more comprehensive evaluation that encompasses a larger and diverse population of individuals with long-COVID symptoms could potentially mitigate the inherent genetic variability and lead to the identification of genetic variations associated with this symptomatology. Additionally, the inclusion of a large number of SNPs and genes can also elucidate potential relationships with specific post-COVID symptoms.

7. Epigenetic Influence on Long-COVID

Together with genetic alterations, epigenetics plays a major role in the natural gene expression and pathophysiological phenotype and has also been investigated in relation to viral infections [111].

Epigenetics is defined as the molecular process that regulates gene expression without altering the DNA sequence including methylation, histone protein modifications and the action of non-coding RNA (ncRNA) [112]. These molecular changes can be influenced by several internal and external factors, such as environmental exposures, stress and nutrition, leading to a specific regulation of protein product production [113]. The effects of epigenetic changes induced by COVID-19 infection are still under investigation, with research looking into possible systemic and cellular modifications induced by SARS-CoV-2 infection [114]. Several research studies have been conducted to investigate methylation patterns in COVID-19 patients [115]. Most research reveals a distinct pattern of hypermethylation in interferon-related genes and hypomethylation in genes responsible for regulating the inflammatory response providing valuable evidence regarding the dynamic epigenetic regulation of genes that play crucial roles in determining COVID-19 severity [116]. Additionally, recent findings have demonstrated that the methylation signatures detected during the acute phase of infection persist even after one year from the initial infection, specifically in circulating leukocytes [117].

Further, an Epigenome-Wide Association Study (EWAS) reported a hypomethylation of three specific CpG islands located on the gene Interferon-induced protein 44 like (IFI44L), involved in the interferon-induced innate viral response and protection against disease, in COVID-19 patients three months after the infection, showing not a clear association with the severity of the infection but reporting the possibility to detect this alteration after some time and hypothesizing an involvement of interferon responsive genes in the pathophysiology of COVID-19 and indicate a possible link to systemic autoimmune diseases [118]. Other epigenetic changes, such as epigenetic aging driven by telomers regulators of cell senescence, have been shown to increase susceptibility to SARS-CoV-2 infection and severe COVID-19 [119]. This molecular mechanism is possibly influenced by SARS-CoV-2 itself, leading to accelerated epigenetic aging and contributing to long-COVID [119]. Epigenetic changes have been also proposed as a potential therapy for COVID-19, with the action of miRNA, derived from mesenchymal stem cells (MSCs) able to block the action of IL-6 demonstrated to be a biomarker of long-lasting post-COVID symptoms, such as fatigue, depression and anxiety in COVID-19 survivors [120,121].

Regarding the identification of biomarkers for the individualization of long-COVID patients, recent systematic reviews have brought attention to a potential subset of serological biomarkers that warrant investigation in the circulation of people with long-COVID. These reviews found elevated levels of inflammatory biomarkers and cytokines, such as C reactive protein (CRP), IL-6, D-dimer, lactate dehydrogenase (LDH) and TNF-α in people with long-COVID [67,122]. Furthermore, in the context of epigenetic changes, miRNA regulation during different stages of acute SARS-CoV-2 infection demonstrated its potential to help in patient stratification allowing for the estimation of heightened risk of long-term health issues following the acute phase [123]. These miRNA profiles also hold promise for identifying informative biomarkers that can be targeted for preventive measures.

Future research direction: Despite the increasing evidence, there is still a lack of results that validate the epigenetic involvement in individuals with long-COVID. In this regard, future studies that explore and compare these processes in various affected populations will provide insight into the effects of this recent pandemic and highlight promising potential targets for understanding long-COVID.

8. SARS-CoV-2 Variants, Re-Infections and Vaccination Status

The fast spread of SARS-CoV-2 resulted in the appearance of several variants in a short period of time [124]. Among all SARS-CoV-2 variants identified after the historical strain (20A.EU2), Alpha (B.1.1.7), Delta (B.1.617.2) and Omicron (B.1.1.529/BA.1) are considered those variants of concern (VOCs) [125]. Current data suggest that the prevalence of long-COVID symptomatology is higher in individuals infected with the historical strain when compared with posterior SARS-CoV-2 variants (e.g., Alpha, Delta, Omicron) and that the risk of long-COVID seems to be lower in individuals infected with the Omicron variant [126,127]. Nevertheless, the presence of these variants has led to an increased number of reinfections. Thus, SARS-CoV-2 reinfections were uncommon until the end of 2021 (when the Delta variant was the predominant) but exponentially increased with Omicron variant (the most transmissible variant) [128].

Although individuals who had been infected with the historical strain had protection against reinfections with other SARS-COV-2 variants such as Alpha or Delta, this protection is lower with the Omicron variant [129]. Secondary infections are common due to organ damage and altered immune status. In fact, evidence shows that SARS-CoV-2 reinfection further increases the risks of death, hospitalization and organ damage [130]. Accordingly, it could be expected that re-infection with different SARS-CoV-2 variants could lead to a higher risk of developing long-COVID in those who did not develop long-lasting symptoms after the first infection, could exacerbate current symptoms or result in the appearance of new symptoms in individuals who developed long-COVID after the first infection [131]. In fact, Peghin et al. have observed that two years after the COVID-19 outbreak, the long-COVID dynamic seems to be not influenced by SARS-CoV-2 immunization status and reinfection [132], although there is evidence that pre-existing humoral immunity protects against long-COVID-19 [27].

In parallel with the appearance of SARS-CoV-2 variants, the development of vaccines has also marked the progression of the disease. It seems clear that vaccinated subjects had a significantly lower likelihood of reinfection than unvaccinated individuals [133]. Accordingly, the topic of reinfections could be prevented by vaccination. However, the effect of SARS-CoV-2 vaccines in long-COVID is different depending on whether vaccination has occurred before or after infection. Notarte et al. found a low level of evidence suggesting that administrating the vaccine before SARS-CoV-2 infection would reduce the risk of long-COVID [134]. However, the effect of vaccination in people with pre-existing long-COVID was not clear [134]. The meta-analysis by Gao et al. confirmed that vaccination had a protective effect against long-COVID if two doses are administered [135]. These authors also found that vaccination was effective against long-COVID independently if the vaccine is administered before or after SARS-CoV-2 acute infection [135]. A more recent meta-analysis confirmed that vaccination before SARS-CoV-2 infection is associated with a lower risk of long-COVID, but that vaccination in patients with ongoing long-COVID is not clear since most studies did not report any change in symptoms [136]. The fact that the impact of vaccines is higher when administered before infection should be expected since most people received the first two doses of COVID-19 vaccines in the first semester of 2021 when the Alpha and Delta SARS-CoV-2 variants were circulating. It therefore makes sense that vaccinated individuals were protected against severe COVID-19 caused by the Alpha and Delta variants and accordingly, lower rates of long-COVID would be expected. However, hybrid immunity did not provide further protection compared to vaccination or natural infection [27].

<u>Future research direction:</u> There is a lack of studies specifically investigating the development or changes in long-COVID symptomatology depending on the number of reinfections and on the specific SARS-CoV-2 variant [137]. Studies considering reinfections and vaccination status are needed to clarify this.

9. Conclusions

Although there has been an increasing advance in the understanding of long-COVID in the recent two years, it remains a not well-understood, underestimated and undertreated condition due to the lack of recognition of the phenomenon and proper knowledge of underlying mechanisms. The current paper discusses past, present and future research directions of long-COVID in different aspects: (1) definition and phenotyping; (2) identification of sub-groups (clusters); (3) risk factors; (4) underlying pathophysiological mechanisms; (5) genetics and epigenetics, and (6) reinfections by SARS-CoV-2 variants and vaccination status. Each section of the current perspective review includes some questions to be answered in future studies based on the identified gaps in the current literature.

Author Contributions: All the authors cited in the manuscript had substantial contributions to the concept and design, the execution of the work, or the analysis and interpretation of data; drafting or revising the manuscript and have read and approved the final version of the paper. C.F.-d.-l.-P.: conceptualization, methodology, validation, writing—original draft, writing—review and editing. A.V.R.: conceptualization, validation, writing—original draft, writing—review and editing. R.G.: methodology, validation, writing—original draft, writing—review and editing. L.A.-N.: conceptualization, methodology, validation, writing—original draft, writing—review and editing. All authors have read and agreed to the published version of the manuscript.

Funding: Center for Neuroplasticity and Pain (CNAP) is supported by the Danish National Research Foundation (DNRF121) and Novo Nordisk Foundation (NNF21OC0067235). The University Rey Juan Carlos (URJC) is supported by a grant associated to the Fondo Europeo De Desarrollo Regional—Recursos REACT-UE del Programa Operativo de Madrid 2014–2020, en la línea de actuación de proyectos de I+D+i en materia de respuesta a COVID 19 (LONG-COVID-EXP-CM).

Institutional Review Board Statement: Not Applicable.

Informed Consent Statement: Not Applicable.

Data Availability Statement: Not Applicable.

Conflicts of Interest: The authors declare no conflict of interest.

References

1. WHO Coronavirus (COVID-19) Dashboard. 2023. Available online: https://covid19.who.int/ (accessed on 1st October 2023).
2. COVID-19 Treatment Guidelines. Available online: https://www.covid19treatmentguidelines.nih.gov/management/clinical-management-of-adults/hospitalized-adults--therapeutic-management/ (accessed on 15 September 2023).
3. Therapeutic Management of Non-Hospitalized Adults with COVID-19. Available online: https://www.covid19treatmentguidelines.nih.gov/management/clinical-management-of-adults/nonhospitalized-adults--therapeutic-management/ (accessed on 15 September 2023).
4. Zheng, C.; Shao, W.; Chen, X.; Zhang, B.; Wang, G.; Zhang, W. Real-world effectiveness of COVID-19 vaccines: A literature review and meta-analysis. *Int. J. Infect. Dis.* **2022**, *114*, 252–260. [CrossRef] [PubMed]
5. Wang, K.; Wang, L.; Li, M.; Xie, B.; He, L.; Wang, M.; Zhang, R.; Hou, N.; Zhang, Y.; Jia, F. Real-word effectiveness of Global COVID-19 vaccines against SARS-CoV-2 Variants: A systematic review and meta-analysis. *Front. Med.* **2022**, *9*, 820544. [CrossRef] [PubMed]
6. Hayes, L.D.; Ingram, J.; Sculthorpe, N.F. More Than 100 Persistent Symptoms of SARS-CoV-2 (Long COVID): A scoping review. *Front. Med.* **2021**, *8*, 750378. [CrossRef] [PubMed]
7. Amdal, C.D.; Pe, M.; Falk, R.S.; Piccinin, C.; Bottomley, A.; Arraras, J.I.; Darlington, A.S.; Hofsø, K.; Holzner, B.; Jørgensen, N.M.H.; et al. Health-related quality of life issues, including symptoms, in patients with active COVID-19 or post COVID-19; a systematic literature review. *Qual. Life Res.* **2021**, *30*, 3367–3381. [CrossRef] [PubMed]
8. Tene, L.; Bergroth, T.; Eisenberg, A.; Ben David, S.S.; Chodick, G. Risk factors, health outcomes, healthcare services utilization, and direct medical costs of long COVID patient. *Int. J. Infect. Dis.* **2023**, *128*, 3–10. [CrossRef] [PubMed]
9. Moens, M.; Duarte, R.V.; De Smedt, A.; Putman, K.; Callens, J.; Billot, M.; Roulaud, M.; Rigoard, P.; Goudman, L. Health-related quality of life in persons post-COVID-19 infection in comparison to normative controls and chronic pain patients. *Front. Public Health* **2022**, *10*, 991572. [CrossRef] [PubMed]
10. Michelen, M.; Manoharan, L.; Elkheir, N.; Cheng, V.; Dagens, A.; Hastie, C.; O'Hara, M.; Suett, J.; Dahmash, D.; Bugaeva, P.; et al. Characterising long COVID: A living systematic review. *BMJ Glob. Health* **2021**, *6*, e005427. [CrossRef]
11. Fernández-De-Las-Peñas, C.; Palacios-Ceña, D.; Gómez-Mayordomo, V.; Florencio, L.L.; Cuadrado, M.L.; Plaza-Manzano, G.; Navarro-Santana, M. Prevalence of post-COVID-19 symptoms in hospitalized and non-hospitalized COVID-19 survivors: A systematic review and meta-analysis. *Eur. J. Intern. Med.* **2021**, *92*, 55–70. [CrossRef]
12. Chen, C.; Haupert, S.R.; Zimmermann, L.; Shi, X.; Fritsche, L.G.; Mukherjee, B. Global prevalence of post COVID-19 condition or long COVID: A meta-analysis and systematic review. *J. Infect. Dis.* **2022**, *226*, 1593–1607. [CrossRef]
13. Alkodaymi, M.S.; Omrani, O.A.; Fawzy, N.A.; Shaar, B.A.; Almamlouk, R.; Riaz, M.; Obeidat, M.; Obeidat, Y.; Gerberi, D.; Taha, R.M.; et al. Prevalence of post-acute COVID-19 syndrome symptoms at different follow-up periods: A systematic review and meta-analysis. *Clin. Microbiol. Infect.* **2022**, *28*, 657–666. [CrossRef]
14. Han, Q.; Zheng, B.; Daines, L.; Sheikh, A. Long-Term Sequelae of COVID-19: A Systematic Review and Meta-Analysis of One-Year Follow-Up Studies on Post-COVID Symptoms. *Pathogens* **2022**, *11*, 269. [CrossRef] [PubMed]
15. Kuodi, P.; Gorelik, Y.; Gausi, B.; Bernstine, T.; Edelstein, M. Characterization of post-COVID syndromes by symptom cluster and time period up to 12 months post-infection: A systematic review and meta-analysis. *Int. J. Infect. Dis.* **2023**, *134*, 1–7. [CrossRef] [PubMed]
16. Global Burden of Disease Long COVID Collaborators; Hanson, S.W.; Abbafati, C.; Aerts, J.G.; Al-Aly, Z.; Ashbaugh, C.; Ballouz, T.; Blyuss, O.; Bobkova, P.; Bonsel, G.; et al. Estimated global proportions of individuals with persistent fatigue, cognitive, and respiratory symptom clusters following symptomatic COVID-19 in 2020 and 2021. *JAMA* **2022**, *328*, 1604–1615.
17. Rahmati, M.; Udeh, R.; Yon, D.K.; Lee, S.W.; Dolja-Gore, X.; McEVoy, M.; Kenna, T.; Jacob, L.; López Sánchez, G.F.; Koyanagi, A.; et al. A systematic review and meta-analysis of long-term sequelae of COVID-19 2-year after SARS-CoV-2 infection: A call to action for neurological, physical, and psychological sciences. *J. Med. Virol.* **2023**, *95*, e28852. [CrossRef] [PubMed]
18. Ji, G.; Chen, C.; Zhou, M.; Wen, W.; Wang, C.; Tang, J.; Cheng, Y.; Wu, Q.; Zhang, X.; Wang, M.; et al. Post-COVID-19 fatigue among COVID-19 in patients discharged from hospital: A meta-analysis. *J. Infect.* **2022**, *84*, 722–746. [CrossRef]

19. Ceban, F.; Ling, S.; Lui, L.M.W.; Lee, Y.; Gill, H.; Teopiz, K.M.; Rodrigues, N.B.; Subramaniapillai, M.; Di Vincenzo, J.D.; Cao, B.; et al. Fatigue and cognitive impairment in Post-COVID-19 Syndrome: A systematic review and meta-analysis. *Brain Behav. Immun.* **2022**, *101*, 93–135. [CrossRef]

20. Fernández-de-las-Peñas, C.; Navarro-Santana, M.; Plaza-Manzano, G.; Palacios-Ceña Arendt-Nielsen, L. Time course prevalence of Post-COVID pain symptoms of musculoskeletal origin in patients who had survived to SARS-CoV-2 infection: A systematic review and meta-analysis. *Pain* **2022**, *163*, 1220–1231. [CrossRef]

21. Marjenberg, Z.; Leng, S.; Tascini, C.; Garg, M.; Misso, K.; El Guerche Seblain, C.; Shaikh, N. Risk of long COVID main symptoms after SARS-CoV-2 infection: A systematic review and meta-analysis. *Sci. Rep.* **2023**, *13*, 15332. [CrossRef]

22. Perumal, R.; Shunmugam, L.; Naidoo, K.; Abdool Karim, S.S.; Wilkins, D.; Garzino-Demo, A.; Brechot, C.; Parthasarathy, S.; Vahlne, A.; Nikolich, J.Ž. Long COVID: A review and proposed visualization of the complexity of long COVID. *Front. Immunol.* **2023**, *14*, 1117464. [CrossRef]

23. Boaventura, P.; Macedo, S.; Ribeiro, F.; Jaconiano, S.; Soares, P. Post-COVID-19 condition: Where are we now? *Life* **2022**, *12*, 517. [CrossRef]

24. Mumoli, N.; Conte, G.; Evangelista, I.; Cei, M.; Mazzone, A.; Colombo, A. Post-COVID or long-COVID: Two different conditions or the same? *J. Infect. Public Health* **2021**, *14*, 1349–1350. [CrossRef]

25. Akbarialiabad, H.; Taghrir, M.H.; Abdollahi, A.; Ghahramani, N.; Kumar, M.; Paydar, S.; Razani, B.; Mwangi, J.; Asadi-Pooya, A.A.; Malekmakan, L.; et al. Long COVID, a comprehensive systematic scoping review. *Infection* **2021**, *49*, 1163–1186. [CrossRef]

26. Soriano, J.B.; Murthy, S.; Marshall, J.C.; Relan, P.; Diaz, J.V.; WHO Clinical Case Definition Working Group on Post-COVID-19 Condition. A clinical case definition of post-COVID-19 condition by a Delphi consensus. *Lancet Infect. Dis.* **2022**, *22*, e102–e107. [CrossRef] [PubMed]

27. Cegolon, L.; Mauro, M.; Sansone, D.; Tassinari, A.; Gobba, F.M.; Modenese, A.; Casolari, L.; Liviero, F.; Pavanello, S.; Scapellato, M.L.; et al. A Multi-center study investigating long COVID-19 in healthcare workers from North-Eastern Italy: Prevalence, risk factors and the impact of pre-existing humoral immunity-ORCHESTRA Project. *Vaccines* **2023**, *11*, 1769. [CrossRef]

28. Zheng, B.; Daines, L.; Han, Q.; Hurst, J.R.; Pfeffer, P.; Shankar-Hari, M.; Elneima, O.; Walker, S.; Brown, J.S.; Siddiqui, S.; et al. Prevalence, risk factors and treatments for post-COVID-19 breathlessness: A systematic review and meta-analysis. *Eur. Respir. Rev.* **2022**, *31*, 220071. [CrossRef]

29. Fernández-de-las-Peñas, C.; Florencio, L.L.; Gómez-Mayordomo, V.; Cuadrado, M.L.; Palacios-Ceña, D.; Raveendran, A.V. Proposed integrative model for post-COVID symptoms. *Diabetes Metab. Syndr.* **2021**, *15*, 102159. [CrossRef]

30. Fernández-de-las-Peñas, C. Are patients exhibiting post-Coronavirus Disease (COVID) symptoms at 12 months the same at 5 or 9 months? The fluctuating nature of Post-COVID. *Clin. Infect. Dis.* **2022**, *75*, e1208. [CrossRef]

31. Korompoki, E.; Gavriatopoulou, M.; Hicklen, R.S.; Ntanasis-Stathopoulos, I.; Kastritis, E.; Fotiou, D.; Stamatelopoulos, K.; Terpos, E.; Kotanidou, A.; Hagberg, C.A.; et al. Epidemiology and organ specific sequelae of post-acute COVID19: A narrative review. *J. Infect.* **2021**, *83*, 1–16. [CrossRef] [PubMed]

32. National Institute for Health and Care Excellence (NICE); Royal College of General Practitioners; Healthcare Improvement Scotland SIGN. COVID-19 Rapid Guideline: Managing the Long-Term Effects of COVID-19. London: National Institute for Health and Care Excellence. 2020. Available online: https://www.nice.org.uk/guidance/ng188 (accessed on 1 October 2023).

33. Baig, A.M. Chronic COVID Syndrome: Need for an appropriate medical terminology for Long-COVID and COVID Long-Haulers. *J. Med. Virol.* **2021**, *93*, 2555–2556. [CrossRef] [PubMed]

34. Halpin, S.; O'Connor, R.; Sivan, M. Long COVID and chronic COVID syndromes. *J. Med. Virol.* **2021**, *93*, 1242–1243. [CrossRef]

35. Marshall, M. The lasting misery of coronavirus long-haulers. *Nature* **2020**, *585*, 339–341. [CrossRef] [PubMed]

36. Fernández-de-las-Peñas, C. Long COVID: Current definition. *Infection* **2022**, *50*, 285–286. [CrossRef]

37. Peter, R.S.; Nieters, A.; Kräusslich, H.G.; Brockmann, S.O.; Göpel, S.; Kindle, G.; Merle, U.; Steinacker, J.M.; Rothenbacher, D.; Kern, W.V.; et al. Post-acute sequelae of COVID-19 six to 12 months after infection: Population-based study. *BMJ* **2022**, *379*, e071050. [CrossRef]

38. Diem, L.; Schwarzwald, A.; Friedli, C.; Hammer, H.; Gomes-Fregolente, L.; Warncke, J.; Weber, L.; Kamber, N.; Chan, A.; Bassetti, C.; et al. Multidimensional phenotyping of the post-COVID-19 syndrome: A Swiss survey study. *CNS Neurosci. Ther.* **2022**, *28*, 1953–1963. [CrossRef]

39. Crook, H.; Raza, S.; Nowell, J.; Young, M.; Edison, P. Long COVID-mechanisms, risk factors, and management. *BMJ* **2021**, *374*, n1648. [CrossRef]

40. Nalbandian, A.; Sehgal, K.; Gupta, A.; Madhavan, M.V.; McGroder, C.; Stevens, J.S.; Cook, J.R.; Nordvig, A.S.; Shalev, D.; Sehrawat, T.S.; et al. Post-acute COVID-19 syndrome. *Nat. Med.* **2021**, *27*, 601–615. [CrossRef]

41. Iqbal, F.M.; Lam, K.; Sounderajah, V.; Clarke, J.M.; Ashrafian, H.; Darzi, A. Characteristics and predictors of acute and chronic post-COVID syndrome: A systematic review and meta-analysis. *EClinicalMedicine* **2021**, *36*, 100899. [CrossRef]

42. Maglietta, G.; Diodati, F.; Puntoni, M.; Lazzarelli, S.; Marcomini, B.; Patrizi, L.; Caminiti, C. Prognostic Factors for Post-COVID-19 Syndrome: A Systematic Review and Meta-Analysis. *J. Clin. Med.* **2022**, *11*, 1541. [CrossRef] [PubMed]

43. Thompson, E.J.; Williams, D.M.; Walker, A.J.; Mitchell, R.E.; Niedzwiedz, C.L.; Yang, T.C.; Huggins, C.F.; Kwong, A.S.F.; Silverwood, R.J.; Di Gessa, G.; et al. Long COVID burden and risk factors in 10 UK longitudinal studies and electronic health records. *Nat. Commun.* **2022**, *13*, 3528.

44. Notarte, K.I.; de Oliveira, M.H.S.; Peligro, P.J.; Velasco, J.V.; Macaranas, I.; Ver, A.T.; Pangilinan, F.C.; Pastrana, A.; Goldrich, N.; Kavteladze, D.; et al. Age, sex and previous comorbidities as risk factors not associated with SARS-CoV-2 infection for long COVID-19: A systematic review and meta-analysis. *J. Clin. Med.* **2022**, *11*, 7314. [CrossRef]
45. Tsampasian, V.; Elghazaly, H.; Chattopadhyay, R.; Debski, M.; Naing, T.K.P.; Garg, P.; Clark, A.; Ntatsaki, E.; Vassiliou, V.S. Risk factors associated with post-COVID-19 condition: A systematic review and meta-analysis. *JAMA Intern. Med.* **2023**, *183*, 566–580. [CrossRef] [PubMed]
46. Bwire, G.M. Coronavirus: Why men are more vulnerable to covid-19 than women? *SN Compr. Clin. Med.* **2020**, *2*, 874–876. [CrossRef] [PubMed]
47. Spicuzza, L.; Campisi, R.; Alia, S.; Prestifilippo, S.; Giuffrida, M.L.; Angileri, L.; Ciancio, N.; Vancheri, C. Female sex affects respiratory function and exercise ability in patients recovered from COVID-19 pneumonia. *J. Womens Health* **2023**, *32*, 18–23. [CrossRef] [PubMed]
48. Sha, J.; Qie, G.; Yao, Q.; Sun, W.; Wang, C.; Zhang, Z.; Wang, X.; Wang, P.; Jiang, J.; Bai, X.; et al. Sex differences on clinical characteristics, severity, and mortality in adult patients with COVID-19: A multicentre retrospective study. *Front. Med.* **2021**, *8*, 607059. [CrossRef] [PubMed]
49. Barek, M.A.; Aziz, M.A.; Islam, M.S. Impact of age, sex, comorbidities and clinical symptoms on the severity of COVID-19 cases: A meta-analysis with 55 studies and 10014 cases. *Heliyon* **2020**, *6*, e05684. [CrossRef]
50. Zheng, Z.; Peng, F.; Xu, B.; Zhao, J.; Liu, H.; Peng, J.; Li, Q.; Jiang, C.; Zhou, Y.; Liu, S.; et al. Risk factors of critical and mortal COVID-19 cases: A systematic literature review and meta-analysis. *J. Infect.* **2020**, *81*, e16–e25. [CrossRef] [PubMed]
51. Sahu, A.K.; Mathew, R.; Aggarwal, P.; Nayer, J.; Bhoi, S.; Satapathy, S.; Ekka, M. Clinical determinants of severe COVID-19 Disease: A systematic review and meta-analysis. *J. Glob. Infect. Dis.* **2021**, *13*, 13–19.
52. Sansone, D.; Tassinari, A.; Valentinotti, R.; Kontogiannis, D.; Ronchese, F.; Centonze, S.; Maggiore, A.; Cegolon, L.; Filon, F.L. Persistence of symptoms 15 months since COVID-19 diagnosis: Prevalence, risk factors and residual work ability. *Life* **2022**, *13*, 97. [CrossRef] [PubMed]
53. Raveendran, A.V. Long COVID-19: Challenges in the diagnosis and proposed diagnostic criteria. *Diabetes Metab. Syndr.* **2021**, *15*, 145–146. [CrossRef]
54. Castanares-Zapatero, D.; Chalon, P.; Kohn, L.; Dauvrin, M.; Detollenaere, J.; Maertens de Noordhout, C.; Primus-de Jong, C.; Cleemput, I.; Van den Heede, K. Pathophysiology and mechanism of long COVID: A comprehensive review. *Ann. Med.* **2022**, *54*, 1473–1487. [CrossRef]
55. Sherif, Z.A.; Gomez, C.R.; Connors, T.J.; Henrich, T.J.; Reeves, W.B.; RECOVER Mechanistic Pathway Task Force. Pathogenic mechanisms of post-acute sequelae of SARS-CoV-2 infection (PASC). *Elife* **2023**, *12*, e86002. [CrossRef]
56. O'Donnell, J.S.; Chappell, K.J. Chronic SARS-CoV-2, a Cause of Post-acute COVID-19 Sequelae (Long-COVID)? *Front. Microbiol.* **2021**, *12*, 724654. [CrossRef] [PubMed]
57. Chen, B.; Julg, B.; Mohandas, S.; Bradfute, S.B.; RECOVER Mechanistic Pathways Task Force. Viral persistence, reactivation, and mechanisms of long COVID. *Elife* **2023**, *12*, e86015. [CrossRef] [PubMed]
58. Proal, A.D.; VanElzakker, M.B.; Aleman, S.; Bach, K.; Boribong, B.P.; Buggert, M.; Cherry, S.; Chertow, D.S.; Davies, H.E.; Dupont, C.L.; et al. SARS-CoV-2 reservoir in post-acute sequelae of COVID-19 (PASC). *Nat. Immunol.* **2023**, *24*, 1616–1627. [CrossRef] [PubMed]
59. Bussani, R.; Zentilin, L.; Correa, R.; Colliva, A.; Silvestri, F.; Zacchigna, S.; Collesi, C.; Giacca, M. Persistent SARS-CoV-2 infection in patients seemingly recovered from COVID-19. *J. Pathol.* **2023**, *259*, 254–263. [CrossRef] [PubMed]
60. Stein, S.R.; Ramelli, S.C.; Grazioli, A.; Chung, J.Y.; Singh, M.; Yinda, C.K.; Winkler, C.W.; Sun, J.; Dickey, J.M.; Ylaya, K.; et al. SARS-CoV-2 infection and persistence in the human body and brain at autopsy. *Nature* **2022**, *612*, 758–763. [CrossRef] [PubMed]
61. Zollner, A.; Koch, R.; Jukic, A.; Pfister, A.; Meyer, M.; Rössler, A.; Kimpel, J.; Adolph, T.E.; Tilg, H. Postacute COVID-19 is characterized by gut viral antigen persistence in inflammatory bowel diseases. *Gastroenterology* **2022**, *163*, 495–506. [CrossRef]
62. Swank, Z.; Senussi, Y.; Manickas-Hill, Z.; Yu, X.G.; Li, J.Z.; Alter, G.; Walt, D.R. Persistent circulating Severe Acute Respiratory Syndrome Coronavirus 2 spike is associated with post-acute coronavirus disease 2019 sequelae. *Clin. Infect. Dis.* **2023**, *76*, e487–e490. [CrossRef]
63. Tian, F.; Chen, Z.; Feng, Q. Nirmatrelvir-ritonavir compared with other antiviral drugs for the treatment of COVID-19 patients: A systematic review and meta-analysis. *J. Med. Virol.* **2023**, *95*, e28732. [CrossRef]
64. Marshall, G.D., Jr. The pathophysiology of post-acute sequelae of COVID-19 (PASC): Possible role for persistent inflammation. *Asia Pac. Allergy* **2023**, *13*, 77–84.
65. PHOSP-COVID Collaborative Group. Clinical characteristics with inflammation profiling of Long-COVID and association with one-year recovery following hospitalisation in the UK: A prospective observational study. *Lancet Respir. Med.* **2022**, *10*, 761–775. [CrossRef]
66. Yin, J.X.; Agbana, Y.L.; Sun, Z.S.; Fei, S.W.; Zhao, H.Q.; Zhou, X.N.; Chen, J.H.; Kassegne, K. Increased interleukin-6 is associated with long COVID-19: A systematic review and meta-analysis. *Infect. Dis. Poverty* **2023**, *12*, 43. [CrossRef]
67. Lai, Y.J.; Liu, S.H.; Manachevakul, S.; Lee, T.A.; Kuo, C.T.; Bello, D. Biomarkers in long COVID-19: A systematic review. *Front. Med.* **2023**, *10*, 1085988. [CrossRef]
68. Williams, E.S.; Martins, T.B.; Shah, K.S.; Hill, H.R.; Coiras, M.; Spivak, A.M.; Planelles, V. Cytokine deficiencies in patients with long-COVID. *J. Clin. Cell. Immunol.* **2022**, *13*, 672.

69. Tavakolpour, S.; Rakhshandehroo, T.; Wei, E.X.; Rashidian, M. Lymphopenia during the COVID-19 infection: What it shows and what can be learned. *Immunol. Lett.* **2020**, *225*, 31–32. [CrossRef]

70. Hawley, H.B. Long COVID: Clinical findings, pathology, and endothelial molecular mechanisms. *Am. J. Med.* **2023**, *in press*. [CrossRef]

71. Griesel, M.; Wagner, C.; Mikolajewska, A.; Stegemann, M.; Fichtner, F.; Metzendorf, M.I.; Nair, A.A.; Daniel, J.; Fischer, A.L.; Skoetz, N. Inhaled corticosteroids for the treatment of COVID-19. *Cochrane Database Syst. Rev.* **2022**, *3*, CD015125.

72. Wagner, C.; Griesel, M.; Mikolajewska, A.; Metzendorf, M.I.; Fischer, A.L.; Stegemann, M.; Spagl, M.; Nair, A.A.; Daniel, J.; Fichtner, F.; et al. Systemic corticosteroids for the treatment of COVID-19: Equity-related analyses and update on evidence. *Cochrane Database Syst. Rev.* **2022**, *11*, CD014963.

73. Badenes Bonet, D.; Caguana Vélez, O.A.; Duran Jordà, X.; Comas Serrano, M.; Posso Rivera, M.; Admetlló, M.; Herranz Blasco, A.; Cuadrado Godia, E.; Marco Navarro, E.; Martin Ezquerra, G.; et al. Treatment of COVID-19 during the acute phase in hospitalized patients decreases post-acute sequelae of COVID-19. *J. Clin. Med.* **2023**, *12*, 4158. [CrossRef]

74. Gao, Z.-W.; Zhang, H.-Z.; Liu, C.; Dong, K. Autoantibodies in COVID-19: Frequency and function. *Autoimmun. Rev.* **2021**, *20*, 102754. [CrossRef]

75. Ehrenfeld, M.; Tincani, A.; Andreoli, L.; Cattalini, M.; Greenbaum, A.; Kanduc, D.; Alijotas-Reig, J.; Zinserling, V.; Semenova, N.; Amital, H.; et al. COVID-19 and autoimmunity. *Autoimmun. Rev.* **2020**, *19*, 102597. [CrossRef]

76. Blagova, O.; Varionchik, N.; Zaidenov, V.; Savina, P.; Sarkisova, N. Anti-heart antibodies levels and their correlation with clinical symptoms and outcomes in patients with confirmed or suspected diagnosis COVID-19. *Eur. J. Immunol.* **2021**, *51*, 893–902. [CrossRef] [PubMed]

77. Harne, R.; Williams, B.; Abdelal, H.F.M.; Baldwin, S.L.; Coler, R.N. SARS-CoV-2 infection and immune responses. *AIMS Microbiol.* **2023**, *9*, 245–276. [CrossRef]

78. Yin, K.; Peluso, M.J.; Luo, X.; Thomas, R.; Shin, M.-G.; Neidleman, J.; Andrew, A.; Young, K.; Ma, T.; Hoh, R.; et al. Long COVID manifests with T cell dysregulation, inflammation, and an uncoordinated adaptive immune response to SARS-CoV-2. *bioRxiv* **2023**. [CrossRef]

79. Peluso, M.J.; Deveau, T.M.; Munter, S.E.; Peluso, M.J.; Deveau, T.-M.; Munter, S.E.; Ryder, D.; Buck, A.; Lu, S.; Goldberg, S.A.; et al. Evidence of recent Epstein-Barr virus reactivation in individuals experiencing long COVID. *medRxiv* **2022**. [CrossRef]

80. Banko, A.; Miljanovic, D.; Cirkovic, A. Systematic review with meta-analysis of active herpesvirus infections in patients with COVID-19: Old players on the new field. *Int. J. Infect. Dis.* **2023**, *130*, 108–125. [CrossRef] [PubMed]

81. Loo, J.; Spittle, D.A.; Newnham, M. COVID-19, immunothrombosis and venous thromboembolism: Biological mechanisms. *Thorax* **2021**, *76*, 412–420. [CrossRef] [PubMed]

82. Santoro, L.; Zaccone, V.; Falsetti, L.; Ruggieri, V.; Danese, M.; Miro, C.; Di Giorgio, A.; Nesci, A.; D'Alessandro, A.; Moroncini, G.; et al. Role of endothelium in cardiovascular sequelae of long COVID. *Biomedicines* **2023**, *11*, 2239. [CrossRef]

83. Georgieva, E.; Ananiev, J.; Yovchev, Y.; Arabadzhiev, G.; Abrashev, H.; Abrasheva, D.; Atanasov, V.; Kostandieva, R.; Mitev, M.; Petkova-Parlapanska, K.; et al. COVID-19 complications: Oxidative stress, inflammation, and mitochondrial and endothelial dysfunction. *Int. J. Mol. Sci.* **2023**, *24*, 14876. [CrossRef]

84. Shabani, Z.; Liu, J.; Su, H. Vascular dysfunctions contribute to the long-term cognitive deficits following COVID-19. *Biology* **2023**, *12*, 1106. [CrossRef]

85. Zanini, G.; Selleri, V.; Roncati, L.; Coppi, F.; Nasi, M.; Farinetti, A.; Manenti, A.; Pinti, M.; Mattioli, A.V. Vascular "Long COVID": A new vessel disease? *Angiology* **2023**, *75*. [CrossRef]

86. Moreno-Corona, N.C.; López-Ortega, O.; Pérez-Martínez, C.A.; Martínez-Castillo, M.; De Jesús-González, L.A.; León-Reyes, G.; León-Juárez, M. Dynamics of the microbiota and its relationship with post-COVID-19 syndrome. *Int. J. Mol. Sci.* **2023**, *24*, 14822. [CrossRef] [PubMed]

87. Plummer, A.M.; Matos, Y.L.; Lin, H.C.; Ryman, S.G.; Birg, A.; Quinn, D.K.; Parada, A.N.; Vakhtin, A.A. Gut-brain pathogenesis of post-acute COVID-19 neurocognitive symptoms. *Front. Neurosci.* **2023**, *17*, 1232480. [CrossRef] [PubMed]

88. Liu, Q.; Mak, J.W.Y.; Su, Q.; Yeoh, Y.K.; Lui, G.C.; Ng, S.S.S.; Zhang, F.; Li, A.Y.L.; Lu, W.; Hui, D.S.; et al. Gut microbiota dynamics in a prospective cohort of patients with post-acute COVID-19 syndrome. *Gut* **2022**, *71*, 544–552. [CrossRef] [PubMed]

89. Settanni, C.R.; Ianiro, G.; Ponziani, F.R.; Bibbò, S.; Segal, J.P.; Cammarota, G.; Gasbarrini, A. COVID-19 as a trigger of irritable bowel syndrome: A review of potential mechanisms. *World J. Gastroenterol.* **2021**, *27*, 7433–7445. [CrossRef] [PubMed]

90. Hall, P.A.; Sheeran, P.; Fong, G.T.; Cheah, C.S.L.; Oremus, M.; Liu-Ambrose, T.; Sakib, M.N.; Butt, Z.A.; Ayaz, H.; Jandu, N.; et al. Biobehavioral Aspects of the COVID-19 Pandemic: A Review. *Psychosom. Med.* **2021**, *83*, 309–321. [CrossRef] [PubMed]

91. Mazza, M.G.; Palladini, M.; Poletti, S.; Benedetti, F. Post-COVID-19 depressive symptoms: Epidemiology, Pathophysiology, and pharmacological treatment. *CNS Drugs* **2022**, *36*, 681–702. [CrossRef]

92. Al-Jassas, H.K.; Al-Hakeim, H.K.; Maes, M. Intersections between pneumonia, lowered oxygen saturation percentage and immune activation mediate depression, anxiety, and chronic fatigue syndrome-like symptoms due to COVID-19: A nomothetic network approach. *J. Affect. Disord.* **2022**, *15*, 233–245. [CrossRef]

93. Bottemanne, H.; Gouraud, C.; Hulot, J.S.; Blanchard, A.; Ranque, B.; Lahlou-Laforêt, K.; Limosin, F.; Günther, S.; Lebeaux, D.; Lemogne, C. Do anxiety and depression predict persistent physical symptoms after a severe COVID-19 episode? A prospective study. *Front. Psychiatry* **2021**, *12*, 757685. [CrossRef]

94. Merikanto, I.; Dauvilliers, Y.; Chung, F.; Wing, Y.K.; De Gennaro, L.; Holzinger, B.; Bjorvatn, B.; Morin, C.M.; Penzel, T.; Benedict, C.; et al. Sleep symptoms are essential features of long-COVID—Comparing healthy controls with COVID-19 cases of different severity in the international COVID sleep study (ICOSS-II). *J. Sleep Res.* **2022**, *32*, e13754. [CrossRef]

95. Pacho-Hernández, J.C.; Fernández-de-las-Peñas, C.; Fuensalida-Novo, S.; Jiménez-Antona, C.; Ortega-Santiago, R.; Cigarán-Mendez, M. Sleep quality mediates the effect of sensitization-associated symptoms, anxiety, and depression on quality of life in individuals with post-COVID-19 pain. *Brain Sci.* **2022**, *12*, 1363. [CrossRef] [PubMed]

96. Aletaha, D. Precision medicine and management of rheumatoid arthritis. *J. Autoimmun.* **2020**, *110*, 102405. [CrossRef] [PubMed]

97. National Research Council Committee on AFfDaNToD. *The National Academies Collection: Reports funded by National Institutes of Health. Toward Precision Medicine: Building a Knowledge Network for Biomedical Research and a New Taxonomy of Disease*; National Academies Press: Washington, DC, USA, 2011.

98. Hetta, H.F.; Muhammad, K.; Algammal, A.M.; Ramadan, H.; Abdel-Rahman, M.S.; Mabrok, M.; Koneru, G.; Elkady, A.A.; El-Saber Batiha, G.; Waheed, Y.; et al. Mapping the effect of drugs on ACE2 as a novel target site for COVID-19 therapy. *Eur. Rev. Med. Pharmacol. Sci.* **2021**, *25*, 3923–3932. [PubMed]

99. de Bruin, N.; Schneider, A.K.; Reus, P.; Talmon, S.; Ciesek, S.; Bojkova, D.; Cinatl, J.; Lodhi, I.; Charlesworth, B.; Sinclair, S.; et al. Ibuprofen, Flurbiprofen, Etoricoxib or Paracetamol do not influence ACE2 expression and activity in vitro or in mice and do not exacerbate in-vitro SARS-CoV-2 infection. *Int. J. Mol. Sci.* **2022**, *23*, 1049. [CrossRef]

100. Darbeheshti, F.; Abolhassani, H.; Bashashati, M.; Ghavami, S.; Shahkarami, S.; Zoghi, S.; Gupta, S.; Orange, J.S.; Ochs, H.D.; Rezaei, N. Coronavirus: Pure infectious disease or genetic predisposition. *Adv. Exp. Med. Biol.* **2021**, *1318*, 91–107.

101. Darbeheshti, F.; Rezaei, N. Genetic Predisposition Models to COVID-19 Infection. *Med. Hypotheses* **2020**, *142*, 109818. [CrossRef]

102. Hou, Y.; Zhao, J.; Martin, W.; Kallianpur, A.; Chung, M.K.; Jehi, L.; Sharifi, N.; Erzurum, S.; Eng, C.; Cheng, F. New insights into genetic susceptibility of COVID-19: An ACE2 and TMPRSS2 polymorphism analysis. *BMC Med.* **2020**, *18*, 216. [CrossRef]

103. Saengsiwaritt, W.; Jittikoon, J.; Chaikledkaew, U.; Udomsinprasert, W. Genetic polymorphisms of ACE1, ACE2, and TMPRSS2 associated with COVID-19 severity: A systematic review with meta-analysis. *Rev. Med. Virol.* **2022**, *8*, e2323. [CrossRef]

104. Gupta, K.; Kaur, G.; Pathak, T.; Banerjee, I. Systematic review and meta-analysis of human genetic variants contributing to COVID-19 susceptibility and severity. *Gene* **2022**, *844*, 146790. [CrossRef]

105. Acosta, P.L.; Byrne, A.B.; Hijano, D.R.; Talarico, L.B. Human type I interferon antiviral effects in respiratory and reemerging viral infections. *J. Immunol. Res.* **2020**, *2020*, 1372494. [CrossRef]

106. Zhang, Y.; Qin, L.; Zhao, Y.; Zhang, P.; Xu, B.; Li, K.; Liang, L.; Zhang, C.; Dai, Y.; Feng, Y.; et al. Interferon-induced transmembrane protein 3 genetic variant Rs12252-C associated with disease severity in Coronavirus Disease 2019. *J. Infect. Dis.* **2020**, *222*, 34–37. [CrossRef]

107. Karcioglu Batur, L.; Hekim, N. Correlation between interleukin gene polymorphisms and current prevalence and mortality rates due to novel coronavirus disease 2019 (COVID-2019) in 23 countries. *J. Med. Virol.* **2021**, *93*, 5853–5863. [CrossRef] [PubMed]

108. Fernández-de-las-Peñas, C.; Arendt-Nielsen, L.; Díaz-Gil, G.; Gómez-Esquer, F.; Gil-Crujera, A.; Gómez-Sánchez, S.M.; Ambite-Quesada, S.; Palomar-Gallego, M.A.; Pellicer-Valero, O.J.; Giordano, R. Genetic association between ACE2 (rs2285666 and rs2074192) and TMPRSS2 (rs12329760 and rs2070788) polymorphisms with post-COVID symptoms in previously hospitalized COVID-19 survivors. *Genes* **2022**, *13*, 1935. [CrossRef]

109. Fernández-de-las-Peñas, C.; Giordano, R.; Díaz-Gil, G.; Gómez-Esquer, F.; Ambite-Quesada, S.; Palomar-Gallego, M.A.; Arendt-Nielsen, L. Post-COVID pain is not associated with inflammatory polymorphisms in people who had been hospitalized by COVID-19. *J. Clin. Med.* **2022**, *11*, 5645. [CrossRef]

110. Fernández-de-las-Peñas, C.; Giordano, R.; Díaz-Gil, G.; Gil-Crujera, A.; Gómez-Sánchez, S.M.; Ambite-Quesada, S.; Arendt-Nielsen, L. Are pain polymorphisms associated with the risk and phenotype of post-COVID pain in previously hospitalized COVID-19 survivors? *Genes* **2022**, *13*, 1336. [CrossRef] [PubMed]

111. Atlante, S.; Mongelli, A.; Barbi, V.; Martelli, F.; Farsetti, A.; Gaetano, C. The epigenetic implication in coronavirus infection and therapy. *Clin. Epigenet.* **2020**, *12*, 156. [CrossRef] [PubMed]

112. Capp, J.P. Interplay between genetic, epigenetic, and gene expression variability: Considering complexity in evolvability. *Evol. Appl.* **2021**, *14*, 893–901. [CrossRef]

113. Mantovani, A.; Netea, M.G. Trained innate immunity, epigenetics, and COVID-19. *N. Engl. J. Med.* **2020**, *383*, 1078–1080. [CrossRef]

114. Corley, M.J.; Pang, A.P.S.; Dody, K.; Mudd, P.A.; Patterson, B.K.; Seethamraju, H.; Bram, Y.; Peluso, M.J.; Torres, L.; Iyer, N.S.; et al. Genome-Wide DNA Methylation profiling of peripheral blood reveals an epigenetic signature associated with severe COVID-19. *J. Leukoc. Biol.* **2021**, *110*, 21–26. [CrossRef]

115. Dey, A.; Vaishak, K.; Deka, D.; Radhakrishnan, A.K.; Paul, S.; Shanmugam, P.; Daniel, A.P.; Pathak, S.; Duttaroy, A.K.; Banerjee, A. Epigenetic perspectives associated with COVID-19 infection and related cytokine storm: An updated review. *Infection* **2023**, *51*, 1603–1618. [CrossRef]

116. Balnis, J.; Madrid, A.; Hogan, K.J.; Drake, L.A.; Chieng, H.C.; Tiwari, A.; Vincent, C.E.; Chopra, A.; Vincent, P.A.; Robek, M.D.; et al. Blood DNA Methylation and COVID-19 outcomes. *Clin. Epigenet.* **2021**, *13*, 118. [CrossRef]

117. Balnis, J.; Madrid, A.; Hogan, K.J.; Drake, L.A.; Adhikari, A.; Vancavage, R.; Singer, H.A.; Alisch, R.S.; Jaitovich, A. Whole-Genome methylation sequencing reveals that COVID-19-induced epigenetic dysregulation remains 1 year after hospital discharge. *Am. J. Respir. Cell Mol. Biol.* **2023**, *68*, 594–597. [CrossRef] [PubMed]

118. Lee, Y.; Riskedal, E.; Kalleberg, K.T.; Istre, M.; Lind, A.; Lund-Johansen, F.; Reiakvam, O.; Søraas, A.V.L.; Harris, J.R.; Dahl, J.A.; et al. EWAS of post-COVID-19 patients shows methylation differences in the immune-response associated gene, IFI44L, three months after COVID-19 infection. *Sci. Rep.* **2022**, *12*, 11478. [CrossRef] [PubMed]

119. Cao, X.; Li, W.; Wang, T.; Ran, D.; Davalos, V.; Planas-Serra, L.; Pujol, A.; Esteller, M.; Wang, X.; Yu, H. Accelerated biological aging in COVID-19 patients. *Nat. Commun.* **2022**, *13*, 2135. [CrossRef] [PubMed]

120. Kappelmann, N.; Dantzer, R.; Khandaker, G.M. Interleukin-6 as potential mediator of long-term neuropsychiatric symptoms of COVID-19. *Psychoneuroendocrinology* **2021**, *131*, 105295. [CrossRef]

121. Schultz, I.C.; Bertoni, A.P.S.; Wink, M.R. MSC-exosomes carrying MiRNA—Could they enhance tocilizumab activity in neuropathology of COVID-19? *Stem Cell Rev. Rep.* **2023**, *19*, 279–283. [CrossRef]

122. Yong, S.J.; Halim, A.; Halim, M.; Liu, S.; Aljeldah, M.; Al Shammari, B.R.; Alwarthan, S.; Alhajri, M.; Alawfi, A.; Alshengeti, A.; et al. Inflammatory and vascular biomarkers in post-COVID-19 syndrome: A systematic review and meta-analysis of over 20 biomarkers. *Rev. Med. Virol.* **2023**, *33*, e2424. [CrossRef]

123. Jankovic, M.; Nikolic, D.; Novakovic, I.; Petrovic, B.; Lackovic, M.; Santric-Milicevic, M. MiRNAs as a potential biomarker in the COVID-19 infection and complications course, severity, and outcome. *Diagnostics* **2023**, *13*, 1091. [CrossRef]

124. Parra-Lucares, A.; Segura, P.; Rojas, V.; Pumarino, C.; Saint-Pierre, G.; Toro, L. Emergence of SARS-CoV-2 variants in the world: How could this happen? *Life* **2022**, *12*, 194. [CrossRef]

125. Thye, A.Y.; Law, J.W.; Pusparajah, P.; Letchumanan, V.; Chan, K.G.; Lee, L.H. Emerging SARS-CoV-2 Variants of Concern (VOCs): An Impending Global Crisis. *Biomedicines* **2021**, *9*, 1303. [CrossRef]

126. Fernández-de-las-Peñas, C.; Notarte, K.I.; Peligro, P.J.; Velasco, J.V.; Ocampo, M.J.; Henry, B.M.; Arendt-Nielsen, L.; Torres-Macho, J.; Plaza-Manzano, G. Long-COVID symptoms in individuals infected with different SARS-CoV-2 variants of concern: A systematic review of the literature. *Viruses* **2022**, *14*, 2629. [CrossRef] [PubMed]

127. Du, M.; Ma, Y.; Deng, J.; Liu, M.; Liu, J. Comparison of long COVID-19 caused by different SARS-CoV-2 strains: A systematic review and meta-analysis. *Int. J. Environ. Res. Public Health* **2022**, *19*, 16010. [CrossRef]

128. Medić, S.; Anastassopoulou, C.; Lozanov-Crvenković, Z.; Vuković, V.; Dragnić, N.; Petrović, V.; Ristić, M.; Pustahija, T.; Gojković, Z.; Tsakris, A.; et al. Risk and severity of SARS-CoV-2 reinfections during 2020–2022 in Vojvodina, Serbia: A population-level observational study. *Lancet Reg. Health-Eur.* **2022**, *20*, 100453. [CrossRef] [PubMed]

129. COVID-19 Forecasting Team. Past SARS-CoV-2 infection protection against re-infection: A systematic review and meta-analysis. *Lancet* **2023**, *401*, 833–842. [CrossRef] [PubMed]

130. Bowe, B.; Xie, Y.; Al-Aly, Z. Acute and postacute sequelae associated with SARS-CoV-2 reinfection. *Nat. Med.* **2022**, *28*, 2398–2405. [CrossRef]

131. Boufidou, F.; Medić, S.; Lampropoulou, V.; Siafakas, N.; Tsakris, A.; Anastassopoulou, C. SARS-CoV-2 reinfections and long COVID in the post-Omicron phase of the pandemic. *Int. J. Mol. Sci.* **2023**, *24*, 12962. [CrossRef]

132. Peghin, M.; De Martino, M.; Palese, A.; Chiappinotto, S.; Fonda, F.; Gerussi, V.; Sartor, A.; Curcio, F.; Grossi, P.A.; Isola, M.; et al. Post-COVID-19 syndrome 2 years after the first wave: The role of humoral response, vaccination and reinfection. *Open Forum Infect. Dis.* **2023**, *10*, ofad364. [CrossRef]

133. Flacco, M.E.; Acuti Martellucci, C.; Baccolini, V.; De Vito, C.; Renzi, E.; Villari, P.; Manzoli, L. COVID-19 vaccines reduce the risk of SARS-CoV-2 reinfection and hospitalization: Meta-analysis. *Front. Med.* **2022**, *9*, 1023507. [CrossRef]

134. Notarte, K.I.; Catahay, J.A.; Velasco, J.V.; Pastrana, A.; Ver, A.T.; Pangilinan, F.C.; Peligro, P.J.; Casimiro, M.; Guerrero, J.J.; Gellaco, M.M.L.; et al. Impact of COVID-19 vaccination on the risk of developing long-COVID and on existing long-COVID symptoms: A systematic review. *EClinicalMedicine* **2022**, *53*, 101624. [CrossRef]

135. Gao, P.; Liu, J.; Liu, M. Effect of COVID-19 vaccines on reducing the risk of long COVID in the realworld: A systematic review and meta-analysis. *Int. J. Environ. Res. Public Health* **2022**, *19*, 12422. [CrossRef]

136. Watanabe, A.; Iwagami, M.; Yasuhara, J.; Takagi, H.; Kuno, T. Protective effect of COVID-19 vaccination against long COVID syndrome: A systematic review and meta-analysis. *Vaccine* **2023**, *41*, 1783–1790. [CrossRef] [PubMed]

137. Orendáčová, M.; Kvašňák, E. Effects of vaccination, new SARS-CoV-2 variants and reinfections on post-COVID-19 complications. *Front. Public Health* **2022**, *10*, 903568. [CrossRef] [PubMed]

MDPI AG
Grosspeteranlage 5
4052 Basel
Switzerland
Tel.: +41 61 683 77 34

Microorganisms Editorial Office
E-mail: microorganisms@mdpi.com
www.mdpi.com/journal/microorganisms

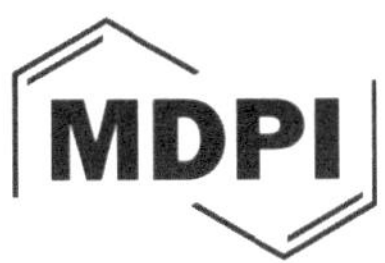